MANUAL OF CLINICAL PROBLEMS IN PULMONARY MEDICINE

Seventh Edition

T0200221

MANUAL OF CLINICAL PROBLEMS IN PULMONARY MEDICINE

Seventh Edition

Editors

Timothy A. Morris, MD, FCCP

Professor of Medicine and Clinical Service Chief,
Division of Pulmonary and Critical Care Medicine, University of California,
San Diego School of Medicine, La Jolla, California;
Medical Director of Respiratory Care and Pulmonary Function Laboratory,
University of California, San Diego Medical Center, San Diego, California

Andrew L. Ries, MD, MPH

Associate Vice Chancellor for Academic Affairs,
Professor of Medicine and Family and Preventive Medicine, University
of California, San Diego School of Medicine, La Jolla, California;
Director of Pulmonary Rehabilitation,
University of California,
San Diego Medical Center, San Diego, California

Richard A. Bordow, MD

Associate Director,
Pulmonary Function Laboratory,
Doctors' Hospital, San Pablo, California

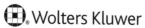
Wolters Kluwer
Health

Philadelphia • Baltimore • New York • London
Buenos Aires • Hong Kong • Sydney • Tokyo

Executive Editor: Rebecca Gaertner
Senior Product Development Editor: Kristina Oberle
Production Project Manager: Bridgett Dougherty
Senior Manufacturing Manager: Beth Welsh
Design Coordinator: Holly McLaughlin
Compositor: S4Carlisle Publishing Services

© 2014 Wolters Kluwer Health | Lippincott Williams & Wilkins
2001 Market Street
Philadelphia, PA 19103 USA
LWW.com

6th edition, © 2005 by Lippincott Williams & Wilkins
5th edition, © 2000 by Lippincott Williams & Wilkins
4th edition, © 1996 by Churchill Livingstone
3rd edition, © 1991 by Little Brown & Co.
2nd edition, © 1985 by Little Brown & Co.
1st edition, © 1980 by Time Warner Books

Printed in China

Library of Congress Cataloging-in-Publication Data

Manual of clinical problems in pulmonary medicine / editors, Timothy A. Morris, Andrew L. Ries, Richard A. Bordow. — Seventh edition.
    p. ; cm.
Includes bibliographical references and index.
ISBN 978-1-4511-1658-8 (alk. paper)
I. Morris, Timothy A., editor of compilation. II. Ries, Andrew L., editor of compilation.
III. Bordow, Richard A., editor of compilation.
[DNLM: 1. Lung Diseases—Handbooks. WF 39]
RC756
616.2'4—dc23

                                                            2013050544

Care has been taken to confirm the accuracy of the information presented and to describe generally accepted practices. However, the authors and publisher are not responsible for errors or omissions or for any consequences from application of the information in this book and make no warranty, expressed or implied, with respect to the currency, completeness, or accuracy of the contents of the publication. Application of this information in a particular situation remains the professional responsibility of the practitioner.

The authors and publisher have exerted every effort to ensure that drug selection and dosage set forth in this text are in accordance with current recommendations and practice at the time of publication. However, in view of ongoing research, changes in government regulations, and the constant flow of information relating to drug therapy and drug reactions, the reader is urged to check the package insert for each drug for any change in indications and dosage and for added warnings and precautions. This is particularly important when the recommended agent is a new or infrequently employed drug.

Some drugs and medical devices presented in this publication have Food and Drug Administration (FDA) clearance for limited use in restricted research settings. It is the responsibility of the health care provider to ascertain the FDA status of each drug or device planned for use in their clinical practice.

To

Prudy

Who remains optimistic, cheerful, and courageous
in the midst of life's adversity. You are loved more than
you will ever know. (TM)

To

Vivian and the UCSD Pulmonary Family

We could not have done this without you. (AR)

To

Liz

Who has encouraged, supported, and sustained me
for the last forty years and seven editions. It has been
a truly wonderful journey! (RB)

And

To

Kenneth Moser (i.e., KM)

A gifted physician and teacher. He was the common
thread among the three of us as well as the inspiration
for creating and perpetuating this manual.

Contributing Authors

Dennis E. Amundson, DO
Staff Physician
Scripps Clinic
Encinitas, California

William R. Auger, MD
Professor of Clinical Medicine
Pulmonary and Critical Care
  Medicine
University of California, San Diego
San Diego, California

Frank D. Bender, MD
Staff Physician
Escondido Pulmonary
  Medicine Group
Escondido, California

Jonathan L. Benumof, MD
Professor of Anesthesia
Department of Anesthesiology
UCSD School of Medicine
San Diego, California

Robert Bercovitch, MD
Staff Physician
Yale–New Haven Hospital
New Haven, Connecticut

Timothy D. Bigby, MD
Professor of Medicine
Pulmonary & Critical
  Care Medicine
University of California, San Diego
La Jolla, California
Section Chief, Pulmonary and Critical Care
  Medicine Service
VA San Diego Healthcare System
San Diego, California

Jennifer Blanchard, MD
Assistant Professor
Department of Medicine
University of California, San Diego
San Diego, California

Richard A. Bordow, MD
Associate Director
Pulmonary Function Laboratory
Doctors' Hospital
San Pablo, California

Shari A. Brazinsky, MD
Staff Physician
Alvarado Hospital Medical
  Center
San Diego, California

David M. Burns, MD
Professor Emeritus
Family and Preventive Medicine
UCSD School of Medicine
San Diego, California

J. Jonas Carmichael, MD
Fellow
Department of Pulmonary/Critical Care Medicine
Naval Medical Center San Diego
San Diego, California

Antonino Catanzaro, MD
Professor of Medicine
Pulmonary and Critical Care Medicine
University of California, San Diego
San Diego, California

Henri G. Colt, MD
Professor of Medicine
Pulmonary & Critical Care
University of California, Irvine
Orange, California

Douglas J. Conrad, MD
Professor of Medicine
Pulmonary and Critical Care Medicine
University of California, San Diego
San Diego, California
Director, UCSD Adult Cystic Fibrosis
  Clinic
Department of Medicine
UCSD Medical Center
La Jolla, California

Laura E. Crotty Alexander, MD
Assistant Professor of Medicine
Pulmonary and Critical Care Medicine
University of California, San Diego
San Diego, California

Konrad L. Davis, MD
Staff Physician
Pulmonary Department
Naval Medical Center San Diego
San Diego, California

David J. De La Zerda, MD
Fellow
Division of Pulmonary and Critical Care
  Medicine
University of California, San Diego
San Diego, California

Asha Devereaux, MD, MPH
Pulmonary Medicine
Sharp-Coronado Hospital
Coronado, California

Jeffrey R. Dichter, MD
Medical Director
Unity Hospital Intensive Care
Allina Health
Minneapolis, Minnesota

David Wayne Dockweiler, MD
Medical Director, Surgical Services
Staff Physician
Scripps Memorial Hospital, La Jolla
La Jolla, California

Richard D. Drucker, MD
Staff Physician
Kaiser Permanente
Woodland Hills, California

Wael ElMaraachli, MD
Assistant Professor of Medicine
Pulmonary and Critical Care Medicine
University of California, San Diego
San Diego, California

Mary Elmasri, MD
Fellow
Pulmonary and Critical Care Medicine
University of California, San Diego
San Diego, California

Steven J. Escobar, MD, FCCP, FACP
Assistant Professor
Internal Medicine
Uniformed Services University
 of the Health Sciences
Bethesda, Maryland
Head
Pulmonary Medicine
Naval Medical Center
San Diego, California

Garner G. Faulkner, RRT
Manager
Respiratory Care Department
University of California, San Diego
 Health System
San Diego, California

Peter F. Fedullo, MD
Clinical Professor of Medicine
Pulmonary and Critical Care Medicine
University of California, San Diego
San Diego, California

Timothy M. Fernandes, MD
Associate Physician
Pulmonary and Critical Care Medicine
University of California, San Diego
San Diego, California

Patricia W. Finn, MD
Professor and Head, Department of Medicine
University of Illinois College of Medicine at Chicago
Chicago, Illinois

Amy L. Firth, PhD
Research Scientist
Salk Institute
Laboratory of Genetics
La Jolla, California

Richard Ford, BS, RRT, FAARC
Administrative Director
Respiratory Care Department
University of California, San Diego Health System
San Diego, California

Michael J. Freudiger, PharmD
Clinical Pharmacist
Saint Agnes Medical Center
Fresno, California

Mark M. Fuster, MD
Assistant Professor of Medicine
Pulmonary and Critical Care Medicine
University of California, San Diego
Staff Physician
Pulmonary & Critical Care Section
VA San Diego Healthcare System
San Diego, California

Eugene M. Golts, MD
Assistant Clinical Professor of Surgery
Department of Surgery
Division of Cardiothoracic Surgery
University of California, San Diego
San Diego, California

Ian R. Grover, MD
Associate Clinical Professor of Medicine
Emergency Medicine
Medical Director
Hyperabaric Medicine Center
University of California, San Diego
 Medical Center
San Diego, California

Tony S. Han, MD
Staff Physician
Department of Pulmonary/Critical
 Care Medicine
Naval Medical Center San Diego
San Diego, California

Carl K. Hoh, MD
Professor of Radiology
Division Chief, Nuclear Medicine
University of California, San Diego
San Diego, California

William G. Hughson, MD, DPhil
Clinical Professor of Medicine
Director, Center for Occupational &
Environmental Medicine
University of California, San Diego
San Diego, California

Tristan J. Huie, MD
Instructor
Medicine
University of Colorado, Denver
Aurora, Colorado
Instructor
Medicine
National Jewish Health
Denver, Colorado

Shazia M. Jamil, MD, FCCP, FAASM
Assistant Clinical Professor
Department of Medicine
University of California, San Diego School
of Medicine
Attending Physician
Pulmonary and Critical Care Medicine
Scripps Clinic, Scripps Green Hospital
La Jolla, California

Lindsay G. Jensen, BA
Research Fellow
Department of Radiation Oncology
Moores Cancer Center
University of California, San Diego
La Jolla, California

Kim M. Kerr, MD
Clinical Professor of Medicine
Director, Medical Intensive Care
Unit–Thornton
Pulmonary and Critical Care Medicine
University of California, San Diego
San Diego, California

Erik B. Kistler, MD, PhD
Assistant Professor of Anesthesiology
Department of Anesthesiology &
Critical Care
University of California, San Diego, & VA
San Diego Healthcare System
San Diego, California

Andrew Kitcher, MD
Fellow
Pulmonary and Critical Care Medicine
University of California, San Diego
San Diego, California

David H. Kupferberg, MD, MPH
Staff Physician
Pulmonary & Critical Care Division
Physician Lead, Health Connect Optimization,
San Diego
San Diego Medical Center–Zion
Southern California Permanente Medical Group
San Diego, California

Judd W. Landsberg, MD
Assistant Professor of Medicine
Pulmonary and Critical Care Medicine
University of California, San Diego
San Diego, California
Staff Physician
Pulmonary & Critical Care Section
VA San Diego Healthcare System
San Diego, California

Deneen A. LeBlanc, RRT, NPS, AE-C
Practice Manager
Mercy Health Physician Partners Southeast
Kentwood, Michigan

Stephen H. Lee, MD
Staff Physician
Sharp Rees-Stealy Medical Group
San Diego, California

Andrew D. Lerner, MD
Fellow
Pulmonary and Critical Care Medicine
University of California, San Diego
San Diego, California

Julian P. Lichter, MD, FCCP
Associate Clinical Professor
Department of Medicine
University of California, San Diego
Director of ICU and Respiratory
Department of Medicine
Scripps Mercy Hospital
San Diego, California

Thuy K. Lin, MD
Staff Physician
Department of Pulmonary/Critical Care Medicine
Naval Medical Center San Diego
San Diego, California

Philip A. LoBue, MD
Associate Director for Science
Division of Tuberculosis Elimination
Centers for Disease Control and Prevention
Atlanta, Georgia

José S. Loredo, MD, MS, MPH
Professor of Clinical Medicine
Pulmonary and Critical Care Medicine
University of California, San Diego
San Diego, California

Bao Q. Luu, MD
Staff Physician
Scripps Clinic
San Diego, California

Marisa Magaña, MD
Assistant Clinical Professor
Pulmonary and Critical Care Medicine
University of California, San Diego
San Diego, California

Samir S. Makani, MD
Associate Clinical Professor
Pulmonary and Critical Care Medicine
University of California, San Diego
San Diego, California

Jess Mandel, MD
Associate Professor of Medicine
Pulmonary and Critical Care Medicine
University of California, San Diego
San Diego, California

Gregory Matwiyoff, MD
Fellowship Program Director
Department of Pulmonary/Critical Care Medicine
Naval Medical Center San Diego
San Diego, California

Russell J. Miller, MD
Fellow
Department of Pulmonary/Critical Care Medicine
Naval Medical Center San Diego
San Diego, California

Omar H. Mohamedaly, MD
Fellow
Pulmonary and Critical Care Medicine
University of California, San Diego
San Diego, California

Philippe R. Montgrain, MD
Assistant Professor
Pulmonary and Critical Care Medicine
University of California, San Diego
Staff Physician
Medicine Service
VA San Diego Healthcare System
San Diego, California

Timothy A. Morris, MD, FCCP
Professor of Medicine and Clinical Service Chief
Division of Pulmonary and Critical Care Medicine
University of California, San Diego School of Medicine
La Jolla, California
Medical Director of Respiratory Care and Pulmonary Function Laboratory
University of California, San Diego Medical Center
San Diego, California

Dominic A. Munafo Jr., MD
Assistant Clinical Professor
Internal Medicine
University of California
Medical Director
Sleep Data, Inc.
San Diego, California

Jennifer M. Namba, PharmD, BCPS
Assistant Professor of Clinical Pharmacy
Skaggs School of Pharmacy
San Diego, California

John Scott Parrish, MD
Associate Fellowship Program Director
Department of Pulmonary/Critical Care Medicine
Naval Medical Center San Diego
San Diego, California

David Poch, MD
Assistant Clinical Professor
Pulmonary and Critical Care Medicine
University of California, San Diego
San Diego, California

Bruce M. Potenza, MD, FACS
Clinical Professor
Department of Surgery
UCSD School of Medicine
San Diego, California

Frank L. Powell, PhD
Professor of Medicine and Chief
Division of Physiology
University of California, San Diego
La Jolla, California

Jennifer M. Radin, MPH
Graduate Student
University of California, San Diego/San Diego State University Joint Doctoral Program in Public Health (Epidemiology)
San Diego, California

Charles A. Read, MD
Professor of Medicine and Surgery
Division of Pulmonary, Critical Care,
  and Sleep Medicine
Vice Chairman, Inpatient Medicine
Director, Adult Critical Care
Director, Pulmonary Fellowship Program
Georgetown University Medical Center
Washington, D.C.

Justin C. Reis, MD
Pulmonary Fellow
Department of Pulmonary/Critical
  Care Medicine
Naval Medical Center San Diego
San Diego, California

Andrew L. Ries, MD, MPH
Associate Vice Chancellor for Academic Affairs
Professor of Medicine and Family and Preventive
  Medicine
University of California, San Diego School of
  Medicine
La Jolla, California
Director of Pulmonary Rehabilitation
University of California, San Diego Medical Center
San Diego, California

David R. Riker, MD
Director, Interventional Pulmonology/Critical Care
San Diego Interventional Procedures & Complex
  Airway Center
San Diego, California

William L. Ring, MD
Pulmonary and Critical Care Medicine
Scripps Clinic Torrey Pines
Co-Director, Intensive Care Unit
Pulmonary and Critical Care Medicine
Green Hospital of Scripps Clinic
La Jolla, California

Omar Saeed, MD
Staff Physician
Department of Pulmonary/Critical
  Care Medicine
Naval Medical Center San Diego
San Diego, California

Ajay P. Sandhu, MD, DMRT
Clinical Professor
Department of Radiation Oncology
University of California, San Diego
Medical Director
Department of Radiation Oncology
Moores Cancer Center
La Jolla, California

Kathleen Sarmiento, MD, MPH
Assistant Professor
Pulmonary and Critical Care Medicine
University of California, San Diego
Staff Physician
Medicine Service
VA San Diego Healthcare System
San Diego, California

Gregory B. Seymann, MD, SFHM
Clinical Professor of Medicine
Division of Hospital Medicine
UCSD School of Medicine
San Diego, California

Kevin D. Shaw, MD
Assistant Clinical Professor
Pulmonary and Critical Care Medicine
University of California, San Diego
San Diego, California

Cecilia M. Smith, DO, FACP, FCCP
Clinical Professor of Medicine
Department of Medicine
Jefferson Medical College
Philadelphia, Pennsylvania
Chair
Department of Medicine
The Reading Hospital and
  Medical Center
West Reading, Pennsylvania

Robert M. Smith, MD
Professor of Medicine
Pulmonary and Critical Care Medicine
University of California, San Diego
Associate Chief of Staff for Research and
  Development
Chief of Staff/Medical Director, VA San Diego
  Healthcare Systems
San Diego, California

Maida V. Soghikian, MD
Staff Physician
Pulmonary and Critical Care Medicine
Scripps Clinic Torrey Pines
Co-director of Respiratory Care
Scripps Green Hospital
Co-chair, Scripps Health Respiratory and Critical
  Care Co-management Group
La Jolla, California

Xavier Soler, MD, PhD
Assistant Professor of Clinical Medicine
Department of Medicine
University of California, San Diego
San Diego, California

Paul Stark, MD
Professor Emeritus of Radiology
Department of Radiology
University of California, San Diego
San Diego, California

Justin P. Stocks, MD
Pulmonary Fellow
Department of Pulmonary/Critical Care Medicine
Naval Medical Center San Diego
San Diego, California

Victor J. Test, MD, FCCP
Professor of Medicine
Pulmonary Medicine, Critical Care
University of Oklahoma
Tulsa, Oklahoma

Michael Tripp, MD, FCCP
Pulmonologist and Intensivist
Staff Physician
Department of Pulmonary/Critical Care Medicine
Naval Medical Center San Diego
San Diego, California

Angela C. Wang, MD
Staff Physician
Scripps Clinic Torrey Pines
La Jolla, California

James H. Williams Jr., MD
Adjunct Professor
University of California, Irvine
Orange, California

Jason X.-J. Yuan, MD, PhD
Professor of Medicine and Vice Chair
*   for Scholarly Activities*
Department of Medicine
University of Illinois College of Medicine
*   at Chicago*
Chicago, Illinois

Gordon L. Yung, MD
Professor of Medicine
Pulmonary and Critical Care Medicine
University of California, San Diego
San Diego, California

Preface

Thirty-four years ago, the first edition of the *Manual of Clinical Problems in Pulmonary Medicine* was published. Inspired by the talented and enthusiastic members of a relatively new Pulmonary Division at the University of California Medical School, San Diego (founded in 1968), the *Manual* emphasized the importance of clear and rational approaches to clinical challenges. Subsequent editions, while acknowledging the "half-life of truth" in clinical medicine, continued to integrate essential fact with well-researched expert opinion and provided an annotated bibliography emphasizing the path to understanding the current "state of the art." Despite the enormous changes in every facet of health technology, the *Manual's* focus on the clinician has remained constant. It has been an invaluable resource for physicians of all skill levels who were faced with a wide variety of pulmonary problems.

Now in its seventh edition, we have endeavored to provide clinicians with concise, clear, and practical essays on topics that are highly relevant to specific situations. The chapters are modeled after collegial conversations, consultations, and teaching sessions, rather than an encyclopedic compendium.

The current edition is divided into three sections. The first section is an up-to-date overview of the various resources and procedures available to the pulmonary physician. The second section, which is a new one for the *Manual*, describes common clinical presentations of respiratory disorders. It emphasizes how the subtleties inherent to respiratory complaints might guide the formulation of differential diagnoses as well as the initiation of treatment. The last, and largest, section contains state-of-the-art information about specific pulmonary disorders.

The editors express their heartfelt appreciation to the faculty, fellows, alumni, and friends of the UCSD Division of Pulmonary and Critical Care Medicine for the many hours they spent authoring these chapters. We are especially grateful to our pulmonary colleagues at the Naval Medical Center San Diego ("Balboa"), who came through in a clutch with their superbly written chapters.

We hope you enjoy reading these chapters as much as we enjoyed authoring and editing them.

Timothy A. Morris
Andrew L. Ries
Richard A. Bordow

Contents

Section I Pulmonary Resources and Procedures 1

1 Radiographic Evaluation of Lung Disease 1
Paul Stark

2 Radioisotopic Techniques 5
Timothy A. Morris • Carl K. Hoh

3 Pulmonary Function Testing 9
Timothy A. Morris

4 Exercise 19
Andrew L. Ries

5 Evaluation of Arterial Blood Gases and Acid–Base Homeostasis 23
Timothy A. Morris

6 Thoracic Ultrasound Uses in Pulmonary Medicine 32
David R. Riker

7 Interventional Pulmonology: Advanced Diagnostic Procedures 40
Andrew D. Lerner • Samir S. Makani

8 Preoperative Pulmonary Evaluation 45
Stephen H. Lee

9 Pharmacotherapy 50
Jennifer M. Namba • Michael J. Freudiger

10 Pulmonary Rehabilitation 57
Andrew L. Ries

11 Interventional Pulmonology Therapeutic Procedures 61
Andrew D. Lerner • Samir S. Makani

12 Pulmonary Therapeutics 64
Garner G. Faulkner • Deneen A. LeBlanc

13 Tobacco Control 69
David M. Burns

14 Disaster Management by the Pulmonologist **74**
Asha Devereaux • Jeffrey R. Dichter • Dennis E. Amundson

15 Mechanical Ventilation: Devices and Methods **84**
Timothy A. Morris

16 Mechanical Ventilation: Complications and Discontinuation **89**
Timothy A. Morris

17 Protocol-Driven Care in Respiratory Therapy **96**
Timothy A. Morris • Ford Richard

18 Techniques for Clinical Quality Improvement and Error Reduction Techniques **100**
Gregory B. Seymann

19 Disability and Medicolegal Evaluation **106**
William G. Hughson

20 Air Travel and High-Altitude Medicine **110**
David J. De La Zerda • Frank L. Powell

Section II Presentations of Respiratory Disorders 120

21 Dyspnea **120**
Victor J. Test

22 Approach to Pulmonary Vascular Disease **124**
David Poch

23 Chronic Cough **128**
Judd W. Landsberg

24 Pleural Effusion **131**
Henri G. Colt

25 Hemoptysis **137**
Henri G. Colt

26 Complications of Pulmonary Resections **143**
Eugene M. Golts

27 Pneumothorax 148
Henri G. Colt

28 Aspiration 155
Shazia M. Jamil

29 The Lung in Pregnancy 159
Kathleen Sarmiento • Andrew Kitcher

30 Lung Disease in the Immunocompromised Patient 167
Shazia M. Jamil

31 The Lung in Drug Abuse 173
Tristan J. Huie • Charles A. Read

32 Pneumonia: General Considerations 180
Maida V. Soghikian • William L. Ring

33 Airway Obstruction 185
Russell J. Miller • Gregory Matwiyoff • John Scott Parrish

34 Acute Hypercapnic Respiratory Failure 190
Timothy A. Morris

35 Bronchiectasis 197
Kevin D. Shaw

36 The Difficult Airway 206
Erik B. Kistler • Jonathan L. Benumof

37 Occupational-Environmental Lung Disease 212
William G. Hughson

38 Solitary Pulmonary Nodule 215
Andrew D. Lerner • Samir S. Makani

39 Mediastinal Masses 222
Timothy M. Fernandes

40 Eosinophilic Lung Disease 228
Timothy M. Fernandes

Section III Diseases 233

41 **Pneumococcal Pneumonia** 233
Julian P. Lichter

42 **Staphylococcal and Streptococcal Pneumonias** 240
Omar H. Mohamedaly • Laura E. Crotty Alexander

43 *Haemophilus influenzae* **Infections** 245
Dennis E. Amundson • Jennifer M. Radin

44 *Klebsiella* **Pneumonia** 250
Steven J. Escobar

45 **Other Gram-Negative Pneumonias:** *Pseudomonas aeruginosa,*
Escherichia coli, Proteus, Serratia, Enterobacter, **and** *Acinetobacter* 253
James H. Williams, Jr.

46 **Anaerobic Lung Infections** 263
Laura E. Crotty Alexander

47 **Atypical Pneumonias:** *Mycoplasma, Chlamydophila* (Chlamydia),
Q Fever, and *Legionella* 267
Maida V. Soghikian

48 **Viral Pneumonia** 273
Bao Q. Luu

49 **Tuberculosis: Epidemiology, Diagnosis, and Treatment of Latent
Infection** 278
Philip A. LoBue

50 **Tuberculosis: Clinical Manifestations and Diagnosis of Disease** 282
Philip A. LoBue

51 **Tuberculosis: Treatment of Disease** 286
Philip A. LoBue

52 **Nontuberculous Mycobacterial Pulmonary Infections** 291
Marisa Magaña • Antonino Catanzaro

53 **Coccidioidomycosis** 297
Robert Bercovitch • Antonino Catanzaro

54 **Histoplasmosis** 303
Omar Saeed • J. Jonas Carmichael

55 Blastomycosis 308
David Wayne Dockweiler

56 *Aspergillus* Lung Disease 311
Judd W. Landsberg

57 Nocardiosis and Actinomycosis 320
Wael ElMaraachli • Antonino Catanzaro

58 Cryptococcosis 325
Wael ElMaraachli • Antonino Catanzaro

59 Nematode and Trematode Diseases of the Lung 331
Konrad L. Davis

60 Amebiasis and Echinococcal Diseases of the Lung 335
William L. Ring

61 Pulmonary Infections and Complications in HIV-Infected Patients 339
Jennifer Blanchard

62 Hospital-Acquired Pneumonia 347
Kim M. Kerr

63 Asthma 353
Timothy D. Bigby • Patricia W. Finn

64 Chronic Obstructive Pulmonary Disease: Definition and Epidemiology 363
Andrew L. Ries

65 Chronic Obstructive Pulmonary Disease: Clinical and Laboratory Manifestations, Pathophysiology, and Prognosis 368
Andrew L. Ries

66 Chronic Obstructive Pulmonary Disease: Management 372
Andrew L. Ries

67 The Acute Respiratory Distress Syndrome 378
Robert M. Smith

68 Thromboembolic Disease: Epidemiology, Natural History, and Diagnosis 385
Timothy A. Morris

69 Thromboembolic Disease: Prophylaxis   393
Timothy M. Fernandes • Timothy A. Morris

70 Thromboembolic Disease: Therapy   399
Mary Elmasri • Timothy A. Morris

71 Chronic Thromboembolic Pulmonary Hypertension   406
Peter F. Fedullo • William R. Auger

72 Unusual Forms of Embolism   413
Peter F. Fedullo

73 Pulmonary Hypertension: Pathogenesis and Etiology   420
Amy L. Firth • Jason X.-J. Yuan

74 Pulmonary Hypertension: Diagnosis and Treatment   425
David Poch • Jess Mandel

75 Lung Transplantation   430
Marisa Magaña • Gordon L. Yung

76 Pulmonary Manifestations of Sickle Cell Disease   439
Marisa Magaña • Jess Mandel

77 Cystic Fibrosis   444
Douglas J. Conrad

78 Disorders of the Thoracic Spine   449
Thuy K. Lin • Justin C. Reis

79 Disorders of the Diaphragm   454
Tony S. Han

80 Neuromuscular Diseases and Spinal Cord Injury   459
Russell J. Miller • John Scott Parrish

81 Sleep Apnea, Alveolar Hypoventilation,
and Obesity-Hypoventilation   466
Kathleen Sarmiento • José S. Loredo

82 Silicosis   474
Richard D. Drucker

83 Coal Workers' Pneumoconiosis 477
William G. Hughson

84 Asbestos-Related Disease 480
William G. Hughson

85 Work-Related Asthma 484
William G. Hughson

86 Pulmonary Injury in Burn Patients 488
Bruce M. Potenza

87 Hypersensitivity Pneumonitis 493
Dominic A. Munafo, Jr.

88 Drowning and Diving Accidents 498
Ian R. Grover

89 Radiation-Induced Lung Disease 504
Lindsay G. Jensen • Mark M. Fuster • Ajay P. Sandhu

90 Sarcoidosis 512
Xavier Soler

91 Granulomatosis with Polyangiitis (Wegener Granulomatosis) 516
Justin P. Stocks • Michael Tripp

92 Goodpasture Syndrome 521
Omar H. Mohamedaly

93 Idiopathic Pulmonary Hemosiderosis 527
William L. Ring

94 Idiopathic Interstitial Pneumonias 530
Gordon L. Yung • Cecilia M. Smith

95 Pulmonary Manifestations of Rheumatoid Arthritis 540
Frank D. Bender

96 The Lungs in Systemic Lupus Erythematosus, Systemic Sclerosis, Polymyositis, Dermatomyositis, and Mixed Connective Tissue Disease 547
Cecilia M. Smith • Gordon L. Yung

97 **Pulmonary Langerhans Cell Histiocytosis** 558
Cecilia M. Smith • Gordon L. Yung

98 **Neurofibromatosis, Lymphangioleiomyomatosis, and Tuberous Sclerosis** 562
Cecilia M. Smith • Gordon L. Yung

99 **Pulmonary Alveolar Proteinosis** 571
Angela C. Wang

100 **Bronchial Carcinoids and Benign Neoplasms of the Lung** 575
David H. Kupferberg

101 **Lung Cancer: Diagnosis, Staging, and Prognosis** 580
Samir S. Makani • Mark M. Fuster

102 **Lung Cancer: Classification, Epidemiology, and Screening** 585
Philippe R. Montgrain

103 **Lung Cancer: Treatment** 590
Mark M. Fuster

104 **Extrathoracic and Endocrine Manifestations of Lung Cancer** 594
Shari A. Brazinsky

105 **Neoplastic Disease of the Pleura** 601
Henri G. Colt

INDEX 607

Pulmonary Resources and Procedures

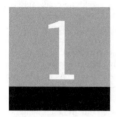

Radiographic Evaluation of Lung Disease

Paul Stark

Chest radiography provides noninvasive information about patient anatomy and pathology, and is invaluable in the assessment of lung, pleural, mediastinal, cardiovascular, and chest wall diseases. Wilhelm Roentgen discovered x-rays in 1895 and until recently the traditional radiographic assessment employed a cassette or dedicated chest unit with intensifying screens to record the x-ray image, and lightboxes to view the films. This has largely been supplanted by electronic imaging, computer manipulation, wide area network distribution, and viewing on computer workstations.

Effective use of imaging modalities in general and of chest radiography in particular depends upon integrating clinical information with the imaging findings. A request for a chest radiograph should convey specific information and questions to the radiologist to get the most useful interpretation. Comparison studies and supplementary views can complement the interpretation of an abnormal radiograph. Knowledge of the limitations, costs, and relative radiation risks are important issues to consider.

TECHNIQUE

Standard chest radiographs are made at a 6-ft or 2-m distance (from x-ray tube focus to image detector), in frontal, usually posteroanterior (PA) and left lateral projections (left side against the image detector). The patient is instructed to take and hold a maximal inspiration. The image detector should have a wide dynamic range and a high sensitivity, in order to display multiple shades of gray and limit the required radiation dose. Using kilovoltage between 120 and 140 kilovolt peak (kVp) makes it possible to display normal anatomy and pathologic findings of the mediastinum and chest wall in tandem with findings in the lungs on the same image. During interpretation of the image, the radiologist can change the window level and window width (contrast and brightness) on the fly and enhance the visibility of different structures on the chest radiograph. A fixed grid is used to absorb x-ray scatter, which otherwise would degrade the quality of the image.

Portable or bedside examinations account for a large proportion of chest radiographs, despite their greater cost and diminished quality. They are more difficult to interpret because of shallow inspiration, which crowds normal structures together to simulate lung parenchymal abnormalities, and lower kilovoltage technique, which can result in overexposed lungs and an underpenetrated mediastinum. Because of the apical lordotic projection of the x-ray beam in bedridden patients, the diaphragm obscures a considerable portion of the lower lobes. Antilordotic projection distorts the configuration of the chest as well. The anteroposterior projection and short tube-cassette distance geometrically magnify the cardiac silhouette, which obscures part of the lungs. On supine radiographs, pleural effusions and pneumothorax are more difficult to detect. It is important to avoid overinterpretation of bedside studies, particularly those of poor quality.

Fluoroscopy of the chest serves mainly as a guide to special procedures or as a means of localizing a lesion seen on only one radiographic view. However, diaphragmatic paralysis, mediastinal shift resulting from air trapping, or tracheobronchial collapse can be detected with fluoroscopy by observing these structures dynamically in deep inspiration, in deep expiration, during coughing, and with sniffing maneuvers.

SUPPLEMENTAL RADIOGRAPHIC STUDIES

In the past, apical lordotic views were used to assess lesions obscured by the clavicle and first rib. In practice, lordotic views are confusing and should be avoided. The pulmonary apices can be adequately visualized with frontal, high kilovolt peak techniques and with oblique chest radiographs.

Oblique views were used formerly to assess cardiac chambers, but are now useful mainly to provide additional tangential projections of the pleura, as in screening for asbestos pleural plaques. Localization of pulmonary nodules and differentiation of lung from chest wall pathology can be facilitated. Oblique views can be useful when abnormalities are located in the costophrenic sulcus or superimposed on the hilar regions. The tracheobronchial tree is best seen on the left anterior oblique projection, since it is unobscured by the thoracic spine. As mentioned, the contralateral oblique views provide the best display of the pulmonary apices: the left anterior oblique view for the right apex and the right anterior oblique view for the left apex.

The lung bases are better visualized on supine views of the abdomen due to better penetration and more favorable orientation of the central x-ray beam. Antilordotic chest radiographs can be utilized in bedridden patients to enhance the visibility of the lung bases.

Lateral decubitus views have a variety of uses. In the case of pleural disease, they have a dual function: to show that an effusion is mobile (not loculated or organized) by layering when it is dependent, and to reveal whether the otherwise obscured lung expands normally when it is nondependent. The decubitus view is named according to the dependent side. The study is often misused to see whether large effusions are mobile (or *layer out*). Additional studies like computed tomography (CT) scanning or ultrasonography are better tools to guide the drainage of such effusions and to determine the optimal site for insertion of needles or tubes.

In the bedridden patient, gas–liquid levels in lung abscesses or pleural pockets can be best demonstrated with the decubitus position, because it requires a horizontal x-ray beam to show a gas–liquid level. This position is also effective for the detection of pneumothorax on the nondependent side in patients who cannot assume the upright position. The decubitus position allows assessment of diaphragmatic mobility by inducing expansion of the lung on the nondependent side, even in uncooperative patients.

Frontal chest radiography in the prone, recumbent position is an examination that expands the posterior lung and shifts pleural effusions, resulting in unobstructed views of the lung base.

Traditionally, an expiratory image has been used to detect a small pneumothorax, because the trapped pleural gas will appear larger in a smaller hemithorax. This procedure is not recommended for several reasons: (1) a pneumothorax so small as to be visible only on an expiratory study is not clinically relevant; (2) prospective studies have shown that virtually every pneumothorax detected on expiratory images can be identified as well on an accompanying inspiratory study; and (3) the expiratory examination cannot be compared with prior or subsequent inspiratory studies to see whether the patient is getting better or worse. A pair of inspiratory and expiratory chest radiographies can test for mediastinal shift or detect subtle findings caused by air trapping. Similarly, a forced expiration, or Valsalva maneuver, will cause a reduction in the size of systemic veins compared to an inspiratory study, and can be used to help distinguish venous vascular structures from enlarged lymph nodes or other solid lesions and may be useful in the detection of large airway collapse as seen in tracheomalacia.

DIGITAL CHEST RADIOGRAPHY

Traditionally, the pattern of x-rays that emerges from the body was captured by intensifying screens whose light directly exposed the film. The developed film negative was then displayed, viewed, and interpreted on a light box. The film itself had three functions: detection, display, and storage.

In 1980, storage phosphor plates were introduced. They are composed of barium halide (Br, J, F) doped with europium. Storage phosphor plates receive and store the x-ray image, which is then decoded by a laser reader which generates an electronic output. CR, or computed radiography, has virtually replaced conventional film and has separated the detection, display, and storage functions, previously unified by conventional film. Today, in most institutions, digitized images are read on the video screen of dedicated workstations (soft copies). Detail resolution has improved such that it is now comparable to conventional radiography. Additionally, the wide latitude of CR leads to a marked reduction in over- or underpenetrated images. CR is most useful for bedside imaging, where the benefits of consistent image quality (by avoiding the frequent under- and over-exposure of conventional films) outweighs the lower spatial resolution of CR.

In the radiology department and in ambulatory settings, dedicated chest units are used. Earlier machines utilize direct digital radiography which employs an electrically charged selenium drum with an electrometer for readout. More recently, flat panel radiography with a phosphor composed of cesium iodide that emits light after interaction with incident x-rays is utilized. The emitted light activates a light-sensitive thin film transistor (TFT) composed of a silicon photodiode matrix that generates electrical charges which are ultimately converted into shades of gray by a processor. The processed image is eventually sent to a picture archiving and communication system (PACS) and from there to a video workstation. This image can be enhanced, manipulated, zoomed, and panned during readout. Dual energy radiography allows for separation of high–atomic number structures (i.e., calcium) from soft tissue structures: thus osseous structures and soft tissues can be visually separated, facilitating the display of nodules, hidden by ribs or other bony structures.

PACS is an important advance that has eliminated the conventional file room. PACS allows for storage of digital images and their distribution throughout the entire enterprise. Retrieval of comparison studies is facilitated, speeding up the radiologic interpretation of current images. Multiple physicians can view the same image simultaneously throughout the health care enterprise at multiple sites. The problem of lost images has been nearly eliminated and duplication of images is only rarely needed.

Computer-Aided Diagnosis

Computer-aided diagnosis (CAD) refers to computerized algorithms designed for the automated detection of lung nodules and interstitial lung disease. Automated nodule detection can be implemented as an advanced PACS application. The location of possible nodules can be indicated as overlays on images. Temporal subtraction techniques subtract a previous chest radiograph from a current chest radiograph in order to enhance interval changes. These algorithms have the potential to improve performance and enhance diagnostic accuracy and work flow, but to date, have limited utility because of a high false-positive rate.

SCREENING

The exception to the concept of carefully planned radiography is the screening examination. Large screening surveys for tuberculosis have been shown to be ineffective with current prevalence rates, although institutions still use routine chest radiography for pregnant women who have positive tuberculin skin tests or have not been tested before delivery, for health-care workers; some states require chest radiographs for teachers or food handlers. Screening radiography for tuberculosis can be justified in patients in whom skin tests are unreliable (e.g., those with AIDS). Usually, just a frontal view is sufficient, since the lateral view doesn't contribute additional useful information in this particular setting.

Screening for occupational lung disease is a well-established practice and has epidemiologic and clinical utility. An elaborate system of classification of pneumoconiosis-related changes in the lungs and pleura has been developed for the International Labor Organization (ILO). A network of readers qualified by examination (so called B-readers) is maintained by the National Institute of Occupational Safety and Health (NIOSH).

Screening for lung cancer has been studied extensively; its efficacy can be expressed in terms of cost per resectable lung cancer discovered, by decrease of disease-specific mortality in the population, or by a favorable stage-shift in detected cancers. The recently completed National Lung Cancer Screening Trial (NLST) demonstrated a 20% lung cancer mortality reduction in individuals after three annual screening rounds with CT compared to chest radiographic screening for lung cancer during an 8-year follow-up. Whereas systematic screening of high-risk groups is of measurable yet still debatable utility, a routine annual chest radiography, as part of an annual physical examination, is of limited value. See Chapter 2 for further discussion of chest CT in lung cancer screening.

Another controversial screening application is the routine admission chest radiograph. Patients with no history or findings related to the heart or lungs are not likely to show abnormalities. Similarly, a routine preoperative screening chest radiography has low efficacy in patients without clinical evidence of heart or lung abnormalities, but in patients older than 60 years, the likelihood of confirming significant pathology increases. Preoperative radiographies can play an important role as reference studies in the postoperative period.

Error

Radiologic evaluation of the chest is accompanied by a significant rate of error. Studies dealing with detection of well-defined, predetermined abnormalities (e.g., lung cancer) have shown an average false-negative rate of 30% to 40%. Part of these errors of omission may be attributed to failure to detect lesions against the background complexity of normal anatomy or due to an incomplete search of the image: satisfaction of search occurs while the reader is distracted by one positive finding and stops investigating the image for further abnormalities.

Errors of commission occur due to mistakes in interpretation of detected abnormalities that are not assigned the appropriate diagnostic significance. It has been shown that the likelihood of reaching a correct diagnosis based on an imaging examination is enhanced by the availability of an appropriate clinical history and by independent double reading of relevant studies.

FURTHER READING

1. Gurney JW, ed. *Diagnostic Imaging of the Chest*. Salt Lake City, UT: Amirsys; 2006.
   Comprehensive review of the subject.
2. Webb WR, Higgins CB. *Thoracic Imaging: Pulmonary and Cardiovascular Radiology*. Baltimore, MD: Lippincott, Williams & Wilkins; 2010.
   Up to date review of chest and cardiac imaging.
3. Reed JC. *Chest Radiology: Plain Film Patterns and Differential Diagnosis*. Philadelphia, PA: Mosby; 2003.
   Practical approach to differential diagnosis and interpretation of chest radiographs.
4. Milne ENC, Pistolesi M. *Reading the Chest Radiograph—A Physiologic Approach*. Philadelphia, PA: Mosby; 1993.
   Detailed review of cardiopulmonary physiology as it pertains to the interpretation of chest radiographs.
5. Friedman PJ. Practical radiology of the hila and mediastinum. *Postgrad Radiol*. 1981;1:269.
   Practical approach to radiographic anatomy as it pertains to interpreting the chest radiograph.
6. International Labour Office. *Guidelines for the Use of the ILO International Classification of Radiographs of Pneumoconiosis*. 2000 ed. Geneva, Switzerland: International Labour Office; 2002.
7. Korner M, Weber CH, Wirth S, et al. Advances in digital radiography: physical principles and system overview. *Radiographics*. 2007;27:675–686.
   Practical review of physics and equipment used in digital radiography.
8. Shiraishi J, Li F, Doi K. Computer-aided diagnosis for improved detection of lung nodules by use of posterior-anterior and lateral chest radiographs. *Acad Radiol*. 2007;14(1):28–37.
   Describes computer-aided diagnosis and the value of lateral chest radiographs in tandem with the frontal chest radiograph, in detecting pulmonary nodules.
9. Mendelson DS, Khilnani N, Wagner LD, et al. Preoperative chest radiography: value as a baseline examination for comparison. *Radiology*. 1987;165(2):341–343.
   Preoperative chest radiographs may have an important role to play when used as reference films for postoperative imaging.
10. Eisenberg RL, Pollock NR. Low yield of chest radiography in a large tuberculosis screening program. *Radiology*. 2010;256(3):998–1004.
    Universal chest radiography in a large pre-employment TB screening program was of low yield in detection of active TB.

Radioisotopic Techniques

Timothy A. Morris and Carl K. Hoh

Lung ventilation and perfusion ($\dot{V}/\dot{Q}$) scanning is a powerful tool for assessing regional pulmonary blood flow and ventilation. Its most common application is for diagnosing pulmonary embolism, strongly suggested by a focal perfusion defect without a matching ventilation defect. Although contrast-enhanced computed tomographic (CT) scanning is becoming more popular for this purpose, nuclear medicine lung scanning remains the most affordable, reliable, and noninvasive diagnostic option for pulmonary embolism. In addition, $\dot{V}/\dot{Q}$ scanning has unique diagnostic properties that make it useful in several other clinical situations.

Perfusion scans are performed after injection of the radioisotope technetium-99m (^{99m}Tc), incorporated into particles of macroaggregated albumin (MAA) or human albumin microspheres (HAM). A typical dose of ^{99m}Tc MAA for a Q scan contains 100,000 particles and 37 to 148 MBq (1–4 mCi) of radioactivity. Because the individual particles are larger than the pulmonary capillary lumen, they become trapped in the lungs on the "first pass." The focal ^{99}Tc radioactivity intensity therefore reflects the proportional distribution (but not the absolute amount) of blood flow to each lung region. The temporary capillary obstruction from the particles is harmless, as only 0.3% of the capillaries are affected and the albumin particles disintegrate by 8 hours.

Because the distribution of pulmonary blood flow is gravity-dependent, the radioisotope ideally should be injected half in the supine and half in the prone position. Injecting in the sitting or standing position can lead to artifactual apical "defects" on the scan. Optimally, the perfusion scan should include at least six views: anterior, posterior, right and left lateral, and two oblique views.

Ventilation scanning can be performed with several different radiopharmaceuticals, either as a gas or as an aerosol. The most commonly used isotopic gas is xenon-133 (^{133}Xe). For ventilation scans, ^{133}Xe is mixed with air or with a suitable concentration of oxygen to obtain a dose of approximately 185 MBq/L (5 mCi/L). After several deep breaths of air, the patient is connected to a shielded spirometer containing the radioactive gas. Usually, an initial breath is taken to total lung capacity and recorded (single-breath scan). Next, the patient breathes tidally while the distribution of gas is recorded (wash-in phase). After the concentration of radioactivity has equilibrated between the patient's lung and spirometer (equilibrium phase), the patient resumes breathing room air (washout phase). Retention of the gas locally during the washout phase is the most sensitive finding for detecting ventilation abnormalities; this phase should be used for interpretation.

Aerosolized radiolabeled particles have become popular alternative agents for ventilation scans. The most widely used of these is ^{99m}Tc DTPA. Because it is an aerosol rather than a gas, ^{99m}Tc DTPA distribution is determined by the mass and inertial properties of the aerosol particles as well as by the patterns of regional ventilation. Turbulent airflow in large airways can lead to deposition on bronchial walls, causing localized "hot spots" that complicate scan interpretation. Although they have some practical advantages, some ventilation scans performed with aerosolized ^{99}Tc particles yield different results than ^{133}Xe scans. Pertechnegas, consisting of very small (<1 μm) aerosolized ^{99m}Tc-labeled carbon particles, avoids some of the disadvantages inherent in other radiolabeled particle ventilation scans. The small Pertechnegas particles travel to the alveoli without being deposited on airway walls. Thus, there is less residual radioactivity superimposed on the perfusion images. It is yet to be determined whether the theoretical advantages of Pertechnegas will translate into improved diagnostic accuracy over more conventional (and less expensive) methods.

While cost and efficiency considerations have led to widespread use of aerosols, at UCSD, we prefer ^{133}Xe for diagnostic ventilation studies. In addition to the more physiologic image of ventilation, there are practical advantages to this method. Because of the much larger dose of xenon gas (740 MBq) compared to ^{99m}Tc-MAA (148 MBq), the (^{133}Xe) ventilation scan can follow the (^{99}Tc) perfusion scan without significant degradation of the ventilation images. In this sequential technique, the ventilation scan can be performed in the view that optimally displays the perfusion defects; also, a normal perfusion scan makes ventilation scanning unnecessary, minimizing scanning cost and radiation exposure. Finally, aerosols do not provide a washout phase, and that phase has additional diagnostic value in several clinical contexts.

The major application of perfusion and ventilation scans has been to exclude or confirm the diagnosis of pulmonary embolism. Multiple clinical trials defining the sensitivity and specificity of lung scans for pulmonary embolism have concluded that the perfusion and ventilation tests should be considered separately. Interpreted alone, the *sensitivity* of the perfusion scan is extremely high. Indeed, a normal perfusion scan excludes the diagnosis of clinically significant embolism, and outcome studies have shown that withholding treatment in patients with a normal scan (and no venous thrombosis) is safe. However, abnormal perfusion scans are nonspecific. To enhance specificity, three key features should be considered: (1) the size of the perfusion defect, (2) matching chest x-ray findings, and, if necessary, (3) corresponding ventilation scan findings (comprising a ventilation/perfusion, or V̇/Q̇ scan). If the perfusion defects are in areas with infiltrates by chest radiograph or if all defects are subsegmental in size, the study is nondiagnostic, and ventilation scanning will add little of diagnostic value. If one or more defects are segmental or larger, without corresponding chest x-ray findings, a ventilation scan is done. If the areas with perfusion defect(s) ventilate normally, the scan is diagnostic for pulmonary arterial occlusion. If they ventilate abnormally, the scan is nondiagnostic.

Unfortunately, a large proportion of patients tested for possible pulmonary embolism will have nondiagnostic V̇/Q̇ scans. Depending on the patient population being investigated, 10% to 20% of scans will disclose normal perfusion and another 15% to 20% will be diagnostic of acute pulmonary embolism; the remainder will be nondiagnostic. Nondiagnostic studies, however, are associated with a significant incidence of embolism. Calling such nondiagnostic studies "intermediate" or "low" probability may, unfortunately, lull the physician into complacency that pulmonary embolism is not present.

In patients with acute symptoms, the V̇/Q̇ scan indicating "pulmonary arterial obstruction" means acute pulmonary embolism in the overwhelming majority of patients. However, any process that blocks blood flow through the pulmonary arteries can produce this pattern. Among such processes are chronic pulmonary thromboembolic disease (where the obstruction is due, at least in part, to fibroblastic organization of a once-active thrombus), Takayasu's arteritis, fibrosing mediastinitis, primary tumors of the pulmonary arteries, pulmonary artery agenesis, and, rarely, invasion or compression of pulmonary arteries by tumors or other mediastinal components (e.g., aorta, lymph nodes).

Another application of V̇/Q̇ scans is in the quantitative measurement of lung function in the presurgical assessment of a patient with limited lung reserve. For example, in a patient considered for lung resection for cancer or bronchiectasis or for bullectomy, the lung scan provides important regional information that spirometry and other function tests cannot. Specifically, it can define whether the proposed area of resection/bullectomy is a major contributor to the patient's overall ventilation and pulmonary blood flow. In these situations, it is helpful to perform "quantitative" scans, in which the proportion of counts from various lung regions (relative to the entire lung) are measured to determine their contribution to the total lung ventilation and perfusion. If, for example, a right lower lobe site of bronchiectasis is poorly ventilated and barely perfused, its removal won't significantly impair gas exchange function; indeed, it may even improve it. If, however, the lobe carries a large percentage of the total blood flow, its resection may have serious hemodynamic and gas exchange consequences. Thus, quantitative V̇/Q̇ scans provide topographic data that, along with indicators of global function such as spirometry, help complete the pulmonary assessment of the surgical candidate.

V̇/Q̇ scanning also offers a means of noninvasively differentiating primary pulmonary hypertension (PPH) from large vessel, chronic thromboembolic pulmonary hypertension (CTEPH). In PPH, perfusion scans are normal or demonstrate a "mottled" appearance, whereas in CTEPH, multiple, segmental or larger perfusion defects are invariably present. It should be noted, however, that the Q̇ scan results in CTEPH often significantly underestimate the actual degree of angiographic obstruction. Patients with unexplained pulmonary hypertension and one or more segmental perfusion defects should undergo further workup, especially if the perfusion defects are mismatched (see Chapter 66).

Modern nuclear medicine imaging hardware and processing software can generate three-dimensional tomographic images (single photon emission computerized tomography, or SPECT scans) of the lungs. Compared to conventional *planar* V̇/Q̇ imaging, SPECT V̇/Q̇ scans provide higher image contrast, which results in higher sensitivity and reduced nondiagnostic interpretations of ventilation/perfusion. In addition, the three-dimensional images improve anatomical localization and correlation of ventilation and perfusion defects. Parametric images of V̇/Q̇ ratios, coregistered images with diagnostic chest CT scans, and fusion images from hybrid SPECT/CT scanners are newer technologies that will provide simultaneous physiologic and anatomic images for research and (eventually) clinical use.

Radioisotope techniques using thrombus-specific targeting agents have also been used, or are under study, for the detection of venous thrombi and pulmonary emboli. The prototype of such approaches, radiolabeled fibrinogen (RLF), is no longer available, but was of great value in prior epidemiologic studies of deep venous thrombosis. Of potentially greater diagnostic value are radiolabeled antibodies and other radiolabeled agents with high affinity for fibrin, platelet receptors, and other components of active thrombi. Radiolabeled antifibrin antibodies, for example, bind to sites on the surface of acute thrombi and allow them to be detected by gamma camera imaging. An important advantage these agents may have over other imaging modalities is the ability to distinguish *acute* thrombi from other causes of vascular obstruction. For example, intravascular "scars" in the deep veins or pulmonary arteries resulting from prior (inactive) thromboembolic disease may be confused with acute thrombi on more conventional "anatomic" tests, such as ultrasound imaging, V̇/Q̇ scanning, helical CT, and even contrast angiography. However, radiolabeled antibodies will bind to vascular lesions only if biological components of thrombosis are present. In addition, because the antibodies bind equally well to both deep vein thrombi and pulmonary emboli, both lesions may be imaged with a single test.

Gallium-67 (^{67}Ga) lung scanning has limited usefulness in pulmonary medicine. After intravenous injection, ^{67}Ga accumulates in tissues with increased metabolic activity (e.g., neoplasm, inflammation). Although capable of detecting roentgenographically inapparent foci of disease, the clinical application of ^{67}Ga scanning is limited by its nonspecificity. Certain "niches" for ^{67}Ga lung scanning are still used by some clinicians. For example, in sarcoidosis, ^{67}Ga scanning is frequently positive and is used in some centers to follow the progression of this condition. Whether ^{67}Ga scanning can predict functional deterioration or response to therapy more accurately than do more standard tests (e.g., chest roentgenogram, spirometry) remains inconclusive.

Finally, radiolabeled white blood cells have been used widely to detect the presence of abscesses in the lungs and solid organs. The technique is imprecise and typically used only if other means of diagnosing infection have failed.

FURTHER READING

1. Alderson PO, Lee H, Summer WR, et al. Comparison of Xe-133 washout and single breath imaging for the detection of ventilation abnormalities. *J Nucl Med.* 1979;20:917.

   Demonstrates the superiority of ^{133}Xe washout imaging over single-breath imaging in the diagnosis of pulmonary embolism.

2. Baughman RP, Shipley R, Eisentrout CE. Predictive value of gallium scan, angiotensin-converting enzyme level, and bronchoalveolar lavage in two-year follow-up of pulmonary sarcoidosis. *Lung.* 1987;165:371.

   The finding of a negative gallium scan suggests a small likelihood that disease activity will worsen after 2 years.

3. Fishman AJ, Moser KM, Fedullo PF. Perfusion lung scans vs pulmonary angiography in evaluation of suspected primary pulmonary hypertension. *Chest.* 1983;84:679.

Patients with primary pulmonary hypertension had normal or "mottled" perfusion scan patterns; those with chronic thromboembolic pulmonary hypertension had scans characterized by multiple, mismatched segmental defects.

4. Keyes JW. Three-dimensional display of SPECT images: advantages and problems. *J Nucl Med.* 1990;31:1428.

   A good discussion of the problems and promise of SPECT.

5. Hull RD, Hirsh J, Carter CJ, et al. Diagnostic value of ventilation-perfusion lung scanning in patients with suspected pulmonary embolism. *Chest.* 1985;88:819.

   The frequency of angiographically documented pulmonary embolism in scans classified as "low probability" ranged from 25% to 40%.

6. Hull RD, Raskob G. Low probability lung scan findings: a need for change. *Ann Intern Med.* 1991;114:142.

   The term "low probability," or even "intermediate," is potentially harmful to proper assessment of embolic suspects. The term "nondiagnostic" is preferable.

7. Kahn D, Bushnell DL, Dean R, et al. Clinical outcome of patients with a "low probability" of pulmonary embolism on ventilation-perfusion lung scan. *Arch Intern Med.* 1989;149:377.

   None of 90 patients with a "low probability" perfusion scan demonstrated clinical evidence of pulmonary embolism subsequent to the V/Q scan.

8. Knight LC. Do we finally have a radiopharmaceutical for rapid, specific imaging of venous thrombosis [editorial]? *J Nucl Med.* 1991;32:791–795.

   Review of the various approaches, with a good reference list; seems to favor antifibrin antibodies over other agents.

9. Kanke M, Matsueda GR, Strauss HW, et al. Localization and visualization of pulmonary emboli with radiolabeled fibrin-specific monoclonal antibody. *J Nucl Med.* 1991;32:1254.

   One of multiple papers describing similar approaches to the diagnosis of venous thromboembolism.

10. Kipper MS, Moser KM, Kortman KE, et al. Longterm follow-up of patients with suspected embolism and a normal lung scan: perfusion scans in embolic suspects. *Chest.* 1982;82:411.

    This report describes long-term follow-up of embolic suspects who had normal perfusion scans and were not treated with anticoagulant drugs. Excellent outcomes indicate that, in the absence of venous thrombosis, anticoagulant therapy can be withheld on the basis of a normal scan.

11. Kipper MS, Alazraki N. The feasibility of performing Xe-133 ventilation imaging following the perfusion study. *Radiology.* 1982;144:581.

    Demonstrates that the ventilation scan can follow the perfusion scan without significant image degradation.

12 Miniati M, Pistolesi M, Marini C, et al. Value of perfusion lung scan in the diagnosis of pulmonary embolism: results of the Prospective Investigative Study of Acute Pulmonary Embolism Diagnosis (PISA-PED). *Am J Respir Crit Care Med.* 1996;154:1387–1393.

    Perfusion scans alone were assessed, without ventilation, for patients suspected of having PE. Characteristic wedge-shaped defects were highly associated with the presence of PE on angiogram, particularly if the clinical suspicion was high prior to the scan itself.

13. Oster ZH, Sum P. Of monoclonal antibodies and thrombus specific imaging. *J Nucl Med.* 1990;31:1055.

    A good review of the past, present, and future of this approach.

14. Pantin CF, Valind SO, Sweatman M, et al. Measures of the inflammatory response in cryptogenic fibrosing alveolitis. *Am Rev Respir Dis.* 1988;138:1234.

    The initial level of gallium-67 uptake did not predict response to therapy.

15. Peters AM. Imaging inflammation: current role of labeled autologous leukocytes. *J Nucl Med.* 1992;33:65.

    The authors review the use of radiolabeled leukocytes in diagnosing inflammatory states.

16. Ramanna L, Alderson PO, Waxman AD, et al. Regional comparison of technetium-99m DTPA aerosol and radioactive gas ventilation (xenon and krypton) studies in patients with suspected pulmonary embolism. *J Nucl Med.* 1986;27:1391.

Discrepancies existed between gas and aerosol ventilation scan findings, but did not impact on the final scintigraphic probability of pulmonary embolism.

17. Ryan KL, Fedullo PF, Davis GB. Perfusion scan findings understate the severity of angiographic and hemodynamic compromise in chronic thromboembolic pulmonary hypertension. *Chest.* 1988;93:1180.

Perfusion scanning can suggest the diagnosis of thromboembolic pulmonary hypertension, but cannot provide information regarding its severity or surgical accessibility.

18. Reinartz P, Wildberger JE, Schaefer W, et al. Tomographic imaging in the diagnosis of pulmonary embolism: a comparison between V/Q lung scintigraphy in SPECT technique and multislice spiral CT. *J Nucl Med.* 2004;45(9):1501–1508.

In this series of 83 patients suspected of having acute PE, V/Q with SPECT and multislice spiral CT had comparable diagnostic accuracies. CT was a little more specific, but SPECT was more sensitive. Both techniques were more sensitive and specific than planar lung VQ.

19. Bajc M, Olsson B, Palmer J, et al. VQ SPECT for diagnostics of pulmonary embolism in clinical practice. *J Intern Med.* 2008;264(4):379–387.

VQ SPECT was feasible in nearly all of 2,328 patients in this retrospective series, VQ SPECT was feasible in 99% of cases. Compared to follow-up clinical data, the sensitivity was 99% (601 positives in 608 PE cases) and specificity was 985 (1,153 negative scans in 1,153 patients without diagnoses of PE).

20. Roach PJ, Thomas P, Bajc M, et al. Merits of V/Q SPECT scintigraphy compared with CTPA in imaging of pulmonary embolism. *J Nucl Med.* 2008;49(1):167–168.

This is an excellent review by a pioneering group in the field of acute PE detection by nuclear medicine scanning.

21. Stein PD, Freeman LM, Sostman HD, et al. SPECT in acute pulmonary embolism. *J Nucl Med.* 2009;50(12):1999–2007.

This is also an excellent review by an authoritative group. They discuss the higher sensitivity of than that of planar V/Q. The specificity of SPECT tended to be higher as well. Nondiagnostic scans, which were the Achilles' heel of planar V/Q scans, are uncommon in SPECT V/Q scans.

22. Soler X, Hoh CK, Test VJ, et al. Single photon emission computed tomography in chronic thromboembolic pulmonary hypertension. *Respirology.* 2011;16(1):131–137.

23. Soler X, Kerr KM, Marsh JJ, et al. Pilot study comparing SPECT perfusion scintigraphy with CT pulmonary angiography in chronic thromboembolic pulmonary hypertension. *Respirology.* 2012;17(1):180–184.

References 22 and 23 emphasize that SPECT V/Q is an accurate method of detecting perfusion defects in patients with CTEPH.

Pulmonary Function Testing

Timothy A. Morris

The pulmonary function laboratory is an invaluable resource for diagnosis and management of patients with respiratory disorders. Pulmonary function tests (PFTs) are best interpreted using the same approach employed for a physical examination: the *pattern* of findings yields the most clinically useful information, rather than any one particular value. PFTs have a variety of clinical uses, including characterizing the type and degree of respiratory dysfunction (even when it is clinically undetected) and diagnosing disease associated with a particular pattern of dysfunction. PFTs can quantify objectively the physiologic severity of disease, to help monitor disease progression and gauge the impact of therapeutic intervention. The accuracy of PFTs and the clinical utility of the results depend on (1) the technical and clinical expertise of the personnel performing and interpreting the studies, (2) the quality of the equipment, (3) the application of consistent and validated testing techniques, (4) the precision of the data collection and reduction, and (5) the selection of appropriate normal predictive data.

Abnormal PFT values are identified in each subject with the use of individualized normal ranges, which are based on empirically derived regression equations that take into account parameters such as age, height, and sex. For some PFT values, weight, race, and altitude of the laboratory should also be considered. Published series for predicted normal values are numerous (see Table 3-1).

For many PFT parameters such as vital capacity (VC) and the forced expiratory volume in the first second (FEV_1), predictive values calculated from equations from different published studies are generally similar. For other tests (e.g., single-breath diffusing capacity for carbon monoxide [D_{LCO}], instantaneous maximal expiratory flows, partial pressure of oxygen in arterial blood [Pa_{O_2}]), predictive values derived from different equations can differ significantly. For such parameters, it is important that each laboratory evaluates its testing methodology and choice of predicted values by comparing measured values in normal subjects (n = 10–20) with the predicted ones. If more normal subjects than expected have test results outside normal limits, then both the testing methodology and choice of predictive values need to be reevaluated. The optimal prediction equations can then be identified from the study that produces the lowest sum of residuals.

Predicted values for some pulmonary function parameters differ by race. Optimal correction factors are controversial and not well defined. For African Americans, the ATS recommends reducing Caucasian predicted values for VC, total lung capacity (TLC), and FEV_1 by 12%. Predictive values for residual volume (RV), functional residual capacity (FRC), and instantaneous flows (e.g., forced expiratory flow [FEF], 50%) are reduced by 7%. For Asians, the issue of race correction is more complex and is affected by the individual's geographical (and hence nutritional) history.

The clinical significance of abnormal PFT results for an individual patient requires an appreciation of the lower limits of normal. Although the mean plus or minus 1.96 times SD (two-tailed t test, $P < .05$) is a commonly used statistical criterion for normally distributed data, the mean *minus* 1.65 times SD (one-tailed t test, $P < .05$) is a more appropriate limit of normal when extreme values in one direction are not considered to be clinically abnormal (e.g., high flow rates or VC). For parameters in which the data are not distributed normally, the lower limits must be defined either by normalizing the regression equation or by observing the actual upper and lower percentile values taken from a large population. Identification of the limits of normal for a specific patient is best accomplished using computer-developed reports that derive the normal limits for each measured parameter from its corresponding prediction equation. As a rule of thumb, approximate lower limits of normal for some parameters (95th percentile) are presented

TABLE 3-1	Suggested References for Normal Values
Test	**References**
Spirometry	6, 7, 10
Flow–volume	8
Lung volumes (RV, FRC, TLC)	9, 10, 22
D_{LCO}	13, 14
Pa_{O_2}, Pa_{CO_2}, pH	12
MIP/MEP	11

RV, residual volume; *FRC*, functional residual capacity; *TLC*, total lung capacity; *D_{LCO}*, carbon monoxide, diffusing capacity; *Pa_{O_2}*, arterial oxygen tension; *Pa_{CO_2}*, partial pressure of carbon dioxide in arterial blood; *MIP*, maximum inspiratory pressure; *MEP*, maximum expiratory pressure.

TABLE 3-2	Approximate Upper and Lower Limits of Normal at the Fifth Percentile Level	
Parameter	**Limits of Normal (% Predicted)**	
VC, FVC	75	
FRC	70, 130	
RV	65, 135	
TLC	80, 120	
FEV_1	75	
FEV_1/FVC (%)	85	
FEF 25/75	65	
MIP	65	

VC, vital capacity; *FVC*, forced vital capacity; *FRC*, functional residual capacity; *RV*, residual volume; *TLC*, total lung capacity; *FEV₁*, one-second forced expiratory volume; *FEF*, forced expiratory flow; *MIP*, maximum inspiratory pressure.

in Table 3-2. It should be noted that, despite rigorous efforts to predict optimal normal values, a relatively wide range of normal is still found for most PFT parameters. Hence, the most useful "normal values" in an individual patient are baseline measurements made when the patient was free of disease.

Individual results from patients with mild disease can widely overlap the range of predicted normal values. For this reason, it is best to interpret such borderline results as reflecting either mild disease or a variant of normal function (*low-normal*). Such findings are best interpreted in the context of other complimentary PFT results and clinical data. They may suggest the need for further testing if clinically indicated.

Selection of the appropriate PFTs to perform in each patient is essential for obtaining the maximal clinical information without unnecessary use of healthcare resources. The clinical situation being evaluated should guide the selection from among the wide variety of PFTs available. A survey of the available tests and their potential applications follows.

Spirometry is used to characterize the pattern of inspiratory and expiratory flow (Fig. 3-1) and to measure certain lung volumes (e.g., VC, FEV_1, expiratory reserve volume, inspiratory capacity, and tidal volume). Spirometry alone can often differentiate obstructive from restrictive pulmonary disorders by measuring VC, FEV_1, and expiratory flow rates. In obstructive disorders, spirometry demonstrates a decrease in flow rates and a normal or decreased VC (Fig. 3-2). If the VC is decreased, however, further testing is often necessary to determine if the defect is attributable to obstruction alone. Asthma, chronic bronchitis, and emphysema are the most common obstructive diseases. Obstruction can also result from a localized lesion (e.g., a tumor, foreign body, granulation tissue, or scarring) anywhere in the tracheobronchial tree.

Restrictive defects typically reduce the TLC, VC, or both. They can be due to a large variety of disorders that reflect five basic pathophysiologic categories (summarized by the mnemonic PAINT): *P*leural disease, *A*lveolar, *I*nterstitial, *N*euromuscular weakness involving ventilatory muscles, and *T*horacic cage abnormalities (e.g., kyphoscoliosis, obesity).

In restrictive disease, spirometry demonstrates a decrease in VC and normal or increased ratio of FEV_1 to forced vital capacity (FVC). Flow rates may be reduced solely because of the reduction of absolute lung volumes in the absence of any identifiable causes of obstructive airway disease (Fig. 3-3). Spirometry alone, however, cannot identify the presence of restriction when a patient has combined obstructive and restrictive disorders; in such patients, direct measurements of TLC are needed to identify, characterize, and quantify the restriction.

The FEV_1 is the most reproducible flow parameter and is particularly useful in diagnosing and monitoring response to therapy in patients with obstructive disease. The FEV_1 as the percent of the predicted value (FEV_1 %pred) has been recommended as a means of grading the severity of ventilatory disease, using somewhat arbitrary threshold values for each gradation.

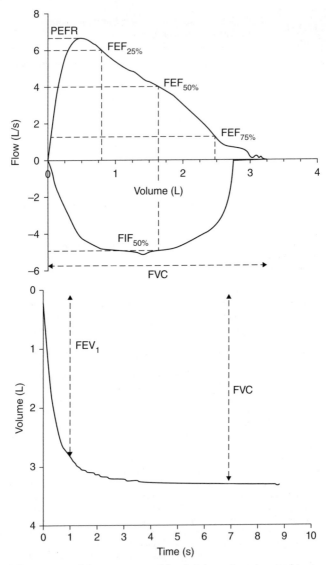

Figure 3-1. Illustration of the measurement of forced vital capacity and maximal inspiratory and expiratory flow parameters in a normal subject, displayed as a flow–volume curve (**top**) or a volume–time curve (**bottom**).

The FEV_1 %pred corresponds reasonably well to disease severity in patients with chronic obstructive pulmonary disease (COPD) (see Chapter 64) and is endorsed for this purpose by the American Thoracic Society/European Respiratory Society (ATS/ERS) guidelines as well as the Global Initiative for Chronic Obstructive Lung Disease (GOLD). Although the ATS/ERS guidelines also endorse the FEV_1 %pred to grade the severity of restrictive diseases, there is less

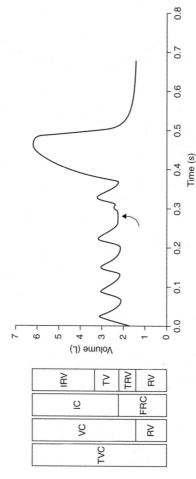

Figure 3-2. Left panel: The static lung volumes are derived from standard spirometry and from a measurement of functional residual capacity, by body plethysmography, gas dilution, or washout. They include TLC (total lung capacity), VC (vital capacity), RV (residual volume), FRC (functional residual capacity), TV (tidal volume), IRV (inspiratory reserve volume), ERV (expiratory reserve volume), and IC (inspiratory capacity). **Right panel:** Illustration of lung volume measurement in a normal subject by body plethysmography.

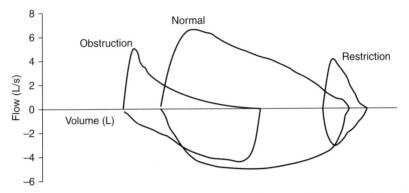

Figure 3-3. Examples of flow–volume curves in obstructive and restrictive disease, compared to a normal subject. Although it represents data from the same respiratory maneuver as the standard volume–time plot, the flow–volume loop provides a more graphic demonstration of the relationship between flow rates and lung volumes. Although flow rates referenced to forced vital capacity are lower than normal in the patient with restriction, when referenced to the absolute lung volumes, the flows are actually higher than in a normal subject.

evidence to support that recommendation. A wide variety of diseases fall into the category of restriction, with many different manifestations and natural histories that may not be consistently quantified by reductions in FEV_1 %pred. Patients with combined restriction and obstruction pose an additional challenge of rating the severity of each component. In those cases, adjustment of the FEV_1 %pred by the TLC %pred may help grade the severity of the obstruction.

The FEF measured during expiration of 25% to 75% of the VC ($FEF_{25\%-75\%}$), also called the *maximum mid-expiratory flow rate*, can be decreased in diseases of the small airways that are manifested by dynamic airway compression during exhalation. The $FEF_{25\%-75\%}$ may be more sensitive than the FEV_1 in detecting mild dysfunction of the small airways. However, other types of lung defects may also lower the $FEF_{25\%-75\%}$, and the clinical significance of an isolated finding of decreased $FEF_{25\%-75\%}$ is uncertain. The wide range of normal values for $FEF_{25\%-75\%}$ and related instantaneous flows such as $FEF_{50\%}$ and $FEF_{75\%}$ also limit the clinical usefulness of these parameters.

In an effort to obviate the need for prolonged forced expiration in patients with obstructive lung disease, the FEV expired in the first 6.0 seconds (FEV_6) has been proposed as a surrogate for FVC. Analyses indicate that the FEV_1/FEV_6 is comparable to the FEV_1/FVC ratio for identifying obstructive lung disease, is reasonably comparable to FVC for diagnosing restrictive disease, and that its reproducibility is superior to FVC. Volume-based flow parameters (e.g., $FEF_{25\%-75\%}$), however, may differ significantly if based on the FEV_6 rather than the FVC, necessitating new reference values based on the FEV_6.

Spirometry performed before and after exercise is useful for confirming the diagnosis of exercise-induced asthma. In patients undergoing evaluation for hypersensitivity lung disease (bronchospastic or restrictive), physiologic testing after inhalation of cholinergic agents or of the suspected antigenic material is often useful in identifying a specific cause. In addition to serial measurements of VC and expiratory flow rates, it is often useful to monitor other pulmonary measurements, such as airway resistance, specific conductance, and lung volume increases.

In contrast to the volume–time graph, the flow–volume loop (Figs. 3-1, 3-3, and 3-4) displays flow rates in relation to lung volume during maximum inspiration from RV and maximum expiration from TLC. The principal advantage of the flow–volume loop is that the relationship between flows and lung volume is more readily recognized. Common obstructive diseases such as asthma and COPD manifest markedly decelerating flows as the lung volumes decrease during exhalation. A hyperbolic-appearing concave shape to the expiratory portion of the flow–volume

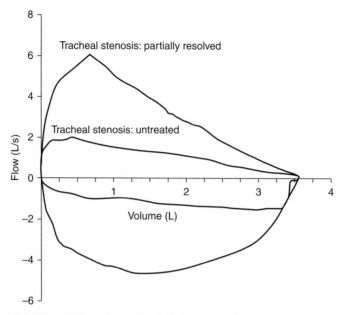

Figure 3-4. Effects of different degrees of tracheal obstruction on flow–volume loops. Prior to treatment, a patient with a tracheal web displays a squared loop, characteristic of localized fixed obstruction of central airways. After partial treatment, the stenosis is difficult to appreciate from the flow–volume loop, despite residual stenosis resulting in a tracheal diameter of 9 mm. The stenosis is even more difficult to appreciate on volume–time displays (not shown).

curve represents this phenomenon (Fig. 3-3). Although marked blunting of peak flows and the resultant square loop shape of flow–volume curves are commonly taught to be characteristic of localized upper airway obstruction (e.g., tracheal stenosis), it is important to note that these are relatively insensitive signs of localized obstruction and usually signify severe localized airway narrowing (Fig. 3-4).

The "absolute" lung volumes are typically evaluated at three specific respiratory states: TLC (the volume after maximal use of the inspiratory muscles), RV (the volume after maximal use of the expiratory muscles), and FRC (the "resting volume" during minimal use of the ventilatory musculature) (Fig. 3-3). Gas dilution (or washout) techniques, body plethysmography, and radiographic planimetry can be used to measure lung volumes directly or indirectly. Although all three techniques give comparable results in normal subjects, this is frequently not the case in patients with lung disease. Gas dilution techniques (e.g., helium dilution, nitrogen washout) are the most commonly available methods for measuring absolute lung volume, but often underestimate the true TLC in patients with obstructive disease. Because they measure only the lung volume that communicates freely with all air spaces within the lungs, poorly ventilated lung regions (such as the superior regions in typical COPD patients) can be largely underrepresented. Body plethysmography measures the compressible gas volume within the thorax and gives more accurate TLC measurements in COPD, although under some conditions plethysmography may overestimate lung volumes in patients with severe obstruction. TLC can also be measured from conventional posteroanterior chest radiographs using planimetric or ellipsoid techniques; although averages of radiographic volumes from groups of normal subjects have shown remarkable correspondence to plethysmographically measured TLC, the accuracy of the measurements in individual patients can limit the clinical usefulness of these measurements to serial studies. In patients with severe reduction in lung volumes from space-occupying abnormalities, radiographic TLC can be significantly larger than plethysmographic measurements. Assuming the patient has made an adequate effort (an often overlooked assumption), a reduced TLC indicates the presence of a restrictive disorder.

Measurements of DLCO by either the single-breath or the steady-state method are relatively sensitive, albeit nonspecific, indicators of respiratory dysfunction and loss of alveolar–capillary surface area. Decreases in the single-breath DLCO correlate well with loss of lung tissue secondary to emphysema; however, in contrast to the steady-state method, the single-breath method occasionally gives false-negative results. Because of the wide range of normal values, both the single-breath and steady-state techniques are of limited use for early detection of emphysema. The DLCO is also reduced in a variety of restrictive diseases involving the lung parenchyma, such as sarcoidosis, interstitial fibrosis, and drug toxicity. It can also be low in pulmonary vascular diseases such as pulmonary emboli; hence, the specificity of the abnormal DLCO is low. The test may be most useful in the evaluation of a patient complaining of dyspnea who has normal spirometry and arterial blood gases. In such patients, a low DLCO strongly suggests the presence of significant lung disease, although a normal DLCO does not exclude the presence of disease. Recent data also indicate that serial measurements of DLCO are useful in treating patients with Goodpasture syndrome, in which an occult pulmonary hemorrhage is mirrored by an increase in DLCO.

Maximum inspiratory pressure (MIP) is determined during maximum inspiratory effort against a closed system, usually at RV, while maximum expiratory pressure (MEP) is typically measured at TLC. MIP and MEP are useful direct tests of respiratory muscle strength in patients with suspected neuromuscular disease or in those with dyspnea, restricted lung volumes, and an absence of parenchymal or thoracic cage abnormalities on chest roentgenograms. Measurement of MIP and MEP is nonspecific in that it cannot distinguish among lack of effort, muscle weakness or dysfunction, and neural disease. Nonetheless, the test is useful for following the course of the disease. Tests to assess respiratory muscle fatigue have improved but are too complex for widespread clinical use. The contributions of respiratory muscle fatigue to dyspnea and respiratory failure remain poorly defined.

Exercise testing is useful for diagnosis and assessment of dysfunction in patients with lung and heart disease (see Chapter 4). Its measured parameters include respiratory rate and tidal volumes, arterial blood gases, expired gas concentrations, and, frequently, heart rate and blood pressure. Abnormalities in gas exchange (e.g., hypoxemia or hypercapnia) can occur in patients who are normal at rest. Exercise testing can be valuable in detecting lung disease, assessing the impact on exercise, establishing the need for supplementary oxygen, and assessing the impact of therapy, including rehabilitation programs for patients with chronic lung diseases.

Assessments of changes in FRC and flow limitation of tidal volumes during exercise can help to identify causes of dyspnea during exercise and exercise limitation not otherwise detected during conventional exercise testing. Such testing is currently available in relatively few centers, and its clinical usefulness remains to be fully defined. Assessing changes in tidal breathing flow–volume curves during the application of negative pressures can be useful also in identifying patients for whom airway collapse may play an important role in the genesis of dyspnea at rest or during exercise.

Pulse oximeters expand the ability to monitor arterial oxygenation in a variety of situations (e.g., during general anesthesia or bronchoscopy and in intensive care units). However, the absolute accuracy of these devices for measuring oxygen saturation ($\pm 3\% - 5\%$) limits their usefulness when accurate assessments of oxygenation are needed (e.g., prescribing long-term ambulatory oxygen therapy, detecting changes in arterial oxygenation with exercise).

Causes of hypoxemia include hypoventilation, diffusion abnormalities, ventilation–perfusion mismatches, right-to-left shunts, and decreased oxygen in inspired gases. Gas exchange abnormalities leading to hypoxemia and hypercapnia occur as a result of (1) wasted ventilation, when lung units are ventilated but not perfused, (2) shunted pulmonary blood flow, when lung units are perfused but not ventilated, and, more commonly, (3) other less extreme forms of ventilation–perfusion mismatch. The alveolar–arterial oxygen difference ($P[A-a]O_2$) estimates the degree of shunt and *low* mismatch. More specific tests are available to quantify and define the topography of such mismatching within the lungs. Wasted ventilation can be calculated by determining the dead space ratio (dead space per unit of tidal ventilation) using the Bohr equation:

$$\frac{\dot{V}_D}{\dot{V}_T} = \frac{Pa_{CO_2} - Pe_{CO_2}}{Pa_{CO_2}}$$

where Pe_{CO_2} is the end-tidal expiratory concentration of carbon dioxide and Pa_{CO_2} is the arterial carbon dioxide concentration. An elevated dead space ratio (>0.45), in the absence of restrictive or obstructive lung disease, may suggest pulmonary vascular disease.

The degree of right to left shunt can be assessed by determining the arterial oxygen tension (Pa_{O_2}) while the patient breathes 100% oxygen; this technique does not distinguish between intracardiac and intrapulmonary shunts. A Pa_{O_2} of less than 550 mmHg suggests the presence of a shunt. However, resorptive atelectasis induced by breathing 100% oxygen for prolonged periods of time may convert areas of low oxygen into areas of temporary shunting. Quantitative information regarding the spectrum of mismatch can be derived by elegant but complicated multiple inert gas methods, which remain a tool of the research laboratory. The topography of relationships can be displayed in a semiquantitative fashion by ventilation and perfusion scintiphotography.

The importance of disturbances of respiration during sleep has been increasingly recognized. Comprehensive sleep studies, including electromyographically and electroencephalographically defined stages of sleep and arousals, are important for understanding the relationship between disturbances of respiration and sleep, daytime fatigue, and excessive daytime sleepiness. The increasing availability of miniaturized, portable multichannel recorders provide a much less-expensive option for the detection of nocturnal desaturation, alterations in inspiratory airflow and ventilatory effort, and cardiac arrhythmias that may occur only during sleep (see Chapter 81).

FURTHER READING

1. Miller MR, Crapo R, Hankinson J, et al. General considerations for lung function testing. *Eur Respir J.* 2005;26(1):153–161.
2. Pellegrino R, Viegi G, Brusasco V, et al. Interpretative strategies for lung function tests. *Eur Respir J.* 2005;26(5):948–968.
3. MacIntyre N, Crapo RO, Viegi G, et al. Standardisation of the single-breath determination of carbon monoxide uptake in the lung. *Eur Respir J.* 2005;26(4):720–735.
4. Wanger J, Clausen JL, Coates A, et al. Standardisation of the measurement of lung volumes. *Eur Respir J.* 2005;26(3):511–522.
5. Miller MR, Hankinson J, Brusasco V, et al. Standardisation of spirometry. *Eur Respir J.* 2005;26(2):319–338.

   The first five references are from a very well-written and well-referenced consensus series that contains recommendations regarding the performance of various pulmonary function tests, use of predicted values, and the evidence-based strategies for interpretation.

6. Cerveri I, Dore R, Corsico A, et al. Assessment of emphysema in COPD: a functional and radiologic study. *Chest.* 2004;125(5):1714–1718.

   Comparison of PFTs and high-resolution CT (HRCT) scans for assessing the extent of emphysema. FRC, $FEV_{50\%}/FIV_{50\%}$ ratio, and D_{LCO}/VA correlated with extent of emphysema as determined by HRCT.

7. Coates AL, Peslin R, Rodenstein D, et al. Measurement of lung volumes by plethysmography. *Eur Respir J.* 1997;10(6):1415–1427.

   Comprehensive review of these demanding measurements by experts experienced with both pediatric and adult applications.

8. Hankinson JL, Odencrantz JR, Fedan KB. Spirometric reference values from a sample of the general U.S. population. *Am J Respir Crit Care Med.* 1999;159(1):179–187.

   An important contribution because of the inclusion of significant numbers of Blacks and Hispanics in the subjects.

9. Crapo RO, Morris AH, Gardner RM. Reference spirometric values using techniques and equipment that meet ATS recommendations. *Am Rev Respir Dis.* 1981;123(6):659–664.

   Sophisticated statistical analyses and comparisons with other published studies.

10. Bass H. The flow volume loop: normal standards and abnormalities in chronic obstructive pulmonary disease. *Chest*. 1973;63(2):171–176.

    Contains predictive equations for both inspiratory and expiratory flow rates derived from 247 nonsmoking adults.

11. Crapo RO, Morris AH, Clayton PD, et al. Lung volumes in healthy nonsmoking adults. *Bull Eur Physiopathol Respir*. 1982;18(3):419–425.

    Although measured by the single-breath helium dilution technique, which may result in volumes in healthy subjects slightly smaller (e.g., 0.3 L) than those with plethysmography, the predicted values from these equations were among the best when testing normals and equations in our laboratory.

12. Black LF, Hyatt RE. Maximal static respiratory pressures in generalized neuromuscular disease. *Am Rev Respir Dis*. 1971;103(5):641–650.

    Includes references for normal values.

13. Crapo RO, Jensen RL, Hegewald M, et al. Arterial blood gas reference values for sea level and an altitude of 1,400 meters. *Am J Respir Crit Care Med*. 1999;160(5, pt 1):1525–1531.

    A meticulous and comprehensive contribution that includes well-defined confidence limits. The predicted values for PaO$_2$ are significantly higher than those of Sorbini et al. Respiration. 1968;25:3, a reference used commonly in the past.

14. Crapo RO, Morris AH. Standardized single breath normal values for carbon monoxide diffusing capacity. *Am Rev Respir Dis*. 1981;123(2):185–189.

    Although widely used for predictive values for D$_{LCO}$, for many laboratories the values are inappropriately high, perhaps related to the 1,400-m elevation of the study sample.

15. Miller A, Thornton JC, Warshaw R, et al. Single breath diffusing capacity in a representative sample of the population of Michigan, a large industrial state. Predicted values, lower limits of normal, and frequencies of abnormality by smoking history. *Am Rev Respir Dis*. 1983;127(3):270–277.

    An important source because it includes predictive equations for both nonsmokers and smokers and represents data from adults living at sea-level altitudes.

16. Shade D Jr, Cordova F, Lando Y, et al. Relationship between resting hypercapnia and physiologic parameters before and after lung volume reduction surgery in severe chronic obstructive pulmonary disease. *Am J Respir Crit Care Med*. 1999;159(5, pt 1):1405–1411.

    In addition to illustrating the important role that PFT is playing in selecting patients for and assessing the benefits of lung volume reduction surgery, this article challenges the convention of labeling patients with CO$_2$ retention as high risk for thoracic surgery.

17. Crapo RO, Casaburi R, Coates AL, et al. Guidelines for methacholine and exercise challenge testing-1999. This official statement of the American Thoracic Society was adopted by the ATS Board of Directors, July 1999. *Am J Respir Crit Care Med*. 2000;161(1):309–329.

    Guidelines adopted by the ATS in 1999. Standardization of these complex tests is long overdue. However, the usefulness of these guidelines is diluted somewhat by a number of controversial issues being resolved by approving alternative methods for which scientific evidence of equivalency is not always available.

18. Carlin BW, Clausen JL, Ries AL. The use of cutaneous oximetry in the prescription of long-term oxygen therapy. *Chest*. 1988;94(2):239–241.

    An important example of the limitations of cutaneous oximetry. More than 80% of patients who would qualify for home oxygen therapy based on measurement of PaO$_2$ did not qualify based on pulse oximetry.

19. Munoz X, Torres F, Sampol G, et al. Accuracy and reliability of pulse oximetry at different arterial carbon dioxide pressure levels. *Eur Respir J*. 2008;32(4):1053–1059.

    Hypoxemia and hypercarbia increased the difference between oxyhemoglobin saturations estimated from pulse oximetry and those from simultaneously measured arterial blood gas co-oximetry.

20. Hart N, Kearney MT, Pride NB, et al. Inspiratory muscle load and capacity in chronic heart failure. *Thorax*. 2004;59(6):477–482.

    Illustrates current methodology for assessing inspiratory muscle strength and endurance.

21. Babb TG, Rodarte JR. Exercise capacity and breathing mechanics in patients with airflow limitation. *Med Sci Sports Exerc*. 1992;24(9):967–974.

    Illustrates the greater sensitivity of analyses of tidal breathing flow limitation during exercise to limitations in exercise when compared with the expired volume per unit time:maximum voluntary ventilation ratio.

22. Swanney MP, Jensen RL, Crichton DA, et al. FEV(6) is an acceptable surrogate for FVC in the spirometric diagnosis of airway obstruction and restriction. *Am J Respir Crit Care Med.* 2000;162 (3, pt 1):917–919.

   This study supports the termination of FVC efforts after 6.0 seconds, thereby obviating the need for prolonged maximal expiratory efforts in patients with obstructive lung disease. Normal values for the FEV_6 are being published.

23. Eltayara L, Becklake MR, Volta CA, et al. Relationship between chronic dyspnea and expiratory flow limitation in patients with chronic obstructive pulmonary disease. *Am J Respir Crit Care Med.* 1996;154(6, pt 1):1726–1734.

24. Aggarwal AN, Agarwal R. The new ATS/ERS guidelines for assessing the spirometric severity of restrictive lung disease differ from previous standards. *Respirology.* 2007;12(5):759–762.

   The ATS/ERS recommended interpretive strategy (ref. 4) focuses on FEV_1 %pred rather than FVC %pred to grade the severity of restrictive lung diseases. In about half the patients, the two methods yielded different gradation categories. The trend was inconsistent: the (newer) FEV_1 %pred method results in lower severity scores for some and higher scores for others.

25. Gardner ZS, Ruppel GL, Kaminsky DA. Grading the severity of obstruction in mixed obstructive-restrictive lung disease. *Chest.* 2011;140(3):598–603.

   The FEV_1 %pred commonly overestimated the degree of obstruction in patients with combinations of obstruction and restriction. Adjusting the FEV_1 %pred by accounting for the TLC %pred (FEV_1 %pred/ TLC %pred) resulted in a more believable distribution in the severities of obstruction.

26. Culver BH. Obstructive? Restrictive? Or a ventilatory impairment? *Chest.* 2011;140(3):568–569.

   Interesting comment on the above paper (Gardner 2000), suggesting that severities might best be assigned to the "ventilatory impairment," rather than attempting to partition the severities of restriction and obstruction separately.

Exercise

Andrew L. Ries

Exercise is a physiologic stimulus that stresses the body's capability to increase metabolic activity and gas transport in response to higher work demand. Diseases that adversely impact cardio-pulmonary organ function and limit respiratory reserves may produce exertional symptoms not present at rest. Dyspnea on exertion is among the most common complaints leading patients to seek medical advice. Because dyspnea is a subjective symptom, with multiple potential origins, evaluation during exercise is useful in reproducing a patient's symptoms and characterizing the physiologic responses. Exercise testing should be used for evaluating patients complaining of exercise limitation and may have several objectives:

1. Measure an individual's work capacity (e.g., to guide exercise training, follow the course of disease, prognostic indicator of risk)
2. Assess the factors limiting exercise tolerance (e.g., evaluate unexplained dyspnea, assess respiratory disability)
3. Evaluate changes in gas exchange with physical activity (e.g., detect exercise-induced hypoxemia, prescribe supplemental oxygen)
4. Evaluate exercise-induced bronchospasm/asthma (e.g., assess changes with disease or the effects of therapeutic interventions)

There are differences in the physiologic principles and appropriate techniques used for exercise testing of different populations, such as normal individuals, cardiac patients, and patients with pulmonary disease. These differences reflect the reason(s) for exercise limitation in each of these groups. Therefore, to be safe and informative, exercise testing should be planned with consideration of these limiting factors.

In the normal individual, maximum exercise capacity is limited by the level to which cardiac output can be elevated to meet the metabolic demands of the muscle and by the ability of the muscles to generate sufficient metabolic energy. No limitations are imposed by ventilatory reserves or pulmonary gas exchange in healthy persons, except with extreme exercise levels in trained athletes.

In normal subjects, low-level exercise results in an increase in cardiac output (primarily due to an increase in heart rate), widening of the arterial-mixed venous oxygen difference (a–vo_2), and increase in oxygen consumption ($\dot{V}o_2$) and carbon dioxide production ($\dot{V}co_2$). Minute ventilation increases sufficiently to maintain the alveolar ventilation at a level sufficient to remove all the carbon dioxide produced; therefore, the $Paco_2$ remains normal. The $P(A–a)o_2$ gradient may decrease slightly with exercise because of improvement in ventilation–perfusion ($\dot{V}/\dot{Q}$) relationships as pulmonary blood flow increases and pulmonary perfusion becomes more evenly distributed.

As the exercise level is increased further, the blood flow to the exercising muscles ultimately becomes inadequate to provide sufficient oxygen to maintain pure aerobic metabolism. At that point, anaerobic glycolytic metabolism occurs (anaerobic threshold). Lactic acid enters the venous circulation, is buffered by bicarbonate, and an additional amount of carbon dioxide is produced. In response to this nonoxidative carbon dioxide production, minute ventilation ($\dot{V}E$) rises disproportionately to the $\dot{V}o_2$—a signal that the anaerobic threshold has been reached. At higher exercise levels, lactic acidosis decreases the pH level sufficiently to drive $\dot{V}E$ higher, out of proportion to carbon dioxide production, causing a fall in $Paco_2$. This classic sequence of response to exercise has been characterized carefully in normal subjects. For example, at lower "aerobic" levels of exercise, the physiologic variables reflecting increased metabolic demand are related closely, e.g., $\dot{V}o_2$, $\dot{V}co_2$, $\dot{V}E$, heart rate, cardiac output, and a–vo_2. The patterns of physiologic response to exercise stress can be used to detect abnormalities in patients with cardiac or pulmonary dysfunction. In patients with left ventricular failure and reduced stroke volume, for instance, the heart rate increases and the a–vo_2 difference widens more at a given level of $\dot{V}o_2$ than in normal subjects.

In many patients with lung diseases, the classic physiologic pattern of exercise limitation described in normals does not occur because pulmonary patients generally are not limited by cardiac output but, rather, by ventilatory limitations, pulmonary gas exchange compromise, or both. Recent evidence suggests that peripheral muscle dysfunction also may contribute to the limitations in maximum exercise tolerance in patients with chronic lung disease. Ventilatory limitations are imposed by factors such as disordered respiratory mechanics, an increase in the work of breathing, disturbances of $\dot{V}/\dot{Q}$ relationships (e.g., large dead space ventilation), and respiratory muscle fatigue. Recent work emphasizes the important role of dynamic hyperinflation in end-tidal lung volume in patients with chronic obstructive pulmonary disease (COPD) as a cause of exertional dyspnea and exercise limitation. Gas exchange limitations may be a consequence of alveolar hypoventilation, shunting, and right heart failure, or $\dot{V}/\dot{Q}$ mismatch. Because the limitation to exercise in many pulmonary patients is not of hemodynamic origin, the use of heart rate, for example, to guide "maximum exercise" or training targets is often not useful. Furthermore, many patients with moderate to severe lung disease may not achieve a definable anaerobic threshold because they are forced by dyspnea to discontinue exercise before this point is reached.

Thus, it is characteristic in pulmonary patients for exercise limitation to occur at $\dot{V}o_2$ and heart rate levels well below those predicted from nomograms developed in normal populations. Furthermore, to test exercise tolerance safely in pulmonary patients, it is important to monitor arterial oxygenation; hypoxemia is not a consequence of exercise in normal subjects, except at extreme levels of exertion.

The practical details of exercise testing in the pulmonary patient depend on the purpose for which such testing is done. For example, if the exercise testing is a prelude to developing an exercise training program for a patient with chronic lung disease, testing is best accomplished on an apparatus (e.g., treadmill) that requires exercise comparable to that used during training (e.g., walking). This is because muscle conditioning is most specific for the type of exercise used in training and may not be transferable directly to another form of exercise. For example, tolerance for walking is not improved by training on a supine bicycle or by arm exercises.

The specific measurements made also depend on the purposes of the test. For instance, if the question relates to whether the patient requires supplemental oxygen during exercise, then measurement of arterial blood gases (ABGs) (or cutaneous oximetry) at rest and during exercise is necessary, and the exercise level should be appropriate to the patient's daily activities. Furthermore, if arterial hypoxemia appears with exercise, the test may be repeated with supplemental oxygen provided at known flow rates, to ensure that the flow rate selected prevents hypoxemia.

Laboratory exercise testing is most commonly performed using either (1) rapid, progressive, incremental levels to a symptom-limited maximum or (2) defined steady-state levels. The former is most useful for determining exercise tolerance and the limitations to maximum performance. The latter may be preferred for assessing training prescriptions (e.g., heart rate target for endurance exercise) or for accurately measuring physiologic variables requiring a steady state (e.g., AGSs, cardiac output, or dead space ventilation). Simpler exercise tests, such as the 6-minute walk test and the shuttle walk test (SWT), have been used increasingly in recent years to measure exercise tolerance outside of a laboratory setting. Timed distance walk tests measure the maximum distance a person can walk within a defined period (e.g., 6 minutes). In the SWT, the subject walks back and forth between two traffic cones placed 10 m apart on a flat course. The incremental SWT uses a recorded metronome to pace the walking speed, which is increased every minute until the subject is unable to keep up with the pace or stops because of symptoms. The endurance SWT measures the maximum time (up to 20 minutes) that the subject can walk at a constant speed, set at 85% of the maximum speed from the incremental SWT. Such field tests have the advantage of requiring less equipment and technical expertise; however, attention must be paid to the details of testing procedures because variations in factors such as the walking course, patient instructions, encouragement during tests, use of oxygen or monitoring devices, and number of tests performed will influence the results. If these tests are to be used widely, then better standardization of procedures is needed. Also, these tests do not provide the detailed physiologic data typically included in more formal laboratory exercise tests.

Two common errors in the use of exercise tests in pulmonary patients are to assume that (1) normal ABG values at rest obviate the need for exercise measurements and (2) one can judge from resting pulmonary function and ABG testing that the patient will or will not have serious gas exchange deterioration with exercise. Neither of these assumptions is correct. Also, it is often difficult to relate a patient's report of dyspnea on exertion to his or her actual physiologic performance during exercise—not a surprising fact, as dyspnea, like pain, is a largely subjective sensation.

In exercise training for the pulmonary patient, another common error is to select target training levels that are too low. In normal subjects or cardiac patients, training levels typically are chosen at submaximum percentages (e.g., 60%–70%) of maximum $\dot{V}o_2$ or heart rate. Many patients with chronic lung disease, however, are often ventilatory limited at low levels of exercise, which may be below their anaerobic threshold. Such individuals are able to sustain exercise levels at higher percentages of maximum (e.g., 90% or above), even though the absolute levels are low.

Exercise testing has become an increasingly important component of the diagnostic-management approach to the patient with pulmonary disease. Familiarity with the techniques used and with the utility of the data derived is essential to proper patient care.

FURTHER READING

1. American Thoracic Society/American College of Chest Physicians. ATS/ACCP statement on cardiopulmonary exercise testing. *Am J Respir Crit Care Med.* 2003;167:211–277.

   Comprehensive review of current state of exercise testing, including sections on Indications, Methodology, Physiologic Basis of Measurements, Reference Values, Normal Response, Limitation in Cardiopulmonary Patients, and Interpretation.

2. Palange P, Ward SA, Carlsen K-H, et al. Recommendations on the use of exercise testing in clinical practice. *Eur Respir J.* 2007;29:185–209.

   Recommendations of a European Respiratory Society Task Force on the use of cardiopulmonary exercise testing in the evaluation of patients with lung and heart diseases. Includes discussion of the assessment of exercise intolerance, prognostic assessment, and the evaluation of therapeutic interventions.

3. Jones NL. *Clinical Exercise Testing.* 4th ed. Philadelphia, PA: WB Saunders; 1997.

A practical guide to clinical exercise testing. Discussion of physiologic basis, clinical uses, methods, and interpretation including normal standards.

4. Wasserman K, Hansen JE, Sue DY, et al, eds. *Principles of Exercise Testing and Interpretation.* 4th ed. Philadelphia, PA: Lea & Febiger; 2004.

   A well known textbook that reviews physiological principles of exercise and the use of cardiopulmonary exercise testing.

5. Ries AL. The role of exercise testing in pulmonary diagnosis. *Clin Chest Med.* 1987;8:81–89.

   Review of principles of exercise testing for pulmonary patients including discussion of methods, protocols, and indications.

6. O'Donnell DE, Revill SM, Webb KA. Dynamic hyperinflation and exercise intolerance in chronic obstructive pulmonary disease. *Am J Respir Crit Care Med.* 2001;164:770–777.

   Demonstration of the key role of dynamic hyperinflation of end-tidal lung volume as a determinant of exercise intolerance in patients with COPD.

7. Mahler DA. The measurement of dyspnea during exercise in patients with lung disease. *Chest.* 1992;101(suppl 5):242S–247S.

   Review of techniques of measuring dyspnea during exercise in pulmonary patients. The Borg and visual analog scales are used most commonly. Breathlessness ratings are generally reliable over time and sensitive to change with interventions.

8. American Thoracic Society. Guidelines for the six-minute walk test. *Am J Respir Crit Care Med.* 2002;166:111–117.

9. Sciurba FC, Slivka WA. Six-minute walk testing. *Semin Respir Crit Care Med.* 1998;9:383–391.

10. Brown CD, Wise RA. Field tests of exercise in COPD: the six-minute walk test and the shuttle walk test. *COPD.* 2007;4:217–223.

11. Singh SJ, Morgan MDL, Scott S, et al. Development of the shuttle walking test of disability in patients with chronic airways obstruction. *Thorax.* 1992;47:1019–1024.

12. Revill SM, Morgan MDL, Singh SJ, et al. The endurance shuttle walk: a new field test for the assessment of endurance capacity in chronic obstructive pulmonary disease. *Thorax.* 1999;54:213–222.

References 8–12 provide a review of the use of timed distance walk and shuttle walk tests for evaluating exercise tolerance.

13. American Thoracic Society/European Respiratory Society. Skeletal muscle dysfunction in chronic obstructive pulmonary disease. *Am J Respir Crit Care Med.* 1999;159(4, pt 2):S1–S40.

   Comprehensive summary of skeletal muscle dysfunction in patients with chronic lung disease, including discussion of principles of normal muscle function, skeletal muscle abnormalities in COPD, and effects of interventions on muscle dysfunction.

14. Casaburi R. Exercise training in chronic obstructive lung disease. In: Casaburi R, Petty TL, eds. *Principles and Practice of Pulmonary Rehabilitation.* Philadelphia, PA: WB Saunders; 1993:204–224.

   Review of principles and benefits of exercise training in patients with COPD. Comprehensive table summarizing 37 published studies in 933 patients with overwhelmingly positive results.

15. Ries AL, Farrow JT, Clausen JL. Pulmonary function tests cannot predict exercise-induced hypoxemia in chronic obstructive pulmonary disease. *Chest.* 1988;93:454–459.

16. Owens GR, Rogers RM, Pennock BE, et al. The diffusing capacity as a predictor of arterial oxygen desaturation during exercise in patients with chronic obstructive pulmonary disease. *N Engl J Med.* 1984;310:1218–1221.

   References 11 and 12 highlight the variability of changes of arterial oxygenation with exercise in patients with COPD. Although titles and focus of the two articles differ, both demonstrate that in patients with mild obstructive disease, oxygenation does not worsen with exercise (tends to improve or stay the same), whereas in those with moderate to severe disease, it changes unpredictably (i.e., worsens, improves, or is unchanged).

17. Ries AL, Farrow JT, Clausen JL. Accuracy of two ear oximeters at rest and during exercise in pulmonary patients. *Am Rev Respir Dis.* 1985;132:685–689.

   Accuracy of ear oximeters (95% confidence limits) ±4% to 5% compared to direct measurement of SaO_2. More accurate in measuring change in SaO_2 (±2.5%–3.5%).

18. Storms WW. Review of exercise-induced asthma. *Med Sci Sports Exerc.* 2003;35:1464–1470.

   Succinct review of exercise-induced asthma.

5 Evaluation of Arterial Blood Gases and Acid–Base Homeostasis

Timothy A. Morris

Arterial blood gas (ABG) measurements allow the assessment of pulmonary gas exchange and the presence and severity of acid–base disturbances. The information they provide, such as oxyhemoglobin saturation, arterial oxygen and carbon dioxide tension (PaO$_2$ and PaCO$_2$), and pH values, is best considered in light of other relevant clinical information. Proper interpretation requires knowledge of the clinical state, the therapy being applied, and, frequently, other data such as mixed venous oxygen saturation, hemoglobin concentration, and cardiac output.

To provide accurate information, the arterial blood gas specimen must be collected, handled, and analyzed properly. Typically, blood from the radial artery is collected into a heparinized syringe by direct puncture with a 20G (or smaller) needle or, when repeated sampling is necessary, an indwelling arterial catheter. Arterial catheters must be carefully monitored for local complications, including infection, thrombus formation, occlusion of arterial flow, and distal microemboli. The radial artery or (less commonly) the dorsalis pedis artery is the preferred site for monitoring, since the ulnar or posterior tibial arteries provide redundant circulation in case of arterial blood flow compromise. The brachial and femoral arteries do not have collateral arteries and are less desirable, but can be used when circumstances warrant.

The ABG specimen should be collected without exposure to ambient air, usually by allowing arterial pressure to force blood into the syringe. Many devices have been designed specifically for this purpose and facilitate good sampling technique. Any bubbles introduced into the syringe during collection should be promptly expelled; the sample should then be mixed to ensure complete anticoagulation and placed in ice water. Analysis should take place within minutes using an instrument system that has been recently calibrated against commercially available standards for each blood gas electrode (PO$_2$, PCO$_2$, and pH). The electrodes and sampling chambers are maintained at 37°C, and the results must be corrected to the patient's body temperature if it is abnormal. PaO$_2$ and PaCO$_2$ are expressed in terms of pressure, typically as mmHg or kilopascal (kPa) (1 torr = 1 mmHg = 7.5 kPa).

In addition to the directly measured values (oxyhemoglobin saturation, PO$_2$, PCO$_2$, and pH), ABG results often include calculated values that depend on the accurate measurement of PO$_2$, PCO$_2$, and pH. The electrodes are extremely accurate when calibrated correctly (PO$_2$ and PCO$_2$ ± 2 torr, pH ± 0.01 units), and the calculated values are equally precise. The most common calculated values are the bicarbonate level, base excess or deficit, and alveolar–arterial oxygen difference. A common misconception is that the [HCO$_3^-$] value calculated from ABG analysis (via the Henderson–Hasselbalch equation, described in the "Arterial pH, Bicarbonate and Acid–Base Homeostasis" section) is less accurate than that measured in the chemistry laboratory. With modern analytical techniques, the measured and calculated values rarely differ significantly, provided they are in the normal range. However, venous blood is typically measured in a chemistry analyzer after dissipation of the CO$_2$, and the assumptions about the original PaCO$_2$ when the sample was obtained render the chemistry laboratory's measurement inaccurate in the presence of a respiratory disturbance. The alveolar–arterial oxygen gradient requires knowledge of the inspired oxygen (FIO$_2$) and typically relies on an assumed respiratory exchange ratio (R or RER), which may be abnormal in disease states or non–steady state conditions (e.g., hyperventilation).

The initial evaluation of an ABG measurement should include consideration of its technical adequacy. A few simple rules can help: (1) PO$_2$ above 48 is unlikely to have been collected from a venous sample; (2) the sum of the PaO$_2$ and PaCO$_2$ should be less than 140 mmHg if the patient is breathing room air; and (3) a rapid large change in the calculated bicarbonate by more than 5 mEq suggests an error in the PaCO$_2$ or pH, or the presence of excessive amounts of heparin (an acid) in the collection syringe in the absence of a primary metabolic disturbance.

OXYGEN

The normal value of Pao_2 decreases with age and is influenced by barometric pressure (P_B) and, therefore, by altitude. A Pao_2 less than 80 mmHg is abnormal at sea level. However, the predicted value for Pao_2 in Denver (where ambient barometric pressure is 625 mmHg) for a young person is typically about 80 mmHg and is lower for elderly persons (60–65 mmHg).

The classification of hypoxemia severity based on Pao_2 is somewhat arbitrary: at sea level, reduced values down to 60 mmHg are usually considered mild hypoxemia; 45 to 59 mmHg, moderate; and below 45 mmHg, severe. The major causes of hypoxemia are (1) a decrease in the oxygen content of the inhaled gas (e.g., from reduced barometric pressure with altitude or a hypoxemic gas mixture), (2) global hypoventilation, (3) ventilation–perfusion ($\dot{V}/\dot{Q}$) imbalance, and (4) right-to-left shunt (intrapulmonary or intracardiac). Decreased mixed venous oxygen content by itself, as can occur when cardiac output is severely reduced, does not typically cause hypoxemia directly. However, it will markedly worsen the effects of shunt or $\dot{V}/\dot{Q}$ imbalance (Table 5-1).

The first two mechanisms can be differentiated from the latter two by the calculation of the alveolar–arterial oxygen difference (A–a)Do_2 using the simplified alveolar gas equation:

$$Pao_2 = \frac{Pio_2 - Paco_2}{R} \tag{5.1}$$

where $R = \dot{V}co_2/\dot{V}o_2$ and (A–a)$Do_2 = Pao_2 - Pao_2$.

The (A–a)Do_2 (also known as the [A–a] gradient or the [A–a] Po_2 difference) is normally less than 20 mmHg. Patients with hypoxemia resulting from a decreased Fio_2 (e.g., altitude) or from hypoventilation (elevated $Paco_2$) have a normal $P(A-a)o_2$, whereas the other processes lead to a widened $P(A-a)o_2$.

Characteristically, patients with hypoventilation or $\dot{V}/\dot{Q}$ mismatch show a 3- to 5-mmHg rise in Pao_2 for each 1% increment in Fio_2; those with a shunt show a less than 2-mmHg rise for each 1% increment in Fio_2. Alternatives to the (A–a)Do_2 calculation are the Pao_2/Pao_2 or Pao_2/Fio_2 ratios; these values are easier to compute but are more highly dependent on changes in Fio_2.

The Pao_2 accounts for only the small amount of oxygen transported in solution in the plasma. The bulk of the oxygen-carrying capacity of blood resides in hemoglobin contained in red blood cells. The relationship between the Pao_2 and hemoglobin oxygen saturation (Sao_2) is depicted in a sigmoid-shaped oxyhemoglobin dissociation curve. At relatively high Pao_2 values, a decrease in Pao_2 corresponds to a minimal decline in Sao_2. If the Pao_2 drops to 60 mmHg (corresponding to an Sao_2 of 90%), the Sao_2 falls more rapidly with further drops in Pao_2. For this reason, efforts to elevate the Pao_2 much above 60 to 65 mmHg rarely provide significant clinical benefit in the management of hypoxemic patients. The oxyhemoglobin dissociation curve depends on many factors, and may change depending on clinical conditions. For example, the dissociation curve is shifted to the right in acidosis and to the left in alkalosis: a Pao_2 of 60 at pH of 7.30 corresponds to a saturation of 87.7%, whereas an identical Pao_2 at pH of 7.50 corresponds to an oxygen saturation of 93.4%.

The pulse oximeter is a popular and relatively low-cost method for estimating oxyhemoglobin saturation. It is invaluable for monitoring patients continuously, and it can reduce the number of ABG analyses required when treating a patient on a ventilator or with respiratory failure.

TABLE 5-1	Guidelines for Assessing Hypoxemia		
Status	**(A–a)Do_2**	**Pao_2/Pao_2**	**Pao_2/Fio_2**
Normal	5–20	>0.80	>500
Low $\dot{V}/\dot{Q}$	30–50	0.65–0.70	300–450
Shunt	>60	<0.55	<250

The accuracy of oximetry is reasonably good if one assumes no significant carboxyhemoglobin or methemoglobin. In addition, the agreement between oximetry- and ABG-derived oxyhemoglobin saturation is not as strong when patients are significantly hypercarbic or hypoxemic. Oximetry, of course, gives no information about alveolar ventilation or about the acid–base status; so ABG analysis must be performed to gain information about those processes.

CARBON DIOXIDE

The $Paco_2$ reflects the balance between carbon dioxide production and carbon dioxide elimination by ventilation. This is stated by the following equation:

$$Paco_2 = \frac{k \times \dot{V}co_2}{\dot{V}A} \tag{5.2}$$

where $\dot{V}co_2$ = carbon dioxide production per minute, $\dot{V}A$ = alveolar ventilation, and k is a constant. If $\dot{V}A$ decreases, $Paco_2$ will rise (hypercapnia), whereas a rise in $\dot{V}A$ will result in a fall in $Paco_2$ (hypocapnia).

The normal range for $Paco_2$ is 37 to 43 mmHg, regardless of age. $Paco_2$ values of 30 to 37 mmHg are regarded as mild hypocapnia, 26 to 29 mmHg as moderate, and below 25 mmHg as severe. Mild hypercapnia is in the 44- to 50-mmHg range; moderate, 51 to 60 mmHg; and severe, above 60 mmHg. These numbers should also be compared with baseline values, as any sudden change from the baseline $Paco_2$ may portend a serious change in pulmonary function.

Hypercapnea may be further divided into conditions where the total amount of ventilation itself is decreased versus those in which the total ventilation is normal, but the proportion of ventilation resulting in gas exchange, the *effective* ventilation, is low. Decreased total ventilation may be due to disorders of the control of breathing (e.g., opiate overdose, hypothyroidism, brainstem strokes, etc.) or to weakness of the muscles of ventilation (e.g., myasthenia gravis, organophosphate poisoning, etc.). Decreased effective ventilation typically occurs in disorders that increase dead space ventilation (e.g., chronic obstructive airway disease).

ARTERIAL pH, BICARBONATE AND ACID–BASE HOMEOSTASIS

Two major principles of physical chemistry govern our understanding of acid–base balance. The first principle is that dissociation constants describe the equilibrium between a weak acid (HA) and its conjugate base:

$$HA \leftrightarrow H^+ + HA^-$$

or expressed mathematically:

$$K_A = \frac{[H^+][A^-]}{[HA]} \tag{5.3}$$

The primary buffer in blood is the carbonate–bicarbonate base pair. Carbon dioxide is hydrated to carbonic acid and this dissociates to bicarbonate and $[H^+]$, according to the following relationship:

$$CO_2 + H_2O \leftrightarrow H_2CO_3 \leftrightarrow H^+ + HCO_3^-$$

$$pK = 6.1 \tag{5.4}$$

Mathematically, this is expressed as:

$$K = \frac{[H^+][HCO_3^-]}{[H_2CO_3]} \text{ or, since } H_2CO_3 \text{ is ine quilibrium with } CO_2,$$

$$K = \frac{[H^+][HCO_3^-]}{[CO_2]} \tag{5.5}$$

Rearranging and supplying the correct constants gives the Henderson equation, whereas taking the negative log of each side and rearranging gives the Henderson–Hasselbalch equation:

$$[H^+] = \frac{24[P_{CO_2}]}{[HCO_3^-]} \quad pH = 6.1 + \log \frac{[HCO_3^-]}{[0.03 \times P_{CO_2}]} \quad (5.6)$$

Henderson equation   Henderson–Hasselbalch equation

The Hendersen–Hasselbalch equation is represented graphically in curve (a) of Figure 5-1 as the inverse logarithmic relationship between P_{aCO_2} and pH when the $[^-HCO_3] = 24$ mEq/L. The relationship becomes much more "user-friendly" when one realizes that, within the ranges of pH 7.1 to 7.45, the relationship can be approximated by line (b), which has a slope of 0.08 decrease in pH for each 10-torr increase in P_{aCO_2}.

Although pH is the usual form of reporting the ABG, it may be illustrative to convert logarithm-based pH units to $[H^+]$ in nanoequivalents per liter (nEq/L). A normal pH (between 7.37 and 7.43) converts to $[H^+]$ of 43 to 37 nEq/L. A change in pH of 1 unit corresponds to a tenfold change in concentration, and a 0.3-unit pH change corresponds to a twofold concentration change ($\log[10] = 1$, and $\log[2] = 0.3$). On this basis, it is easy to construct a conversion table even when a scientific calculator is not available (Table 5-2). This conversion permits easier calculation of acid–base relationships using the simplified Henderson formula.

An elevation of blood pH (decrease in blood $[H^+]$) is called alkalemia, whereas a decrease in pH (increase in $[H^+]$) is called acidemia. A condition that leads to acidemia or alkalemia is an acidosis or alkalosis, respectively, but compensatory mechanisms may actually leave the patient with a normal pH.

THE ANION GAP

The second principle that governs acid–base homeostasis is that a solution must contain equal numbers of positively and negatively charged ions. For biologic systems, this can be expressed as:

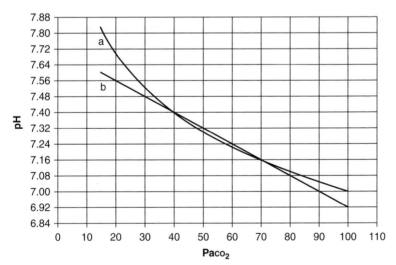

Figure 5-1. Graphical illustration of the relationship between pH and P_{aCO_2} if the $[HCO_3]$ were normal (24 mEq/L). The curve *(a)* represents the negative inverse logarithmic relationship predicted by the Hendersen–Hasselbalch equation (see text). The line *(b)* represent the portion of the relationship where P_{aCO_2} ranges from 30 to 80 torr, which is well approximated by a line with a slope of 0.08 pH decrease for every 10 torr P_{aCO_2} increase.

TABLE 5-2	Conversion between pH and Hydrogen Ion Concentration		
Alkalemia		**Acidemia**	
pH	[H⁺] (nEq/L)	pH	[H⁺] (nEq/L)
8.00	10	7.30	50
7.90	12.5	7.20	63
7.80	16	7.10	79
7.70	20	7.00	100
7.60	25	6.90	125
7.50	32	6.80	160
		6.70	200
Normal			
7.40	40		

Total cations – Total anions = 0, or

$$[Na^+] + [K^+] - [Cl^-] - [HCO_3^-] - [A^-] - [Unmeasured\ anions] = 0$$
$$140 + 4 - 102 - 25 - 15 - 2 = 0 \tag{5.7}$$

The concentration of the unmeasured anions that are normally present (e.g., So_4^{2-} or Po_4^{2-}) is only 1 to 3 mEq/L, and the [H⁺] concentration is so low relative to other charged species that it can be neglected. [A⁻] represents the base pairs of other weak acids in blood. These consist predominantly of charged amino acid residues on plasma proteins. The pK of these charged groups is typically 6.6 to 6.8, and so they are 90% dissociated at pH 7.4. The total concentration of these protein-based weak acids in blood (A_{TOT} in mEq/L) is typically 2.4 times the protein concentration (g/dL). Thus:

$$A^- = A_{TOT} \times 0.90 = [protein\ g/dL] \times 2.4 \times 0.90\ (normal = 11-16) \tag{5.8}$$

This equation allows calculation of [A⁻] and fosters an understanding of the effect of hypoproteinemia on its magnitude. This concept is also the basis for the more common calculation of the "anion gap" in which [A⁻] and [K⁺] are assumed to be constant. With that assumption, a shortened version of the equation is:

$$Anion\ gap = [Na^+] - [Cl^-] - [HCO_3^-]\ (normal\ range = 10-15) \tag{5.9}$$

Here, increases in the anion gap above the normal range reflect the presence of unmeasured anions, but there is no provision for changes resulting from hypoproteinemia or for changes in [A⁻] caused by pH (which changes the dissociation state of the buffer groups). Correct estimation of the amount of unmeasured anions in solution is essential, as an elevation indicates the presence of a metabolic acidosis.

APPROACHES TO ACIDOSES AND ALKALOSES

As noted, the hydrogen ion concentration [H⁺] is controlled to a very narrow concentration range between 10 and 100 nEq/L. To maintain the [H⁺] within this range, acid generation must closely match acid elimination. This extremely low concentration range (six orders of magnitude less than that of most other electrolytes) is even more remarkable relative to those overall rates of acid production. More than 100 mEq of "fixed" nonvolatile acids (e.g., sulfates or phosphates) and approximately 13,000 mEq of volatile acid are generated daily as byproducts of metabolism. The kidney excretes nonvolatile acids while the lungs eliminate the volatile acid load as CO_2 (equivalent to 200 mL/minute).

Disorders that alter CO_2 elimination (e.g., ventilatory changes that affect $Paco_2$) are reflected in the denominator of the Henderson–Hasselbalch equation. These are referred to as respiratory derangements of acid–base balance. Conversely, if the excretion of fixed acids slows or accelerates in relationship to production, or if there is abnormal intake of acid or alkali, a metabolic disturbance in acid–base balance is said to develop. These changes are largely reflected in the numerator of the Henderson–Hasselbalch equation.

If the bicarbonate–carbonate system were the only buffer in blood, then changes in pH as a result of acute changes in $Paco_2$ should not cause any change in bicarbonate levels. However, the presence of other blood buffers with a pK that is different from that of bicarbonate means that changes in pH will generate or use $[H^+]$ with a resulting small change in $[HCO_3^-]$.

The magnitude of the changes in pH and in bicarbonate as a result of acute changes in $Paco_2$ can be quantified in three different ways. First, the Henderson–Hasselbalch relationship illustrated in Figure 5-1 can be simplified (within ranges of $Paco_2$ 30–70 torr) as an expected decrease in pH of 0.08 for every 10 torr increase in $Paco_2$. A nomogram of the expected relationship can also be used, or it can be estimated from prediction equations (Table 5-3). For example, elevation of $Paco_2$ from 40 to 60 mmHg (an acute respiratory acidosis) produces a fall in pH (20×0.008) of 0.16 unit to 7.24 and a 2-mEq rise (0.1×20) in $[HCO_3^-]$. An acute respiratory alkalosis, characterized by a decrease in $Paco_2$, produces a rise in pH of the same magnitude as that in acute respiratory acidosis, but bicarbonate falls 0.2 mEq for every 1-mmHg decrease in $Paco_2$.

The ability to predict pH and bicarbonate changes in response to ventilation is the basis of the concept of "base excess" and "base deficit." Base excess (or deficit) is the difference between the measured bicarbonate and the bicarbonate level that would be predicted on the basis of the measured Pco_2 change alone. In other words, the base excess represents the amount of strong acid that would have to be added to the blood to return the pH to 7.40 if the $Paco_2$ were 40 torr, while the base deficit (or a negative number for base excess) represents the amount of strong base that would have to be added. Base excess is often reported with the directly measured ABG results. While it uses essentially the same information as the Henderson–Hasselbalch equation, it is a useful means of estimating the metabolic processes that are present in combination with respiratory changes. However, the calculations assume normal values for electrolytes and serum protein that may not be valid. Thus, uncritical use of base excess or deficit values can lead to error.

Although a great idea of variability exists in clinical situations, the response of an otherwise healthy person to a chronic (more than several days) change in $Paco_2$ is compensation through increased elimination or retention of bicarbonate by the kidney. These compensatory mechanisms act to restore the pH toward, but not quite to, normal values. The magnitude of these compensatory metabolic changes in otherwise healthy persons are well established from clinical observation (Table 5-3). For every 10 mmHg elevation of $Paco_2$ in chronic CO_2 retention, bicarbonate retention results in an increase in levels by 4 mEq/L, blunting the pH change to 0.03 units for every 10 torr change in $Paco_2$. With chronic hyperventilation, there is renal bicarbonate elimination until levels fall by 5 mEq for every 10 torr fall in $Paco_2$ with full compensation. However, it is important to keep in mind that the determination of whether a process can be attributed to "normal compensation" or whether it represents an independent process (i.e., other pathology, response to medications, etc.) is a clinical decision. An appreciation of the expected magnitude of compensation in normal subjects may support this clinical decision, but it is not a substitute for it.

Metabolic acidosis and alkalosis occur when there is a primary disturbance in the bicarbonate concentration of the blood. Respiratory responses occur to moderate the acidemia or

TABLE 5-3	Predicted Changes in Response to Processes Causing Acidosis or Alkalosis

Respiratory Acidosis (Primary Disorder, ↑ $Paco_2$; Compensation, ↑ [HCO_3^-])

	Acute	Chronic
ΔpH	$-0.008 \times \Delta Pco_2^a$	$-0.003 \times \Delta Pco_2$
ΔH^+	$0.8 \times \Delta Pco_2$	$0.3 \times \Delta Pco_2$
ΔHCO_3^-	$0.1 \times \Delta Pco_2$	$0.4 \times \Delta Pco_2$
H^+	$0.8 \times Pco_2 + 8$	$0.3 \times Pco_2 + 27$

Respiratory Alkalosis (Primary Disorder, ↓ $Paco_2$; Compensation, ↓ [HCO_3^-])

	Acute	Chronic
ΔpH	$-0.01 \times \Delta Pco_2^a$	$-0.003 \times \Delta Pco_2$
ΔH^+	$0.75 \times \Delta Pco_2$	$0.3 \times \Delta Pco_2$
ΔHCO_3^-	$0.2 \times Pco_2$	$0.5 \times \Delta Pco_2$
H^+	$0.75 \times Pco_2 + 10$	$0.3 \times Pco_2 + 28$

Metabolic Acidosis (Primary Disorder, ↓ [HCO_3^-]; Compensation, ↓ $Paco_2$)

ΔPco_2	$1.1–1.3 \times \Delta HCO_3$
Pco_2	$1.5 \times [HCO_3] + 8$
Pco_2	Last two digits of the pH

Metabolic Alkalosis (Primary Disorder, ↑ [HCO_3^-]; Compensation, ↑ $Paco_2$)

ΔPco_2	$0.6–0.8 \times \Delta HCO_3$
Pco_2	$0.7 \times [HCO_3] + 21$

^{a}Applicable for Pco_2 between 40 and 80 mmHg.

alkalemia (Table 5-3). A quick rule of thumb is that the $Paco_2$ in response to a metabolic acidosis should equal the last two digits of the pH, although maximum respiratory compensation will only reduce the $Paco_2$ to 12 to 15 mmHg. If significant underlying respiratory disease is present, adequate compensation may not occur, and the pH will be lower than anticipated. For example, a $Paco_2$ of 35 mmHg in the presence of a pH of 7.20 suggests an inadequate respiratory compensation caused either by underlying respiratory disease or by altered respiratory drive from a central nervous system (CNS) process. An individual with normal lungs would reduce his $Paco_2$ to approximately 20 mmHg. Significant hypoventilation ($Paco_2 > 45$) resulting from metabolic alkalosis also occurs, but less consistently. The best "rule of thumb" in metabolic alkalosis is that $Paco_2$ rises by 0.7 for every 1-mEq rise in [HCO_3^-].

When independent metabolic and respiratory processes affect the pH, a mixed acid–base disturbance is said to exist. It is most easily recognized when both processes drive the pH in the same direction, so there is no confusion regarding one compensating for the other. For instance, during cardiac arrest, respiratory acidosis and metabolic acidosis coexist in a combined acid–base disturbance and result in a greater reduction in pH than expected from the $Paco_2$ elevation alone. Combined metabolic and respiratory alkaloses can lead to a marked elevation of pH with cardiac arrhythmia, fall in cardiac output, or seizures.

In contrast, a mixed metabolic and respiratory disturbance exists when a process leading to acidosis is superimposed on an alkalosis, or vice versa. These are common in clinical practice and tend to be a little more difficult to recognize because the pH tends to be more normal. For instance, patients with chronic respiratory acidosis from obstructive pulmonary disease will develop a compensatory metabolic alkalosis. If treated with corticosteroids or diuretics, they may develop a further metabolic alkalosis resulting in a normal or slightly alkalemic pH. One specific condition to be aware of is the mixed metabolic acidosis and respiratory alkalosis of salicylate intoxication. The characteristic pattern of low pH, elevated anion gap, and a lower $Paco_2$ than predicted from the compensation rules points to such a diagnosis.

Common conditions leading to acid–base derangements are listed in Table 5-4. In general, therapy should be directed at the underlying condition and not simply at correcting the pH toward a normal value.

To understand fully acid–base derangements, it is valuable to use a systematic approach to the analyses of the ABG results (Table 5-5). Most approaches begin by identifying any respiratory component to the derangement. If the entire abnormality is explained on the basis of acute respiratory changes, then a primary respiratory disorder is said to be present. If there is change in $[HCO_3^-]$ beyond that predicted for an acute respiratory disturbance, one may ask if the change of a magnitude appropriate to compensation for a chronic respiratory disturbance. Metabolic compensation that is greater than the predicted value suggests a combined acid–base disturbance, whereas compensation that is less that the predicted range indicates either a

TABLE 5-4	Common Causes of Disturbances of Acid–Base Balance
Respiratory Acidosis	**Respiratory Alkalosis**
• Diminished ventilatory drive • Sedatives • Central hypoventilation syndromes • Severe CNS depression or injury • Diminished respiratory muscle function • Guillain–Barré syndrome • Myasthenia gravis • Severe hypokalemia • Diminished pulmonary function • Chronic obstructive pulmonary disease • Status asthmaticus • Severe restrictive disease	• Catastrophic CNS event • Drug with direct stimulation of respiration (salicylates, progesterone) • Sepsis (early) • Cirrhosis • Pregnancy (third trimester) • Decreased lung compliance (J receptor) • Anxiety
Metabolic Acidosis	**Metabolic Alkalosis**
With normal anion "gap" • GI bicarbonate loss • Renal tubular acidosis • Ureteral diversion • NH_4Cl or HCl infusion • Rehydration • Hyperalimentation • Compensation for respiratory alkalosis With elevated anion "gap" • Ketoacidosis • Lactic acidosis • Salicylate intoxication • Methanol ingestion • Ethylene glycol ingestion	• Hypochloremia (often with volume contraction) • Hypokalemia • Mineralocorticoid excess • Bartter syndrome • Administration of alkali • Compensation for respiratory acidosis

CNS, central nervous system.

TABLE 5-5	Approaches to the Interpretation of Blood Gases

Step-by-Step

1. Is the patient acidemic or alkalemic?
2. If the P_{CO_2} is abnormal, estimate whether an acute change in P_{CO_2} is sufficient to explain the pH change. If so, then the disturbance is predominantly a respiratory disturbance in acid–base balance.
3. If an acute change in P_{CO_2} is insufficient to explain all of the pH change, evaluate the nature of the additional metabolic disorder. Is the metabolic disturbance consistent with the predicted compensation for a chronic respiratory change?

4. If the disturbance appears primarily metabolic, evaluate the adequacy of respiratory compensation. The absence of complete respiratory compensation or of excessive respiratory compensation for a metabolic disturbance implies a secondary respiratory disturbance.
5. If a metabolic acidosis is present, ascertain the presence or absence of unmeasured anions using the anion gap or charge neutrality equations.
6. Identify other metabolic disturbances present in the patient with an anion gap metabolic acidosis.

"Quick and Dirty"

1. Determine the predicted pH if all of the abnormality were due to changes in ventilation (i.e., if the P_{CO_2} were corrected to 40).
2. Determine the difference between the measured and predicted pH.
3. Estimate the base deficit or excess: multiply the difference between the measured and predicted pH and move the decimal point two places to the right (answer is in milliequivalent per liter).

4. Calculate the anion gap to estimate the contribution of strong ions to any base deficit.

mixed disorder or incomplete compensation. A similar analytic approach should be used if the primary disorder is metabolic. Finally, the presence of increased amounts of unmeasured anions determines the presence of a metabolic acidosis even when [HCO_3^-] is normal.

FURTHER READING

1. Albert MS, Dell RB, Winters RW. Quantitative displacement of acid–base equilibrium in metabolic acidosis. *Ann Intern Med.* 1967;66:312–322.

   Classic article that establishes confidence limits for metabolic acidosis.

2. Adrogue HJ, Madias NE. Management of life-threatening acid–base disorders: part one. *N Engl J Med.* 1998;338:26–34.

3. Adrogue HJ, Madias NE. Management of life-threatening acid–base disorders: part two. *N Engl J Med.* 1998;338:107–111.

   A two-part comprehensive review of acid–base homeostasis (153 references).

4. Forsythe SM, Schmidt GA. Sodium bicarbonate for the treatment of lactic acidosis. *Chest.* 2000;117:260–267.

   A review of the literature supporting bicarbonate administration in lactic acidosis. The absence of evidence suggesting improved outcomes prompts the authors to recommend that it not be used (91 references).

5. Gilfix BM, Bique M, Magder S. A physical chemical approach to the analysis of acid–base balance in the clinical setting. *J Crit Care.* 1993;8:187–197.

   A discussion of an alternative approach to estimating unmeasured anions and comparing with the classical anion "gap" approach.

6. Inman KJ, Sibbald WJ, Rutledge FS, et al. Does implementing pulse oximetry in a critical care unit result in substantial arterial blood gas savings? *Chest.* 1993;104:542–546.

    Compares the practice relating to obtaining ABG on 300 patients in the critical care unit, before and after the availability of oximetry.

7. McCurdy DK. Mixed metabolic and respiratory acid base disturbances: diagnosis and treatment. *Chest.* 1972;62:35S–44S.

    One of the best reviews of metabolic acid–base disorders with the classic graphic relationship of P_{aCO_2} to $[H^+]$.

8. Morris LR, Murphy MB, Kitabchi AE. Bicarbonate therapy in severe diabetic ketoacidosis. *Ann Intern Med.* 1986;105:836–840.

    This article sparked a controversy over the use of bicarbonate in metabolic acid–base disturbances.

9. Narins RG. Diagnostic strategies in disorders of fluid, electrolyte, and acid–base homeostasis. *Am J Med.* 1982;72:496–520.

    An excellent review with clinical case studies.

10. Palmer BF, Alpern RJ. Metabolic alkalosis. *J Am Soc Nephrol.* 1997;8:1462–1469.

    A review of the manifestations and approach to the management of metabolic alkalosis in the critical care environment.

11. Peris LV, Boix JH, Salom JV, et al. Clinical use of the arterial/alveolar oxygen tension ratio. *Crit Care Med.* 1983;11:888–891.

    Review of the use of the P_{aO_2}/P_{AO_2} ratio and how it also can be used to predict the F_{IO_2} level needed to provide desired P_{aO_2}.

12. Kumar V, Karon BS. Comparison of measured and calculated bicarbonate values. *Clin Chem.* 2008;54:1586–1587.

    In nearly 18,000 clinical instances in which $[^-HCO_3]$ was simultaneously measured (in the chemistry laboratory) and calculated (from the ABG), there was excellent agreement when the $[^-HCO_3]$ values were within normal range (96% of values). However, among the 4% (513) measured $[^-HCO_3]$ values outside the normal range, only 10 of the matched calculated $[^-HCO_3]$ values were outside the normal range.

13. Munoz X, Torres F, Sampol G, et al. Accuracy and reliability of pulse oximetry at different arterial carbon dioxide pressure levels. *Eur Respir J.* 2008;32(4):1053–1059.

    The agreement between pulse oximetry and co-oximetry measured with an ABG is not as tight during hypoxemia or hypercapnea.

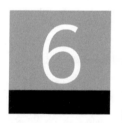

Thoracic Ultrasound Uses in Pulmonary Medicine

David R. Riker

Ultrasound (US) technology is an important tool in pulmonary medicine, especially in the intensive care unit (ICU) setting where it can facilitate accurate and safe vascular access and help determine a cause for shock. It is also important in evaluating pulmonary and pleural disease. The value of an US option rests in its associated absence of radiation, low cost, bedside availability, and short examination time. Although US among current pulmonary and critical care practitioners remains underutilized, the standard of care is quickly swinging toward routine utilization in medical practice.

TECHNICAL ASPECTS AND PHYSICS OF ULTRASOUND

US images are generated by ceramic crystals located in the ultrasound transducer. The crystals are electronically stimulated to produce sound pulses, which contact the tissue and are reflected, refracted, adsorbed, or scattered. Echoes returning from tissues distort the crystal elements, producing an electric pulse, which is processed into a gray scale image. When no sound wave is reflected, as found with a transudative pleural effusion, the image is termed "anechoic" and appears black. The term "isoechoic" is used when echoes display comparable amplitude with surrounding tissue, like the liver or spleen, and the term "hyperechoic" is used when the echo display is stronger than surrounding tissue, as with the diaphragm and pleura. "Hypoechoic" refers to echoes weaker than surrounding tissue.

When sound waves strike a moving object such as blood traversing a vessel, frequency changes occur and an alteration in sound waves create a Doppler effect which may be used to determine blood flow velocity and direction. Color Doppler sonography is sensitive to Doppler signals in the field and shows flow in color. Standard color changes include (1) red signal as flow moves toward the transducer and (2) blue signal when flow travels away from the transducer.

PREPARING FOR EXAMINATION

Frequency—Higher-frequency transducers (5 or 7.5 MHz) provide improved resolution for structures like chest wall and pleura. For deeper (e.g., lung tissue) imaging, a 3.5-MHz transducer is more suitable. Frequency is directly related to resolution: as frequency increases, resolution increases as well. However, frequency and penetration are inversely related.

Probe—For the chest ultrasound, curvilinear or convex probes are appropriate. For chest survey and a wider view of the thoracic and abdominal cavities, convex probes are preferred. The linear probe gives better resolution and can be used in patients with a thin thoracic chest wall. A sector transducer should be considered for lesions with a small US window or in patients with narrowed intercostal spaces.

Gain and power—These are manually adjusted to give sharpness to the image.

Mode—B-mode (brightness mode or bidimensional mode) converts sound waves into real-time gray scale anatomical images. M-mode is motion modulation, and it offers less information in thoracic ultrasound imaging.

Color Doppler sonography—Allows visualization and delineation of vascular structures in the ultrasound field.

NORMAL FINDINGS

Layers of chest wall muscle and fascia are represented by linear shadows of soft tissue echogenicity. Positioning the transducer in a longitudinal (perpendicular) direction to the ribs creates a "batwing" sign where the ribs appear as curvilinear echogenic interfaces with prominent acoustic shadowing. When using the high-frequency probe, the parietal pleura and visceral pleura are seen as two thin bright echogenic lines, normally measuring no more than 2 mm in thickness. The space between the visceral and parietal pleura is about 0.3 to 0.4 mm. Normally, the visceral pleura slides over the parietal pleura during the respiratory cycle; this phenomenon is termed "sliding sign." Using M-mode, it is possible to confirm the lung sliding by the "seashore sign": the visceral pleura moving during respiration resembles the "sand" and the immobile parietal pleura and chest wall tissue the "sea." The normal diaphragm is seen through the lower intercostal spaces as an echogenic 1- to 2-mm-thick and curved line which contracts with inspiration. The costodiaphragmatic angle may disclose the "curtain sign," which describes how the normal air-filled lung during inspiration moves downward in front of the probe and temporarily obscures the sonographic window. In normal conditions, US cannot discern the lung, but the sound pulse distortion caused by chest wall structures originates horizontal artifacts that are seen as a series of echogenic parallel lines equidistant from one another below the pleura. These lines are known as reverberation artifacts or "A lines" and diminish in intensity with increasing distance from the pleura. In the presence of lung sliding, A lines correlate with normal aeration pattern. B lines are also reverberation artifacts and originate from the pleural surface and extend vertically in a ray-like pattern to the bottom of the screen. B lines are also known as "lung rockets" or "comet tails" and may be seen in lateral chest walls in normal subjects, but more often are associated with lung diseases.

US is a valuable tool in managing pleural disease. It is more sensitive than clinical examination or chest x-rays (including lateral decubitus film) in diagnosing a pleural effusion. It can detect as little as 50 mL of pleural fluid. In addition, US can estimate the amount of fluid, determine whether it is free flowing or encapsulated, and suggest the nature of the effusion. Pleural effusion displays as an echo-free space between visceral and parietal pleuras. When effusions are large enough to cause compression atelectasis, the lung may display as a hyperechoic tongue-like structure within the effusion (the "jellyfish" or "tongue" sign). On M-mode, it is possible to see visceral pleura moving toward the chest wall during respiration, creating the sinusoid sign.

US may help define anatomy when a radiograph suggests hemidiaphragmatic elevation. It can differentiate between subpulmonary effusion, subphrenic fluid collection, and diaphragmatic paralysis by defining the diaphragm's position and real-time motion. US is also useful in the evaluation of unilateral "white lung" in chest x-ray because it can distinguish between fluid and solid lesions.

US may also disclose the nature of a pleural effusion and define one of four typical patterns: (a) homogeneously anechoic, (b) complex nonseptated with heterogeneously hyperechoic spots inside the effusion, (c) complex septated with septa or fibrin strands, and (d) homogeneously echogenic. Transudates have a homogeneously anechoic appearance, while patterns b, c, and d corresponded to exudates. Pleural nodules are highly specific for exudates and often indicate malignancy. Pleural thickening and parenchymal lesions strongly suggest exudates. The homogeneously echogenic pattern may be due to hemorrhagic effusion or empyema.

Pleural thickening is defined as a focal echogenic lesion arising from either pleura that is greater than 3 mm in width and usually indicates empyema, hemothorax, or iatrogenic pleurodesis. The thickened pleura may contain high-echogenic lesions that indicate calcification. Small pleural effusions have similar ultrasonographic characteristics to pleural thickening.

Primary or metastatic pleural tumors may appear as echogenic or hypoechoic nodules located within the visceral or parietal pleura. The presence of nodules highly suggests a malignant pleural effusion. However, the observation of lung consolidation adjacent to pleural fluid suggests a parapneumonic effusion.

Organized effusions like complex parapneumonic effusions, empyemas, and hemorrhagic effusions are characterized by the presence of floating weblike structures within pleural fluid corresponding to fibrinous septa or by echogenic particles that move with respiration or heart beats ("plankton sign") or by increased echogenicity. Contrast enhanced CT scans are less sensitive for clearly defining strandings or septations in the evaluation of complex pleural effusions.

THORACENTESIS, CHEST DRAINAGE CATHETERS, AND BIOPSIES

The Society of Critical Care Medicine recommends the use of thoracic US guidance for all pleural procedures. Thoracic US reduces procedure failures (dry taps) and complication rates. A recent chest x-ray or CT scan should be available in order to confirm the indication of the procedure and the affected side.

Lower-frequency probes (3.5–5 MHz) are the most appropriate to guide pleural fluid drainage because it is possible to evaluate deeper structures as well as to avoid vital organs such as the liver, spleen, or blood vessels. Higher-frequency transducers (7.5–10 MHz) have a better resolution in evaluating pleural thickening/nodules and to guide pleural biopsies. The patient should be placed in the most appropriate position to evaluate the site of interest. The seated position is often the most appropriate but patients on mechanical ventilation or in the ICU cannot tolerate this position. In those cases, lateral decubitus or oblique positioning is required. For free-flowing effusion drainage or pleural biopsy in ICU patients, a posterior axillary line approach optimizes the point of entry by raising the head of the bed and adducting the ipsilateral arm. An alternative option requires the patient turned to a lateral decubitus position with the target hemithorax up.

With the patient in the optimal position, US localizes the effusion and ensures that the diaphragm or lung are not in the projected path of the thoracentesis needle. The operator should measure the depth of the pleura or pleural effusion from the skin surface and mark the skin site of entry. When the needle is inserted, it should enter the skin at the same angle of the US probe. While real-time needle visualization can be used for thoracentesis, it may not improve yield or safety. However, when considering pleural or lung biopsy, this method of active ultrasound guidance is preferred.

Ultrasound-guided thoracentesis improves procedural success and safety. The risk of pneumothorax using US guidance is 2.7% to 3.6% compared to 5% to 18% without. In a large (n = 523) retrospective study of complication rates during thoracentesis, US guidance was associated with a lower rate of pneumothoraces (4.9% vs 10.3%) and need for chest drainage tube insertion (0.7% vs 4.1%) than thoracentesis without ultrasound. While there is a higher risk of pneumothorax in mechanically ventilated patients undergoing thoracentesis compared to spontaneously breathing patients, the rates of pneumothoraces are low (1.3%–2%) when US guidance is utilized.

Closed Pleural Biopsy

Thoracic ultrasound allows detection of focal pleural abnormalities with higher sensitivity than chest CT imaging. The presence of pleural fluid or pleural air is required for a closed blind pleural biopsy in order to avoid lung perforation; US guidance may reduce the risk of lung laceration in patients with small or no pleural effusion. In malignant disease, pleural biopsy by US guidance has a sensitivity between 77% and 86% and a specificity of 100%. Blind closed pleural biopsy has a sensitivity of 65% for malignant disease and 90% for tuberculosis. For this procedure, most studies favor the use of core needle biopsy (Tru-Cut) over pleural biopsy needles (Abrams or Cope) and fine-needle aspiration. Complication rates of image guided pleural biopsies are less than 5% (pneumothorax, hemothorax, and vasovagal reaction), whereas closed pleural biopsy without US may have complication rates as high as 11%.

Chest Drain Insertion

Thoracic US is a useful tool during chest tube insertion to locate the most appropriate site for drain placement. For loculated effusions, US may enhance the success of chest tube drainage by isolating the largest locule or largest separate collections in the case of multiple locules. US allows the precise insertion of small bore catheters (8–14 F) to treat pleural disease with high efficacy (resolution in 73%–94% of cases) and low risk of complications. Empyema can also be successfully treated without the need for larger chest tubes. In patients with empyema failing conventional management (large bore chest tube insertion), 76.5% of cases were successfully treated with US-guided small pleural catheters. US can reduce complication rates of chest tube placement in the emergent ICU setting equal to rates comparable to nonemergent situations.

US IN SPECIFIC LUNG DISEASES
Consolidation

Consolidated areas of the lung are hypoechoic or isoechoic in relation to the liver, hence the term "hepatization sign" (tissue like pattern). When the transducer is parallel to the long axes of bronchi, air bronchograms can be seen as linear hyperechoic patterns which converge toward the hilum. When the transducer is in short axis, air bronchograms may be seen as scattered round or elongated hyperechoic structures. They may move cranio-caudally within the respiratory cycle, depending on lung compliance. These "dynamic air bronchograms" differentiate lung consolidation from resorptive atelectasis. Another sonographic finding of consolidation is a fluid bronchogram that is characterized by US as flow signal-free tubular structures, corresponding to exudate-filled airways. C lines or "shred sign" can be observed in incomplete lobar consolidation. These findings are similar to B lines; however, the artifact arises from the region of consolidation, not from the pleural line. Thoracic US has superior sensitivity and specificity in the diagnosis of pneumonia in ER patients compared to chest x-ray (99% and 95% vs 67% and 85% respectively). Thoracic US compares favorably with chest CT as a gold standard for detecting consolidation, with 90% sensitivity and 98% specificity. The US finding of consolidation, however, is nonspecific and must be interpreted for each clinical situation. ARDS, lung contusion, pulmonary embolus, and infiltrating tumors such as bronchoalveolar carcinoma may all show consolidation patterns.

Pneumothorax

Pneumothorax can present in an emergent fashion, requiring rapid identification. Relying on radiographic modalities such as chest x-ray and CT imaging may cause a delay in pneumothorax diagnosis and treatment. US can be used to rapidly rule out pneumothorax. Pre- and post-procedure US scanning during thoracentesis, transbronchial biopsy, and central line placement can exclude large pneumothoraces. Lung sliding reflects the normal interaction of lung and chest wall; its presence rules out pneumothorax and its absence is highly predictive of pneumothorax. Difficulty with pneumothorax exclusion or absence of lung sliding can occur with subcutaneous emphysema and low lung compliance conditions such as ARDS and pulmonary fibrosis. Other conditions with absence of lung sliding are large consolidations and contusions, emphysema, hyperinflated lungs, and pleural adhesions. In the case of low lung compliance diseases with absent lung sliding, the presence of B lines ("comet tail artifacts") excludes a pneumothorax. The absence of lung sliding and B lines in the presence of A lines is highly suggestive of pneumothorax. With a pneumothorax, the "seashore sign" on M-mode is absent and instead the "stratosphere sign" (or "barcode sign") is observed. Stratosphere sign is composed of horizontal and parallel lines without the presence of a pleural line. The pleural line divides the "sea" and the "shore" when a pneumothorax is not observed. Rarely, a "lung point" is detected, which is the area of transition between the pneumothorax and aerated lung that intermittently contacts the chest wall with inspiration. Using M-mode, "lung point" appears as "seashore sign" combined with the "stratosphere sign." The lung point confirms the presence of pneumothorax with a 79% sensitive but a 100% specific for pneumothorax. Thoracic US using these methods is more sensitive than chest radiography for detecting pneumothorax.

Alveolo-Interstitial Edema

In the setting of acute dyspnea, the US presence of diffuse B lines in the anterior chest wall reliably differentiates patients with pulmonary edema from those with COPD having a sensitivity of 100% and specificity of 92%. Lung comet artifacts detect early pulmonary edema before clinical manifestations are apparent, which may support the use of US as a noninvasive modality for the hemodynamic management of critically ill patients. Ultrasound may also have a role in detecting interstitial lung disease such as pulmonary fibrosis, sarcoidosis, viral pneumonia, lymphangitic carcinomatosis, silicosis, and radiation pneumonitis. Interestingly, ILD patients may also show pleural surface alterations such as pleural thickening (85%) and irregular pleural architecture (98%).

TRANSTHORACIC BIOPSIES OF LUNG LESIONS

Biopsy of peripheral tumors abutting the pleura or invading the chest wall can be sampled with US guidance using fine needle aspiration (FNA) with a 22 G spinal needle or core needle biopsy (CNB). Both procedures offer a high diagnostic yield and a low rate of pneumothorax. Lung carcinomas usually present as a homogeneous hypoechoic rounded or pleomorphic shape lesions.

Necrosis within the tumor gives an anechoic signal. Lung lesions have respirophasic movement that is absent when infiltration of the chest wall occurs.

Transthoracic biopsies can also be considered in the diagnosis of lung consolidation, particularly in immunocompromised patients. Lung abscess are observed on US imaging as oval hypoechoic lesions with hyperechoic and irregular margins. About 90% of US-guided lung aspirates yield pathogenic organisms.

CENTRAL VENOUS CATHETER ACCESS

US-guided central vein cannulation (CVC) with a linear high-frequency probe (7.5–10 MHz), compared to the anatomic landmark method, can reduce the numbers of failed catheter placements and complications. The benefits are more apparent in critically ill patients: access time, number of attempts as well as complications such as carotid artery puncture, hematoma, hemothorax, pneumothorax, catheter-associated blood stream infections are significantly reduced with US.

There are two methods for central line placement using US: indirect and direct. In the indirect method, US is used to establish the puncture site and angle of needle insertion and visualize the associated surrounding vessels, including arteries. The direct method uses real-time US guidance to direct the needle into the vein. A sterile cover or sheath is applied to the US probe. Both direct and indirect approaches are superior to the traditional landmark method. Although the indirect method can be used, the direct method is preferred to maximize procedural success while minimizing complications.

MEDIASTINAL ULTRASOUND

The greatest role of medistinal US is interrogation of the anterior superior mediastinum. Tumors adjacent to the sternum can be biopsied under US guidance, with reduction in bleeding risk because surrounding vessels or tumor vessels can be easily evaluated during the procedure. US can be used in the evaluation of patients with superior vena cava syndrome, allowing evaluation of the superior vena cava, adjacent veins, as well as collateral vessels. Pericardial effusion is easily detected by mean of US, with subcostal and parasternal views being most useful. Pericardiocentesis can also be performed under US guidance. EBUS (endobronchial ultrasound) has rapidly become the modality of choice to assess and stage mediastinal, paratracheal, and subcarinal lymph nodes (see Chapter 7).

FURTHER READING

1. Beckh S, Bolcskei PL, Lessnau KD. Real-time chest ultrasonography: a comprehensive review for the pulmonologist. *Chest.* 2002;122:1759–1773.
   Concise review of chest ultrasound.
2. Yang PC, Luh KT, Chang DB, et al. Value of sonography in determining the nature of pleural effusion: analysis of 320 cases. *AJR Am J Roentgenol.* 1992;159:29–33.
   Categorization of sonographic findings in pleural effusions.
3. McLoud TC, Flower CD. Imaging the pleura: sonography, CT, and MR imaging. *AJR Am J Roentgenol.* 1991;156:1145–1153.
   Provides description of pleural imaging modalities.
4. Barnes TW, Morgenthaler TI, Olson EJ, et al. Sonographically guided thoracentesis and rate of pneumothorax. *J Clin Ultrasound.* 2005;33:442–446.
   Reduction of thoracentesis complications using ultrasound.
5. Gervan DA, Petersen A, Lee MJ, et al. US guided thoracentesis: requirement for postprocedure chest radiography in patients who receive mechanical ventilation versus patients who breathe spontaneously. *Radiology.* 1997;204:503–506.
   Limited utility of post procedure chest x-ray after US thoracentesis.

6. Mayo PH, Goltz HR, Tafreshi M, et al. Safety of ultrasound guided thoracentesis in patients receiving mechanical ventilation. *Chest.* 2004;125(3):1059–1062.
   Low complications associated with US-guided thoracentesis in intubated ICU patients.

7. Rahman NM, Gleeson FV. Image-guided pleural biopsy. *Curr Opin Pulm Med.* 2008;14:331–336.
   Overview of pleural biopsy with image guidance.

8. Liu CM, Hang LW, Chen WK, et al. Pigtail tube drainage in the treatment of spontaneous pneumothorax. *Am J Emerg Med.* 2003;21:241–244.
   Use of small bore chest tube catheters for pneumothorax.

9. vanSonnenberg E, Nakamoto SK, Mueller PR, et al. CT- and ultrasound-guided catheter drainage of empyemas after chest-tube failure. *Radiology.* 1984;151:349–353.
   Comparison of US and CT placed pleural catheters for empyema management.

10. Havelock T, Teoh R, Laws D, et al. Pleural procedures and thoracic ultrasound: British Thoracic Society pleural disease guideline 2010. *Thorax.* 2010;65(suppl 2):ii61–ii76.
    BTS guidelines reviewing pleural disease and pleural procedures.

11. Weinberg B, Diakoumakis EE, Kass EG, et al. The air bronchogram: sonographic demonstration. *AJR Am J Roentgenol.* 1986;147(3):593–595.
    Air bronchogram sonographic sign and clinical implications.

12. Lichtenstein DA, Lascols N, Meziere G, et al. Ultrasound diagnosis of alveolar consolidation in the critically ill. *Intensive Care Med.* 2004;30(2):276–281.
    ICU finding of alveolar consolidation on US and overview of US techinques.

13. Nalos M, Kot M, McLean AS, et al. Bedside lung ultrasound in the care of the critically ill. *Curr Respir Med Rev.* 2010;6:271–278.
    Clinical implications of using US in routine ICU patient care.

14. Cortellaro F, Colombo S, Coen D, et al. Lung ultrasound is an accurate diagnostic tool for the diagnosis of pneumonia in the emergency department. *Emerg Med J.* 2012;29(1):19–23. doi:10.1136/emj.2010.101584.
    Diagnosis of pneumonia without chest x-ray in ER patients.

15. Miller LD, Joyner CR, Dudrick SJ, et al. Clinical use of ultrasound in the detection of pulmonary embolism. *Trans Assoc Am Phys.* 1966;166:381–392.
    Alternative options for PE diagnosis using US.

16. Reissig A, Heyne JP, Koegel C. Sonography of lung and pleura in pulmonary embolism: sonomorphologic characterization and comparison with spiral CT scanning. *Chest.* 2001;120:1977–1983.
    CT scan compared with US in the diagnosis of PE.

17. Mathis G. Ultrasound diagnosis of pulmonary embolism. *Eur J Ultrasound.* 1996;3:153–160.
    Review of US use and PE diagnosis emphasizing clinical implications.

18. Mathis G, Blank W, Reissig A, et al. Thoracic ultrasound for diagnosing pulmonary embolism: a prospective multicenter study of 352 patients. *Chest.* 2005;128(3):1531–1538.
    Large prospective study identifying US for PE based on pretest probability.

19. Lichtenstein DA, Menu Y. A bedside ultrasound sign ruling out pneumothorax in the critically ill: lung sliding. *Chest.* 1995;108(5):1345–1348.
    Lung sliding US sign with 100% negative predictive value for pneumothorax.

20. Lichtenstein D, Meziere G, Biderman P, et al. The comet tail artifact: an ultrasound sign ruling out pneumothorax. *Intensive Care Med.* 1999;25(4):383–388.
    Negative predicting US findings in patients suspected of having pneumothorax.

21. Lichtenstein DA, Meziere G, Lascols N, et al. Ultrasound diagnosis of occult pneumothorax. *Crit Care Med.* 2005;33(6):1231–1238.
    Discussion of occult pneumothorax in the critically ill.

22. Blaivas M, Lyon M, Duggal S. A prospective comparison of supine chest radiography and bedside ultrasound for the diagnosis of traumatic pneumothorax. *Acad Emerg Med.* 2005;12(9):844–849.
    US in the care of trauma patients.

23. Soldati G, Copetti R, Sher S. Sonographic interstitial syndrome: the sound of lung water. *J Ultrasound Med.* 2009;28(2):163–174.

Overview of sonographic interstitial syndrome.

24. Lichtenstein D, Goldstein I, Mourgeon E, et al. Comparative diagnostic performances of auscultation chest radiography, and lung ultrasonography in acute respiratory distress syndrome. *Anesthesiology.* 2004;100(1):9–15.

Lung ultrasonography as a bedside tool in ARDS patients.

25. Volpicelli G, Mussa A, Garofalo G, et al. Bedside lung ultrasound in the assessment of alveolar-interstitial syndrome. *Am J Emerg Med.* 2006;24(6):689–696.

Interstitial pulmonary disease diagnosed using bedside ultrasound.

26. Lichtenstein D, Meziere G. A lung ultrasound sign allowing bedside distinction between pulmonary edema and COPD: the comet-tail artifact. *Intensive Care Med.* 1998;24(12):1331–1334.

Distinguishing US findings to determine SOB in patients with CHF or COPD.

27. Lichtenstein DA, Meziere G, Lagoueyte JF, et al. A-lines and B-lines: lung ultrasound as a bedside tool for predicting pulmonary artery occlusion pressure in the critically ill. *Chest.* 2009;136(4):1014–1020.

Clinical utility of US artifacts in patients with elevated left atrial pressures.

28. Agricola E, Bove T, Oppizzi M, et al. "Ultrasound comet-tail images": a marker of pulmonary edema: a comparative study with wedge pressure and extravascular lung water. *Chest.* 2005;127(5):1690–1695.

Pulmonary edema, interstitial findings and US comet tail imaging.

29. Reissig A, Kroegel C. Transthoracic sonography of diffuse parenchymal lung disease. *J Ultrasound Med.* 2003;22(2):173–180.

Discussion of thoracic ultrasound and several common lung diseases.

30. Bouhemad B, Liu ZH, Arbelot C, et al. Ultrasound assessment of antibiotic-induced pulmonary reaeration in ventilator-associated pneumonia. *Crit Care Med.* 2010;38(1):84–92.

VAP and response to treatment based on thoracic ultrasound.

31. Bouhemad B, Brisson H, Le-Guen M, et al. Bedside ultrasound assessment of positive end-expiratory pressure-induced lung recruitment. *Am J Respir Crit Care Med.* 2011;183(3):341–347.

PEEP and alveolar changes based on US interpretation.

32. Diacon AH, Schuurmans MM, Theron J, et al. Safety and yield of ultrasound-assisted transthoracic biopsy performed by pulmonologist. *Respiration.* 2004;71(5):519–522.

Procedural assisted ultrasound, technique, safety and yield.

33. Yang PC, Chang DB, Yu CJ, et al. Ultrasound guided percutaneous cutting biopsy for the diagnosis of pulmonary consolidations of unknown aetiology. *Thorax.* 1992;47(6):457–460.

Discussion of CNB for pulmonary parenchymal disease.

34. Chen HJ, Yu YH, Tu CY, et al. Ultrasound in peripheral pulmonary air-fluid lesions: color Doppler imaging as an aid in differentiating empyema and abscess. *Chest.* 2009;135(6):1426–1432.

Ultrasound improves the diagnostic challenge of differentiating empyema and pulmonary abscess.

35. Hind D, Calvert N, McWilliams R, et al. Ultrasonic locating devices for central venous cannulation: a meta-analysis. *BMJ.* 2003;327:361.

Concise overview of US and vascular access.

36. Karakistos D, Labropoulos N, De Groot E, et al. Real-time ultrasound-guided catheterisation of the internal jugular vein: a prospective comparison with the landmark technique in critical care patients. *Crit Care.* 2006;10(6):R162.

Provides comparison of US and landmarks for CVC insertion.

37. Blaivas M, Brannam L, Fernandez E. Short-axis versus long-axis approaches for teaching ultrasound-guided vascular access on a new inanimate model. *Acad Emerg Med.* 2003;10(12):1307–1311.

Summerizes different techniques for teaching vascular US use.

38. Wernecke K, Vassallo P, Potter R, et al. Mediastinal tumors: sensitivity of detection with sonography compared with CT and radiography. *Radiology.* 1990;175:135–143.

Concurrent review of mediastinal imaging.

39. Soldati G, Testa A, Silva FR, et al. Chest ultrasonography in lung contusion. *Chest.* 2006; 130(2):533–538.

   Discussion of the role of US in trauma patients with lung contusion.

40. Breikreutz R, Walcher F, Seeger FH. Focused echocardiographic evaluation in resuscitation management: concept of an advanced life support-conformed algorithm. *Crit Care Med.* 2007;35(suppl 5): S150–S161.

   US evaluation and management implications in advanced life support.

41. Elmer J, Noble V. An evidence-based approach for integrating bedside ultrasound into routine practice in the assessment of undifferentiated shock. *ICU Director.* 2010;1(3):163–174.

   Incorporation of US in management of shock.

42. Feissel M, Michard F, Faller JP, et al. The respiratory variation in inferior vena cava diameter as a guide to fluid therapy. *Intensive Care Med.* 2004;30(9):1834–1837.

   Summarizes fluid resuscitation based on inferior vena cava US findings.

43. Bolliger CT, Herth FJF, Mayo PH, et al., eds. *Clinical Chest Ultrasound: From the ICU to the Bronchoscopy Suite.* Vol 37. Basel, Switzerland: Karger; 2009:208–217.

   Comprehensive discussion and review of pulmonary applications of chest ultrasound.

7 Interventional Pulmonology: Advanced Diagnostic Procedures

Andrew D. Lerner and Samir S. Makani

Exciting advances in bronchoscopy over the last 10 years have improved the diagnosis and treatment of lung disease. New technologies have diminished invasiveness, increased diagnostic yields, and decreased risks. And as a corollary, patients have benefited from lower health care costs and more streamlined transitions to appropriate care. Improved diagnostic yields from advanced pulmonary procedures such as endobronchial ultrasound and navigational bronchoscopy have revolutionized the approach to lung cancer staging and to the diagnosis of peripheral pulmonary lesions.

FLEXIBLE FIBEROPTIC BRONCHOSCOPY

Flexible bronchoscopy consists of inserting a bronchoscope into the airways via the nares or oral pharynx to visualize the airways from the larynx to the subsegments of the tracheobronchial tree. Flexible bronchoscopy accounts for 97% of all airway interventions performed by pulmonologists. The most common indications for flexible bronchoscopy are (1) for assessing lung masses, lung cancer staging, undiagnosed pulmonary infiltrates, mediastinal lymphadenopathy, hemoptysis, disorders affecting the central airways, endobronchial lesions; (2) for placing an endotracheal tube; and (3) for therapeutic suctioning of secretions and mucus plugs.

Flexible bronchoscopy carries a very low complication rate. Temporary hypoxemia is the most common complication and may be avoided in most cases by using supplemental oxygen during the procedure. Significant bleeding occurs in 1% to 4% of bronchoscopies. It usually is associated with transbronchial biopsies, brushings, or endobronchial biopsies. For this reason, most authorities recommend that a patient's platelet count be above 50,000 per µL for a bronchoscopy that will include a biopsy. Aspirin does not increase the risk of bleeding after a transbronchial biopsy, provided there are no other risk factors. One study, however, demonstrated an increased risk of bronchoscopy-associated bleeding with other antiplatelet agents, such as clopidogrel. For these reasons, we do not delay bronchoscopy merely because a patient has used aspirin, but we will delay elective bronchoscopy until other antiplatelet agents have been discontinued for 7 days. Warfarin should be held for 5 days prior to bronchoscopy, but certain patient populations may require "bridging" with heparin or low–molecular-weight heparin in the interim before procedure. With these precautions, mortality associated with flexible bronchoscopy is typically less than 0.04%. The deaths result from hemorrhage, cardiovascular events, bronchospasm, aspiration pneumonia, or medication reactions.

A variety of sampling techniques, including bronchial washing, bronchial brushing, bronchoalveolar lavage, endobronchial or transbronchial forceps biopsy, and endobronchial or transbronchial needle aspiration, allows the operator to collect specimens from the respiratory tract. Selected paratracheal and parabronchial lymph nodes or other lesions also can be sampled by transbronchial needle aspiration techniques. Fluoroscopy or computed tomography (CT) guidance can help localize lesions during the procedure.

Flexible bronchoscopy is limited by the fact that it allows visualization only of the lumen and internal surface of the airways. The bronchoscopist cannot see lung diseases within the interior bronchial wall or the parabronchial structures. Indirect signs, such as mucosal and anatomical wall changes, may be used to assess pathology outside of the airway, but they are often inaccurate. Radiological imaging prior to the procedure provides valuable information, although it is unreliable for defining the pathological characteristics of lung lesions. For these reasons, tissue sampling of lesions outside the airways via flexible bronchoscopy had been limited by low yield and dependent on user experience. In some cases, mediastinoscopy has higher yields, but is limited by its highly invasive nature.

ENDOBRONCHIAL ULTRASOUND BRONCHOSCOPY

Endobronchial ultrasound (EBUS) has greatly advanced the bronchoscopist's ability to precisely visualize and biopsy extrabronchial lesions as well as lymph nodes. It has greatly enhanced the ability to accurately diagnose and stage thoracic cancers, without the costs and complications inherent to thoracic surgery.

EBUS uses an ultrasound probe at the end of a flexible bronchoscope. The ultrasound creates images of tissues beyond the airway lumen (e.g., endoluminal, intramural, and parabronchial structures) based on their differences in resistance to sound waves. It is valuable for evaluating endobronchial and peripheral lesions, for lung cancer staging with lymph node biopsy, and for distinguishing masses from their surrounding tissues and vascular structures.

EBUS bronchoscopy, like conventional bronchoscopy, is performed with a flexible scope fitted with a standard camera, a working channel, and a suction channel. In addition, the EBUS bronchoscope includes a convex ultrasound probe. Although the scope can be flexed and rotated in a way similar to a conventional flexible bronchoscope, the camera is at an oblique angle. The ultrasound probe is surrounded by a saline-filled balloon to help create close contact with the airway mucosa and to remove the air-interface which otherwise would cause artifact. The ultrasound probe has a biopsy channel that allows a biopsy needle to be inserted with a real-time view of its orientation and depth into the tissue or lesion.

The most common indication for EBUS bronchoscopy is the evaluation and staging of lung cancer and of other masses external to the endobronchial wall. In lung cancer staging,

EBUS has been essential for mediastinal and hilar lymph node sampling and for evaluating mediastinal invasion by tumor. Suspicious mediastinal and hilar lymph nodes can be accurately biopsied via EBUS guided transbronchial needle aspiration (TBNA) with sensitivities recorded up to 90%. In fact, EBUS-TBNA is not different from mediastinoscopy in sensitivity, negative predictive value, and diagnostic accuracy of lymph node staging of non–small cell lung cancer.

EBUS-TBNA alone has been found to have a sensitivity of 0.93 (95% CI, 0.91–0.94) and a specificity of 1.00 (95% CI, 0.99–1.00) in diagnosing cancer spread to the lymph nodes. The sensitivity is increased when selecting for lymph nodes that are suspicious on CT or positron-emission tomography (PET) scan. Previous prospective studies have found no significant differences between mediastinoscopy and EBUS bronchoscopy in determining the true pathologic nodal stage. In another review study, mediastinoscopy would have changed the tumor stage and treatment planning in only 2 (2.7%) of 73 patients.

Besides facilitating biopsies, EBUS also can evaluate tumor depth, disclose the relationship of vessels to the surrounding structures, and precisely localize a lesion's borders prior to brachytherapy.

Benefits of EBUS include (1) avoidance of a surgical incision, (2) increased comfort for the patient, (3) enhanced ability for repeat sampling of lymph nodes, and (4) safety. In a meta-analysis of 11 studies with 1,299 patients, only two complications occurred with EBUS (0.15%, one case of pneumothorax requiring chest tube placement; one case of transient hypoxemia). In a study of 153 patients undergoing EBUS-TBNA of mediastinal lymph nodes, there were no major or minor complications seen with EBUS.

Limitations of EBUS-TBNA are its decreased yield when sampling lymph nodes under 5 mm and difficulty in accessing all of the lymph node zones in the chest. However, most small lymph nodes are typically benign. Furthermore, EBUS can typically sample more lymph node areas with less risk of complications than can mediastinoscopy.

EBUS is a safe, cost-effective, and accurate procedure for the work up and staging of lung cancer, as well as the characterization of lung lesions. Although the performance of EBUS bronchoscopy is not yet part of standard pulmonary fellowship training, its use is expanding and more programs are recognizing its importance.

NAVIGATIONAL BRONCHOSCOPY

The incidental detection of peripheral pulmonary lesions is on the rise, as CT imaging for lung cancer screening becomes more popular. Determining the etiology of asymptomatic peripheral lesions is often a challenge. They are frequently unreachable by conventional bronchoscopy, and the yield of transbronchial lung biopsy, even under fluoroscopy, has been poor. Historically, the diagnostic approach ranged from watchful waiting, with possible delays in the treatment of malignancy, to surgical resection, with relatively high associated morbidity. Although transthoracic needle aspiration biopsy (TTNA) is commonly used to sample solitary peripheral nodules, it is frequently unable to access them.

Navigational bronchoscopy is a form of bronchoscopy that uses a virtual, three-dimensional computerized map of the airways to guide the bronchoscope and biopsy tools to the exact location of a peripheral lesion. This "road map" of the airways is first constructed with specialized computer software that uses data from a recently completed CT scan of the chest. Once the airways are mapped out, the patient is brought back to the bronchoscopy suite and placed in an electromagnetic field. A conventional bronchoscope is then placed into the airways, with a modification that allows real-time images from the bronchoscope to be superimposed over the previously developed virtual map. A special catheter is inserted through the working channel of the bronchoscope. This small steerable catheter has a location sensor at its tip and its position is visualized in the electromagnetic field within the body. The catheter is then guided by hand through the small airways to the lesion based on directions made by the virtual map. Once the lesion is reached by the catheter, standard bronchoscopic tools inserted through the channel can sample the lesion.

Navigational bronchoscopy is improved even further when combined with radial probe endobronchial ultrasound (RP-EBUS). RP-EBUS uses a radial ultrasound probe that, when inserted through an extended guide sheath during navigational bronchoscopy, can confirm visually that the lesion has been reached. After the steerable catheter reaches the target on the road map, the RP-EBUS probe is inserted to the area to further confirm the presence and location of the lesion. The real-time images significantly improve the accuracy and yield of biopsies.

Navigational bronchoscopy is most helpful for localizing peripheral lesions in the distal airways. A "bronchus sign," a radiographically visualized airway leading to the target lesion, is a good indication that navigational bronchoscopy would be useful. Although CT-guided transthoracic biopsy has higher yields for peripheral lesions, navigational bronchoscopy has significantly less risk of pneumothorax.

A drawback of the computer generated "virtual map" is the lack of finely detailed information about the airway. However, the image data are becoming more comprehensive as technology improves. It is noteworthy that the imaging data are not captured in real time. It is taken from the prior CT scan images, so the bronchoscopist must assume that the images reflect the patient's current condition. Bronchoscopy performed under navigation also can be obscured by imaging artifact. These limitations, as well as the need for specialized training, somewhat hinder the widespread use of navigational bronchoscopy. Nevertheless, navigational bronchoscopy with the addition of RP-EBUS is a promising, low-risk tool for obtaining tissue from peripheral lung lesions.

FURTHER READING

1. Silvestri GA, Feller-Kopman D, Chen A, et al. Latest advances in advanced diagnostic and therapeutic pulmonary procedures. *Chest.* 2012;142(6):1636–1644.

   Good recent review article of advanced procedures.

2. Becker HD. *A Short History of Bronchoscopy.* New York, NY: Cambridge University Press; 2009.

3. Wang KP, Mehta AC. *Flexible Bronchoscopy.* Cambridge, MA: Blackwell Scientific; 1995.

   This text covers all the clinical aspects of flexible bronchoscopy.

4. Borchers SD, Beamis JF Jr. Flexible bronchoscopy. *Chest Surg Clin N Am.* 1996;6:169–192.

   References 2 to 38 are almost exclusively review articles.

5. Arroliga AC, Matthay RA. The role of bronchoscopy in lung cancer. *Clin Chest Med.* 1993;14:87–98.

6. Dasgupta A, Mehta AC. Transbronchial needle aspiration: an underused diagnostic technique. *Clin Chest Med.* 1999;20:39–51.

   This entire issue of Clinics in Chest Medicine is devoted to aspects of flexible bronchoscopy.

7. Sharafkhaneh A, Baaklini W, Gorin AB, et al. Yield of transbronchial needle aspiration in diagnosis of mediastinal lesions. *Chest.* 2003;124:2131–2135.

8. Ernst A, Eberhardt R, Wahidi M, et al. Effect of routine clopidogrel use on bleeding complications after transbronchial biopsy in humans. *Chest.* 2006;129:734–737.

9. Wahidi MM, Garland R, Feller-Kopman D, et al. Effect of clopidogrel with and without aspirin on bleeding following transbronchial lung biopsy. *Chest.* 2005;127(3):961–964.

10. Mares DC, Wilkes DS. Bronchoscopy in the diagnosis of respiratory infections. *Curr Opin Pulm Med.* 1998;4:123–129.

    A brief review.

11. Yasufuku K, Pierre A, Darling G, et al. A prospective controlled trial of endobronchial ultrasound-guided transbronchial needle aspiration compared with mediastinoscopy for mediastinal lymph node staging of lung cancer. *J Thorac Cardiovasc Surg.* 2011;142(6):1393.e1–1400.e1.

    Landmark trial comparing EBUS to mediastinoscopy for cancer staging.

12. Herth F, Becker HD. Endobronchial ultrasound. In: Simoff MJ, Sterman DH, Ernst A, eds. *Thoracic Endoscopy: Advances in Interventional Pulmonology.* Malden, MA: Blackwell Futura; 2006:33–43.

13. Yung RC, Lawler LP. Advances in diagnostic bronchoscopy: virtual bronchoscopy and advanced airway imaging. In: Simoff MJ, Sterman DH, Ernst A, eds. *Thoracic Endoscopy: Advances in Interventional Pulmonology.* Malden, MA: Blackwell Futura; 2006:44–75.

14. Annema JT, van Meerbeeck JP, Rintoul RC. Mediastinoscopy vs endosonography for mediastinal nodal staging of lung cancer: a randomized trial. *JAMA*. 2010;304(20):2245–2252.

15. Gu P, Zhao YZ, Jiang LY, et al. Endobronchial ultrasound-guided transbronchial needle aspiration for staging of lung cancer: a systematic review and meta-analysis. *Eur J Cancer*. 2009; 45(8):1389–1396.

16. Lee BE, Kletsman E, Rutledge JR, et al. Utility of endobronchial ultrasound-guided mediastinal lymph node biopsy in patients with non-small cell lung cancer. *J Thorac Cardiovasc Surg*. 2012; 143(3):585–590.

17. Kurimoto N, Murayama M, Yoshioka S, et al. Assessment of usefulness of endobronchial ultrasonography in determination of depth of tracheobronchial tumor invasion. *Chest*. 1999;115: 1500–1506.

18. Bülzebruck H, Bopp R, Drings P. New aspects in the staging of lung cancer: prospective validation of the International Union against Cancer TNM classification. *Cancer*. 1992;70(5):1102–1110.

19. Herth F, Becker HD, Ernst A. Conventional vs endobronchial ultrasound-guided transbronchial needle aspiration: a randomized trial. *Chest*. 2004;125(1):322–325.

20. Herth FJ, Becker HD, Ernst A. Ultrasound-guided transbronchial needle aspiration: an experience in 242 patients. *Chest*. 2003;123(2):604–607.

21. Shannon JJ, Bude RO, Orens JB, et al. Endobronchial ultrasound-guided needle aspiration of mediastinal adenopathy. *Am J Respir Crit Care Med*. 1996;153(4, pt 1):1424–1430.

22. Varela-Lema L, Fernandez-Villar A, Ruano-Ravina A. Effectiveness and safety of endobronchial ultrasound-transbronchial needle aspiration: a systemic review. *Eur Respir J*. 2009;33(5):1156–1164.

23. Wang Memoli JS, Nietert PJ, Silvestri GA. Meta-analysis of guided bronchoscopy for the evaluation of the pulmonary nodule. *Chest*. 2012;142(2):385–393.

    A good recent meta-analysis evaluating the utility of navigational bronchoscopy.

24. Gould MK, Fletcher J, Iannettoni MD, et al. Evaluation of patients with pulmonary nodules: when is it lung cancer? ACCP evidence-based clinical practice guidelines (2nd edition). *Chest*. 2007;132(3)(suppl):108S–130S.

25. Eberhardt R, Anantham D, Ernst A. Multimodality bronchoscopic diagnosis of peripheral lung lesions: a randomized controlled trial. *Am J Respir Crit Care Med*. 2007;176(1):36–41.

26. Ernst A, Silvestri GA, Johnstone D, et al. Interventional pulmonary procedures: guidelines from the American College of Chest Physicians. *Chest*. 2003;123:1693–1717.

27. Yasufuku K, Chiyo M, Sekine Y, et al. Real-time endobronchial ultrasound guided transbronchial needle aspiration of mediastinal and hilar lymph nodes. *Chest*. 2004;126:122–128.

28. Kurimoto N, Miyazawa T, Okimasa S. Endobronchial ultrasonography using a guide sheath increases the ability to diagnose peripheral pulmonary lesions endoscopically. *Chest*. 2004;126:959–965.

29. Lacasse Y, Martel S, Hebert A, et al. Accuracy of virtual bronchoscopy to detect endobronchial lesions. *Ann Thorac Surg*. 2004;77:1774–1780.

    A prospective evaluation of the sensitivity, specificity, positive predictive value, and negative predictive value, and a review of prior studies evaluating virtual bronchoscopy.

30. Seijo LM, de Torres JP, Lozano MD, et al. Diagnostic yield of electromagnetic navigation bronchoscopy is highly dependent on the presence of a Bronchus sign on CT imaging: results from a prospective study. *Chest*. 2010;138(6):1316–1321.

Preoperative Pulmonary Evaluation

Stephen H. Lee

Postoperative pulmonary complications (PPCs) are major contributors to increased hospitalization costs, morbidity, and mortality. The goal of preoperative pulmonary evaluation is to assess and identify individuals who are at increased risk for PPCs. This evaluation is accomplished by carefully reviewing the specific characteristics of the patient and the details of the operative procedure. Recently, sleep apnea has been focused on as an emerging risk factor for PPCs.

PPCs are variably defined in the literature and encompass outcomes such as pneumonia, atelectasis, bronchospasm, pneumothorax, pleural effusion, hypoxemia, prolonged mechanical ventilation, and need for reintubation. The reported incidence of PPCs varies widely, depending on the patient population, type of surgery, and criteria used to define a PPC. No one standard exists.

The most important operative risk factor for a PPC is the anatomic location of the procedure. Surgeries close to the diaphragm (i.e., thoracic and upper abdominal) are associated with a much higher risk of PPCs versus those further away from the diaphragm. Neurosurgical and orofacial operations are exceptions to this rule, in view of a higher risk for aspiration pneumonia and airway compromise. Chest and upper abdominal surgeries are associated with significant decreases in both vital capacity and functional residual capacity (FRC). FRC decreases by about 30% after upper abdominal surgery and by 35% after thoracotomy, compared to about 10% to 15% reduction for lower abdominal surgery. Postoperative diaphragmatic dysfunction may contribute significantly to restrictive pulmonary physiology. Maintaining an adequate FRC is important to prevent atelectasis and subsequent ventilation–perfusion mismatch. Other surgical factors associated with increased PPC risk are increased duration of surgery and complexity of the operation. PPCs are very uncommon in extremity surgery.

Data about the reduced risk of PPCs with laparoscopic versus open techniques in a variety of surgeries such as splenectomy, cholecystectomy, colectomy, and, recently, bariatric surgery continue to emerge. Compared to open approaches, laparoscopic procedures are associated with less impairment in postoperative lung function, possibly due to decreased postoperative pain. Interestingly, the decreased PPC risk with laparoscopic procedures appears to hold despite the fact that operative times are usually longer than for open approaches.

General anesthesia can lead to pulmonary complications by several mechanisms. Endotracheal intubation may be complicated by aspiration or bronchospasm. Anesthetic gases attenuate hypoxic vasoconstriction, impair mucociliary function and clearance of secretions, abolish the cough reflex and periodic sighs, and impair diaphragmatic function. The consequences are ventilation–perfusion mismatch, atelectasis, and decrease in FRC. There is some evidence that regional neuraxial (spinal, epidural) anesthesia results in fewer PPCs than general anesthesia. A systematic review of randomized trials showed that the odds of postoperative pneumonia are reduced by 39% with neuraxial blockade compared to general anesthesia. When comparing procedures using a combination of regional and general anesthesia versus general anesthesia alone, the odds of respiratory depression are reduced by 57% and pneumonia by 47%. Thus, regional anesthesia, with or without general anesthesia, appears to be associated with lower risk of PPCs.

The impact of increasing age on PPCs has been difficult to determine since aging is accompanied by additional comorbidities that impact the risk of PPCs and other postoperative complications. One large meta-analysis that included only studies using multivariate analyses reported that not only is age an independent risk factor for PPCs, but also that this risk increased with advancing age. This same analysis also showed that higher American Society of Anesthesiologists (ASA) class and level of functional dependence were associated with significantly increased PPC risk.

Chronic obstructive pulmonary disease (COPD) is a consistent risk factor for PPC. The incidence of PPC increases with the severity of underlying disease and likely results from perioperative changes in lung volumes, diaphragmatic function, and chest wall mechanics, as well as the effects of anesthesia. Acute exacerbations should be treated before any elective or nonemergent surgery. For those with chronic, stable COPD, lung function should be optimized as much as possible. The routine use of prophylactic antibiotics is not recommended. It may be necessary to delay surgery to achieve these goals. Those with active, symptomatic asthma are prone to more PPCs; therefore, like COPD exacerbations, uncontrolled asthma should be treated appropriately before surgery. If needed, a short course of preoperative corticosteroids does not appear to increase the incidence of postoperative complications. During induction of anesthesia, the use of thiobarbiturates and oxybarbiturates is associated with a much higher incidence of wheezing in asthmatics compared with nonasthmatics. Propofol does not appear to cause wheezing in either population. Well-controlled asthma does not appear to be a risk factor for PPCs.

Smoking, whether active or past, is an important risk factor for PPCs. Compared to never smokers, current smokers have greater odds of postoperative pneumonia, unplanned intubation, and prolonged mechanical ventilation. It also appears that the risk of these respiratory events increases with greater pack-year history. Former smokers also have increased risk of PPCs, but not as high as current smokers. Quitting should be a goal for any smoker, but the optimal timing of smoking cessation in relation to surgery to reduce PPCs remains unclear. Expert consensus generally recommends smoking cessation as early as possible and, whenever possible, at least 4 to 8 weeks before surgery.

Counterintuitively, obesity does not appear to increase the risk of PPCs when confounding variables are considered. Obstructive sleep apnea (OSA), however, a condition strongly associated with obesity and increasing age, is being recognized as a likely risk factor for PPCs. Patients with sleep apnea are predisposed to difficult to manage airways, postoperative hypoxemia, and upper airway collapse, the risk of which increases with medications with sedative and muscle relaxant properties that are used commonly in the postoperative period. Anesthesiologists should now be well aware of the perioperative risks for patients with sleep apnea. The ASA has established practice guidelines for the perioperative management of patients with OSA. Certainly, careful clinical monitoring is warranted in such patients, given the potential impact that pain, diaphragmatic and chest wall dysfunction, sedatives, and analgesics may have on upper and lower airway respiratory function during the postoperative period. For those with known sleep apnea already on positive pressure therapy preoperatively, it should be continued in the postoperative period. For those without a definitive preoperative diagnosis of sleep apnea, but who are strongly suspected of having OSA, empiric therapy with positive pressure should be considered in the postoperative period.

There is growing awareness of pulmonary hypertension (PH) as a potential risk factor for increased PPC (e.g., prolonged mechanical ventilation), but the data are relatively scant and complicated by the varied ways in which PH is diagnosed. Currently, the link of PH to increased risk of postoperative mortality is well established.

Preoperative evaluation should include a through history and physical examination. Although physical examination findings themselves do not appear to be significant predictors of PPCs, abnormalities may lead to further investigation that uncovers underlying conditions that are linked to higher PPC risk. In otherwise healthy patients, routine preoperative chest radiography to detect occult disease are not recommended since they rarely alter the choice of anesthetic technique or the surgical approach. For those with cardiopulmonary disease, a chest radiography before high-risk surgery may be helpful as a baseline against which postoperative imaging studies may be compared. Routine arterial blood gases (ABG) are also not recommended. Although several older case series identify $Paco_2$ higher than 45 mmHg as a significant risk factor for PPCs, a recent review of blinded trials did not find hypercarbia to be a significant risk factor in either univariate or multivariate analyses. Furthermore, hypercarbia is usually found in patients with severe underlying lung disease that can be suspected on clinical grounds and confirmed by pulmonary function testing.

Methodologic differences in studies about preoperative pulmonary function testing (PFT) make it difficult to draw firm conclusions about the value of these tests. Several reviews suggest that the information from the clinical evaluation (e.g., history, physical examination, functional/ASA class) is just as informative PFTs for purposes of preoperative evaluation. Nevertheless, in patients undergoing high-risk surgery, it may be reasonable to perform PFTs in those with a history of unexplained dyspnea, chronic lung disease, or significant smoking. In such patients, the PFT results may influence preoperative pulmonary care and other perioperative management strategies.

Several multivariate risk factor indices have been developed and validated to help clinicians stratify risk of different PPCs such as pneumonia and respiratory failure. Some of these indices, while comprehensive, are not practical in daily practice because of the number of variables included. Practical risk indices use variables that can be easily assessed and/or acquired preoperatively. Canet and coworkers have developed a simple-to-calculate predictive index for a composite PPC end-point that includes respiratory infection, respiratory failure, bronchospasm, atelectasis, pleural effusion, pneumothorax, and aspiration pneumonia. Gupta et al. and Arozullah et al. have published risk indices using only five and seven simple variables, respectively, that are specific for postoperative respiratory failure as defined by failure to extubate within 48 hours after surgery or unplanned reintubation.

The preoperative physiologic evaluation of patients undergoing lung resection surgery requires additional considerations. All patients should undergo evaluation to determine whether they can withstand the loss of resected lung tissue without significantly increasing morbidity or mortality risk. Candidates for lung resection surgery should undergo spirometry and testing for diffusion capacity in order to calculate the percent predicted postoperative (PPO) pulmonary reserve remaining after resection. The percent PPO FEV_1 may be calculated by using the following formula:

$$\frac{\text{Preoperative } FEV_1 \times (\text{No. of segments remaining after surgery/Total no. of segments})}{\text{Predicted } FEV_1}$$

There are a total of 19 bronchopulmonary segments: RUL (3), RML (2), RLL (5), LUL (5), and LLL (4). The percent PPO diffusing capacity is calculated in a similar fashion. Both the PPO FEV_1 and diffusing capacity may also be calculated based on the results of quantitative perfusion scanning. There are several published evidence-based guidelines for lung resection candidates. The American College of Chest Physicians recommends no further testing if both the percent PPO FEV_1 and diffusing capacity are greater than 60% predicted. If either value is between 30% and 60% predicted, simple exercise testing is recommended for further risk stratification. If either value is lesser than 30% predicted, formal cardiopulmonary exercise testing is recommended. These patients are at high risk for PPCs.

FURTHER READING

1. Ferguson MK. Preoperative assessment of pulmonary risk. *Chest*. 1999;115:58S–63S.

   A concise review of PPCs related to different types of surgeries with a particular focus on the pathophysiology underlying the increased risk.

2. Simonneau G, Vivien A, Sartene R, et al. Diaphragm dysfunction induced by upper abdominal surgery: role of postoperative pain. *Am Rev Respir Dis*. 1983;128:899–903.

   Small study showing marked diaphragmatic dysfunction after upper abdominal surgery resulting in restrictive physiology.

3. Winslow ER, Brunt ML. Perioperative outcomes of laparoscopic versus open splenectomy: a meta-analysis with an emphasis on complications. *Surgery*. 2003;134:647–655.

   Laparoscopic splenectomy is associated with a threefold decreased risk of PPCs compared with open splenectomy (3.1% vs 9.0%, respectively).

4. Hall JC, Tarala RA, Hall JL. A case-control study of postoperative pulmonary complications after laparoscopic and open cholecystectomy. *J Laparoendosc Surg*. 1996;6:87–92.

   Open cholecystectomy is associated with a 6.4 times higher risk of PPCs compared with laparoscopic cholecystectomy (17.2% vs 2.7%, respectively).

5. Weller WE, Rosati C. Comparing outcomes of laparoscopic versus open bariatric surgery. *Ann Surg.* 2008;248(1):10–15.

   Open gastric bypass is associated with an OR of 1.92 for PPCs versus laparoscopic gastric bypass.

6. Rodgers A, Walker N, Schug S, et al. Reduction of postoperative mortality and morbidity with epidural or spinal anaesthesia: results from overview of randomized trials. *BMJ.* 2000;321:1–12.

   The use of regional, neuraxial (spinal, epidural) anesthesia, with or without general anesthesia, is associated with decreased risk of postoperative pneumonia and respiratory depression.

7. Smetana GW, Lawrence VA, Cornell JE. Preoperative pulmonary risk stratification for noncardiothoracic surgery: systematic review for the American College of Physicians. *Ann Intern Med.* 2006;144:581–595.

8. Girish M, Trayner E Jr, Dammann O, et al. Symptom-limited stair climbing as a predictor of postoperative complications after high-risk surgery. *Chest.* 2001;120:1147–1151.

   In this prospective study of patients undergoing high-risk surgeries, the positive predictive values for a postoperative cardiopulmonary complication were 89%, 80%, 63%, 52%, and 32% for those unable to climb at least one, two, three, four, and five flights of stairs, respectively. Overall, pulmonary complications were nearly three times as common as cardiac complications (30% vs 11%, respectively).

9. Wong DH, Weber EC, Schell MJ, et al. Factors associated with postoperative pulmonary complications in patients with severe chronic obstructive pulmonary disease. *Anesth Analg.* 1995;80:276–284.

   In this retrospective review of patients with severe underlying COPD undergoing nonthoracic surgery, the odds of a PPC were 14 times higher for those in ASA class IV or higher compared with those in ASA class III or lower (multivariate analysis).

10. Kroenke K, Lawrence VA, Theroux JF, et al. Postoperative complications after thoracic and major abdominal surgery in patients with and without obstructive lung disease. *Chest.* 1993;104:1445–1451.

    The incidence of serious, postoperative pulmonary complications increased with increasing severity of the underlying COPD. For those with no, mild–moderate, and severe COPD, the incidence of severe PPCs was 4% versus 10% versus 23%, respectively.

11. Kabalin CS, Yarnold PR, Grammer LC. Low complication rate of corticosteroid-treated asthmatics undergoing surgical procedures. *Arch Intern Med.* 1995;155:1379–1384.

    Preoperative treatment with corticosteroids in asthmatics does not increase the risk of postoperative infection.

12. Pizov R, Brown RH, Weiss YS, et al. Wheezing during induction of general anesthesia in patients with and without asthma: a randomized, blinded trial. *Anesthesiology.* 1995;82:1111–1116.

    Wheezing during induction of anesthesia occurred in 45% versus 26% of asthmatics receiving thiobarbiturates and oxybarbiturates, respectively, compared with 16% versus 3% of nonasthmatics, respectively. There was no wheezing in either group when propofol was used as the induction agent.

13. Nagagawa M, Tanaka H, Tsukuma H, et al. Relationship between the duration of the preoperative smoke-free period and the incidence of postoperative pulmonary complications after pulmonary surgery. *Chest.* 2001;120:705–710.

    Among patients who quit smoking before surgery, the incidence of PPCs does not start to decline until the smoke-free period is at least 5 to 8 weeks, and reaches the incidence of never-smokers with 8 to 11 weeks of a smoke-free period.

14. Warner MA, Offord KP, Warner ME, et al. Role of preoperative cessation of smoking and other factors in postoperative pulmonary complications: a blinded prospective study of coronary artery bypass patients. *Mayo Clin Proc.* 1989;64:609–616.

    The PPC rate was four times greater for those who stopped smoking for 2 months or less compared with those who stopped for more than 2 months. With 6 months of smoking cessation, the PPC rate was similar to that of nonsmokers.

15. Turan A, Mascha EJ, Roberman D, et al. Smoking and perioperative outcomes. *Anesthesiology.* 2011;114(4):837–846.

    Current smokers have higher risk of postoperative pneumonia (OR 2.1), unplanned intubation (OR 1.9), and prolonged mechanical ventilation (OR 1.5) compared to never smokers.

16. Musallam KM, Rosendaal FR, Zaatari G, et al. Smoking and the risk of mortality and vascular and respiratory events in patients undergoing major surgery. *JAMA Surg.* 2013;148(8):755–762.

Compared to never smokers, current smokers and prior smokers have higher risk of postoperative respiratory events, with the risk of current smokers being higher than prior smokers.

17. Wong J, Lam DP, Abrishami A, et al. Short-term preoperative smoking cessation and postoperative complications: a systematic review and meta-analysis. *Can J Anaesth.* 2012;59(3):268–279.

Smoking cessation at least 4 weeks prior to surgery reduced postoperative respiratory complications.

18. Mills E, Eyawo O, Lockhart I, et al. Smoking cessation reduces postoperative complications: a systematic review and meta-analysis. *Am J Med.* 2011;124:144–154.

Smoking cessation prior to surgery is associated with reduced risk of PPCs.

19. Kaw R, Pasululeti V, Walker E, et al. Postoperative complications in patients with obstructive sleep apnea. *Chest.* 2012;141(2):436–441.

The risk of postoperative hypoxemia was higher in patients with OSA than without (OR 7.9). The risk for postoperative respiratory failure also appeared higher in patients with OSA than without (OR 4.3), but the statistical significance of this could not be computed because of inadequate sample size.

20. Kaw A, Chung F, Pasupuleti V, et al. Meta-analysis of the association between obstructive sleep apnoea and postoperative outcome. *Br J Anaesth.* 2012;109:897–906.

A meta-analysis of 13 studies showing that patients with OSA had higher odds for postoperative acute respiratory failure (OR 2.4) and desaturation (OR 2.8) compared to patients without OSA.

21. Practice guidelines for the perioperative management of patients with obstructive sleep apnea. *Anesthesiology.* 2006;104:1081–1093.

22. Lai HC, Lai HC, Wang KY, et al. Severe pulmonary hypertension complicates postoperative outcome of noncardiac surgery. *Br J Anaesth.* 2007;99(2):184–190.

This case-control study showed that those with echocardiogram-defined severe pulmonary hypertension had a higher rate of "delayed tracheal extubation" compared to controls, 21% versus 3%, respectively.

23. Gupta H, Gupta PK, Fang X, et al. Development and validation of a risk calculator predicting postoperative respiratory failure. *Chest.* 2011;140:1207–1215.

This risk calculator provides an exact risk estimate of postoperative respiratory failure based on five preoperative variables: type of surgery, ASA class, emergency case, functional status, and sepsis. The calculator can be accessed on-line at: http://surgicalriskcalculator.com/prf-risk.calculator. The on-line calculator also provides a link to download it as a mobile app.

24. Arozullah AH, Daley J, Henderson WG, et al. Multifactorial risk index for predicting postoperative respiratory failure in men after major noncardiac surgery. *Ann Surg.* 2000;232(3):242–253.

This index uses seven variables to stratify patients into five risk groups for postoperative respiratory failure (0.5%, 1.8%, 4.2%, 10.1%, 26.6%): type of surgery, emergency surgery, albumin, BUN, functional status, history of COPD, and age. While the derivation and validation samples were very large, women were not included in the study.

25. Canet J, Gallart L, Gomar C, et al. Prediction of postoperative pulmonary complications in a population-based surgical cohort. *Anesthesiology.* 2010;113:1338–1350.

Stratification for PPC risk into low (1.6%), intermediate (13.3%), and high (42.1%) risk groups are based on seven variables: age, preoperative SpO_2, respiratory infection in the last month, preoperative anemia, site of surgical incision, duration of surgery, and emergency procedure. Data were derived from close to 2,500 patients from a broad range of 59 Spanish hospitals.

26. Brunelli A, Kim AW, Berger KI, et al. Physiologic evaluation of the patient with lung cancer being considered for resectional surgery: diagnosis and management of lung cancer, 3rd ed: American College of Chest Physicians evidence-based clinical practice guidelines. *Chest.* 2013;143(5)(suppl):e166S–e190S.

An evidence-based guideline on the physiologic evaluation of lung resection candidates.

Pharmacotherapy

Jennifer M. Namba and Michael J. Freudiger

The many exciting advances in the pharmacotherapy of airway diseases and of pulmonary hypertension have resulted in marked improvements in quality of life, and at least in pulmonary hypertension, they have improved prognosis as well.

AIRWAY DISEASES

The pharmacotherapy of asthma and chronic obstructive pulmonary disease (COPD) includes similar medication classes. In both, drug selection, doses, and therapeutic combinations are adjusted according to a stepwise approach that is based on the severity of a patient's current symptoms. Important differences exist between the therapeutic strategies for the two diseases: for example, pharmacological therapy improves symptoms of COPD but not long-term morbidity and mortality.

Short-acting beta-2 agonists (SABAs) are bronchodilators that provide rapid symptomatic relief from acute bronchospasm and improve lung function for up to 6 hours. Inhaled SABAs (albuterol, levalbuterol, pirbuterol) delivered via metered dose inhalers (MDIs) or nebulizers are preferred over oral forms (isoproterenol, metaproterenol) because of their faster onset (5–15 minutes), their greater efficacy and tolerability, and their reduced potential for cardiac stimulation. Possible adverse reactions to SABAs include tremor, tachycardia, and electrolyte disturbances. Levalbuterol is the *R*-enantiomer of albuterol; it may cause less tachycardia than albuterol but is more expensive and typically is reserved for patients with significant risks for adverse effects from albuterol. The use of terbutaline is limited because of the greater incidence of tachycardia.

Ipratropium is a *short-acting anticholinergic* bronchodilator that is beneficial for patients with increased mucus gland secretions, acute asthma exacerbations, and COPD. It is similar to a SABA and has a rapid onset (15–20 minutes) and short duration (2–8 hours). Its anticholinergic properties warrant caution in patients with narrow-angle glaucoma or urinary obstructive disorders. Ipratropium is commonly given in combination with albuterol (DuoNeb®, Combivent® RESPIMAT®) to provide additive benefits, primarily in COPD. Combivent RESPIMAT® is safe in patients with soy and peanut allergies, but Combivent® MDI is contraindicated because of the soy lecithin used as a suspending agent.

Long-acting bronchodilators provide sustained control in patients with moderate to severe asthma or COPD symptoms. They are commonly used along with short-acting agents for symptomatic relief. *Long-acting beta-2 agonists* (LABAs), such as salmeterol, formoterol, and arformoterol, have a slower onset than SABA and a long (12–24 hour) duration. Indacaterol (75–300 mcg/day) is a very long-acting beta-2 agonist that lasts an entire day and is approved only for COPD.

Many authorities are against LABAs as monotherapy for asthma, without the addition of corticosteroids, because of an increased risk of asthma-related death. Tiotropium is a once-daily, *long-acting anticholinergic* bronchodilator approved for COPD. Tiotropium (18 mcg) inhaled daily has been shown to be more effective than salmeterol in preventing exacerbations in moderate to severe COPD. It also may be efficacious as supplemental therapy in poorly controlled asthma.

Inhaled corticosteroids (fluticasone, beclomethasone, budesonide, flunisolide, triamcinolone) reduce airway hyperresponsiveness and prevent long-term inflammation. The onset of improvement is 5 to 7 days, and further improvements may occur for several subsequent weeks. Patients should rinse their mouths with water following each inhalation in order to avoid oral thrush.

Inhalation is the preferred route because of the risk of adverse effects observed with *systemic corticosteroids* (prednisone, prednisolone, methylprednisolone, triamcinolone IM). The systemic agents are typically reserved for acute exacerbations, during which they are given in high-dose "burst" therapy, followed by tapering doses over 3 to 10 days. Side effects from short-term systemic corticosteroids include hyperglycemia, increased appetite, edema, weight gain, mood alterations, hypertension, and peptic ulcers. Long-term use may lead to adrenal axis suppression, dermal striae, diabetes, osteoporosis, and heart failure exacerbation. There is evidence of growth suppression in children that leads to minor reductions in adult height with the use of inhaled glucocorticoids.

Roflumilast (Daliresp®) is an oral *phosphodiesterase-4* (PDE-4) *inhibitor* with anti-inflammatory effects that inhibit lung infiltration by neutrophils and leukocytes. At a dose of 500 mcg PO daily, it improves lung function and reduces the risk of COPD exacerbations associated with chronic bronchitis. Roflumilast is contraindicated in moderate to severe liver impairment and in nursing mothers. Noteworthy adverse effects include weight loss, diarrhea, and neuropsychiatric effects that may contribute to suicidal ideations. It is metabolized via CYP3A4 and CYP1A2, so drug–drug interactions may occur with other inducers/inhibitors.

Methylxanthines, such as theophylline, inhibit phosphodiesterase and relax bronchial smooth muscle, reduce infiltration of eosinophils into the bronchial mucosa, increase diaphragm contractility, and improve mucociliary clearance for up to 24 hours. Theophylline is an alternative agent for asthma, but is not a preferred first-line therapy because of its narrow therapeutic index and lower efficacy for acute exacerbations. For COPD, theophylline is generally regarded as third-line therapy, after inhaled anticholinergics and beta-2 agonists. Peak drug levels should be drawn at steady state 2 to 4 hours after an oral dose or 1 hour after an IV dose, with a goal of 5 to 15 mcg/mL. Dose-related toxicities include tachycardia, nausea, vomiting, seizures, central nervous system stimulation, hyperglycemia, and hypokalemia. Adverse effects at therapeutic doses include insomnia, dysuria, and aggravation of gastroesophageal reflux disease and peptic ulcer disease from relaxation of the lower esophageal sphincter. Theophylline is a major substrate of CYP1A2, CYP2E1, and CYP3A4, which can cause numerous drug interactions.

Mast cell stabilizers (cromolyn) block the early and late reactions to allergens by stabilizing mast cell membranes and inhibiting the subsequent activation and release of inflammatory mediators from eosinophils and epithelial cells. They are indicated in mild persistent asthma. It is inhaled at a dose of 20 mg nebulized or 2 MDI puffs three to four times daily. Its advantages include its safety during pregnancy and the absence of known significant drug interactions. Therapeutic response is achieved within 2 weeks, and a maximal response occurs at 4 to 6 weeks. The most common adverse effects include cough, mouth/throat irritation, and unpleasant taste.

Leukotriene modifiers inhibit the leukotriene pathway that causes airway edema, smooth muscle contraction, and the inflammatory processes associated with allergen response in asthma. Leukotriene modifiers are divided into two classes: (1) leukotriene-receptor antagonists (zafirlukast and montelukast), which prevent leukotriene binding; and (2) leukotriene-receptor inhibitors (zileuton), which inhibit their synthesis. They are indicated in mild to moderate persistent asthma, and may be beneficial as supplemental therapy as alternatives to increased doses of inhaled corticosteroids. The benefits, however, are less pronounced in elderly populations. Montelukast is approved for adults at 10 mg PO once daily and children aged 1 year and older at 4 to 5 mg PO once daily, but it has been used in patients as young as 6 months. Zafirlukast is dosed 20 mg PO BID in adults and 10 mg PO BID for children aged 5 years and older. Zileuton is dosed 600 mg PO four times daily or 1,200 mg PO BID (ER formulation) for adults and children aged 12 years and older. They are all administered on an empty stomach in order to increase bioavailability. Liver function is typically monitored at baseline, monthly for 3 months, then every 2 to 3 months for one year. Headache and GI upset are the most common side effects, but mood alteration, aggression, agitation, hallucinations, depression, suicidal ideation, and tremor may occur. There have been reports of Churg–Strauss syndrome occurring when leukotriene modifiers are begun concurrent with rapid systemic corticosteroid tapering, although a cause–effect relationship has not been established definitively. The leukotriene modifiers are metabolized principally through CYP3A4, CYP2C9, and CYP1A2 (especially zileuton), which increases the risk of drug interactions with agents such as warfarin and theophylline.

Omalizumab is an *IgG1 monoclonal antibody* specific for IgE that prevents its binding to IgE receptors on mast cells and basophils. The resulting reduction in allergic response pathways is efficacious in patients prone to allergic asthma exacerbations, even those that are poorly controlled with high-dose corticosteroids and LABAs. Clinical responses, however, may take several weeks to occur. It is typically used only in patients who are at least 12 years old. The dose ranges from 150 to 375 mg subcutaneously every 2 to 4 weeks, depending on body weight and pretreatment IgE serum levels. Adverse reactions include pain and/or bruising at the injection site and upper respiratory tract infections. There is a small, but finite risk of hypersensitivity and anaphylactoid reactions, so administration and monitoring are typically performed in a physician's office.

Macrolides are a class of antibiotics that can have beneficial anti-inflammatory and immune modulatory effects in asthma, including decreased airway mucus secretions and reduced bacterial adhesion biofilms. Prophylactic therapy with macrolides may also play a role in reducing pneumonia-related exacerbations of COPD. In recent studies, azithromycin 250 mg daily or three times weekly for 1 year decreased the frequency of exacerbations in patients with COPD. While current guidelines do not recommend prophylactic antimicrobial therapy at this time, criteria for their use in preventing acute exacerbations have been proposed.

PULMONARY VASCULAR DISEASES

The pharmacologic treatment of pulmonary arterial hypertension includes supportive medications such as diuretics, anticoagulants, and digoxin, as well as therapy that is targeted toward the pulmonary vasculature itself ("advanced therapy"). This section only describes the latter group of agents. Their selection is based on clinical factors such as the severity of each patient's illness, as described in detail in Chapter 74.

Calcium channel blockers have been associated with prolonged survival, sustained functional and hemodynamic improvement only in patients who respond to acute vasoreactivity testing.[26] Calcium channel blockers should be titrated to the maximal tolerated dose (diltiazem 120–960 mg/day, nifedipine 30–240 mg/day, amlodipine 2.5–30 mg/day) with close monitoring of blood pressure, heart rate, and oxygen saturation. Verapamil is not typically used because of its more pronounced negative inotropic effects. Hypotension and peripheral edema are often reported at the doses required to alleviate pulmonary arterial hypertension symptoms, and ventilation–perfusion mismatching and decreased right ventricular function can also occur. Calcium channel blockers are not recommended in patients with significant right heart failure, hemodynamic instability, or portopulmonary hypertension and have no role in patients who do not respond to acute vasodilators.

Prostanoids have vasodilatory and antiproliferative effects, and improve hemodynamics and functional capacity in patients with pulmonary arterial hypertension. They are typically reserved for more seriously ill patients due to their complicated administration and side effects. Parenteral prostanoids (epoprostenol, treprostinil) require continuous infusion and adverse effects include headache, jaw pain, flushing, nausea, diarrhea, rash, arthralgias, hypotension, and injection site pain or infection. Inhaled prostanoids (iloprost, treprostinil) have fewer systemic and infusion-related side effects, but can cause cough, throat irritation, and may exacerbate underlying lung disease.

Epoprostenol (Flolan®, Veletri®) has the most evidence for improving survival and is considered first line in functional class IV patients (see Chapter 74). Epoprostenol administration is complex due to a half-life of only 3 to 5 minutes. Patients must manage a continuous infusion through a central venous catheter, prepare doses and back-up supplies daily, and maintain most formulations on ice. Initiation is done in a closely monitored setting with trained personnel. Dosing is started at 1 to 2 ng/kg/min and titrated to symptom control and adverse effects. There is no absolute maximum dose, but adverse effects are often dose-limiting. Recommendations for dose conversion between epoprostenol brands are not currently available.

Treprostinil (Remodulin®) can be administered intravenously, subcutaneously, or by inhalation for functional classes II, III, and IV patients (see Chapter 74). The advantages of treprostinil over epoprostenol include a longer half-life of 4 hours, the option of subcutaneous administration, and greater stability at room temperature. Parenteral doses are initiated at 1.25 ng/kg/min and titrated weekly. Infusion site pain is a common limitation of the subcutaneous route. Transition from epoprostenol can be initiated at 10% of the epoprostenol dose and titrated up in increments of 20% while the epoprostenol is titrated down.

Inhaled prostanoids may provide additional symptomatic and functional benefits in combination with other oral agents. *Inhaled iloprost* (Ventavis®) is initiated at 2.5 mcg and titrated up to a target dose of 5 mcg six to nine times per day. Each treatment requires about 10 minutes to administer. *Inhaled treprostinil* is initiated at three breaths (54 mcg) four times daily and titrated every 1 to 2 weeks to a target dose of nine breaths four times daily. Inhaled treprostinil offers advantages such as less frequent dosing, shorter treatment times, and once-daily dose preparation.

Endothelin-receptor antagonists are oral agents that improve hemodynamics, exercise capacity, and time to clinical worsening in group I pulmonary arterial hypertension, functional classes II, III, and possibly selected class IV patients (see Chapter 74). *Bosentan* (Tracleer®) is also approved for class IV patients. Endothelin-receptor antagonists are only available through limited distribution programs due to the risk of hepatotoxicity and teratogenicity. Endothelin-receptor antagonists are not recommended in moderate to severe hepatic impairment or with other medications that may cause liver impairment. Liver-associated enzymes must be monitored monthly during bosentan therapy, but routine monitoring is not required with *ambrisentan* (Letairis®). The FDA classifies endothelin-receptor antagonists as "pregnancy category X," in which the risks involved for pregnant women clearly outweigh the potential benefits. For this reason, women of child-bearing potential must use two forms of effective birth control and check monthly pregnancy tests while taking endothelin-receptor antagonists and for 1 month after therapy is discontinued. Other adverse effects include peripheral edema and anemia. Hemoglobin is monitored every 3 months with bosentan.

Bosentan is a non-selective ETA and ETB antagonist that is initiated at 62.5 mg twice daily for 4 weeks and titrated up to 125 mg twice daily. Ambrisentan is a selective ETA antagonist that is initiated at 5 mg and increased to 10 mg daily if tolerated. Use of either agent at the same time as potent CYP3A4 or 2C9 inhibitors (e.g., cyclosporine, ritonavir) or inducers (e.g., rifampin) should be avoided or done cautiously. Bosentan is also a CYP3A4 and 2C9 inducer, so closer monitoring of other CYP3A4 or 2C9 substrates (e.g., warfarin, sildenafil) may be warranted.

Phosphodiesterase-5 inhibitors (sildenafil, tadalafil) are oral agents that improve exercise capacity, hemodynamics, and delay clinical worsening in group 1 pulmonary arterial hypertension, functional classes II and III. Headache, flushing, nausea, diarrhea, dyspepsia, epistaxis, and nasal congestion are the most common side effects. Serious adverse effects include hypotension, loss of vision or hearing, priapism and vaso-occlusive crisis. Phosphodiesterase-5 inhibitors are contraindicated with nitrates because of the risk of severe hypotension and death. Combination with other antihypertensives, particularly alpha-blockers, should be initiated at the lowest dose and carefully monitored. Use with potent 3A4 inducers or inhibitors should be avoided or done with caution.

Sildenafil (Revatio®) is FDA approved at a dose of 20 mg orally three times daily, but has been studied in doses up to 240 mg/day. For patients who are temporarily unable to tolerate oral medications, sildenafil can be given in an intravenous dose of 10 mg three times daily. The use of sildenafil in children and adolescents is not recommended due to reports of increased mortality at higher doses. Tadalafil (Adcirca®) is dosed at 40 mg orally once per day, but reduced doses of 20 mg daily are recommended in the presence of hepatic or renal impairment.

FURTHER READING

1. *National Asthma Education and Prevention Program Guidelines (NAEPP): NAEPP Expert Panel Report 3*. Washington, DC: US Department of Health and Human Services; 2007. NIH publication 08–5846.

   The 2007 updated DHHS asthma guidelines with a new focus on monitoring control, assessment measures, patient education, and modified treatment strategies for asthma exacerbations, and the stepwise approach to long-term asthma management.

2. *The Global Strategy for Asthma Management and Prevention.* Vancouver, WA: Global Initiative for Asthma; 2012. http://www.ginasthma.org/.

   Includes an impact summary of 19 landmark papers from a literature search of 386 articles providing enough evidence for updates to the guidelines in 2012.

3. *The Global Strategy for the Diagnosis, Management and Prevention of COPD.* Vancouver, WA: Global Initiative for Chronic Obstructive Lung Disease; 2013. http://www.goldcopd.org/.

   Classifies COPD severity and management with updated pharmacotherapy options.

4. Qaseem A, Wilt TJ, Weinberger SE, et al. Diagnosis and management of stable chronic obstructive pulmonary disease: a clinical practice guideline update from the American College of Physicians, American College of Chest Physicians, American Thoracic Society, and European Respiratory Society (ACP/ACCP/ATS/ERS guidelines). *Ann Intern Med.* 2011;155:179–191.

   Includes seven major recommendation updates for the management of stable COPD.

5. Fanta CH. Asthma. *N Engl J Med.* 2009;360:1002.

   A review and comparison of available pharmacotherapy in the management of asthma.

6. Hubbard RC, Crystal RG. Alpha-1-antitrypsin augmentation therapy for alpha-1-antitrypsin deficiency. *Am J Med.* 1988;84:52.

   Characterizes alpha-1-antitrypsin deficiency and treatment options.

7. Ram FS, Sestini P. Regular inhaled short acting beta-2 agonists for the management of stable chronic obstructive pulmonary disease: Cochrane systematic review and meta-analysis. *Thorax.* 2003;58:580.

   A meta-analysis showing that inhaled short-acting beta-2 agonists used regularly for greater than 7 days in moderate to severe COPD improves post-bronchodilator lung function and decreases symptoms of breathlessness.

8. Bone R, Boyars M, Braun SR, et al. In chronic obstructive pulmonary disease, a combination of ipratropium and albuterol is more effective than either agent alone. An 85-day multicenter trial. COMBIVENT Inhalation Aerosol Study Group. *Chest.* 1994;105:1411.

   A multicenter, prospective, double-blind, parallel study showing the combination treatment of ipratropium and albuterol was more effective than either agent alone.

9. Jaeschke R, O'Bryne PM, Mejza F, et al. The safety of long-acting β-agonists among patients with asthma using inhaled corticosteroids. *Am J Respir Crit Care Med.* 2008;178(10):1009–1016.

   A systemic review demonstrating the addition of LABA to ICS therapy in asthma patients did not increase the risk of asthma-related hospitalizations or death.

10. Kerstjens HAM, Engel M, Dahl R, et al. Tiotropium in asthma poorly controlled with standard combination therapy. *N Engl J Med.* 2012;367:1198–1207.

    The addition of tiotropium significantly reduced the risk of worsening asthma and asthma exacerbations in patients poorly controlled on ICS and LABA.

11. Vogelmeier C, Hederer B, Glaab T, et al. Tiotropium versus salmeterol for the prevention of exacerbations of COPD. *N Engl J Med.* 2011;364:1093.

    A randomized, double-blind, double-dummy, parallel-group trial demonstrating tiotropium was more effective than salmeterol in preventing exacerbations in patients with moderate-to-very severe COPD.

12. Kelly HW, Sternberg AL, Lescher R, et al. Effect of inhaled glucocorticoids in childhood on adult height. *N Engl J Med.* 2012;367:904–912.

    The reductions in growth velocity in prepubertal children using inhaled glucocorticoids over 4 to 6 years impacted adult height but were not cumulative or progressive.

13. Giembycz MA, Field SK. Roflumilast: first phosphodiesterase 4 inhibitor approved for treatment of COPD. *Drug Des Devel Ther.* 2010;4:147–158.

    Roflumilast improves lung function either as monotherapy or in combination with long-acting bronchodilators in patients with more severe COPD, chronic bronchitis, recent exacerbations, or patients requiring frequent rescue inhalers.

14. Ram FS, Jones PW, Castro AA, et al. Oral theophylline for chronic obstructive pulmonary disease. *Cochrane Database Syst Rev.* 2002;(4):CD003902.

    Theophylline has a role in moderate to severe COPD by providing modest effect on FEV_1 and FVC and slightly improved arterial blood gas tensions.

15. Korenblat PE, Kemp JP, Scherger JE, et al. Effect of age on response to zafirlukast in patients with asthma in the Accolate Clinical Experience and Pharmacoepidemiology Trial (ACCEPT). *Ann Allergy Asthma Immunol.* 2000;84:217.

    A 4-week open-label trial of zafirlukast demonstrating that improvements in pulmonary function with less reliance on SABA rescue inhalers decreased with age, but improvements in symptom response were recorded in all age groups.

16. Hanania NA, Alpan O, Hamilos DL, et al. Omalizumab in severe allergic asthma inadequately controlled with standard therapy. *Ann Intern Med.* 2001;154(9):573–582.

    A 48-week prospective, double-blind, placebo-controlled trial showing patients with severe allergic asthma inadequately controlled with high dose ICS and LABA therapy may benefit from omalizumab.

17. Strunk RC, Bloomberg GR. Omalizumab for asthma. *N Engl J Med.* 2006;354:2689–2695.

    A pathophysiological review of allergen mediated asthma exacerbations with a case vignette outlining omalizumab's place in therapy.

18. Hatipoglu U, Rubinstein I. Low-dose, long-term macrolide therapy in asthma: an overview. *Clin Mol Allergy.* 2004;2:4.

    An overview of the immunomodulatory effects of macrolide antibiotics in addition to their anti-infective properties that impart additional benefits in asthma.

19. Hernando-Sastre V. Macrolide antibiotics in the treatment of asthma: an update. *Allergol Immunopathol (Madr).* 2010;38(2):92–98.

    Examines the role of Mycoplasma pneumoniae *and* Chlamydia pneumoniae *in patients with stable asthma, including the anti-inflammatory and immune modulatory effects of macrolide antibiotics. The authors express the need for more randomized clinical trials with larger study populations to assess if the extra benefits of macrolides are clinically relevant in asthma.*

20. Albert RK, Connett J, Bailey WC, et al. Azithromycin for prevention of exacerbations of COPD. *N Engl J Med.* 2011;365:689–698.

    Azithromycin 250 mg taken for 1 year in addition to usual treatment reduced acute exacerbations in patients at risk. Mild hearing impairment was seen in some patients. The authors noted patients are more likely to be colonized by macrolide-resistant organisms, but found no evidence. This increased the incidence of acute exacerbations. The possible increased risk of macrolide-resistant organisms in the community was not studied.

21. Wenzel RP, Fowler AA, Edmond MB. Antibiotic prevention of acute exacerbations of COPD. *N Engl J Med.* 2012;367:340–347.

    Reviews the current evidence for antibiotic prophylaxis in COPD and proposes criteria for selecting COPD patients eligible for long-term azithromycin prophylaxis. The patient in the case vignette is prescribed azithromycin 250 mg three times weekly for one year.

22. McLaughlin VV, Archer SL, Badesch DB, et al. ACCF/AHA 2009 expert consensus document on pulmonary hypertension: a report of the American College of Cardiology Foundation task force on expert consensus documents and the American Heart Association. *Circulation.* 2009;119:2250–2294.

    Comprehensive US guidelines on the diagnosis and management of pulmonary hypertension.

23. Barst RJ, Gibbs JS, Ghofrani HA, et al. Updated evidence-based treatment algorithm in pulmonary arterial hypertension. *J Am Coll Cardiol.* 2009;54:S78–S84.

    Review of medication therapy that proposes a treatment algorithm for PAH, including the strength of recommendation by WHO class.

24. Johnson SR, Mehta S, Granton JT. Anticoagulation in pulmonary arterial hypertension: a qualitative systematic review. *Eur Respir J.* 2006;28:999.

    Review of seven observational studies suggesting that warfarin may be effective for IPAH. Five studies demonstrated improved mortality with anticoagulation, whereas two did not.

25. Mathur PN, Powles P, Pugsley SO, et al. Effect of digoxin on right ventricular function in severe chronic airflow obstruction. *Ann Intern Med.* 1981;95:283.

    Selected hemodynamics improved with digoxin, but the study did not address other outcomes.

26. Sitbon O, Humbert M, Jais X, et al. Long-term response to calcium channel blockers in idiopathic pulmonary arterial hypertension. *Circulation.* 2005;111:3105–3111.

Seminal study responsible for the current guidelines for calcium channel blocker use in the treatment of pulmonary arterial hypertension.

27. Barst RJ, Rubin LJ, Long WA, et al. A comparison of continuous intravenous epoprostenol (prostacyclin) with conventional therapy for primary pulmonary hypertension: the primary pulmonary hypertension study group. *N Engl J Med.* 1996;334:296–302.
28. Badesch DB, Tapson VF, McGoon MD, et al. Continuous intravenous epoprostenol for pulmonary hypertension due to the scleroderma spectrum of disease: a randomized, controlled trial. *Ann Intern Med.* 2000;132:425–434.

References 27 and 28 are open-label, randomized trials showing that IV epoprostenol reduced symptoms and improved hemodynamics over 12 weeks. Improved survival was only seen in patients with IPAH and HPAH (reference 27).

29. Simonneau G, Barst RJ, Galie N, et al. Continuous subcutaneous infusion of treprostinil, a prostacyclin analogue, in patients with pulmonary arterial hypertension: a double-blind, randomized, placebo-controlled trial. *Am J Respir Crit Care Med.* 2002;165:800–804.
30. Hiremath J, Thanikachalam S, Parikh K, et al. Exercise improvement and plasma biomarker changes with intravenous treprostinil therapy for pulmonary arterial hypertension: a placebo-controlled trial. *J Heart Lung Transplant.* 2010;29:137–149.
31. Olschewski H, Simonneau G, Galiè N, et al. Inhaled iloprost for severe pulmonary hypertension. *N Engl J Med.* 2002;347:322.

References 29 to 31 showed that other prostacyclins can effectively decrease symptoms, improve exercise capacity and hemodynamics. Treprostinil and iloprost offer administration advantages vs epoprostenol and may be considered as alternatives for some patients.

32. McLaughlin VV, Benza RL, Rubin LJ, et al. Addition of inhaled treprostinil to oral therapy for pulmonary arterial hypertension: a randomized controlled clinical trial. *J Am Coll Cardiol.* 2010;55:1915–1922.

    Adding inhaled treprostinil was safe and effective for improving exercise capacity and quality of life in NYHA class III and IV patients symptomatic on bosentan or sildenafil alone.

33. Channick RN, Simonneau G, Sitbon O, et al. Effects of the dual endothelin-receptor antagonist bosentan in patients with pulmonary hypertension: a randomised placebo-controlled study. *Lancet.* 2001;358:1119.
34. Rubin LJ, Badesch DB, Barst RJ, et al. Bosentan therapy for pulmonary arterial hypertension. *N Engl J Med.* 2002;346:896.
35. Galie N, Rubin LJ, Hoepper MM, et al. Treatment of patients with mildly symptomatic pulmonary arterial hypertension with bosentan (EARLY study): a double-blind, randomised controlled trial. *Lancet.* 2008;371:2093–2100.

References 33 to 35 showed that bosentan improved exercise capacity, hemodynamics, functional class, and increased time to clinical worsening in PAH, NYHA classes II–IV.

36. Galiè N, Olschewski H, Oudiz RJ, et al. Ambrisentan for the treatment of pulmonary arterial hypertension: results of the ambrisentan in pulmonary arterial hypertension, randomized, double-blind, placebo-controlled, multicenter, efficacy (ARIES) study 1 and 2. *Circulation.* 2008;117:3010.

    Ambrisentan was safe and effective for improving exercise capacity. Significant liver enzyme elevation was not observed, which may suggest a better safety profile versus bosentan.

37. Galiè N, Ghofrani HA, Torbicki A, et al. Sildenafil citrate therapy for pulmonary arterial hypertension. *N Engl J Med.* 2005;353:2148–2157.
38. Galiè N, Brundage BH, Ghofrani HA, et al. Tadalafil therapy for pulmonary arterial hypertension. *Circulation.* 2009;119:2894–2903.

References 37 and 38 showed that sildenafil and tadalafil improve exercise capacity and hemodynamics in symptomatic PAH with minimal side effects (~50% of tadalafil patients were already on bosentan). Tadalafil also delayed time to clinical worsening.

10 Pulmonary Rehabilitation

Andrew L. Ries

Comprehensive pulmonary rehabilitation (PR) programs are well established as a means to enhance standard medical therapy, control and alleviate symptoms, optimize functional capacity, and reduce disability for patients with chronic lung diseases. The primary goal is to restore the patient to the highest possible level of independent function. This can be accomplished by helping patients to become (1) more knowledgeable about their disease, (2) more actively involved in their own healthcare, and (3) more independent in performing daily care activities. Consequently, patients do much better and become less dependent on family, friends, health professionals, and expensive medical resources.

The typical program includes multidisciplinary participation by physicians and allied health professionals such as nurses, respiratory and physical therapists, exercise specialists, psychologists, and others with a particular expertise. The program should be tailored to the needs of the individual patient. To be successful, it should address important emotional and psychosocial problems and optimize medical therapy to improve lung function. The goal of the rehabilitation program is to provide support for the patient, family, and primary care physician. Any patient with symptomatic chronic lung disease is a candidate for PR. The greatest experience with PR has been in patients with chronic obstructive pulmonary disease (COPD); however, patients with other chronic lung diseases are also appropriate candidates. PR has also been found to be a beneficial adjunct to surgical programs such as lung transplantation and lung-volume reduction surgery. In these settings, PR not only helps to better prepare patients for surgery and facilitate their recovery but also aids in selection by assisting both patients and staff to better understand and weigh the risks and potential benefits.

Appropriate patients for PR are those who recognize that their symptoms are caused by lung disease, perceive impairment or disability related to that disease, and are motivated to be active participants in their own care to improve their health status. Patients should be stabilized on standard medical therapy and evaluated carefully before entering a program so that appropriate and realistic goals can be set. Pulmonary function tests are used to characterize the lung disease and quantify its severity; however, patient selection should be based on symptoms and disability, not on arbitrary criteria based on lung function alone. Exercise testing helps to assess initial exercise tolerance, evaluate possible blood gas changes (e.g., exercise-induced hypoxemia), and plan a safe and appropriate training program.

The components of a comprehensive PR program include education, instruction in respiratory chest physiotherapy techniques, psychosocial support, and exercise training. Educating patients and significant others about lung disease and teaching them specific ways to deal with problems are essential. Educated patients are better able to cope with their disease, easier to deal with, and more likely to avoid unnecessary visits to physicians' offices, emergency departments, and hospitals. Patients should be taught appropriate chest and respiratory therapy techniques. Proper coughing and postural drainage techniques are important for all patients, especially those with excess mucus production. Techniques of pursed-lip and diaphragmatic breathing and relaxation training help to improve ventilatory efficiency and assist patients in gaining control over the frightening symptom of dyspnea. Patients with respiratory therapy equipment should be instructed in its proper use, care, and cleaning. Patients with significant hypoxemia should be evaluated for optimal methods of continuous oxygen therapy and instructed in its proper use because oxygen therapy has been shown to improve survival and to reduce morbidity for these patients. Lightweight portable oxygen systems should be emphasized for ambulatory patients.

Patients with chronic lung disease have significant psychosocial problems as they struggle to cope with symptoms that they often poorly understand. They become depressed, frightened, anxious, and dependent on others to care for their needs. Progressive breathlessness leads to a vicious fear–dyspnea cycle in which increasing dyspnea produces more fear and anxiety, which, in turn, leads to more dyspnea. In PR, these problems can be dealt with effectively by enthusiastic and supportive staff who can communicate with, understand, and motivate these patients. Important family members and friends should be included in program activities. Support groups and group therapy sessions are also effective. Patients with severe psychiatric disorders may benefit from individual counseling and psychotherapy. Psychotropic drugs should generally be reserved for patients with severe levels of psychological dysfunction.

Exercise training provides both physiologic and psychological benefits and is an ideal opportunity for patients to practice methods for controlling dyspnea. The exercise program should be safe and designed appropriately for each patient's interest, environment, and level of function. Walking programs are particularly useful and have the added benefit of encouraging patients to expand their social horizons. Other types of exercise (e.g., cycling, swimming) are also effective. Because many patients with chronic lung disease have limited exercise tolerance, emphasis during training should be placed on increasing *endurance*, the time of sustained activity. Exercise training of the upper extremities may be beneficial for the many pulmonary patients who report disabling dyspnea for daily care activities involving the arms (e.g., lifting, grooming) at work levels much lower than for the legs.

In recent years, increased attention has been drawn to peripheral muscle dysfunction in patients with chronic lung disease and the role of muscle fatigue as a limitation to exercise tolerance. This has stimulated new research initiatives in this area. Specific peripheral muscle strength and endurance training regimens have been developed and incorporated into PR programs. The potential role of respiratory muscle fatigue in pulmonary patients has led to attempts to train the ventilatory muscles. Although ventilatory muscles can be trained successfully, the role of this type of training in improving exercise performance has not been clearly established.

Exercise-induced hypoxemia occurs unpredictably in patients with COPD who may not be hypoxemic at rest. Hypoxemia is not a contraindication to exercise training. Patients with exercise-induced hypoxemia can be given convenient, lightweight portable systems for ambulatory oxygen so that exercise can be performed safely.

There is now a substantial body of evidence with well-designed trials that demonstrate the benefits of PR. As an effective, preventive healthcare intervention, PR has proved to be cost effective in decreasing both hospitalization days and the use of expensive medical resources. After rehabilitation, patients have an improved quality of life, reduced symptoms, increased exercise tolerance, more independence, increased ability to perform activities of daily living, and improvement in psychological function, with less anxiety and depression and increased feelings of hope, control, and self-esteem. Even after a short-term intervention, benefits typically last for at least 1 to 2 years.

FURTHER READING

1. Ries AL, Bauldoff GS, Carlin BW, et al. Pulmonary rehabilitation: joint ACCP/AACVPR evidence-based clinical practice guidelines. *Chest.* 2007;131(5 suppl):4S–42S.
2. Ries AL, Carlin BW, Carrieri-Kohlman V, et al; ACCP/AACVPR Pulmonary Rehabilitation Guidelines Panel. Pulmonary rehabilitation: joint ACCP/AACVPR evidence-based guidelines. *Chest.* 1997;112:1363 and *J Cardiopulm Rehab.* 1997;17:371.

References 1 and 2 are the most recent evidenced-based guidelines developed jointly by the American College of Chest Physicians and American Association of Cardiovascular and PR that review the available scientific evidence for PR. Recommendations are supported by evidence tables summarizing published clinical trials.

3. American Association of Cardiovascular and Pulmonary Rehabilitation. *Guidelines for Pulmonary Rehabilitation Programs.* 4th ed. Champaign, IL: Human Kinetics; 2011.
   Updated reference that provides recommended guidelines for practice.
4. American Thoracic Society, European Respiratory Society. ATS/ERS statement on pulmonary rehabilitation. *Am J Respir Crit Care Med.* 2006;173·1390.

Official statement of the American Thoracic Society (ATS) and European Respiratory Society (ERS) summarizing the benefits and describing the current practice of PR.

5. Qaseem A, Wilt TJ, Weinberger SE, et al. Diagnosis and management of stable chronic obstructive pulmonary disease: a clinical practice guideline update from the American College of Physicians, American College of Chest Physicians, American Thoracic Society, and European Respiratory Society. *Ann Intern Med.* 2011;155:179.

Official statement of the ACP, ACCP, ATS, and ERS providing standards for the management of patients with COPD. Includes recommendation for pulmonary rehabilitation for patients with symptomatic COPD.

6. Hodgkin JE, Celli BR, Connors GL. *Pulmonary Rehabilitation: Guidelines to Success.* 4th ed. St Louis, MO: Mosby Elsevier; 2009.

7. Fishman AP. *Pulmonary Rehabilitation.* New York, NY: Marcel Dekker; 1996.

References 6 and 7 are excellent comprehensive books that review all aspects of PR.

8. Birnbaum S. Pulmonary rehabilitation: a classic tune with a new beat, but is anyone listening? *Chest.* 2011;139:1498.

Summary of Medicare regulations implemented in 2010 in response to 2008 Congressional mandate for national coverage of PR in the US for patients with COPD.

9. Lacasse Y, Martin S, Lasserson TJ, et al. Meta-analysis of respiratory rehabilitation in chronic obstructive pulmonary disease: a Cochrane systematic review. *Eura Medicophys.* 2007;43:475.

Meta-analyses and Cochrane review of 31 randomized clinical trials that evaluated the effect of PR on quality of life and/or exercise capacity. Concluded that PR produced moderately large and clinically significant improvements in important aspects of quality of life and increase in exercise tolerance.

10. Puhan M, Scharplatz M, Troosters T, et al. Pulmonary rehabilitation following exacerbations of chronic obstructive pulmonary disease. *Cochrane Database Syst Rev.* 2009;(1):CD005305. doi:10.1002/14651858.

Cochrane review of six randomized controlled trials including 219 patients suggesting that PR reduces hospital admissions and mortality and improves quality of life in patients with COPD after an acute exacerbation.

11. Ries AL, Kaplan RM, Limberg TM, et al. Effects of pulmonary rehabilitation on physiologic and psychosocial outcomes in patients with chronic obstructive pulmonary disease. *Ann Intern Med.* 1995;122:823.

12. Ries AL, Kaplan RM, Myers R, et al. Maintenance after pulmonary rehabilitation in chronic lung disease: a randomized trial. *Am J Respir Crit Care Med.* 2003;167:880.

Two randomized clinical trials evaluating PR. Reference 11 demonstrates significant improvements after a short-term intervention that lasts 1 to 2 years. Reference 12 evaluates a postrehabilitation maintenance program and emphasizes the importance of looking at rehabilitation strategies as longer term interventions and an integral part of chronic disease management.

13. Griffiths TL, Phillips CJ, Davies S, et al. Cost effectiveness of an outpatient multidisciplinary pulmonary rehabilitation programme. *Thorax.* 2001;56:779.

Randomized controlled trial of 200 patients with COPD demonstrating that PR produces cost-effective benefits (cost per QALY).

14. O'Shea SD, Taylor NF, Paratz JD. Progressive resistance exercise improves muscle strength and may improve elements of performance of daily activities for people with COPD: a systematic review. *Chest.* 2009;136:1269.

Review of 18 controlled trials demonstrating moderate effects for increases in muscle strength from resistance training in patients with COPD. Resistance training is commonly included in PR programs and is thought to be important for performance of daily activities.

15. Costi S, Crisafulli E, Antoni FD, et al. Effects of unsupported upper extremity exercise training in patients with COPD: a randomized controlled trial. *Chest.* 2009;136:387.

Randomized trial that corroborates previous trials and confirms the benefits of upper extremity exercise training that is included commonly in PR and thought to be important for many activities of daily living involving the arms.

16. Salhi B, Troosters T, Behaegel M, et al. Effects of pulmonary rehabilitation in patients with restrictive lung diseases. *Chest.* 2010;137:273.

17. Varadi RG, Goldstein RS. Pulmonary rehabilitation for restrictive lung diseases. *Chest.* 2010; 137:247.

References 16 and 17 are a recent observational study and accompanying editorial that discuss the use of PR for patients with restrictive lung diseases. Improvements in symptoms, quality of life, and exercise tolerance were similar to those observed in patients with COPD.

18. Palmer SM, Tapson VF. Pulmonary rehabilitation in the surgical patient: lung transplantation and lung volume reduction surgery. *Respir Care Clin N Am.* 1998;4:71.

19. Ries AL. Pulmonary rehabilitation and lung volume reduction surgery. In: Fessler HE, Reilly JJ Jr, Sugarbaker DJ, eds. *Lung Volume Reduction Surgery for Emphysema.* New York, NY: Marcel Dekker; 2004:123.

20. Ries AL, Make BJ, Lee SM, et al. The effects of pulmonary rehabilitation in the National Emphysema Treatment Trial. *Chest.* 2005;128:3799.

References 18, 19, and 20 discuss the role of PR as an adjunct to surgical programs like lung transplantation and lung volume reduction surgery. Reference 14 demonstrates that PR administered through a large number of both university and community-based programs was effective in patients with severe emphysema.

21. Ries AL, Bullock PJ, Larsen CA, et al. *Shortness of Breath: A Guide to Better Living and Breathing.* 6th ed. St Louis, MO: Mosby; 2001.

    An excellent book for patient education.

22. Dudley DL, Glaser EM, Jorgenson BN, et al. Psychosocial concomitants to rehabilitation in chronic obstructive pulmonary disease: part 1, psychosocial and psychological considerations; part 2, psychosocial treatment; part 3, dealing with psychiatric disease (as distinguished from psychosocial or psychophysiologic problems). *Chest.* 1980;77:413, 544, 677.

    A comprehensive three-part review of the psychosocial problems of patients with COPD, including a review of the literature and recommendations for evaluation and treatment.

23. Casaburi R. Exercise training in chronic obstructive lung disease. In: Casaburi R, Petty TL, eds. *Principles and Practice of Pulmonary Rehabilitation.* Philadelphia, PA: WB Saunders; 1993.

    An excellent review of exercise training issues in patients with COPD. Includes a table summarizing literature review of 37 published studies with 933 patients.

24. California Pulmonary Rehabilitation Collaborative Group. Effects of pulmonary rehabilitation on dyspnea, quality of life and health care costs in California. *J Cardiopulm Rehabil.* 2004;24:52.

    Collaborative study of 647 patients in 10 centers in California that demonstrated significant improvements in dyspnea and quality of life with substantial reduction in health care utilization over 18 months of follow-up.

25. Ries AL, Farrow JT, Clausen JL. Pulmonary function tests cannot predict exercise-induced hypoxemia in chronic obstructive pulmonary disease. *Chest.* 1988;93:454.

    Reports on blood gas changes with exercise in 40 patients with COPD, indicating that exercise-induced hypoxemia is unpredictable from resting measurements of pulmonary spirometry and gas exchange.

26. Petty TL, Casaburi R. Recommendations of the Fifth Oxygen Consensus Conference. *Respir Care.* 2000;45:940.

    Discussion of use of long-term oxygen therapy for patients with chronic lung disease. Review of scientific rationale based on two classic randomized trials (Nocturnal Oxygen Therapy trial and British Medical Research Council studies).

11 Interventional Pulmonology Therapeutic Procedures

Andrew D. Lerner and Samir S. Makani

Advanced minimally invasive therapeutic procedures have a unique role in the management of airway obstruction and stenosis, as well as in asthma. Examples include tumor ablation and airway stenting techniques via rigid bronchoscopy, as well as bronchial thermoplasty. These procedures provide physicians with opportunities to make marked improvements in patients' quality of life.

RIGID BRONCHOSCOPY WITH ADVANCED THERAPEUTIC TECHNIQUES

Rigid bronchoscopy is especially suited to help manage diseases of the central airways. The rigid bronchoscope is a nonflexible metal tube. The lumen is sufficient to permit mechanical ventilation during general anesthesia and to visualize and pass instruments into the airways. It is especially useful for the management of large airway obstructions and for massive hemoptysis. Although rigid bronchoscopy is more invasive than flexible bronchoscopy and requires general anesthesia, the ability to control the airway and ventilate a patient during the procedure offer distinct advantages over fiberoptic bronchoscopy. The large lumen of the tube allows removal of large amounts of tissue and clotted blood. Its rigid distal edge can be used to "core out" lesions or, if manipulated properly, to dilate stenotic airways or to place airway stents. Flexible bronchoscopy can be performed through the lumen of a rigid bronchoscope; in fact, rigid bronchoscopy is rarely used without some flexible bronchoscopy.

Rigid bronchoscopy is essential in the treatment of large airway obstruction from benign or malignant causes. Benign airway stenosis is associated with a wide variety of disorders, including sarcoidosis, amyloidosis, broncholithiasis, relapsing polychondritis, Wegener's granulomatosis, lung transplantation, pill aspiration, and postintubation tracheal stenosis. Bronchoscopic techniques commonly used for these conditions include laser excision, dilatational therapy, and stent placement.

Malignant obstruction of the central airways is a common indication for rigid bronchoscopy. Malignant airway obstruction comes in three forms: (1) endobronchial tumor, (2) pure extrinsic tumors with external compression, or (3) a combination of the above. The therapeutic goal is usually palliation, since cure of malignancies at stages advanced enough to obstruct the central airways is rare. The therapeutic modality used with the rigid bronchoscope depends on the form of obstruction and the tumor type. Techniques used during rigid bronchoscopy to manage malignant airway obstruction include (1) endobronchial ablative techniques such as Nd:YAG laser therapy, argon plasma coagulation, electrocautery, and cryotherapy; (2) dilatational therapy using the rigid bronchoscope itself or inflated balloons; (3) airway stents; (4) brachytherapy; and (5) photodynamic therapy.

Endobronchial ablative therapies are used to destroy endobronchial lesions. The Nd:YAG laser is the most commonly used ablative techniques. It produces a variety of effects, including coagulation, carbonization, and vaporization of malignant tissue. Tissue penetration is approximately 6 mm. The most appropriate indications for Nd:YAG laser therapy are short endobronchial obstructing lesions with patent airways and functional lung distal to the obstruction. The best results are achieved in the large central airways (trachea, main bronchi, and bronchus intermedius). Airway patency can be established in approximately 80% to 90% of patients with obstructing lesions in those airways. Besides palliating a variety of symptoms, Nd:YAG laser therapy usually improves functional status. It should be emphasized that airway obstruction from purely *extrinsic* airway compression is a contraindication to all the endobronchial ablative methods, including Nd:YAG laser therapy. Major complications are rare (~1%) and include perforations (tracheobronchial wall, blood vessels), arrhythmia, myocardial infarction, air embolism, and death. Safety and training guidelines for laser therapy have been published.

Other endobronchial ablative techniques are relatively new in interventional pulmonology, including argon plasma coagulation, a form of electrocautery using argon gas. The advantage of argon plasma coagulation is the ability to treat lesions at right angles to the probe, which facilitates therapy directed at the upper lobes. Tissue penetration is generally limited to 3 mm, and complications are rare. A disadvantage of argon plasma coagulation is that it is time-consuming, making it unsuitable for debulking large tumors. Standard electrocautery can be used in most situations in which laser is used. Its main advantage is cost savings for the institution. However, electrocautery, especially in the presence of supplemental oxygen, carries the risk of developing endotracheal fire.

Cryotherapy uses cold temperatures to destroy tissue. It requires successive freezing cycles during the same treatment session. Unfortunately, the resulting depth of tissue destruction is hard to predict and cell death happens progressively over a 1- to 2-week period. This requires a second "clean-up" bronchoscopy after the initial treatment to remove necrotic debris. It is not suitable for emergency management of central airway obstruction. In addition to its application in tumor destruction, cryotherapy is also useful for the removal of foreign bodies, large mucus plugs, and blood clots.

Dilatational therapy for benign airway stenosis is performed with either the rigid bronchoscope itself or with a variety of angioplasty and valvuloplasty balloons. Sequentially larger diameter scopes or balloons are introduced into the airways for progressive dilatation. The risk of a tracheobronchial tear is minimized with an experienced and cautious operator. For this reason, several treatment sessions may be necessary to achieve the desired airway diameter.

Endobronchial stents are invaluable tools to help maintain airway patency. Indications include (1) extrinsic large airway compression from benign or malignant causes; (2) preparation for subsequent therapy in patients with malignancy (e.g., radiation therapy after tumor debulking by laser); (3) benign airway obstruction, such as tracheobronchomalacia; and (4) tracheoesophageal fistulas. A variety of different silicone stents are available. These include Silastic™ stents, nitinol metal stents, and hybrid stents. Important features of Silastic™ stents include external studs that impede migration and smooth edges. Placement and removal of Silastic™ stents requires rigid bronchoscopy. Metal stents can be placed under bronchoscopic or fluoroscopic guidance and may not require rigid bronchoscopy.

Possible stent complications include migration, the development of granulation tissue at the stent margins, and impacted secretions. Stent migration in the subglottic space is a particularly difficult problem that can be prevented by a percutaneous suturing technique or Y stent placement. Metal stents carry unique complications including stent fracture and difficulty with removal secondary to epithelialization through the metal mesh surfaces. Consequently, the FDA has issued a black box warning against the use of pure metal stents in benign disease.

Brachytherapy (endoluminal radiotherapy) is an additional treatment option for malignant airway lesions. The procedure is used mainly for palliation, although cure is possible for certain lesions (e.g., carcinoma in situ).

BRONCHIAL THERMOPLASTY

Bronchial thermoplasty is a relatively new therapy approved by the FDA in 2010 for patients with severe asthma. It is a bronchoscopic procedure that uses a special radiofrequency catheter to apply controlled thermal energy to the smooth muscle of the airways. Airway smooth muscle is felt to play a key role in the bronchoconstriction during asthma attacks as well as in the remodeling and narrowing of the airways from chronic inflammation. Smooth muscle destruction with thermal energy leads to its replacement with connective tissue that has less capacity for bronchoconstriction and continued remodeling. In theory, this mechanism of bronchial thermoplasty reduces symptoms in patients with severe asthma.

Bronchial thermoplasty is considered a viable option in patients with severe asthma that is not controlled with inhaled corticosteroids and long-acting beta agonists. A complete treatment course requires three sequential bronchoscopic procedures performed 3 weeks apart from each other: one procedure for each lower lobe individually, and one procedure for the two upper lobes together. A special "Alair" radiofrequency catheter delivers a series of 10-second heated bursts of thermal energy to the lining of the lungs.

Two multicenter randomized controlled trials (AIR and RISA) have reported improved quality of life and improved asthma symptoms with bronchial thermoplasty, when compared to patients on standard pharmacologic therapy. However, both trials were limited by the possibility of placebo effects from the procedures themselves. In a large multinational, randomized, prospective, double-blinded, sham-controlled trial (AIR II) of 288 patients comparing bronchial thermoplasty with a sham bronchoscopic procedure, there were significantly fewer emergency room visits, severe exacerbations, and days missed from school or work in those who underwent bronchial thermoplasty. The benefits persisted for at least 2 years. However, none of the studies have shown any significant effect on FEV_1, peak flow, rescue medication use, or airway hyperresponsiveness.

Bronchial thermoplasty appears to be a relatively safe and well-tolerated procedure. Adverse events typically include transient increases in respiratory symptoms (cough, wheezing, and chest discomfort) due to a brief increases in airway inflammation following the procedure. Most symptoms are mild to moderate and require only temporary increases in asthma inhaler therapy. A small proportion of patients may require temporary hospitalization. Symptoms generally resolve within 1 week. In the AIR II trial, there were no severe adverse events attributed to bronchial thermoplasty and no late occurring adverse events up to 5 years on follow up.

With the currently available information, the role of bronchial thermoplasty is still unclear in the management of asthma. Additional studies are needed to define the exact patient population who would benefit from this innovative form of therapy.

FURTHER READING

1. Silvestri GA, Feller-Kopman D, Chen A, et al. Latest advances in advanced diagnostic and therapeutic pulmonary procedures. *Chest*. 2012;142(6):1636–1644.

   Good recent review article of advanced procedures.

2. Becker HD. *A Short History of Bronchoscopy*. Cambridge: Cambridge University Press; 2009.

3. Wang KP, Mehta AC. *Flexible Bronchoscopy*. Cambridge: Blackwell Scientific; 2012.

   This text covers all the clinical aspects of flexible bronchoscopy.

4. Borchers SD, Beamis JF Jr. Flexible bronchoscopy. *Chest Surg Clin N Am*. 1996;6:169.

   References 2 to 38 are almost exclusively review articles.

5. Arroliga AC, Matthay RA. The role of bronchoscopy in lung cancer. *Clin Chest Med*. 1993;14:87.

6. Ernst A, Silvestri GA, Johnstone D, et al. Interventional pulmonary procedures: guidelines from the American College of Chest Physicians. *Chest*. 2003;123:1693–1717.

7. Wain JC. Rigid bronchoscopy: the value of a venerable procedure. *Chest Surg Clin N Am*. 2001;11:735–748.

   A concise review.

8. Duhamel DR, Harrell JH II. Laser bronchoscopy. *Chest Surg Clin N Am*. 2001;11:769–789.

   A concise review.

9. Ciccone AM, De Giacomo T, Venuta F. Operative and non-operative treatment of benign subglottic laryngotracheal stenosis. *Eur J Cardiothorac Surg*. 2004;26:818–922.

   A comparison of surgical and nonsurgical therapies for subglottic stenosis with a discussion of complications.

10. Wood DE. Airway stenting. *Chest Surg Clin N Am*. 2001;11:841–860.

    A general review of airway stents.

11. Unger M. Endobronchial therapy of neoplasms. *Chest Surg Clin N Am.* 2003;13:129–147.
    Review of interventional techniques in the management of endobronchial neoplasms.
12. Dweik RA, Stoller JK. Role of bronchoscopy in massive hemoptysis. *Clin Chest Med.* 1999;20:89.
13. Swanson KL, Edell ES. Tracheobronchial foreign bodies. *Chest Surg Clin N Am.* 2001;11:861–872.
14. Yasufuku K, Chiyo M, Sekine Y, et al. Real-time endobronchial ultrasound guided transbronchial needle aspiration of mediastinal and hilar lymph nodes. *Chest.* 2004;126:122–128.
15. Makani S, Simoff MJ. Bronchial thermoplasty. In: Wang K-P, Mehta AC, Turner JC, eds. *Flexible Bronchoscopy.* 3rd ed. Oxford: Blackwell; 2012.
    Excellent comprehensive review article on bronchial thermoplasty.
16. Wahidi MM, Kraft M. Bronchial thermoplasty for severe asthma. *Am J Respir Crit Care Med.* 2012;185(7):709–714.
17. Castro M, Rubin AS, Laviolette M, et al. Effectiveness and safety of bronchial thermoplasty in the treatment of severe asthma: a multicenter, randomized, double-blind, sham-controlled clinical trial. *Am J Respir Crit Care Med.* 2010;181(2):116–124.
    AIR II trial.
18. Cox G, Thomson N, Rubin A, et al. Asthma control during the year after bronchial thermoplasty. *N Engl J Med.* 2007;356:1327–1337.
    AIR trial study group.
19. Pavord I, Cox G, Thomson N, et al. Safety and efficacy of bronchial thermoplasty in symptomatic, severe asthma. *Am J Respir Crit Care Med.* 2007;176:1185–1191.
    RISA trial study group.

Pulmonary Therapeutics

Garner G. Faulkner and Deneen A. LeBlanc

Pulmonary therapeutics encompass a wide range of treatment options ranging from oxygen therapy to advanced airway management. This chapter describes the modalities and devices that deliver oxygen, enhance airway humidity, provide bronchial hygiene, and expand the lung.

OXYGEN DELIVERY

Supplemental oxygen to maintain oxygen saturation above a safe threshold is frequently necessary in patients with pulmonary disease. The initial step in determining an appropriate oxygen delivery method is to assess whether a low-flow or a high-flow system is required to maintain saturation. Low-flow oxygen systems supply 100% oxygen from either a 50-psi outlet or a cylinder tank and deliver gas flow at rates substantially less than the patient's peak inspiratory flow rate. As the patient inhales, inspiratory flow mixes ambient air with the low flow of supplemental oxygen, thereby increasing the fraction of inspired oxygen (FIO_2) delivered to the airway and the alveoli, but the actual partial pressure delivered to the alveoli is determined by the alveolar gas equation ($PaO_2 \approx FIO_2(P_{atm} - PH_2O) - PaCO_2/RQ$). The resulting FIO_2 is somewhat variable, depending on the proportion of the inspired flow that comes from the fixed, low flow of supplemental oxygen versus the remainder of the flow that comes from ambient air. If the supplemental oxygen flows are lower, more ambient air is entrained, the supplemental oxygen is diluted, and the FIO_2 is relatively small. At higher flows, less air tends to be entrained and the FIO_2 is higher.

TABLE 12-1	Approximate NC F_{IO_2}, Delivery Conversion
Nasal Cannula Liter Flow	Delivered F_{IO_2}% (Approximation)
1	24
2	28
3	32
4	36
5	40
6	44

Low-flow delivery devices include (1) nasal cannulas, (2) simple masks, (3) non-rebreather masks, and (4) reservoir cannulas. Nasal cannulas are simple nasal prong devices that typically allow flows from 1 to 6 liters per minute (Lpm), although some varieties allow 6 to 15 Lpm. Pediatric nasal cannulas support flow rates less than 1 Lpm. Nasal cannulas typically increase the F_{IO_2} by about 4% for every Lpm of supplemental oxygen, although precise F_{IO_2} also depends on the patient's own inspiratory flow rate (Table 12-1).

Reservoir cannulas are nasal prong devices similar to standard nasal cannulas but with an additional oxygen reservoir designed to store and conserve gas. There are two common varieties, the *pendant* and *mustache*. The reservoirs on both devices store 100% oxygen, but the mustache stores 18 to 20 mL, while the pendant holds nearly 40 mL. They also differ in the placement of the reservoir along the cannula. The mustache reservoir (e.g., *Oxymizer*) extends from the nasal prong region of the device and sits directly on the patient's upper lip. Some patients may be reluctant to use them, however, because of their cosmetic appearance and their heaviness on the face. Some patients prefer the pendant reservoir, which hangs from the cannula tubing at chest level. It can be concealed more easily and lies lighter on the face. Both devices contain an internal diaphragm within the reservoir housing that regulates the flow of gas and air-entrainment during inspiration. They provide the patient with a higher F_{IO_2} than what would be delivered at the same flow rate with a standard nasal cannula. This feature conserves gas, which could be important for long-term (home) users. The reservoir cannulas, however, require the patient to generate adequate inspiratory pressures to open their internal diaphragms. They are ideal for patients with higher-than-normal oxygen requirements such as those with pulmonary fibrosis and pulmonary hypertension, provided they can generate adequate inspiratory pressures.

Simple masks are conical plastic face masks that cover the nose and mouth. Similar to nasal cannula, they work by mixing a low flow of supplemental (100%) oxygen with inspired ambient air. They can raise the F_{IO_2} to approximately 35% to 50%, using oxygen flow rates of 5 to 10 Lpm. Open ports on both sides of the mask allow the inflow of ambient air during inhalation and the release of expired gas during exhalation. Because of the volume between the mask and the face, supplemental oxygen flows greater than or equal to 5 Lpm are needed to prevent the build-up of expired carbon dioxide within the mask itself. This property can be problematic if the oxygen flow rate is erroneously titrated below the threshold of 5 Lpm as a patient's oxygenation improves. If the oxygen requirement falls below 35%, the simple face mask should be discontinued and a nasal cannula should be used to deliver the lower F_{IO_2}. For this reason, simple face masks are often used as short-term devices, in areas such as postoperative recovery units.

A non-rebreather mask is a face mask with a construction similar to that of a *simple mask* with the addition of an oxygen reservoir bag attached to the base of the mask. The reservoir bag holds a supply of 100% oxygen, which is separated from the mask by a one-way valve. As the patient inhales, the one-way valve opens, allowing oxygen from the bag to flow into the mask. During exhalation, the valve closes and prevents expired carbon dioxide from contaminating the oxygen reserve. Additionally, the mask contains side ports, one of which is covered with a one-way valve that operates in a different manner from the reservoir valve. The side valve closes during inspiration to minimize air entrainment and dilution of inhaled oxygen, and opens on exhalation to release exhaled gas from the mask. It is often assumed that a non-rebreather mask provides 100% F_{IO_2}, but this is false. The delivery range for the mask is typically 60% to 80%; the precise amount depends on the integrity of the seal achieved between the patient's face and mask borders as well as the patient's inspiratory flow. In addition to delivering *relatively* high F_{IO_2} to hypoxemic patients, non-rebreather masks are commonly used to treat small pneumothoraces by washing out nitrogen (see Chapter 27) and to deliver helium–oxygen (Heliox) therapy to treat airway obstruction (see Chapter 33).

High-flow oxygen devices deliver gas at flow rates that approximate the patient's peak inspiratory flow, so less ambient air is haphazardly entrained from around the mask or cannula. This feature allows them to control the entrainment of air and the resulting oxygen-to-air ratio. They deliver a more constant and predictable F_{IO_2} to the patient than do low-flow devices. Depending on the specific device used, the resulting F_{IO_2} delivery may range from 21% to 100%. High-flow delivery devices include (1) air-entrainment masks; (2) large volume entrainment nebulizers; and (3) humidified, heated high-flow nasal cannulas. Although they all use some degree of high-flow oxygen, they have very different properties and clinical uses.

An air-entrainment mask (e.g., *VentiMask*) is typically cone-shaped and is similar to a simple mask, but with the addition of a jet nozzle adapter that creates a Venturi effect to mix the supplemental oxygen with ambient air. The Venturi effect is the reduction in pressure that occurs at a site where the high-flow oxygen travels through a constricted section of the tubing. At that site, specific-sized air-entrainment ports allow the system to regulate the air-to-oxygen dilution ratio precisely. Each mask is packaged with various-sized jet nozzles that are color-coded to correspond to a specific F_{IO_2}. *VentiMasks* deliver 24% to 50% F_{IO_2} at flow rates that approximate the patient's peak inspiratory flow. They are most often used when patients require consistent delivery of low to moderate F_{IO_2} levels, for example, COPD patients at risk for carbon dioxide retention. The *VentiMask* can be modified for tracheostomy patients who require supplemental oxygen during transport.

A large volume entrainment nebulizer operates under the same principle as the *VentiMask*, but it also supplies moisture to the airways. The system consists of a self-contained Venturi device with an adjustable air-entrainment port, as well as a capillary tube that feeds sterile water into the system. A nebulizer aerosolizes the water and the system delivers it along with the entrained air–oxygen mixture to the patient. Large volume entrainment nebulizers can work with aerosol facemasks or tracheostomy masks. They come in a variety of styles and F_{IO_2} delivery ranges, typically between 28% and 100% F_{IO_2}. They are excellent for patients with high oxygen requirements or tracheostomy patients who need supplemental airway hydration.

A humidified heated high-flow nasal cannula (e.g., *Comfortflow*™, *Optiflow*™) is a relatively new technology that consists of a very high-flow nasal cannula, a servo-controlled humidifier, and a heated wire circuit. The combination of features delivers extraordinarily high air flows (20–50 Lpm) that enter the respiratory system at body temperature, fully saturated with water. Humidification and heating allow delivery of much higher flows than would be tolerable otherwise. Colder, drier air would rapidly evaporate the moisture from airway membranes, which would be painful, retard mucocilliary airway clearance, and lead to tracheobronchial obstruction. The unique properties of humidified heated high-flow nasal cannula systems differentiate them from the "high-flow" devices described above. One notable difference is that the 20- to 50-Lpm flow is typically very close to the patient's actual peak inspiratory flow. For that reason, nearly all of the patient's breath is from the system itself, with virtually no haphazard entrainment of ambient air. The system connects to a high-pressure gas source that delivers oxygen along with an air blender, the combination of which can deliver a precise F_{IO_2} in the range of 21% to 100%. Humidified heated high-flow nasal cannula systems are most often used for patients with high peak inspiratory demand, high F_{IO_2} requirements, or those who cannot tolerate facemask devices. It also serves as an excellent transition device for patients liberated from noninvasive mechanical ventilation but still demanding high inspiratory flow delivery. The very high flows also flush air from some of the anatomical dead space and supply small amounts of airway positive-end expiratory pressure (PEEP), although the clinical significance of those actions is uncertain.

HUMIDIFICATION

Humidification adds water vapor to gas, and may play an important role in the delivery of oxygen and other medical gases. Moisturization of otherwise dry inhaled gases helps to maintain the integrity of mucus membranes and normal mucociliary airway clearance. Dry mucus membranes with impaired ciliary action can lead to retained secretions and the potential for airway obstruction by thick mucus plugs. In general, flows in excess of 4 Lpm should be humidified. It is especially important that gas delivered through an artificial airway such as an endotracheal tube be properly humidified since that method bypasses the upper airway (the primary physiological mechanism for moistening and heating inspired air). Three common devices to humidify inspired oxygen and other medical gases are (1) bubblers, (2) passovers, and heat-moisture exchangers.

A bubbler is a simple unheated device that consists of a capillary tube extending into a water reservoir. Gas passes through the capillary tube into the water and then bubbles to the surface. The bubbles have a relatively high surface area, which allows the water to moisturize the gas as it ascends to the surface. However, since the water vapor capacity of air is dependent on temperature, the unheated air has a limited potential to be humidified. As the patient's respiratory system heats the room-temperature gas to body temperature, the water carrying capacity increases. The warming air evaporates water from the airways, which may dry the mucous membranes.

A passover device directs the gas source over a container of water before delivering it to the patient. As the gas passes over the water surface, water vapor is pulled into the gas current. The passover systems may also provide heat as the air passes over the water, which increase the water content of the air. If the flowing air remains heated at approximately body temperature until it reaches the patient, the inspired gas will be fully saturated with water as it traverses the airways and will not dry them out. Heated passovers are commonly used in conjunction with invasive and noninvasive ventilator circuits as well as humidified, heated high-flow nasal cannula systems.

A heat moisture exchanger (HME) captures the patient's expired breath and uses its temperature and moisture to heat and humidify inspired gas. As the patient exhales, a membrane in the HME captures the expired heat and water vapor, which are then added to the next inspiratory breath. Referred to as an "artificial nose," the HME is designed to mimic the action of the nasal membranes and turbinates. They are most often used with nonheated ventilator circuits that are employed for short periods of time (e.g., postoperative mechanical ventilation and ventilator transports).

BRONCHIAL HYGIENE

Bronchial hygiene therapy, also known as secretion clearance, embodies a variety of noninvasive techniques that help mobilize and remove secretions to improve gas exchange. In the past, handclapping, postural drainage, and directed coughing were the only modalities available. These techniques had many drawbacks, and have been largely replaced with newer, more efficacious modalities such as: (1) percussion; (2) mechanical insufflation and exsufflation; (3) airway oscillation; (4) high-frequency airway oscillation; and (5) high-frequency chest wall oscillation.

Percussion is performed with handheld electrical or pneumatic devices that generate vibrational and percussive energy waves. The device interface is placed over specific regions on the patient's chest wall that correspond to lung segments and lobes. The vibration and percussion loosens secretions, liquefies them, and moves them into the larger airways. The concurrent use of percussion, postural drainage (the use of positioning and gravity to drain segmental areas of the lung), and directed coughing/breathing techniques is especially efficacious. An example of a percussor device is the G5 Percussor™. The small size and portability of these devices make them ideal therapeutic choices to target specific lung segments. Unfortunately, the external pressure that must be applied to the chest wall during therapy can be very uncomfortable to the patient (and the respiratory care practitioner administering it).

Mechanical insufflation and exsufflation devices (e.g., The *CoughAssist Mechanical Insufflation/Exsufflation*™) simulate coughing by mechanically applying positive and then negative pressures during a breath cycle. Positive pressure (20 to 50 cm H_2O) is gradually applied to the airway via a face mask, mouthpiece, or tracheostomy adapter during a 2- to 3-second inhalation.

Negative pressure is then applied for 2 to 3 seconds of exhalation. The rapid change from positive to negative pressure creates an abrupt expiratory flow that mimics an actual cough. A typical treatment consists of five cycles of inspiration/expiration. Secretions move into the upper airway where they can be physically expelled by the patient or suctioned out by the clinician. Patients with chronic neuromuscular disorders that result in a weak or absent cough, such as amyotrophic lateral sclerosis or quadriplegia, may particularly benefit from this therapy at home and in the hospital to maintain effective bronchial hygiene.

Airway oscillation devices (e.g., the Acapella™ and the Flutter Valve™) are handheld instruments that provide oscillation (movement of small amounts of air back-and-forth with rapid vibratory energy) as well as an expiratory flow resistance. The patient exhales into the device, which generates oscillations that travel through the airways and loosen secretions. Expiratory resistance from the device also creates back pressure to stent open the airways and promote lung expansion. Airway oscillation devices are useful in long-term treatment of chronic pulmonary disease (bronchiectasis, cystic fibrosis, etc.) as well as for acute disease where the patient cannot tolerate more aggressive forms of secretion clearance.

High-frequency airway oscillation devices (e.g., *Percussionaire, Intrapulmonary Percussive Ventilation*™) generate internal high-frequency (12–25 Hz) percussions within the airway. It is performed with a pneumatically driven device that also incorporates a nebulizer to deliver aerosolized water or medications during treatment. Oscillatory frequencies are manipulated from slow to fast in order to break up secretions and move them up into the large airways for expulsion.

High-frequency chest wall oscillation devices generate oscillatory vibrations externally on the patient's chest wall. The two of the most common ones are the *Frequencer*™ and the *ThairapyVest*™. The *Frequencer*™ is handheld and uses acoustic frequencies to generate gentle chest wall vibrations. As the sound waves penetrate the chest wall, secretions are loosened, liquefied, and moved into the large airways. It is particularly helpful for patients who cannot tolerate traditional percussive secretion clearance therapy. The *ThairapyVest*™ is an inflatable vest attached to a variable air-pulse generator that delivers external chest wall vibrations through pressure pulses. The pressure pulses loosen secretions, which travel into the large airways. The vest is particularly helpful for patients with widespread retained secretions, such as those with cystic fibrosis.

LUNG EXPANSION

Lung expansion therapy includes a variety of modalities focused on preventing or correcting atelectasis. Incentive spirometry encourages patients to take slow deep and prolonged inhalations that mimic yawns or sighs. Intermittent Positive Pressure Breathing (IPPB) delivers positive pressure to spontaneously breathing patients during inspiration in order to increase FRC. Positive Airway Pressure (e.g., the EZ Pap™) expands the lungs with positive pressure during exhalation. The patient exhales against a resistance threshold, which can be adjusted for the desired effect. The back pressure stents open the airways and increases lung volume. It is a good alternative for patients who do not improve with standard incentive spirometry or who require supplemental oxygen during lung expansion therapy.

FURTHER READING

1. Cairo JM. Administering medical gases: regulators, flowmeters, and controlling devices. In: Cairo JM, Pilbeam SP, eds. *Mosby's Respiratory Care Equipment.* 7th ed. St Louis, MO: Mosby; 2004.

   A comprehensive textbook of respiratory care equipment, this specific chapter focuses on O_2/gas administration.

2. Cairo JM. Lung expansion device. In: Cairo JM, Pilbeam SP, eds. *Mosby's Respiratory Care Equipment.* 7th ed. St Louis, MO: Mosby; 2004.

   A comprehensive textbook of respiratory care equipment, this specific chapter focuses on lung expansion techniques.

3. Fink J. Humidity and bland aerosol therapy. In: Wilkins RL, Stoller JK, Kacmarek RM, eds. *Fundamentals of Respiratory Care.* 9th ed. St Louis, MO: Mosby; 2009.

A comprehensive textbook covering fundamentals of respiratory care, this specific chapter reviews humidi-fication and delivery of bland aerosol.

4. Dymedso website. *The Frequencer, Acoustical Airway Clearance Device User Manual.* http://www .dymedso.com/pdf/manuel_V2_ENG_US-CAN_v11-02-04.pdf. Accessed May 4, 2011.

   Thorough overview of the Frequencer airway clearance device.

5. Heuer AJ, Scanlan CL. Medical gas therapy. In: Wilkins RL, Stoller JK, Kacmarek RM, eds. *Funda-mentals of Respiratory Care.* 9th ed. St Louis, MO: Mosby; 2009.

   A review of medical gases and their administration, specifically oxygen therapy.

6. Myslinski MJ, Scanlan CL. Bronchial hygiene therapy. In: Wilkins RL, Stoller JK, Kacmarek RM, eds. *Fundamentals of Respiratory Care.* 9th ed. St Louis, MO: Mosby; 2009.

   A comprehensive textbook covering fundamentals of respiratory care, this specific chapter discusses the various therapies encompassing bronchial hygiene.

7. Oakes D. *Clinical Practitioner's Pocket Guide to Respiratory Care.* 4th ed. Old Town, ME: Health Educator Publications; 1996.

   A thorough overview of respiratory care and techniques for the bedside practitioner.

8. Wilkins RL. Lung expansion therapy. In: Wilkins RL, Stoller JK, Kacmarek RM, eds. *Fundamentals of Respiratory Care.* 9th ed. St Louis, MO: Mosby; 2009.

   A comprehensive textbook covering fundamentals of respiratory care, this specific chapter reviews lung expansion therapy.

9. Wissing DR. Humidity and aerosol therapy. In: Cairo JM, Pilbeam SP, eds. *Mosby's Respiratory Care Equipment.* 7th ed. St Louis, MO: Mosby; 2004.

   A comprehensive textbook of respiratory care equipment, this specific chapter focuses on review of humidi-fication and delivery of aerosols.

Tobacco Control

David M. Burns

Cigarette smoking causes lung cancer, oral cancer, laryngeal cancer, esophageal cancer, kidney cancer, bladder cancer, pancreatic cancer, leukemia, cervical cancer, stomach cancer, abdominal aortic aneurysm, atherosclerotic peripheral vascular disease, cerebrovascular disease, coronary heart disease, and chronic obstructive pulmonary disease. The use of oral contraceptives in-creases the risk of vascular disease in women who smoke, and there are higher fetal and maternal complications of pregnancy if women smoke during the last 6 months of pregnancy. In addi-tion, there is sufficient evidence to suggest that smoking causes cataracts, hip fractures, low bone density, peptic ulcer disease, and adverse surgical outcomes resulting from poor wound healing and postoperative respiratory complications.

The major goals of tobacco control interventions are prevention of tobacco initiation, cessa-tion of tobacco use, and prevention of exposure to second-hand tobacco smoke. Prevention of smoking initiation is a crucial public health goal in itself, but near-term reduction in smoking-related disease rates in the total population can only be achieved by smoking cessation. Prevent-ing adolescents from smoking contributes little to reduction in disease rates until 30 years or more after the point at which they would have started to smoke.

Tobacco control efforts are intended to influence individual tobacco use. Tobacco con-trol interventions may be focused on the individual smoker (e.g., pharmacologic treatment), the environment (e.g., restrictions on where smoking is allowed). They may also focus on the product itself and its marketing, now that the Food and Drug Administration has been given jurisdiction over tobacco products. Since the 1960s, tobacco control strategies have gradually transitioned from being focused exclusively on education and interventions with the individual smoker toward an understanding of the role of environmental factors in promoting and enhancing cessation and preventing initiation. Efforts to educate the smoker and clinic-based cessation assistance have been supplemented by efforts to change community norms, to increase the cost of cigarettes, to restrict where smoking is allowed, to limit tobacco industry marketing practices, and to provide societal-based persistent and inescapable messages to quit coupled with support for cessation. The current belief is that an effective program utilizes a multilayered approach that combines a multitude of options for cessation assistance supported by environmental changes denormalizing tobacco use, including restrictions on smoking behavior and increasing the psychological and financial cost of tobacco use.

Changes in public policies about tobacco use can affect large numbers of individuals at minimal cost. Increasing the price of cigarettes is the most powerful tool in altering smoking behavior, and tax increases result in lowered total and per capita cigarette consumption, higher cessation rates, and reduced initiation levels. Most studies demonstrate a relatively consistent decline in consumption of 4% for each 10% increase in price. Increases in the cost of cigarettes can influence both short-term cessation attempts and long-term cessation success.

Changes in public policies on where tobacco use is allowed also affect large numbers of individuals at minimal cost. There has been a marked increase in the fraction of the working population protected by total bans on smoking in the workplace, from 3% in 1986 to 77% by 2003. Multiple workplace observations have demonstrated that instituting a change in workplace smoking restrictions is accompanied by an increase in cessation attempts and a reduction in number of cigarettes smoked per day. Once restrictions on smoking in the workplace have been successfully implemented, smokers continue to reduce the number of cigarettes smoked per day and there is an increase in the success rate of smokers attempting to quit. The current widespread implementation of restrictions on where smoking is allowed is felt to be a principal factor in the marked fall in the percentage of smokers who smoke more than a pack per day and the recent decline in the average number of cigarettes smoked per day by daily smokers.

The healthcare system is a logical and potentially productive means of reaching smokers, with cessation messages increasing the chances of successful cessations. Approximately 70% of smokers see a physician each year, offering the potential to reach large numbers of smokers with advice to quit. The fraction of patients who report receiving cessation advice in the last year from their physician remains too low, but it has been increasing over time and now exceeds 60% of all smokers who have seen a physician. The U.S. Food and Drug Administration has approved a variety of pharmacologic approaches to smoking cessation over the last two decades, including nicotine replacement therapy with gum, patches, nasal and oral inhalers; clonidine; bupropion; and varenicline. Nicotine patches and gum have been approved for over-the-counter sale since 1996. Use of nicotine replacement in conjunction with buproprion further improves cessation rates compared to either used singly. Use of long-term (6 months or longer) nicotine replacement and pretreatment with nicotine replacement for several weeks prior to the cessation date look promising as improvements in pharmacological management.

Multiple controlled clinical trials have demonstrated that both physician advice and pharmacologic treatment have substantial effects on long-term successful smoking cessation. In their offices, physicians should record a patient's smoking history, motivate the smoker to quit, negotiate a quit date, follow up the quit attempt, and notify the smoker about additional cessation assistance. Current recommendations suggest that all patients interested in making a quit attempt be offered some form of pharmacological assistance. When physicians provide this type of intervention, they can double the rate of long-term successful cessation in their patients. In addition, physician encouragement can also double the likelihood that a patient will participate in more structured cessation assistance, such as a smoking clinic or telephone counseling, which provides additional improvements achieving long-term abstinence. Once these interventions move beyond the controlled investigational setting, and are used in isolation without the structure and support provided by a clinical trial, they have less impact on the smoker.

The gap between the effect achieved in clinical trials and population-based data defines the potential that can be achieved if these strategies are delivered in a more comprehensive, organized manner and integrated with other available cessation resources.

The natural history of achieving successful abstinence commonly includes multiple cessation failures prior to achieving successful abstinence, and this should be recognized in clinical practice. Cessation should be viewed as a long-term process that will require continued monitoring and motivation for repetitive cessation attempts as a normal part of treatment. There is a high rate of relapse back to smoking for at least 2 years following cessation, and as with most addictions, former smokers need to be abstinent for 5 or more years in order to be confident of continued success. This reality emphasizes the need for continued monitoring of the smoking status of former smokers.

Improving the effectiveness of individual interventions requires integrating tobacco control resources so that they support the availability and effectiveness of cessation messages and assistance. This can be accomplished by reducing healthcare system barriers to access (particularly cost) of cessation aids and counseling, and linking physician or other practitioner advice with telephone hotline counseling. It is particularly useful to encourage healthcare systems to view cessation as a population-based intervention utilizing messages delivered by various media and multiple personnel rather than having messages come exclusively from physicians. To obtain maximal benefit, we need to integrate tobacco control interventions into healthcare delivery systems, link them to community cessation resources, and create an environment that encourages access. When this is done, marked improvements in population-based rates of cessation are possible.

There is concern that successful cessation by more than half those who have ever smoked has left behind a residual population of smokers who have more difficulty quitting and are more resistant to tobacco control interventions. Despite the compelling logic of this concern, the evidence shows that current smokers are quitting at higher rates and there is little evidence that tax increases or other tobacco control efforts are losing their effect on increasing cessation.

Two common components of most comprehensive tobacco control programs are mass media and self-help materials. They share the ability to reach large numbers of individuals at relatively low cost. However, they also share the misconception that they are autonomous interventions whereby cessation goals are achieved simply by delivering self-help materials or exposing the smoker to the media message. It is clear that both of these tobacco control channels are just that: channels. They are methods by which other tobacco control interventions can be facilitated, reinforced, and publicized and by which agendas can be set. However, in isolation, without integration into a more comprehensive approach, they have little effect.

Changing the environment in which the smoker lives and smokes to provide persistent and inescapable messages to quit while giving support for cessation has been a goal of most comprehensive tobacco control approaches, but accomplishing this goal has been problematic. Comprehensive statewide programs in California and Massachusetts have reduced smoking behaviors and disease risks, and are models for programs in other states. Unfortunately, downturns in tax revenue and political pressures have markedly reduced or eliminated the funding for many state tobacco control efforts and are likely to continue to minimize their future impact.

Telephone counseling services are effective in promoting long-term successful cessation both independently and in conjunction with healthcare system interventions. Several approaches to individualized counseling are available to provide assistance to the general population of smokers.

Computer-based interactive software can tailor the intervention and counseling provided to an individual smoker. The possibility of providing this kind of customized intervention over the Internet, in public locations where smokers have access, on home computers, or in hand-held devices can overcome some of the traditional resistance of smokers, particularly younger smokers, to the more intensive, but more effective, smoking cessation interventions.

Current models of smoking behavior postulate that smokers cycle through stages during which they are disinterested in cessation, contemplate quitting, make a quit attempt, and are either successful or relapse back to smoking. Smoking relapse can be followed by a period of disinterest in cessation or the smoker may think about making an additional cessation attempt. Individual components of a comprehensive tobacco control program may affect the process of cessation at different stages. For example, public information campaigns can help smokers think about the need to quit, physician advice may trigger a cessation attempt, and working in a smoke-free environment may facilitate abstinence once the attempt is made. Public information about the risks of smoking, negative images of the smoker, and physician warnings about risks can all convince a smoker to attempt to quit. In addition, the desire to set a good example for children and concern about being dependent on smoking are reasons smokers give for wanting to quit. Acute illness can also trigger cessation activity and provides a teachable moment for cessation in healthcare interactions.

Forces influencing smoking cessation attempts may be different from those that lead to longer-term successful cessation. For example, older smokers are less likely to report making a cessation attempt in the last 12 months, but they are more likely to quit successfully for 3 or more months based on that attempt. This observation suggests that efforts to promote cessation among older smokers can yield important benefits.

FURTHER READING

1. Agency for Health Care Policy and Research. *Treating Tobacco Use and Dependence: 2008. Update.* Rockville, MD: US Department of Public Health and Human Services, Public Health Service, Agency for Health Care Policy and Research; 2008. http://www.ncbi.nlm.nih.gov/books/NBK12193/.

   A comprehensive evidence based review of what is effective in interventions for the clinical practice setting, based on comprehensive meta-analyses of existing literature and best judgment of experts.

2. Patnode CD, O'Connor E, Whitlock EP, et al. *Primary care relevant interventions for tobacco use prevention and cessation in children and adolescents: A systematic evidence review for the U.S. Preventive Services Task Force.* Rockville, MD: Agency for Healthcare Research and Quality (US); December 2012. Report No 12-05175-EF-1.

   A comprehensive evidence based review of interventions to prevent smoking uptake or encourage cessation among children or adolescents.

   http://www.cdc.gov/mmwr/PDF/wk/mm6044.pdf.

3. Centers for Disease Control and Prevention. *Best Practices for Comprehensive Tobacco Control Programs—2007.* Atlanta, GA: U.S. Department of Health and Human Services, Centers for Disease Control and Prevention, National Center for Chronic Disease Prevention and Health Promotion, Office on Smoking and Health; 2007. http://www.cdc.gov/tobacco/stateandcommunity/best_practices/pdfs/2007/BestPractices_Complete.pdf.

   Recommendations for the components that should be part of a comprehensive state tobacco control campaign with recommended budgets for each state.

4. Centers for Disease Control and Prevention. *Tobacco Control State Highlights, 2010.* Atlanta, GA: U.S. Department of Health and Human Services, Centers for Disease Control and Prevention, National Center for Chronic Disease Prevention and Health Promotion, Office on Smoking and Health; 2010. www.cdc.gov/tobacco/data_statistics/state_data/state_highlights/2010/.

   Provided state-specific data on smoking behaviors, policies, and funding in relation to the recommended best practices.

5. Centers for Disease Control and Prevention. Current cigarette smoking among adults aged—United States. *MMWR Morb Mortal Wkly Rep.* 2011;61(44):889–894. http://www.cdc.gov/mmwr/preview/mmwrhtml/mm6144a2.htm?s_cid=mm6144a2_w.

   Recent data on the prevalence of smoking in the United States from the National Health interview survey.

6. Centers for Disease Control and Prevention. Quitting smoking among adults—United States, 2001–2010. *MMWR Morb Mortal Wkly Rep.* 2011;60(44):1513–1519.

   Recent data showing that cessation is increasing in the U.S. population.

7. Curry SJ, Grothaus LC, McAfee T, et al. Use and cost effectiveness of smoking-cessation services under four insurance plans in a health maintenance organization. *N Engl J Med.* 1998;339:673.

   An older but still relevant description of the effectiveness of a comprehensive healthcare, systems-based smoking cessation program, which increased successful cessation by 2.4-fold and demonstrated the importance of removing financial barriers to accessing cessation assistance for increasing participation in cessation assistance programs.

8. Johnston LD, O'Malley PM, Bachman JG, et al. *Monitoring the Future National Survey Results on Drug Use, 1975–2011. Volume II: College Students and Adults Ages 19–50.* Ann Arbor, MI:

Institute for Social Research, The University of Michigan; 2012. http://www.monitoringthefuture
.org/pubs/monographs/mtf-vol2_2011.pdf.

Demonstrates the recent national trends of adolescent initiation of cigarette smoking in the context of other adolescent drug use.

9. Morris CD, Waxmonsky JA, May MG, et al. Smoking reduction for persons with mental illnesses: 6-month results from community-based interventions. *Community Ment Health J.* 2011;47(6):694–702.

Demonstration of the effectiveness of telephone counseling and group therapy for individuals with mental illness who may represent a growing portion of the remaining current daily smokers.

10. National Cancer Institute. *Those Who Continue to Smoke: Is Achieving Abstinence Harder and Do We Need to Change Our Interventions?* Smoking and Tobacco Control Monograph No 15. USDHHS, NIH, NCI, NIH publication No 03-5370; 2003. http://cancercontrol.cancer.gov/tcrb/monographs/15/index.html.

A review of the trends in cessation demonstrating that existing tobacco control efforts continue to work and that the residual smoking population continues to be influenced by them.

11. National Cancer Institute. *Risks Associated With Smoking Cigarettes With Low Machine-Measured Yields of Tar and Nicotine.* Smoking and Tobacco Control Monograph No 13. USDHHS, PHS, NIH, NCI; 2001. http://cancercontrol.cancer.gov/tcrb/monographs/13/.

A review of existing evidence, which reaches the conclusion that the changes in cigarette design over the past 50 years have not reduced the disease risks of smoking.

12. US Department of Health and Human Services. *How Tobacco Smoke Causes Disease: The Biology and Behavioral Basis for Smoking-Attributable Disease A Report of the Surgeon General 2010.* Atlanta, GA: US Department of Health and Human Services, Public Health Service, Centers for Disease Control and Prevention, National Center for Chronic Disease Prevention and Health Promotion, Office on Smoking and Health; 2010. http://www.cdc.gov/tobacco/data_statistics/sgr/2010/index.htm.

A comprehensive review of the mechanisms by which smoking causes disease.

13. US Department of Health and Human Services. *The Health Consequences of Smoking: A Report of the Surgeon General.* Atlanta, GA: US Department of Health and Human Services, Public Health Service, Centers for Disease Control and Prevention, National Center for Chronic Disease Prevention and Health Promotion, Office on Smoking and Health; 2004. http://www.cdc.gov/tobacco/sgr/sgr_2004/index.htm.

An encyclopedic description of the disease consequences of smoking and the evidence supporting a causal relationship with smoking.

14. US Department of Health and Human Services. *The Health Consequences of Involuntary Exposure to Tobacco Smoke.* Atlanta, GA: US Department of Health and Human Services, Public Health Service, Centers for Disease Control and Prevention, National Center for Chronic Disease Prevention and Health Promotion, Office on Smoking and Health; 2006.

Extensively documented review of the disease consequences of environmental tobacco smoke exposure.

Useful Web Sites

CDC web site for state-specific tobacco control information

http://www.cdc.gov/tobacco/data_statistics/state_data/

American Legacy Foundation cessation resources

http://www.legacyforhealth.org/ex.aspx

Agency for Health Care Policy Research web site for clinical practice guidelines

http://www.ncbi.nlm.nih.gov/books/NBK12193/

National Cancer Institute Smoking and Tobacco Control monograph series

http://cancercontrol.cancer.gov/tcrb/monographs/

14 Disaster Management by the Pulmonologist

Asha Devereaux, Jeffrey R. Dichter,
and Dennis E. Amundson

According to a report published in March 2011 by the Centers for Disease Control and Prevention, nearly a third of hospitals are unprepared for the six types of mass-casualty disasters that public health officials fear most. A comprehensive approach to disaster medicine requires a blend of emergency and public health medicine principles. Planning for disasters ranges from preparing for isolated incidents such as power outages, accidents, chlorine gas spills, or building collapse to higher-impact occurrences, such as nuclear catastrophes, earthquakes, wildfires, hurricanes, and tsunamis. Most disasters result from natural events and produce injuries familiar to acute care physicians. However, acts of terrorism involving chemical, biological, and nuclear agents present unique situations beyond the practical experience of most healthcare providers. Because these exposures either impact the respiratory system or require intensive care, pulmonologists will play a prominent role in managing these patients. Catastrophic events may lead to a mass-casualty incident in which an overwhelming number and severity of casualties present to a medical system. Multiple challenges must be considered, including surge capacity, triage, crisis standards of care, and allocation of scarce resources. Personal protection equipment (PPE) and decontamination are beyond the scope of this chapter, but references to this subject are provided in the annotated bibliography.

BASIC PRINCIPLES
Surge Capacity and Management in Disaster Planning

Surge capacity may be defined *as the ability to manage and adapt to a large and unexpected influx of patients*. This may range from the usual ebb and flow of a routine busy hospital up to a major disaster where emergency mass critical care (EMCC) may need to be invoked. Surge management includes the processes and strategies used to adapt patient care capacity to higher than usual numbers. As a pulmonologist involved with disaster planning, it is crucial to understand your resources, available treatment and disaster response strategies, personal protection, and communication methods with internal and external chains of command.

To simplify, surge capacity planning can be divided into four broad categories of consideration:

1. Personnel ("staff," including all critical care and hospital based professionals)
2. Hospital environment ("space," such as intensive care units [ICUs], step-down units, and wards)
3. Equipment ("stuff," such as ventilators, medications, etc.)
4. "System" (processes required for communication and coordination)

For each resource, there are six key strategies that are used to adapt to a disaster surge, listed with examples:

1. *Prepare:* planning for likely disasters ahead of time, stockpiling supplies and cross-training personnel.
2. *Substitute:* using equivalent medications for narcotics or antibiotics, rather than the specific ones desired; having a coronary care unit (CCU) nurse caring for a sick medical intensive care unit (MICU) patient.
3. *Conserve:* accepting lower oxygen saturations to conserve oxygen, managing some patients with higher nurse/patient ratios.
4. *Adapt:* using anesthesia machines instead of standard ventilators in "low risk" patients.

5. *Reuse:* reusing lines or tubes, possibly after some effort at sterilization.

6. *Reallocate:* providing life-saving care, such as a ventilator or an ICU bed/level of care, only to those patients with the best chance of survival.

When planning for the continuum of potential disasters, mass casualty standards of care can be divided based on the severity of the disaster:

1. *Conventional:* the staff, space, stuff, and systems are all consistent with routine daily practices and with preserved normal standard of care, but toward the limits of usual care. An example would be the normal "competition" that may happen in any ICU, where patients may have to wait in other areas such as the emergency room (ER) or postanesthesia care unit (PACU) while ICU beds are "opened up."

2. *Contingency:* the staff, space, stuff, and systems are used in ways that are not consistent with usual practices, but have little, if any, impact on the normal standard of care. An example would be where a PACU or intermediate care unit had to be urgently repurposed to function as an ICU for days or weeks. This occurred in NYC's Bellevue Hospital following Hurricane Sandy, where patients were relocated based on the availability of generator power.

3. *Crisis capacity:* the staff, space, stuff, and systems are not consistent with a usual standard of care, but likely provide the best care possible given the magnitude of the disaster and available resources. An example would be the events involving Memorial Medical Center in New Orleans after Hurricane Katrina in 2005, where healthcare staff, under conditions without power and of nearly exhausted resources, was ultimately required to make triage decisions regarding which patients had the best chance of survival. At least 34 patients died during or immediately after the hurricane.

It is imperative that any limitation of usual care during a disaster is coordinated with local, county, and/or state partners depending upon the extent and duration of the event. Mutual aid agreements should be in place with neighboring facilities during disaster planning so that resources and patient transfers can be effectively managed and tracked. Medical and legal policies are currently in place in many states with some federal guidance, but still in active evolution.

EARTHQUAKES

Since 2006, there have been an increasing number of earthquakes throughout the world. Medical casualties usually result from the secondary damage caused by structural collapse, flooding, and, most recently in Japan, nuclear radiation exposure. Experiences in both Haiti and the Philippines demonstrate that care of disaster victims following an earthquake is difficult because of the destruction of existing medical, transportation, and communication system infrastructure. The pulmonologist/intensivist will likely be involved in stabilizing trauma patients from injuries such as long-bone fractures, open femur fractures, pelvic fractures, gangrene, skull or spinal fractures as they await or recover from surgical intervention. Medical issues from entrapment, weather extremes, and dehydration also should be anticipated. Complications from crush injuries, including infection, renal failure, anemia, and cardiomyopathy, are common and require intensive support. Coordination of care during a chaotic influx of patients is challenging and requires enhanced and redundant communication and triage of resources and staff. Nursing and physician ratios are expanded, while lab and radiology utilization will be limited. Some useful tools to the provider in order to rapidly assess patients include portable ultrasonography, digital x-rays, and communication devices (including GPS systems) to coordinate transfer and locations of alternate echelons of care. Situational awareness and cross training of staff are key recommendations following every disaster where communication and access are limited. It is important to convene a multidisciplinary ethics committee that will help coordinate and support difficult decisions during allocation of scarce resources in conjunction with the incident command system internally and external to the healthcare facility using the steps outlined above.

IONIZING RADIATION EXPOSURE

Ionizing radiation exposure arising from nuclear accidents (e.g., Chernobyl), sequelae of earthquakes (e.g., Fukishima), or possible acts of terrorism has the potential for creating catastrophic mass casualties. Significant human exposure to ionizing radiation may result from a single point source (e.g., radiation dispersal device [RDD] or "dirty bomb"), accident or sabotage in a nuclear power plant, or detonation of a nuclear weapon, which may also result in additional injury patterns due to the blast, thermal, light, and electromagnetic pulse (affects communication and electronic equipment) energy emissions. The clinical effects following exposure can be predicted from the method of detonation, weather conditions, physical environment, and duration of exposure. An individual's radiation dose can be estimated by determining the time of onset and severity of prodromal symptoms (nausea and vomiting), the decline in absolute lymphocyte count over the first 48 hours, and the appearance of chromosome aberrations in peripheral blood lymphocytes. Exposure can be in the form of local irradiation, whole-body irradiation, external contamination, internal contamination, or a combination. Frequently, the adverse effects of radiation exposure are seen in association with traumatic injuries. Regardless of the scenario, the principles of decontamination and treatment of casualties arising from radiation events remain the same.

The management of radiation exposure initially should consist of actions to (1) minimize exposure time, (2) increase distance from the source, and (3) maximize shielding. Decontamination efforts should be initiated in the field. All uninjured but externally contaminated individuals can be decontaminated without medical interventions. Simply removing clothing and washing the skin with soap and warm water is effective in removing more than 99% of external contamination. Injured contaminated patients pose unique problems for the healthcare facility. Treatment of life-threatening injuries always takes precedence over decontamination (i.e., pay attention to the ABCs first). All casualties with non–life-threatening injuries should be decontaminated before treatment. This should be followed by a radiologic survey to determine the dose, assess prodromal symptoms, and collect samples for biodosimetry. Patients can then be triaged based on the estimated dose received and the presence or absence of other injuries. Surgery for traumatic injuries, if indicated, should be performed within 36 hours of exposure. Further surgery should be delayed for 6 weeks to allow recovery of immune function and normalization of wound healing. Internal contamination can result from wounds, ingestion, or inhalation of radioactive material. Wounds can be decontaminated by irrigation and removal of foreign material. Debridement should be limited to devitalized tissue. Gastrointestinal decontamination may include the use of cathartics or chelating agents. Whole-lung lavage can potentially remove as much as 50% of the radioactivity after inhalation of significant amounts of material. This reduction in radioactivity is accomplished primarily through the removal of alveolar macrophages, which have engulfed contaminated particles in the alveoli and alveolar ducts.

Acute Radiation Syndrome

Acute radiation syndrome (ARS) may develop after systemic irradiation. Generally, ARS results from acute whole-body doses above 1 gray (Gy). With exposures exceeding 10 Gy, survival is unlikely and treatment should be limited to comfort care. The syndrome progresses through four distinct phases: prodromal, latent, manifest illness, and recovery/death. After exposure, prodromal symptoms may develop within hours, but also may develop as late as 6 days after exposure. Prodromal symptoms classically consist of nausea, vomiting, and diarrhea. The duration to onset of these symptoms depends upon the dose received. Rapid onset of prodromal symptoms suggests shorter latency and predicts a more severe acute illness (usually >6 Gy exposure). After the prodromal phase, symptoms may remit for hours to days, which may appear to suggest recovery, but this transient latent phase is followed by the manifest-illness phase. This stage may last for weeks and is characterized by profound immune suppression. The time course and severity of ARS depends upon the degree of exposure. A person exposed to a supra-lethal dose of radiation may experience all phases within hours before death. At lower doses, ARS may consist predominantly of a hematopoietic syndrome. With increasing exposure, gastrointestinal, cardiac, and cerebrovascular syndromes will be seen. After significant exposure, interstitial radiation pneumonitis can develop, which can progress to fibrosis. Patients who develop acute lung injury requiring mechanical ventilation should be treated with usual ICU care with attention to a lung-protective strategy using the lowest FIO_2, in order to maintain oxygen saturation greater than 90% so as to decrease the possibility of additional oxygen toxicity. Monoclonal antibodies, vitamin A, interleukin 11, fibroblast growth factors, and pentoxifylline are currently considered experimental therapies for radiation-induced lung injury. Angiotensin II receptor blockers, angiotensin-converting enzyme inhibitors, and penicillamine may attenuate radiation-induced lung injury in rat models.

Depending upon the severity of the hematopoietic syndrome, treatment with cytokines, transfusions, or stem cell transplantation may be indicated. Supportive care may include administration of antibiotics, antiemetics, antidiarrheal medications, fluids, electrolytes, and analgesics. Because there will likely be many casualties following radiation injury, the US National Marrow Donor Program, the US Navy, and the American Society for Blood and Marrow Transplantation collaboratively developed the *Radiation Injury Treatment Network (RITN)*, which comprises 55 hematopoietic stem cell transplant centers, donor centers, and umbilical cord blood banks across the United States with the goal of providing surge capacity and guidelines for the management of radiation exposure. Critical care should be provided for patients who develop multiorgan failure days to weeks after exposure, as their dose received is likely to have been less than 10 Gy. Patients who experience multiorgan failure within hours of exposure (>6 Gy) should receive expectant care.

CHEMICAL EXPOSURE

After intentional chemical exposure, patients most frequently present with symptoms similar to toxic inhalation of common industrial agents, such as chlorine, organophosphate products, or combustion. Chemical substances can be classified as (1) inhalational toxins that primarily affect the lungs or (2) neurotoxic agents that primarily involve the central nervous system. If appropriate hazardous materials (HAZMAT) assessment is available, prompt identification of the agent will allow the clinician to prepare specific antidotes and treatment supplies before the patient's arrival.

Inhalational Toxins

Inhalational toxins may be classified as (1) direct respiratory irritants and (2) airway vesicants. Chemical asphyxiants such as carbon monoxide, hydrogen cyanide, and hydrogen sulfide may produce significant morbidity, but do not usually cause pulmonary injury unless exposure is overwhelming, as occurred in 1984 with the accidental release of 30 to 40 tons of methylisocyanite in Bhopal, India. Over 2,000 people died, with autopsy findings consistent with acute respiratory disease syndrome (ARDS) and overwhelming pulmonary toxicity. Chronic lung diseases, such as chronic obstructive pulmonary disease (COPD) and pulmonary fibrosis, prevail in survivors.

Direct Respiratory Irritants (Chlorine, Phosgene)

Chlorine is a highly reactive greenish yellow gas that is 2.5 times as dense as air. It is used in the production of chemicals, bleaching and plastics processing, and in a variety of recreational and household settings (e.g., swimming pools, cleaning solutions). Previously it was thought that chlorine reacted with tissue water to form hydrochloric acid and oxygen radicals and caused significant mucosal irritation. However, hydrochloric acid is much less toxic than chlorine, and recent animal studies demonstrate that chlorine directly damages the respiratory system via oxidative injury of epithelial proteins. Symptoms range from mild to moderate chest burning, chest tightness, cough, throat irritation, dyspnea, and ocular irritation. Severe or prolonged exposures can result in ulcerative tracheobronchitis, diffuse alveolar damage with hyaline membrane formation, and pulmonary edema. Treatment includes supplemental humidified oxygen and inhaled/nebulized bronchodilators. Nebulized sodium bicarbonate and inhaled budesonide have been used with mass chlorine exposures from swimming pools and from exposure to mixing cleaning fluids with a suggestion that symptom duration and pulmonary sequela are reduced.

Phosgene and diphosgene have been used in chemical warfare. These agents are poorly soluble in water and, thus, have a delayed onset of action (30 minutes–8 hours). Initial exposure produces a burning sensation of the mucus membranes of the eyes, nose, throat, and upper respiratory tract. More severe exposures can result in cough, wheezing, stridor, dyspnea, hypotension, and noncardiogenic pulmonary edema. Development of acute lung injury after exposure to phosgene carries a poor prognosis. Treatment of respiratory irritant exposure is supportive with bronchodilators and local care. The use of steroids has been advocated, but is of unproven benefit.

Vesicants (Mustards)

The mustard compounds are a family of similar agents that have had significant use on the battlefield, either alone or in combination with other chemical and biological agents. The most common agent is sulfur mustard, which has a simple structure and is easily produced with ingredients typically used to manufacture plastics. Mustard vapor, which smells like garlic, is heavier than air and concentrates in low-lying areas. Because of its low volatility, mustard can persist in an environment for up to 5 days. Liquid mustard is rapidly absorbed and hydrolyzed in extracellular fluid. Within 2 minutes of exposure, mustard can irreversibly alkylate cellular DNA, resulting in necrotic cell death. Also, within minutes target organs irreversibly bind the chemical agent, making delayed elimination difficult, if not impossible. Skin, eye, airway, bone marrow, gastrointestinal, and nervous system findings predominate. The clinical effects of mustard toxicity typically begin 2 to 48 hours after exposure. More severe exposures are heralded by earlier onset of signs and symptoms. Typical manifestations include skin blistering and eye and airway symptoms resulting from direct irritant effects. Incapacitating respiratory tract injury can occur at vapor exposures significantly lower than those that cause skin blistering. A sore throat or productive cough that begins within 4 hours of exposure implies lower respiratory tract involvement and should prompt immediate airway evaluation and intervention. Sloughing and ulceration of the trachea and bronchi can lead to obstruction. Pseudomembrane formation may cause necrotic obstruction that can complicate airway management. Mortality soon after exposure is most often related to pulmonary complications. Later mortality is usually due to bone marrow suppression and septic complications of lung injury and superficial skin lesions.

The initial approach to mustard gas contact is to minimize further exposure. Primary preventive techniques with barriers, such as protective clothing and lotions, may provide limited protection. Effective and early decontamination maneuvers (within 5 minutes) can remove residual agents on the skin. In contrast to treatment of thermal burns, care of chemical dermal wounds should include addressing large blisters or bullae with frequent irrigation and application of topical antibiotics. Because of the superficial nature of chemical burns compared with heat-related burns, skin grafting is seldom needed and initial fluid requirements are not as great. Pain management includes the judicious use of oral or systemic narcotics. Topical mydriatics, lubricating ocular gels, and local anesthetics can help relieve irritant ocular pain and later scarring. Humidified air and cough suppressants help soothe inhalational injury. Bronchodilator therapy is the mainstay of treatment. Airway control should be considered if dysphonia, cough, or respiratory distress occurs soon after exposure. The role of corticosteroids is controversial; however, they may be useful in severe cases. Antibiotics should be reserved for confirmed cases of infectious pneumonia. Sulfur-containing drugs should be avoided because they may potentiate the cellular injury caused by sulfur mustard exposure. In some animal studies, pretreatment or treatment within 20 minutes of exposure with *N*-acetylcysteine (Mucomyst, Mucosil-20) eliminated some of the organ damage. Some experts recommend post exposure treatment with intravenous sodium thiosulfate (500 mg/kg/day) for 48 hours, followed by 10 days of oral *N*-acetylcysteine and vitamin C. Although sulfates are contraindicated with mustard exposure, preparations that act as sulfur donors have minimized systemic effects and elevated the lethal dose in research animals. Persons who have been exposed to mustard are at significant risk for long-term effects, particularly lung and upper airway cancers. Persons with respiratory exposure may experience asthma or syndromes similar to COPD.

Neurotoxic Agents

In the 1930s, German scientists developed toxic "nerve agents" in industrial organophosphate factories. The four major compounds are tabun, sarin, soman, and VX. These agents inhibit the ability of acetylcholinesterase to hydrolyze acetylcholine. The accumulation of acetylcholine produces excess stimulation of nicotinic and muscarinic receptors.

The attachment of the nerve agent to the enzyme becomes permanent through a process called "aging" when acetylcholinesterase cleaves a portion of the bound nerve agent to produce a stable bond. The time required for aging varies, ranging from 2 minutes for soman to hours for other nerve agents. If administered prior to aging, several compounds can remove the nerve agent from the enzyme. The most important group of such compounds is the oximes. Nerve agents are liquids that may constitute both a liquid hazard and a vapor hazard during dispersal. All nerve agents rapidly penetrate clothing, skin, and mucous membranes. They may be absorbed by inhalation, ingestion, or dermal contact. Symptoms depend on the route of exposure and dose. After dermal contact, symptoms may be delayed for up to 18 hours; however, after inhalation, symptoms occur within seconds to minutes.

The clinical manifestations of nerve agent toxicity reflect the hyperstimulation of muscarinic and nicotinic receptors in the nervous system. Muscarinic effects include rhinorrhea, pinpoint pupils, blurred vision, hypersecretion by glands (e.g., salivary, lacrimal, sweat, respiratory), bronchospasm, nausea, vomiting, diarrhea, bradycardia, abdominal pain, and bowel and bladder incontinence. Nicotinic effects include skeletal muscle twitching, cramping, weakness, tachycardia, and hypertension. Mild exposure results in rhinorrhea, pinpoint pupils, bronchospasm, increased secretions, and dyspnea. More severe exposures cause muscle fasciculations, nausea, vomiting, diarrhea, unconsciousness, seizures, paralysis, apnea, and death. Patients who survive exposure to nerve agents may experience fatigue, irritability, and memory impairment for weeks after recovery from the short-term effects.

The management of patients begins with a careful assessment of airway, breathing, and circulation. Victims should be separated from the source of exposure and rapidly decontaminated. Clothing should be removed, eyes flushed with water for 5 to 10 minutes, and skin washed with soap and water. Antidotes for nerve agent poisoning are atropine sulfate and pralidoxime chloride (2-PAM or Protopam chloride). The initial dose of atropine is 2 to 6 mg intramuscularly (IM), depending on the severity of exposure, followed by 2 mg IM every 5 to 10 minutes until secretions and dyspnea or airway obstruction are minimized. As an oxime, 2-PAM acts as an acetylcholinesterase reactivator that binds the nerve agent and removes it from the enzyme. The initial dose is 600 to 1,800 mg IM, depending on the severity of exposure. Lorazepam or diazepam can be used as an adjunct to control seizures.

Providing medical care to a contaminated patient will tax even the most practiced clinician. PPE such as gas masks, respirators, and thick overgarments lead to heat stress within 30 minutes and make adequate communication with the patient and staff nearly impossible. Manual dexterity is also compromised. It should be noted that chemical agents traverse latex gloves readily and double gloves should be changed every 20 minutes. Wash the patient with lukewarm water and mild soap rather than hypochlorite bleach solution because bleach can potentiate further chemical injury. Eyes, mucus membranes, and wounds should be irrigated for at least 2 minutes with normal saline. There are a variety of commercial decontamination solutions that are effective and non-toxic.

Biologic Agents

The biologic agents that concern pulmonary physicians include "biologic toxins" (ricin and botulinum), "infecting zoonoses" (anthrax, plague, tularemia), and communicable viruses (smallpox or viral encephalitides). The agents that pose the most likely threat include anthrax, smallpox, plague, and ricin. In 2002, anthrax and ricin had been intentionally released, while smallpox and plague still present a substantial communicable risk to the population.

Anthrax

Anthrax is caused by the spore-forming *Bacillus anthracis*. Historically it is a disease of skin contamination (Woolsorter disease). In 2001, it had been used as an aerosolized bioweapon killing

5 and infecting 22 others via the US mail. There are three forms of anthrax infection depending on the route of exposure: cutaneous, gastrointestinal, or inhalational. To produce respiratory infection, 3,000 to 5,000 airborne spores (1–1.5 μm in size) must be inhaled, phagocytosed by pulmonary macrophages, and transported via lymphatics to hilar and mediastinal lymph nodes, where they may remain dormant as "vegetative cells" for approximately 10 to 60 days or longer. Rapid germination in the lymph nodes to the bacillary form leads to massive toxin production by the replicating bacteria resulting in hemorrhagic mediastinitis. Acute disease initially resembles a severe influenza-like illness, followed by rapid progression to sepsis, shock, multiorgan failure, and death. Inhalational anthrax has a high fatality rate (50%–70%), but number of spores inhaled, underlying clinical status, and age of patient impact the clinical course of disease. Diagnosis requires clinical suspicion and assessment for mediastinal widening in severely ill patients. *B. anthracis* is easily cultured from blood, CSF, ascites, and vesicular fluid using Biosafety Level-2 precautions. Rapid detection via immunohistochemistry and polymerase chain reaction (PCR) is also available through the laboratory response network. Treatment is predicated on the early use of effective antibiotics (usually a combination of intravenous ciprofloxacin, rifampin, and/or clindamycin), complete pleural drainage, and meticulous ICU care. A vaccine (AVA-Biothrax) against the bacterial toxin is the only licensed human anthrax vaccine in the United States, but is currently only available to the Department of Defense. Prolonged chemoprophylaxis with ciprofloxacin (500 mg twice daily), levofloxacin (500 mg daily) or doxycycline (100 mg twice daily) for 60 days, with or without vaccine, has been used in potentially exposed patients.

Plague

Plague is caused by *Yersinia pestis*, a Gram-negative coccobacillus of the Enterobacteriaceae family. It holds a historic place in pandemic human diseases and as an intentional agent of warfare since the 1300s. A rodent reservoir zoonosis, plague occurs naturally in endemic areas and is transmitted by all species of fleas. There are three clinical forms: (1) bubonic (lymphadenitis), (2) septicemic (usually from hematogenous spread), and (3) pneumonic (the greatest threat as a biowarfare agent). Pneumonic plague produces a severe, overwhelming pneumonia with hemoptysis, fever, cough, chest pain, dyspnea, and tachycardia. Chest radiographs show bilateral alveolar opacities, pleural effusions, and cavitations. Hilar lymphadenopathy is often present, but mediastinal widening is not, which can help distinguish the presentation from inhalational anthrax. Shock and death occur within 2 to 6 days with mortality approaching 60%. Diagnosis is via culture of sputum or body fluid showing *Y. pestis*, direct fluorescent antibody (DFA), PCR, or IgM assays. Treatment is with IM streptomycin 1 gm twice daily or gentamycin (5 mg/kg IV/IM once daily). Alternative agents include doxycycline (100 mg IV twice daily or 200 mg once daily), ciprofloxacin (400 mg IV twice daily), or chloramphenicol (25 mg/kg IV 4 times/day). Antibiotics must be administered early to improve survival. Persons with possible exposure should receive chemoprophylaxis with oral doxycycline or ciprofloxacin. No plague vaccine is currently available.

Smallpox

Smallpox is caused by the *Variola* virus and is believed to have been eradicated in 1980, with the last case of endemic smallpox occurring in Somalia in 1977. It is likely that it still exists in bioweapons arsenals in some countries. Smallpox is extremely contagious and clinical disease carries a 30% mortality rate. Clinical manifestations appear in a series of distinct phases: incubation phase (7–17 days), prodrome phase (lasts 2–4 days), eruption phase, vesicular phase, pustular phase, crust phase, and desquamation phase. Rash and fever syndrome occurs after a prolonged incubation period. The rash is similar to chickenpox and any severe case of "chickenpox" should be suspect for smallpox. Respiratory symptoms can occur owing to mucosal lesions or secondary infection. Confirmation of smallpox can be performed by PCR analysis of skin scrapings, body fluids, and oropharyngeal swabs and processed using Biosafety Level 4. Currently, there is no FDA approved treatment for acute infections. The public health approach is predicated on prevention and control by isolation, cohorting, and ring vaccination strategies. An antiretroviral agent, cidofovir, shows promise in animal studies and is being tested for therapy. Vaccinia immune globulin decreases pulmonary viral loads and pneumonitis in animals with vaccinia or cowpox, but there is no evidence that it offers any survival or therapeutic benefits in patients infected with smallpox.

Ricin

Ricin is a biologic toxin consisting of a protein extracted from the seed of the castor bean plant. It is easy to produce and highly toxic. Exposure to the freeze-dried powder can occur through inhalation, ingestion, or injection. Ricin causes ribosomal inactivation in cells to produce necrotic cell death. Inhaled ricin (based upon animal data) causes rapidly progressive, severe respiratory failure with pulmonary edema within 3 hours and is frequently fatal. Diagnosis is by enzyme-linked immunosorbent assay (ELISA) analysis of nasal mucosal swabs taken within 24 hours of exposure. Specific ricin antigen testing or immunochemical staining of serum and respiratory secretions can also be done. Acute and convalescent titers are recommended. Management is mainly supportive. There is currently no effective antidote, although a vaccine is under development.

FURTHER READING

1. Amundson D, Dadekian G, Etienne M, et al. Practicing internal medicine onboard the USNS comfort in the aftermath of the Haitian earthquake. *Ann Intern Med.* 2010;152:733–737.

   This article offers practical knowledge regarding the surge of patients and injury patterns following massive earthquake.

2. Amundson D, Lane D, Ferrara E. Operation aftershock: the US military disaster response to the Yogyakarta earthquake May through June 2006. *Mil Med.* 2008;173(3):236.

   Discussion of military response, language and cultural aspects of disaster response, medical diplomacy during a disaster.

3. Borak J, Sidell FR. Agents of chemical warfare: sulfur mustard. *Ann Emerg Med.* 1992;21:303–308.

   One of the first reviews and often-cited complete works on chemical and biologic agents.

4. Cevik Y, Akmaz I, Sezigen S. Mass casualties from acute inhalation of chlorine gas. *South Med J.* 2009;102(12):1209–1213.

   Description of chlorine exposure in 25 Turkish soldiers exposed to mixed cleaning solutions.

5. Christian MD, Devereaux AV, Dichter JR, et al. Definitive care for the critically ill during a disaster: current capabilities and limitations : from a Task Force for Mass Critical Care summit meeting, January 26-27, 2007, Chicago, IL. *Chest.* 2008;133:8S–17S.

   Discussion of the framework and infrastructure for mass critical care delivery during a disaster.

6. Daugherty EL. Health care worker protection in mass casualty respiratory failure: infection control, decontamination, and personal protective equipment. *Respir Care.* 2008;53:201–212.

   Excellent resource regarding PPE, infection control, and decontamination.

7. Dean A, Ku B, Zeserson E. The utility of handheld ultrasound in an austere medical setting in Guatemala after a natural disaster. *Am J Disaster Med.* 2007;2(5):249–256.

   Adaptation of technology to meet medical needs during a disaster.

8. Devereaux A, Amundson DE, Parrish JS, et al. Vesicants and nerve agents in chemical warfare. *Postgrad Med.* 2002;112:90–96.

   Review of chemicals used in military warfare and the clinical approach to management.

9. Devereaux A, Jeffrey R, Dichter MD, et al. Definitive care for the critically ill during a disaster: a framework for allocation of scarce resources in mass critical care. *Chest.* 2008;S51–S66.

   First consensus-based document to address triage of scarce resources during a disaster.

10. Etienne M, Powell C, Amundson D. Healthcare ethics: the experience after the Haitian earthquake. *Am J Disaster Med.* 2010;5(3):141–147.

    Practical application of triage algorithms and establishment of an ethics committee to assist with resource allocation.

11. Feldman KA, Russel EE, Lathrop SL. An outbreak of primary pneumonic tularemia on Martha's vineyard. *N Engl J Med.* 2001;345:1601–1606.

    Clinical experience with tularemia is discussed in this article.

12. Hick JL, Barbera J, Kelen G. Refining surge capacity: conventional, contingency, and crisis capacity. *Disaster Med Public Health Prep.* 2009;3(2):S59–S67.

    One of the first articles published formally, establishing and defining a method to increase capacity during a disaster.

13. Kales S, Christiani DC. Acute chemical emergencies. *N Engl J Med*. 2004;350(8):800–808.
    An excellent and concise review of likely chemical agents and treatments.

14. Knebel A, Coleman N, Cliffer K, et al. Allocation of scarce resources after a nuclear detonation: setting the context. *Disaster Med Public Health Prep*. 2011;5:S20–S31.
    Excellent supplement encompassing the breadth of care following a catastrophic nuclear event.

15. Lazarus A, Deveraux AV. Potential agents of chemical warfare. *Postgrad Med*. 2002;112:133–140.
    Brief review of chemical warfare agents based upon military field manual and training.

16. Lazarus AA, Devereaux A, Mohr LC. Biological agents of mass destruction. In: Irwin RS, Rippe JM, eds. *Intensive Care Medicine*. 7th ed. Philadelphia, PA: Lippincott Williams & Wilkins; 2011.
    Detailed chapter regarding the diagnosis, treatment, and management of patients exposed to biological zoonosis.

17. Lehavi O, Leiba D, Schwartz D, et al. Lessons learned from chlorine intoxications in swimming pools: the challenge of pediatric mass toxicological events. *Prehosp Disaster Med*. 2008;23(1):90–95.
    Information gathered from this articles helps address treatment approach to large number impacted by chlorine inhalation and may offers some clinical lessons that could be of use in the event of acute inhalational catastrophe due to chlorine.

18. Martin J, Campbell HR, Iijima H, et al. Chlorine-induced injury to the airways in mice. *Am J Respir Crit Care Med*. 2003;168:568–574.
    Discussion of the pathophysiologic mechanism of chlorine injury.

19. Armed Forces Radiology Research Institute. *Medical Management of Radiological Casualties Handbook*. 2nd ed. Bethesda, MD: Armed Forces Radiology Research Institute; 2003.
    The primary source of concise treatment and management of radiological emergencies in the field setting for the military.

20. Mettler FA, Voelz GL. Major radiation exposure—what to expect and how to respond. *N Engl J Med*. 2002;346(20):1554–1561.
    A concise and thorough review regarding radiation exposure, physiology, and treatment.

21. Moores LK, Geiling JA, Devereaux A, et al. Respiratory illnesses related to the intentional release of chemicals and biological agents of terror. In: Fein A, Kamholz S, Ost D, eds. *Respiratory Emergencies*. Boca Raton, FL: CRC Press; 2006.
    Chapter discussing in detail pulmonary effects of biological and chemical agents.

22. Manthous CA, Jackson WL. The 9–11 Commission's invitation to imagine: a pathophysiology-based approach to critical care of nuclear explosion victims. *Crit Care Med*. 2007;35:716–723.
    ICU management of nuclear victims.

23. Mishrai P, Samarthi R, Pathaki N, et al. Bhopal gas tragedy: review of clinical and experimental findings after 25 years. *Int J Occup Med Environ Health*. 2009;22(3):193–202.
    Good discussion of long-term sequela from Bhopal disaster.

24. Okie S. Dr. Pou and the hurricane—implications for patient care during disasters. *N Engl J Med*. 2008;358(1):1–5.
    Important discussion regarding physicians caught in disaster situation without resources or support.

25. Ricks RC, Berger ME, O'Hara FM Jr, eds. *The Medical Basis for Radiation-Accident-Preparedness. The Clinical Care of Victims*. Boca Raton, FL: CRC Press; 2002.
    A good discussion of dose assessment and correlation of medical treatment for radiation victims.

26. Robinson B, Alatas MF, Robertson A, et al. Natural disasters and the lung. *Respirology*. 2011; 16(3):386–395.
    Review of the pulmonary effects of natural disasters and how this could inform planning for future disasters.

27. Rorison D, McPherson SJ. Acute toxic inhalations. *Emerg Med Clin North Am*. 1992;10:409–435.
    Scientific discussion of mechanisms of toxic inhalation injury.

28. Rubinson L, Hick J, Hanfling DG, et al. Definitive care for the critically ill during a disaster: a framework for optimizing critical care surge capacity. *Chest*. 2008;133:18S–31S.

29. Rubinson L, Hick J, Curtis JR, et al. Definitive care for the critically ill during a disaster: medical resources for surge capacity. *Chest*. 2008;133:32S–51S.

References 28 and 29 are excellent as a guide to help prepare ICU for surge capacity.

30. Swartz MN. Recognition and management of anthrax: an update. *N Engl J Med*. 2001;345: 1621–1626.

Good update on management of anthrax.

31. USAMRICD. *The Medical Management of Chemical Casualties Handbook*. 4th ed. Bethesda, MD: Office of the Army Surgeon General; 2007.

Small handbook used in the field for military management of chemical casualties.

32. Waselenko JK, MacVittie TJ, Blakely WF, et al. Medical management of the acute radiation syndrome: recommendations of the Strategic National Stockpile Radiation Working Group. *Ann Intern Med*. 2004;140:1037–1051.

Excellent resource that provides specific guidance for the triage and management of radiation casualties (91 references).

Useful Web Sites

United States Army Office of the Surgeon General. This site offers detailed military-relevant information on chemical and nerve agents.

http://sis.nlm.nih.gov/Tox/ChemWar.html

REAC/TS Radiation Emergency Assistance: Center/Training Site. Provides support to the US Department of Energy, WHO, and the International Atomic Energy Agency in the medical management of radiation accidents. Web site contains information for management of radiation emergencies and guidance for initial hospital medical management.

www.orau.gov/reacts

Armed Forces Radiobiology Research Institute. Multiple references available at this web site for download including (1) *Medical Management of Radiological Casualties Handbook*, (2) *Pocket Guide for Responders to Ionizing Radiation Terrorism*, and (3) *Textbook of Military Medicine: Consequences of Nuclear Warfare*.

www.afrri.usuhs.mil

Center for Disease Control and Prevention—Emergency Preparedness and Response. Excellent web site geared toward both natural disasters and acts of terrorism.

www.bt.cdc.gov

American College of Radiology. Provides access to the handbook *Disaster Preparedness for Radiology Professionals*.

www.acr.org

Institute of Medicine of the National Academies. Guidance for establishing crisis standards of care for use in disaster situations.

http://www.iom.edu/Reports/2012/Crisis-Standards-of-Care-A-Systems-Framework-for-Catastrophic-Disaster-Response.aspx

15 Mechanical Ventilation: Devices and Methods

Timothy A. Morris

The introduction of microprocessor-controlled algorithms to manage ventilator performance has markedly expanded the ability to provide a variety of modes for ventilatory support. In *mandatory ventilation*, the most commonly used type, the ventilator delivers an inhaled breath for a set time, during which a number of parameters are controlled. A variety of inspiratory flow patterns may be delivered in order to target specific tidal volumes, or inspiratory flow may be adjusted based on the pressure during inspiration. The ratio of inspiratory to expiratory time may be inverted to produce very long inspiratory times, very short expiratory times, or both. Positive end-expiratory pressure (PEEP) may be applied to the airway to keep alveoli open throughout exhalation. The choice of appropriate modalities for ventilatory support is determined by the respiratory objectives for the patient at a given point in the disease course (e.g., improving oxygenation, optimizing CO_2 clearance, resting respiratory muscles, etc.). One of the advantages of the newer generation of microprocessor-based mechanical ventilators is that the same ventilator can deliver markedly different types of ventilatory support as the patient's requirements change.

The wide variety of mandatory ventilation modalities may be categorized according to how the following functions are handled: (1) control and adjustment of air movement into the lungs during inspiration, (2) function during exhalation, (3) initiation and termination of mandatory (machine-controlled) breaths, and (4) function during spontaneous (patient-driven) breaths. Each function has the goal of improving arterial oxygenation, protecting the alveoli from overdistension, or reducing the work of breathing by synchronization with spontaneous patient effort.

CONTROL: VOLUME VS PRESSURE

The most fundamental aspect of mandatory modes of mechanical ventilation is how air movement into the lungs is controlled and adjusted during an inspiration. The basic choice is either to control pressure or to control flow (and hence, volume). The most straightforward model to conceptualize pressure control (PC) is a simple pressure-driven system. In this idealized situation, the patient's airway would be connected to a large source of air maintained at a specific pressure. At the start of inspiration, pressurized air from the source enters the lungs at a flow rate determined by the resistance and compliance of the patient's respiratory system. As the lung pressure approaches equilibrium with the pressure from the source, flow decelerates at a rate determined by the respiratory system's resistance and compliance. In this model, the pressure in the airways would be "controlled" at a constant level, while at any given instant, the flow rate would depend on the resistance and compliance of the respiratory system.

In volume control (VC), the ventilator supplies a predetermined pattern of air flow to the lungs and it is the airway pressure that changes, depending on the respiratory system's resistance and compliance. The volume of air delivered to the lungs is determined by the flow rate and duration of the breath delivered. A simple, idealized model to conceptualize VC is a highly pressurized tank of air connected to the patient's airway by a resistor valve to control airflow, a setup similar to the high-pressure pump used to inflate one's car tires at a filling station. In this idealized system, flow is held constant, and the intrapulmonary pressure at any given instant depends on the resistance and compliance of the lungs. The lungs (like car tires) are not allowed to reach equilibrium with the high-pressure tanks.

These two idealized systems are, of course, too cumbersome and inflexible for actual clinical use. However, modern ventilator modalities simulate either one of these two basic models by using microprocessor-controlled valves to regulate the output from high-pressure solenoid pumps. The ventilator generates a "volume-controlled" breath by repetitively sampling the flow it is delivering during inspiration and adjusting the solenoid output to provide a precise flow pattern for a specific duration of time (volume = flow × time). To generate a pressure-controlled breath, the microprocessor samples the pressure it is delivering and adjusts the solenoid pump output to achieve and maintain a constant pressure in the airways.

During any single breath, the ventilator may control airway pressure (PC) or airflow (VC), but not both simultaneously. However, a ventilator mode entitled "volume-targeted pressure control" or "pressure-regulated volume control" is designed to provide the benefits of both PC and VC. In this mode, any single inhalation is a pressure-controlled breath, so the airflow and volume during that inhalation depend on the patient's characteristics. However, the amount of pressure is adjusted from breath to breath in order to target a specific tidal volume. The clinician sets a target volume, similar to VC. The ventilator targets this volume during each breath by adjusting the pressure-control setting up or down according to the tidal volumes delivered during the previous few breaths. This mode enhances the ventilator's synchrony with the patient's ventilatory muscles, as does PC, and also promotes the delivery of specified tidal volumes, as does VC.

As modern ventilators develop faster methods of monitoring and adjusting their output, as well as more complete control over airway pressure and flow, they increase their versatility and applicability to a variety of clinical needs. For example, if a patient who coughs or "bucks" when an older-style ventilator is delivering an inhaled breath (in pressure-control or volume-control mode), the airway pressure may rise rapidly, exposing the lungs to barotrauma before the ventilator detects the high pressure and ends the breath. Modern ventilators, however, can adapt to rapid changes in lung compliance (such as coughing or bucking) by (1) increasing the rapidity with which the flow and pressure in the airway is monitored and (2) using the microprocessor to constantly adjust both the inhalation valves and exhalation valves in the airway circuit without ending the inspired breath. Thus, barotrauma is minimized, minute ventilation is preserved, and the work of breathing is reduced.

BREATH SEQUENCE IN MANDATORY VENTILATION

Ventilator modes also differ in scheduling when mandatory breaths (driven entirely by the ventilator) are given. Mandatory breaths can be delivered at a set rate (controlled*) or they may be triggered by the patient's effort (assisted). With intermittent mandatory ventilation (IMV) or synchronized intermittent mandatory ventilation (SIMV), mandatory breaths are delivered only at specific time intervals, resulting in a set number of breaths per minute. With continuous mandatory ventilation (CMV) or assist/control (AC), the ventilator assists with a mandatory breath every spontaneous inhalation effort that it detects. In addition, if the patient does not trigger an assisted breath within a specified time interval, the machine delivers a mandatory breath, similar to IMV. In CMV or AC, the patient may receive some combination of assisted and controlled breaths, depending on set ventilator rate and his own intrinsic respiratory rate. Patients receiving only assisted (self-initiated) breaths may become fatigued because, although assisting the breath decreases the work of breathing, it does not entirely rest the ventilatory muscles. Once the diaphragm begins an inhalation, it continues to contract throughout the entire inspiratory cycle. One approach to resting the diaphragm is to set the ventilator rate such that a majority of breaths are controlled (machine initiated).

Whatever modality is chosen, matching the ventilator response to the patient's demand reduces the work performed by the respiratory muscles and may prevent respiratory muscle fatigue. The patient perceives the ventilator's response on each breath in four ways: (1) the energy necessary to begin inspiratory flow, (2) the rate at which inspiration flow actually occurs given the level of muscle effort expended, (3) the duration of inspiratory flow (inspiratory time), and (4) the volume inspired. When the response of the ventilator fails to match the patient's demand in one or

---

Unfortunately, the term "control" has two unrelated meanings in ventilator literature. "Volume control" and "pressure control" refer to the adjustment of airflow and pressure, respectively, during inhalation. When referring to breath sequencing, a "controlled" breath is one initiated by the ventilator, independent of any triggering by the patient."

more of these aspects, the work performed by the patient increases, the ventilatory drive increases, and the patient becomes uncomfortable and may begin to fight the mechanical ventilator.

TRIGGERING INHALATION

Mechanical ventilators differ in their responsiveness to patient effort in their inspiratory triggering mechanisms, their inspiratory demand values, and their mechanisms of ending the inspired breath. When a mechanical ventilator is assisting the patient's breath, it must "sense" that the patient has begun inhaling and initiate the machine-driven breath using an inspiratory triggering mechanism. For many ventilators, the breath is triggered once the patient's spontaneous efforts exceed a preset negative pressure. For earlier generations of mechanical ventilators, this threshold was –2 cm H_2O or more. Newer generations of mechanical ventilators have thresholds that can be set as slow as –0.5 cm H_2O. In addition, ventilators also can be triggered by a drop in the flow passing by the endotracheal tube. Flow triggering may make the ventilator more sensitive to the patient's inspiratory effort and, by using software to drive the pressure at the airway opening to a slightly positive value, further reduces patient work during spontaneous breathing. The result is a virtual elimination of the ventilatory work added by the mechanical ventilator circuit during spontaneous breathing.

The work performed by the patient increases when the flow provided by the mechanical ventilator lags behind that demanded by the patient. Inspiratory demand valves on older models of many mechanical ventilators required greater effort to produce higher flows. More recently, ventilator inspiratory flow valves have been designed to increase flows with much smaller effort.

DURATION OF INHALATION AND EXHALATION

Modern ventilators also may vary the duration of the inspiratory and expiratory phases of breathing to suit the needs of the patient. Conscious patients, for example, tolerate mechanical ventilation more readily with relatively brief inhalation times, allowing more time for exhalation (similar to the normal cadence of spontaneous breathing). However, if severe hypoxemia occurs, the patient may require long inspiratory and short expiratory times: a reversal of the normal inspiratory-to-expiratory (I/E) time ratio, termed *inverse ratio ventilation* (IRV). The IRV mode is commonly used with pressure-controlled ventilation, but can be used with volume control as well. The inspiratory time, respiratory rate, and I/E ratio are, of course, interdependent. Some ventilators allow the setting of two parameters (such as I/E and rate) directly; the other parameter is adjusted as needed. Because IRV so distorts the normal pattern of ventilation, the patient usually requires sedation, neuromuscular blockade, or both to avoid patient–ventilator dyssynchrony. This mode of ventilation is able to achieve acceptable levels of arterial oxygenation at lower peak and end-expiratory airway pressure. It remains controversial whether this effect is the result of the inspiratory pressure plateau preventing alveolar collapse or whether the short expiratory times, which do not allow expiration flow to finish before inspiration begins, simply provide PEEP at the alveolar level that is not measured at the airway opening (alveolar or intrinsic PEEP).

PEEP

During exhalation, the ventilator may either allow the lungs to reach atmospheric pressure or it may provide a continuous source of positive pressure throughout exhalation (positive end-expiratory pressure, or PEEP). The most common use of PEEP is to prevent damaged alveoli from collapsing during exhalation, increasing the proportion of ventilated lung units and decreasing the amount of shunt. Because a large component of gas exchange dysfunction in lung injury is attributed to intrapulmonary shunting, PEEP may relieve hypoxemia in these cases without requiring the use of high oxygen concentrations. Some clinicians also use PEEP for other uses, such as (1) reducing the work of breathing in patients manifesting intrinsic PEEP from obstructive lung disease; and (2) decreasing intrathoracic venous return (preload) in patients with congestive heart failure.

While the ventilator is in the PEEP mode, pressure support (PS) may be used to reduce inspiration work. PS is triggered by inspiratory efforts in the same way that assisted breaths are triggered. Once this occurs, PS increases the airflow to maintain a positive pressure higher than the PEEP pressure, allowing the ventilator to provide some of the work of inhalation without controlling the patient's breathing pattern.

BILEVEL VENTILATION AND AIRWAY-PRESSURE RELEASE VENTILATION

Bilevel ventilation and airway-pressure release ventilation (APRV) both describe a mode in which mandatory breaths per se are not delivered, but the ventilator alternates between two different pressure levels. The two pressure levels are referred to as $PEEP_{high}$ and $PEEP_{low}$, but the term "PEEP" in this circumstance refers to the ventilator's method of maintaining airway pressure, and does not refer to a particular phase of respiration. As with the PEEP used during mandatory ventilation, spontaneous breathing is permitted, and even encouraged through the use of small amounts of PS.

APRV is a subset of bilevel ventilation in which $PEEP_{high}$ is sustained for a majority of the time, in order to enhance alveolar recruitment and subsequent oxygenation. CO_2 clearance is achieved by periodically releasing the airway pressure down to $PEEP_{low}$, which is typically kept at zero (atmospheric) pressure. After a fraction of a second, before the alveoli have fully equilibrated with the $PEEP_{low}$ pressure, the airway pressure is returned to the $PEEP_{high}$ value and optimal oxygenation resumes. Although this pattern is similar to IRV with PC, APRV has the advantage of permitting spontaneous ventilation throughout the cycle, reducing the requirement for pharmacological paralysis and deep sedation.

HIGH-FREQUENCY OSCILLATING VENTILATION

High-frequency oscillating ventilation (HFOV) is an intriguing form of mechanical ventilation that does not deliver mandatory breaths. As in APRV, maintenance of relatively high mean airway pressures optimizes oxygenation. In HFOV, however, CO_2 clearance without alveolar deflation is achieved by rapid (5–6 Hz) oscillations in airway pressure. Manipulation of the amplitude, frequency, and "inspiratory" proportion of the oscillations may enhance CO_2 clearance. HFOV offers potential physiological benefits in certain cases of severe respiratory failure. However clinical studies have not identified a population in which HFOV consistently provide better outcomes than more conventional forms of mechanical ventilation.

PROPORTIONAL ASSIST VENTILATION

Synchronization between the patient and the mechanical ventilator may be enhanced in a new generation of mechanical ventilators. Complex software algorithms and rapid feedback mechanisms to control airway pressure and flow allow these ventilators a great deal of flexibility to adjust their function to patient demands. One such strategy made possible by these developments is proportional assist ventilation, which is designed to provide a fixed proportion of the energy required for ventilation regardless of the size of the tidal volume generated or minute ventilation required. The energy required to move the respiratory system during ventilation can be divided into that part required to overcome the elastic recoil of the lung and chest wall, and that part required to overcome the resistance to airflow through the airways. A proportional assist mechanical ventilator continuously adjusts the pressure it provides throughout inspiration, calculating at each adjustment both the pressure required to drive the instantaneous airflow and the pressure required to support the current inspired volume. The clinical benefits of proportional assist ventilation and other new modes of mechanical ventilation are unclear and are topics of ongoing research.

FURTHER READING

1. Chatburn RL. Classification of ventilator modes: update and proposal for implementation. *Respir Care.* 2007;52:301–323.

   A useful classification terminology for mechanical ventilators.

2. Chan K, Abraham E. Effects of inverse ratio ventilation on cardiorespiratory parameters in severe respiratory failure. *Chest.* 1992;102:1556.

   In 10 patients with severe respiratory failure, pressure-controlled IRV was associated with significant increases in PaO_2, arterial pH, and mean airway pressure. Significant decreases in pulmonary shunt fraction, $PaCO_2$, and cardiac index were also found in comparison to pressure-controlled ventilation without inverse ratios.

3. Downs J, Klein EF, Desautels D, et al. Intermittent mandatory ventilation: a new approach to weaning patients from mechanical ventilators. *Chest.* 1973;64:331.

   Describes the rationale, circuitry, and advantages of this ventilator mode.

4. Duncan SR, Riak NW, Raffin TA. Inverse ratio ventilation PEEP in disguise. *Chest.* 1987;92:390.

   Editorial that raises the question whether IRV is effective because of prolonged inspiratory plateaus or because of alveolar PEEP.

5. Forese A, Bryan AC. Effects of anesthesia and paralysis on diaphragmatic mechanics in man. *Anesthesiology.* 1974;41:242.

   An often-quoted and controversial paper describing use of a fluoroscopic technique to compare diaphragmatic function in mechanical ventilation and spontaneous ventilation.

6. Hinson JR, Marini JJ. Principles of mechanical ventilator use in respiratory failure. *Annu Rev Med.* 1992;43:341.

   Review of the physiology of respiratory failure and its treatment using mechanical ventilation.

7. MacIntyre NR. Respiratory function during pressure support ventilation. *Chest.* 1986;89:677.

   Pressure support ventilation improves patient comfort, reduces ventilatory work, and tends to normalize the pressure–volume change characteristics of the remaining work of breathing in stable patients recovering from acute respiratory failure.

8. MacIntyre NR. Clinically available new strategies for mechanical ventilatory support. *Chest.* 1993;104:560.

   Recent review of strategies for mechanical ventilation.

9. Marini JJ, Smith TC, Lamb VJ. External work output and force generation during synchronized intermittent mechanical ventilation. *Am Rev Respir Dis.* 1988;138:1169.

   Respiratory muscle work in the synchronized intermittent mechanical ventilation mode is similar for the assisted and the spontaneous breaths.

10. Marini JJ, Rodriguez RM, Lamb VJ. The inspiration workload of patient-initiated mechanical ventilation. *Am Rev Respir Dis.* 1986;134:902.

    Substantial respiratory muscle effort occurs in patients on mechanical ventilators even when the ventilator is set to assist each breath, particularly for older ventilators with less responsive inspiratory flow values.

11. Slutsky AS. Non-conventional methods of ventilation. *Am Rev Respir Dis.* 1988;138:175.

    An excellent review of apneic oxygenation, high-frequency ventilation, and low-frequency positive pressure ventilation with extracorporeal carbon dioxide removal.

12. Suter PM, Fairley HB, Isenberg MD. Effect of tidal volume and positive end-expiratory pressure on compliance during mechanical ventilation. *Chest.* 1978;73:158.

    During mechanical ventilation, both static and dynamic lung compliance are affected by changes in tidal volume and PEEP. Measurements of lung compliance must be made at constant mechanical ventilation settings.

13. Tharratt RS, Roblee PA, Albertson TE. Pressure controlled inverse ratio ventilation in severe adult respiratory failure. *Chest.* 1988;94:755.

    A description of this mode of mechanical ventilation in comparison to conventional ventilation with results that suggest that comparable gas exchange can be achieved with lower minute volume, peak airway pressure, and PEEP.

14. Tobin MJ. Mechanical ventilation. *N Engl J Med.* 1994;330:1056.

    An excellent review of mechanical ventilation.

15. Putensen C, Mutz NI, Putensen-Himmer G, et al. Spontaneous breathing during ventilatory support improves ventilation-perfusion distributions in patients with acute respiratory distress syndrome. *Am J Respir Crit Care Med.* 1999;159:1241–1248.

    Spontaneous breathing, as permitted during airway-pressure release ventilation, may provide physiological benefits to patients, such as improved matching of ventilation and perfusion as well as higher RVEDV, SV, CI, PaO_2, DO_2, and PvO_2. However, the effect on clinical outcome is not as well established.

16. Sydow M, Burchardi H, Ephraim E, et al. Long-term effects of two different ventilatory modes on oxygenation in acute lung injury. Comparison of airway pressure release ventilation and volume-controlled inverse ratio ventilation. *Am J Respir Crit Care Med.* 1994;149(6):1550–1556.

    Hemodynamic variables and oxygen uptake was similar during both ventilatory modes. However, APRV allowed lower sedation and spontaneous breathing. In addition, there was physiological evidence of progressive alveolar recruitment over 24 hours during ventilation with APRV.

17. Derdak S, Mehta S, Stewart TE, et al. High-frequency oscillatory ventilation for acute respiratory distress syndrome in adults: a randomized, controlled trial. *Am J Respir Crit Care Med.* 2002;166(6):801–808.

    High-frequency oscillatory ventilation used higher applied mean airway pressure than conventional ventilation and showed an early improvement in oxygenation that did not persist beyond the first day. No significant differences in subsequent oxygenation, mortality, hemodynamic variables, ventilation failure, barotraumas, or mucus plugging compared to conventional ventilation.

18. Hurst JM, Branson RD, Davis K Jr, et al. Comparison of conventional mechanical ventilation and high-frequency ventilation. A prospective, randomized trial in patients with respiratory failure. *Ann Surg.* 1990;211(4):486–491.

    Outcomes of acute respiratory failure were comparable between high-frequency oscillatory ventilation and conventional mandatory ventilation.

19. Younes M. Proportional assist ventilation: a new approach to ventilatory support. *Am Rev Respir Dis.* 1992;145:114.

    Presents the theoretic justification for proportional assist ventilation and an experimental prototype to implement this form of ventilation.

20. Younes M, Puddy A, Roberts D, et al. Proportional assist ventilation: results of an initial clinical trial. *Am Rev Respir Dis.* 1992;145:121.

    Proportional assist mechanical ventilation was well tolerated in four patients with a 50% reduction in peak airway pressure and a reduction in the spontaneous respiratory rate when compared to synchronized intermittent mechanical ventilation.

Mechanical Ventilation: Complications and Discontinuation

Timothy A. Morris

Mechanical ventilation itself poses an increased risk for serious complications and should be discontinued as soon as it is safe to do so. Unnecessarily prolonged mechanical ventilation may be minimized by (1) frequently assessing the ventilated patient to determine when the patient is capable of breathing without mechanical assistance and (2) progressing the transition to unassisted breathing as rapidly as tolerated by the patient. The term *weaning*, which implies a mandatory stepwise reduction in support, is more appropriately referred to as *liberation* from mechanical ventilation, which implies no such requirement.

In general, the reasons for mechanical ventilation dictate both the complications of mechanical ventilation and the method of liberation. Patients are placed on mechanical ventilators because of (1) failure to maintain adequate arterial oxygenation on supplemental oxygen, (2) failure to maintain adequate alveolar ventilation (excrete carbon dioxide), or (3) therapeutic objectives not directly related to gas exchange (e.g., hyperventilation for head trauma, paralysis for tetanus). More than one indication may coexist; however, one indication usually predominates.

COMPLICATIONS

Complications associated with endotracheal intubation are common to all ventilated patients and include sinusitis, laryngeal injury, and tracheomalacia (see Chapter 33). In addition, patients with hypoxic ventilatory failure are at higher risk because they often require high fractional inspiratory oxygen concentrations (FiO_2) and elevated peak and end-expiratory ventilatory pressures. The inhalation of an FiO_2 above 0.5 for extended periods of time increases the risk of oxygen toxicity and pulmonary fibrosis. The use of an FiO_2 of 1.0 (i.e., 100% oxygen) can result in an increased shunt fraction because of resorption atelectasis involving segments of the lung containing low ventilation–perfusion ($\dot{V}/\dot{Q}$) units.

Hemodynamic Compromise and Barotrauma

Hemodynamic compromise and barotrauma are associated with high inspiratory and expiratory pressures. High inspiratory pressure and positive end-expiratory pressure (PEEP) may unpredictably diminish cardiac output and blood pressure. Although PEEP typically reduces intrapulmonary shunting due to alveolar collapse, it also may lead to (1) a fall in left ventricular compliance and right atrial venous return; (2) an increase or decrease in pulmonary vascular resistance; and (3) overdistention and injury of unimpaired ("normal") alveolar units. The net effect on cardiac output and gas exchange is usually impossible to predict for an individual patient. Therefore, some patients with severe hypoxic ventilatory failure who receive high levels of PEEP may benefit from systemic arterial and pulmonary artery catheterization for repeated measurements of hemodynamic parameters and gas tensions. However, these invasive methods of hemodynamic monitoring carry their own complication risks, which must be weighed against their potential to guide PEEP, intravascular volume expansion, and drug therapy. When hemodynamic stability and oxygen delivery can be achieved, efforts should be aimed at decreasing the FiO_2 to a safer level (below 0.7).

Hemodynamic compromise also may occur in the setting of an increase in intrathoracic pressure inherent in mechanical ventilation by reducing the venous return from the rest of the body and, in some cases, by decreasing ventricular filling and cardiac output. Naturally, patients with low venous pressure or tenuous right ventricular function are especially vulnerable to this effect, while volume expansion may help mitigate it. Patients with obstructive diseases such as chronic obstructive pulmonary disease (COPD) and asthma are at particular risk for hemodynamic deterioration from intrathoracic pressure increases during mechanical ventilation. Those patients may be incapable of fully exhaling during the ventilator cycle, and can build up dangerous levels of end-expiratory pressure, termed "intrinsic PEEP" or "auto-PEEP." Although difficult to measure precisely, intrinsic PEEP is often reflected on the ventilator's flow-time graph by the failure of the expiratory flow to return to zero prior to the initiation of the next inhalation.

The risk of barotrauma in mechanically ventilated patients is high and correlates with mean and peak airway pressures. Pneumothorax may be unpredictable in presentation. A tension pneumothorax, in which the intrapleural pressure becomes markedly positive, may cause catastrophic vascular collapse. However, a pneumothorax also may be manifest as a subtle radiographic finding because of the limited potential for some severely damaged lungs to collapse. The presence of a chest tube (either prophylactic or therapeutic) does not guarantee that another pneumothorax will not develop in the same hemithorax; in fact, patients with severe adult respiratory distress syndrome (ARDS) may require multiple chest tubes bilaterally. If a bronchopleural fistula develops, ventilation may be further compromised. Patients with hypoxic ventilatory failure are at increased risk for barotrauma; this is probably related to localized differentials in alveolar pressure and distention, rather than to absolute transpulmonary pressure. The markedly distorted lung architecture in these patients may lead to barotrauma at much lower pressures.

Although it occurs less abruptly than barotraumas, damage to alveoli from repeated overinflation during mechanical ventilation ("volutrauma") is arguably a much higher risk for patients with acute lung injury or ARDS (see Chapter 67). The insidious and progressive damage to the lungs by volutrauma is illustrated by the higher mortality observed in the multicenter ARDS-net trial for patients ventilated with higher tidal volumes, despite the fact that their oxygenation was significantly better early-on than those ventilated with lower tidal volumes.

Infection

Intubated patients of all types are at an increased risk of infection. Bacterial overgrowth of gastric contents, following adjustment of gastric pH with antacid or H_2-blocking agents, is a major source of nosocomial pneumonias. Whether the risk can be minimized by substitution of sucralfate for these agents as prophylaxis for gastric bleeding remains controversial. Malnutrition can be a major problem in patients requiring prolonged ventilatory support. Nutritional support should begin as soon as possible in any patient in whom prolonged ventilatory support is contemplated.

In some mechanically ventilated patients, respiratory complications are related to the therapeutic modalities that necessitated mechanical ventilation, rather than to the ventilator per se. Some of these patients enter the intensive care unit (ICU) with relatively normal lungs. Paralyzed patients, for example, are at very high risk if disconnected from mechanical ventilation, even briefly. Appropriate safeguards, including carefully tested apneic alarms, should be initiated in this situation. The application of barbiturate coma for head trauma patients, particularly in conjunction with rigorous maintenance of the head-up posture, may lead to problems maintaining bronchial secretion clearance, even in patients with normal lungs. This group may develop lobar collapse and Gram-negative pneumonia if careful prophylactic measures are not initiated (see Chapter 12).

In addition to respiratory complications, patients on mechanical ventilation also may experience cardiac arrhythmias, seizures, and gastrointestinal bleeding. Arrhythmias may be related to hypoxemia, hypokalemia, or other electrolyte disturbances and the use of drugs (e.g., beta agonists, aminophylline) with an arrhythmogenic potential. Seizures may occur because of hypoxemia, rapid reversion of chronic hypercapnia, or drugs such as theophylline. Gastrointestinal bleeding from gastritis or frank gastric ulceration is common; however, the mechanisms responsible are not clear. Antacids and H_2-receptor blockers appear to reduce the incidence of bleeding, particularly in patients with acute central nervous system disease (e.g., head trauma, cerebrovascular accidents).

DISCONTINUATION

Mechanical ventilation should be discontinued as soon as it is safe to do so. Although this usually requires the reversal, to some degree, of the primary causes for mechanical ventilation, the causes need not be entirely resolved before patients can be safely extubated. The phrase *liberation from mechanical ventilation* has largely replaced the term *weaning* to describe the process of ventilator discontinuation, in recognition that gradual tapering of ventilator support is typically not necessary. Procedures to liberate patients from mechanical ventilation have the general purpose of assuring the medical team that mechanical ventilation is no longer necessary. Somewhat more controversial is the potential for the process to gradually train the respiratory muscles in some patients to assume the entire work of breathing.

As much as 40% of the time on mechanical ventilation is spent after gas exchange itself has improved to the point that spontaneous breathing could be possible. Methods to decrease the time it takes to liberate patients from mechanical ventilation may reduce complication rates and save considerable expense. Timing is a major issue. The patient who is extubated too early, requiring reintubation, is subject to difficulties obtaining an airway, laryngeal injury, aspiration pneumonia, and cardiac ischemia, all of which lead to a higher mortality. Conversely, the patient who is left on mechanical ventilation too long risks nosocomial pneumonia, tracheal injury, and the other complications mentioned.

Successful extubation requires that the work required for breathing be substantially less than the capacity to breathe. The work of breathing depends on factors such as (1) the amount of gas exchange required, which in turn depends on O_2 consumption and CO_2 production; (2) gas exchange efficiency, including the (A–a) O_2 gradient and $\dot{V}_D/\dot{V}_T$; and (3) the physical work required to inflate the lungs, such as lung and chest wall compliance. The capacity to breathe, in turn, depends on (1) neurologic mechanisms to control breathing, (2) respiratory muscle strength, and (3) endurance. Despite a great deal of clinical investigation, it is still difficult to predict when the balance of these factors permits discontinuation of mechanical ventilation in particular patients.

Indications

The good news for clinicians is that complex, time-consuming, and often inconsistent methods of weaning are largely being replaced by simpler algorithms that are at least as effective. In our center, we use a protocol represented by the acronym STEER, for *s*creening, *t*esting, *e*xercising, *e*valuating and *r*eporting on the progress of patients being liberated from mechanical ventilation. Essential to the process is the classification of patients into one of four basic categories: (1) those in whom immediate extubation is likely to be successful; (2) those in whom weaning is progressing toward the goal of extubation; (3) those who are not progressing, in whom further investigation is necessary; and (4) those in whom weaning of any type is contraindicated.

Screen: The first step is to identify patients in whom initiation of the liberation process would likely cause harm (described above as category 4). This group generally has one or more of the following problems: (1) inadequate gas exchange, evidenced by a low Po_2/Fio_2 ratio or the requirement for high levels of PEEP; (2) inability to cough or clear secretions during spontaneous breathing; (3) instability such as shock or hypotension; (4) severe muscle weakness or paralysis; (5) sedation or obtundation; (6) major procedures planned in the near future; (7) unstable myocardial ischemia; or (8) elevated intracranial pressure. Patients with these contraindications to weaning are monitored daily for signs of their resolution. Others begin the process of liberation. This aggressive approach is safe and shortens the duration of mechanical ventilation.

Test: The next step is to distinguish those patients who are ready for immediate discontinuation of mechanical ventilation from those in whom intermediate steps are necessary. The patient's respiratory performance (while receiving minimal support from the ventilator) may predict when extubation will be tolerated. A variety of "weaning parameters" have become popular, such as minute ventilation, respiratory rate, and inspiratory pressures. A simple and accurate predictor is the "rapid shallow breathing index," representing the ratio of the respiratory rate to the tidal volume ($f/\dot{V}_T$). Our preference is to test the $f/\dot{V}_T$ during brief periods of spontaneous breathing (on T-piece or with low amount of pressure support) at least once daily. Patients with low $f/\dot{V}_T$ ratios are allowed to continue spontaneous breathing and, if they tolerate the "sprint" for 1 to 2 hours, are extubated. Those in whom the initial $f/\dot{V}_T$ is high require further steps to be liberated from mechanical ventilation.

Exercise: For those patients who cannot be extubated immediately, intermediate steps may be necessary. Whether the patient's performance during these weaning steps is the cause of or the result of improved respiratory status is controversial. Options include (1) periodically "sprinting" the patient with intervals where the ventilator provides lower levels of assistance, using IMV, pressure support, or T-piece with humidified oxygen flowing past; or (2) intermittently decreasing the assistance from the ventilator allowing the patient to gradually assume the burden of ventilation, using IMV, pressure support, or a combination. Although there is no general consensus on the relative merits of these two strategies, recent evidence appears to favor periodic sprinting.

Evaluate: Whatever the modality chosen, a few points should be considered when designing a weaning program. First, patients may improve faster than expected, and any liberation process should include processes to identify those who have developed the ability to breathe without mechanical assistance. Conversely, during the sprint, the patient should not be allowed to work the respiratory muscles to exhaustion, because a prolonged period of rest may then be necessary before the next attempt. If possible, the intensity of each sprint should be more demanding than the previous one, until the patient is eventually performing unassisted spontaneous ventilation. Finally, the clinician must routinely evaluate the patients' progress during weaning, and identify those who are not advancing toward extubation (category 3).

Report: The STEER protocol ensures that the clinician is expeditiously informed when the patients is capable of spontaneous ventilation, and can be extubated. On the other hand, patients who fail to progress during weaning can be systematically evaluated to disclose any reversible causes of prolonged dependency on the ventilator (see "Procedure" section).

Procedure

The STEER protocol is best begun early in the morning when the patient is rested and the ICU staff count is maximal. The patient should be observed clinically and with oximetry. Clinical evidence of respiratory muscle fatigue includes tachycardia, an increase in the respiratory rate to 35 or above, or complaints of severe dyspnea. In most patients, these signs indicate the need to return to the prior level of ventilatory support regardless of blood gases. However, a PaO_2 of less than 60 mmHg or a pH less than 7.25 is also an indication to stop the weaning interval.

Psychological factors can be a major problem for some patients during weaning. An attempt should be made to carefully explain to the patient the weaning process and the likely sensations. The development of trust between the patient and staff is particularly important. Continued reassurance and confidence often achieve the best results.

Failure to advance toward liberation from the ventilator (category 3) typically can be traced to insufficiencies of gas exchange, ventilatory drive, muscle strength, or endurance. In general, a PaO_2 greater than 60 mmHg on 35% oxygen or less should be enough to permit spontaneous breathing. True neurologic abnormalities of ventilatory drive are rare and, when present, are usually inconsistent with successful weaning. However, secondary abnormalities of respiratory drive are common and usually reversible. The most common secondary abnormalities are metabolic alkalosis and oversedation. One hallmark of a suppressed respiratory drive is the presence of an elevated $PaCO_2$ during weaning without a corresponding increase in respiratory rate. Mechanical advantage and muscle strength also are critical to successful weaning, and should be considered in relation to the work the muscles are obligated to perform. The maximum inspiratory pressure (MIP) is a simple measure of muscle strength, and the peak pressure needed by the ventilator to move a tidal volume breath provides a gross approximation of the work the muscles will have to perform. Useful rules of thumb are that the MIP should equal the ventilatory peak pressure and that the vital capacity should at least equal the tidal volume provided by the ventilator.

Careful examination of the patient during the liberation process may help explain the reasons for failure to progress. The pattern of muscle fatigue during weaning is usually characterized by a decreasing tidal volume and an increasing respiratory rate. An important warning sign is the development of paradoxical motion of chest and abdomen, in which the abdomen moves inward during inspiration, suggesting diaphragmatic fatigue. These changes may precede $PaCO_2$ elevation and indicate the need to return the patient to a higher level of ventilatory support. A number of factors may contribute to muscle weakness and fatigue: inadequate nutrition, respiratory muscle deconditioning and atrophy, electrolyte depletion (potassium, phosphate, magnesium, and calcium), hormonal imbalance (thyroid or steroid), neural and neuromuscular lesions (including spinal cord lesions), and increased lung volume. Many of these problems are easily detected once they are considered. Correcting them can make a profound difference in a patient's ability to be liberated from mechanical ventilation.

FURTHER READING

1. Antonelli M, Moro ML, Capelli O, et al. Risk factors for early onset pneumonia in trauma patients. *Chest.* 1994;105(1):224–228.

   In 124 trauma patients, combined severe abdominal and thoracic trauma represented a major risk factor for early-onset pneumonia. Mechanical ventilation administered during the first days after trauma seems to reduce the risk of early-onset pneumonia. Mechanical ventilatory support lasting more than 5 days is associated with an increased risk of late-onset pneumonia.

2. Beach T, Millen E, Grenvik A. Hemodynamic response to discontinuance of mechanical ventilation. *Crit Care Med.* 1973;1(2):85–90.

   Approximately 50% of cases showed an increase and 50% showed a decrease in cardiac output, possibly reflecting differences in "myocardial reserve."

3. Bellemare F, Grassino A. Evaluation of human diaphragm fatigue. *J Appl Physiol.* 1982;53(5): 1196–1206.

   Two determinants of respiratory muscle fatigue are the percentage of time spent in inspiration (Ti/Tt) and the strength of muscle contraction on a breath as a fraction of maximal contraction.

4. Craven DE, Kunches LM, Kilinsky V, et al. Risk factors for pneumonia and fatality in patients receiving continuous mechanical ventilation. *Am Rev Respir Dis*. 1986;133(5):792–796.

The use of H_2-blocking agents increased the risk of nosocomial pneumonia, possibly by altering the pH of the stomach contents in patient on mechanical ventilation.

5. Douglass JA, Tuxen DV, Horne M, et al. Myopathy in severe asthma. *Am Rev Respir Dis*. 1992;146(2):517–519.

In 19 of 25 (76%) patients mechanically ventilated for exacerbation of asthma who received corticosteroids and aminophylline intravenously and salbutamol both nebulized and intravenously, there was elevation of creatine kinase (CK) levels to a median of 1,575 U/L, occurring 3.6 ± 1.5 days after admission. In nine patients, there was clinically detectable myopathy. The presence of either myopathy or CK enzyme rise was associated with a significant prolongation of ventilation time.

6. Elpern EH, Scott MG, Petro L, et al. Pulmonary aspiration in mechanically ventilated patients with tracheostomies. *Chest*. 1994;105(2):563–566.

Feeding-related aspiration is seen frequently in patients with tracheostomies receiving prolonged positive pressure mechanical ventilation. Advanced age increases the risk of aspiration in this population, and episodes of aspiration are not consistently accompanied by clinical symptoms of distress to alert the bedside observer to their occurrence.

7. Ely EW, Baker AM, Dunagan DP, et al. Effect on the duration of mechanical ventilation of identifying patients capable of breathing spontaneously. *N Engl J Med*. 1996;335(25):1864–1869.

8. Esteban A, Alia I, Ibanez J, et al; The Spanish Lung Failure Collaborative Group. Modes of mechanical ventilation and weaning. A national survey of Spanish hospitals. *Chest*. 1994;106(4):1188–1193.

Weaning may account for more than 40% of the time patients spend on mechanical ventilation.

9. Esteban A, Frutos F, Tobin MJ, et al; Spanish Lung Failure Collaborative Group. A comparison of four methods of weaning patients from mechanical ventilation. *N Engl J Med*. 1995;332(6): 345–350.

10. Esteban A, Alia I, Tobin MJ, et al; Spanish Lung Failure Collaborative Group. Effect of spontaneous breathing trial duration on outcome of attempts to discontinue mechanical ventilation. *Am J Respir Crit Care Med*. 1999;159(2):512–518.

Thirty-minute sprints may be just as good a test as 2-hour sprints for predicting the ability to tolerate discontinuing mechanical ventilation.

11. Field S, Kelly SM, Macklem PT. The oxygen cost of breathing in patients with cardiorespiratory disease. *Am Rev Respir Dis*. 1982;126(1):9–13.

The average oxygen cost of taking over spontaneous ventilation was 75 mL of oxygen per minute and ranged up to 286 mL/min.

12. Mitsuoka M, Kinninger KH, Johnson FW, et al. Utility of measurements of oxygen cost of breathing in predicting success or failure in trials of reduced mechanical ventilatory support. *Respir Care*. 2001;46(9):902–910.

13. Gandia F, Blanco J. Evaluation of indexes predicting the outcome of ventilator weaning and value of adding supplemental inspiratory load. *Intensive Care Med*. 1992;18(6):327–333.

The ratio of inspiratory airway occlusion pressure at 0.1 second to MIP and the ratio of respiratory frequency to tidal volume were accurate, early predictors of weaning outcome.

14. Gracey DR, Viggiano RW, Naessens JM, et al. Outcomes of patients admitted to a chronic ventilator-dependent unit in an acute-care hospital. *Mayo Clin Proc*. 1992;67(2):131–136.

The outcomes in 61 patients admitted to a chronic ventilator-dependent unit are reviewed. Of 58 who survived, 53 weaned from the mechanical ventilator and 35 were discharged home (5 of these patients required nocturnal mechanical ventilation). COPD was the most common reason for admission to the unit.

15. Kumar A, Pontoppidan H, Falke KJ, et al. Pulmonary barotrauma during mechanical ventilation. *Crit Care Med*. 1973;1(4):181–186.

Pulmonary barotrauma (e.g., pneumothorax, pneumomediastinum, subcutaneous emphysema) correlated with the presence of chronic lung disease and with peak airway pressure (>35 cm H_2O), but not with PEEP per se.

16. Laggner AN, Tryba M, Georgopoulos A, et al. Oropharyngeal decontamination with gentamicin for long-term ventilated patients on stress ulcer prophylaxis with sucralfate? *Wien Klin Wochenschr.* 1994;106(1):15–19.

    Despite reduction of bacterial colonization rates of pharyngeal and tracheal secretions, gentamicin administered topically to the oropharynx did not seem to offer additional clinical benefits in long-term mechanically ventilated patients on stress ulcer prophylaxis with sucralfate.

17. Liebler JM, Benner K, Putnam T, et al. Respiratory complications in critically ill medical patients with acute upper gastrointestinal bleeding. *Crit Care Med.* 1991;19(9):1152–1157.

    Respiratory complications occurred during 22% of serious upper gastrointestinal bleeding episodes.

18. Pingleton SK, Hinthorn DR, Liu C. Enteral nutrition in patients receiving mechanical ventilation. Multiple sources of tracheal colonization include the stomach. *Am J Med.* 1986;80(5):827–832.

    Seventy-five percent of the bacteria contaminating the respiratory tract originated in the oropharynx or stomach and suggests that the high gastric pH due to tube feeding may increase gastric colonization.

19. Prod'hom G, Leuenberger P, Koerfer J, et al. Nosocomial pneumonia in mechanically ventilated patients receiving antacid, ranitidine, or sucralfate as prophylaxis for stress ulcer. A randomized controlled trial. *Ann Intern Med.* 1994;120(8):653–662.

    Stress ulcer prophylaxis with sucralfate reduces the risk for late-onset pneumonia in ventilated patients compared with antacid or ranitidine.

20. Rouby JJ, Lherm T, Martin de Lassale E, et al. Histologic aspects of pulmonary barotrauma in critically ill patients with acute respiratory failure. *Intensive Care Med.* 1993;19(7):383–389.

    Air space enlargement, defined as the presence of either alveolar overdistention in aerated lung areas or intraparenchymal pseudocysts in nonaerated lung areas, was found in 26 of 30 lungs of young critically ill patients (mean age, 34 ± 10 years) that were histologically examined in the immediate postmortem period. Patients with severe air space enlargement had a significantly greater incidence of pneumothorax, were ventilated using higher peak airway pressures and tidal volumes, were exposed significantly longer to toxic levels of oxygen, and lost more weight than patients with mild air space enlargement.

21. Tobin MJ, Guenther SM, Perez W, et al. Konno-Mead analysis of ribcage-abdominal motion during successful and unsuccessful trials of weaning from mechanical ventilation. *Am Rev Respir Dis.* 1987;135(6):1320–1328.

    Paradoxical motion of the rib cage and abdomen can occur due to increased airway resistance or decreased compliance and is not specific for respiratory muscle fatigue. Asynchronous motion with a phase difference between rib cage and abdominal motion was a more sensitive indicator.

22. Tobin MJ, Perez W, Guenther SM, et al. The pattern of breathing during successful and unsuccessful trials of weaning from mechanical ventilation. *Am Rev Respir Dis.* 1986;134(6):1111–1118.

    Patients who failed a weaning trial developed rapid shallow breathing.

23. Warner MA, Warner ME, Weber JG. Clinical significance of pulmonary aspiration during the perioperative period. *Anesthesiology.* 1993;78(1):56–62.

    Patients with clinically apparent aspiration who do not develop symptoms within 2 hours are unlikely to have respiratory sequelae.

24. Yang KL, Tobin MJ. A prospective study of indexes predicting the outcome of trials of weaning from mechanical ventilation. *N Engl J Med.* 1991;324(21):1445–1450.

    Rapid shallow breathing, reflected by the ratio, was the most accurate predictor of failure, and its absence the most accurate predictor of success, in weaning 64 patients from mechanical ventilation.

25. Zwillich CW, Pierson DJ, Creagh CE, et al. Complications of assisted ventilation. A prospective study of 354 consecutive episodes. *Am J Med.* 1974;57(2):161–170.

    Reports that 314 consecutive patients on mechanical ventilation were studied prospectively for complications. Intubation of right mainstem bronchus, endotracheal tube malfunction, and alveolar hypoventilation were associated with decreased survival.

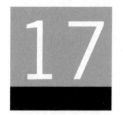

17 Protocol-Driven Care in Respiratory Therapy

Timothy A. Morris and Ford Richard

Patient-driven protocols are a set of medical staff-approved care plans driven by the patient's condition and response to therapy that allow respiratory care practitioners (RCPs) to initiate, change, discontinue, or restart treatments and services. RCPs provide cardiopulmonary interventions and treatment that can improve patient outcomes and reduce morbidity, mortality, and costs. RCPs are licensed within each State to provide treatment, support, and monitoring. The scope of practice for RCPs includes protocol-directed care, however, and requires supervision by a medical director. The medical director is ultimately responsible for the content of protocol-directed care plans and is accountable for the competency of RCPs performing protocol-based treatment. The use of established protocols may help respiratory therapists deliver appropriate and efficient care under conditions of an increased workload. Protocols are based on scientific evidence and include guidelines and options at decision points. The use of protocols can help assure that all treatments have established indicators, but are also highly effective in reducing the volume of unnecessary care. Data suggest that 25% to 60% of respiratory therapy treatments may be misallocated. Evidence-based literature exists supporting the use of protocols to minimize unnecessary treatments and provides self-administration options for patients who demonstrate their ability to do so as documented by the respiratory therapists. It is important to note that numerous studies have concluded that protocols can reduce the volume of unneeded care, and, therefore, contribute to an overall reduction in workload. For patients who require bronchodilator therapy, protocols can be effective in switching patients from small volume nebulizers to the less time-consuming metered dose inhalers administered via hand-held spacer devices.

Early and sustained experience at the University of California, San Diego (UCSD) demonstrated that when protocols were implemented in 1993, up to 60% reduction occurred in routine medicated aerosol and chest physiotherapy. Such reductions are attributed to reducing variation in treatment, providing guidelines for medical necessity, allowing the RCP to refine the care plan based on response to therapy, and providing the RCP with guidelines on when it is imperative to contact the MD when further evaluation is necessary. Although today's healthcare system demands increased efficiency, it is imperative to balance that demand with the need for appropriate, effective, and skilled patient care. In order to provide safe, cost-effective care, the concept of patient-driven protocol evolved.

The success of patient-driven protocols depends on a clear understanding of the elements by all healthcare practitioners charged with implementing them. Protocols ensure that (1) the physician's intentions are realized; (2) care is appropriate, timely, and driven by the patient's condition; (3) lower cost alternatives are implemented when appropriate; and (4) most important, clinical conditions requiring physician notification are clear. Protocols are simply algorithmic paths that specify what care will be delivered, when it will be discontinued or altered, and when the physician will be contacted for changes in management. They cover only those alterations in care that the hospital physicians agree should always occur when the protocol criteria are fulfilled.

Once the physician establishes the need for treatment, protocols provide a means to ensure that what is supposed to happen to the patient does happen. Access to the program may be structured so the physician can request a specific therapy, specific protocol, or simply "respiratory care protocol." If the therapist identifies the opportunity to use a protocol of care that differs from the initial physician request, he or she contacts the physician to review and approve new or additional care plans. The protocols supplement, but never override, physician instructions; orders that deviate from the protocols continue to define the care delivered.

Physicians who use protocols should be familiar with the protocol path or algorithms and understand the ability of the protocol program to achieve the desired outcomes. On the other hand, they should also recognize exceptionally complicated cases for which protocols may be inappropriate. Protocols should contain clear decision points defining when the therapist should apprise the physician of changes in patient status, both directly if there is any acute deterioration in a patient's condition or indirectly for the inability of the patient to achieve the desired outcomes. Advantages to physicians include: (1) the ability to write flexible orders that can adapt to predictable changes in the patient's condition; (2) assurance that the care provided is state of the art; (3) notification when the patient's status changes significantly; (4) freedom from documentation; and (5) the ability to exempt patients who do not fit the protocols.

DEVELOPMENT

In a 1992 consensus paper the American College of Chest Physicians (ACCP) was among the first physician groups to endorse and promote the use of patient-driven protocols. They identified the following elements of successful respiratory care protocols:

1. Clearly stated objectives.
2. Outline of the protocol including a decision tree or algorithm.
3. Description of alternative choices at decision and action points.
4. Description of potential complications and corrections.
5. Description of end points and decision points where the physician must be contacted.

The ACCP also identified that implementation and maintenance of respiratory care protocols requires:

1. Use of written protocols with sound scientific basis.
2. Strong medical director support.
3. Intensive education of RCPs.
4. Medical staff approval and confidence in the protocol.
5. Frequent auditing of outcomes and continuing education.
6. Adjustment of protocol to meet needs and new scientific evidence.

Respiratory care protocols are developed by physicians, RCPs, and other members of the medical team as a group process and depend on a thorough review of published literature and the savvy of experienced clinicians. Tailored to the specifics of each hospital, the protocols reflect the consensus of the medical team regarding the optimal care plans to be used in most cases for specific respiratory conditions. Protocols allow a physician to have active input into evaluation and treatment algorithms, as well as to specify when a protocol should be stopped and when he or she should be notified. The clarity and detail with which these plans are made far exceed what is possible through written orders for each individual patient. Similarly, the respiratory care practitioner becomes much less an "ancillary service" and more an agent of the physician, ensuring that patients receive timely and appropriate interventions as outlined in the protocol. The respiratory care practitioner is trained to evaluate and quantify the physiologic effects of treatment on each patient. Round-the-clock documentation of physiologic parameters can be invaluable to the care of patients with respiratory conditions. Furthermore, the therapist is able to follow a clear consensus plan on how to adjust therapy based on the "real-time" condition of the patient and previous response to treatment.

ADVANTAGES

Although the hospital or department administrator may realize that protocols have the ability to significantly reduce expenses, the creation of respiratory care protocols more than 20 years ago had little to do with cost reduction. The need arose as technology to support mechanical ventilation was developed and devices were designed to treat and support patients with respiratory impairments. As treatment became more complex and dynamic, caring for the respiratory patient was like hitting a moving target. Patient condition changed continuously, requiring ongoing modifications to treatment. The observation and feedback from the bedside therapist became an important asset to the physician, who could not always be in the room.

Initiating and maintaining a respiratory care protocol program requires a team effort among (1) the medical director of respiratory care; (2) a program leader to oversee planning and keep the program on track; (3) interested physicians to plan and utilize the protocols; and (4) the therapists who will execute them. Step-by-step instructions on how to plan and initiate respiratory care protocol programs, as well as detailed examples of specific protocols, are referenced below. The number of protocols implemented and the timeline for program expansion likely depend on the readiness of the respiratory care (RC) department and physician staff. It is essential to provide specific training and competency assessment prior to implementing any protocol. Program development extends well beyond drafting a set of protocols. It includes defining related policies, identifying responsibilities, determining competencies and required training, and establishing mechanisms to monitor activities.

Protocols must be considered statements of what everyone agrees should happen when certain conditions occur. All of the "stakeholders" must be offered the opportunity to modify the protocols prior to acceptance. Although attempts to gain some consensus among physicians in the institution regarding the complex aspects of RC delivery may take considerable time (4–12 months), the early "buy-in" is critical. All suggestions should be incorporated or addressed in some way. All applicable medical staff committees should review protocols in the developmental stage, and a one-on-one conference should be conducted with key stakeholders to foster the support needed for implementation. An understanding of the medical center environment, medical staff objectives, and incentives for change may assist in developing a strategy to gain medical staff support of protocols.

CONSIDERATIONS

Many barriers are encountered during implementation of complex programs such as these. Despite known benefits of protocol-driven care, therapists can view them as too much work and physicians can perceive them as loss of control over the patient. Such barriers need to be addressed and can be overcome through education, participation, and sharing in the positive outcomes of the program. Establishing a high level of support and intrinsic motivation among RC staff is the most important aspect of implementation and can also be the most difficult, particularly in a program that demands that the therapists learn new skills, enhance communication abilities, and adapt to change. Workgroups and teams consisting of members of the department accelerates planning and implementation.

The adage that "the best evidence of life is growth" is particularly true for RC protocols. To be effective and to reflect the true state of the art in therapy, the protocols must be regularly reappraised. The protocols must be routinely updated as new medical information relevant to RC becomes available. In addition, routine feedback from physicians and other staff members during protocol updating helps to ensure that the protocols remain practical while fostering communication with the entire healthcare team.

Overall, the available evidence regarding RC protocols suggests that they can confer several benefits, including (1) Enhanced allocation of RC services, including arterial blood gas (ABG) sampling, arterial line placement, use of supplemental oxygen, bronchial hygiene therapies, and bronchodilators. The advantage of enhanced allocation can be achieved either by implementing protocols for individual respiratory treatments or by using a comprehensive protocol service, in which protocols guide the choice of respiratory treatments and the specific RC plan. (2) In the case of weaning, protocols can accelerate patients' liberation from mechanical ventilation, with associated benefits of shorter ICU stay and cost savings. As hospitals continue to struggle with the myriad of challenges they face as a result of the nation's continuing healthcare crises, protocol-based care offers a refreshing and practical strategy for improving the level and intensity of all RC services.

FURTHER READING

1. American Association for Respiratory Care. 2011. Resources for Patient-Driven Protocols. http://www.aarc.org/resources/protocols.
2. AARC Position Statement. Respiratory Therapy Protocol: position statement. May 16, 2001. http://www.aarc.org/resources/position_statements.
3. Kollef MH, Shapiro SD, Clinkscale D, et al. The effect of respiratory therapist-initiated treatment protocols on patient outcomes and resource utilization. *Chest.* 2000;117:467–475.

4. Jasper A, Kahan S, Goldberg H, et al. Cost-benefit comparison of aerosol bronchodilator delivery methods in hospitalized patients. *Chest.* 1987;91:414–418.

5. Stoller JK, Haney D, Burkhart J, et al. Physician-ordered respiratory care vs. physician-ordered use of a respiratory therapy consult service: early experience at The Cleveland Clinic Foundation. *Respir Care.* 1993;38(11):1143–1154.

6. Stoller JK, Mascha EJ, Kester L, et al. Randomized controlled trial of physician-directed versus respiratory therapy consult service-directed respiratory care to adult non-ICU inpatients. *Am J Respir Crit Care Med.* 1998;158:1066–1075

7. Ford RM, Phillips-Clar JE, Burns DM. Implementing therapist-driven protocols. *Respir Care Clin N Am.* 1996;2:51–76.

   Excellent compendium of information, including the rationale for protocols, logistics for implementing them, and legal considerations. The chapter authored by the UCSD team specifically describes the UCSD experience and the results of implementing a hospital-wide program.

8. Burton GG. A short history of therapist-driven respiratory care protocols. *Respir Care Clin N Am.* 1996;2(1):15–26.

   Dr. Burton is credited with creating the first formalized protocols for RC nearly 20 years ago. This lecture provides his unique insight regarding the value of such programs. A tape of this lecture can be obtained from the American Association for Respiratory Care offices in Dallas, Texas.

9. Kester L, Stoller JK. Ordering respiratory care services for hospitalized patients: practices of overuse and underuse. *Cleve Clin J Med.* 1992;59:581–585

   While the focus of protocols is often to reduce unnecessary care, this study found that 20% of patients needed more intensive respiratory treatment. This demonstrates an important aspect of respiratory care "consult services" in recognizing the need for additional interventions.

10. Hess D. The AARC (American Association for Respiratory Care) clinical practice guidelines. *Respir Care.* 1991;36(12):1398–1401.

11. The AARC (American Association for Respiratory Care) clinical practice guidelines *Respir Care.* 1992;37(8):882–922.

    National standards available through American Association for Respiratory Care (AARC) that list the indications, hazards, and considerations in the delivery of many RC procedures. These standards, developed by experts, provide an evidence-based reference to develop protocol programs.

12. Browning JA, Kiaser DL, Durbin CG Jr. The effect of guidelines on the appropriate use of arterial blood gas analysis in the intensive care unit. *Respir Care.* 1989;34:269–276.

    Browning was one of the first to evaluate the impact of RC protocol programs. In an ICU setting, a reduction in the number of blood gases per patient was demonstrated in his early work.

13. Albin RJ, Criner JG, Thomas S, et al. Pattern of non-ICU inpatient supplemental oxygen utilization in a university hospital. *Chest.* 1992;102:1672–1675.

    Demonstrates that programs can be designed specific for oxygen therapy in which respiratory practitioners can insure improved compliance with indications for therapy.

14. Tenholder MF, Bryson MJ, Whitlock WL. A model for conversion from small volume nebulizer to metered dose inhaler aerosol therapy. *Chest.* 1992;101:634–637.

    When lower cost alternatives are available to achieve similar clinical outcomes, they should be considered. This reference is one of the first of many to demonstrate a successful program in which patients were converted from small volume nebulizers to metered dose inhalers.

15. Nielson-Tietsort J, Poole B, Creagh CE, et al. Respiratory care protocol: an approach to in-hospital respiratory therapy. *Respir Care.* 1981;26:430–436.

    Few protocol programs existed in the early 1980s and this review of the impact of such programs suggested that protocols should be the approach to the delivery of RC.

16. Burns DM. When information is key to survival: breathing life into respiratory care. *Healthc Inform.* 1994;11:24–30.

    Protocol programs require that significant information be captured and that reports be available to assist in tracking clinical and cost outcomes. A department information system provides a valuable tool in the development, implementation, and surveillance of protocol programs.

17. Ford R, Phillips J, Burns D. Early results of implementing a patient driven protocol system [abstract]. *Respir Care.* 1993;38:1306.

Significant reductions in both aerosol therapy and CPT were experienced at UCSD within 90 days of implementing protocols on a single Pulmonary Intensive floor. The results of the pilot program are presented.

18. Phillips JE, Ford RM, Morris TA. *UCSD Patient Driven Protocols*. Ann Arbor, MI: Daedalus Enterprises Inc; 1998.

A detailed view of 23 protocols, developed at the UCSD Department of Respiratory Care, including algorithms, policies, and one-page reference guidelines.

19. Burton GG, Tietsort JA. *Therapist-Driven Respiratory Care Protocols: A Practitioner's Guide.* Oregon, OR: Academy Medical Systems; 1993.

Early protocols were assembled from RC departments throughout the country and assembled in this text for review.

20. Stoller J, Kester L, eds. Therapist-driven protocols. *Respir Care Clin N Am.* 1996;2(1, special issue).

This issue is an excellent compendium of information, including the rationale for protocols, the logistics for implementing them, and legal considerations.

21. Durbin CG Jr. 2006 Philip Kittredge Memorial Lecture. What to do when protocols fail. *Respir Care.* 2007;52(3):324–326.

Describe the observations made in centers that have not been successful in implementing protocol systems, the barriers at the physician and practitioner level, and how these barriers can be overcome.

22. Stoller JK. The effectiveness of respiratory care protocols. *Respir Care.* 2004;49(7):761–765.

Provides an overview of the success and impact of protocols and the characteristics and qualities of centers with effective programs. Specifically identifies the evidence-based effectiveness of protocols related to aerosol administration, bronchial hygiene, oxygen administration, and ventilator management.

Techniques for Clinical Quality Improvement and Error Reduction Techniques

Gregory B. Seymann

BACKGROUND

Generations of physicians have been raised with the notion that the practice of medicine is based on science as well as art. This traditional thesis suggests that science provides an understanding of pathophysiology, justifies its application to technology and pharmacology, and enables clinicians to heal patients. The "art of medicine" has been relegated to the individual practitioner who forges a unique relationship with his or her patient, and chooses how best to apply the scientific data to each case. This process has been deemed an "art" ideally practiced by a seasoned clinician who is capable of creating a customized treatment plan.

This conception of the practice of medicine has changed markedly since the Institute of Medicine (IOM) published its seminal report in 1999, *To Err Is Human*, declaring, "medicine is not as safe as it should be—and can be." It referenced two studies suggesting, "At least 44,000 people, and perhaps as many as 98,000 people, die in hospitals each year as a result of medical errors that could have been prevented…," an annual mortality rate that exceeded AIDS or breast cancer. This information awakened the public and the medical community to the fact that despite the exponential increase in the volume of scientific discoveries, the US healthcare system was not performing optimally for all patients.

The early advocates of the patient safety and quality improvement movements realized that the data from the IOM might represent only the tip of the iceberg and suggested that many more nonfatal errors resulting in temporary harm or in "near misses" must go unreported. Subsequently, a follow-up study by the Office of the Inspector General (OIG) in the Department of Health and Human Services disclosed that during the month of October 2008, the adverse event rate among hospitalized Medicare beneficiaries was 27%. Of these events, only 1.5% led to death. The remainder of the events led to serious or temporary harm, or prolongation of the hospital stay. Most importantly, physician reviewers in this study determined that 44% of the events were clearly or likely preventable. These events impacted 270,000 patients per month, at an additional annual cost to Medicare of $4.4 billion.

The nature and frequency of the events defined as "errors" are fairly broad. The OIG study confirmed that, despite significant media attention, drastic errors such as wrong-site surgery remain exceedingly rare. The majority were attributed to medications (e.g., excessive bleeding due to anticoagulants, delirium due to psychoactive drugs, and renal insufficiency due to nephrotoxins). Other studies consistently demonstrate that medical errors commonly involve underuse of interventions proven to be beneficial. McGlynn and colleagues reviewed the care provided to a large, geographically diverse group of patients over a 2-year period. They found that overall adherence to a group of well-developed, standardized measures of quality (e.g., vaccination for influenza in the elderly, treatment of uncontrolled hypertension, treatment of elevated cholesterol in patients with known coronary artery disease) was 54.9%. In other words, patients received evidence-based standard of care approximately half the time. The majority of the deficiencies involved underuse of proven interventions.

The fiscal impact of these errors alone is staggering and has energized the entities that pay for healthcare to call for change. In addition to the $4 billion in expenditures for inpatient medical errors, preventable hospital readmissions cost the US healthcare system $25 billion annually. Increasingly, healthcare advocacy groups, private and public payers have created incentives for hospitals and physicians to improve the quality and safety of patient care.

SYSTEMS IMPROVEMENT: EXAMPLES

Revisiting the concept of the "art of medicine" reveals that its role is more limited than physicians who have been trained to believe. In reviewing some examples of the errors listed above, it is apparent that many interventions that are well-supported by evidence don't reliably reach the patients who need them. Why can't the scientific method be applied to the "art of medicine" too? In other words, rigorous investigation to discover better ways to ensure consistent application of appropriate medical interventions to eligible patients may add as much benefit to patient outcomes as the discovery of new knowledge. The adage becomes: "We don't need to do better things, we need to do things better."

It was clear to the authors of the IOM report that high error rates in healthcare are not linked primarily to negligent or poorly trained physicians. Other industries, notably the automotive and aviation industries, have achieved decades of success in improving the reliability of their products and services, and offer excellent models for medicine. In contrast to medicine, these industries have not put the primary culpability for error on the individual employee. Instead, they have accepted the inherent fallibility of the individual worker, and have sought ways to improve their systems to account for it. Leaders in the fields of patient safety and quality improvement have spent the past two decades exploring ways to apply such concepts to medicine, and to energize the healthcare community to accept this approach.

There have been many success stories among those who embrace the idea that we can transform healthcare into a highly reliable industry. It is instructive to review several examples of how the scientific method was employed to yield innovative changes in local hospitals.

The Keystone Project focused on the application of a simple intervention to eliminate central venous catheter (CVC)-related bloodstream infections in their intensive care unit (ICU).

Data suggested that CVCs were responsible for 80,000 bloodstream infections annually and up to 28,000 deaths in ICUs, at a cost of $2.3 billion. Secondly, they identified a set of evidence-based best practices to reduce CVC-related bloodstream infections:

1. Strict adherence to handwashing
2. Full sterile barrier precautions during CVC insertion (cap, gown, mask, drape)
3. Skin preparation with chlorhexidine
4. Avoidance of the femoral insertion site when possible
5. Prompt removal of unnecessary catheters.

These best practices were known to most clinicians who practiced in the ICU at the time of the study, but it was unclear how strict adherence would improve outcomes. More importantly, the investigators recognized that a systematic change was needed to ensure that these practices were followed reliably; counting on physicians and nurses to remember each step every time was not sufficient to effect a change in practice technique.

As part of the study, a physician and nurse champion were recruited for every ICU. These local leaders were tasked with educating their colleagues about the changes, and exerted influence in their units to facilitate acceptance of the intervention. A procedure cart with necessary equipment was created to ensure that compliance with sterile precautions was easy for physicians, and a checklist was created to facilitate adherence with all five steps. Unit staff was empowered to stop practitioners in non-emergent situations if the listed practices were not being followed, and daily rounds included a discussion of catheter removal on every patient. Teams were given feedback on a regular basis about their rates of CVC-related bloodstream infection.

Using this straightforward model, the median number of ICU bloodstream infections in the study hospitals dropped from 2.7 infections per 1,000 catheter days to 0 within 3 months of implementation. Remarkably, the median infection rate remained at 0 for a full 18 months of observation. The overall incidence of bloodstream infections was reduced by 66%. The study population encompassed 85% of the available ICU beds in the state of Michigan, and thus the impact was widespread. Extrapolation of these practices to ICU's across the country has major implications for patient safety.

Prevention of hospital-acquired venous thromboembolism (VTE) is another subject in which performance lags far behind evidence. It is estimated that 100,000 deaths annually are attributable to VTE in the United States. Despite well-established evidence and widely disseminated national guidelines, rates of appropriate pharmacologic prophylaxis among hospitalized patients fall between 30% and 50%. Clinicians at a San Diego, California University hospital understood that this poor performance represented an opportunity for improvement. With development and implementation of a simplified risk assessment tool, they increased and sustained rates of appropriate VTE prophylaxis to 98%. The investigators recognized that physicians needed reminders to ensure reliable performance of the risk assessment. They organized a multidisciplinary team, consisting of hospitalists, pulmonologists with expertise in VTE, pharmacists, nurses, and information systems specialists to develop an evidence-based protocol. Their risk assessment tool stood apart from others in existence because it was simple to use. Rather than a numerical point-based scoring system, the tool was designed such that clinicians could quickly review criteria and classify patients as low, moderate, or high risk for VTE.

An equally important facet of the intervention was the "forcing" of the risk assessment on admitting physicians by its inclusion in routine admission orders. Physicians could not finalize their hospital admission orders without completing the VTE risk assessment, which prompted ordering of the appropriate anticoagulant prophylaxis. An advantage at the study hospital was the presence of a computerized order entry system, which made dissemination of the risk assessment more seamless; however, it could have easily been incorporated in preprinted handwritten admit order checklists.

Finally, the remarkable success was also attributable to the investigators ongoing re-evaluation of their results, which allowed them to achieve "continuous quality improvement." For example, shortly after implementation, rates of appropriate VTE prophylaxis rose from 50%

to 80%. Realizing that this laudable improvement left 20% of patients without adequate protection from VTE, the investigators reviewed utilization data for the protocol. They discovered that physicians occasionally misclassified patients with significant VTE risk factors as low-risk. After modifications to reduce this error were implemented, improvement was again noted, to 98% by the end of the study period.

SYSTEMS IMPROVEMENT: KEY CONCEPTS

These two straightforward interventions are illustrative of some of the broader concepts that drive successful quality improvement. A solid grasp of such concepts will be useful for all clinicians who are motivated to effect positive change in their practice, unit, hospital, or health system (Table 18-1).

The first concept is to *keep it simple*. Healthcare providers are busy, and changes to workflow that are burdensome or complicated are unlikely to be adopted. The Pneumonia Severity Index, developed by Fine and colleagues and published over a decade ago, was a rigorously developed and well-validated prediction tool that allowed clinicians to estimate 30-day mortality risk for patients with community-acquired pneumonia. In addition, it has been validated as a safe and effective tool to be used to determine site of care for such patients. Although it is a central part of the risk adjustment methodology in most clinical studies of pneumonia, in actual practice it is rarely used, because it requires a complex scoring system that integrates data from 19 different variables. Similarly, models for VTE risk stratification predating the San Diego study had been cumbersome and required point systems to risk stratify patients. In contrast, the simplified tool was adopted quickly at the local institution, with powerful results. The model is now being disseminated widely across the country.

The Keystone Project beautifully illustrates that something as simple as a checklist can have dramatic impact on patient outcomes. Interventions such as this must not only be simple, but must *integrate smoothly into the workflow of the practitioner*. In the case of the Keystone Project, if the checklist were not located conveniently on the procedure cart, the likelihood of compliance would have been markedly less. Any impediment to an already busy workload is an opportunity to skip a step; it is unlikely a physician or nurse would have gone searching for the checklist during the process of CVC insertion. In the case of the VTE study, the protocol was embedded in the admission orders, which could not be completed without it. If the setup required the physician to actively seek out the orderset, again an opportunity to bypass this critical step would have arisen. These "workarounds" are the enemy of any good quality improvement effort, thus it is critical to ensure that the intervention provides minimal interruption to the otherwise routine workflow of the practitioner.

Both the Keystone Project and the VTE prophylaxis project are examples of the power of *standardization of a process*. Prior to the interventions, each physician approached the practice of insertion of a CVC or selecting VTE prophylaxis according to his own individual preference. This variation in practice allowed room for error. Through the CVC checklist and the VTE

TABLE 18-1	Key Concepts for Successful Quality Improvement Interventions

- Keep interventions simple for users
- Ensure interventions integrate into the standard workflow, so interruptions are minimized
- Attempt to standardize processes when possible
- Provide timely feedback on performance
- Make efforts to secure "buy-in" from the primary users of any new process
- Create a culture of safety in your organization
- Once improvement is realized, continue ongoing monitoring to ensure it is maintained
- Set high thresholds for achievement and continue to strive for further improvement

orderset, clinicians were reminded of evidence-based best practices every time the decision point arose. The fact that the majority of physicians did things the same then allowed investigators to study the effect of the process itself, and in the case of the VTE prophylaxis protocol, flaws were identified early on that were addressed to increase the power of the intervention.

Timely feedback on performance serves as a motivator for change. Medical training selects for people who are inherently motivated to perform at a high level, and so regular feedback drives improvement. In the Keystone Project, teams were given monthly reports of their rates of CVC infections, which in this case, served to reinforce the power of the checklist and strengthen the adherence by physicians and nurses.

Ensuring that there is *buy-in from the primary users* of the quality improvement intervention is another critical key to success. The VTE prophylaxis effort achieved this by involving a multidisciplinary team consisting of key stakeholders, with broad representation to ensure that issues that affect all users were considered before implementation. The Keystone Project accomplished this by assigning local clinical "champions," in this case from medicine and nursing, to lead the effort. When workers see an initiative embraced by their colleagues, it is often easier to garner support than when it is viewed as a "top down" mandate from administrators.

Creating a *"culture of safety"* is another key concept that all institutions seeking systematic error reduction must strive to achieve. One component of such a culture is the abolition of traditional chains of authority when issues of patient safety arise. In the Keystone Project, a priori agreement that the administration at each participating hospital would empower and support the nursing staff to enforce physician compliance with the CVC best practice measures was essential for success. This concept has been used successfully in the aviation industry, where it is standard practice that anyone on the flight crew may challenge a superior if there is a perceived or potential deviation from safety procedures. Without such a team approach in healthcare, significant progress in error reduction cannot be achieved.

It is important that leaders of positive change do not rest on their laurels after a successful effort. The term "quality improvement" should more realistically be replaced with "continuous quality improvement," because we can *always look for ways to do better*. The VTE project achieved a significant improvement in outcomes after the protocol was rolled out; however, the investigators were not satisfied with a performance of 80%, even though it represented over a 50% relative increase. With the concept of "continuous quality improvement" firmly in mind, they reassessed the structure of their protocol and, with minor revisions, improved their results further.

Finally, it is important to *ensure that early success is maintained over time*. As many frustrated smokers and dieters are aware, it is difficult to maintain positive behavioral changes over time without ongoing accountability. "Holding the gains" is a central goal for realistic and lasting improvement, and ongoing audits of successful interventions remain important. The investigators in the Keystone Project monitored the effectiveness of their checklist for 18 months before reporting their data, and both the VTE and CVC infection prevention initiatives continue to perform active surveillance to ensure their successes are retained.

CONCLUSIONS

The practice environment for healthcare providers has shifted to move quality and safety to the forefront. Advances in the understanding of the techniques required to improve the delivery of healthcare have moved the industry closer toward achieving the goal of providing the right care to the right patient at the right time, every time.

External forces will make it increasingly difficult for the individual clinician to avoid incorporating some of the tools required to integrate quality improvement techniques into practice. Public reporting of performance on quality measures for hospitals has been in effect since 2003, and reporting of physician performance is on the horizon. "Pay for performance" methodologies are being actively implemented by the federal government and private payers, with the intention of redesigning reimbursement strategies to reward quality rather than quantity of care. Maintenance of certification from the American Board of Internal Medicine in all specialties requires concrete demonstration of facility with quality improvement techniques, in addition to the written exam.

The increasing momentum to engage clinicians, patients, payers, and regulators of the healthcare delivered in the United States in optimizing performance will ultimately serve to maximize the health and welfare of our population. Raising awareness of the topic among consumers and providers of care is essential, and nurturing physicians to lead the charge will ensure that the quality agenda moves forward in a direction that benefits both. For those inspired to learn more, the references provide opportunities for more in-depth study.

FURTHER READING

1. Corrigan J, Kohn LT, Donaldson MS, eds. *To Err Is Human: Building a Safer Health System.* Washington, DC: National Academy Press; 1999.

   The landmark report by the IOM has helped revolutionize the approach to improving quality and patient safety in the US healthcare system for more than a decade, and sets the agenda for ongoing healthcare reform.

2. Department of Health and Human Services, Office of Inspector General. *Adverse Events in Hospitals: National Incidence Among Medicare Beneficiaries.* Washington, DC: Government Printing Office; 2010.

   This report enhances information discussed by the IOM a decade earlier by estimating the rates of nonfatal medical errors affecting Medicare patients in US hospitals, revealing a more robust picture of the scope of errors in healthcare.

3. McGlynn E, Asch S, Adams J, et al. The quality of health care delivered to adults in the United States. *N Engl J Med.* 2003;348:2635–2645.

   This large study reveals significant deficiencies in the delivery of standardized evidence-based indicators of quality care. It is informative for skeptics to review the indicators chosen, as they consist of uniformly well-accepted practices that were notably underused.

4. National Priorities Partnership. "Preventing hospital readmissions: a $25 billion opportunity." Compact action brief: a roadmap for increasing value in healthcare. http://www.nehi.net/publications/51/compact_action_brief_preventing_hospital_readmissions. Accessed August 3, 2011.

   This document compiles data from various sources to estimate the financial burden of preventable hospital readmissions, currently a major target for incentivizing quality by the federal government.

5. Pronovost P, Needham D, Berenholtz S, et al. An intervention to decrease catheter-related bloodstream infections in the ICU. *N Engl J Med.* 2006;355:2725–2732.

   This seminal study showed that simple interventions could have remarkable impact on patient outcomes. A revision of the processes of care in Michigan ICU's led to a 66% reduction in catheter-related bloodstream infections statewide.

6. Gawande A. The checklist. *The New Yorker.* December 10, 2007. http://www.newyorker.com/reporting/2007/12/10/071210fa_fact_gawande. Accessed March 15, 2011.

   A prosaic but insightful treatise on the impact of simple interventions on quality by one of the most important authors about health issues for the lay public. He expands on the impact of Pronovost's work and the barriers to broader implementation.

7. Geerts W, Bergqvist D, Pineo G, et al. Prevention of venous thromboembolism: American College of Chest Physicians Evidence-Based Clinical Practice Guidelines (8th ed.). *Chest.* 2008;133(S6):381S–453S.

   This edition of an ongoing and regularly updated systematic review published by the American College of Chest Physicians (ACCP) provides a thorough review of the evidence for VTE prophylaxis in various clinical settings.

8. Maynard G, Morris T, Jenkins I, et al. Optimizing prevention of hospital-acquired venous thromboembolism (VTE): prospective validation of a VTE risk assessment model. *J Hosp Med.* 2010;5:10–18.

   This study nicely illustrates how front line clinicians can employ quality improvement techniques to achieve powerful results. As discussed in the text, investigators were able to increase rates of appropriate VTE prophylaxis to 98% at their institution.

9. Fine M, Auble T, Yealy D, et al. A prediction rule to identify low-risk patients with community-acquired pneumonia. *N Engl J Med.* 1997;336:243–250.

   Investigators in this study derived and validated an accurate, reliable tool that is useful in predicting pneumonia mortality rates and also in determining the need for inpatient care, but is too complex to have practical applications at the bedside. It highlights the difficulties in applying good science to patient care.

10. Motykie G, Zebala L, Caprini J, et al. A guide to venous thromboembolism risk factor assessment. *J Thromb Thrombolysis.* 2000;9(3):253–262.

    See this review and notably the appendix for an example of the complexity of some of the proposed VTE risk stratification systems predating the San Diego study. It is evident that these systems would be challenging for busy clinicians to adopt.

11. Berwick D; The Commonwealth Fund. *Escape Fire: Lessons for the Future of Health Care.* New York, NY: The Commonwealth Fund; 2002.

    The CEO of the Institute of Healthcare Improvement and acting administrator of the Center for Medicare and Medicaid Services offers an eloquent discussion of opportunities to redesign the US health care system to better meet the needs of patients.

12. Chassin M. Is health care ready for six sigma quality? *Milbank Q.* 1998;76(4):565–591.

    A call to arms for organized medicine to follow the lead of high performance industries who have achieved reliable performance at levels far beyond what the healthcare industry has accomplished by using the "six-sigma" approach to quality.

13. Leape L. Error in medicine. *JAMA.* 1994;272(23):1851–1857.

    An in-depth discussion of the science of human error from the perspective of cognitive and human factors psychology, and of the application of systems redesign to improve safety in the workplace. The essay, by one of the pioneers in patient safety research, reviews key concepts from high reliability industries like aviation which informed the changes adopted in healthcare in the decade that followed.

14. Gawande A. *Better: A Surgeon's Notes on Performance.* New York, NY: Picador Books (Henry Holt and Company); 2007.

    For readers interested in further examples of innovation in healthcare quality improvement, Gawande provides fascinating stories of various individuals who focused on making health care better in their communities. He encourages readers to become "positive deviants," and shares his thoughts about ways to make an individual career in medicine have a larger impact.

19 Disability and Medicolegal Evaluation

William G. Hughson

Many physicians dislike writing medicolegal reports. They are more comfortable with their traditional role of diagnosing and treating disease. However, providing clearly written reports is essential in ensuring that their patients receive appropriate workers' compensation and other benefits following work-related disease and injury. These reports are read by nonmedical personnel such as disability raters, insurance claims adjusters, and workers' compensation judges and often require the use of special forms and obscure terms to achieve specific legal and administrative goals.

It is important to distinguish between impairment and disability. *Impairment* describes an anatomic or functional loss caused by a disease process. *Disability* describes the effects of the impairment on the patient's life, including the ability to work. It can be defined as the inability to perform at a specified level of activity, or as undue distress during the performance of that task. The degree of disability is directly related to the physical requirements of the job. For example, a teacher with a forced expiratory volume in 1 second (FEV_1) of 1 L might have no disability, whereas a general laborer would need retraining for another job. Nonmedical people who rely on the physician's opinions make the final decision regarding disability.

The medicolegal report should contain all of the sections found in a typical medical consultation plus a detailed occupational history. A patient-generated form that is completed before an examination can facilitate the latter. The assessment section of the report should contain answers to all of the questions listed in Table 19-1. We favor a question-and-answer format because it saves time and allows a clearer explanation of the issues and the physician's opinion. The key points that should be discussed require a very specific vocabulary with legal implications.

WHAT IS THE DIAGNOSIS?

This is generally the easiest question to answer. Each lung condition should be listed along with the evidence supporting its diagnosis. For example, the diagnosis of asbestosis is based on a history of exposure, appropriate latency, the presence of interstitial markings on the chest radiograph, pulmonary function tests showing a restrictive pattern and reduction in the diffusing capacity, and crackles on physical examination. Nonpulmonary diagnoses should also be listed, particularly those affecting impairment or disability.

IS THE DIAGNOSIS WORK-RELATED?

This requires a judgment that the disease was caused, aggravated, accelerated, or precipitated by a workplace exposure. This opinion must be expressed in terms of *reasonable medical probability*, which means it is more likely than not (i.e., >50% probability) that the diagnosis is work-related. The legal system understands that there will always be some uncertainty, but failure to express your opinion in terms of reasonable medical probability renders it useless for resolving the legal issues for the patient. *Causation* is defined as a new disease that has been caused by work (e.g., an insulator with asbestosis). *Aggravation* means a preexisting condition that did not interfere with work or usual activities is now worse because of employment (e.g., chronic obstructive pulmonary disease in a smoker exposed to industrial dusts). *Acceleration* means a preexisting condition that would naturally worsen with time deteriorated more rapidly because of employment (e.g., airway obstruction in a patient with emphysema exposed to fumes). *Precipitation* means a preexisting condition that became manifest for the first time because of employment (e.g., asthma in an atopic patient exposed to flour). The time sequence

---

TABLE 19-1	**Questions to Be Answered in a Disability Evaluation Report**

1. What is the diagnosis?
2. Is the diagnosis work-related by causation, aggravation, acceleration, or precipitation?
3. Is there evidence of impairment? If so, how severe is the impairment? What rating system is used, and how do the patient's findings correspond to this system?
4. Is temporary disability present? If so, is it partial or total? What is the anticipated time of recovery?
5. Can the patient return to his or her previous occupation? Could the patient return to the job if it were modified? Are there any work restrictions or preclusions?
6. Is permanent disability present? If so, is the patient stationary for rating purposes? When did the patient become permanent and stationary?
7. How severe is the permanent disability? What rating system is used, and how do the patient's findings correspond to this system?
8. Are there permanent work restrictions? If so, what are they?
9. Is there any basis for apportionment of the permanent disability? If the work injury had not occurred, would a preexisting condition contribute to the disability?
10. Is vocational retraining indicated? If so, which types of jobs are appropriate?
11. Is further medical treatment needed? If so, what is the nature, frequency, and duration of the treatment?

of the disease in relation to employment is very important. For example, pneumoconiosis takes years to develop, and immune-mediated reactions require weeks to months before sensitization occurs. It is important to note whether symptoms are worse at work, and then improve on weekends or vacations. The presence of similar problems in coworkers is highly suggestive. The nature and severity of exposure should be determined by obtaining Material Safety Data Sheets and available industrial hygiene information. The use of protective devices (e.g., respirators) and adequacy of ventilation should be described.

IS THERE EVIDENCE OF IMPAIRMENT? IF SO, HOW SEVERE IS THE IMPAIRMENT?

Subjective data (e.g., dyspnea, weakness, and pain) must be differentiated from objective data because symptoms are often unreliable measures of disease in the setting of litigation. The physical examination and chest radiographs provide diagnostic information, but are not useful in measuring function. Basic spirometry remains the cornerstone for assessing impairment. Other techniques (e.g., exercise testing) are added as necessary. It is important to know which rating system applies to the patient's case. The American Medical Association's (AMA) *Guides to the Evaluation of Permanent Impairment* is the one most commonly used. The referral source should give clear instructions and provide the rating system to the physician when necessary.

IS DISABILITY PRESENT?

If so, is it partial or total, temporary or permanent? The key question is "Can the patient return to the usual and customary activities of employment?" This requires a clear understanding of the patient's work, including the physical effort needed and the potentially harmful exposures. The work history can be obtained from the patient, and supplemented with a written job description provided by the employer. Partial disability exists when the patient can perform some, but not all, of the usual job responsibilities. Useful questions include: Could the patient return to the job if it were modified? Are there any work restrictions or preclusions? In most states, the employer is required to make reasonable accommodations. However, job modification is often difficult, and the definition of *reasonable* can be contentious. Total disability exists if the patient is completely unable to perform the job, even with accommodation. If the disability is temporary (either partial or total), it is important to provide both the patient and the employer with an estimate of the time needed for recovery. This allows assignment of tasks to other workers. If permanent disability is likely, it is wise to advise both the employer and patient as soon as possible. This facilitates realistic planning for the patient's future.

IS DISABILITY PERMANENT?

If permanent disability is present, is the patient stationary for rating purposes? How severe is the disability? The patient is permanent and stationary for rating purposes after maximal medical improvement has been achieved and no prospect is seen for further recovery. The report should include a lucid description of the patient's impairment and its impact on work capacity. This includes any permanent restrictions and preclusions, but caution is warranted. Sweeping statements such as "No further exposure to dusts or fumes" may make the patient unemployable. Precision is needed, with a description of any specific precluded exposures (e.g., allergens or sensitizers) and consideration of dose (e.g., respirator use, ventilation requirements, Occupational Safety and Health Administration-permissible exposure limits). For example, an insulator with mild asbestosis might be able to continue working under current regulations, because permissible dust levels are now very low. The description of permanent disability must contain terminology appropriate for the rating system that applies. For example, in California, words such as *minimal* or *moderate, occasional* or *frequent* have specific meanings when used to describe dyspnea. The California Labor Code has categories such as *Disability precluding heavy work* and *Standard ratings* with percent disability caused by pulmonary disease. Copies of rating systems can be obtained from the referral source or from state and federal regulatory agencies.

IS THERE ANY BASIS FOR APPORTIONMENT?

Apportionment is only considered when permanent disability is present. It is used to describe the relative contribution of occupational and nonoccupational lung diseases to the total disability. However, the medical concept of apportionment differs from the legal principle, just as impairment differs from disability. For example, whereas most physicians would consider preexisting asthma as a factor in a painter with pulmonary impairment, the legal concept of apportionment is concerned only with preexisting disability. A useful question is: If the work injury had not occurred, would the preexisting condition contribute to disability? In the case of the painter, if no evidence was found of disability before the injury at work (e.g., work restrictions, prior job loss because of the condition), no basis would be seen for apportionment, and the entire disability would be considered work-related. If a preexisting condition causing disability is aggravated or accelerated by employment, the increment in disability is apportioned and is compensable. The best way to deal with apportionment is to dictate two paragraphs describing the permanent disability. The first describes existing disability factors (subjective and objective) and work restrictions. The second describes disability factors and work restrictions that would have existed without the occupational injury. The hearing officer then decides the extent of disability represented by each of the two paragraphs and, by subtraction, allocates the disability caused by employment.

IS VOCATIONAL RETRAINING APPROPRIATE?

Patients with severe impairment may be totally disabled from any type of employment. Those with better function are suitable for retraining, which is a worker's compensation benefit. The physician should describe the types of jobs and work preclusions suitable for the patient. The physician may be asked to communicate with vocational rehabilitation counselors regarding the patient's condition.

IS FURTHER MEDICAL TREATMENT NEEDED?

It is important to describe the nature, frequency, and anticipated duration of all treatment. In most instances, the cost of medical care is paid by workers' compensation if employment has contributed to disability, even when nonoccupational factors are present. Apportionment of medical costs is usually not allowed.

FURTHER READING

1. Brigham CR, Babitsky S. Independent medical evaluations and impairment ratings. *Occup Med.* 1998;13:325–343.

   A detailed review of medicolegal report writing.

2. Cowl CT. Occupational asthma: review of assessment, treatment and compensation. *Chest.* 2011;139:674–681.

   Good review which includes discussion of impairment, disability, workers' compensation, and insurance systems.

3. Demeter SL. Disability evaluation. *Occup Med.* 1998;13:315–323.

   Discusses various rating systems, including the AMA Guides.

4. Guidotti TL, Martin CJ. Evaluation of the worker with suspected occupational lung disease. *Occup Med.* 1998;13:279–288.

   Reviews the approach to occupational lung diseases, including issues of causation and disability.

5. Lentz G, Christian JH, Tierman SN. Disability prevention and management. In: Ladou J, ed. *Current Occupational and Environmental Medicine.* 4th ed. New York, NY: McGraw-Hill; 2007:21–35.

   Good review of the concept of disability, and the general approach to its assessment and management. Other chapters in this book deal with the occupational history and worker's compensation.

6. Plumb JM, Cowell JWF. An overview of workers' compensation. *Occup Med.* 1998;13:241–272.

   A detailed review of all aspects of workers' compensation.

7. Rondinelli RD, Beller TA. Impairment rating and disability evaluation of the pulmonary system. *Phys Med Rehabil Clin N Am.* 2001;12:667–679.

   A review of the diagnostic procedures and assessment criteria for pulmonary disability evaluations.

8. Rondinelli R, Genovese E, Mueller KL, eds. *Guides to the Evaluation of Permanent Impairment.* 6th ed. Chicago, IL: American Medical Association; 2007.

    This book describes the AMA rating system.

9. Sood A, Beckett WS. Determination of disability for patients with advanced lung disease. *Clin Chest Med.* 1997;18:471–482.

    Discusses various rating systems and the approach to report writing.

10. Sood A, Redlich CA. Pulmonary function tests at work. *Clin Chest Med.* 2001;22:783–793.

    Excellent review of pulmonary function tests used to diagnose occupational lung diseases and assess impairment.

11. Taiwo OA, Cain HC. Pulmonary impairment and disability. *Clin Chest Med.* 2002;23:841–851.

    Detailed review article, including a discussion of pulmonary function tests and disability rating systems.

Air Travel and High-Altitude Medicine

David J. De La Zerda and Frank L. Powell

INTRODUCTION

The most common medical emergency elicited by ascending to high altitude is hypobaric hypoxia from a low partial pressure of inspired oxygen (PIO_2). The decrease in PIO_2 at high altitude is predicted by the formula: $PIO_2 = FIO_2 \times (P_{baro} - PH_2O)$. FIO_2 is the fraction of inspired oxygen and remains constant at 21% regardless of the altitude. P_{baro} is the atmospheric pressure (e.g., 760 mmHg at sea level). PH_2O is the partial pressure of water vapor when the air is fully humidified, as it is in the alveoli. P_{baro} is the major factor that determines PIO_2 because at body temperature (37°C), PH_2O is 47 mmHg and FIO_2 and PH_2O are constant. Table 20-1 shows the PIO_2 at various altitudes. The drop in P_{baro} at high altitudes causes hypobaric hypoxia. In patients with preexisting hypoxemia from lung disease, either air travel or activities at high altitude (e.g., skiing and mountaineering) can increase the risk of developing severe hypoxemia.

AIR TRAVEL

Although most commercial flights cruise between 22,000 and 44,000 ft (6,700–13,400 m), the Federal Aviation Administration mandates that cabins should be pressurized to simulate an altitude below 8,000 ft (2,438 m). At that altitude, the partial pressure of oxygen in arterial blood (PaO_2) in normal individuals is typically between 75 and 53 mmHg, which corresponds to a decrease in oxygen saturation of 3% to 5% from sea level.

According to the Centers for Disease Control and Prevention (CDC), in-flight medical emergencies are rare. One in 10,000 to 40,000 air travelers have a medical incident, 1 in 150,000 require the use of medical equipment or drugs, and 0.3 of 1,000,000 die (and two-thirds of these deaths are due to cardiac disease). The most common medical problems are vasovagal, gastrointestinal, respiratory, cardiac, and neurologic incidents. Prescreening patients appears to be valuable in assuring healthy flying. In a study of 1,115 patients referred for screening, 1,011 were cleared for travel and none had significant in-flight problems. The

TABLE 20-1	Barometric Pressure, Altitude and Oxygen				
Barometric pressure (mmHg)	590	460	300	270	215
Altitude (ft)	6,500	13,000	20,000	26,000	32,000
Arterial oxygen (mmHg)	150	90	65	55	45
Arterial oxygen saturation (%)	95	90	80	65	55

remaining 104 patients had a variety of unstable and stable conditions that precluded air travel. Preflight evaluations and management requires some understanding of the risks involved for a variety of specific disease states. Even with preflight screening, a few problems can be anticipated.

Most, but not all, patients with chronic obstructive pulmonary disease (COPD) can fly safely with little or no intervention. There is considerable individual variation, since even the moderate altitudes reached in commercial aircraft can lead to changes in ventilatory function. After 60 minutes at 8,000 ft (2,438 m, Pb = 565 mmHg), pulmonary function changes reported in both healthy persons and patients with severe COPD include a fall in forced vital capacity (FVC), increase in residual volume, and variable changes in airway resistance. In a small cohort of 44 COPD patients with FEV_1 of 34% ($\pm$9%) of predicted who flew for a median time of 3 hours over a 28-day period, 18.2% reported symptoms and signs during their flight. Complaints were primarily dyspnea, edema, wheezing, and cyanosis. Only two patients requested supplemental oxygen, and none required hospital admission. Other studies have shown similar results.

Patients with pulmonary hypertension have an increased risk of hypoxia during air travel because lower inspired oxygen tension induces pulmonary artery vasoconstriction. The subsequent elevation in pulmonary vascular resistance may increase the stress on the already compromised right ventricle. For this reason, patients with functional class III or IV should probably avoid unnecessary flights. Ideally, patients in functional class I and II should receive a formal evaluation with a hypoxia-altitude simulation test before air travel. If, after a thorough evaluation, a patient is deemed fit to fly, the Aerospace Medical Association recommends that exercise be limited during the flight.

Asthma is a common pulmonary condition that poses a risk of exacerbation during air travel. Most flight-associated exacerbations can be managed with inhaled bronchodilators alone. While it is most convenient for the patients themselves to bring their own bronchodilators on board, emergency-use bronchodilators are part of the standard in-flight emergency medical kits on commercial planes. The Aerospace Medical Association recommends that all asthmatic patients bring a course of oral prednisone on board for use in an emergency during the flight.

Pneumothorax poses a special risk during flight. Before air travel, the etiology of a pneumothorax must be established and corrected. A recent pneumothorax may expand during air travel and progress to become a tension pneumothorax. The presence of a pneumothorax, therefore, is an absolute contraindication for air travel. It may be reasonable to travel 3 weeks after successful drainage of a pneumothorax, provided complete resolution is confirmed radiographically prior the flight.

Extrapulmonary air in the chest cavity (e.g., following thoracic surgery) also may pose significant risk and should delay air travel. If the cabin pressure was to abruptly decrease, the entrapped air may rapidly expand and increase the risk of life-threatening tension pneumothorax.

Commercial air travel is associated with an increased risk for the development of deep vein thrombosis (DVT). Extrinsic risk factors include immobility, dehydration, increased venous pressure from cramped seating, endothelial damage from seat edges, and hemoconcentration from fluid shifts to the interstitial space from decreased cabin pressure. Intrinsic risk factors that contribute to the development of DVT from air travel include history of DVT or pulmonary embolism (PE), postthrombotic syndromes, malignancy, pregnancy, and chronic venous insufficiency. In high-risk patients, the American College of Chest Physicians (ACCP) recommends frequent ambulation (when permitted by the aircrew), isometric calf muscle exercise, aisle seating, and graduated compression stockings (below-knee, 15–30 mmHg of pressure at the ankle). ACCP recommends against the use of aspirin or anticoagulants to prevent DVT during air travel, but anticoagulant treatment for other purposes should not be discontinued.

The primary cardiac response to moderate hypobaric hypoxia that occurs during flight is an increase in heart rate with a subsequent reduction in stroke volume. These processes may increase the risk of coronary events in patients with previous histories of coronary artery disease. Stable cardiac disorders, however, do not preclude flight. For example, stable angina requires little, if any, change in management, but air travel within 2 weeks of myocardial infarction would be advisable only if there is no angina or dyspnea at rest, the passenger is not alone or rushed, and nitroglycerin is readily available. Complicated myocardial infarction or limited ambulatory ability requires further cardiology evaluation and perhaps stress testing before air travel.

The Aerospace Medical Association considers the following cardiovascular conditions as contraindications for commercial flights: uncomplicated myocardial infarction within 2 to 3 weeks, complicated myocardial infarction within 6 weeks, unstable angina, decompensated or severe congestive heart failure, uncontrolled hypertension, coronary artery bypass grafts (CABG) within 10 to 14 days, cerebrovascular accident (CVA) within 2 weeks, uncontrolled ventricular or supraventricular tachycardia, Eisenmenger syndrome, and severe symptomatic valvular heart disease. Further recommendations regarding these conditions are beyond the scope of this review, but cardiology evaluation is strongly recommended before air travel.

Supplemental oxygen may circumvent most barriers to flight among patients with limited cardiopulmonary function. The sea level Pao_2 is a useful screen to predict which patients might require supplemental oxygen in flight. Oxygen should be considered for patients with a sea level Pao_2 of less than 70 mmHg. For those with a Pao_2 more than 70 mmHg, a number of preflight evaluations have been used to predict oxygen requirements during flight. For those who already require supplemental oxygen, some authors suggest simply adding 2 L/min of flow to baseline requirements. Others use more complicated prediction equations. Such equations should be used with caution, because they are derived from specific populations. More subjective issues such as cardiopulmonary reserve or muscle weakness are not included in the equations. Prediction equations also tend to overestimate Pao_2 values for healthy controls. Below is one such equation that resulted in a high predictive value ($r^2 = .99$, $P < .001$) at moderate altitude:

$$Pao_2 \text{ alt} = 0.19(FEV_1 \times Pao_2 \text{ grnd}) - 11.51[\ln(\text{max alt} - \text{grnd alt})]$$

where Pao_2 alt = Pao_2 at expected altitude achieved, Pao_2 grnd = Pao_2 at baseline elevation, max alt = maximum altitude achieved in meters, and grnd alt = baseline elevation in meters.

In 1984, Gong et al. described the use of the hypoxia-altitude simulation test (HAST) or hypoxia inhalation test, to objectively evaluate at sea level the oxygen demands in patients with pulmonary diseases. Their initial report included 22 patients with COPD who were asked to breathe a low Fio_2 (high nitrogen) mixture of gases from a tight-fitting mask for 15 minutes. Three different Fio_2 are typically used: 0.209 (baseline), 0.17 (simulating 5,000 ft), and 0.15 (simulating 8,000 ft). These conditions are comparable to the results achieved in hypobaric chambers, but are much simpler to perform.

HAST is a relatively simple test. Initially a baseline arterial blood gas is obtained to measure Pao_2 and $Paco_2$. The inhaled gas mixture is then changed to an Fio_2 of 0.15. The patient's vital signs, oximetry, and symptoms (e.g., dyspnea or chest pain) are closely monitored. If worrisome symptoms or physical signs occur, or if pulse oximetry readings fall below 85%, then arterial blood gases are repeated and the test is stopped. If the saturation remains greater than or equal to 88% for 20 minutes, then the test is completed and arterial blood gases are repeated. If Pao_2 at the end of the test is greater than 55 mmHg, then supplemental oxygen typically is not required for air travel. If it is less than 50 mmHg, then supplemental oxygen would be warranted. A borderline test result (Pao_2 between 50 and 55 mmHg) may be supplemented by an additional arterial blood gas sample taken while the patient is walking and breathing an Fio_2 of 0.15.

In summary, several medical problems may occur during air travel. At-risk patients should be carefully evaluated prior to travel and appropriate recommendations should be made based upon their underlying conditions. Hypoxia associated with reduced cabin barometric pressure can be prevented by supplemental oxygen. Patients with preexisting needs for supplemental oxygen may increase their oxygen flow by 2 L/min above their baseline requirements during air travel. For those with milder hypoxemia, HAST or several prediction equations may help guide the decision to supply supplemental oxygen for air travel. Arrangements should be made by the patient with the airline way in advance of the travel date to determine method of administration, stopping points at elevated altitudes, and length of travel time during which supplemental oxygen may be needed. In more challenging situations, discussion with the airline's flight surgeon may be needed to complete the arrangements.

HIGH-ALTITUDE ILLNESS

Altitudes exceeding those typically simulated by pressurized cabins can produce a unique set of disorders that range from benign to fatal. Fortunately, the more serious problems arise with considerable less frequency. However, increasingly publicized accidents in remote locales reflect a surge of interest in high-altitude adventure and a corresponding risk of high-altitude illness. Most high-altitude illnesses occur among the 12 million skiers traveling to mountainous areas each year. However, increasing numbers of people are adventuring into extreme altitudes where more serious problems can occur.

Altitudes can be defined physiologically as "high altitude" (5,000–11,500 ft, or 1,500–3,500 m) above sea level, "very high altitude" (11,500–18,000 ft, or 3,500–5,500 m) and "extreme altitude" (>18,000 ft or 5,500 m). Altitudes above 20,000 ft have been called the "death zone" as permanent life is not sustainable at such heights. Ascent to high altitudes can produce a continuum of altitude-related illnesses. Acute mountain sickness (AMS) is most common at high altitudes (5,000–11,500 ft), while high-altitude pulmonary edema (HAPE) and high-altitude cerebral edema (HACE) are more serious high-altitude illnesses that may result in death but occur only rarely at very high and extreme altitudes. A number of other altitude disorders can arise, but exceed the scope of this review. These include snow blindness, retinal hemorrhages, hypothermia, and high-altitude flatus expulsion (a serious concern for climbers trapped in the closed confines of a tent during inclement weather), and problems associated with chronic exposure.

Ski resorts constitute the bulk of recreational destinations at high altitude. Many resorts are located at or above 10,000 ft (3,000 m), and they can be accessed very rapidly by motorized transport. There are also commercial and research activities at high altitudes, such as copper mines at 19,520 ft (5,950 m) in Chile and astronomy at 13,779 ft (4,200 m) at the Mauna Kea Observatory in Hawaii. Some 6,000 people climb Mt. Rainier at 14,408 ft (4,392 m) per year, and 800 climbers summit Denali, the highest peak in North America at 20,320 ft (6,193 m). Nearly 50% of all travelers to these altitudes experience some symptoms. Altitude illness is reported by 66% of climbers on Mt. Rainier, 47% on Mt. Everest, and 30% on Denali.

Factors contributing to the development of altitude-related illnesses include the maximum altitude achieved, rate of ascent, intensity of exercise, viral illnesses, alcohol consumption, sleep-enhancement drugs, and individual susceptibility. Other factors may include age and gender. However, there is no good predictor of who will, and who will not suffer altitude illness except a subject's previous history at high altitude. Considerable evidence suggests that the incidence of mountain sickness increases substantially above 10,000 ft (3,000 m) and with rates of ascent greater than approximately 1,000 ft (300 m) per day. A number of extrinsic factors may also contribute by way of lowering the barometric pressure below what would be predicted by altitude alone. Latitude, temperature, low-pressure storm systems, and winter season may result in lower barometric pressure than expected and, therefore, predispose to altitude-related illness.

Acute adaptation to high altitude and to moderate altitude is similar. At higher altitudes, FVC declines by about 4% at 15,000 ft (4,572 m) and about 13% at 29,000 ft (8,839 m), probably due to increases in interstitial edema. Other changes occurring as a result of acute exposure include increased minute ventilation and decreased lung compliance. At rest, ventilation/perfusion matching becomes more homogenous, but probably worsens with exercise. Diffusion limitation becomes a major determinant to adaptation, especially at extreme altitudes. Hemodynamically, cardiac output and cerebral blood flow increase, as does pulmonary vascular resistance from hypoxia-induced vasoconstriction. Hemoglobin concentrations rise within 1 to 2 days from hemoconcentration. Changes in hemoglobin–oxygen affinity are mainly a result of changes in blood pH and Pco_2, which tend to offset any effects of 2,3-diphosphoglycerate. Acute hypobaric hypoxia results in a significant decrease in maximum oxygen consumption and exercise performance, and this never fully recovers to sea level values even with full acclimatization.

AMS represents the most common altitude-related illness. Upon rapid ascent, symptoms may appear immediately on arrival at altitude and usually resolve spontaneously over a few days. However, AMS can develop as many as 3 days after ascent. Headache, the most common complaint, occurs in as many as 70% of visitors above 8,000 ft (2,438 m). Sleep disturbances and sleep-disordered breathing (e.g., Cheyne–Stokes respirations) occur in 60% to 80% of travelers to altitude and may contribute to worsening disease. Other symptoms of AMS include nausea, vomiting, dyspnea, peripheral edema, malaise, anorexia, and fatigue. The most common method for diagnosing AMS is the Lake Louise system with five self-reported scores (headache, GI symptoms, fatigue, dizziness/lightheadedness, and difficulty sleeping rated 0–3 points each) and three clinical scores (change in mental status, 0–3 points; ataxia, 0–4 points; and peripheral edema, 0–2 points). AMS is defined as a headache plus a score of at least 3 points from the self-reports or 5 points if the clinical assessment is included too. There is some discussion in the literature about the role of headache in AMS, but it is noteworthy that headache is required for AMS diagnosis with the Lake Louise scoring system.

The mechanism behind AMS is quite likely multifactorial. Chief among them are hypobaric hypoxia and the individual response to the insult. Many people suffering from AMS have a low hypoxic ventilatory response, although this is not a universal finding. In addition, many people experience an alteration in body fluid mechanics with retention and redistribution. Evidence continues to mount for increased cerebral blood flow and, possibly, capillary leak as the main cause of headache and AMS. This theory is consistent with AMS representing the least dangerous end of a spectrum of high-altitude illnesses, which ends with HACE that can be fatal (see below). There are no specific laboratory markers of AMS, leaving the diagnosis to historical details in the appropriate setting.

The self-limited nature of AMS usually requires only conservative management, even allowing for continued ascent after brief recovery periods. Treatment of AMS consists primarily of symptomatic measures, using acetaminophen or nonsteroidal antiinflammatory drugs for headache or antiemetics (preferably prochloperazine, because it increases hypoxic ventilatory response). For refractory or more severe cases, further ascent should be postponed and descent of at least 1,000 ft (300 m) considered. Dexamethasone has been used successfully in treating symptoms of AMS, usually at doses of 4 mg every 6 hours (some suggest a loading dose of 8 mg). Failure to resolve after 1 to 2 days of conservative or medical management could indicate progression to more serious high-altitude pulmonary or cerebral edema (see below), which require prompt attention and descent by whatever means possible, including helicopter evacuation as necessary.

To prevent AMS, a gradual rate of ascent (<1,000 ft per day to above 10,000 ft) that allows time for the body to acclimatize is the best approach. Alcohol and other soporifics should be avoided. Acetazolamide, the most effective pharmacological prophylaxis, acts by creating a metabolic acidosis. It augments the normal response of the kidneys to compensate for the respiratory alkalosis that accompanies hyperventilation from hypoxia at high altitude. Most studies suggest 125 to 250 mg of acetazolamide twice per day, starting before ascent and continuing for a few days at high altitude. Acetazolamide is a diuretic, so it is essential to remain hydrated. People with sulfa allergy cannot use acetazolamide. Recent studies have not supported *Ginko biloba* as an effective prophylactic for AMS.

At altitudes above 10,000 ft (3,000 m), HAPE can occur. HAPE is more serious but also more rare than AMS. For example, in workers on the high-altitude railroad at 3,500 to 5,000 m in Tibet, over 50% had AMS but HAPE occurred only in about 0.5%. The pathogenesis of HAPE is not fully understood, but quite likely involves a variety of changes in the pulmonary vascular system. Among them are uneven hypoxic pulmonary vasoconstriction, altered pulmonary hemodynamics, blood flow heterogeneity, and increased capillary permeability. These changes lead to extravasation of proteins, blood, and fluid from the pulmonary capillaries into interstitial tissue and alveolar units, causing a potentially cascading scenario of worsening inflammation and alveolar flooding.

Clinically, patients with HAPE invariably have symptoms of AMS, but will also have progressive dyspnea on exertion or at rest, and, initially, a nonproductive cough that may progress to pink frothy sputum. Signs include increasing tachypnea, tachycardia, and cyanosis. Rales typically arise first in the right midaxillary line and spread diffusely with worsening disease, especially while sleeping. Chest radiographs reveal diffuse patchy infiltrates, with prominence of pulmonary arteries. Notably absent are Kerley B lines or other evidence of pulmonary venous congestion, because pulmonary capillary wedge pressures typically remain normal.

HAPE is the most common cause of death due to altitude-related illnesses, and, therefore, requires immediate treatment. Numerous studies have attempted to delineate methods to prevent HAPE, but only AMS prevention strategies have been advocated until recently. Descent remains the most important aspect of successful treatment of HAPE, with most authors recommending descent to 2,000 to 3,000 ft (600 to 1,000 m). Supplemental oxygen also plays a major role in the treatment of HAPE, if it is available. Unfortunatley, HAPE victims are often unable to descend because of their physical condition or because of poor weather. In these cases, the calcium-channel blockers (nifedipine at 20–30 mg orally every 6–8 hours) or phosphodiesterase inhibitors (tadalafil 10 mg every 12 hours, sildenafil 50 mg every 8 hours) can be used to reduce pulmonary hypertension. Dexamethasone (2 mg every 6 hours or 4 mg every 2 hours) can be helpful too. Portable hyperbaric chambers (e.g., the Gamow bag) can also simulate a descent of about 1,476 ft (450 m), but are usually only found on large expeditions to very remote destinations.

Patients with preexisting pulmonary hypertension are at risk of worsening at high altitude. Those with mean pulmonary artery (PA) pressure greater than 35 mmHg or systolic PA pressure greater than 50 mmHg at baseline should typically avoid travel to greater than 2,000 m; but if such travel is necessary or strongly desired, they should use supplemental oxygen during the sojourn. Patients with milder degrees of pulmonary hypertension may travel to altitudes less than 3,000 m, but should consider pulmonary vasodilators or supplemental oxygen.

The most serious illness for high-altitude visitors is HACE, which occurs even more rarely than HAPE but may be a harbinger of death. Symptoms indicating HACE include worsening ataxia, changes in level of consciousness, coma, severe lassitude, seizures, cranial nerve palsies, retinal hemorrhages, cyanosis, and hallucinations superimposed on symptoms of AMS or HAPE. Studies have shown elevated cerebral spinal fluid pressures (up to 300 mmHg). Autopsies have also often revealed clinically indolent pulmonary edema. The disorder requires prompt recognition and immediate descent, if possible. In addition, dexamethasone (4 mg, intravenously, intramuscularly, or orally, followed by 4 mg every 6 hours) and oxygen remain important adjuncts. Portable hyperbaric chambers are also useful, when available.

In summary, increasing numbers of people are traveling to high altitude for a variety of reasons. Many of these travelers suffer symptoms of AMS, which resolves over a few days as acclimatization progresses and can be reduced by gradual ascent or acetazolamide. Fewer travelers at higher altitudes may experience HAPE or HACE, which require prompt attention and descent to prevent life-threatening progression. Patients with pulmonary hypertension should be evaluated for travel to high altitude.

FURTHER READING

1. Aerospace Medical Association, Air Transport Medicine Committee. Medical guidelines for air travel. *Aviat Space Environ Med.* 2003;74(5, suppl):A1–A19.

   A comprehensive monograph of current recommendations regarding air travel for the most common disease states thought to be potentially exacerbated by commercial aviation. Thoroughly referenced.

2. Gong HJ. Air travel and oxygen therapy in cardiopulmonary patients. *Chest.* 1992;101:1104–1113.

   A concise review of flight pathophysiology, medical clearance procedures, and in-flight oxygen issues.

3. Gong HJ, Mark JA, Cowan MN. Preflight medical screenings of patients. Analysis of health and flight characteristics. *Chest.* 1993;104:788–794.

   Analysis of patient characteristics referred for preflight screening based on 1,115 patients mostly referred for in-flight oxygen use.

4. Rosenberg CA, Pak F. Emergencies in the air: problems, management, and prevention. *J Emerg Med.* 1997;15:159–164.

   Reviews the incidence of in-flight emergencies, the onboard medical kit, and some in-flight medical problems and treatments.

5. Dillard TA, Beninati WA, Berg BW. Air travel in patients with chronic obstructive pulmonary disease. *Arch Intern Med.* 1991;151:1793–1795.

   A prospective study of the frequency and outcome of air travel among a cohort of military COPD patients. The authors noted an 18.9% annual frequency of air travel with an 18.2% incidence of transient in-flight complaints.

6. Dillard TA, Rosenberg AP, Berg BW. Hypoxemia during altitude exposure. A meta-analysis of chronic obstructive pulmonary disease. *Chest.* 1993;103:422–425.

   Meta-analysis that reviewed evidence regarding the use of altitude simulation chamber to predict in-flight PaO_2 among patients with severe COPD using sea level PaO_2 and FEV_1.

7. Schwartz JS, Bencowitz HZ, Moser KM. Air travel hypoxemia with chronic obstructive pulmonary disease. *Ann Intern Med.* 1984;100:473–477.

   Correlation between 17% oxygen arterial blood gas and direct measurement in unpressurized cabin at 5,000 ft (1,650 m) in patients with severe COPD. Validates HAST in this cohort.

8. Vohra KP, Klocke RA. Detection and correction of hypoxemia associated with air travel. *Am Rev Respir Dis.* 1993;148:1215–1219.

   Used Venturi device to assess in-flight oxygen requirement in COPD patients.

9. Cramer D, Ward S, Geddes D. Assessment of oxygen supplementation during air travel. *Thorax.* 1996;51:202–203.

   Used body plethysmograph to determine in-flight oxygen requirements for normals and those with either obstructive or restrictive lung disease. The authors found that 2 to 3 L/min supplemental O_2 corrected PaO_2 values obtained in 15% FiO_2 to that obtained in room air in all subjects.

10. Mercer A, Brown JD. Venous thromboembolism associated with air travel: a report of 33 patients. *Aviat Space Environ Med.* 1998;69:154–157.

    Recent chart review of 134 patients admitted for DVT. Among them, air travel was the only risk factor for 12 subjects (36%); all experienced at least 4 hours of flight time within the preceding 31 days prior to admission.

11. Gong HJ, Tashkin DP, Lee EY, et al. Hypoxia-altitude simulation test. Evaluation of patients with chronic airway obstruction. *Am Rev Respir Dis.* 1984;130:980–986.

    Classic study outlining design and validation of simulation test using hypoxic gas mixtures. The authors also derived a regression equation and nomogram to estimate PaO_2 at altitudes between 5,000 to 10,000 ft in patients with normocapnic COPD.

12. Dillard TA, Berg BW, Rajagopal KR, et al. Hypoxemia during air travel in patients with chronic obstructive pulmonary disease. *Ann Intern Med.* 1989;111:362–367.

   Increased sensitivity of in-flight PaO$_2$ prediction equation by combining FEV$_1$ with ground-level PaO$_2$ in hypobaric chamber in patients with severe COPD (FEV$_1$ 31 ± 10% of predicted) to aid in supplemental oxygen requirement prediction.

13. Berg BW, Dillard TA, Rajagopal KR, et al. Oxygen supplementation during air travel in patients with chronic obstructive lung disease. *Chest.* 1992;101:638–641.

   The authors outline the capability of oxygen delivery devices to increase PaO$_2$ to levels sufficient for tissue oxygenation in severe COPD patients during acute moderate simulated altitude exposure (8,000 ft, 2,438 m).

14. Dillard TA, Rajagopal KR, Slivka WA, et al. Lung function during moderate hypobaric hypoxia in normal subjects and patients with chronic obstructive pulmonary disease. *Aviat Space Environ Med.* 1998;69:979–985.

   The authors found a slight change in FVC in some, but not all, normals and COPD patients following exposure to a simulated 8,000 ft (2,438 m).

15. Kramer MR, Jakobson DJ, Springer C, et al. The safety of air transportation of patients with advanced lung disease. Experience with 21 patients requiring lung transplantation or pulmonary thromboendarterectomy. *Chest.* 1995;108:1292–1296.

   Outcomes of patients traveling by air with severe lung disease.

16. Naughton MT, Rochford PD, Pretto JJ, et al. Is normobaric simulation of hypobaric hypoxia accurate in chronic airflow limitation? *Am J Respir Crit Care Med.* 1995;152:1956–1960.

   Study showing no significant difference between normobaric and hypobaric hypoxia-altitude simulation tests.

17. Gong HJ. Advising patients with pulmonary diseases on air travel. *Ann Intern Med.* 1989;111: 349–351.

   Editorial with practical advice.

18. Ling IT, Singh B, James AL, et al. Vital capacity and oxygen saturation at rest and after exercise predict hypoxaemia during hypoxic inhalation test in patients with respiratory disease. *Respirology.* 2013;18:507–513.

   Evaluate the use of post-exercise SpO(2) ≥95% on room air to exclude the need for hypoxic inhalation test (HIT) to assess oxygen requirement for air travel.

19. Hampson NB, Kregenow DA, Mahoney AM, et al. Altitude exposures during commercial flight: a reappraisal. *Aviat Space Environ Med.* 2013;84:27–31.

   Report in cabin altitude in flights of shorter distance and the need of supplemental oxygen.

20. Smith D, Toff W, Joy M, et al. Fitness to fly for passengers with cardiovascular disease. *Heart.* 2010;96(suppl 2):ii1–ii16.

   Report about heart diseases and air travel

21. Ahmedzai S, Balfour-Lynn IM, Bewick T, et al. Managing passengers with stable respiratory disease planning air travel: British Thoracic Society recommendations. *Thorax.* 2011;66(suppl 1):i1–i30.

   British Thoracic Society (BTS) guidelines for air travel in patient with different pulmonary diseases.

22. Am A, Singh P, Ensor JE, et al. Air travel after biopsy-related pneumothorax: is it safe to fly? *J Vasc Interv Radiol.* 2011;22:595.

   Report concerning pneumothorax and air travel.

23. Walker J, Kelly PT, Beckert L. Airline policies for passengers with obstructive sleep apnoea who require in-flight continuous positive airways pressure. *Respirology.* 2010;15:556–561.

   Study about current policies of Australian and New Zealand airlines on the use of in-flight continuous positive airway pressure (CPAP) by passengers with OSA (obstructive sleep apnea).

24. Humphreys S, Deyermond R, Bali I, et al. The effect of high altitude commercial air travel on oxygen saturation. *Anaesthesia.* 2005;60:458–460.

   Case control study consisted of anaesthetists and their traveling companions, each passenger acted as their own control (none of the passenger have history of heart disease). Different hemodynamic variables were measured before and during air travel in both short and long flights.

25. Antman EM, Anbe DT, Armstrong PW, et al. ACC/AHA guidelines for the management of patients with ST-elevation myocardial infarction. A Report of the American College of Cardiology/ American Heart Association Task Force on Practice Guidelines (Committee to revise the 1999 guidelines for the management of patients with acute myocardial infarction). *J Am Coll Cardiol.* 2004;44:E1–E211.

Current ACC/AHA guidelines for the management of myocardial infarction.

26. Guyatt GH, Akl EA, Crowther M, et al. Executive summary: antithrombotic therapy and prevention of thrombosis, 9th ed. American College of Chest Physicians Evidence-Based Clinical Practice Guidelines. *Chest.* 2012;141(2, suppl):7S–47S.

Guidelines from ACCP regarding prevention of thrombosis.

27. Mohr LC. Hypoxia during air travel in adults with pulmonary disease. *Am J Med Sci.* 2008;335(1):71.

Review article related to clinical evaluation of patient with pulmonary diseases before air travel.

28. Marienau KJ, Illig PA, Kozarsky PE, et al. Air travel. In: Brunette GW, ed. *CDC Health Information for International Travel 2014.* New York, NY: Oxford University Press; 2014.

This is an excellent chapter in a reference source published by the CDC every 2 years, which is commonly referred to as the "Yellow Book." It is targeted to healthcare professionals who advise international travelers about health risks, but is written in plain language and can be a direct resource for patients as well.

High-Altitude Medicine

29. Hackett PH, Roach RC, Sutton JR. High altitude medicine. In: Auerbach PS, Geehr EC, eds. *Management of Wilderness and Environmental Emergencies.* 2nd ed. St Louis, MO: Mosby; 1989:1–34.

Textbook chapter with comprehensive review of adaptation, pathophysiology, and altitude-related illnesses. Includes practical advice and thorough references.

30. Luks A, Swenson ER, Schoene RB. High altitude. In: Murray JF, Nadel JA, eds. *Textbook of Respiratory Medicine.* 6th ed. Philadelphia, PA: WB Saunders; 2013: chap 77.

Textbook chapter detailing the physiology of adaptation to high altitude. Very thorough with extensive references.

31. Hultgren HN, Spickard WB, Hellriegel K, et al. High altitude pulmonary edema. *Medicine.* 1961;40:289–313.

First detailed account and classic characterization of the disorder.

32. Houston CS. Operation Everest one and two. Studies of acclimatization to simulated high altitude. *Respiration.* 1997;64:398–406.

Review of the classic physiologic studies of acclimatization conducted first on Mt. Everest and later in a hypobaric altitude simulation chamber with comprehensive analysis of the results.

33. Wagner PD, Sutton JR, Reeves JT, et al. Operation Everest II: pulmonary gas exchange during a simulated ascent of Mt. Everest. *J Appl Physiol.* 1987;63:2348–2359.

Classic physiologic study showing increasing ventilation–perfusion mismatch with long-term exposure to both altitude and exercise, thought to be related to interstitial edema because of the relationship to pulmonary arterial pressure.

34. Hackett PH, Rennie D, Grover RF, et al. Acute mountain sickness and the edemas of high altitude: a common pathogenesis? *Respir Physiol.* 1981;46:383–390.

Study of Nepal trekkers looking at body weight correlations with AMS symptom scores as a gauge of fluid retention. The authors conclude that rapid ascent combined with fluid retention may identify a common pathogenesis for peripheral, pulmonary, and cerebral edema.

35. Schoene RB, Lahiri S, Hackett PH, et al. Relationship of hypoxic ventilatory response to exercise performance on Mount Everest. *J Appl Physiol.* 1984;56:1478–1483.

Study examined the change in ventilation at sea level, 5,400 m and 6,300 m. The authors conclude that hypoxic ventilatory response (HVR) predicts exercise ventilation at sea level and high altitude; that the drop in $SaO_2\%$ that occurs with exercise is inversely related to HVR; and persons with a high HVR may perform better at extreme altitude.

36. Hackett PH, Rennie D, Hofmeister SE, et al. Fluid retention and relative hypoventilation in acute mountain sickness. *Respiration.* 1982;43:321–329

Study showing correlation between fluid retention and AMS scores in 42 healthy subjects between Katmandu, Nepal (4,518 ft, 1,377 m) and Pheriche (13,921 ft, 4,243 m) within 6 days of exposure.

37. Eldridge MW, Podolsky A, Richardson RS, et al. Pulmonary hemodynamic response to exercise in subjects with prior high-altitude pulmonary edema. *J Appl Physiol*. 1996;81:911–921.

   The authors develop a multiple regression analysis showing a greater pulmonary arterial pressure reactivity to exercise in HAPE-susceptible compared to controls at sea level. The response, however, was not affected by ascent to an altitude of 3,810 m, suggesting an intrinsic pattern among HAPE-susceptible individuals.

38. Podolsky A, Eldridge MW, Richardson RS, et al. Exercise-induced VA/Q inequality in subjects with prior high-altitude pulmonary edema. *J Appl Physiol*. 1996;81:922–932.

   The authors found a higher exercise-induced ventilation–perfusion mismatch (assessed by log standard deviation of perfusion distribution) at sea level, but not at 3,810 m, among HAPE-susceptible individuals.

39. Schoene RB, Hackett PH, Henderson WR, et al. High-altitude pulmonary edema. Characteristics of lung lavage fluid. *JAMA*. 1986;256:63–69.

   Classic description showing elevated total proteins and products of inflammation in lung lavage fluid among patients with HAPE. Direct evidence characterizing HAPE as a high-permeability, rather than hydrostatic, form of pulmonary edema.

40. Hackett PH, Rennie D. The incidence, importance, and prophylaxis of acute mountain sickness. *Lancet*. 1976;2:1149–1155.

   Landmark study of AMS and prevention with gradual ascent or acetazolamide.

41. Johnson TS, Rock PB, Fulco CS, et al. Prevention of acute mountain sickness by dexamethasone. *N Engl J Med*. 1984;310:683–686.

   Key study documenting effectiveness of dexamethasone vs placebo in preventing AMS in a simulated ascent to 15,000 ft (4,570 m) as determined by questionnaire.

42. Hornbein TF, Townes BD, Schoene RB, et al. The cost to the central nervous system of climbing to extremely high altitude. *N Engl J Med*. 1989;321:1714–1719.

   Landmark study of neurobehavioral changes after either actual or simulated ascent to altitudes between 18,005 ft (5,488 m) and 29,028 ft (8,848 m) at 1 to 30 days. The authors found a decline in visual long-term memory and twice as many aphasic errors compared to controls. Interestingly, both correlated with a more vigorous ventilatory response to hypoxia after returning to lower elevations.

43. Honigman B, Theis MK, Koziol-McLain J, et al. Acute mountain sickness in a general tourist population at moderate altitudes. *Ann Intern Med*. 1993;118:587–592.

   Documents incidence of altitude-related disorders among cohort of travelers to Colorado sleeping between 6,300 and 9,700 ft (1,920 and 2,957 m).

44. Gilbert DL. The first documented report of mountain sickness: the China or Headache Mountain story. *Respir Physiol*. 1983;52:315–326.

   Detailed historical account of widely believed first documented reports of altitude-related sickness.

45. Netzer N, Strohl K, Faulhaber M, et al. Hypoxia-related altitude illnesses. *J Trav Med*. 2013;20:247–255.

   Recent review of studies identified in Medline (1965 to May 2012).

46. Hackett PH, Oelz O. The Lake Louise consensus on the definition and quantification of altitude illness. In: Sutton JR, Coates G, Houston CS, eds. *Hypoxia and Mountain Medicine*. Burlington, VT: Queen City Printers; 1992:327–330.

   Scoring system for AMS.

47. West JB, Schoene RB, Luks AM, et al. *High Altitude Medicine and Physiology*. 5th ed. Boca Raton, FL: CRC Press; 2013.

   Up-to-date textbook with chapters on AMS, HAPE, HACE, and other aspects of high-altitude medicine and physiology.

48. Dubowitz DJ, Dyer EA, Thelmann RJ, et al. Early brain swelling in acute hypoxia. *J Appl Physiol*. 2009;107:244–252.

   Research report on how changes in cerebral blood flow may contribute to AMS.

49. Luks AM. Can patients with pulmonary hypertension travel to high altitude? *High Alt Med Biol*. 2009;10(3):215.

   A thorough review regarding pulmonary vascular responses to high altitude related acute hypoxia.

Presentations of Respiratory Disorders

21 Dyspnea
Victor J. Test

INTRODUCTION

Breathing is an involuntary action, controlled by the subconscious and normally does not prompt recognition by the conscious mind. Dyspnea is defined as an uncomfortable awareness or sensation associated with breathing. However, awareness of breathing is not synonymous with dyspnea, since the context of the awareness is crucial to determining if the sensation is uncomfortable or not. For example, a sprinter who completes a 400-m race may breathe quite hard; however, the work of breathing is expected in this setting and is not in itself an uncomfortable sensation.

Dyspnea is one of the more common complaints in pulmonary medicine and is more common in women and obese and older patients. The complaint of dyspnea is often difficult to elicit in clinical practice, since patients may provide disparate descriptions use such as "I can't breathe," "I am smothering," "I get tired," "I am puffed," and "I am panting." In addition, the evaluation of dyspnea may be delayed when patients and physicians attribute the symptom to aging, obesity, deconditioning, and/or smoking.

PRESENTATION

Dyspnea is an alarming symptom, even when compared to chest pain. Among patients who present with dyspnea and/or chest pain, all-cause mortality is much higher when dyspnea or dyspnea and chest pain are the presenting symptoms. In this group, mortality due to myocardial infarction and coronary revascularization is much higher when compared to patients who presented with chest pain alone.

Dyspnea is affected by numerous receptors and factors, as well as by one's perceptions. The cerebral cortex interprets dyspnea-related data from chemoreceptors, muscles, skin, and the lung in order to place them in context. The medulla and subcortex receive input from the afferent receptors and central chemoreceptors as part of the control of breathing. The chest wall has mechanoreceptors in muscle spindles and tendon organs that are innervated by the anterior horn cells and project to the somatosensory cortex. The vagus nerve also has afferent nerves that relay information about lung inflation and volume changes. Chemorecepters in the carotid body and the medulla detect changes in pH, Pco_2, and Po_2. Myelinated nerves and unmyelinated C-fibers in the lung conduct information from the lungs, larynx, and trachea and send information via the vagus nerve regarding pulmonary stretch and air movement. Even the skin of the face and mucous membranes of the nasopharynx detect air flow and affect the sensation of dyspnea.

The differential diagnosis of acute onset of dyspnea is quite broad and includes asthma, anxiety-related hyperventilation, pneumothorax, pulmonary embolism, exacerbation of chronic lung disease, pulmonary edema, and myocardial ischemia. The evaluation of acute dyspnea should be guided by the history, physical examination, and judicious diagnostic testing. Basic diagnostic evaluation may include an electrocardiogram, chest radiography, complete blood count, and arterial blood gases. History and physical examination in conjunction with these diagnostic tests should establish the diagnosis of pulmonary edema, pneumothorax, and chest trauma. In a pure hyperventilation syndrome, arterial blood gases demonstrate respiratory alkalosis and normal alveolar–arterial gradient. The detection of myocardial ischemia and pulmonary embolism may be more difficult and generally mandates additional testing such as cardiac enzymes, D-dimer measurement, echocardiography, and thoracic imaging: either by contrast-enhanced computed tomography (CT) or ventilation–perfusion scanning. The Well's Score or Geneva Score can help stratify the patient's probability of having pulmonary embolism. Spirometry can identify airflow obstruction. The brain natriuretic peptide (BNP) and N-terminal pro-brain natriuretic peptide (NT-pro-BNP) are useful in identifying decompensated heart failure, although, it can increase in other conditions such as pulmonary embolism.

Chronic dyspnea is shortness of breath that has persisted for more than 3 weeks. As is the case in acute dyspnea, the diagnosis of chronic dyspnea can usually be identified with a careful history, physical examination, and a few basic tests such as chest radiography, electrocardiography, spirometry, and simple laboratory testing (complete blood count, chemistry, and thyroid testing). Elements of the history such as previous diagnoses may, however, be misleading in patients with chronic dyspnea. One study demonstrated that a historical diagnosis of reactive airway disease was associated with a positive predictive value (PPV) of only 0.55 for the final diagnosis of asthma. Similarly, a patient's report of chronic obstructive pulmonary disease (COPD) was associated with a PPV of 0.45 for COPD. A history of smoking in patients with chronic dyspnea carried a PPV of 0.40 for COPD.

ETIOLOGY AND DIFFERENTIAL DIAGNOSES

The etiology of chronic dyspnea may be difficult to identify. The initial clinical impression is reported to be correct 55% of the time and correct 72% of the time when pulmonary function testing was utilized in the decision making. However, a systematic evaluation of the patient can identify the diagnosis with a high degree of accuracy. Laboratory testing (complete blood count, comprehensive metabolic profile, thyroid stimulating hormone [TSH] and BNP) can be helpful. A recent study found that 14% of the patients presenting with chronic dyspnea had significant anemia. This same study evaluated the BNP and found that it had a strong negative predictive value for cardiomyopathy but a very poor PPV for it.

Chronic unexplained dyspnea exists if the diagnosis is not apparent after basic testing. There are a number of approaches to this diagnosis; two studies have disclosed the clinical benefits of algorithmic approaches. The algorithmic approaches to dyspnea usually employ early challenge by methacholine to test for subtle airway hyperactivity. Not surprisingly, the diagnosis of chronic dyspnea is most commonly pulmonary, but the more common diagnosis vary according to age (see Table 21-1). Younger populations tend to have higher percentages of asthma and vocal cord dysfunction when

TABLE 21-1	Diagnoses Associated with Chronic Dyspnea					
	Pratter 1989	Depaso 1991	Martinez 1994	Flaherty 2001	Morris 2001	Pratter 2011
Average age (years)	52	59	55	36.9	29	60.2
Asthma (%)	29	17	24	31	47	29
COPD (%)	14	5	0	—	3	9
ILD (%)	14	5	8	15	8	8
Cardiac (%)	9	14	14	18	16	16

compared to studies in older patients. The most common diagnosis is reactive airway disease. It accounts for the final diagnosis in between 17% and 55% of patients with chronic dyspnea.

In patients diagnosed with reactive airway disease, methacholine challenge is required for the diagnosis in 41% to 72% of cases. A decreased diffusion capacity is helpful in clarifying the diagnosis of obstructive lung disease from asthma and is universally decreased in patients with interstitial lung disease. In addition, a decrease in the diffusion capacity can be useful in identifying patients with pulmonary vascular disease, and additional testing such as echocardiography and imaging for thromboembolism may be helpful. A decrease in vital capacity or lung volumes should trigger a search for interstitial lung disease or neuromuscular disease with a mandatory minute volume (MVV) and maximal inspiratory pressure and maximal expiratory pressures.

Two other diagnoses may be more difficult to identify. One study identified a surprising number of young patients with mitochondrial myopathy that was detected with a decreased MMV and confirmed with muscle biopsy. In this population, the maximal inspiratory and expiratory pressures were often normal. Morris et al. studied a military population and found that vocal cord dysfunction was the etiology of chronic dyspnea in 10% of patients. About 20% of patients with vocal cord dysfunction may be identified by a truncated inspiratory limb on the flow-volume loop in the absence of other evidence of significant air flow obstruction. Fiberoptic laryngoscopy during exercise may be required to diagnose the patient with vocal cord dysfunction; many may have a false positive methacholine inhalation challenge test.

Cardiopulmonary exercise testing may be very useful in identifying the organ system responsible for dyspnea as well as identifying deconditioning, obesity, and nonphysiologic dyspnea as the cause of the symptom. Further, cardiopulmonary exercise testing was able to direct invasive testing when indicated. After a diagnosis is made through diagnostic testing, it is usually recommended that the diagnosis be confirmed with a positive response to therapy.

QUANTIFICATION OF DYSPNEA

After a diagnosis of dyspnea has been established and therapy is being contemplated, it is often useful to quantify the degree of dyspnea with a detailed description of the amount of activity that stimulates the symptoms. As patients improve, it is typical for them to continue to complain of dyspnea. This may represent failure to improve or it may represent an increase in activity. Good documentation and objective measures of exercise levels are very useful in this setting.

In addition, there are a variety of patient-assessment tools available to quantify patients' symptoms. These include the Visual Analogue Scale, the Borg Dyspnea Index, and the Mahler Dyspnea Score. Each of these tests can be repeated as an objective measure of the patient's symptoms. The Visual Analogue Scale and the Borg Index are also useful during exercise testing for the patient to rate their degree of symptoms.

CONCLUSION

The clinical complaint of shortness of breath is a common complaint that is associated with difficulty in diagnosis and significant implications for the patient. With a systematic approach, the diagnosis can be identified and treatment begun with a high degree of success.

FURTHER READING

1. Irwin RS, Curlee FJ, Grossman RF, eds. *Diagnosis and Treatment of Symptoms of the Respiratory Tract.* Hoboken, NJ: Wiley-Blackwell; 1997.

   An outstanding book chapter and summary on the mechanisms of dyspnea, evaluation, and treatment.

2. Simon PM, Schwartstein RM, Weiss JM, et al. Distinguishable sensations of breathlessness induced in normal volunteers. *Am Rev Respir Dis.* 1989;140:121–127.

   A study that describes in depth the ways that patients describe dyspnea.

3. Bergeron S, Ommen SR, Bailey KR, et al. Exercise echocardiography and the outcome of patients referred for evaluation of dyspnea. *J Am Coll Cardiol.* 2004;43:2242–2246.

   A large study that demonstrates the importance of dyspnea as a symptom and its implications on mortality.

4. Burki NK, Lee L-Y. Mechanisms of dyspnea. *Chest.* 2010;138(5):1196–1201.

   A recent update on the mechanisms of shortness of breath.

5. Cherniak NS, Altose MD. Mechanisms of dyspnea. *Clin Chest Med.* 1987;8(2):207–214.

 A classic paper on the mechanisms of dyspnea.

6. Schwartstein RM. Dyspnea: mechanisms, assessment, and management. A consensus statement. *Am J Respir Crit Care Med.* 1999;159(1):321–340.

 An outstanding review of the mechanisms of dyspnea.

7. Mahler DA. Dyspnea: diagnosis and management. *Clin Chest Med.* 1987;8(2):215–228.

8. Pratter MA, Curlee F, Dubois J, et al. Cause and evaluation of dyspnea in a pulmonary clinic. *Arch Intern Med.* 1989;149:2277–2282.

 The classic article that first described a systematic approach to the evaluation and treatment of dyspnea.

9. Ray P, Delerme S, Jourdain P, et al. Differential diagnosis of acute dyspnea in the emergency department: the utility of the BNP and NT-pro-BNP. *QJM.* 2008;101:831–843.

10. Pratter MA, Abouzgheib W, Akers S, et al. An algorithmic approach to chronic dyspnea. *Respir Med.* 2011;105(7):1014–1021.

 This paper describes a highly successful algorithmic approach to the evaluation of chronic dyspnea.

11. Morris MJ, Grbach VX, Deal LE, et al. Evaluation of exertional dyspnea in the active duty patient: the diagnostic approach and the utility of clinical testing. *Mili Med.* 2002;167:281–288.

 An excellent paper that describes a systematic evaluation of exertional dyspnea in a population of younger patients.

12. Martinez FJ, Stanopoulos J, Acero R, et al. Graded comprehensive cardiopulmonary exercise testing in the evaluation of dyspnea unexplained by routine evaluation. *Chest.* 1994;105:168–175.

13. DePaso WJ, Winterbauer RH, Lusk JA, et al. Chronic dyspnea unexplained by history, physical examination, chest roentgenogram, and spirometry. Analysis of a seven-year experience. *Chest.* 1991;100:1293–1299.

14. Flaherty KR, Wald J, Weisman IM, et al. Unexplained exertional limitation: characterization of patients with a mitochondrial myopathy. *Am J Respir Crit Care Med.* 2001;164:425–432.

 This paper examines a series of patients who present to a dyspnea clinic and the surprising incidence of mitochondrial myopathy.

15. Morris MJ, Christopher MD. Diagnostic criteria for the classification of vocal cord dysfunction. *Chest.* 2010;138(5):1213–1223.

 An outstanding review of vocal cord dysfunction.

16. Abidov A, Rozank A, Hachamovic R, et al. *Prognostic significance of dyspnea in patients referred for cardiac stress testing. N Eng J Med.* 2005;353:1889–1898.

17. Klok FA, Kruisman E, Spaan J, et al. Comparison of the revised Geneva score with the Wells rule for assessing clinical probability of pulmonary embolism. *J Thromb Haemost.* 2008;6(1):40–44.

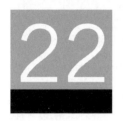

22 Approach to Pulmonary Vascular Disease

David Poch

INTRODUCTION: THE PULMONARY VASCULAR SYSTEM

Under normal conditions, the pulmonary vascular bed is a low resistance and high compliance circuit that accommodates the entire cardiac output at pressures that are 20% to 25% of systemic pressures. Normal pulmonary artery pressures are as follows: for systolic, 15 to 30 mmHg; for diastolic, 4 to 12 mmHg; and for mean, 9 to 18 mmHg. Even during exercise, when the cardiac output increases by 2- to 4-fold, the normal pulmonary vascular bed can accommodate increased flow with only modest increases in pressure and minimal effects on pulmonary vascular resistance.

Disruption of the normal pulmonary vascular bed can occur as a result of a primary vasculopathy of the pulmonary vessels, diseases of the lung parenchyma, thromboembolic disease, and pulmonary venous hypertension secondary to left heart dysfunction. Identification of the anatomic location of the diseased portion of the pulmonary vascular bed is paramount in the evaluation of pulmonary vascular disease. Diseases that involve the precapillary pulmonary arterial bed have a very different natural history and treatment strategy as compared to primary parenchymal lung disorders and diseases affecting the postcapillary, pulmonary venous compartment.

Pulmonary hypertension (PH) is present when the mean pulmonary artery pressure is greater than 25 mmHg. Pulmonary *arterial* hypertension (PAH) is present when the mean pulmonary artery pressure is greater than 25 mmHg and the pulmonary capillary wedge pressure or left ventricular end-diastolic pressure is less than or equal to 15 mmHg. The pressure gradient from the mean pulmonary artery pressure to the pulmonary capillary wedge pressure is the transpulmonary gradient; elevation of the gradient distinguishes PAH from other causes of elevated pulmonary pressures. Despite the fact that PAH is defined clinically by elevated pressures, it is truly a disease of increased pulmonary vascular resistance. Pulmonary vascular resistance is equal to the transpulmonary gradient divided by cardiac output. It is the pulmonary vascular resistance that determines disease severity. Normal pulmonary vascular resistance is less than 3 WU, and if there is significant PAH, the pulmonary vascular resistance must be higher than this. The right ventricle, unlike the left ventricle, is ill-equipped to maintain cardiac output against an increased afterload. As destruction of the precapillary vessels progresses, pulmonary vascular resistance increases and the right ventricle fails. A patient may experience dyspnea, chest pain, fluid retention, and syncope.

While increased pulmonary vascular resistance and right heart failure account for the majority of morbidity and mortality in PAH, alterations in ventilation and perfusion matching and impairments in oxygen diffusion also play a role. Increased dead space ventilation, particularly in patients with chronic thromboembolic PH, may account for symptoms of dyspnea that seem to exceed what alterations in hemodynamics alone might predict.

DETECTION OF PULMONARY HYPERTENSION

The majority of PH is due to heart diseases associated with elevated pulmonary arterial pressures due to increased pulmonary venous pressures (e.g., congestive heart failure, valvular heart disease) and to parenchymal lung disease (e.g., chronic obstructive pulmonary disease and interstitial lung disease). PAH is rare and has a prevalence of 15 to 40 cases per million. Before treatment can be properly planned, it is essential to identify the etiology of elevated pulmonary arterial pressure because pulmonary vasodilators used to treat PAH are not helpful in most other causes of PH.

The most common presenting symptom in PAH is dyspnea (>85%) which is often initially attributed to more common cardiopulmonary disorders leading to a sometimes problematic delay in diagnosis. Data from multicenter PAH registries indicate that more than 20% of patients report symptoms for more than 2 years before the correct diagnosis is made. Other symptoms that may help suggest the diagnosis of PAH include fatigue (26%), chest pain (22%), presyncope/syncope (17%), edema (20%), and palpitations (12%).

Cardiac exam findings consistent with PAH include elevated jugular venous distention, a right ventricular heave, a loud P2, a fixed split S2, a right sided S3, and a tricuspid regurgitation murmur. The absence of physical examination findings of left heart disease is important to a diagnosis of PAH. The presence of pulmonary edema or pleural effusions should raise suspicion for left heart disease or, in the correct setting, rare conditions such as pulmonary veno-occlusive disease. Exam findings consistent with alternative causes of dyspnea such as obstructive lung disease or sleep disordered breathing should prompt further evaluation.

EPIDEMIOLOGY OF PULMONARY VASCULAR DISEASE

The current World Health Organization classification of PH (see Table 22-1) provides an excellent outline of populations at risk for developing PAH. The idiopathic form of the disease (IPAH)

TABLE 22-1	Revised WHO Classification of PH17

Basis for Current Classification Schema of Pulmonary Hypertension

Group I
1. Pulmonary arterial hypertension (PAH)
   - 1.1. Idiopathic (IPAH)
   - 1.2. Familial (FPAH)
   - 1.3. Associated with (APAH):
     - 1.3.1. Connective tissue disorder
     - 1.3.2. Congenital systemic-to-pulmonary shunts
     - 1.3.3. Portal hypertension
     - 1.3.4. HIV infection
     - 1.3.5. Drugs and toxins
     - 1.3.6. Other (thyroid disorders, glycogen storage disease, Gaucher disease, hereditary hemorrhagic telangiectasia, hemoglobinopathies, chronic myeloproliferative disorders, splenectomy)
   - 1.4. Associated with significant venous or capillary involvement
     - 1.4.1. Pulmonary veno-occlusive disease (PVOD)
     - 1.4.2. Pulmonary capillary hemangiomatosis (PCH)
   - 1.5. Persistent pulmonary hypertension of the newborn

Group II
2. Pulmonary hypertension with left heart disease
   - 2.1. Left-sided atrial or ventricular heart disease
   - 2.2. Left-sided valvular heart disease

Group III
3. Pulmonary hypertension associated with lung diseases and/or hypoxemia
   - 3.1. Chronic obstructive pulmonary disease
   - 3.2. Interstitial lung disease
   - 3.3. Sleep disordered breathing
   - 3.4. Alveolar hypoventilation disorders
   - 3.5. Chronic exposure to high altitude
   - 3.6. Developmental abnormalities

Group IV
4. Pulmonary hypertension due to chronic thrombotic and/or embolic disease (CTEPH)
   - 4.1. Thromboembolic obstruction of proximal pulmonary arteries
   - 4.2. Thromboembolic obstruction of distal pulmonary arteries
   - 4.3. Nonthrombotic pulmonary embolism (tumor, parasites, foreign material)

Group V
5. Miscellaneous
   Sarcoidosis, histiocytosis X, lymphangiomatosis, compression of pulmonary vessels (adenopathy, tumor, fibrosing mediastinitis)

accounts for nearly half of the prevalent PAH in recent published registries; it affects women more frequently than men (1.7:1) and presents most often in the third decade of life.

Other specific populations at risk for developing PAH include patients with associated diseases such as connective tissue diseases, congenital heart diseases, portal hypertension, and stimulant use.

Familial forms of PAH have been identified with gene mutations in two receptors of the transforming growth factor-b family, bone morphogenic protein receptor-2 (BMPR2) and activin-like kinase type-1 (ALK-1). Penetrance is incomplete, so the mutation is not useful for screening the general population.

The majority of patients with chronic obstructive pulmonary disease (COPD) have mild to moderate elevations in pulmonary pressures. Dyspnea is due to altered lung mechanics, hypoxia, and impaired ventilation rather than elevations in pulmonary vascular resistance. Severe, "out-of-proportion" elevation of pulmonary pressure and pulmonary vascular resistance occurs in a small subset of patients with COPD who have a relatively high mortality. Pulmonary vasodilator therapy is not helpful in this population. The only therapy that has proven helpful for reducing pulmonary artery pressures is long-term oxygen therapy.

The true prevalence of chronic thromboembolic PH is unknown, but occurs in less than 5% of patients after acute pulmonary embolism. In up to two-thirds of patients with chronic thromboembolic PH, there is no antecedent diagnosis of acute pulmonary embolism. One may speculate that the acute pulmonary embolism diagnosis was missed in those cases. Risk factors for the development of chronic thromboembolic PH following an acute pulmonary embolism include systolic pulmonary pressure greater than 50 mmHg at the time of presentation and a large clot burden.

RIGHT HEART CATHETERIZATION IN THE EVALUATION OF PULMONARY VASCULAR DISEASE

Right heart catheterization is mandatory in the diagnosis of PH and must be performed prior to initiating pulmonary vasodilator therapy. It is a safe procedure in patients with PH. Complication rates are only 1.1% and are most frequently related to venous access, arrhythmias, and hypotension from vagal episodes. Overall procedure-related mortality is rare and is reported in 0.05% of cases.

During right heart catheterization, assessment for intracardiac left to right shunts is made with measurement of oxygen saturations in the great vessels and cardiac chambers. Hemodynamics are measured with particular attention toward the accurate measurement of pulmonary capillary wedge pressure. To eliminate the impact of respiration on measured pressures, all measurements including pulmonary capillary wedge pressure should be made at the end of exhalation. Cardiac output can be measured using the Fick method or with thermodilution. Each method has unique limitations, but both have proven reliable in the diagnosis of PAH.

For patients in whom pulmonary venous hypertension is suspected but pulmonary capillary wedge pressure measurements are less than 15 mmHg, maneuvers such as fluid challenge, exercise challenge, or inotropic challenge can be used during right heart catheterization to elicit elevated pulmonary capillary wedge pressure.

In addition to accurate measurement of hemodynamics, right heart catheterization allows for vasoreactivity testing. During the right heart catheterization, a pulmonary vasodilator such as nitric oxide, epoprostenol, or adenosine is used to identify a small subgroup of patients who respond well to treatment with high-dose calcium channel blockers. The current criteria for patients who are "vasoreactive" is a fall in mean pulmonary artery pressures of more than 10 mmHg to an absolute value of less than 40 mmHg while maintaining cardiac output.

PAH is a rare disorder of the small precapillary pulmonary vessels. There are a number of associated conditions that confer increased risk for developing PAH. The primary treatment is with specific pulmonary vasodilator therapy.

Chronic thromboembolic pulmonary hypertension occurs following acute pulmonary embolism in a small number of patients. While medical therapy for chronic thromboembolic pulmonary hypertension can improve hemodynamics, there is limited clinical outcome data to support their use in chronic thromboembolic pulmonary hypertension. Surgical thromboendarterctomy remains the treatment of choice.

FURTHER READING

1. McLaughlin VV, Archer SL, Badesch DB, et al. ACCF/AHA 2009 expert consensus document on pulmonary hypertension: a report of the American College of Cardiology Foundation Task Force on Expert Consensus Documents and the American Heart Association, developed in collaboration with the American College of Chest Physicians, American Thoracic Society, Inc., and the Pulmonary Hypertension Association. *Circulation.* 2009;119(16):2250–2294.

   Comprehensive US guidelines on the diagnosis and management of pulmonary hypertension.

2. Waxman AB. Exercise physiology and pulmonary arterial hypertension. *Prog Cardiovasc Dis.* 2012;55(2):172–179.

3. Kovacs G, Berghold A, Scheidl S, et al. Pulmonary arterial pressure during rest and exercise in healthy subjects: a systematic review. *Eur Respir J.* 2009;34(4):888–894.

   References 2 and 3 are excellent references describing the effects of exercise on the pulmonary circulation.

4. Zhai Z, Murphy K, Tighe H, et al. Differences in ventilatory inefficiency between pulmonary arterial hypertension and chronic thromboembolic pulmonary hypertension. *Chest.* 2011;140(5): 1284–1291.

5. van der Plas MN, Reesink HJ, Roos CM, et al. Pulmonary endarterectomy improves dyspnea by the relief of dead space ventilation. *Ann Thorac Surg.* 2010;89(2):347–352.

6. Brown LM, Chen H, Halpern S, et al. Delay in recognition of pulmonary arterial hypertension: factors identified from the REVEAL Registry. *Chest.* 2011;140(1):19–26.

7. Badesch DB, Raskob GE, Elliott CG, et al. Pulmonary arterial hypertension: baseline characteristics from the REVEAL Registry. *Chest.* 2010;137(2):376–387.

   References 6 and 7 are derived from the REVEAL Registry, a large US database of patients with PAH treated at referral centers.

8. Montani D, Price LC, Dorfmuller P, et al. Pulmonary veno-occlusive disease. *Eur Respir J.* 2009;33(1):189–200.

   Comprehensive review of pulmonary veno-occlusive disease.

9. Rich S, Dantzker DR, Ayres SM, et al. Primary pulmonary hypertension. A national prospective study. *Ann Intern Med.* 1987;107(2):216–223.

   Baseline characteristics of patients with PAH in the first NIH registry.

10. Newman JH, Trembath RC, Morse JA, et al. Genetic basis of pulmonary arterial hypertension: current understanding and future directions. *J Am Coll Cardiol.* 2004;43(12, suppl S):33S–39S.

11. Chaouat A, Naeije R, Weitzenblum E. Pulmonary hypertension in COPD. *Eur Respir J.* 2008;32(5):1371–1385.

12. Hoeper MM, Lee SH, Voswinckel R, et al. Complications of right heart catheterization procedures in patients with pulmonary hypertension in experienced centers. *J Am Coll Cardiol.* 2006;48(12):2546–2552.

13. Hoeper MM, Maier R, Tongers J, et al. Determination of cardiac output by the Fick method, thermodilution, and acetylene rebreathing in pulmonary hypertension. *Am J Respir Crit Care Med.* 1999;160(2):535–541.

14. Rich S, Rabinovitch M. Diagnosis and treatment of secondary (non–category 1) pulmonary hypertension. *Circulation.* 2008;118(21):2190–2199.

   Excellent review of the approach to diagnosis and treatment of non-WHO group I PAH.

15. Nootens M, Wolfkiel CJ, Chomka EV, et al. Understanding right and left ventricular systolic function and interactions at rest and with exercise in primary pulmonary hypertension. *Am J Cardiol.* 1995;75(5):374–377.

16. Sitbon O, Humbert M, Jais X, et al. Long-term response to calcium channel blockers in idiopathic pulmonary arterial hypertension. *Circulation.* 2005;111(23):3105–3111

   Seminal study responsible for the current guidelines for calcium channel blocker use in the treatment of pulmonary arterial hypertension.

17. Simonneau G, Galiè N, Rubin LJ, et al. Clinical classification of pulmonary hypertension. *J Am Coll Cardiol.* 2004;43(12, suppl S):5S–12S.

23

Chronic Cough

Judd W. Landsberg

The cough reflex arc usually begins with stimulation of irritant receptors located primarily in the vocal cords, trachea, and airways. These sites are sensitive to mechanical, thermal, chemical, and pH disturbances commonly caused by mucus or aspiration. Afferent impulses then travel to the brain via the trigeminal, glossopharyngeal, superior laryngeal, and vagus nerves and are processed in the cough center located in the medulla. Efferent impulses are then transmitted via the vagus, phrenic, and spinal motor nerves to the glottis, diaphragm, intercostals, and abdominal muscles, culminating in a choreographed sequence of (1) inspiration, (2) glottic closure, (3) diaphragmatic relaxation, (4) forceful expiratory muscle contraction (raising intrapleural pressure up to 200 mmHg), followed by (5) sudden glottic opening, explosively releasing the large transpulmonary pressure gradient between the pleura and the airway. Expiratory volume is no greater than during a forced exhalation, but extreme narrowing of the airway caused by the pressure gradient leads to higher linear velocities (close to the speed of sound), which are generally effective in dislodging mucus and foreign materials. Patients with chronic airway obstruction produce appropriate intrathoracic pressures but generate lower linear velocities and a less effective cough because of pathologic airway collapse.

Occasional cough caused by minor irritations (e.g., aspiration of oral secretions) is normal. Cough remaining after upper or lower respiratory tract infections (typically viral, mycoplasma, chlamydia, or pertussis) may continue for 8 weeks or more. This type of postinfectious cough is the most common cause of subacute cough (lasting 3–8 weeks). An empiric course of macrolide antibiotics is usually warranted in this clinical setting, though treatment after the first 2 weeks is of unproven benefit, and the course should be self-limited. Chronic cough (lasting more than 8 weeks) can cause complications, distress, and be debilitating to the individual. Most chronic cough is attributable to upper airway cough syndrome (UACS) from postnasal drip (PND), asthma (often cough variant), or gastroesophageal reflux disease (GERD), alone or in combination.

The initial step in the evaluation of chronic cough is screening for special situations (e.g., ACE inhibitor therapy) and identifying high-risk patients, namely the immunosuppressed, smokers, and those with purulent sputum or hemoptysis. Immunosuppressed patients need an aggressive workup to exclude atypical bacterial and fungal infection usually requiring sputum culture, a noncontrast chest computed tomography (CT) scan, and a bronchoscopic evaluation if parenchymal abnormalities are discovered. Although chronic cough occurs in up to 75% of cigarette smokers, the majority do not seek treatment. Those who do should get a posteroanterior (PA) and lateral chest radiograph to screen for obvious lung cancer with most abnormalities mandating timely CT characterization and outpatient pulmonary evaluation and follow-up. Smokers must also be repeatedly counseled about smoking cessation, especially during the evaluation of potential lung cancer. Individuals with a chronic cough productive of purulent sputum with or without hemoptysis need to have the etiology established, that is, bronchiectasis, sinusitis, atypical lung infection, or chronic bronchitis (active smokers). Such individuals need cultures (for typical and atypical organisms), antibiotic therapy, and a PA and lateral chest radiograph. If parenchymal abnormalities exist, further investigation with a noncontrast chest CT scan and serologies may be appropriate to rule out an atypical lung infection requiring specific therapy (e.g., fungal or mycobacterial infection), as well as an appropriate bronchiectasis work up.

Patients on angiotensin-converting enzyme (ACE) inhibitor therapy complaining of a chronic dry cough should be switched to an angiotensin receptor blocker (ARB). Up to 15% of patients on ACE inhibitors experience an irritant-mediated cough (typically within the first

6 months of therapy) quite likely secondary to bradykinin accumulation (also broken down by the ACE).

The next step in the evaluation and management of chronic cough involves a diagnostic, therapeutic medication trial using history and physical examination to establish whether obvious symptoms of UACS, asthma, or GERD exist (e.g., PND, episodic wheeze, sour taste in the mouth). If no obvious symptoms exist, UACS can be inferred on physical exam if signs of chronic sinusitis are present, or upper airway examination demonstrates upper airway secretions, cobblestoning, and laryngeal inflammation. Ultimately, the practitioner and the patient must decide to pursue a stepwise approach in which UACS, GERD, and asthma are treated sequentially, or an aggressive approach where all three conditions are treated at once, with medications then sequentially pulled away after the cough abates. People who are fearful of medications usually prefer a stepwise approach, whereas individuals debilitated by coughing will try everything (at once) to make the cough stop. While many practitioners (as scientists) prefer a stepwise approach, many times all three diseases require maximal therapy in order for a chronic cough to resolve.

UACS describes cough due to the irritation, inflammation, and sensitization that occurs in the upper airway in the setting of PND. Individuals may or may not be aware of a dripping sensation or sinusitis symptoms. Occasionally, upper airway laryngoscopic examination and sinus CT scan are indicated, but generally a trial of an oral, potent (first generation) antihistamine (e.g., diphenhydramine, cetirizine) is the appropriate initial step. A nasal steroid can be used as an alternative for those intolerant to the drowsiness of antihistamines, but therapeutic effect may take longer to be achieved. Oral leukotriene antagonists and nasal cromolyn are alternatives. In general, if the cough fails to improve despite maximal therapy as outlined above in 2 to 4 weeks, the diagnosis of UACS should be considered less likely.

GERD, like UACS, may be obvious on history or occult, with patients experiencing no symptoms referable to reflux. A nocturnal cough is often seen in GERD as well as asthma. While overnight pH studies can provide a definitive diagnosis, the standard of care involves a more pragmatic trial of lifestyle changes (weight loss, head of bed elevation, smoking cessation, and dietary modification) with once-daily proton pump inhibitor therapy. GERD-related cough should generally improve after 8 weeks of the above interventions.

Traditional asthma (i.e., accompanied by wheezing) or cough variant asthma (positive bronchoprovocation test without the clinical syndrome of asthma) is another common cause of chronic cough. Often these patients have a personal or family history of atopy, and will demonstrate sputum eosinophilia. Recently, a distinction has been made between cough variant asthma and eosinophilic bronchitis, a more appropriate term for individuals with cough, atopy, sputum eosinophilia, and a negative result for the bronchoprovocation test. Bronchoprovocation testing should not be performed within 2 months of a respiratory illness because hyperreactivity may be a normal consequence in the postinfectious period. As with the other common causes of chronic cough, an empiric diagnostic, therapeutic trial often obviates the need for advanced testing. Inhaled glucocorticoids are the first-line therapy for both cough variant asthma and nonasthmatic eosinophilic bronchitis. Improvement in cough should occur in 2 to 4 weeks.

When combined therapy for UACS, GERD, and asthma fail to improve chronic cough, other less common causes should be entertained. While bronchoscopy has no role in the routine evaluation of chronic cough, it should be considered in patients who fail empiric therapy to exclude an endobronchial cause (e.g., tumor, foreign body, broncholith). Occasionally, bronchoscopy will reveal significant lower airway purulence not suspected by the dry nature of the cough and the bland nature of imaging. These patients benefit from cultures (looking for pseudomonas), antibiotics, and chest physiotherapy.

Occasionally, cough remains unexplained and may be labeled chronic idiopathic cough or, more appropriately, cough hypersensitivity syndrome since it is believed to be caused by increased sensitivity of the mucosal irritant receptors (and their coupled ion channels). There is no specific therapy for this syndrome. The diagnosis of psychogenic cough, where cough like a tic, is one of exclusion and should only be considered when emotional stress is the predominant trigger and all other diagnoses have been excluded. Speech therapy may be of some benefit.

With intrapleural pressures rising as high as 300 mmHg, chronic cough can cause severe complications, including sleep disruption, multiple rib fractures, emesis, stress incontinence, social isolation, and syncope. While cough is one of many causes of vasovagal syncope, cough syncope is not vasovagal. Instead, it is a direct consequence of extremely forceful coughing, leading to increased intracranial pressure and reversal of middle cerebral artery blood flow during diastole. Treatment is aimed at the cough.

Nonspecific antitussive therapies are occasionally required. Central acting medications like dextromethorphan (DM) or codeine may effectively control symptoms, but the latter therapy's abuse potential makes it a second-line choice. Sedation may be a limiting side effect for some. Gabapentin at doses from 300 to 1,800 mg daily showed benefit in a study of 62 patients with chronic refractory cough, but side effects were common (30%) and cough worsened for some after discontinuation. In the occasional patient with persistent cough, oral benzonatate (e.g., Perles) or nebulized lidocaine (e.g., 5 mL of 4% solution) may provide substantial relief.

FURTHER READING

1. Birkebaek NH, Kristiansen M, Seefeldt T, et al. Bordetella pertussis infection and chronic cough in adults. *Clin Infect Dis.* 1999;29:1239–1242.

   Articles, suggesting approximately 20% of patients with persistent cough have culture or serologic evidence of B. pertussis infection. These infections usually respond to macrolide therapy.

2. Brightling CE, Ward R, Goh KL, et al. Eosinophilic bronchitis is an important cause of chronic cough. *Am J Respir Crit Care Med.* 1999;160:406.

   Eosinophilic bronchitis is an important, recently recognized cause of cough. It presents with chronic cough and sputum eosinophilia (>3%) without abnormal spirometry or bronchial hyperreactivity and responds to inhaled corticosteroids. In this study, eosinophilic bronchitis was the final diagnosis in 12 of 91 patients referred for unexplained cough. After treatment with inhaled budesonide (400 μg twice daily), cough improved and sputum eosinophilia fell from 16.8% to 1.6%.

3. Corrao WM, Braman SS, Irwin RS. Chronic cough as the sole presenting manifestation of bronchial asthma. *N Engl J Med.* 1979;300:633.

   Classic description of the cough variant of asthma, established by demonstration of bronchial hyperreactivity and response to bronchodilators in the absence of the usual stigmata of asthma (e.g., wheezing, airflow limitation).

4. Dykewicz MS. Cough and angioedema from angiotensin-converting enzyme inhibitors: new insights into mechanisms and management. *Curr Opin Allergy Clin Immunol.* 2004;4(4):267.

   ACE inhibitors cause cough and angioedema through accumulation of kinins. Most patients who develop either cough or angioedema from ACE inhibitors can tolerate angiotensin-II receptor blocking agents.

5. Groneberg DA, Niimi A, Dinh QT, et al. Increased expression of transient receptor potential vanilloid-1 in airway nerves of chronic cough. *Am J Respir Crit Care Med.* 2004;170(12):1276.

   Transient receptor potential vanniloid-1 (TRPV-1) mediates the irritant cough response. The group obtained airway mucosal biopsies by fiberoptic bronchoscopy in 29 patients with chronic cough and 16 healthy volunteers without a cough. Immunostaining showed a 5-fold increase of TRPV-1 staining in chronic persistent cough (P < .001).

6. Irwin RS, Baumann MH, Bolser DC, et al; for American College of Chest Physicians (ACCP). Diagnosis and management of cough executive summary: ACCP evidence-based clinical practice guidelines. *Chest.* 2006;129(1 suppl):1S.

   Consensus panel report on the diagnosis and treatment of cough.

7. Irwin RS, Curley FJ, French CL. Chronic cough. The spectrum and frequency of causes, key components of the diagnostic evaluation, and outcome of specific therapy. *Am Rev Respir Dis.* 1990;141:640.

   The classic and enthusiastic presentation of the anatomic diagnostic protocol made famous by the lead author. A specific cause of cough was determined in 101 of 102 patients: one cause in 73%, two in 23%, and three in 3%. Postnasal drip syndrome was a cause 41% of the time, asthma 24%, gastroesophageal reflux 21%, chronic bronchitis 5%, and bronchiectasis 4%. Cough was often the sole presenting manifestation of asthma (28%) and reflux (43%). Of note, methacholine challenge was falsely positive 22% of the time, although our experience has not been as encouraging.

8. Irwin RS, Madison JM. The persistently troublesome cough. *Am J Respir Crit Care Med.* 2002;165:1469.

   Two excellent articles that are highly recommended reading. The first is a comprehensive approach to acute and chronic cough, with an algorithm for diagnosis and treatment. The second emphasizes a novel approach to the patient with chronic cough, particularly the one in whom a diagnostic and therapeutic workup has been unrevealing.

9. Irwin RS. The diagnosis and treatment of cough. *N Engl J Med.* 2000;343:1715.

10. Palombini BC, Villanova CA, Araujo E, et al. A pathogenic triad in chronic cough: asthma, post-nasal drip syndrome, and gastroesophageal reflux disease. *Chest.* 1999;116:279.

   Yet another group finds that some combination of asthma, gastroesophageal reflux, and postnasal drip explains most (i.e., here 93.6%) chronic coughs and suggests that this be known as the pathogenic triad for chronic cough.

11. Pratter MR. Chronic upper airway cough syndrome secondary to rhinosinus diseases (previously referred to as postnasal drip syndrome): ACCP evidence-based clinical practice guidelines. *Chest.* 2006;129(1, suppl):63S.

   The original description of UACS, the most common cause of chronic cough, with practice guidelines.

12. Sen RP, Walsh TE. Fiberoptic bronchoscopy for refractory cough. *Chest.* 1991;99:33.

   Bronchoscopy provided a diagnosis in seven of 25 patients with chronic unexplained cough.

13. Trochtenberg S. Nebulized lidocaine in the treatment of refractory cough. *Chest.* 1994;105:1592.

   Convincing case report of prolonged treatment of refractory cough with nebulized lidocaine. Mild dysphonia was the only side effect.

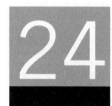

Pleural Effusion

Henri G. Colt

Pleural fluid serves as a lubricating film between the visceral and parietal pleural surfaces. A few milliliters of pleural fluid are present normally within the pleural space. In normal individuals, thoracentesis may yield less than 1 mL of fluid, although quantities of 3 to 20 mL have been obtained in as many as 10% of healthy individuals in some series. The protein content of pleural fluid is below 1.5 g/dL, and the protein electrophoretic pattern is qualitatively similar to plasma, although the content of albumin is slightly higher and that of fibrinogen slightly lower.

The volume and composition of pleural fluid are maintained virtually constant in healthy individuals by an intricate balance of hydrostatic and oncotic pressures and by the relative permeabilities of the pleural capillaries and lymphatics. Systemic arteries supply the parietal pleura and bronchial arteries do the same for the visceral pleura. Fluid and protein exchange in the pleural space is almost exclusively achieved through the parietal pleura. Fluid may accumulate as a result of any process that obstructs lymphatic drainage.

Pleural effusion is defined as the abnormal accumulation of fluid within the pleural space. It may be caused by either excess fluid production or decreased absorption; in some conditions, both mechanisms may be operative. Effusions are a common manifestation of both systemic and intrathoracic diseases. Factors that determine whether pleural fluid accumulates include (1) oncotic pressure in the pleural fluid, pleural microcirculation, and lymphatics; (2) permeability of the pleural microcirculation; and (3) pressures in the systemic and pulmonary veins. The most common cause of a pleural effusion is congestive heart failure with elevation of the pulmonary venous pressure. Whether elevation of systemic venous pressure alone (pure right heart failure) prompts pleural effusions remains controversial, but elevations of both systemic and pulmonary venous pressures appear to result in larger effusions.

Peritoneal fluid can gain access to the pleural space via diaphragmatic defects and transdiaphragmatic lymphatics. Simple transfer of ascitic fluid across diaphragmatic defects has been invoked as a mechanism for pleural effusions that accompany ascites, as occurs in cirrhosis and Meig syndrome (i.e., benign ovarian fibroma, ascites, and pleural effusion). A similar mechanism has been proposed for fluid accumulation in pancreatitis or subdiaphragmatic abscess, although enhanced transdiaphragmatic lymph flow also can play a role.

From a pathophysiolgic perspective, increased negative pressure in the pleural space enhances fluid accumulation (as occurs in patients with atelectasis). While decreased plasma oncotic pressure favors pleural fluid accumulation, it is unlikely to be sufficient, since effusions are rare in congenitally hypoalbuminemic individuals. Increased capillary permeability caused by local inflammation, circulating toxins, or vasoactive substances play a role in pleural fluid accumulation associated with collagen-vascular diseases, pancreatitis, pulmonary emboli, and pneumonitis. Furthermore, as pleural space oncotic pressure approaches that of plasma (32 cm H_2O), fluid resorption is impaired. An increase in pleural oncotic pressure also contributes to some effusions. This occurs as a consequence of (1) enhanced capillary protein leak, (2) protein exudation from local pleural inflammation or tumor, or (3) defective lymphatic resorption.

On physical examination, patients may have dullness to percussion, diminished breath sounds, and reduced tactile and vocal fremitus over the involved hemithorax. Altering the patient's position will occasionally *shift* these physical findings to dependent regions. Large effusions (>1,500 mL) are frequently associated with an appreciable inspiratory lag, bulging intercostal margins, contralateral mediastinal shift, or atelectasis (e.g., egophony, bronchial breath sounds). Nonthoracic signs might suggest the cause of the effusion; pedal edema, distended neck veins, and an S_3 gallop, for example indicate possible congestive heart failure.

Often, the chest roentgenogram is the only clue to the presence of an effusion. It also may suggest its cause (e.g., cardiomegaly and redistribution of pulmonary veins in heart failure, lung or pleural-based masses, atelectasis, rib erosions signifying metastatic carcinoma, or an elevated hemidiaphragm suggesting subdiaphragmatic abscess, volume loss, or bronchial obstruction). At least 150 mL of fluid is required to detect an effusion on a standard posteroanterior and lateral chest roentgenogram. Today, pleural ultrasonography is increasingly used to image both large and small effusions. Typically, fluid initially collects between the anteroinferior lung surface and the diaphragm. It then obliterates the costophrenic angle on the frontal view of the chest radiograph, or creates a triangular density that obscures the ipsilateral diaphragm and posterior costophrenic sulcus on a lateral film. Further accumulation obliterates the hemidiaphragm and opacifies the hemithorax with an upward concavity that extends higher laterally than medially. On the lateral view, pleural fluid ascends obliquely along the posterior chest wall. Significantly smaller quantities of pleural fluid are detectable on lateral decubitus views. On lateral decubitus films, fluid layers along the dependent chest wall. On the opposite decubitus view, fluid shift allows examination of underlying parenchyma. However, decubitus films often are not necessary because both loculated and free flowing fluid are detected by pleural ultrasonography before thoracentesis. A very large effusion should cause a contralateral mediastinal shift. When this shift does not occur, parenchymal collapse or mediastinal fixation, often from a tumor, may be present.

When underlying parenchymal abnormalities or adhesions between pleural layers exist, atypical patterns of fluid accumulation result. A subpulmonic effusion can harbor more than 1,000 mL of fluid and may resemble merely an elevated hemidiaphragm. However, the "diaphragmatic" contour is often more horizontal than usual, with a steep angulation laterally that creates a shallow costophrenic angle. A lateral decubitus film may layer the fluid and reveal the true diaphragmatic shadow. When pleural fluid becomes loculated (or entrapped) within an interlobar fissure, it can create the appearance of an elliptic opacity, or *pseudotumor*, on the posteroanterior film and a spindle-shaped opacity tapering into fissure lines on the lateral film. For unknown reasons, this appearance is especially common with congestive heart failure and resolves as hemodynamics improve. Fluid that is loculated laterally can result in a smooth, contoured, semicircular opacity abutting a pleural surface, which can simulate a mass lesion on a posteroanterior film. Loculations are frequently seen in patients with evolving parapneumonic effusions or empyema after either thoracic surgery or pleurodesis. It is noteworthy that computed tomography (CT) scans often exaggerate the amount of fluid actually present.

The information from chest radiographs can be supplemented by pleural ultrasonography and CT scans. Bedside ultrasound, which is now commonplace, visualizes the effusion as well as loculations, diaphragmatic movements, and the underlying lung. CT scans should be performed in the investigation of unexplained exudative effusions, and can be useful in distinguishing malignant from benign pleural thickening. CT scans should be performed with contrast enhancement, and before complete drainage of the effusion. Scans also are performed in cases of complicated pleural infections, especially if initial tube drainage has been unsuccessful, magnetic resonance imaging (MRI) may also help distinguish malignant from benign disease, particularly if chest wall or diaphragmatic involvement is suspected. Positron emission tomography–computed tomography (PET–CT), in combination with MRI may have a role to monitor response to chemotherapy in the treatment of malignant mesothelioma.

The differential diagnosis of pleural effusion should reflect the clinical context and ancillary findings, but thoracentesis and careful examination of the pleural fluid are indicated in nearly every instance. Thoracentesis has low morbidity in experienced hands. Precautions should be used in patients with a bleeding diathesis, a very small effusions, or an obliterated pleural space, as well as in patients taking anticoagulant drugs, those who are uncooperative, and those for whom even a small pneumothorax could be extremely hazardous. Ultrasound guidance increases the likelihood of successful sampling, and reduces the risk of complications. Furthermore, ultrasound has a specificity similar to that of CT in differentiating malignant from benign effusions, and identifies exudative effusions through detection of septations (loculations) or echogenicity. It is traditionally suggested that no more than 1,000 mL of fluid be removed at any one sitting to avoid reexpansion pulmonary edema, but this complication is unusual. The procedure should probably be halted, however, if the patient begins to cough, has chest pain, or other possible signs of increasingly negative pleural pressure. Regardless, fluid should be removed slowly.

Numerous laboratory examinations can be performed on pleural fluid; those required are largely dictated by the clinical context. If foul-smelling pus is obtained, for example, extensive biochemical analysis is not required; only Gram stain and culture are needed. Pleural fluid differential cell count abnormalities are not disease specific, and any long-standing effusion may be populated by lymphocytes, although very high lymphocytic effusions (>80%) are most commonly seen in patients with tuberculosis, lymphoma, chronic rheumatoid pleurisy, sarcoidosis, and postcoronary artery bypass graft.

In most situations, fluid analysis is needed to distinguish a transudate from an exudate, an important distinction necessary for differential diagnosis of the cause of the effusion. An exudate is defined by any one of the following: ratio of pleural fluid to serum protein greater than 0.5; lactate dehydrogenase (LDH) ratio greater than 0.6; or LDH greater than two-thirds of the *normal* serum value. These represent Light criteria. Other key measures are white blood count and differential, glucose, and pleural pH. A hematocrit is useful in the diagnosis of hemithorax.

Exudates are characteristic of malignancy, parapneumonic effusions, and a variety of infectious and noninfectious inflammatory states. Acidosis (pH < 7.30) and reduced glucose (<60 µg/dL) are characteristic of empyema and rheumatoid pleurisy, but can occur in other conditions, such as pleural carcinomatosis and evolving parapneumonic effusions. Measurement of amylase is warranted in clinical settings in which an elevated pleural fluid amylase would suggest conditions such as esophageal rupture, pancreatitis, pancreatic pseudocyst, and, rarely, certain malignancies. The use of pleural cholesterol levels is still investigative, and no set of measures has yet replaced Light criteria (LDH, protein) to differentiate exudates from transudates. If chylothorax is suspected, triglycerides and chylomicron analysis (by lipoprotein electrophoresis) should be requested; fluid is not always turbid or milky in these instances. Serologies are useful, since antinuclear antibodies (ANA) titers >1:320 are suggestive of systemic Lupus and rheumatoid factor (RF) titers >1:320 are suggestive of rheumatoid arthritis. However, neither of these serological tests are sufficient by themselves to make the diagnosis. Pleural adenosine deaminase (ADA) is elevated (>70 U/L) in tuberculosis, but is also elevated in rheumatoid arthritis, malignancy, and empyema. Pleural fluid cytologic examination is indicated whenever neoplasm is suspected. The yield for malignancy increases if cell blocks and smears are prepared from the sample. If lymphoma is suspected, a specimen should be sent for flow cytometry or immunocytochemistry. Tumor markers are not routinely indicated, but a positive pleural fluid mesothelin is highly suggestive of pleural malignancy, such as mesothelioma and metastases from ovarian, pancreatic, and bronchogenic adenocarcinoma.

One point of particular interest has been the differentiation between a benign parapneumonic effusion that requires no chest tube drainage and one that does (increasingly referred to as a *complicated parapneumonic effusion*). The need for drainage, in addition to antibiotic therapy, is indicated by a positive Gram's stain, culture, or the presence of pus in the pleural space (empyema). Drainage also should be considered if pleural fluid pH is below 7.10 or if pleural glucose is low and LDH is greater than 1,000 g/L after excluding other diagnoses for these abnormalities (e.g., tuberculosis, rheumatoid arthritis, and pleural carcinomatosis).

The procedures described above, along with the results of cultures for bacteria, fungi, and tuberculosis, will yield a diagnosis for most pleural effusions. In some instances, however, additional evaluation is warranted. A closed needle biopsy of the pleura might be considered in cases in which granulomatous diseases or a neoplasm are suspected. The British Thoracic Society guidelines, however, suggest Abrams or Cope needle biopsy only in areas with a high incidence of tuberculosis, although thoracoscopic and image-guided cutting needles have a higher diagnostic yield. If malignancy is suspected and there is evidence of pleural nodularity on contrast-enhanced CT, image-guided percutaneous pleural biopsy is warranted. Routine flexible bronchoscopy is of no demonstrated value unless imaging studies demonstrates a parenchymal or nodal abnormality or are suggestive of bronchial obstruction, or if the patient has hemoptysis.

In patients with an undiagnosed exudative effusion, or one in which malignancy is suspected, thoracoscopy is a remarkably safe and commonly used diagnostic procedure. Thoracoscopy can be performed through a single access site, often under local anesthesia or using spontaneous ventilation and intravenous sedation in the operating room setting. General anesthesia and tracheal intubation are desirable in some cases in which adhesions, loculations, or infection are suspected. Thoracoscopy permits direct visualization of the pleura and external surface of the lung, lysis of adhesions, biopsy of pleura and lung, pleural fluid removal, and pleurodesis. If necessary, indwelling pleural catheters can be inserted using thoracoscopic or flex-rigid pleuroscopic guidance.

Open pleural biopsy under general anesthesia may be required for patients in whom other procedures have failed to provide a diagnosis or when contemplated lung biopsy poses special risk (e.g., pulmonary hypertension) and open exposure is required to assure hemostasis. Despite proceeding to thoracoscopy or open biopsy, a small number of effusions remain undiagnosed and either resolve or, subsequently, express themselves as neoplasm. This may particularly be the case for malignant mesothelioma.

Treatment of pleural effusions is usually focused on the underlying disease. Repeat therapeutic thoracentesis may be necessary in cases of a large effusion, when the patient has significant underlying parenchymal lung disease, or when prognosis is poor and the patient refuses pleurodesis or indwelling pleural catheter. Symptoms such as dyspnea, chest pain, or cough should resolve after evacuation of the effusion. If not, repeat therapeutic thoracentesis is probably not warranted. Patients with symptoms that coincide with recurrent fluid accumulation should be considered for pleurodesis or for insertion of an indwelling, tunneled percutaneous pleural catheter for periodic drainage. This may be particularly helpful in patients with malignant mesothelioma or pleural carcinomatosis. Patients with trapped lung may also benefit from indwelling pleural catheters. Patients with empyema, tuberculosis effusions, or hemithorax may require a multidisciplinary approach to care, with considerations for image-guided, thoracoscopic, or open surgical exploration and drainage.

FURTHER READING

1. Alexandrakis MG, Passam FH, Kyriakou DS, et al. Pleural effusions in hematologic malignancies. *Chest.* 2004;125:1546–1555.

   Hodgkin and non-Hodgkin lymphoma are the most frequent, but also 10% to 20% of patient's status postbone marrow transplant develop effusions. In all patients, drug toxicity should be considered.

2. Azoulay E. Pleural effusions in the intensive care unit. *Curr Opin Pulm Med.* 2003;9:291–297.

   Incidence of effusions depends on screening methods (8% for physical examination to 60% using ultrasonography). This article reviews etiologies and workup strategies.

3. Bielsa S, Esquarda A, Salud A, et al. High level of tumor markers in pleural fluid correlate with poor survival in patients with adenocarcinomatous or squamous malignant effusion. *Eur J Intern Med.* 2009;20(4):383–386.

   Malignant pleural effusion of CA-125 greater than 1,000 and ck-19 greater than 100 ng/mL have poor outcome and is independent risk factor.

4. Brown NE, Zamel N, Aberman A. Changes in pulmonary mechanics and gas exchange following thoracocentesis. *Chest.* 1978;74:540.

   The changes in pulmonary mechanics and gas exchange, which occurred in the first 3 hours after removal of 600 to 1,800 mL in nine patients, did correlate with subjective improvement by the patients.

5. Burrows CM, Mathews WC, Colt HG. Predicting survival in patients with recurrent symptomatic malignant pleural effusions: an assessment of the prognostic values of physiologic, morphologic, and quality of life measures of extent of disease. *Chest.* 2000;117:73–78.

   A study that questions the predictive value of pH and demonstrates the importance of quality of life assessment.

6. Cugell DW, Kamp DW. Asbestos and the pleura. *Chest.* 2004;125:1103–1117.

   A great review of history, mineralogy, and clinical significance of asbestos-related pleural disease.

7. Colt HG, Brewer N, Barbur E. Evaluation of patient-related and procedure-related factors contributing to pneumothorax following thoracentesis. *Chest.* 1999;116:134.

   Pneumothorax is rare and not easily predictable, even when procedures are performed by experienced operators.

8. Colt HG, Mathur PN. *Manual of Pleural Procedures.* Philadelphia, PA: Lippincott Williams & Williams; 1999.

   A 200-page guide to performing procedures, including ultrasound, chest tubes pleurodesis, and thoracoscopy (with useful hints and many black and white photos).

9. Doyle JJ, Hnatiuk OW, Torrington KG, et al. Necessity of routine chest roentgenography after thoracentesis. *Ann Intern Med.* 1996;124:816.

   Answers an age-old question: Are chest films needed in patients, even though the risk of thoracentesis-related pneumothorax is low in experienced hands?

10. Duysinx B, Corhay JL, Larock MP, et al. Contribution of positron emission tomography in pleural disease. *Rev Mal Respir.* 2010;27(8):e47–e53.

    PET is useful in characterizing malignant pleural etiology, staging of lung CA and prognosis for mesothelioma. PET-CT should be used for undiagnosed pleural disease prior to invasive diagnostic procedure as PET/CT scan has 100% sensitivity, 94.8% specificity, and 97.5% accuracy. There were no false negatives.

11. Fysh E, Smith NA, Lee YCG. Optimal chest drain size: the rise of the small bore pleural catheter. *Semin Respir Crit Care Med.* 2010;31(6):760–768.

    Small bore catheter is increasingly used for pleural effusion drainage and efficacy is good.

12. Goto M, Noguchi Y, Koyama H. Diagnostic value of adenosine deaminase in tuberculous pleural effusions: a meta-analysis. *Ann Clin Biochem.* 2003;40:374–381.

    Adenosine deaminase may be useful and could allow avoidance of pleural biopsy, especially in countries where tuberculosis prevalence is high.

13. Heffner JE, Highland K, Brown LK. A meta-analysis derivation of continuous likelihood ratios for diagnosing pleural fluid exudates. *Am J Respir Crit Care Med.* 2003;167:1591–1599.

    Logistic regression of a multicenter registry of pleural effusions demonstrates that diagnostic accuracy for Light criteria decreased to as low as 65% to 86% as any one of the criteria reached its binary cutoff point.

14. Huggins JT. Chylothorax and cholesterol pleural effusion. *Semin Respir Crit Care Med.* 2010;31(6):743–750.

    For chylous ascites, TG greater than 110 mg/dL is diagnostic, chylomicron confirms the diagnosis.

15. Jantz MA, Antony VB. Pathophysiology of the pleura. *Respiration*. 2008;75:121–133.

    Another excellent review.

16. Jones PW, Moyers JP, Rogers JT, et al. Ultrasound-guided thoracentesis: is it a safer method? *Chest*. 2003;123:418–423.

    Prospective descriptive study of 941 thoracenteses performed by interventional radiologists using ultrasound guidance resulted in fewer complications that those reported with non–image-guided thoracentesis.

17. Kalokairinou-Motogna M, Maratou K, Paianid I, et al. Application of color Doppler ultrasound in the study of small pleural effusion. *Med Ultrason*. 2010;12(1):12–16.

    US detection of pleural effusion has 60% specificity, 100% sensitivity, and 88.37% accuracy. Adding color Doppler adds specificity to 100%, sensitivity to 96.72%, and accuracy of 97.57%.

18. Lee P, Colt HG. Using diagnostic thoracoscopy to optimal effect. *J Resp Illn*. 2003;24:503–509.

    A review of therapeutic modalities and indications, especially geared to nonsurgeon thoracoscopists.

19. Lee P, Hsu A, Lo C, et al. Prospective evaluation of flex-rigid pleuroscopy for indeterminate pleural effusion: accuracy, safety and outcome. *Respirology*. 2007;12:881–886.

    Excellent yield similar to rigid thoracoscopy.

20. Lee P, Mathur NP, Colt HG. Advances in thoracoscopy: 100 years since Jacobaeus. *Respiration*. 2010;79:177–186

    Review of new results pertaining to this technique.

21. Lee MH, Nahm CH, Choi JW. Thrombin-antithrombin III complex, proinflammatory cytokines, and fibrinolytic indices for assessing the severity of inflammation in pleural effusions. *Ann Clin Lab Sci*. 2010;40(4):342–347.

    TB pleurisy has higher concentration of TNF-alpha and PAI-1.

22. Light RW, MacGregor I, Luchsinger PC. Pleural effusions: the diagnostic separation of transudates and exudates. *Ann Intern Med*. 1972;77:507.

    The Classic. A prospective study of 150 pleural effusions, exploring the utility of cell counts, protein, and LDH determinations in pleural fluid.

23. Mahon RT, Colt HG. Bedside thoracentesis in critically ill patients: the "rolled bedsheet" technique. *J Bronchol*. 2000;7:340–342.

    Description of a technique that facilitates thoracentesis in mechanically ventilated patients.

24. Morelock SY, Sahn SA. Drugs and the pleura. *Chest*. 1999;116:212.

    Small numbers of drugs cause effusions when compared with the large number of drugs that can cause pulmonary parenchymal abnormalities. A concise, review.

25. Maskell NA, Butland RJ; Pleural Diseases Group, Standards of Care Committee, British Thoracic Society. BTS guidelines for the investigation of a unilateral pleural effusion in adults. *Thorax*. 2003;58(suppl 2):ii8–ii17.

    An incredibly informative "state of the art" review of pleural effusions: clinical workup, algorithms, differential diagnosis.

26. Mcgrath EE, Anderson PB. Diagnosis of pleural effusion: a systematic approach. *Am J Crit Care*. 2011;20(2):119–128.

    Light criteria is 100% sensitive for exudates.

27. Moisiuc FV, Colt HG. Thoracoscopy: origins revisted. *Respiration*. 2007;74:344–355.

    History of the procedure.

28. Pien GW, Gant MJ, Washam CL. Use of an implantable pleural catheter for trapped lung syndrome in patients with malignant pleural effusion. *Chest*. 2001;119:1641–1646.

    A series of patients with trapped lung treated successfully using the PleurRx pleural catheter, a 15.5-F silicone catheter that allows periodic drainage.

29. Porcel JM. Pleural fluid tests to identify complicated parapneumonic effusions. *Curr Opin Pulm Med*. 2010;16(4):357–361.

    Promising biomarkers for detecting nonpurulent complicated parapneumonic effusions are TNF-Alpha, myeloperoxidase, Matrix metalloproteinase 2, neutrophil elastase, IL-8, lipopolysaccharide binding protein, terminal complement complex SC5b-9 and CRP 37.

30. Porcel JM, Esquerda A, Bielsa S. Diagnostic performance of adenosine deaminase activity in pleural fluid: a single-center experience with over 2100 consecutive patients. *Eur J Intern Med.* 2010;21(5):419–423.

    Pleural ADA's positive predictive value may be as low as 7% in area of low prevalence, but the negative predictive value remains high.

31. Du Rand I, Maskell N. Introduction and methods: British Thoracic Society pleural disease guideline 2010. *Thorax.* 2010;65:ii1–ii16.

    Excellent set of guidelines with more than 150 references.

32. Sallach SM, Sallach JA, Vasquez E, et al. Volume of pleural fluid required for diagnosis of pleural malignancy. *Chest.* 2002;122:1913–1917.

    Retrospective review of 282 patients showed that the sensitivity for diagnosis of pleural malignancy was not dependent on volume of fluid removed by thoracentesis.

33. Sioris T, Sihvo E, Salo J, et al. Long-term indwelling pleural catheter (pleurx) for malignant pleural effusion unsuitable for talc pleurodesis. *Eur J Surg Oncol.* 2009;35(5):546–551.

    For patients who are too unstable to undergo talc pleurodesis, pleurx catheter is a safe alternative and spontaneous pleural fusion could be obtained in 21% of the patients.

34. Stathopoulos GT, Zhu Z, Everhart MB, et al. Translational advances in pleural diseases. *Respirology.* 2011;16:53–63.

    Calretinin, soluble mesothelin-related peptide, and osteopontin are helpful markers for mesothelioma.

Hemoptysis
Henri G. Colt

Hemoptysis (i.e., coughing up blood) is a frightening event for both healthcare provider and patient and may occur in a variety of clinical conditions. The amount and quality can range from blood-streaked sputum to several cups of blood or even massive bleeding leading to exsanguination. Death is rare, but may occur as a consequence of asphyxiation and respiratory arrest associated with flooding of the tracheobronchial tree. Massive hemoptysis is a life-threatening medical emergency that may not be controllable even by endotracheal intubation and mechanical ventilation.

The incidence of hemoptysis reflects the type of population studied (e.g., surgical vs medical or cancer center vs tuberculosis clinic). In the United States, the most common causes are chronic bronchitis, bronchiectasis, and bronchogenic carcinoma, followed by tuberculosis, fungal infections (especially aspergillosis or aspergilloma), bacterial pneumonia and abscess, and pulmonary infarction. Less common causes of hemoptysis include mitral stenosis, Goodpasture syndrome, endobronchial foreign bodies, bronchial adenoma, pulmonary arteriovenous (AV) fistulas, Behçet disease, lung parasites (ascariasis, paragonimiasis, and schistosomiasis), Wegener granulomatosis, drugs (cocaine, anticoagulants, penicillamine), cystic fibrosis, lymphangioleiomyomatosis, pulmonary artery injury from a balloon-tipped catheter, coagulopathies, and even bioterrorism (pneumonic plague, tularemia, and tricothecene mycotoxin). Hemoptysis also may be caused by airway inflammation, granulation tissue overgrowth, and erosion of tracheobronchial mucosa from indwelling metal, hybrid, and silicone airway stents. When a diagnosis is not found, hemoptysis is said to be cryptogenic. This should be a diagnosis of exclusion, although it has been reported in up to 40% of cases, usually in tobacco smokers.

The approach to the diagnosis and initial management focuses on the following questions:

1. What is the origin of the bleeding (lungs, the airways, nasopharynx, or digestive tract)?
2. Can the bleeding be stopped?
3. Will the bleeding recur at some time in the future?
4. Does the patient have a systemic disease that predisposes to bleeding?
5. Is emergency intervention needed? If so, what kind of surveillance should be instituted, and what might be done to prevent recurrent bleeding?

The anatomic source of bleeding depends on the specific pathologic process. However, bronchial arteries and collaterals from axillary, intercostal, diaphragmatic, and other systemic arteries of the thorax are the source of bleeding in most cases. Inflammation associated with infection and carcinoma can cause reactive hypervascularity of bronchial arteries and stimulation of collaterals. Localized inflammation can result in bleeding by erosion of these hypervascular networks of vessels. Chronic inflammation may encourage enlargement of the bronchial arteries as a result of enhanced abnormal communication with pulmonary arterioles. Furthermore, angiogenic growth factors can be released that promote neovascularization and recruitment of collateral circulation from systemic blood vessels. Pulmonary arteries, capillaries, and veins are the source of hemoptysis in fewer than 10% of cases.

Hemoptysis associated with chronic bronchitis accounts for more than 50% of hemoptysis cases in the United States and arises from superficial vessels in the bronchial mucosa. Hemoptysis associated with chronic fibrocavitary disorders such as tuberculosis, is caused by rupture or erosion of enlarged bronchial arteries and bronchopulmonary anastomoses. Pulmonary artery aneurysms and vessel rupture secondary to wall invasion can also occur. In mitral stenosis, the primary sites of bleeding are bronchial veins with blood supplied from both bronchial arteries and reversed blood flow from pulmonary veins.

Recent world events warrant special emphasis on potential bioterrorist causes of hemoptysis. Pneumonic plague is caused by *Yersinia pestis*, a Gram-negative bacillus that can be weaponized and spread by aerosolized droplets, causing rapidly progressive pneumonia, chest pain, and hemoptysis. Treatment includes oral doxycycline or ciprofloxacin. Tularemia, caused by the aerobic Gram-negative coccobacillus *Francisella tularensis,* has also been weaponized. Its aerosolization causes influenzae-like symptoms with rapidly progressive pneumonia and hemoptysis. The treatment of choice is intravenous gentamicin. Finally, tricothecene mycotoxin, also known as "yellow rain" in its aerosolized form, causes sore throat, skin necrosis, and hemoptysis. An oily residue on the facial skin of victims of biologic attacks might lead one to suspect the diagnosis. Treatment is, for the most part, supportive.

All instances of hemoptysis require careful evaluation to determine the cause and site of bleeding. The history is invaluable and establishes the duration and extent of bleeding, prior episodes, and the presence of known cardiopulmonary or other diseases. Hemoptysis must be differentiated from hematemesis and nasopharyngeal bleeding. The physical examination provides specific clues to the diagnosis (e.g., oronasopharyngeal bleeding site, microtelangiectasia, pulmonary or cardiac findings). The chest radiograph may suggest the cause and location of the hemoptysis in up to 50% of cases. A "negative" radiograph is not reassuring: one study suggested that the radiographs of 25% of patients with hemoptysis due to lung cancer provided no clues to this diagnosis. The characteristic radiographic finding of blood in the air spaces is a confluent or patchy alveolar filling pattern that becomes reticular over days and clears in 3 to 10 days. However, the pattern may represent blood aspirated from another bleeding site elsewhere in the lungs, making precise localization of a bleeding site challenging. Computed tomography (CT) scans, including multidetector CT with angiography (MDCTA) (high resolution angiographic studies performed with a single breath hold to reduce scanning time and respiratory motion artifacts) can identify underlying disease, assist in the diagnosis and mapping of bronchiectasis, usually precluding surgical resection if bronchiectasis is bilateral or diffuse, as well as direct surgical interventions in case focal pulmonary or vascular abnormalities are identified. More importantly, CT may detect vascular lesions such as aneurysms and arteriovenous malformations, and has a high accuracy predicting involvement of nonbronchial systemic arteries in patients with massive bleeding. Information from MDCTA is essential for planning arterial embolization, providing more accurate information about bronchial and nonbronchial systemic arteries than conventional angiography.

Other relevant laboratory studies include a complete blood count; smear, culture, and cytologic examination of the sputum; and, when appropriate, arterial blood gas analysis, as well as ventilation/perfusion $(\dot{V})/(\dot{Q})$ lung scans if pulmonary emboli are suspected. Perfusion scans are not, however useful in localizing a bleeding site. Several studies have found an elevated single-breath diffusion capacity (D_{LCO}) in patients with intrapulmonary bleeding, although it does not appear that D_{LCO} plays a useful role in the diagnosis or care of most patients (except, possibly, in patients with suspected Goodpasture syndrome).

Flexible bronchoscopy is indicated for a patient with hemoptysis of uncertain cause. Bronchogenic carcinoma has been detected bronchoscopically in at least 2% to 13% of patients with hemoptysis and a normal chest radiograph. Foreign bodies, bronchial adenoma, and other causes of bleeding are also readily identified. Furthermore, the site of the bleeding can usually be determined if a careful, systematic bronchoscopic inspection is performed, or if patients have previously undergone biopsy of endobronchial abnormalities.

The need for diagnostic flexible bronchoscopy in evaluating hemoptysis is clear, but whether it should be performed emergently or after bleeding has ceased remains controversial. A report from the American College of Chest Physicians stated that 64% of physicians favored performing bronchoscopy in the first 24 hours after an episode. Although early bronchoscopy is desirable because it minimizes the likelihood that the site will go undiscovered when bleeding has stopped, no evidence indicates that delaying bronchoscopy for 24 or 48 hours will adversely affect the ultimate outcome (e.g., detection of operable carcinoma). Flexible bronchoscopy should be performed carefully, however, and operators should be ready to handle massive bleeding by having large-channel bronchoscopes available for suctioning; equipment for emergency intubation, sedation, and ventilation; and, preferably, the capacity and ability to perform rigid bronchoscopy. Operators should be familiar with the use of tamponade balloons and endobronchial blockade balloon devices. They should recognize that cough induced by the procedure can promote more bleeding and that blood can easily spread throughout the tracheobronchial tree during the procedure, completely filling the central airway, obscuring the bleeding site, and causing asphyxiation. A bronchoscopy team that is well-versed in their response to emergencies should be available. Overall, bronchoscopy in a moderately or massively bleeding patient should not be taken lightly. Patients should be hospitalized in the intensive care unit, and the threshold for intubation with a large endotracheal tube should be low.

Arteriography and embolization of bronchial and related collateral vasculature (e.g., intercostal, axillary, and subclavian arteries) are increasingly useful in the treatment of hemoptysis that is not responsive to conservative measures. As mentioned previously, MDCTA is oftentimes favored over conventional angiography. Initially, bronchial artery embolization (BAE) was a temporizing measure until patients could undergo definitive surgical management by lung resection or to repair vascular injury. Many experienced clinicians now believe BAE plays a primary role for long-term control of recurrent or persistent hemoptysis (e.g., recurrent episodes of more than 200 mL/day) even in patients who might be candidates for resectional surgery. Patients who are particularly suitable include those with diffuse lung disease in whom bleeding can arise from more than one site, and those who are not candidates for surgery (which is often the case because of preexisting comorbidities and poor respiratory reserve).

Since the first bronchial artery embolization for hemoptysis in the 1970s, many physicians have successfully used this technique to stop hemoptysis and prevent its recurrence. Actual visualization of a *bleeding blush* during arteriography is rare. Localization is inferential from the visualization of the abnormal vascularity of reactive bronchial arterial networks; hence, previous specific localization by flexible bronchoscopy can be important. Bronchial arteries usually present as nodular or linear structures within the mediastinum and around the central airways on contrast-enhanced CT. Vessels greater than 2 mm in diameter are considered abnormal. They are often found in the retrotracheal, retroesophageal, and aortopulmonary window regions as well as along the posterior wall of the main bronchi. Collateral blood supply from nonbronchial systemic arteries should not be overlooked, and can be a cause for recurrence, even in the event of presumed successful bronchial artery embolization. Pleural thickening greater than 3 mm in an area adjacent to a pulmonary abnormality and tortuous enhancing vascular structures within hypertrophic extrapleural fat are signs of abnormality. Pseudoaneurysms should also be searched for specifically, as they may be seen in up to 10% of patients undergoing arteriography for hemoptysis, particularly those with underlying tuberculosis.

Inadvertent embolization of spinal arteries is a significant complication of bronchial artery embolizaton. However, it is uncommon if care is exercised in identifying possible spinal arteries branching from vessels considered for embolization. A number of investigators have reported initial control of bleeding in 80% to 90% of cases, with long-term recurrences in 10% to 55%. Recanalization or growth of new bronchial vessels can limit the long-term effectiveness of this therapeutic procedure in some patients. Embolization materials include Gelfoam, steel coils, polyvinyl alcohol, and isobutyl-2-cyanoacrylate. Increasingly, gelatin cross-linked particles called tris-acryl microspheres are used. Although infusion of sclerosing liquids or small embolic particles is appealing because of the theoretic advantages of occlusion of flow distal to collateral feeder vessels, the incidence of bronchial wall necrosis, spinal artery occlusion, and intense acute chest pain sometimes precludes the use of these agents. Early recurrence after bronchial artery embolization is usually the result of incomplete embolization. Rebleeding has been reported in up to 30% of cases. Late recurrence, on the other hand, is probably due to recanalization of previously embolized vessels, revascularization, or disease progression. Rebleeding can often be controlled by reembolization. Patients with aspergilloma or malignancy seem to have the worst outcomes, with greater chances for recurrence and higher mortality than patients with other benign causes for hemoptysis, including tuberculosis.

Therapy for hemoptysis, therefore, depends on the bleeding severity, the specific cause of the bleeding, and the patient's overall condition. The four goals of therapy are to prevent asphyxiation (often by protection of the contralateral airway), stop the bleeding, treat the primary cause, and prevent recurrence. If the volume of hemoptysis is large (>200 mL/day), or if the patient has minimal respiratory reserve, an emergency exists. The first goal of therapy is to identify the bleeding site, stop the bleeding, and prevent aspiration of blood into other major airways. In experienced hands, flexible bronchoscopy will identify the bleeding site. MDCTA is helpful, especially if embolization is being considered. In some cases of massive bleeding, rigid bronchoscopy may be necessary. Tamponade balloons or endobronchial balloon blockade devices can be inserted and left in place for hours or days while the patient is stabilized and readied for resectional therapy. Coughing, however, can dislodge the balloon. If therapeutic embolization of bronchial arteries is contemplated, placing a Fogarty tamponade balloon may allow time for the prerequisite angiographic or CT studies. Bronchoscopists should avoid removing newly formed clot from the secured segmental bronchial airway once bleeding has ceased. Clot removal in these instances may lead to recurrent bleeding.

Another approach to protecting functional airways involves placing a special endotracheal tube with an inflatable distal cuff into the nonbleeding right or left main stem bronchus. The use of a double-lumen tube permits adequate suctioning of blood. However, placement of the tube requires experienced personnel, and tube insertion can be difficult, especially in the actively bleeding patient. It may be wise to first insert a large endodtrachceal tube and, if necessary, selectively intubate the patient's good lung while turning the patient on the lateral decubitus position (bleeding site downwards). A suction catheter or even the flexible bronchoscope can be inserted adjacent to the endotracheal tube to help suction blood from the bleeding bronchus. Increasingly, bronchial arteriography with embolization is advocated for patients with massive hemoptysis who do not respond to more conservative measures, and in patients with moderate hemoptysis to help prevent recurrence. Recent improvements in angiographic techniques have minimized its potential complications. The efficacy of temporizing measures such as iced saline lavage, epinephrine, and Fogarty balloon placement is not well documented, and dependent on local expertise. The role of intravascular infusions or topical applications of vasoconstrictor agents (e.g., vasopressin) has not been established. Reports of successful treatment of bleeding pulmonary aspergilloma by percutaneous intracavitary infusion of amphotericin are anecdotal.

Surgical resection of any bleeding site requires its identification and a patient able to tolerate thoracotomy. Occasionally, patients require emergency surgery before a diagnosis has been established, particularly in cases of massive hemoptysis. In an often-quoted older study, Crocco et al. found that the mortality of patients with massive hemoptysis (i.e., 600 mL of blood/16-hour period) treated medically was 75%. Among similar patients treated by surgical resection, the mortality was 23%. An especially high mortality rate in patients treated medically was also observed in the setting of massive hemoptysis associated with lung abscesses. The high mortality rate associated with conservative medical therapy may reflect the bias of a nonrandomized study and a patient population with advanced tuberculosis and multiple disease processes. Other studies have found comparable mortality rates between conservative medical management and surgical resection. Surgery, especially in an emergency setting, has a mortality rate as high as 40%, and has a high risk of fistula formation, intraoperative bleeding, and postoperative respiratory failure. In a report from the American College of Chest Physicians, the majority of those surveyed preferred bronchial artery embolization over conservative or surgical management for controlling hemoptysis. Nevertheless, experience supports the role for surgical resection if all efforts to control bleeding medically (e.g., strict bed rest, no chest percussion or spirometric testing, aggressive cough suppression, bronchoscopic intervention) are unsuccessful and embolization of bronchial artery and related vessels is either not available or unsuccessful.

FURTHER READING

1. Bobrowitz ID, Ramakrishna S, Shim YS. Comparison of medical versus surgical treatment of major hemoptysis. *Arch Intern Med.* 1983;143:1343.

   This classic article reviews the course of 113 patients with substantial hemoptysis and argues the case for conservative management.

2. Bruzzi JF, Remy-Jardin M, Delhaye D, et al. Multi-detector row CT of hemoptysis. *Radiographics.* 2006;26:3–22.

   Detailed explanation of technology and technique.

3. Chun JY, Morgan R, Belli AM. Radiological management of hemoptysis: a comprehensive review of diagnostic imaging and bronchial artery embolization. *Cardiovasc Intervent Radiol.* 2010;33:240–250.

   A top-notch recent review of technique and anatomy. A must-read.

4. Colice GL. Detecting lung cancer as a cause of hemoptysis in patients with normal chest radiograph: bronchoscopy versus CT. *Chest.* 1997;111:877.

   Proposes using sputum cytology first or repeat chest radiographies to select patients for bronchoscopy.

5. Corder R. Hemoptysis. *Emerg Med Clin North Am.* 2003;21:421–435.

   A great review of current differential diagnosis and the role of the emergency room physician facing the patient coughing up blood.

6. Crocco JA, Rooney JJ, Fankushen DS, et al. Massive hemoptysis. *Arch Intern Med.* 1968;121:495.

   A classic. Compares medical and surgical therapy of 67 patients with massive hemoptysis.

7. DiLeo MD, Amedee RG, Butcher RB. Hemoptysis and pseudohemoptysis: the patient expectorating blood. *Ear Nose Throat J.* 1995;74:822.

   Exclude a pulmonary source, but in this retrospective review of 471 cases, 10% had an upper airway cause and 2% had an upper airway malignancy (primary tumor or metastasis) as the site of their bleeding.

8. Eddy JB. Clinical assessment and management of massive hemoptysis. *Crit Care Med.* 2000;28:1642–1647.

   This review argues need for CT scanning and flexible bronchoscopy. Also presents an algorithm for managing massive bleeding.

9. Freitag L, Tekolf E, Stamatis G, et al. Three year experience with a new balloon catheter for the management of hemoptysis. *Eur Respir J.* 1994;7:2033–2037.

   Describes bronchoscopic balloon insertion.

10. Gong H Jr, Salvatierra C. Clinical efficacy of early and delayed fiberoptic bronchoscopy in patients with hemoptysis. *Am Rev Respir Dis.* 1981;124:221.

    Of historical interest. A classic review of 129 patients, focusing on the pros and cons of early versus late bronchoscopy. The debate is still ongoing.

11. Greening AP, Hughes JM. Serial estimations of carbon monoxide diffusing capacity in intrapulmonary haemorrhage. *Clin Sci (Lond).* 1981;60:507.

    Serial measurements were much more sensitive than requiring a single measurement to be above the upper limit of predicted. Of intrapulmonary blood, 200 mL may be the sensitivity for serial measurements of D$_{LCO}$.

12. Gross AM, Diacon AH, van den Heuvel MM. Management of life-threatening hemoptysis in an area of high tuberculosis incidence. *Int J Tuberc Lung Dis.* 2009;13:875–880.

    Prospective study of more than 100 patients with one-year follow-up in South Africa. Validated previous work by the same group identifying four selection criteria for surgery: lack of cessation of bleeding 7 days after BAE, absence of active TB, presence of aspergilloma, and need for blood transfusion.

13. Haponik EF, Chin R. Hemoptysis: clinicians' perspectives. *Chest.* 1990;97:469–475.

    Pulmonary physicians surveyed prefer radiologic intervention to surgical intervention!

14. Hiyama J, Horita N, Shiota Y, et al. Cryptogenic hemoptysis and smoking. *Chest.* 2002; 121:1375–1376.

    Defining hemoptysis of unclear origin.

15. Jolliet P, Soccal P, Chevrolet JC. Control of massive hemoptysis by endobronchial tampoade with a pulmonary artery balloon catheter. *Crit Care Med.* 1992;20:1730–1732.

    Describes this technique, in case you don't have the other balloons available.

16. Katoh O, Yamada H, Hiura K, et al. Bronchoscopic and angiographic comparison of bronchial arterial lesions in patients with hemoptysis. *Chest.* 1987;91:486.

    Presents bronchoscopic appearances of vascular lesions noted on bronchial artery angiography.

17. Keeling AN, Costello R, Lee MJ. Rasmussen's aneurysm: a forgotten entity? *Cardiovasc Intervent Radiol.* 2008;31:196–200.

    A source of pulmonary arterial bleeding that used to be reported in up to 5% of patients with cavitary tuberculosis.

18. Kvale PA, Simoff M, Prakash UB; American College of Chest Physicians. Lung cancer: palliative care. *Chest.* 2003;123:284S–311S.

    Ten percent to 20% of patients with lung cancer may actually present with symptoms of hemoptysis. This is an excellent overview of palliative care in patients with lung cancer, also addressing treatment of chest pain, dyspnea, cough, and distal metastases.

19. Liebow AA, Hales MR, Lindshog GE. Enlargement of the bronchial arteries and their anastomoses with the pulmonary arteries in bronchiectasis. *Am J Pathol.* 1949;25:211.

    An excellent pathologic study of the changes in vasculature of the lung in bronchiectasis.

20. Lee S, Chan JW, Chan SC, et al. Bronchial artery embolization can be equally safe and effective in the management of chronic recurrent hemoptysis. *Hong Kong Med J.* 2008;14:14–20.

    Seventy patients of which 28 had chronic recurring hemoptysis. Self-limiting complications occurred in 13% overall, and of the 28 with chronic hemoptysis, rebleeding occurred in 47%.

21. Lordan JL, Gascoigne A, Corris PA. The pulmonary physician in critical care. *Thorax.* 2003;58:814–819.

    Excellent recent review based on single case report. Excellent images and description of therapeutic modalities, including Fogarty catheter placement and endotracheal intubation.

22. McGuinness G, Naidich DP. CT of airways disease and bronchiectasis. *Radiol Clin North Am.* 2002;40:1–19.

    A careful description of radiographic findings with numerous examples.

23. Sakr L, Dutau H. Massive hemoptysis: an update on the role of bronchoscopy in diaganosis and management. *Respiration.* 2010;80:38–58.

    Nice review of many of the bronchoscopic techniques used, in addition to an overview of recent studies of surgical results and outcomes after embolization.

24. Swanson KL, Johnson CM, Prakash UB, et al. Bronchial artery embolization: experience with 54 patients. *Chest.* 2002;121:789–795.

    Greater than 85% immediate response with cessation of bleeding for up to 30 days or more, and a 10% recurrence rate.

25. Taylor JR, Ryu J, Colby TV, et al. Lymphangioleiomyomatosis. *N Engl J Med.* 1990;323:1254.

    Of 32 patients, 44% had hemoptysis during the course of their lymphangioleiomyomatosis. The actual prevalence is probably much higher; infiltrates from hemorrhage are often misdiagnosed as pneumonia, as they can occur without hemoptysis.

Complications of Pulmonary Resections

Eugene M. Golts

Complications of thoracic surgery fall into two broad categories: those common to any surgical procedure and those unique to pulmonary resection. This chapter focuses on the latter for which the risk of postoperative complications ranges from 38% for major pulmonary resections to 0% in patients undergoing wedge thoracoscopic resection. Thorough knowledge of the topic should serve as the basis for successful avoidance of complications and complete recovery of the patients.

Most complications can be prevented, or at least attenuated, by comprehensive preoperative preparation and meticulous intraoperative technique. Prevention of complications begins preoperatively. Surgeons should rely on (1) the comprehensive assessment of the patient's pulmonary functional status; (2) correction, or improvement in the disease states associated with impaired healing; and (3) optimization of the patient's functional status by pulmonary rehabilitation and smoking cessation.

Preoperative evaluation of pulmonary function is one of the most extensively studied topics for assessing and risk-stratifying postoperative risk among patients undergoing pulmonary resections. Although controversy exists about those cutoff values that convey higher risk, some points are broadly accepted. All patients regardless of age, physical status, or extent of the lesion should have preoperative pulmonary-specific evaluation. Patients are at lower risk of complications and should be able to withstand pulmonary resection including pneumonectomy, if the FEV_1 and D_{LCO} are greater than or equal to 60% of predicted. Further testing, including the quantitative V/Q scan and VO_2 max testing may be helpful to assess resectability if the FEV_1 and D_{LCO} are lower than the above-mentioned cutoff point.

Optimizing nutrition and diminishing and discontinuing immunosuppressive medications can maximize a patient's healing potential. Patients need to stop smoking, since smoking cessation improves outcomes following surgical procedures. The ratio of actual postoperative to predictive postoperative FEV_1, has been shown to be better in patients undergoing perioperative rehabilitation. Pulmonary rehabilitation of several weeks' duration is advisable, in cases when the timing of the operation is elective.

Despite careful preoperative evaluation and training, postoperative pulmonary complications occur frequently after pulmonary resection in 14.5% to 38% of patients. Atelectasis is common early after surgery and may progress to pneumonia and even respiratory failure if left untreated. Patients commonly present within the first 48 hours after surgery with nonspecific symptoms such as low-grade fever, shortness of breath, tachypnea, and tachycardia. Radiographic evaluation is usually diagnostic. Incidence can be lowered by preoperative smoking cessation and training in the use of incentive spirometry. Postoperatively, aggressive pain management, particularly the use of the regional anesthesia, allows for the maintenance of adequate respiratory volumes. Adequate pain management along with the use of bronchodilators and mucolytics can help with effective secretion clearance. When massive atelectasis is present, fiberoptic bronchoscopy provides rapid and effective evacuation of secretions as well as evaluation for possible anatomic abnormalities of the airways.

Postoperative hemorrhage is relatively uncommon after pulmonary resection, with reported incidences between 2.4% and 8%. Pulmonary vessels, systemic sources such as intercostal vessels, bronchial arteries, and large systemic vessels are all potential sources of bleeding in any operative scenario. Intraoperative compromise of these blood vessels can occur during dissection, or due to a stapler malfunction. Thorough knowledge of the intraparenchymal vascular anatomy and meticulous dissection help to decrease the incidence of these complications. In addition, bleeding from adhesions and vessels in the inferior pulmonary ligament as well as from dissected lymph node beds can create problems in the immediate postoperative period.

Bloody chest tube output of 200 mL/hour for 2 hours postoperatively, and/or hemodynamic instability suggests significant hemorrhage and warrants prompt further investigation. However, one should never rely solely on the chest tube drainage for determination of the amount of bleeding. Blood clots or adjacent pulmonary parenchyma can obstruct and diminish drainage thereby misleading the observer about the severity of the problem. Serial chest radiographs are useful in detecting an incompletely drained hemothorax. In cases where there is a suspicion of bleeding, the chest tube insertion sites should be examined for presence of the bloody drainage around the chest tubes.

Prompt reexploration is warranted if there is (1) failure to achieve hemodynamic stability despite seemingly adequate resuscitation with blood products, (2) continued excessive drainage from chest drains, or (3) a significant undrained hemothorax on the chest radiograph. Coagulopathies should be aggressively corrected, but this action should not delay potentially life-saving surgery.

When bleeding is suspected, the thoracic cavity should be inspected systematically to evaluate all the above-mentioned sources of bleeding. Sudden massive hemorrhage after pulmonary resection is almost always due to a problem with the major vascular stump, such as a slipped ligature, and requires emergency re-do thoracotomy.

Although postoperative pleural effusion is relatively common after pulmonary resection, high chest tube output in the immediate postoperative period should raise the suspicion of postoperative hemorrhage. Determining the hematocrit of the chest tube drainage may be helpful in differentiating bleeding from innocuous "blood tinged" drainage.

Large amounts of chest tube drainage that occur later in the postoperative course may signify development of chylothorax. The incidence is reported to be less than 2%. One should suspect chylothorax when a large amount of milky drainage is present in the chest tubes after lobectomy, or smaller pulmonary resections, or when there is a rapid accumulation of fluid in the postpneumonectomy space. Occasionally, tension chylothorax can develop, which is manifested by respiratory and circulatory compromise. Chylothorax is best diagnosed by testing pleural fluid for chylomicrons. Lymphangiography can sometimes pinpoint an area of the injury. Treatment should be conservative with cessation of all oral intake and initiation of parenteral nutrition. Somatostatin analogues can be added to decrease chyle production. Presence of excessive drainage despite institution of conservative measures signifies the need for the reoperation which is usually successful.

In the absence of chylothorax, or bleeding, a conservative approach to even large volumes of chest tube output is warranted. In many institutions, including University of California, San Diego (UCSD), chest tubes are removed when the drainage decreases to less than 200 mL/day. Other surgeons accept significantly higher rates of pleural drainage. Most small pleural effusions that recur after the removal of the chest drains can be observed safely. Large or symptomatic effusions should be drained by thoracentesis as the first step. Tube thoracostomy should be considered, if fluid reaccumulates after thoracentesis.

Postoperative air leaks occur commonly after pulmonary resection and usually are small and arise from lung parenchyma denuded of a pleural cover. The reported incidence after resections other than pneumonectomy ranges from 7.6% to above 50%. Variability is largely due to differences in the definition of an "air leak." In general, an air leak that persists for longer than 7 days is considered a complication. There is no single variable that predicts a higher incidence but low FEV_1, steroid use, lobectomy, upper lobe resections, and the presence of adhesions are touted as risk factors. The incidence can be lowered by adherence to a meticulous operative technique. Dissection should be localized to fissures whenever possible. Lung parenchyma should be handled gently with atraumatic instruments. Areas of exposed parenchyma, such as windows for the passage of the staplers, should be over-sewn with the fine absorbable suture or covered with pleural or pericardial fat flaps. Although not airtight, these flaps along with parenchymal expansion allow for closure of potential air leaks. Test inflation of the remaining lung to 25 to 30 cm H_2O pressure, while submerged under a layer of saline pinpoints the location of occult air leaks. Use of staplers for the division of the lung parenchyma helps decrease the severity of the prolonged air leaks. Pericardial and synthetic strips used for reinforcement of the staple line may reduce the incidence of the air leaks even further, especially in patients with emphysema. Recently, various surgical sealants have been used successfully for the same purpose. However, none of these devices should be considered as substitutes for meticulous surgical technique.

Prolonged air leaks can be prevented by routine placement of chest tubes to water seal, rather to traditional -20 cm of H_2O suction.

Should a prolonged air leak develop, the chest tube outside of the patient should be checked as a possible source of the leak. If still undetected, the chest tube should be withdrawn a few centimeters to change the position of the suction holes relative to the lung tissue and to allow the opposition of parenchymal surfaces; this may promote closure of the air leak. Prolonged air leaks can be treated with the instillation of talc or other sclerosants into the pleural space, to incite an inflammatory reaction and to obliterate the alveolopleural fistulae. Finally, many patients with prolonged air leaks can be discharged home with a Heimlich valve and followed weekly on an outpatient basis with removal of the chest drain in a few weeks. These maneuvers allow for the management of the vast majority of the air leaks and avoid a return to the operating room.

Postresectional space is the result of the inevitable reduction in the volume of the lung after any resection. Management of the space depends on the extent of the resection. It is expected to occur after the pneumonectomy and can safely be left to fill with fluid in the postoperative period. Most of the parenchymal volume reduction after surgery is offset by a combination of hemidiaphragm elevation, reexpansion of the remaining lung, mediastinal shift to the side of resection, and narrowing of the intercostal spaces on the operated side. These mechanisms can be inadequate in cases of large resections, in the presence of visceral and/or parenchymal restriction due to inflammatory process, or when the mediastinum has decreased mobility due to infection, prior radiation, or surgery. Anywhere between 20% and 40% of patients after pulmonary resection will have residual space in the chest at the completion of surgery, as demonstrated by immediate postoperative chest radiography. The proportions would most likely be even higher, if more sensitive imaging techniques, such as thoracic computed tomography (CT) scans, were utilized.

Fortunately, the great majority of postresectional spaces do not create any problems and resorb in the postoperative period. However, it would be unwise to assume that all of the residual spaces are harmless. At least some of the spaces contribute to the development of prolonged air leaks or empyema.

Several intraoperative maneuvers such as complete mobilization of the inferior pulmonary ligament and careful placement of chest drains to allow for the excellent drainage of the postresectional space should help to avoid problems postoperatively. Surgeons should recognize the potential for the development of large postresectional space intraoperatively. In the cases of lobar or bilobar resections, and in resections for infectious processes, preemptive interventions should be undertaken. Pleural tenting is easily performed, adds little time to the operation, and has been shown to decrease the duration of air leaks and chest tube drainage. Intraoperative, or postoperative creation of a pneumoperitoneum by insufflation of 1 to 2 L of air in the peritoneal cavity either percutaneously, or transdiaphragmatically can help in the obliteration of the space. More aggressive interventions, such as thoracoplasty, phrenic nerve crush, and diaphragmatic transfer achieve good results at the expense of decreases in the pulmonary mechanical function postoperatively. In the postoperative period, a brief trial of increased suction on the chest tubes to -30 to 40 cm of H_2O can help in the obliteration of the space. Aggressive secretion management, incentive spirometry use, and early bronchoscopy for the management of secretions allows for maximal reexpansion of the residual lung tissue. In general, many residual postresectional spaces can be observed. Should they become infected, they should be drained completely and obliterated by muscle flaps, or by means of thoracoplasty.

Bronchopleural fistula is a known complication of pulmonary resection. The incidence varies widely, ranging from almost 10% in cases of pneumonectomy for infections to much less than 1% for sublobar resections performed for oncologic reasons. Bronchopleural fistula is more common after a right-sided pneumonectomy. Risk factors for the development of bronchopleural fistulae are associated with risk factors portending poor healing. Consequently, each patient's condition should be optimized preoperatively to maximize his or her healing potential. Intraoperatively, surgeons should avoid extensive devascularization of the bronchial stump as well as aggressive lymph node dissection in peribronchial planes next to the resection margin. The stump should be trimmed close to the next proximal bifurcation of the bronchial tree prior to closure in order to prevent pooling of secretions. Finally, coverage of the stump with pedicled muscle, or a pericardial flap may prevent the development of this complication.

The clinical presentation of a bronchopleural fistula depends on size and extent of the resection and ranges from very subtle signs of infection to severe respiratory compromise and overwhelming sepsis. After a pneumonectomy, the combination of a sudden drop in pleural effusion and a sudden increase in watery sputum should suggest a bronchopleural fistula. Air leak is usually present when a chest tube is reinserted. Bronchoscopy should be performed urgently to diagnose the bronchopleural fistula and to possibly treat small fistulae by the application of fibrin sealant. The patient should be positioned with the head of the bed elevated and operated side in the dependent position to minimize soiling of the bronchial tree by pleural fluids. The chest cavity should be emergently drained as completely as possible. If a bronchopleural fistula occurs within the first postoperative week, a technical error should be suspected requiring possible revision of the stump and flap reinforcement. In cases of late bronchopleural fistula formation, a common problem is rupture of an empyema through the bronchial stump. In these cases, open debridement by means of creation of an Eloesser flap and long-term packing of the chest cavity may be the only option. Eventually, these patients might become candidates for chest cavity obliteration by means of pedicle skeletal muscle flaps.

Some complications develop due to changes in anatomic relations of the intrathoracic structures after pulmonary resections. Lobar torsion results from rotation of the remaining lobe around the longitudinal axis of the bronchovascular pedicle. Torsion of the right middle lobe after right upper lobectomy is most common, but any lobe can be affected. It progresses to the lung gangrene, if left untreated. This complication is prevented by fixing the right middle lobe to the right lower lobe in appropriate anatomic position and observing proper lung reinflation prior to closure of the chest. Diagnosis is usually made based on symptoms of systemic toxicity, chest radiography with lobar consolidation, bronchial cut-off and bronchoscopic evidence of a partial bronchial obstruction that recurs after the bronchoscope is withdrawn. This condition mimics development of lung gangrene as the result of compromised circulation of the remaining parenchyma. Fortunately, prompt reexploration with relief of torsion, inspection of the pulmonary vasculature, and resection of the devitalized parenchyma is indicated in both of these conditions.

Cardiac herniation may occur as the result of the heart protruding into the pleural cavity through a residual pericardial defect. It can happen on either side. Herniation usually happens in the immediate postoperative period and is precipitated by changes in the patient's position or by changes in the relative pressures between the right and left hemithorax. Circulatory compromise ensues and patients may die unless prompt exploration is undertaken. This complication can be avoided by preemptive closure of pericardial defects, either primarily or with a variety of patches. Definitive treatment consists of closure of the pericardium during the reexploration.

Postpneumonectomy syndrome occurs infrequently after pneumonectomy and is much common after right pneumonectomy. The cause of this late and rare complication is the compression of the left mainstem bronchus or trachea between the aorta and left pulmonary artery. Similar compression of the right mainstem bronchus has been described in the cases of left pneumonectomy in the patients with the right-sided aortic arch. Patients usually present with respiratory symptoms and recurrent pulmonary infections. Bronchoscopy and CT scan of the chest are diagnostic. Treatment consists of dissection of adhesions around the compressed segment of the airway and movement of the heart back to the midline. It can be accomplished by filling the operated side with various types of prosthetic material.

Postpneumonectomy pulmonary edema is a very serious complication that occurs at a rate of 2% to 4%. It is more common after right pneumonectomy than left. Mortality varies from 40% to 90%. Several events have been implicated as potential triggers for the development of this complication, including fluid overload, unbalanced suction causing overinflation of the remaining lung, interruption of the lymphatic drainage from the remaining lung during aggressive subcarinal dissection, and administration of blood products perioperatively. Postpneumonectomy pulmonary edema develops 2 to 4 days after pneumonectomy. Symptoms are those of progressive respiratory insufficiency with the clinical picture closely resembling rapid development of acute respiratory distress syndrome (ARDS). Prompt diagnostic workup focused on other treatable causes of ARDS should be undertaken. Treatment is directed at maintenance of acceptable oxygenation levels and prevention of secondary complications. Institution of extracorporeal membrane oxygenation may be necessary. Prevention efforts are centered on adherence to protective lung strategies throughout the operation, minimizing fluid administration perioperatively, avoiding transfusion of blood/blood products transfusion, and liberal use of pressors and diuretics once adequate fluid status has been achieved.

In summary, complications after pulmonary resections are relatively common due to the typically poor overall health status of the patient requiring resections and due to the complexity of the operations themselves. The incidence of most complications can be lowered, or their severity lessened, by meticulous preoperative preparation, careful intraoperative conduct, and attention to postoperative recovery.

FURTHER READING

1. Allen MS, Darling GE, Pechet TT, et al. Morbidity and mortality of major pulmonary resections in patients with early-stage lung cancer: initial results of the randomized, prospective ACOSOG Z0030 trial. *Ann Thorac Surg.* 2006;81(3):1013–1019; discussion 1019–1020.

   Complications occurred in 38% of cases in this large contemporary cohort of patients undergoing lung resections. This number serves as the somber reminder of high incidence of postoperative complications after pulmonary resections.

2. Harpole DH Jr, DeCamp MM Jr, Daley J, et al. Prognostic models of thirty-day mortality and morbidity after major pulmonary resection. *J Thorac Cardiovasc Surg.* 1999;117(5):969–979.

   Study with the one of the largest datasets to-date aimed at development of algorithm to predict postoperative complications, based on several preoperative variables.

3. Datta D, Lahiri B. Preoperative evaluation of patients undergoing lung resection surgery. *Chest.* 2003;123(6):2096–2103.

   Authors describe stepwise approach to preoperative evaluation of lung function prior to resection.

4. Mills E, Eyawo O, Lockhart I, et al. Smoking cessation reduces postoperative complications: a systematic review and meta-analysis. *Am J Med.* 2011;124(2):144–154.e8.

   Comprehensive review of currently available literature on the topic of preoperative smoking cessation.

5. Agostini P, Cieslik H, Rathinam S, et al. Postoperative pulmonary complications following thoracic surgery: are there any modifiable risk factors? *Thorax.* 2010;65(9):815–818.

   Body Mass Index, smoking status, and chronic obstructive pulmonary disease (COPD) are identified as potentially modifiable risk factors for prevention of complications.

6. Peterffy A, Henze A. Haemorrhagic complications during pulmonary resection: a retrospective review of 1428 resections with 113 haemorrhagic episodes. *Scand J Thorac Cardiovasc Surg.* 1983;17(3):283–287.

   Results of the study emphasize the need for meticulous surgical hemostasis. Most of the hemorrhagic complications were attributed to variations in technique.

7. Sivrikoz MC, Tulay CM. Variations of lobar branches of pulmonary arteries in thoracic surgery patients. *Surg Radiol Anat.* 2011;33(6):509–514.

   Review of surgical anatomy of vascular structures of the lung. Knowledge of this topic is essential for avoiding catastrophic vascular complications intraoperatively.

8. Terzi A, Furlan G, Magnanelli G, et al. Chylothorax after pleuro-pulmonary surgery: a rare but unavoidable complication. *Thorac Cardiovasc Surg.* 1994;42(2):81–84.

9. Shimizu K, Yoshida J, Nishimura M, et al. Treatment strategy for chylothorax after pulmonary resection and lymph node dissection for lung cancer. *J Thorac Cardiovasc Surg.* 2002;124(3):499–502.

   Surgical and conservative ways for management of postoperative chylothorax discussed in references 8 and 9.

10. Younes RN, Gross JL, Aguiar S, et al. When to remove a chest tube? A randomized study with subsequent prospective consecutive validation. *J Am Coll Surg.* 2002;195(5):658–662.

11. Cerfolio RJ, Bryant AS. Results of a prospective algorithm to remove chest tubes after pulmonary resection with high output. *J Thorac Cardiovasc Surg.* 2008;135(2):269–273.

    Two papers mentioned above, answer the question of timing of chest tubes' removal after pulmonary resections.

12. Fabian T, Federico JA, Ponn RB. Fibrin glue in pulmonary resection: a prospective, randomized, blinded study. *Ann Thorac Surg.* 2003;75(5):1587–1592.

13. Malapert G, Hanna HA, Pages PB, et al. Surgical sealant for the prevention of prolonged air leak after lung resection: meta-analysis. *Ann Thorac Surg.* 2010;90(6):1779–1785.

Surgical sealants continue to gain popularity among thoracic surgeons as the means for reducing postoperative air leaks. References 12 and 13 provide evidence for the effectiveness and safety of surgical sealants in prevention of prolonged air leaks.

14. Cerfolio RJ, Bass C, Katholi CR. Prospective randomized trial compares suction versus water seal for air leaks. *Ann Thorac Surg.* 2001;71(5):1613–1617.

15. Marshall MB, Deeb ME, Bleier JI, et al. Suction vs water seal after pulmonary resection: a randomized prospective study. *Chest.* 2002;121(3):831–835.

Results of the above-mentioned two trials challenge common practice of prolonged suction on the chest tubes after pulmonary resections.

16. Robinson LA, Preksto D. Pleural tenting during upper lobectomy decreases chest tube time and total hospitalization days. *J Thorac Cardiovasc Surg.* 1998;115(2):319–326; discussion 326–327.

17. De Giacomo T, Rendina EA, Venuta F, et al. Pneumoperitoneum for the management of pleural air space problems associated with major pulmonary resections. *Ann Thorac Surg.* 2001;72(5):1716–1719.

Complementary ways of management of residual pleural air space discussed in references 16 and 17.

18. Hurvitz RJ, Tucker BL. The Eloesser flap: past and present. *J Thorac Cardiovasc Surg.* 1986;92(5):958–961.

Detailed, comprehensive discussion of major surgical technique for the management of infected pleural space.

19. Demir A, Akin H, Olcmen A, et al. Lobar torsion after pulmonary resection; report of two cases. *Ann Thorac Cardiovasc Surg.* 2006;12(1):63–65.

Prompt recognition and intervention are key to the treatment of postoperative lobar torsion. Surgical strategy for the prevention, diagnostic clues for recognition and surgical treatment are discussed.

20. Mehran RJ, Deslauriers J. Late complications: postpneumonectomy syndrome. *Chest Surg Clin N Am.* 1999;9(3):655–673.

Comprehensive reference for management of this serious complication.

21. Grichnik KP, D'Amico TA. Acute lung injury and acute respiratory distress syndrome after pulmonary resection. *Semin Cardiothorac Vasc Anesth.* 2004;8(4):317–334.

Thorough review of these potentially lethal postoperative complications with detailed emphasis on the prevention and treatment.

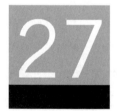

Pneumothorax
Henri G. Colt

The pleural space is located between the visceral pleura surrounding the lung and the parietal pleura lining the inside of the rib cage and is occupied by a small amount of lubricating pleural fluid. Pleural pressure is negative compared with atmospheric pressure, which helps maintain lung inflation. If the parietal or visceral pleura is breached and the pleural space is exposed to atmospheric (positive) pressure, air enters the pleural space (i.e., pneumothorax occurs), and the lung collapses inward toward the mediastinum. Any condition that impairs the structural integrity of either pleural membrane can produce a pneumothorax. This entity presents a true healthcare problem, affecting more than 20,000 individuals each year in the United States and costing more than $130 million in healthcare expenditures. The prognosis and management depend on the underlying cause. Pneumothorax is often categorized as (1) idiopathic or spontaneous, (2) iatrogenic, or (3) traumatic. Within each category, pneumothoraces can be either uncomplicated (usually unaccompanied by symptoms or prolonged air leak) or complicated (accompanied by symptoms, radiographic evidence of mediastinal shift, bleeding, or prolonged air leak). Pneumothorax can also be categorized as "primary" (no underlying lung disease, estimated to occur in 18 to 28 per 100,000 men each year in Great Britain), and "secondary" (presence of underlying lung disease). Primary spontaneous pneumothorax has an estimated yearly incidence of 6 per 100,000 in men and 2 per 100,000 in women. It rarely produces a prolonged air leak. Secondary spontaneous pneumothorax, on the other hand, especially in patients with chronic obstructive pulmonary disease (COPD) occurs in approximately 26 per 100,000 persons per year. Extrapolated to the entire population, this results in about 4,500 cases each year in the United States. At least 20% of these patients will have prolonged air leaks encompassing greater risk of increased morbidity, prolonged hospital stays, and increased used of healthcare resources.

In regard to anatomic abnormalities and other possible risk factors for pneumothorax, smoking has been identified as being associated with a 12% increased risk as compared to 0.1% risk for nonsmoking healthy men. Patients with spontaneous pneumothorax also tend to be taller, suggesting that greater distending pressures at the apex of the lung as compared to the base of the lung might be a contributing factor, especially for the development of apical blebs. Indeed, subapical blebs and bullae have been noticed during thoracoscopy and by computed tomography (CT) in a majority of patients with primary spontaneous pneumothorax, although no significant correlation has been found between existence of these abnormalities and the need to remove them by stapler resection to prevent recurrence. Pleural porosities invisible to white light but detectable on autofluorescent examination, as well as inflammation-mediated small airways obstruction with emphysema-like changes are also suggested etiologic mechanisms. Overall, the risk of recurrence after a primary spontaneous pneumothorax is about 50%. The absence of recurrence in about 50%, and the absence of a firm cause and effect relationship between unruptured blebs or bullae noted on CT scan, makes treatment decisions problematic. Risks for recurrence is increased in the presence of underlying disease such as COPD and pulmonary fibrosis, and age greater than 60 years, but contrary to what was once believed, physical activity has not been identified as a risk factor.

Spontaneous (*idiopathic*) *pneumothorax* (SP) occurs in patients without a history of any event known to cause pneumothorax (e.g., trauma or intervention). It generally occurs unexpectedly in an apparently healthy individual. Patients usually have no evidence of bullous lung disease on radiographic, thoracoscopic, or open surgical examination. Spontaneous pneumothoraces should be categorized as secondary, however, when abnormal lung parenchyma is noted, either from underlying lung disease or by identifying bulla or blebs during radiographic or direct examination.

At least two different mechanisms can lead to spontaneous pneumothorax. One is a visceral pleural *tear* (i.e., a bronchopleural fistula) caused by rupture of a subpleural bleb or bulla or by a parenchymal process that erodes through the visceral pleura (e.g., necrotizing pneumonia). Blebs are found in up to 90% of patients with presumed primary pneumothorax. Another mechanism is partial bronchial obstruction that acts as a *check valve*. Subsequent progressive hyperinflation of distal air spaces occurs until air eventually dissects along bronchovascular spaces into the hilus and mediastinum, leading to pneumomediastinum. From there, air can also dissect through fascial planes in the neck, resulting in subcutaneous emphysema, or through visceral pleura into one (usually the right) or both pleural cavities, resulting in pneumothorax.

In a young, otherwise healthy individual without radiographic evidence of lung disease, SP usually results from the rupture of subpleural apical blebs or bullae. The peak incidence is between the ages of 20 and 30 with a 4:1 male predominance, and as mentioned previously, with a predilection for tall, thin individuals. The incidence of SP has been reported to be increased in cigarette smokers, but this remains controversial. Interestingly, most patients who smoke continue to do so after a first episode of pneumothorax, even though the recurrence rate is more than 50% during the first 4 years after a first episode.

In most cases, symptoms develop at rest; however, onset can be associated with strenuous activity in up to 20% of cases and with a forceful cough or sneeze in at least 5%. Spontaneous pneumothorax should always convey a high index of suspicion for the presence of intrinsic lung disease, particularly if pneumomediastinum also is present. Among the lung conditions often associated with pneumothorax are emphysema (particularly bullous emphysema), diffuse interstitial processes (e.g., eosinophilic granuloma, sarcoidosis, usual interstitial pneumonia, desquamative interstitial pneumonia, and the pneumoconioses), necrotizing pneumonias (including tuberculosis), endometriosis (catamenial pneumothorax in women during menses), and acquired immune deficiency syndrome (related to malnutrition or *Pneumocystis carinii* pneumonia and associated with prolonged air leaks and decreased survival).

Iatrogenic pneumothorax most commonly occurs after invasive thoracic procedures, such as thoracentesis, transbronchial lung biopsy, and subclavian vein catheterization; however, it also can complicate virtually any invasive procedure involving the neck or abdomen (e.g., liver biopsy, transtracheal aspiration, intercostal nerve block, and even acupuncture). A very infrequent cause may be tracheotomy, where iatrogenic tracheal laceration should be suspected in the presence of otherwise unexplained pneumothorax, pneumomediastinum, or even pneumoperitoneum. Iatrogenic pneumothorax can complicate positive pressure ventilation and, in this setting, can be life threatening. The mechanism is usually a combination of partial bronchial obstruction caused by edema, secretions, and check-valve air entry leading to progressive alveolar expansion and rupture.

Traumatic pneumothorax can occur in the setting of penetrating or nonpenetrating chest trauma. The former generally presents no diagnostic problem; however, the latter should prompt a careful search for rib fracture, bronchial rupture, and esophageal injury. Rib fractures are associated with tears of the visceral pleura and pneumothorax; bronchial rupture is associated with deceleration injury; and esophageal rupture is often associated with mediastinal air entry. Pneumothorax can also result from abdominal trauma (e.g., abdominal stab wound, bullet wound) and diaphragmatic tears.

The clinical manifestations of pneumothorax depend on its size, the clinical context in which it occurs, and the mechanism(s) involved. Chest pain and dyspnea are common presenting symptoms. The pain is usually of sudden onset and initially pleuritic in character. After a few hours, it often changes to a dull ache, and spontaneous resolution of the pain can occur within 2 to 3 days. At least 10% of patients do not experience pain. Dyspnea occurs in 80%, often with spontaneous resolution within 24 hours despite persistence of the pneumothorax. Prominent coughing occurs in 10%; occasionally, it is the major or only symptom. Less than 5% of patients are asymptomatic. Symptoms can be transient and do not always correlate well with the radiographic size of the pneumothorax.

The most common physical findings are tachypnea, splinting, and decreased inspiratory expansion of the involved hemithorax, a tympanitic percussion note, decreased fremitus, and decreased breath sounds on the involved side. In patients with a check-valve mechanism, the initial complaint of substernal pressure or discomfort is often interpreted as cardiac in origin. Subsequently, the patient can experience chest pain, dyspnea, and relief of the substernal symptoms if pneumothorax or decompression into cervical subcutaneous tissues occurs. Mediastinal emphysema can be detected on auscultation by the presence of a mediastinal *crunch* (Hamman sign) coincident with cardiac systole and diastole. Similarly, subcutaneous emphysema may be noted on palpation of the anterior chest, axilla, shoulders, and neck. Subcutaneous infiltration of air may not always be readily visible, but can often be felt. Dyspnea can be exaggerated and persistent when underlying lung disease is present. In severely traumatized or mechanically ventilated patients, symptoms and signs can be obscured or difficult to interpret. This also is the case in patients with emphysema who have severe hyperinflation and diminished breath sounds. An electrocardiogram may show nonspecific ST–T wave changes and axis shifts, suggesting myocardial or thromboembolic disease.

The diagnosis of pneumothorax is usually made on clinical history and review of chest radiographs. In some cases, it may be necessary to obtain end-expiratory chest films to visualize the pleural reflection of the collapsed lung, but standard erect chest radiographs usually suffice for initial diagnosis. Comparisons may be necessary with previous films, particularly in the case of small loculated abnormalities, and in patients on mechanical ventilation; or with known bullous lung disease. CT scanning is helpful to document or identify unilateral or bilateral bullous abnormalities during or after episodes of pneumothorax, as well as to guide chest tube drainage in patients with complex, uniloculated, or multiloculated pneumothoraces. Pleural and bullous air collections can be distinguished to avoid inadvertently inserting chest tubes into lung bullae. An American College of Chest Physicians (ACCP) consensus report did not recommend routine CT scanning after a first episode of pneumothorax and did not achieve consensus regarding the role of CT scanning for recurrent pneumothorax or for planning surgical intervention. The value of ultrasound imaging remains to be determined, although ultrasonographic features can be helpful, particularly in supine trauma victims. Both chest radiographs and CT scans can be used to ascertain the size of the pneumothorax, although distinguishing whether the abnormality is large or small differs between British and American Guidelines. (Both use a distance >2 cm between the lung margin and the chest wall. British Thoracic Society [BTS] guidelines measure this at the level of the hilum, and American guidelines measure this from the apex to the cupola.) Another way to evaluate patients with pneumothorax, particularly after a chest tube has been inserted, is to document the volume, duration, and trend of the air leak. The Cerfolio classification System is based on observation of the timing of the air leak in the respiratory cycle (graded 1–4 according to whether the air leak is continuous, inspiratory only, expiratory only, or present during forced expiration only).

Complications of pneumothorax are classified as *acute* and *long term* and can occur in all types. Acute complications include tension pneumothorax, acute respiratory failure, bilateral pneumothorax, hemothorax, and pyothorax. Long-term complications include failure to reexpand (i.e., persistent pneumothorax) and recurrence. Prolonged air leaks contribute to respiratory failure by increasing work of breathing, and are associated with significant other comorbidities such as pneumonia, pulmonary embolus, empyema, atelectasis, nosocomial infections, and subcutaneous emphysema. Furthermore, prolonged air leak is associated with increased hospital stay, as noted in the National Emphysema Treatment Trial and in numerous studies of outcomes after lung resection.

Tension pneumothorax, which can appear rapidly and, if untreated, result in death, is caused by continued air entry into the pleural space. The persistent accumulation of positive pressure within the pleural cavity results in substantial lung collapse, mediastinal shift toward the contralateral side, and possible compression of the uninvolved lung. This situation can occur after rupture of an apical bleb if the visceral pleural tear forms a *flap* (i.e., opening with inspiration and closing with expiration). Tension pneumothorax also can occur after rupture of the mediastinal pleura caused by an intrapulmonary check valve if air continues to be pumped into the mediastinum. This situation is made worse if the patient is on mechanical ventilation and in some cases of cardiopulmonary resuscitation. It can also occur after penetrating chest wounds when air continues to enter the chest with each inspiration, especially if check-valving at the site of chest wall injury prevents expulsion of air during expiration. Patients with indwelling chest tubes for pneumothorax with acute deterioration also may have suspected tension. In these cases, the chest tube may not be communicating adequately with the area of air leakage (because of adhesions, plugging of the chest tube itself, or chest tube malfunction).

A diagnosis of tension pneumothorax should be considered in the setting of (1) progressive dyspnea and tachycardia, (2) shift of the trachea and mediastinal structures away from the involved side, and (3) increasing tympany of the involved side. Roentgenograms can confirm those events, but, if suspected, immediate decompression by transthoracic insertion of a needle attached to a syringe may be indicated. If a patient has a chest tube in place already and the development of a tension pneumothorax is suspected, all bandages should be removed and the tube carefully inspected. Waiting for radiographic confirmation may be fatal.

Bilateral pneumothorax is a rare event that usually is not detected without a chest roentgenogram. Reinflating one lung with a chest tube usually maintains patient stability until this complication is recognized.

Pneumothorax can be accompanied by hemothorax and pyothorax. In these cases, patients are said to have a *hydropneumothorax*. Evacuation of the pneumothorax and evaluation of the pleural effusion are mandatory. Hemothorax, often caused by adhesion rupture, lung parenchyma, or vascular structures, is potentially lethal because the pleural space easily accommodates a large amount of blood and because tamponade of the bleeding site may not occur. In the presumably healthy individual who develops an SP, discovery of pleural effusion is an indication for diagnostic thoracentesis to exclude bleeding. Effusions occur in about 20% of patients and are nonbloody; however, radiographic obscuring (i.e., blunting) of the costophrenic angle requires at least 100 mL of fluid. In the otherwise healthy individual, bleeding is more common with recurrent pneumothorax and is caused by rupture of vascular adhesions between visceral and parietal pleura. If tamponade does not occur, a patient can exsanguinate rapidly from such a benign source. Bleeding sites in other forms of pneumothorax are much more variable, but the same rule applies—thoracentesis should be performed on all effusions to exclude hemothorax.

Pyothorax, on the other hand, usually results from the entry of organisms along with air. Remember that a persistent pneumothorax noted radiographically, particularly in the presence of a thick visceral pleural peel, suggests chronic bronchopleural fistula, which may require special procedures (such as interposed muscle flaps) for surgical correction. Rare in SP not associated with preexisting lung disease, it is much more common with lung rupture caused by necrotizing pneumonia or penetrating trauma. The symptoms and findings are the same as those of an empyema.

The management of pneumothorax depends on the setting in which it occurs. Patients with uncomplicated SP and no underlying lung disease have four reasonable treatment options: (1) observation (inpatient or outpatient); (2) aspiration by needle or by a small lumen catheter; (3) insertion of a small chest tube or catheter attached to a one-way flutter valve; or (4) insertion of a chest tube attached to water seal (*closed*) or suction drainage. Of these, needle aspiration using a 14G to 16G needle, which is a favored therapeutic technique by the British, is the least desirable, although associated with decreased length of stay, and may lacerate the lung and introduce infection. The traditional practice in the United States is either to hospitalize for observation of complications or to insert a chest tube for 1 to 3 days, or both. In case of observation, the rate of resolution is between 1.25% and 2.2% of the volume of the hemithorax per day. Both large- and small-bore chest tubes can be attached to one-way flutter devices (Heimlich valves) that allow ambulation and rapid discharge if breathless or other symptoms make simple observations unwarranted. Patients with hydropneumothorax, should not be treated with one-way valves because of the risk of obstruction from viscous fluid or blood. Careful exclusion of patients at risk for developing significant complications (e.g., the presence of underlying lung disease, heart disease, and advanced age) is essential for the safety of such outpatient approaches.

Insertion of a small catheter followed by aspiration may be all that is needed for therapy of a pneumothorax attributed to introduction of air during a procedure involving the chest wall (e.g., thoracentesis, central venous pressure insertion). In most other categories of pneumothorax, prompt chest tube insertion and closed drainage of the abnormal air collection is indicated. The more severe the underlying lung disease and clinical dysfunction, the more urgent the need for tube drainage. Some guidelines suggest avoiding suction because of the risk of reexpansion pulmonary edema. When suction is applied, it should usually not exceed -20 cm H_2O. Reexpansion pulmonary edema, particularly in young, otherwise healthy individuals, results in increased breathlessness and chest pain. Alveolar-filling type infiltrates are usually noted in the ipsilateral or contralateral lung on chest radiograph.

Patients with unexplained recurrent spontaneous pneumothoraces, persistent bleeding into the pleural space, or unsuccessful chest tube drainage (not resulting in reexpansion of the lung), probably warrant thoracoscopic examination of the pleura and lung. This procedure allows complete inspection of underlying lung parenchyma, identification of air leaks, and closure using endoscopic stapling devices, loop ligation, or electrocauterization of blebs and bullae. Pleurodesis also can be performed using talc insufflation, chemicals, or pleural abrasion. Most experts agree that chest tube drainage is warranted before referral for thoracoscopy, regardless of whether a patient is clinically stable or unstable. Large-bore chest tubes (28 Fr) are warranted in patients who are clinically unstable, have large air leaks, or are on mechanical ventilation with a high risk of large air leaks. In general, both the BTS and ACCP guidelines recommend treatment decisions based on severity of clinical symptoms and the degree of lung collapse on chest radiographs. Patients with prolonged air leaks should be discussed with thoracic surgery colleagues, but considerations can also be given to bronchoscopic approaches, especially if the patient is a poor candidate for surgical repair. Bronchoscopists may help localize the air leak by performing selective airway occlusion using a balloon catheter, and attempt closing the fistula using gel foam, gludes, adheseives, Watanbe spigots, cautery, laser, or bronchial valves.

Thoracotomy may be necessary for some patients with pneumothorax. In these cases, a muscle-sparing axillary thoracotomy is usually possible. Hemothorax may also require exploration or repair of the bleeding site. Failure to reexpand the collapsed lung with tube drainage is another indication for thoracoscopy or thoracotomy. The length of time necessary for a visceral pleural tear to heal and for lung reexpansion to occur during tube drainage depends on the particular patient and the severity of underlying disease. For example, patients with advanced COPD, interstitial fibrosis, cystic fibrosis, or bullous emphysema as well as patients with the human immunodeficiency virus, active *P. carinii* pneumonia, and on corticosteroids are at increased risk for prolonged air leak with its associated increased risk for morbidity and mortality. In general, leaks persisting for more than 7 to 10 days rarely seal without surgical intervention. Open thoracotomy with pleurectomy remains the procedure associated with the lowest recurrence rate (1%), which compares favorably to video-assisted thoracic surgery with pleurectomy and pleural abrasion or pleurodesis (5% recurrence rate).

As mentioned previously, recurrence rates in otherwise healthy patients range from 10% to 50%. Approximately 60% of patients with a second recurrence will develop a third episode; after three episodes, recurrence exceeds 85%. Therefore, thoracoscopy or thoracotomy usually is recommended after the first recurrence and, increasingly, in patients with air leaks persisting for more than 3 to 5 days despite chest tube drainage, or failure of lung reexpansion despite chest tube drainage, as well as in patients with first contralateral pneumothorax, spontaneous hemopneumothorax, professions at risk such as pilots and scuba divers. Because of known increased risks for pneumothorax in pregnancy and parturition, some experts recommend a video-assisted thoracoscopic society (VATS) procedure after delivery to prevent recurrence in pregnant patients with pneumothorax.

FURTHER READING

1. Bense L, Eklund G, Wiman LG. Smoking and the increased risk of contracting spontaneous pneumothorax. *Chest.* 1987;92:1009.

   Smoking increased the relative risk of SP approximately 9 times among women and 22 times among men. A dose-response relationship between number of cigarettes smoked per day and risk of SP was also noted.

2. Baumann MH, Strange C, Heffner JE, et al. Management of spontaneous pneumothorax: an American College of Chest Physicians Delphi consensus statement. *Chest.* 2001;119:590–602.

   Agreement exists for general principles of care, with observation of small pneumothoraces being appropriate only for primary pneumothoraces.

3. Bauman MH. Do blebs cause primary spontaneous pneumothorax? Pro–con debate. *J Bronchol.* 2002;9:313–318.

   A debate with Dr. Noppen that reviews pathogenesis of SP.

4. Colt HG, Mathur PN. *Manual of Pleural Procedures.* Philadelphia, PA: Lippincott Williams & Wilkins; 1999:127.

   Practical, pocket-size reference manual with photographs and text that walks readers through diagnostic and therapeutic pleural procedures, such as chest tube insertion, bedside pleurodesis, chest drainage devices, and thoracoscopy.

5. Colt HG, Murgu SD. Closure of pneumonectomy stump fistula using custom Y and cuff-link shaped silicone prostheses. *Ann Thorac Cardiovasc Surg.* 2009;15(5):339–342.

   An example of an interventional technique to repair prolonged air leak and infection.

6. Green R, McLoud TC, Stark P. Pneumothorax. *Semin Roentgenol.* 1977;12:313.

   An excellent review of roentgenographic manifestations of pneumothorax.

7. Heffner JH, Huggins JT. Management of secondary spontaneous pneumothorax: there's confusion in the air. *Chest.* 2004;125:1190–1192.

   An editorial that explicitly describes many controversial areas pertaining to pneumothorax management and differences between the early 21st century ACCP and BTS guidelines.

8. Janssen JP, van Mourik J, Valentin MC, et al. Treatment of patients with spontaneous pneumothorax during videothoracoscopy. *Eur Respir J.* 1994;7:1281.

   Of patients examined, 34% had normal thoracoscopic inspections, with bullae larger than 2 cm noted in 54% of cases.

9. Kelly AM, Weldon D, Tsang AYL, et al. Comparison between two methods for estimating pneumothorax size from chest x-rays. *Respir Med.* 2006;100:1356–1359.

   Step by step description.

10. Lee P, Yap WS, Pek WY, et al. An audit of medical thoracoscopy and talc poudrage for pneumothorax in advanced COPD. *Chest.* 2004;125:1315–1320.

    A study of 41 patients showing 95% success after a median follow-up of 35 months, although mortality was 10% at 30 days (each in a patient with baseline forced expiratory volume in 1 second [FEV₁] <40% predicted).

11. Lee P, Colt HG. *Flex-Rigid Pleuroscopy Step-by-Step.* Singapore: CMP Medica Asia; 2005.

    In addition to describing pleuroscopy, it provides detailed analysis of numerous different procedure-related and disease-related algorithms.

12. Lal A, Anderson G, Cowen M, et al. Pneumothorax and pregnancy. *Chest.* 2007;132:1044–1048.

    A well-written review paper.

13. Lee P, Mathur NP, Colt HG. Advances in thoracoscopy: 100 years since Jacobaeus. *Respiration.* 2010;79:177–186.

    Another review paper that addresses numerous techniques and instruments and indications.

14. Lee P, Yap W, Pek W, et al. An audit of medical thoracoscopy and talc poudrage for pneumothorax prevention in advanced COPD. *Chest.* 2004;125:1315–1320.

    Talc pleurodesis works quite well, even in patients with large air leaks.

15. MacDuff A, Arnold A, Harvey J, et al. Management of spontaneous pneumothorax: British Thoracic Society Pleural Disease Guideline 2010. *Thorax.* 2010;65:ii17–ii30.

    A great review with management guidelines.

16. Munnell ER. Thoracic drainage. *Ann Thorac Surg.* 1997;63:1497.

    Reviews the advantages and disadvantages of various chest tube insertion techniques and drainage devices.

17. Noppen M. Management of primary spontaneous pneumothorax. *Curr Opin Pulm Med.* 2003;9:272–275.

    Also includes an excellent discussion of management guidelines and whether they are actually being followed.

18. Noppen M, Alexander P, Driesen P, et al. Manual aspiration versus chest tube drainage in first episodes of primary spontaneous pneumothorax. *Am J Respir Crit Care Med.* 2002;165:1240–1244.

    A prospective randomized study in a homogenous population.

19. Sewell RW, Fewel JG, Grover FL, et al. Experimental evaluation of reexpansion pulmonary edema. *Ann Thorac Surg.* 1978;26:126.

    Anatomic and functional changes were seen in the reexpanded lung after relief of pneumothorax. The longer the time of collapse, the greater the pulmonary intravascular water volume after reexpansion.

20. Shen KR, Cerfolio RJ. Decision making in the making of secondary spontaneous pneumothorax in patients with severe emphysema. *Thorac Surg Clin.* 2009;19:233–238.

    Mainly a surgical paper.

21. Traveline JM, McKenna RJ, DeGiacomo T, et al. Treatment of persistent pulmonary air leaks using endobronchial valves. *Chest.* 2009;136:355–360.

    Good review of new technology.

22. Tshopp JM, Rami-Porta, Noppen M, et al. Management of spontaneous pneumothorax: state of the art. *Eur Respir J.* 2006;28:637–650.

    Classic in Europe. Also covers thoracoscopic treatments and pleurodesis.

23. Tschopp JM, Brutsche M, Frey JG. Treatment of complicated spontaneous pneumothorax by simple talc pleurodesis under thoracoscopy and local anesthesia. *Thorax.* 1997;52:329.

    In this study of 93 patients undergoing thoracoscopic talc pleurodesis under local anesthesia, the major predictor for treatment failure was the presence of bullae larger than 2 cm.

24. Tschopp JM, Boutin C, Astoul P, et al. Talcage by medical thoracoscopy for primary sponta-neous pneumothorax is more cost-effective than drainage: a randomized study. *Eur Respir J.* 2002;20:1003–1009.

   Multinational international study that warrants consideration as an example of international collaboration.

25. Wagaruddin M, Bernstein A. Reexpansion pulmonary edema. *Thorax.* 1975;30:54.

   A good discussion of the mechanisms and clinical manifestations of pulmonary edema occurring after reexpansion of pneumothoraces.

26. Wakai A, O'Sullivan RG, McCabe G. Simple aspiration versus intercostal tube drainage for pri-mary spontaneous pneumothorax in adults. *Cochrane Database Syst Rev.* 2007;(1):CD004479.

   Despite good results for simple aspiration, this technique is not widely applied in the United States, and does carry some risks.

27. Wood DE, Cerfolio RJ, Gonzalez X, et al. Bronchoscopic management of prolonged air leak. *Clin Chest Med.* 2010;31:127–133.

   Concise review of bronchoscopic therapies, including valves and spigots.

28. Zhang H, Liu ZH, Yang JX, et al. Rapid detection of pneumothorax by ultrasonography in patients with multiple trauma. *Crit Care.* 2006;10:R112.

   Pleural ultrasonography may have a growing role at the bedside especially in the ICU and trauma.

Aspiration

Shazia M. Jamil

Aspiration is defined as the inhalation of oropharyngeal secretions or gastric contents into the lar-ynx, trachea, or the lower respiratory tract. The aspirate may be characterized into three distinct entities: oropharyngeal secretions colonized with bacterial pathogens, acidified gastric contents, and particulate material. Aspiration may be silent or witnessed. Several pulmonary syndromes may result from aspiration and include aspiration pneumonitis (Mendelson syndrome), aspira-tion pneumonia, acute lung injury/acute respiratory distress syndrome (ALI/ARDS), airway ob-struction, lung abscess, empyema, exogenous lipoid pneumonia, and chronic interstitial fibrosis.

The most common risk factors for aspiration are (1) depressed level of consciousness such as that seen with alcohol intoxication, sedatives, stroke, encephalopathy, and seizures; (2) dyspha-gia due to esophageal motility disorders and due to neuromuscular disorders; (3) impaired gag and cough reflex such as that seen in elderly debilitated patients or those with bulbar paralysis; (4) impaired swallowing or cough reflex secondary to medications; (5) use of nasogastric or endotracheal tubes; (6) sustained supine position as in critically ill, mechanically ventilated, or debilitated patients; (7) trauma; (8) emergency surgery and anesthesia in the absence of preop-erative starvation and upper gastrointestinal endoscopy; (9) anatomic abnormalities, such as tracheoesophageal fistula, gastroesophageal reflux, gastroparesis, gastric outlet obstruction and ileus; and (10) mechanical factors such as obesity and labor.

Half of all healthy adults aspirate some amount of oropharyngeal secretions while they are asleep. That degree of aspiration, however, is of minimal consequence because of the low viru-lence of bacteria in normal secretions, and the protective effect of the cough reflex and active ciliary transport, as well as the normal cellular and humoral immune mechanisms. The most important defense mechanisms preventing aspiration are the intact swallowing function and the cough reflex, both of which are vulnerable to medications and medical conditions. Sedatives impair consciousness, diminish protective airway reflexes, and increase the risk of aspiration pneumonia. Phenothiazines and haloperidol can reduce oropharyngeal swallowing coordination and cause dysphagia; medications that decrease saliva such as anticholinergics and antihistamines make swallowing more difficult. These medications should be used carefully in the elderly. Aspiration occurs in approximately 40% to 50% of stroke patients with dysphagia, which increases their increased risk for aspiration pneumonia.

Aspiration pneumonitis is a chemical injury caused by the inhalation of sterile gastric contents. The classic form of acid aspiration pneumonitis is Mendelson syndrome, which was first described in pregnant women. A pH of less than 2.5 and a volume of gastric aspirate greater than 0.3 mL/kg body weight (20–25 mL in adults) are usually required for its development. Aspiration of gastric contents initially results in a chemical burn of the airways and the pulmonary parenchyma followed by acute inflammation involving the lung interstitium and alveoli. Since gastric acid prevents the growth of bacteria, infection does not typically play a major role. However, high gastric pH, as has been observed in recent years from antacids, histamine-2 receptor antagonists, and proton pump inhibitors, may lead to colonization of gastric contents by pathogenic microbes. Aspiration in this setting may cause both an inflammatory and infectious processes. Aspiration pneumonitis can occur in approximately 1 of 3,000 operations involving anesthesia and accounts for 10% to 30% of all anesthesia associated deaths. Most patients who aspirate sterile gastric contents may present with acute cough or wheezing. Others who aspirate silently may only manifest desaturation, or they may present with fever, dyspnea, cyanosis, pulmonary edema, hypoxemia, leucocytosis, and lung infiltrates. The syndrome may progress rapidly to severe ARDS and death. For this reason, early recognition is crucial.

The management of aspiration pneumonitis is supportive, especially early in the course. The immediate care includes upper airway suctioning (if possible), endotracheal intubation if the patient is unable to protect his airway, humidified oxygen, bronchodilators and, to prevent recurrence, elevation of the head of the bed. Flexible bronchoscopy to facilitate suctioning may be performed if particulate aspiration is visualized or suspected. Bronchioalveolar lavage, however, is of no therapeutic benefit, since the effect of acid is immediate and its absorption occurs within minutes. Despite being a common practice, the prophylactic use of antibiotics in suspected or witnessed aspiration is not helpful. Empiric antibiotics however may be appropriate for patients who have small bowel obstruction or other conditions associated with colonization of the gastric contents, if signs and symptoms last for more than 48 hours or if evidence of infection supervenes (e.g., persistent fever, purulent sputum, progressive abnormality on chest roentgenogram). Human and animal studies have failed to demonstrate a beneficial effect of corticosteroids on pulmonary function, lung injury, alveolar-capillary permeability, or outcome after acid aspiration.

Aspiration pneumonia refers to the development of pneumonia after aspiration of colonized oropharyngeal material. This may be acute, chronic, or recurrent depending on the time of onset, nature of aspirated material, and individual host responses. Any condition that increases the volume or bacterial burden of oropharyngeal secretions in patients with impaired defense mechanism may lead to aspiration pneumonia. For example, the risk of aspiration pneumonia is lower in patients without teeth (i.e., with gingivodental recesses) and in elderly institutionalized patients receiving aggressive oral care. The bacterial pathogens generally reflect the patient's location (i.e., community-acquired vs nosocomial aspiration pneumonia). The most frequently isolated organisms found in community-dwelling patients are anaerobic bacteria resembling mouth flora (e.g., *Fusobacterium nucleatum*, *Peptostreptococcus* spp., and *Prevotella melaninogenicus*), *Streptococcus pneumoniae*, and *Haemophilus influenzae*). Among hospitalized and nursing home patients, anaerobes, nosocomially acquired pathogens such as *Staphylococcus aureus*, and mixed aerobic and facultative Gram-negative bacilli, particularly *Klebsiella pneumoniae*, are common. Patients with acid aspiration can also develop secondary bacterial infections caused by aerobic Gram-positive and Gram-negative organisms, such as *S. aureus* and *Pseudomonas aeruginosa*.

Oral and dental hygiene are especially important for prevention in elderly, hospitalized, debilitated, and nursing home patients who are dependent on caregivers to provide this care.

Chronic infections in the gingivodental crevice increase the concentration of anaerobic bacteria and other pathogens in the mouth. Nasogastric and endotracheal tubes should be removed as soon as possible. Frequent subglottic suctioning of secretions (in patients with nasogastric and endotracheal tubes) and aggressive oral hygiene have been indicated as additional prevention tools in this group of patients. When suspected, dysphagia should be confirmed with swallow studies.

Common clinical features of aspiration pneumonia are dyspnea, fever, wheezing, crackles, rhonchi, hypoxia, tachycardia, leukocytosis, and respiratory failure. Severe hypoxemia is common, occurring in association with a normal or low arterial partial pressure of carbon dioxide in alveolar gas ($Paco_2$), a wide alveolararterial oxygen difference, and a significant reduction in chest compliance. The diagnosis is likely when a predisposed patient develops a radiographically evident infiltrate. Chest roentgenograms early in the course may be entirely normal or may reveal either localized or diffuse (multilobar) alveolar or interstitial infiltrates. All forms of aspiration pneumonia are more common in the dependent portions of the lung, as might be predicted; however, the body position at the time of the aspiration determines the exact location of the infiltrates. For example, involvement of the posterior segments of the upper lobes and apical segments of lower lobes are seen when patients aspirate in the recumbent position, whereas the basal segments of the lower lobes are usually involved when patients aspirate in upright or semi-recumbent positions. Mortality of aspiration pneumonia can be as high as 70% in some groups; for example, it is the most common cause of death in advanced Alzheimer disease.

Treatment includes endotracheal intubation in patients with altered consciousness, aggressive pulmonary toilet to enhance lung volume and clear secretions, and bronchodilators in patients with bronchospasm. Those who do not require endotracheal intubation should not be fed through the mouth or placed in a supine position if there is continued concern about airway control; sedatives and narcotics should be avoided or used with caution. Nasogastric tubes should not be placed without good airway control. Patients with gastroparesis (e.g., diabetics) or intestinal ileus may be either continuously drained through nasogastric tubes or started on pro-motility agents. Sputum should be sent for Gram stain and culture. Bronchoscopy, bronchoalveolar lavage, and quantitative cultures are usually performed in intubated, critically ill patients suspected of developing aspiration pneumonia. Antibiotic use should be guided by appropriate bacteriologic studies; however, in clinical practice they are often started empirically, especially in the critically ill and those with severe pneumonia. The patients suspected of having aspiration pneumonia in community setting may benefit from levofloxacin or ceftriaxone, those residing in long-term facility may benefit from levofloxacin, piperacillin–tazobactam or ceftazidime, while patients with severe periodontal disease, putrid sputum, or alcoholism may be served better with either piperacillin–tazobactam or imipenem or combination of either levofloxacin, ciprofloxacin, or ceftriaxone with either clindamycin or metronidazole. De-escalation or adjustment of antibiotic is based on culture results.

Aspiration pneumonia is common in critically ill patients and deserves special mention. Such patients often have multiple factors predisposing them to aspiration, including sustained supine position, use of nasogastric and endotracheal tubes, use of sedatives and narcotics, swallowing dysfunction, impaired consciousness, exposure to nosocomial environment, and increased risk of bacterial colonization of oropharynx. Nasogastric and endotracheal tubes predispose to aspiration owing to compromise of upper aerodigestive protective mechanisms. Nasogastric tubes themselves have been associated with pathogen colonization and aspiration leading to a high incidence of Gram-negative pneumonia in patients on enteral nutrition. Newly designed endotracheal tubes with an independent dorsal lumen that permits the continuous aspiration of secretions in the subglottic space may decrease the incidence of ventilator-associated aspiration pneumonia. Narcotic antagonists, frequently used in drug overdose, can induce vomiting; consequently, airway control should be secured before their administration in comatose patients.

Many patients with dysphagia have a normal gag reflex, whereas others with an absent gag reflex have normal swallowing function. Therefore, the gag reflex is a poor indicator of swallowing function and its absence does not predict aspiration. A number of tests exist to evaluate swallowing, including videofluoroscopic examination or videoendoscopic examination and simple swallowing provocation test. The swallowing provocation test has limited applicability as a screening tool for aspiration or silent aspiration because of its low sensitivity. This test may be useful for patients who cannot undergo other tests due to cognitive and/or linguistic dysfunction.

Aspiration of mineral and vegetable oils can lead to a chronic form of lipoid pneumonia. Patients are frequently elderly individuals who use oil-containing agents or children with constipation treated with mineral oil. These agents may not elicit a normal protective cough reflex and can impair mucociliary clearance mechanisms. A thorough history regarding the use of nose drops and laxatives may suggest the diagnosis. The chest roentgenogram reveals interstitial infiltrates or solitary or multiple mass lesions that may suggest tumor. Pathologic examination may demonstrate oil- or fat-laden macrophages, but these are nonspecific findings. Bronchoalveolar lavage samples tested by gas chromatography or mass spectrometry may demonstrate the exogenous origin of the lipid. Appropriate therapy includes withdrawal of the offending agent and treatment of secondary infection.

Aspiration of foreign objects can obstruct airways, depending on the object's size, and lead to necrotizing pneumonia. Large objects can obstruct airways and cause rapid suffocation and death. The Heimlich maneuver has been widely publicized as an effective method to dislodge foreign material. Smaller objects (teeth, peanuts, food particles) can occlude smaller bronchi and result in an acute pneumonia or a chronic inflammatory process simulating a lung tumor, distal to the obstruction. Early bronchoscopy by either flexible or rigid instrumentation is indicated for removal of the foreign body; since after a few days, inflammation and fibrotic organization make these procedures less successful. Particulate matter aspiration is a more common cause of lung infiltrates and nodules than generally appreciated. In a clinicopathological study of 59 cases of pulmonary disease due to aspiration of food and other particulate material, the histological finding of bronchiolitis obliterans and organizing pneumonia was present in 52 (88%) cases, usually in combination with multinucleated giant cells, acute bronchopneumonia, bronchiolitis, and/or suppurative granulomas. Foreign materials were identified in all cases, most commonly vegetable or food remnants, and less often talc or microcrystalline cellulose, crospovidone, and kayexalate.

FURTHER READING

1. Mendelson C. The aspiration of stomach contents into the lung during obstetric anesthesia. *Am J Obstet Gynecol.* 1946;52:191.

   This is the classic description of acid aspiration as seen in obstetric patients.

2. DePaso WJ. Aspiration pneumonia. *Clin Chest Med.* 1991;12:269.
3. Wynne J, Modell J. Respiratory aspiration of stomach contents. *Ann Intern Med.* 1977;87:466.
4. Zaloga GP. Aspiration-related illnesses: definitions and diagnosis. *JPEN J Parenter Enteral Nutr.* 2002;26(suppl):S2–S7.

   References 2–4 provide excellent reviews of the subject and recommendations regarding prevention and treatment.

5. Addington WR, Stephens RE, Gilliland KA. Assessing the laryngeal cough reflex and the risk of developing pneumonia after stroke: an interhospital comparison. *Stroke.* 1999;30:1203.

   In 604 acute stroke patients (prospectively studied), a normal reflex cough test was associated with a low risk for developing aspiration pneumonia with oral feeding.

6. Marik P, Kaplan D. Aspiration pneumonia and dysphagia in the elderly. *Chest.* 2003;124:328.

   The article reviews the magnitude of problem and discusses ways to diagnose and treat dysphagia with the potential of preventing aspiration pneumonia.

7. Bynum L, Pierce A. Pulmonary aspiration of gastric contents. *Am Rev Respir Dis.* 1976;114:1129.

   A study concluding that prophylactic antibiotics and steroids are not beneficial.

8. Marik PE. Aspiration pneumonitis and aspiration pneumonia. *N Engl J Med.* 2001;344:665–671.
9. Kalia M. Dysphagia and aspiration pneumonia in patients with Alzheimer's disease. *Metabolism.* 2003;52:36.

   An excellent review article that discusses etiology of dysphagia and factors predisposing to high prevalence of aspiration pneumonia in Alzheimer patients.

10. Loeb M, McGeer A, McArthur M, et al. Risk factors for pneumonia and other lower respiratory tract infections in elderly residents of long-term care facilities. *Arch Intern Med.* 1999;159:2058.

11. Johnson LF, Rajagopal KR. Aspiration resulting from gastroesophageal reflux: a cause of broncho-pulmonary disease. *Chest.* 1988;93:676.

    This article discusses the importance of gastroesophageal reflux and pulmonary aspiration in perpetuating or initiating chronic lung disease.

12. Ramsey DJ, Smithard DG, Kalra L. Early assessments of dysphagia and aspiration risk in acute stroke patients. *Stroke.* 2003;34:1252.

    A comprehensive review of existing swallowing assessment methods, including sensitivity, specificity, and limitations in the diagnosis of aspiration.

13. Spickard A III, Hirschmann JV. Exogenous lipoid pneumonia. *Arch Intern Med.* 1994;154:686.

14. Kallar SK, Everett LL. Potential risks and preventive measures for pulmonary aspiration: new concepts in preoperative fasting guidelines. *Anesth Analg.* 1993;77:171.

    A review with recommendations from a preoperative perspective.

15. Teramoto S. High incidence of aspiration pneumonia in community- and hospital-acquired pneumonia in hospitalized patients: a multicenter, prospective study in Japan. *J Am Geriatr Soc.* 2008;56(3):577–579.

16. Mukhopadhyay S. Pulmonary disease due to aspiration of food and other particulate matter: a clinicopathologic study of 59 cases diagnosed on biopsy or resection specimens. *Am J Surg Pathol.* 2007;31(5):752–759.

17. Raghavendran K. Aspiration-induced lung injury. *Crit Care Med.* 2011;39(4):818–826.

    An excellent review that addresses challenges a clinician faces in differentiating aspiration pneumonia from aspiration pneumonitis.

18. Moore FA. Treatment of aspiration in intensive care unit patients. *JPEN J Parenter Enteral Nutr.* 2002;26:S69.

19. Scolapio JS. Methods for decreasing risk of aspiration pneumonia in critically ill patients. *JPEN J Parenter Enteral Nutr.* 2002;26:S58.

20. McClave SA, DeMeo MT, DeLegge MH, et al. North American summit on aspiration in the critically ill patient: consensus statement. *JPEN J Parenter Enteral Nutr.* 2002;26:S80.

21. Pace CC. The association between oral microorgansims and aspiration pneumonia in the institutionalized elderly: review and recommendations. *Dysphagia.* 2010;25(4):307–322.

22. Paintal HS. Aspiration syndromes: 10 clinical pearls every physician should know. *Int J Clin Pract.* 2007;61(5):846–852.

23. Kagaya H. Simple swallowing provocation test has limited applicability as a screening tool for detecting aspiration, silent aspiration, or penetration. *Dysphagia.* 2010;25(1):6–10.

24. Bouza E. Continuous aspiration of subglottic secretions in the prevention of ventilator-associated pneumonia in the postoperative period of major heart surgery. *Chest.* 2008;134(5):938–946.

The Lung in Pregnancy

Kathleen Sarmiento and Andrew Kitcher

Pregnancy causes dynamic physiologic changes in multiple organ systems including the lungs. These changes can adversely impact preexisting pulmonary disease and increase the likelihood of developing new disorders. Moreover, the normal diagnostic and therapeutic tools of the pulmonologist may be limited in the pregnant patient due to fetal safety concerns.

Pulmonary physiologic changes of pregnancy include increases in (a) the level of the diaphragm (3–4 cm); (b) the anterior-posterior and transverse diameters of the chest (2 cm); and (c) the subcostal angle (68°–103°). These changes take place earlier than can be accounted for by the enlarging uterus itself. Progesterone, estrogen, prostaglandin, corticosteroid, and cyclic nucleotide levels rise during the course of pregnancy. While the multiple functional consequences of these alterations are not clear, increased progesterone is thought to be responsible for the hyperventilation observed during pregnancy. Elevated estrogen levels and capillary engorgement from mucosal edema and hyperemia frequently cause symptoms of rhinitis.

Pulmonary function tests reflect the mechanical changes of pregnancy: diaphragmatic elevation causes a decrease in functional residual capacity (FRC) of 10% to 30%, which is associated with an 8% to 20% fall in expiratory reserve volume and a 7% to 25% fall in residual volume. Flow rates and total lung capacity (TLC) are typically normal throughout most of pregnancy. At term, patients may experience a slight drop in TLC, which may be more pronounced in obese patients. Forced vital capacity (FVC) may increase slightly (4%) after 14 to 16 weeks gestation. The increase tends to be higher in multiparous women than in primigravid women, which suggests that the pregnancy-associated increase in FVC persists following delivery. Diaphragmatic and inspiratory muscle strength are preserved, and inspiratory capacity increases 5% to 10%. Minute ventilation (V_E) increases 20% to 50% compared to nonpregnant values, which is primarily attributable to a 30% to 50% increase in tidal volume. Consequently, the resting $Paco_2$ drops to 27 to 34 mmHg, with compensatory increased renal excretion of bicarbonate and fall in serum bicarbonate to 18 to 22 mEq/L to maintain normal pH. The decline in $Paco_2$ leads to a rise in Pao_2. $DLco$ decreases after the first trimester. It increases appropriately with exercise, but it does not increase in the supine position as it does in normal nonpregnant individuals. This results in a significant reduction in Pao_2 of 10 mmHg in the supine position in late pregnancy.

Dyspnea is a common complaint in healthy pregnant women and may affect 60% to 70% of gravid women in late pregnancy (>30 weeks gestation). Dyspnea, however, must be evaluated carefully to distinguish more serious conditions from the dyspnea that occurs physiologically during pregnancy. Although V_E and chemosensitivity are both increased, the sensation of dyspnea is not due to a difference in progesterone levels, which are similar between dyspneic and nondyspneic pregnant women. Dyspnea usually improves near term, which suggests that the mechanical effect of the gravid uterus itself is not responsible. It appears instead to be related to an increased awareness of the drive to breathe.

Pregnant women suffer from respiratory diseases more than their age-matched, nonpregnant counterparts. Pregnancy does not increase the risk of bacterial pneumonia itself, but it does increase the risk of pneumonia complications, including respiratory failure requiring mechanical ventilation, empyema, bacteremia, and preterm delivery. Community acquired pneumonia is predominantly due to organisms such as *Streptoccocus pneumonia, Haemophilus influenza,* and *Mycoplasma pneumonia,* just as it is in nonpregnant patients. Viral pneumonia is a serious concern in pregnancy, as reflected by the increased mortality of pregnant women (up to 50%) in the influenza pandemic of 1918, as well as the increased morbidity and mortality noted with the more recent epidemic of H1N1 influenza in 2009. Influenza vaccination using the inactivated killed virus is recommended for nearly all pregnant women. It is safe for the fetus and effective in stimulating an immunologic response in the mother. Pregnancy itself is not currently an indication for pneumococcal vaccination, unless there are other recognized indications for receiving it. Varicella pneumonia is also associated with increased mortality in pregnant women compared to nonpregnant adults. Assessment of varicella immunity by history or by IgG titers is recommended prior to pregnancy. If it is indicated, varicella vaccination can be administered 1 to 3 months before pregnancy or in the postpartum period. Disseminated Coccidioides infection complicates 1/5,000 pregnancies in the southwestern United States. Neither tuberculosis nor fungal pneumonias are particularly associated with or influenced by the course of pregnancy. The major implication for pregnancy is that it limits the therapeutic options in tuberculosis and fungal pneumonias due to teratogenic effects of medications. Finally, aspiration pneumonitis due to the increased intra-abdominal pressure and the relaxing effect of progesterone on the esophageal sphincter is also a recognized cause of morbidity and mortality in pregnant women.

Asthma affects up to 8% of pregnant women and can have a variable course during pregnancy. In a review of 2,186 pregnant women with asthma, 39% experienced no change in their disease during pregnancy, 29% improved, 30% worsened, and 2% were undefined. Asthma, especially severe asthma, is associated with worse pregnancy outcomes, including increased risk of preeclampsia, preterm birth, intrauterine growth restriction, and perinatal death. Most medications used to treat asthma (Table 29-1) are considered safe, but individual drug profiles should be considered when selecting individual therapies. It is clear, however, that untreated asthma has a more deleterious effect on the outcome of pregnancy than the judicious use of these drugs. Known triggers should be avoided, and counseling on smoking cessation and second-hand smoke avoidance should be provided.

Infiltrative lung diseases are rare in women of reproductive age, but they can be related to connective tissue disorders, pulmonary vasculitis, sarcoidosis, lymphangioleiomyomatosis (LAM), idiopathic interstitial pneumonias, eosinophilic pneumonias, drug-induced lung disease, and other rare conditions. Pleural effusions, infiltrates, and acute respiratory distress syndrome (ARDS) have been reported to occur following administration of drugs used in ovarian hyperstimulation. The role of sex hormones in LAM remains controversial, since pregnancy is believed to accelerate disease progression due to increased estrogen levels. Pulmonary complications of

TABLE 29-1   Asthma/COPD Medications

Class	Medications	Risk Category	TERIS Rating[a]	Lactation Profile
Short-acting β-agonists	Albuterol[b], Metaproterenol	C	Undetermined/limited	Unknown
	Levalbuterol, Pirbuterol	C	Not available	Unknown
	Terbutaline	C		Compatible
Long-acting β-agonists	Formoterol	C	Not available	Caution
	Salmeterol	C	Undetermined/limited	Caution
Inhaled corticosteroids	Beclomethasone, Flunisolide, Mometasone, Triamcinolone	C	Unlikely/limited to fair	Compatible
	Budesonide	B	Unlikely/limited to fair	Compatible
	Fluticasone	C	Not available	Compatible
ICS/LABA combinations[c]		C	Not available	Caution
Anticholinergics	Ipratropium[d]	B		Unknown
	Tiotropium	C		Caution
Corticosteroids[e]	Prednisone	C		Compatible
Cromones	Cromolyn[d]	B	Unlikely/fair to good	Unknown
	Nedocromil	B	Undetermined/limited	Unknown
Leukotriene modifiers	Montelukast[b]	B	Minimal/very limited	Unknown
	Zafirlukast	B	Undetermined/limited	Unsafe
	Zileuton	C	Not available	Unsafe
Other	Theophylline	C	None/fair to good	Compatible
	Omalizumab	B		Unknown

[a]Magnitude of teratogenic risk/quality and quantity of Data; [b]Preferred in its class; [c]Safety based on profile of least safe components; [d]Not first line therapy; [e]Use lowest effective dose, only as long-term therapy for severe persistent asthma, at higher doses consider prednisolone, avoid breastfeeding for 3 to 4 hours after a dose.

LAM during pregnancy include pneumothorax, preterm birth, chylous effusion, and decline in lung function. Sarcoidosis tends to improve or remain unchanged during pregnancy. In general, the risk of pulmonary complications related to pregnancy increases with progressive impairment of baseline pulmonary function. Women with infiltrative lung disease should be counseled prior to conception about the risks of pregnancy. Successful maternal and fetal outcomes are possible with careful planning and a multidisciplinary approach.

Cystic fibrosis (CF) reduces female fertility through a variety of mechanisms, but as care has improved patients are surviving longer and pregnancy has become increasingly common. Up to 4% of female CF patients of childbearing age are pregnant at any given time. Prepregnancy FEV_1 and BMI are important predictors of maternal and fetal outcomes, with FEV_1 less than 60% and BMI less than 20 kg/m^2 portending poorer prognoses. Complications include preterm birth, gestational diabetes, and cesarean section. In a review by Thorpe-Beeston and colleagues of 48 pregnancies, women with severe prepregnancy lung function defects were observed to have shortened life expectancies; three of seven women with an FEV_1 less than 40% died within 18 months of delivery, and four of eight women with an FEV_1 between 40% and 50% died within 2 to 8 years after delivery. Thus, prepregnancy counseling is imperative and should include the discussion of possible reduced life expectancy in women with more severe disease.

Pregnancy can also be successful following lung transplantation. The National Transplantation Pregnancy Registry reported the outcomes of 30 pregnancies in 21 transplant recipients. There were 18 live births (11 premature), 5 therapeutic abortions, and 9 spontaneous abortions. Two neonatal deaths occurred after preterm birth at 22 weeks. The surviving 16 children were reported to be healthy at follow up. Maternal comorbidities included hypertension, infection, diabetes, preeclampsia, and rejection. At follow up, 13 women had adequate function, 2 had reduced function, 5 had died, and 1 had a nonfunctioning transplant.

Sleep disordered breathing, which includes both snoring and sleep apnea, is more common in pregnant women than in nonpregnant women. Changes in the upper airway that facilitate sleep disordered breathing include increased estrogen levels, glandular hypersecretion, edema, and hyperemia, frequently leading to rhinitis with nasal obstruction. Neck circumference and Mallampati scores have also been shown to increase over the duration of pregnancy. Sleep disordered breathing may be related to adverse maternal and fetal outcomes, including pregnancy induced hypertension, preeclampsia, gestational diabetes, and intrauterine growth restriction. Sleep studies and treatment with continuous positive airway pressure (CPAP) have been demonstrated to be safe during pregnancy. Sleep disordered breathing that develops during pregnancy generally resolves within 3 months postpartum.

Pulmonary embolism (PE) is the leading cause of maternal mortality in the developed world and venous thromboembolism (VTE) a major cause of maternal morbidity. Incidence of VTE during pregnancy is between 0.6 and 1.3/1,000 deliveries. Two-thirds of deep venous thromboses occur antepartum, and one to two-thirds of pulmonary emboli occur within 6 weeks postpartum. Diagnosis can be challenging. D-dimer is often elevated during pregnancy in the absence of deep venous thrombosis (DVT) or PE, and false negatives have also been reported. Doppler ultrasonography of the lower extremities is the first recommending imaging test. Pelvic MRI is an additional complementary technique to ultrasonography due to lack of ionizing radiation, but is highly dependent on local expertise. If initial testing is normal, pulmonary CT angiography or perfusion scintigraphy can be performed, though controversy exists over fetal radiation doses and diagnostic accuracy between the two studies. Prospective Investigation of Pulmonary Embolism Diagnosis III (PIOPED III) demonstrated utility of pulmonary arterial MR angiography and magnetic resonance venography (MRV) for the workup of patients suspected of having VTE, but again, results are dependent on local expertise. A missed diagnosis of PE in pregnant women is associated with a 30% mortality, which decreases to 8% with treatment. Warfarin crosses the placenta, producing both fetal hemorrhage and congenital abnormalities. Heparin can be safely used up to and immediately after labor, however risk of bleeding remains a consideration.

Pulmonary hypertension in pregnant patients carries a high mortality rate: between 30% and 56%. Physiologic changes with major clinical implications include expansion of blood volume by 50% above prepregnant levels, increased heart rate and stroke volume, and decreased systemic vascular resistance. Pulmonary vascular resistance normally decreases during pregnancy, but in women with pulmonary vascular disease this may not occur, resulting in a further rise in pulmonary vascular resistance and cardiac output. Therapies for pulmonary hypertension have been used in pregnant women, but there are few data to help determine their safety profiles. Most complications occur during labor and delivery. Hemodynamic instability can result from a prolonged second stage of labor during vaginal deliveries (bearing down, uterine contractions), decreased preload related to blood loss and anesthetics, increased preload from relief of caval obstruction by the gravid uterus, increase in systemic vascular resistance and pulmonary vascular resistance to prepregnancy levels, and reduced cardiac contractility.

Amniotic fluid embolism carries a mortality risk of greater than 80% and accounts for 4% to 10% of total maternal mortality. Death is often immediate or within several hours of labor and delivery. Clinical features include respiratory distress syndrome, cardiovascular collapse, and disseminated intravascular coagulation. Predisposing factors include a tumultuous labor, the use of intrauterine stimulants, the presence of meconium in the amniotic fluid, advanced maternal age, multiparity, and intrauterine fetal death. Treatment is supportive, as no specific therapy yet exists.

Noncardiogenic pulmonary edema has been reported with most tocolytic agents, including magnesium sulfate, terbutaline, and ritodrine. The incidence is low, approximately 3%, but it appears to be higher in the presence of coexisting maternal infection. Other risk factors include multiple gestations, hydramnios, hypertension, and the use of glucocorticoid steroids. Treatment involves cessation of tocolytic therapy, antibiotics, if clinically indicated, and aggressive support. Peripartum cardiomyopathy should be considered in the patient with signs and symptoms of heart failure in the last month of pregnancy up to 5 months postdelivery.

Pregnancy is not a contraindication to chest imaging and pulmonary procedures, though pregnant women should receive counseling on risks and benefits prior to all procedures. Table 29-2 lists the radiation doses associated with common diagnostic chest imaging. The commonly cited threshold radiation doses are 1 to 5 cGy for increased risk of childhood leukemias and 5 to 10 cGy for teratogenicity. For reference, the developing fetus absorbs 0.5 to 1 mGy of background radiation. All chest imaging modalities result in exposure significantly lower than direct radiation during abdominopelvic imaging, and far below the accepted 5 cGy threshold for increased risk of miscarriage, malignancy, or malformation.

TABLE 29-2	Other Pulmonary Medications			
Indication: Class	**Medications**	**Risk Category**	**Lactation Profile**	**Comments**
Transplant: Antimetabolite	Azathioprine	D	Compatible	Avoid breastfeeding for 4–6 h after therapy is stopped.
	Mycophenolate	D	Unsafe	Use contraception and avoid breastfeeding during treatment and for 6 wk after therapy is stopped.
	Leflunomide	X	Unsafe	Contraindicated in pregnancy or childbearing potential not on contraception.
Transplant: Calcineurin inhibitors	Cyclosporine, Tacrolimus	C	Caution	

(Continued)

TABLE 29-2	Other Pulmonary Medications *(Continued)*			
Indication: Class	Medications	Risk Category	Lactation Profile	Comments
Transplant: mTor inhibitors	Sirolimus	C	Unknown	
	Everolimus	D	Unknown	
Transplant: Alkylation	Cyclophosphamide	D	Unsafe	
PE: Heparins	Unfractionated heparin	C	Compatible	All heparins: Use only preservative-free.
	Enoxaparin, Dalteparin	B	Compatible	Pregnancy: LMWH is the preferred agent. Recommend twice daily dosing.
PE: Vit. K antagonist	Warfarin	X	Compatible	Contraindicated first trimester. Risk category D if valve.
PE: Direct thrombin inhibitors	Dabigatran	C	Unknown	Breastfeeding: consider warfarin/heparin.
	Argatroban	B	Unknown	
	Lepirudin	B	Compatible	Preferred IV DTI; short half-life.
	Bivalirudin	B	Caution	Should be digested in infant's GI tract.
PE: Anti-Xa inhibitors	Fondaparinux	B	Unknown	Use limited to women with contraindications to heparin.
	Rivaroxaban	C	Unknown	
PE: Thrombolytic	Alteplase, tPA	C	Caution	Benefits must be carefully weighed.
CF: Inhaled antibiotics[a]	Tobramycin	D	Caution	Poorly absorbed when given orally.
	Ceftazidime	B	Compatible	Not absorbed when given orally.
	Colistin	C	Unknown	Poorly absorbed when given orally.
CF: Enzymatic	Dornase alfa	B	Caution	

Tables 29-1 and 29-2 created by Catherine Hong, PharmD and Maria Stubbs, RPH, Veterans Administration San Diego Healthcare System, Pharmacy Service.
[a]May alter gut flora, causing diarrhea.

Bronchoscopy has been demonstrated to be safe in pregnancy, but should be deferred until after pregnancy if possible. Complications may be reduced by positioning the patient in the left lateral decubitus or sitting positions, avoiding class D sedatives such as midazolam, and consulting with anesthesiologists and obstetricians preprocedurally to have in place management strategies for complications

FURTHER READING

1. Alaily AB, Carroll KB. Pulmonary ventilation in pregnancy. *Br J Obstet Gynaecol.* 1978;85:518.

   A well-done study comparing pulmonary function testing results during pregnancy and postpartum.

2. Hegewald MJ, Crapo RO. Respiratory physiology in pregnancy. *Clin Chest Med.* 2011;32:1–13.

   An excellent review of changes in respiratory physiology and pulmonary function during pregnancy.

3. Grindheim G, Toska K, Estensen M-E, et al. Changes in pulmonary function during pregnancy: a longitudinal cohort study. *Br J Obstet Gynaecol.* 2012;119:94–101.

   This study evaluates spirometric changes during the first, second, and third trimesters, and at 6 months postpartum in healthy pregnancies. The effects of parity, pregestational weight, and excessive weight gain during pregnancy are also addressed.

4. Gee JB, Packer BS, Millen JE, et al. Pulmonary mechanics during pregnancy. *J Clin Invest.* 1967;46:945.

   A study of compliance and resistance.

5. Cugell DW, Frank NR, Gaensler EA, et al. Pulmonary function in pregnancy, I: serial observations in normal women. *Am Rev Tuberc.* 1953;67:568.

   Considered a classic reference.

6. Goodnight WH, Soper DE. Pneumonia in pregnancy. *Crit Care Med.* 2005;33:S390–S397.

   A detailed overview of the various pneumonias, therapeutics, and vaccinations.

7. American College of Obstetricians and Gynecologists Committee on Obstetric Practice. ACOG committee opinion no 468: influenza vaccination during pregnancy. *Obstet Gynecol.* 2010;116:1006–1007.

8. Martin A, Cox S, Jamieson DJ, et al. Respiratory illness hospitalizations among pregnant women during influenza season, 1998–2008. *Matern Child Health J.* 2012;17(7):1325–1331.

   This study reviewed data from the Healthcare Cost and Utilization Project (HCUP) Nationwide Inpatient Database (NIS) to evaluate healthcare burden, pregnancy outcomes, and impact of high risk medical conditions among pregnancy hospitalizations during influenza season.

9. American Thoracic Society, Centers for Disease Control and Prevention, Infectious Diseases Society of America. Treatment of tuberculosis *MMWR Morb Mortal Wkly Rep.* 2003;52(RR-11):13.

   Current recommendations for treatment of tuberculosis during pregnancy.

10. Yawn B, Knudtson M. Treating asthma and comorbid allergic rhinitis in pregnancy. *J Am Board Fam Med.* 2007;20:289–298.

    A review of safety profiles of pharmacologic options used to treat asthma and allergic rhinitis during pregnancy.

11. Maselli DJ, Adams SG, Peters JI, et al. Management of asthma during pregnancy. *Ther Adv Respir Dis.* 2012;7(2):87–100. doi:10.1177/1753465812464287.

    An excellent review of the epidemiology, immunology, and therapeutics used in asthma management.

12. Freymond N, Cottin V, Cordier JF. Infiltrative lung diseases in pregnancy. *Clin Chest Med.* 2011;32:133–146.

    An eloquent and comprehensive review of infiltrative lung diseases as they relate to pregnancy.

13. Lau EM, Barnes DJ, Moriarty C, et al. Pregnancy outcomes in the current era of cystic fibrosis care: a 15-year experience. *Aust N Z J Obstet Gynaecol.* 2011;51:220–224.

    A review of maternal and fetal outcomes in 20 pregnancies between 1995 and 2009, concluding BMI less than 20 and FEV_1 less than 60% are associated with poorer maternal and fetal outcomes.

14. Thorpe-Beeston JG, Madge S, Gyi K, et al. The outcome of pregnancies in women with cystic fibrosis-single center experience 1998–2011. *BJOG.* 2012;119:1–8.

    A review of outcomes in 48 pregnancies with similar conclusions to reference 12.

15. Bates SM, Greer IA, Pabinger I, et al. Venous thromboembolism, thrombophilia, antithrombotic therapy, and pregnancy: American College of Chest Physicians Evidence-Based Clinical Practice Guidelines (8th edition). *Chest.* 2008;133:844S–886S.

    An overview of therapies used to treat VTE in pregnancy.

16. Shaner J, Coscia LA, Constantinescu S, et al. Pregnancy after lung transplant. *Prog Transplant.* 2012;22:134–140.

   A unique review of maternal and fetal outcomes following lung transplantation, with immunosuppressive regimens, maternal indications for transplant, and neonatal complications also described.

17. Bassily-Marcus AM, Yuan C, Oropello J, et al. Pulmonary hypertension in pregnancy: critical care management. *Pulm Med.* 2012;2012:709407.

   A review article summarizing physiologic changes occurring during pregnancy in women with pulmonary hypertension, evaluation considerations, and intensive care management.

18. Wang PI, Chong ST, Kielar AZ, et al. Imaging of pregnant and lactating patients, part 1: evidence-based review and recommendations. *AJR Am J Roentgenol.* 2012;198:778–784.

   A review of basic concepts of ionizing radiation and safety in pregnancy.

19. Wang PI, Chong ST, Kielar AZ, et al. Imaging of pregnant and lactating patients, part 2: evidence-based review and recommendations. *AJR Am J Roentgenol.* 2012;198:785–792.

   A review of diagnostic imaging techniques in various acute disease processes, including acute PE.

20. Bahhady IJ, Ernst A. Risks of and recommendations for flexible bronchoscopy in pregnancy: a review. *Chest.* 2004;126:1974–1981.

   One of only a few reviews discussing bronchoscopy during pregnancy.

21. Briggs G, Freeman RK, Yaffe SJ. *Drugs in Pregnancy and Lactation: A Reference Guide to Fetal and Neonatal Risk?* Philadelphia, PA: Lippincott Williams & Wilkins; 2011.

   An excellent textbook of monographs providing information on pregnancy and breastfeeding recommendations, fetal risk, and summaries for pregnancy, breast feeding, and fetal risk. Drugs are listed by both generic and trade names.

22. Cutts BA, Dasgupta D, Hunt BJ, et al. New directions in the diagnosis and treatment of pulmonary embolism in pregnancy. *Am J Obstet Gynecol.* 2013;208(2):102–108.

   An overview of current methods in PE diagnostics and anticoagulant profiles during pregnancy.

23. Flume PA, O'Sullivan BP, Robinson KA, et al. Cystic fibrosis pulmonary guidelines. *Am J Respir Crit Care Med.* 2007;176:957–969.

   A systematic review by the CF Foundation of the safety and efficacy of drugs used in chronic CF.

24. *Clinical Pharmacology* [database online]. Tampa, FL: Gold Standard. http://www.clinicalpharmacology.com. Accessed March 2013.

   A point-of-care reference recognized by CMS and state Boards of Pharmacy to determine appropriate uses of drugs and biologics.

25. *DRUGDEX® System* [Internet database]. Greenwood Village, CO: Thomson (Healthcare).

   Updated periodically. An online database of FDA-approved, investigational, prescription, nonprescription, and non-US preparation medications. This database provides information on pharmacokinetics, safety profiles, comparative efficacy, and interactions.

26. *LACTMED–Drugs and Lactation Database.* http://toxnet.nlm.nih.gov/cgi-bin/sis/htmlgen? LACT.

   An online database providing information on drugs and lactation, including breast milk drug levels, infant blood drug levels, and potential effects on lactation and in breastfeeding infants.

30 Lung Disease in the Immunocompromised Patient

Shazia M. Jamil

The immunocompromised patient has an increased susceptibility to infection as a result of qualitative or quantitative defects in inflammatory and immunologic host defenses. These defects are caused by a wide range of processes and diseases that include, but are not limited to, primary congenital syndromes, cancer, rheumatologic diseases, retroviral infection, malnutrition, alcoholism, cirrhosis, diabetes mellitus, and immunosuppressive therapy. Pulmonary complications in immunocompromised patients are becoming more common, owing to increases in solid organ transplantation, hematopoietic stem cell transplantation, the use of more potent chemotherapeutic regimens in cancer, and immunosuppressive therapy in rheumatologic disorders. Lung involvement in this group may be either infectious or noninfectious; however, infectious causes are reported in the majority (50%–75%) of cases. They carry a high risk of morbidity and mortality, which warrants a careful diagnostic and therapeutic approach. Immunocompromised hosts are susceptible to pulmonary infections because of decreased granulocyte number and function, compromised immune function (i.e., lymphocyte activity), mechanical barriers to colonization/infection, and exposure to pathogens.

Infections in immunocompromised patients can be bacterial, viral, fungal, parasitic, or mycobacterial. Bacterial pneumonia is the most common cause of focal pulmonary infiltrates in patients with AIDS or leukemia (before, during, and after chemotherapy). Pneumococcus and Haemophilus are as common in the general population as they are in immunocompromised hosts, while encapsulated Gram-positive cocci (e.g., *Staphylococcus aureus*) and the Enterobacteriaceae species (e.g., *Escherichia coli*, *Klebsiella*, and *Pseudomonas* species) are more prevalent among those with granulocytopenia (<500/mm^3) and hospitalized patients. Nosocomially acquired Legionella infection has also been reported in immunocompromised patients. *Rhodococcus equi*, a Gram-positive coccobacilli, has been increasingly reported to cause pneumonia and lung abscesses in AIDS patients and in solid organ transplant recipients, especially those with heart transplant. Due to its variable acid-fast staining and pleomorphic appearance, it has been misdiagnosed as "diphtheroids" and mistaken as a contaminant.

Fungal infections common in immunocompromised patients include both the filamentous fungi (e.g., *Aspergillus* species and the mucormycosis) and the dimorphic fungi (e.g., *Candida* species, *Cryptococcus neoformans*, *Blastomyces dermatitidis*, *Coccidioides immitis*, and *Histoplasma capsulatum*). Other fungi, including *Ochroconis*, *Trichosporon*, *Fusarium*, *Zygomycetes*, and *Scedosporium apiospermum* and *Scedosporium prolificans* are involving the lung with increasing frequency. *Scedosporium* carries a high mortality rate, particularly in transplant recipients and is resistant to amphotericin B and most other antifungals.

Aspergillus is the most common cause of fungal pneumonia; patients with hematopoietic stem cell transplantation are particularly prone to invasive aspergillosis. *A. fumigatus* and *A. flavus* are the two most common. Recently, *A. ustus* and *A. terrus* are being recognized among severely immunocompromised transplant recipients and frequently involve the lung. Early differentiation of the later two from the more common aspergillus infections is important since these species are resistant to amphotericin B.

Local overgrowth of normal flora such as *Candida albicans* in the mouth (thrush) and esophagus is frequent in patients with deficient granulocyte number or function and those receiving broad-spectrum antibiotics. Candida pneumonia however is rare, with the exception of lung transplant recipients. Prophylactic fluconazole is increasingly being used in immunocompromised patients, a practice that leads to a decreased incidence of *C. albicans* infection, but a rise in more antifungal-resistant *C. krausei* and *C. glabrata*.

The fungus *Ochroconis gallopavum* is a dematiaceous hyphomycete that produces characteristic darkly pigmented, septate hyphae and is an emerging opportunistic and possibly fatal fungal infection that occurs almost exclusively in immunocompromised patients. Brain, lung, and spleen involvement is reported and surgical excision in combination with amphotericin B has been utilized.

Fusarium species are important causes of opportunistic fungal infections, risk factors of which include prolonged neutropenia and T-cell immunodeficiency, especially in hematopoietic stem cell transplantation with severe graft-versus-host disease and lung transplant recipients. *F. solani* is the most virulent species. The principal portal of entry is the airways. The clinical presentation mimics aspergillosis. However, clues to the diagnosis include the pattern of new pulmonary infiltrates (interstitial, nodular or cavitary), sinusitis especially with periorbital cellulitis, cutaneous lesions, and positive 1-3-β-D glucan test but negative aspergillus galactomannin test. Recommended empirical treatment includes voriconazole and amphotericin B as first line, and posaconazole for refractory disease. Since *Fusarium* species have intrinsic resistance to caspofungin and micafungin, susceptibility testing should be performed. Immunotherapy with growth factors (G-CSF) for neutropenic patients and gamma interferon and/or GM-CSF for patients with adequate neutrophil counts is also recommended since nearly ubiquitous mortality is observed in patients with persistent neutropenia and disseminated disease.

Commonly recognized respiratory viruses in immunocompromised patients include influenza A and B, parainfluenza 1 to 4, respiratory syncytial virus (RSV), and adenovirus. In the last decade, novel coronaviruses, enteroviruses, rhinovirus, and human metapneumovirus (hMPV) have also been recognized as pathogens. Newly emerged viruses such as bocavirus, parvovirus 4 and 5, KI and WU polyomaviruses, and mimivirus have been reported to involve lung, however currently there is very limited literature in immunocompromised patients. Herpes simplex, varicella, and cytomegalovirus infections may occur, either as newly acquired infections or as reactivations of dormant processes. Cytomegalovirus is the most common viral respiratory pathogen in non-HIV immunocompromised patients.

After transplantation, the risk of cytomegalovirus is closely related to the donor and recipient's prior cytomegalovirus serostatus. RSV is possibly the most important cause of morbidity and mortality of all respiratory viruses affecting the transplant recipient. Several cases of coronavirus-associated severe acute respiratory syndrome (SARS) were diagnosed among solid organ transplant and hematopoietic stem cell transplantation recipients during the 2003 epidemic. The prevalence of respiratory viruses in a given season depends on exposure, virulence, the types of circulating viruses, and the detection methods used.

The outcome of respiratory viral infections in hematopoietic stem cell transplantation recipients depends on several factors including whether the transplant was myeloablative versus nonmyeloablative, the presence of lymphopenia, and the intensity of immunosuppression. Lung transplant recipients have a greater frequency of respiratory viral infections than other transplant recipients. This may be due to direct communication of the allograft with the environment and the poor immune response in the allograft. Respiratory viral infections occurring after lung transplantation has been associated with greater incidence of acute rejection and bronchiolitis obliterans syndrome. One possible mechanism could be a cytokine-mediated inflammatory cascade that recruits T cells to the allograft, further resulting in intraluminal proliferation of fibroblasts. Treatment consists of specific antiviral therapy for symptomatic infections regardless of the duration of symptoms and if possible a decrease in immunosuppression. Some centers also use high-dose steroids (5–10 mg/kg/day for 3 consecutive days) in addition to specific antiviral therapy to prevent acute rejection and progression to bronchiolitis obliterans syndrome.

Pneumocystis jiroveci (previously *P. carinii*) is an opportunistic infection that can cause fulminant and fatal pneumonia in AIDS patients and other immunocompromised patients. Although its incidence is decreased in at-risk patients who use trimethoprim–sulfamethoxazole for prophylaxis, cases still arise in those with adjustments in immunosuppressives (e.g., tapering of corticosteroids), those noncompliant with prophylaxis, and patients with lymphoid malignancies treated with fludarabine.

Mycobacterium tuberculosis (MTD) infections are particularly common in AIDS patients and recipients of solid organ transplant (especially renal transplant recipients), compared with other immunocompromised hosts. The infection is either newly acquired (in endemic areas) or a reactivation of a latent infection. Tuberculosis may involve the lung very early during HIV infection, whereas extrapulmonary or atypical manifestations are associated with more profound immunodeficiency. Immunocompromised patients may present with mycobacteremia and multidrug resistance. In AIDS patients with relatively high $CD4^+$ T-cell counts, a typical pattern of pulmonary reactivation occurs with fever, cough, weight loss, night sweats, and a radiograph revealing cavitary apical upper lobe disease. Disseminated tuberculosis infection is more common in patients with low $CD4^+$ T-cell counts and appears as diffuse bilateral reticulonodular infiltrates consistent with miliary spread, pleural effusions, and hilar and/or mediastinal adenopathy.

The nontuberculous mycobacteria are seen frequently in the AIDS population and usually appear as disseminated disease. *Mycobacterium avium-intracellulare* (MAC) and *Mycobacterium kansasii* are the most common causes of lung infection. Others include *M. abscessus, M. fortuitum, M. chelonae, M. bovis, M xenopi,* and *M. marinum.* Chest radiographs may show hilar or mediastinal adenopathy, cavitation, and/or pleural effusion. *M. abscessus* infection is usually confined to lungs in cystic fibrosis patients; however, dissemination has been reported in immunocompromised patients especially in transplant recipients, which usually portends a poor prognosis. Treatment is complex due to its resistance to most antimycobacterial agents. It is imperative to identify colonization of airways by resistant mycobacteria before lung transplantation due to the potential of allograft infection posttransplantation.

Noninfectious etiologies involving the lung in immunocompromised patients can be very challenging as they may have similar clinical and radiological presentations as infectious etiologies. Common examples are cardiogenic pulmonary edema, acute lung injury/acute respiratory distress syndrome (ALI/ARDS), transfusion-related acute lung injury (TRALI), diffuse alveolar hemorrhage, alveolar hemorrhage secondary to thrombocytopenia, lung involvement by the hematopoietic malignancies (such as leukemic lung infiltration) and solid organ metastasis, posttransplant lymphoproliferative disease, drug-induced lung disease, engraftment syndrome, radiation toxicity, idiopathic pneumonia syndrome, and bronchiolitis obliterans organizing pneumonia. Large-volume fluid infusion (as can occur with chemotherapy and transfusion) or direct cardiotoxicity from chemotherapeutic agents (e.g., anthracyclines) can lead to pulmonary edema. On the other hand, sepsis, chemotherapeutic agents (such as interleukin-2 and cytarabine), and transfusion may cause noncardiogenic pulmonary edema (e.g., ARDS) by increasing capillary leak.

Posttransplant lymphoproliferative disease, diffuse alveolar hemorrhage, idiopathic pneumonia syndrome, and engraftment syndrome are seen more commonly after hematopoietic stem cell transplantation. The majority of posttransplant lymphoproliferative disease is of B cell origin and is related to immunosuppressive regimen and infection with Epstein–Barr virus. Diffuse alveolar hemorrhage complicates about 2% to 14% of hematopoietic stem cell transplantation. The diagnosis is one of exclusion. Pulmonary infection must be ruled out as the etiology of the hemorrhage, as well as alveolar hemorrhage related to thrombocytopenia, uremia, or endogenous anticoagulants. Idiopathic pneumonia syndrome is a noninfectious, frequent, and often fatal complication of allogenic bone marrow transplantation. It usually develops from 1 to over 3 months after bone marrow transplantation and must be distinguished from cytomegalovirus (CMV) pneumonitis. The pathogenesis has not been fully elucidated, but possible contributing factors include lung injury caused by reactive oxygen and nitrogen intermediates during preconditioning and development of graft-versus-host disease. Engraftment syndrome occurs during neutrophil recovery after hematopoietic stem cell transplantation and is difficult to differentiate from ALI/ARDS and pulmonary edema.

The first approach to diagnosis of respiratory illness in the immunocompromised patient is a thorough assessment of the clinical history, including infection risk, and a detailed physical examination. The history should clarify the exact timing of the onset of symptoms, the progression and the relationship of symptoms to the institution of immunosuppression or transplantation. Other relevant facts include previous and current use of chemotherapeutic agents and other medications, immunization history, place of birth and residence (to explore the possibility of exposure to endemic fungi or mycobacteria), and history of positive tuberculosis skin test and positive CMV serology. Common clinical features include fever, dry or productive cough, hemoptysis, dyspnea, wheezing, chest pain with or without pleurisy, hypoxemia, tachycardia, hypotension, and respiratory failure. Sputum production may be scant due to granulocytopenia, even in patients with bacterial pneumonia. Leukocyte count can be completely normal even during infections and hence cannot be relied upon. Viruses such as herpes and CMV may cause tracheobronchitis or bronchiolitis, and may present with wheezing alone.

Key factors in evaluation are (1) rapidity of onset, (2) severity of illness, (3) relationship with immunosuppression, (5) radiologic pattern, and (6) presence of extrapulmonary manifestations. Bacterial, herpes virus, and *P. jiroveci* lung infections have the most rapid onsets and can progress to respiratory failure in a matter of days. Insidious onset is frequently seen with fungi, Nocardia, and mycobacteria. Gradual onset of symptoms is more common with noninfectious etiologies, such as leukemic infiltration and drug-related lung injury, though notable exceptions to this maxim are cardiogenic pulmonary edema, ALI/ARDS, and pulmonary hemorrhage.

The time after transplantation may help predict the most likely etiologies of infectious and noninfectious pulmonary complications. For example, nosocomial pathogens, bacterial and invasive fungal pneumonia usually presents within a month, whereas the risk of developing most opportunistic infections such as Herpes, MTB, Nocardia, and CMV is highest between 1 and 6 months: the period of most intense immunosuppression. Noninfectious etiologies such as diffuse alveolar hemorrhage, ALI/ARDS, and cardiogenic pulmonary edema should be strongly considered when pulmonary manifestations appear shortly after the procedure or within the first month.

Chest radiographs may be entirely normal early in the course and may remain normal during viral infections that have a predilection for airways. A diffuse interstitial or alveolar filling process is highly suggestive of either an opportunistic infection or a noninfectious cause of lung injury. Herpes viruses, *P. jiroveci*, and dimorphic fungi (e.g., *Histoplasma*, *Coccidioides*) often result in diffuse pneumonias without pleural effusions. Drug-induced injury, ALI/ARDS, cardiogenic pulmonary edema, diffuse alveolar hemorrhage, and pulmonary leukostasis are the usual noninfectious causes of diffuse lung involvement. The most frequent cause of focal consolidation is bacterial pneumonia. Cavitation suggests a diagnosis of *S. aureus*, *Pseudomonas*, *Klebsiella*, *E. coli*, anaerobes, *Legionella*, *Nocardia*, *Mycobacterium* species, or *Rhodococcus equi*. Mycobacterial infection appears as either a focal infiltrate or miliary process. Mass-like lesions (especially those with cavitation), which expand without constraint by lobar fissures and tissue plains, are suggestive of invasive filamentous fungi. Common noninfectious causes of focal infiltrate are local hemorrhage and focal leukemic infiltrates. Extrapulmonary manifestations, such as pleural effusions, cardiomegaly, extrapulmonary soft-tissue masses, and bony lesions, may point to endemic fungi, mycobacterium, and *Nocardia* infections.

Initial laboratory investigation should include complete blood counts with manual differential, electrolytes, liver enzyme and function, blood urea nitrogen, serum creatinine, urinalysis, and a good quality postero-anterior and lateral chest radiograph. Microbiologic evaluation is crucial. Depending upon the presentation, specimens from sites such as blood, urine, sputum, bronchoalveolar lavage, transbronchial biopsy, pleural fluid, needle aspirate from abscess, or suspicious skin lesions should be examined on Gram's stain, acid-fast stain, and fungal stain, and sent for respective culture on appropriate medium. Methenamine silver, Wright–Giemsa, and modified acid-fast stains should also be included for patients with high suspicion of fungal, *P. jiroveci*, or *Nocardia* infection. AIDS and solid organ transplant patients with insidious onset pneumonia or lung abscess should have mycolic acid staining of specimens to rule out *R. equi* if Gram's stain or culture suggests diphtheroids. Aspergillus galactomannin is a polysacharride cell wall antigen that is released during fungal growth. Quantitative detection in serum, urine and bronchoalveolar lavage (BAL) fluid is being used increasingly in immunocompromised hosts for rapid diagnosis of invasive pulmonary aspergillosis, since traditional fungal culture may take weeks. Unilateral pleural effusion should be sampled by thoracentesis. Rapid *Legionella* and *Pneumococcal* urinary antigen detection is being widely utilized as an adjunct to culture. Direct fluorescent antibody (DFA) testing of influenza A and B, parainfluenza 1, 2, and 3, RSV, and AdV using a nasopharyngeal swab provides a rapid result, however is limited in its sensitivity. Nucleic acid amplification testing has taken a leading role in the diagnosis of coronavirus, human metapneumovirus, and rhinovirus. Rapid viral culture and fluorescent antibody stains for herpes viruses and influenza should also be considered.

Although chest radiographs may be more conveniently performed, the chest CT scan is more sensitive and specific and should be considered early in the work up. Up to 50% of immunocompromised patients with lung disease on thin section chest CT may have a normal chest radiograph. The CT scan also provides an anatomic map to help guide invasive procedures, such as sampling of a peripheral lung mass, drainage of pleural effusion, bronchoalveolar lavage, transbronchial biopsy and surgical lung biopsy. Early detection of a pulmonary pathology and early institution of specific therapy can increase the likelihood of survival; therefore, diagnostic procedures to obtain respiratory secretions, washings, or even lung tissue should be considered in a timely fashion. Flexible bronchoscopy is the procedure of choice for sampling areas of radiographic abnormality by telescoping (protected-specimen) brush, bronchoalveolar lavage, transbronchial biopsy for diagnosis. Although the yield of culture in patients receiving antibiotics may be low, a positive culture is highly suggestive of infection and may warrant immediate treatment. Transbronchial biopsy adds significantly in detecting tissue-invasive fungi such as *Candida* and *Aspergillus*, leukemic infiltration, bronchiolitis obliterans and graft-versus-host disease. Percutaneous fine needle aspiration is a useful technique for sampling peripheral lesions. However, a larger lung sample can be achieved via thoracotomy with an open lung biopsy or via video-assisted thoracoscopic surgery, which offers a less morbid approach. Lung biopsy is indicated in (1) rapidly progressive severe pneumonia with insufficient time to wait for response from empiric therapy (or when empirical therapy is relatively contraindicated), and (2) persistent, undiagnosed lung disease, despite attempts at less invasive diagnostic procedures and empiric therapy. Immunocompromised hosts with rapidly deteriorating pulmonary status often are placed on empiric antibacterial and antifungal agents until the results of medical evaluation are completed. Increasingly, immunocompromised hosts with respiratory failure are being successfully managed with noninvasive mechanical ventilation in the hospital and ICU setting.

Prevention of infection should be a high priority in immunocompromised patients. Those presenting with respiratory symptoms have a very broad differential diagnosis that encompasses infectious and noninfectious etiologies as well as emerging resistant pathogens. Early interventions may be necessary to establish a diagnosis rapidly, to institute targeted antimicrobial therapy and to avoid multiple unnecessary toxic antimicrobials. Early bronchoscopy with bronchoalveolar lavage is highly recommended if noninvasive investigations are inconclusive, while thoracoscopic or surgical biopsy should be considered early when bronchoscopy is unrevealing.

FURTHER READING

1. Schmitt J, Adam D. Pulmonary infiltrations in febrile patients with neutropenia: risk factors and outcome under empirical antimicrobial therapy in a randomized multicenter study. *Cancer*. 1994;73:2296.

   Reports on the high risk of fungal infection in patients with febrile neutropenia and pneumonia.

2. Rodriguez-Tudela JL, Berenguer J, Guarro J, et al. Epidemiology and outcome of *Scedosporium prolificans* infection: a review of 162 cases. *Med Mycol*. 2009;47(4):359–370.

   An excellent review of this emergent fungal pathogen.

3. Gerson SL, Talbot GH, Hurwitz S, et al. Prolonged granulocytopenia: the major risk factor for invasive pulmonary aspergillosis in patients with acute leukemia. *Ann Intern Med*. 1984;100:345.

   A classic study of risks for invasive aspergillosis.

4. Nucci M, Anaissie E. Fusarium infections in immunocompromised patients. *Clin Microbiol Rev*. 2007;20(4):695–704.

5. Becker MJ, Lugtenburg EJ, Cornelissen JJ, et al. Galactomannan detection in computerized tomography-based bronchoalveolar lavage fluid and serum in haematological patients at risk for invasive pulmonary aspergillosis. *Br J Haematol*. 2003;121(3):448–457.

   A report showing a high sensitivity, specificity, positive predictive value, and negative predictive value when aspergillus galactomannin is detected in CT guided BAL.

6. Hopkins P, McNeil K, Kermeen F, et al. Human metapneumovirus in lung transplant recipients and comparison to respiratory syncytial virus. *Am J Respir Crit Care Med*. 2008;178(8):876–881.

7. Kumar D, Humar A. Respiratory viral infections in transplant and oncology patients. *Infect Dis Clin North Am.* 2010;24(2):395–412.

   Excellent review of known and emerging respiratory viruses in solid organ transplant, hematopoietic stem cell transplant, and oncology setting.

8. Singh N, Paterson DL. Mycobacterium tuberculosis infection in solid organ transplant recipients: impact and implications for management. *Clin Infect Dis.* 1998;27:1266.

9. Aronchick JM, Miller WT Jr. Disseminated nontuberculous mycobacterial infections in immunosuppressed patients. *Semin Roentgenol.* 1993;28:150–157.

   Comprehensive clinical/radiologic presentation of tuberculous and nontuberculous mycobacterial infection in the immunocompromised host.

10. Steinbach WJ, Benjamin DK Jr, Kontoyiannis DP, et al. Infections due to *Aspergillus terreus*: a multicenter retrospective analysis of 83 cases. *Clin Infect Dis.* 2004;39(2):192–198.

11. Perez MGV, Vassal T, Kemmerly SA. *Rhodococcus equi* infection in transplant recipients: a case of mistaken identity and review of literature. *Transpl Infect Dis.* 2002;4:52.

12. Wang TK, Chiu W, Chim S, et al. Disseminated *Ochroconis gallopavum* infection in a renal transplant recipient: the first reported case and a review of literature. *Clin Nephrol.* 2003;60:415.

13. Chernenko SM, Humar A, Hutcheon M, et al. Mycobacterium abscessus infections in lung transplant recipients: the international experience. *J Heart Lung Transplant.* 2006;25(12):1447–1455.

14. Pyrgos V, Shoham S, Walsh TJ. Pulmonary zygomycosis. *Semin Respir Crit Care Med.* 2008;29(2):111–120.

15. Saito H, Anaissie EJ, Morice RC, et al. Bronchoalveolar lavage in the diagnosis of pulmonary infiltrates in patients with acute leukemia. *Chest.* 1988;94:745.

   Contains a discussion of the relevance of detection of Candida in BAL.

16. Crawford SW. Noninfectious lung disease in the immunocompromised host. *Respiration.* 1999;66:385–395.

   Excellent detailed review of possible noninfectious etiologies of lung disease in immunocompromised hosts.

17. Shorr AF, Susla GM, O'Grady NP. Pulmonary infiltrates in the non-HIV infected immunocompromised patient. *Chest.* 2004;125:260.

   Excellent review of etiologies, diagnostic strategies, and outcomes of lung infiltrates in immunocompromised hosts.

18. Rano A, Agusti C, Jimenez P, et al. Pulmonary infiltrates in non-HIV immunocompromised patients: a diagnostic approach using noninvasive and bronchoscopic procedures. *Thorax.* 2001;56:379.

   Infectious etiologies were responsible for more than three fourths of pulmonary infiltrates in a prospective study of 200 immunocompromised patients.

19. Yen KT, Lee AS, Krowka MJ, et al. Pulmonary complications in bone marrow transplantation: a practical approach to diagnosis and treatment. *Clin Chest Med.* 2004;25:189–120.

20. Heussel CP, Kauczor HU, Heussel G, et al. Early detection of pneumonia in febrile neutropenic patients: use of thin-section CT. *AJR Am J Roentgenol.* 1997;169:1347.

   Reported increased sensitivity of CT scan in detecting lung lesions compared with chest radiograph.

21. White DA, Wong PW, Downey R. The utility of open lung biopsy in patients with hematological malignancies. *Am J Respir Crit Care Med.* 2000;161:723.

   High utility of this procedure prompting changes in therapy in about 57% of such patients.

22. Hilbert G, Gruson D, Vargas F, et al. Noninvasive ventilation in immunosuppressed patients with pulmonary infiltrates, fever, and acute respiratory failure. *N Engl J Med.* 2001;344:481.

   A randomized trial of immunocompromised hosts with pulmonary infiltrates and early respiratory failure showed that patients managed with noninvasive ventilation had decreased mortality compared with those who received standard care (endotracheal intubation).

23. Nishi SP, Valentine VG, Duncan S. Emerging bacterial, fungal, and viral respiratory infections in transplantation. *Infect Dis Clin North Am.* 2010;24(3):541–555.

24. Linden PK. Approach to the immunocompromised host with infection in the intensive care unit. *Infect Dis Clin North Am.* 2009;23(3):535–556.

   An excellent review of diagnostic approaches to various opportunistic infections.

31 The Lung in Drug Abuse

Tristan J. Huie and Charles A. Read

The lungs are particularly vulnerable to medical complications in drug abuse because the most common routes of administration are inhalation and intravenous (IV) injection. Drug abuse may cause infectious and noninfectious lung disorders (Table 31-1). Knowledge of the epidemiology and typical presentation may facilitate timely diagnosis and appropriate treatment.

Illicit drug users are susceptible to numerous infections that arise because the host's immune defenses are suppressed or bypassed. The increased prevalence of HIV infection among drug abusers leads to infectious and noninfectious complications, including community-acquired bacterial pneumonia, pneumocystis pneumonia, tuberculosis, and Kaposi sarcoma (see Chapter 61). In addition to the immune suppression that occurs with HIV infection, the drug user's immune system may be suppressed by the direct effects of the drug itself. Studies in cocaine and marijuana users demonstrate impaired function of alveolar macrophages. Alveolar macrophages exposed to marijuana smoke have reduced phagocytic, bactericidal, and fungicidal activity. Marijuana exposure results in decreased expression of proinflammatory cytokines, such as tumor necrosis factor (TNF)-α and interleukin (IL)-6. T-cell proliferation is shifted from T helper 1 (TH1) cells that are responsible for cell-mediated immunity to T helper 2 (TH2) cells that mediate allergy

TABLE 31-1	Pulmonary Complications of Illicit Drug Use

Infectious
Aspiration pneumonia
Septic emboli
Bacterial pneumonia
Acute bronchitis
Tuberculosis
Fungal pneumonia

Noninfectious
Vascular complications
Noncardiogenic pulmonary edema
Pulmonary hemorrhage
Pulmonary hypertension
Interstitial lung disease
Granulomatous lung disease
Talcosis
Organizing pneumonia (BOOP)
Airway complications
Upper airway injury
Bronchospasm/asthma
Chronic bronchitis
Bullous disease
Bronchiectasis
Pleural complications
Pneumothorax/pneumomediastinum
Pleural effusions/empyema
Respiratory failure
Cancer of upper and lower airway

and atopy. This shift may cause an increased risk of infection and malignancy in marijuana users. Macrophages exposed to crack cocaine are less able to kill bacteria or tumor cells, possibly because of decreased production of reactive oxidant species. Marijuana and cocaine smoking also harm the lungs' primary defenses by replacing ciliated epithelium with nonciliated mucus-secreting cells or metaplastic squamous epithelium. These findings help explain the enhanced susceptibility to infections observed in drug addicts.

Aspiration into the lower respiratory tract commonly occurs after the use of many illicit drugs. Pneumonia complicates heroin overdose in up to half of cases. Sedative overdose depresses consciousness, diminishes protective airway reflexes, and increases the risk for aspiration of oropharyngeal or gastric contents. The initial inflammatory response can result in significant alveolar edema. Patients present with fever, tachypnea, and hypoxia. Radiographs may be normal or may show localized or bilateral diffuse infiltrates, depending on the volume of aspiration and the severity of the inflammatory response. Treatment is generally supportive. The use of antibiotics is controversial, but if used should be directed against the oropharyngeal flora.

Septic pulmonary emboli commonly occur in injection drug users and may occur in up to one quarter of hospitalized drug addicts with pulmonary complaints. Emboli originate from endocarditis, typically of the tricuspid valve, or from thrombophlebitis at the injection site. Presenting symptoms typically include pleuritic chest pain, hemoptysis, and fever. Physical examination in the case of thrombophlebitis reveals erythema, induration, and warmth at the injection site. A palpable cord may be present. In contrast, tricuspid valve endocarditis is often difficult to detect on examination. Tricuspid murmurs are usually soft, and the peripheral stigmata of endocarditis are not present with right-sided lesions. Typical radiographic manifestations include diffuse infiltrates or peripheral nodules, which may cavitate. Sequentially appearing nodules suggest endocarditis. Pleural effusions may occur; hilar and mediastinal lymphadenopathy is rarely seen. Blood cultures are usually positive. *Staphylococcus aureus* causes 80% of cases; Gram-negative bacteria and *Candida* are rarer causes. Complications include lung abscess, empyema, and bronchopleural fistula. Appropriate antimicrobial therapy should be continued for 4 to 6 weeks and is typically effective if compliance is achieved.

Community-acquired pneumonia occurs with increased frequency in drug abusers. There is a 10-fold increased risk of pneumococcal pneumonia in illicit drug users compared to nonusers. The presentation, course of illness, and response to treatment are similar in drug-using and nonusing populations. The usual community-acquired organisms are most common in drug users; however, aspiration is also associated with anaerobes (particularly in the setting of poor dentition), and intravenous drug use is associated with Gram-negative bacilli and *S. aureus*. Drug use increases the risk of methicillin-resistant *S. aureus* infection.

Acute bronchitis develops at an increased frequency in marijuana users. This increased incidence may result in part from the respiratory irritants in marijuana smoke. Although not well studied, other inhaled drugs may also predispose to acute bronchitis. The treatment of acute bronchitis in drug users is similar to that in nonusers.

Pulmonary tuberculosis occurs more frequently in drug users and appears to be related to lower socioeconomic status and the decreased immunity and higher rate of reactivation in this population. Clinically and radiographically, tuberculosis in drug users is indistinguishable from that of nonusers and should be treated with the standard multidrug antimycobacterial regimen. However, directly observed therapy is advisable in drug addicts to ensure compliance and avoid development of resistance.

Fungal pulmonary infections have been linked to illicit drug use. Invasive aspergillosis has been reported in immunocompromised patients who have smoked marijuana contaminated with the fungus. Cases have been described in patients with advanced HIV, chronic granulomatous disease, after bone marrow transplant, and in patients with lung cancer treated with chemotherapy. Aspergillus-laden marijuana has been implicated in *allergic bronchopulmonary aspergillosis*. Lobar candidal pneumonia and systemic candidiasis resulting in the *acute respiratory distress syndrome* (ARDS) have been reported in heroin users. A purported source of candidal infection in this population is the lemon used to acidify the heroin fix. Although severe fungal infections are rare, drug abusers have a high prevalence of serum precipitins against these fungi, suggesting widespread fungal contamination of illicit drugs. Treatment should focus on standard aggressive antifungal therapy.

Illicit substance abuse is also responsible for numerous noninfectious lung disorders that may occur within the pulmonary vasculature, interstitium, airways, or pleura.

Noncardiogenic pulmonary edema is perhaps the most frequent fatal complication of illicit drug abuse. A large number of drugs, including narcotics, cocaine, amphetamines, sedatives, tranquilizers, and hydrocarbons, can acutely produce pulmonary edema. Heroin is a particularly common offender. In one large series, 18% of those with heroin-induced pulmonary edema died. Pulmonary edema has been documented in both the first-time user and the experienced addict; it can occur immediately or up to 24 hours after use. Patients typically are stuporous or comatose, with fever, cyanosis, and crackles. Constricted pupils suggest opiate intoxication. Chest films classically demonstrate fluffy, bilateral alveolar infiltrates without cardiomegaly. The pathophysiology appears to differ depending on the drug involved, but increased permeability is suggested by studies that demonstrate equivalent protein concentrations in the alveolar fluid and serum. Treatment is generally supportive with supplemental oxygen and mechanical ventilation as needed. Naloxone should be considered in opiate-induced edema to reverse respiratory depression. Typically, the edema resolves within 24 to 72 hours, but it can take several weeks until the lung volumes, compliance, and diffusing capacity normalize. This suggests a component of acute lung injury has occurred in these cases.

Crack lung is a form of acute lung injury that presents with fever, cough, chest pain, wheezing, and hypoxia. The radiograph shows diffuse alveolar infiltrates. Eosinophilia is often present in both peripheral blood and bronchoalveolar lavage. Crack lung can develop immediately or up to 48 hours after smoking crack cocaine. It has not been reported after intravenous or intranasal use. Increased neutrophil activation and IL-8 expression may cause the lung injury from cocaine smoking. The infiltrates resolve spontaneously with supportive treatment. Corticosteroid therapy has been used with mixed success, but there is no convincing evidence to support the routine use of steroids.

Pulmonary hemorrhage has been well described in crack cocaine smokers. Volatile hydrocarbons and heroin have also been associated with at least subclinical pulmonary vascular hemorrhage. The amount of pulmonary hemorrhage may be massive or barely detectable. Massive hemoptysis has been associated with pulmonary infarction after cocaine use. Crack users more commonly experience trace hemoptysis; many report black or blood-tinged sputum after crack use. One-third of cocaine smokers have hemosiderin-laden macrophages in their lungs at autopsy, pointing to occult episodes of bleeding. It has been postulated that pulmonary hemorrhage occurs from either the intense vasoconstriction caused by cocaine or the direct alveolar injury. Chest radiographs are usually normal. Treatment depends on the extent of hemoptysis, but is mainly supportive. Bronchoscopy is indicated with significant hemoptysis to investigate for a site of localized bleeding, however, the alveolar hemorrhage is usually diffuse.

Methamphetamine use has been recognized as a significant risk factor in the development of *pulmonary hypertension.* Nearly a third of patients diagnosed with idiopathic pulmonary arterial hypertension had used methamphetamine in a large retrospective cohort. Direct toxicity to the pulmonary arteries via an increase in serotonin release is the suspected mechanism. The treatment is the same as for other causes of idiopathic pulmonary arterial hypertension, although continued drug abuse may complicate these therapies. Pulmonary hypertension may also develop in patients who inject aqueous suspensions of medications intended for oral use only. Addicts often prepare and inject suspensions of tablets containing insoluble filler components such as talc or cellulose. The most frequently crushed and injected tablets include amphetamines, methylphenidate (Ritalin), methadone, and propoxyphene. Heroin and other drugs may be diluted with insoluble adulterants such as starch or inadvertently contaminated with the cotton used to filter the liquid drug. Repeated embolization of insoluble particles results in thrombosis, fibrosis, and ultimately pulmonary vessel occlusion. Progressive loss of pulmonary microcirculation leads to pulmonary hypertension and, if untreated, to cor pulmonale. Treatment options are limited; the most important step is cessation of IV drug use.

Several forms of *interstitial lung disease* have been associated with illicit drug use. The most common is a granulomatous disease that results from the embolization of insoluble particles. Embolized foreign bodies cause endothelial injury in the pulmonary vasculature. Initially a focal inflammatory process develops that leads to damage of the arterial walls. Transvascular migration of the insoluble particles occurs next with the formation of perivascular and interstitial granulomas. *Talcosis* develops after long-term, chronic injection of pills that contain magnesium silicate (i.e., talc). Patients complain of insidious progressive dyspnea, mild cough, and, occasionally, wheezing. Fundoscopic examination often reveals glistening white spots around the macula. Chest radiography is normal in 50% of cases or may have diffuse reticulonodular infiltrates most prominent at the lung bases. Lower lung emphysema appears to characteristically occur with methylphenidate injection. Patients with talcosis classically have an obstructive pattern with decreased diffusing capacity on pulmonary function testing, however, a restrictive pattern may also be seen. Definitive diagnosis requires either a transbronchial or surgical lung biopsy that demonstrates foreign body granulomas containing birefringent talc or other foreign particle. Anecdotal evidence suggests that steroids may be of mild benefit in some patients. A series of six patients, however, showed that all developed severe respiratory insufficiency during long-term follow-up regardless of steroid use, and three died of respiratory failure.

Other forms of interstitial lung disease have been reported in association with drug abuse. *Organizing pneumonia* (formerly called bronchiolitis obliterans organizing pneumonia or BOOP) has been reported following crack cocaine use and heroin use. Pulmonary vasculitis indistinguishable from Wegener granulomatosis developed in the setting of crack cocaine use. *Acute eosinophilic pneumonia* has occurred following cocaine and heroin use. Case reports describe lung disease mimicking pulmonary vasculitis, sarcoidosis, and hypersensitivity pneumonitis following both cocaine and heroin use. Corticosteroids may provide some benefit.

Thermal injury can occur from smoking crack cocaine because of the extremely high temperatures of inhaled chemicals or secondary to ignition of the highly volatile ether residue used in processing the free-base form of cocaine. *Thermal epiglottitis* has been described in a small series of drug abusers who presented with acute epiglottitis. Treatment is supportive with corticosteroids to reduce swelling and airway compromise. Repeated thermal injury to the trachea can lead to *tracheal stenosis*, which has been described in crack cocaine use. Such patients will have wheezing, which may be irreversible, and occasionally with stridor. Severe tracheal stenosis may require a mechanical correction, including tracheostomy placement.

Bronchospasm can occur after the use of a variety of inhaled drugs, with crack cocaine and heroin being the most frequent offenders. The drugs, or their adulterants, induce inflammation of the respiratory epithelium and can result in the direct release of histamine. Bronchospasm is most threatening in patients with poorly controlled asthma. Several case studies have reported that asthma deaths are associated with substance abuse in up to 30% of cases. Treatment involves avoiding the precipitating drug and using standard inhaled steroids and bronchodilators as necessary.

Chronic bronchitis and impaired gas exchange occur with the repeated use of marijuana. Marijuana causes bronchodilation and was once evaluated as a possible therapy for asthma. Bronchodilation results from tetrahydrocannabinol (THC) binding to a cannabinoid receptor that is independent of antimuscarinic or beta-agonistic activity. Unfortunately, these bronchodilatory effects are only transient, and other combustion byproducts tend to worsen asthma. The chronic use of marijuana causes increased cough, sputum production, and wheezing similar to chronic bronchitis.

Bullous lung disease occurs in up to 2% of IV drug users. It is associated with methylphenidate injection and with marijuana use. Bullous disease, predominantly located in the upper lobes, occurs much earlier than expected from cigarette smoking alone. The pathophysiology of bullae formation is uncertain, but is speculated to result from the coalescence of microbullae, which are formed indirectly from either emboli or foreign body granulomas. Barotrauma also appears to play a role. Patients present with obstructive symptoms similar to those of patients with moderate to severe emphysema. Obstructive lung disease can also result from damage to the medium and small airways.

Bronchiectasis has been reported in drug users after one or more episodes of noncardiogenic pulmonary edema. Aspiration, hypoxia, and direct irritant effects may all contribute to the development of bronchiectasis. The best available long-term therapy for bronchiectasis is cessation of drug use. Continued exposure generally leads to progression of the disease.

Pneumothorax or *pneumomediastinum* can result from the use of either IV or inhaled drugs. As sites for peripheral access are exhausted, IV drug abusers may attempt to access the subclavian or internal jugular veins. A "pocket shot" is an injection lateral to the sternocleidomastoid muscle immediately above the clavicle; pneumothorax, pneumomediastinum, pseudoaneurysm formation, and paralysis of the vocal cords because of recurrent laryngeal nerve trauma have been reported. Pneumomediastinum and pneumothorax can also occur with inhalation drug use. This occurs because of weakening of the alveolar walls and from an increased pressure gradient across the alveolar membrane. An increased gradient occurs during "shotgunning," as one person forcibly exhales smoke into another person's mouth, and during a Valsalva maneuver performed after inhalation to increase absorption of the inhaled drug. There have been case reports of pneumothorax and pneumomediastinum after ecstasy use with prolonged dancing.

Respiratory failure, through suppression of the respiratory drive, occurs with many different drug classes. Narcotics and sedatives suppress ventilation; their use may result in carbon dioxide retention, decreased consciousness, respiratory failure, and death. Treatment should be individualized and may include naloxone to antagonize opiates and reverse respiratory depression or, in some cases, flumazenil to antagonize benzodiazepines. Mechanical ventilation may be required. Abuse of volatile inhalants, common among adolescents, may lead to asphyxiation from suppressed respiratory drive and physical displacement of oxygen by the inhalant. Ketamine and gamma hydroxybutyrate may also cause respiratory failure.

Lung cancer occurs with increased frequency in tobacco smokers. The link between various illicit drugs and cancer has been difficult to prove because of the frequent concurrent use of tobacco in drug users and difficulty in enrolling drug users in prospective studies. Indirect evidence suggests that cancers and precancerous changes occur with increased frequency in marijuana and cocaine users. Histologic and molecular alterations linked to carcinogenesis have been identified in the bronchial epithelium of marijuana and cocaine smokers. Epidemiologic evidence also supports a link between drug use and cancer. Marijuana use has been reported at an increased frequency in patients who develop early head and lung cancers. Although not well studied, other illicit substances may have similar carcinogenic effects.

The effects of illicit drug use on the lungs are diverse and most commonly follow smoking or intravenous injection. Many infectious and noninfectious complications may arise acutely or chronically. Patterns of drug abuse frequently change as different drugs gain popularity. Thus, the clinician must maintain a high suspicion for drug use and must remain informed of current drug use trends to provide optimal care for drug users.

FURTHER READING

1. Heffner JE, Harley RA, Schabel SI. Pulmonary reactions from illicit substance abuse. *Clin Chest Med.* 1990;11:151–162.

   A comprehensive review that divides subject material by both drug type and common complications.

2. Hind CR. Pulmonary complications of intravenous drug misuse, I: epidemiology and non-infective complications. *Thorax.* 1990;45:891–898.

3. Hind CR. Pulmonary complications of intravenous drug misuse, II: infective and HIV related complications. *Thorax.* 1990;45:957–961.

   References 2 and 3 provide an excellent review of the subject.

4. Wolff AJ, O'Donnell AE. Pulmonary effects of illicit drug use. *Clin Chest Med.* 2004;25:203–216.

   An excellent, detailed review of the literature.

5. Devlin RJ, Henry JA. Clinical review: major consequences of illicit drug consumption. *Cri Care.* 2008;12:202.

   A review of cardiopulmonary and other critical illnesses that may arise from drug abuse.

6. Tashkin DP. Airway effects of marijuana, cocaine, and other inhaled illicit agents. *Curr Opin Pulm Med.* 2001;7:43–61.

   An excellent review of the pathophysiology and consequences of inhaled drugs.

7. Lee MHS, Hancox RJ. Effects of smoking cannabis on lung function. *Expert Rev Respir Med.* 2011;5:537–546.

   An updated, critical review of the effects of marijuana on respiratory health. Summarizes limitations in the current literature.

8. Haim DY, Lippmann ML, Goldberg SK, et al. The pulmonary complications of crack cocaine: a comprehensive review. *Chest.* 1995;107:233–240.

9. Thadani PV. NIDA conference report on cardiopulmonary complications of crack cocaine use. *Chest.* 1996;110:1072–1076.

10. Restrepo CS, Carrillo JA, Martinez S, et al. Pulmonary complications from cocaine and cocaine-based substances: imaging manifestations. *Radiographics.* 2007;27:941–956.

    An excellent review of pulmonary complications of cocaine use with illustrative imaging.

11. Nguyen ET, Silva CI, Souza CA, et al. Pulmonary complications of illicit use: differential diagnosis based on CT findings. *J Thorac Imaging.* 2007;22:199–206.

    Provides a well-illustrated approach based on radiographic patterns of disease.

12. O'Donnell AE, Pappas LS. Pulmonary complications of intravenous drug abuse: experience at an inner-city hospital. *Chest.* 1988;94:251–253.

13. O'Donnell AE, Selig J, Aravamuthan M, et al. Pulmonary complications associated with illicit drug use: an update. *Chest.* 1995;108:460–463.

    References 12 and 13 catalog the experiences of a pulmonary consult service with an inner city drug-abusing patient population.

14. Jaffe RB, Koschmann EB. Septic pulmonary emboli. *Radiology.* 1970;96:527–532.

    Compilation of the radiographic manifestations of septic pulmonary emboli in 17 patients.

15. Reichman LB, Felton CP, Edsall JR. Drug dependence, a possible new risk factor for tuberculosis disease. *Arch Intern Med.* 1979;139:337–339.

    Demonstrates that drug dependence is a risk factor for the development of active tuberculosis.

16. Hamadeh R, Ardehali A, Locksley RM, et al. Fatal aspergillosis associated with smoking contaminated marijuana, in a marrow transplant recipient. *Chest.* 1988;94:432–433.

    Contaminated marijuana caused invasive aspergillosis in an immunosuppressed host.

17. Llamas R, Hart DR, Schneider NS. Allergic bronchopulmonary aspergillosis associated with smoking moldy marijuana. *Chest.* 1978;73:871–872.

18. Steinberg AD, Karliner JS. The clinical spectrum of heroin pulmonary edema. *Arch Intern Med.* 1968;122:122–127.

    A series of 16 patients that emphasizes the variability in the presentation of heroin-induced noncardiogenic pulmonary edema.

19. Duberstein JL, Kaufman DM. A clinical study of an epidemic of heroin intoxication and heroin-induced pulmonary edema. *Am J Med.* 1971;51:704–714.

    A series of 149 cases of heroin intoxication and its complications.

20. Bishay A, Amchentsev A, Saleh A, et al. A hitherto unreported pulmonary complication in an IV heroin user. *Chest.* 2008;133:549–551.

    A case report of organizing pneumonia that developed while using intravenous heroin.

21. Murray RJ, Albin RJ, Mergner W, et al. Diffuse alveolar hemorrhage temporally related to cocaine smoking. *Chest.* 1988;93:427–429.

    A case report linking cocaine inhalation with life-threatening hemoptysis.

22. Milman N, Smith CD. Cutaneous vasculopathy associated with cocaine use. *Arthritis Care Res.* 2011;63:1195–1202.

    A review of eight cases of cocaine-associated vasculitis. It highlights the clinical presentation and disease course. Cessation of cocaine use was necessary for clinical improvement.

23. Chin KM, Channick RN, Rubin LJ, et al. Is methamphetamine use associated with idiopathic pulmonary arterial hypertension? *Chest*. 2006;130:1657–1663.

    A retrospective study of 340 patients with pulmonary hypertension demonstrating a nearly 30% incidence of stimulant use (methamphetamines, amphetamines, or cocaine) in patients with idiopathic PAH. Accounting for differences in age, patients with idiopathic PAH were 10 times as likely to have used stimulants as patients with identifiable causes of PAH.

24. Waller BF, Brownlee WJ, Roberts WC. Self-induced pulmonary granulomatosis: a consequence of intravenous injection of drugs intended for oral use. *Chest*. 1980;78:90–94.

    An instructive case report that reviews the pathophysiology of pulmonary hypertension and pulmonary granulomatosis.

25. Ward S, Heyneman LE, Reittner P, et al. Talcosis associated with IV abuse of oral medications: CT findings. *AJR Am J Roentgenol*. 2000;174:789–793.

    This report describes the CT findings of 12 patients with talcosis.

26. Marchiori E, Lourenco S, Gasparetto TD, et al. Pulmonary talcosis: imaging findings. *Lung*. 2010;188:165–171.

    A review of various patterns of talcosis.

27. Douglas FG, Kafilmout KJ, Patt NL. Foreign particle embolism in drug addicts: respiratory pathophysiology. *Ann Intern Med*. 1971;75:865–880.

    A series of cases outlining the sequelae of foreign body granulomas.

28. Tashkin DP, Kleerup EC, Koyal SN, et al. Acute effects of inhaled and IV cocaine on airway dynamics. *Chest*. 1996;110:904–910.

29. Goldstein DS, Karpel JP, Appel D, et al. Bullous pulmonary damage in users of intravenous drugs. *Chest*. 1986;89:266–269.

    A retrospective study linking bullous pulmonary disease to use of illicit drugs.

30. Corbridge T, Cygan J, Greenberger P. Substance abuse and acute asthma. *Intensive Care Med*. 2000;26:347–349.

    An overview of several recent studies, including two medical examiner studies, that evaluates the role of substance abuse in fatal asthma.

31. Mayo-Smith MF, Spinale J. Thermal epiglottitis in adults: a new complication of illicit drug use. *J Emerg Med*. 1997;15:483–485.

    Reports four cases of acute epiglottitis caused by thermal injury after crack or marijuana use.

32. Banner AS, Rodriguez J, Sunderrajan EV, et al. Bronchiectasis: a cause of pulmonary symptoms in heroin addicts. *Respiration*. 1979;37:232–237.

    A series of seven case reports linking the development of bronchiectasis to heroin use.

33. Lewis JW Jr, Groux N, Elliott JP Jr, et al. Complications of attempted central venous injections performed by drug abusers. *Chest*. 1980;78:613–617.

    A series of 12 cases illustrating various complications related to central vein injections in IV drug users.

34. Seaman ME. Barotrauma related to inhalational drug abuse. *J Emerg Med*. 1990;8:141–149.

    A case series and literature review related to the presentation and treatment of barotrauma related to inhalational drug abuse.

35. Barsky SH, Roth MD, Kleerup EC, et al. Histopathologic and molecular alterations in bronchial epithelium in habitual smokers of marijuana, cocaine and/or tobacco. *J Natl Cancer Inst*. 1998;90:1198–1205.

36. Baldwin GC, Tashkin DP, Buckley DM, et al. Marijuana and cocaine impair alveolar macrophage function and cytokine production. *Am J Respir Crit Care Med*. 1997;156:1606–1613.

    Alterations in alveolar macrophage function may suggest an increased susceptibility to infection and cancer.

37. Yuan M, Kiertscher SM, Cheng Q, et al. Delta 9-tetrahydrocannabinol regulates Th1/Th2 cytokine balance in activated human T cells. *J Neuroimmunol*. 2002;133:124–131.

    THC was shown to alter T-cell proliferation and decrease T-cell immunity.

32 Pneumonia: General Considerations

Maida V. Soghikian and William L. Ring

Pneumonia is a term generally used to describe inflammation of the lungs from infection. The causative agent can be bacterial, viral, fungal, or even parasitic. However, the term pneumonia is sometimes used interchangeably with the word pneumonitis, which describes a nonspecific state of inflammation of the lungs. Less commonly, the cause of pneumonia/pneumonitis may be unknown (idiopathic) or the result of noninfectious agents such as chemicals, stomach contents, radiation, or autoimmune diseases. The remainder of this chapter will focus on infectious pneumonia.

Pneumonia nomenclature based on where the patient acquired the infection has been used to develop guidelines and determine diagnostic and therapeutic approaches. Community-acquired pneumonia (CAP) refers to infection that develops in a nonhospitalized patient. Hospital-acquired pneumonia (HAP) is an infection occurring 48 hours or more after admission. Health-care-associated pneumonia (HCAP) is defined as pneumonia in patients with at least 2 days of hospitalization in the last 90 days, residence in a nursing home or an extended care facility, chronic hemodialysis within 30 days, home infusion therapy including intravenous (IV) antibiotics, chemotherapy, home wound care, or family member with a multidrug resistant pathogen. Ventilator-associated pneumonia (VAP) is pneumonia arising more than 48 to 72 hours after endotracheal intubation. Although some recent literature has questioned the appropriateness of using these diagnostic categories, this nomenclature continues to be used widely.

Pneumonia is a global public health problem responsible for 1.5 million deaths annually in children younger than 5 years of age, more than any other infectious disease. The Centers for Disease Control (CDC) reported that in 2010 1.1 million people in the United States were hospitalized with pneumonia, more than 50,000 people died of the disease, and it was the fifth most common discharge diagnosis in US hospitals with an average length of stay of 5.2 days.

CAP is not only common but also potentially serious. There tends to be seasonal variation with more cases occurring during the winter months. Although the etiology varies by geographic region, *Streptococcus pneumoniae* remains the most common pathogen identified worldwide. The incidence of CAP in adults is difficult to estimate, but the overall rate is reported between 3 and 40 per 1,000 persons per year, with the highest incidence at the extremes of age. Hospitalization is required in 40% to 60% of patients with CAP, and 10% progress to severe pneumonia requiring ICU admission and with an overall mortality of 10%. Moreover, patients with CAP do poorly long-term, with all-cause mortality approaching 28% in the subsequent year; the highest mortality occurs in those who require hospitalization. Despite the National Hospital Discharge Survey report that the overall rate of hospitalization for pneumonia declined by 20% in the United States from 2000 to 2010, there is concern that the burden of CAP will increase with the aging population.

HAP is the second most common nosocomial infection in the US, occurring in 5 to 10 cases per 1,000 hospital admissions and with a 6- to 20-fold increased incidence in mechanically ventilated patients. Nosocomial pneumonia frequently occurs in the ICU, especially after 48 hours of intubation, with an incidence as high as 20%. These infections are not only responsible for significant increases in hospital stay and cost, but the attributable mortality of HAP has been estimated at 33% to 50%. Aerobic bacteria such as *Pseudomonas aeruginosa* or *Staphylococcus aureus* cause most of these infections, but other pathogens also contribute. Hospitalized patients become colonized with these more virulent organisms and, due to comorbidities such as acute illnesses and immune dysfunction, are more susceptible to developing pneumonia. In the ICU, the presence of invasive lines that may introduce pathogens hematogenously or endotracheal tubes that bypass the natural upper airway barriers to infection contribute to heightened rates of infection. National efforts aimed at decreasing the incidence of ICU related infections have focused on implementation of the Institute for Healthcare Improvement's (IHI) prevention bundles. The National Quality Forum (NQF) and CDC have followed the growing body of literature on these processes closely, and Medicare (CMS) has responded by basing hospital reimbursement strategies on compliance with many of these prevention strategies and the incidence of healthcare acquired infections.

Microbial agents can be introduced into the lungs by several routes including aspiration of oropharyngeal secretions, inhalation, hematogenous spread via the pulmonary or bronchial circulation, and direct spread from surrounding structures. In many cases, breakdown in normal body defenses is responsible for infection. The interplay between body defense mechanisms and microbial inoculation, including the size and virulence of the inoculum, ultimately determines the occurrence and severity of pneumonia. Insufficient immune response can result in life-threatening infection, but an excessive response can also lead to life-threatening inflammatory injury. Further research on immunity, susceptibility, and interaction with specific organisms is necessary to guide the development of prophylactic and therapeutic interventions.

Aspiration including upper airway secretions colonized with a variety of organisms may be the most common mechanism in the pathogenesis of pneumonia. Some bacteria, such as *S. pneumoniae* and *Haemophilus influenzae*, can transiently colonize healthy individuals. Mixed anaerobic flora is often found in those with poor dental hygiene. *S. aureus* and *Pseudomonas* species can be isolated in upper airways of hospitalized patients. It is estimated that 45% of healthy adults experience microaspiration at night, but pulmonary defenses like cough and mucociliary clearance usually prevent bacterial colonization from progressing to infection. These defenses are compromised in patients who are intubated, debilitated, or have altered consciousness.

Legionella species, mycobacteria, endemic fungi, *Mycoplasma pneumoniae, Chlamydia pneumoniae,* and most viral infections are examples of pneumonia resulting from direct inhalation of organisms. Direct inhalation of airborne droplets partially accounts for the geographic and seasonal clustering of cases caused by these organisms.

Hematogenous or embolic causes of pneumonia are uncommon, usually originating from infected heart valves or thrombophlebitis. In these cases, the pulmonary circulation acts as a sieve for venous blood, with microorganisms lodging in the small vessels of the lungs to become the source of infection. Because bacteria are released in clusters from the source, they are likely to reach multiple parts of the pulmonary circulation simultaneously. Hematogenous pneumonia is, therefore, often multifocal and affects the peripheral regions of the lungs.

Patients with infectious pneumonia often present with cough, sputum production, fever, and dyspnea, and, less frequently, with pleuritic chest pain and hemoptysis. However, pneumonitis resulting from noninfectious etiologies, such as malignancy, pulmonary hemorrhage, and drugs can also present with similar symptoms. Certain clinical and radiographic features may suggest specific organisms as the cause of pneumonia. These are discussed in subsequent chapters. In practice, however, such features are often nonspecific and empirical treatment is usually necessary until a definitive diagnosis can be made. Targeted, empiric therapy is a critical principal of pneumonia therapy, highlighting the importance of taking a thorough history of all patients presenting with pneumonia. Historical factors including contacts, geographic location, occupation, travel, habits, hobbies, exposures, specific presenting symptoms, and duration of symptoms should be considered when making empiric antimicrobial choices.

Empiric therapy is generally successful in treating outpatients and, therefore, routine microbiologic testing is not necessary in this population. Most hospitalized patients are also treated empirically without documenting a specific etiologic diagnosis. In hospitalized patients, sputum samples obtained are frequently inadequate. Therefore, the Infectious Diseases Society of America/American Thoracic Society (IDSA/ATS) consensus guidelines recommend that pretreatment sputum Gram stain and culture of sputum only be performed if good quality sputum can be obtained and if hospitalized patients have specific risk factors, such as ICU admission, prior failure of empiric therapy, severe underlying structural lung disease, or immunocompromise. Although Medicare expects facilities to perform blood cultures before administering antibiotics on all patients admitted to the ICU, the clinical value of this inpatient quality reporting measure is controversial.

Numerous noninvasive diagnostic methods are now available to assist with the determination of causative agents in pneumonia, such as sputum direct fluorescence antibody tests (e.g., *Pneumocystis jirovecii, Legionella* species), urinary antigen testing (e.g., *Legionella pneumophila,*

S. pneumonia), serum serologic testing (e.g., *Coccidioidomycosis*), and singleplex and real-time multiplex PCR assays for specific bacterial and viral pathogens. The choice of diagnostic tests should be tailored to the organisms suspected and based on history, clinical and radiographic presentation, and disease course. The frequency of mixed viralbacterial infections and the interactions between these pathogens remain an area of active investigation. There is increasing interest in the use of inflammatory biologic markers in an attempt to distinguish between bacterial and nonbacterial causes of pneumonia. The two most promising are procalcitonin and C-reactive protein.

Invasive testing may be necessary in selected pneumonia cases to improve diagnostic yield when noninvasive testing is unrevealing or the patient is at high risk for multiple opportunistic pathogens, making empiric antimicrobial choices challenging. Flexible fiberoptic bronchoscopy is probably the most common invasive procedure used to diagnose pneumonia. It is particularly useful in patients unable to produce a satisfactory sputum sample. It allows direct sampling of distal airway secretions from selected bronchial segments that correspond to the changes on chest radiographs. Samples can be obtained by either simple washing of a bronchial segment or bronchial alveolar lavage (BAL). Because of potential contamination while passing through the upper airways, a protected brush specimen (PBS) is sometimes obtained. In most cases of bacterial pneumonia, bronchoscopy does not appear to provide any significant advantage over the noninvasive techniques in making a definitive bacterial identification. Some investigators believe that semiquantitative culture by bronchoscopy, defined as PBS greater than 10^3 or BAL greater than 10^4 or 10^5 colony forming units/mL, may improve the diagnostic yield. These results may be affected by prior antibiotic administration, operator skill, and laboratory support. At this time, routine use of PBS or BAL is not recommended. Bronchoscopy does have a role in identifying infection in several conditions, such as tuberculosis when there is a strong clinical suspicion despite negative expectorated sputum, and when there is a clinical suspicion of multiple potential opportunistic organisms in immunocompromised patients. In addition, bronchoscopy allows for direct visualization of the airways and can be useful when bronchial obstruction is suspected. Transbronchial biopsy is rarely indicated in infectious pneumonia, although it may be valuable in distinguishing colonization from invasive disease by demonstrating tissue invasion with microorganisms such as *Aspergillus* species or cytomegalovirus. Bronchoscopy also has been used to diagnose noninfectious causes of pneumonitis. Other invasive techniques to bypass the upper airways, such as percutaneous transthoracic lung aspiration and transtracheal aspiration, have fallen out of favor due to poor specificity and complication risks. Open lung biopsy, by minithoracotomy or thoracoscopy, can provide adequate tissue for histologic examination, but the risks and discomfort of the procedure limit its clinical usefulness. It is typically used in cases of unresolved pneumonia, in which a noninfectious cause or an atypical organism is suspected.

One of the most important treatment decisions in outpatients with pneumonia is whether or not to admit the patient to the hospital and whether that patient requires ICU admission. Several indices and risk stratification methods exist to assist the clinician in making this decision. The most commonly used are the Pneumonia Severity Index (PSI) and CURB-65. They have both been validated and demonstrate reasonable ability to predict 30-day mortality. The PSI, derived and validated as part of the Pneumonia Patient Outcomes Research Team (PORT) study, uses 20 different variables including age, comorbidities, and other clinical variables, and then stratifies patients into five mortality risk classes with associated recommendations for hospitalization. The number of variables and complexity of the scoring can make it difficult to use in the clinical setting. The CURB-65 is modified from British Thoracic Society (BTS) criteria (Confusion, Uremia, Respiratory rate, low BP, age 65 or greater). It is scored by assigning one point for each component. A simplified version is the CRB-65, for use in the event blood urea nitrogen (BUN) is not measured. The 2007 IDSA/ATS consensus statement recommends using the PSI and delineated major and minor criteria for patients admitted with pneumonia to determine who requires ICU admission. The BTS guidelines published in 2009 recommend using the CRB-65. Regardless of the rules utilized, all are intended to supplement and not replace or override the clinician's judgment. The use of procalcitonin (PCT) levels has shown promise in risk stratification for bacterial but not viral pneumonias, and may complement the aforementioned prediction rules with rising PCT correlated with more severe pneumonia and declining levels associated with a better prognosis.

Antimicrobial treatment of pneumonia is typically initiated with an empiric regimen based on the most likely pathogens. Early administration of appropriate antibiotics necessitates assessing the patient's risk of virulent and healthcare acquired infections, atypical or opportunistic pathogens, and resistant organisms. Local and regional patterns of antimicrobial resistance, often reported in antibiograms, provide valuable information to optimize treatment of suspected bacterial pneumonias and minimize inappropriate antimicrobial utilization.

Therapeutic options for outpatients with CAP include respiratory macrolides, beta lactams, doxycycline, and the respiratory fluoroquinolones. The BTS differs from IDSA/ATS and recommends against covering atypical pathogens in patients with low-severity CAP, and reserving fluoroquinolone agents for second-line therapy. IDSA/ATS recommends that patients hospitalized with pneumonia should receive a beta lactam plus a macrolide or doxycycline or a respiratory fluoroquinolone as monotherapy. The BTS recommends the use of broad-spectrum beta lactamase, with clarithromycin added for severe CAP. Some studies have reported improved mortality with macrolide-based regimens and propose that this is a function of immunomodulatory properties of macrolides. HCAP is a distinct pneumonia subset associated with more severe disease, longer hospital stays, and higher mortality. The microbial etiology includes a higher percentage of methicillin-resistant *Staphylococcus aureus* (MRSA) and *Pseudomonas*; therefore recommended empiric therapy is broadened to include coverage of these pathogens. Despite numerous comparisons of different antibiotic regimens, the superiority of one class of medications or combination of medications is primarily dependent on patient-specific risk factors, allergies, drug susceptibilities, and severity of illness. The IDSA/ATS guideline recommendations for pneumonia treatment have come under scrutiny from recent literature suggesting that these distinctions may result in overtreatment in HCAP without any evidence of improved outcome. Due to increasing prevalence of resistant organisms, some have suggested the need for new guidelines to address both risk stratification and empiric treatment of the at-risk populations.

Although it is difficult to define the optimal duration of therapy with currently available data, the IDSA/ATS guidelines recommend CAP treatment for a minimum of 5 days. Longer courses are needed for patients who do not demonstrate clinical improvement in the first 2 to 3 days or have more complicated or unusual infections and sequelae, or significant comorbidities. Patients with VAP that responds to therapy tend to do so within 6 days; studies have shown that one can decrease the duration of therapy from 14 to 8 days without impacting outcomes. Regardless of the anticipated duration of therapy, all therapy needs to be reassessed, targeted, or de-escalated once the results of cultures and other diagnostic tests become available.

Timely administration of appropriate antibiotics to patients with pneumonia has been shown to improve survival in a number of populations, including elderly patients with CAP and patients with pneumonia and severe sepsis. Establishing guidelines for timeliness for all hospitalized patients with pneumonia has proven challenging. The Medicare value-based purchasing program includes a requirement to initiate timely and appropriate antibiotics to patients admitted with a diagnosis of pneumonia. However, the American Academy of Emergency Medicine position statement recommends against measurement of time to first antibiotic due to overuse of antimicrobials and inconsistent results.

Adjuvant therapies aimed at improving immune function and reducing inflammation and coagulation remain controversial. Corticosteroids, GCSF, protein synthesis inhibitors, and a variety of other immunomodulating treatments have been tried without notable differences in outcome. There are studies suggesting that statins, with their inherent anti-inflammatory properties, are associated with reduced risk of pneumonia, particularly fatal pneumonias, but this remains an area of ongoing investigation.

A variety of biomarkers have been used to guide and assist management of CAP. C-reactive protein (CRP) has been used in the evaluation of nonresponders to CAP treatment. Procalcitonin (PCT) has been used to guide management and suggested as a means to minimize antimicrobial exposure, but so far it has not been shown to impact mortality. Further investigation is necessary to define the roles of these biomarkers in the routine care of patients with pneumonia.

Response to therapy can be defined both microbiologically and clinically. Serial assessment of the patient and clinical data will guide treatment modifications and duration of therapy. Failure of the empirically treated pneumonia to respond to appropriate antimicrobial therapy is not uncommon. Factors contributing to lack of response include prior antibiotic therapy, presence of a resistant microorganism, presence of unsuspected organisms, complications of pneumonia (e.g., pleural effusion, cryptogenic organizing pneumonia), or incorrect diagnoses of pneumonia (e.g., CHF, acute lung injury, pulmonary embolism). Patients may also deteriorate as a result of underlying comorbidities that in and of themselves may increase adverse outcomes. In cases non-responsive to therapy, a systematic diagnostic approach that includes further evaluating the history for risk factors and additional radiographic, noninvasive, and possibly invasive procedures should be undertaken. It may be necessary to broaden antimicrobial coverage while awaiting results of additional cultures and diagnostic studies.

Prevention of pneumonia primarily focuses on decreasing or eliminating risk factors. The Joint Commission and Medicare have promoted some simple prevention strategies such as smoking cessation and vaccination. In addition, the bundle outlined by IHI for prevention of ventilator-associated pneumonias has been broadened and widely adopted in most intensive care units. The elements are aimed at minimizing time on the ventilator and reducing both micro-aspiration and bacterial colonization of the respiratory tract. The typical bundle currently used includes the orotracheal route for intubation, a new ventilator circuit for each patient and changing the circuit if it becomes soiled, changing heat and moisture exchanges every 5 to 7 days, a closed endotracheal suctioning system with subglottic secretion drainage, head of bed elevation, oral antiseptic rinses, and rotating beds. The CDC established new surveillance definitions in 2013 for patients receiving mechanical ventilation. The new definitions replace VAP and are designed to achieve two primary goals: (1) broaden the focus of surveillance beyond pneumonia including other common complications of ventilator care; and (2) make surveillance as objective as possible. It remains to be seen whether these new definitions and benchmarking capability will assist in defining the best prevention strategies for this challenging nosocomial infection.

FURTHER READING

1. Rello J, Chastre J. Update in pulmonary infections 2012. *Am J Respir Crit Care Med*. 2013;187:1061.

   An excellent, recent, concise, overall review of pneumonia.

2. Mizgerd J. Mechanisms of disease: acute lower respiratory tract infections. *N Engl J Med*. 2008;358:716.

   A detailed review of the pathophysiology of pneumonia.

3. Niederman MS, Craven DE, Bonten MJ, et al. Guidelines for the management of adults with hospital-acquired, ventilator-associated, and healthcare-associated pneumonia. *Am J Respir Crit Care Med*. 2005;171:388.

   An extensive, official, evidence-based guideline statement by IDSA/ATS on the management of health-care-associated pneumonia that has been widely accepted and utilized.

4. Mandell LA, Wunderink RG, Anzueto A, et al. Infection diseases society of America/American Thoracic Society consensus guidelines on the management of community-acquired pneumonia in adults. *Clin Infect Dis*. 2007;44:S27.

   An extensive, official, evidence-based guideline statement by IDSA/ATS on the management of community-acquired pneumonia that has been widely accepted and utilized.

5. Torres A, Rello J. Update in community and nosocomial pneumonia 2009. *Am J Respir Crit Care Med*. 2010;181:782.

   An update on the 2005 and 2007 IDSA/ATS guideline statements, reporting on new data since the guidelines were published and highlighting some of the areas of controversy, including comparisons with European societies guidelines.

6. Zilberg MD, Shorr AF. Healthcare-associated pneumonia: the state of evidence to date. *Curr Opin Pulm Med*. 2011;17:142.

   A recent update on healthcare-associated pneumonia, reviewing important large studies on HCAP that have been published since the 2005 IDSA/ATS guideline statement.

7. Ewig S, Welte T, Torres A. Is healthcare-associated pneumonia a distinct entity needing specific therapy? *Curr Opin Infect Dis*. 2012;25:166.

One of a number of excellent reviews that bring into focus the question of whether it remains appropriate to divide pneumonias into HCAP and community-acquired pneumonia.

8. Singanayagam A, Chalmers JD, Hill AT. Severity assessment in community-acquired pneumonia: a review. *Q J Med.* 2009;102:379.

A summary of the tools available for the assessment of community-acquired pneumonia severity.

9. Cilloniz C, Ewig S, Polverino E, et al. Microbial aetiology of community-acquired pneumonia and it's relation to severity. *Thorax.* 2011;66:340.

A study of 3,523 patients with community-acquired pneumonia in both ambulatory and hospital-based settings, evaluated the distribution of causative organism based on the clinical setting, the severity score, and outcome, and reported that some organisms are better predicted by the severity index than other organisms.

10. File TM. New diagnostic tests for pneumonia: what is their role in clinical practice. *Clin Chest Med.* 2011;32:417.

A very practical overview of the new tests available for diagnosing and guiding the treatment course of pneumonia.

11. Weyers CM, Leeper KV. Nonresolving pneumonia. *Clin Chest Med.* 2005;26:143.

A review of risk factors and diagnostic steps in the setting of persistent pneumonia.

12. Chopra V, Rogers MA, Buist M, et al. Is statin use associated with reduced mortality after pneumonia? A systematic review and meta-analysis. *Am J Med.* 2012;125:1111.

A review and meta-analysis of the impact statin use has on the outcome of pneumonia patients.

13. Bouadma L, Wolff M, Lucet J-C. Ventilator-associated pneumonia and its prevention. *Curr Opin Infect Dis.* 2012;25:395.

A review of the approaches to prevent the development of pneumonia in ventilated patients.

14. Wip C, Napolitano L. Bundles to prevent ventilator-associated pneumonia: how valuable are they? *Curr Opin Infect Dis.* 2009;22:159.

A review of the various elements included in the care bundles used to prevent ventilator-associated pneumonia.

15. Klompas M. Complications of mechanical ventilation—the CDC's new surveillance paradigm. *N Engl J Med.* 2013;368:1472.

A review of the CDC's surveillance definitions and program for ventilator-associated complications.

Airway Obstruction

Russell J. Miller, Gregory Matwiyoff, and John Scott Parrish

The evaluation and management of obstructive airways disease is the most common out-patient issue faced by pulmonologists. The initial evaluation requires a thorough and focused history and physical examination. Disease processes that cause airflow obstruction increase airways resistance since the flow of air is proportional to the change in pressure divided by the resistance (i.e., Ohm's law). Airway resistance can be increased by a variety of mechanisms such as retained material within the airways (e.g., localized foreign body, secretions, mucous plugs, endobronchial tumors), hypertrophy of airway walls (e.g., chronic inflammation, edema, or smooth muscle hypertrophy), external compression (e.g., malignancy, vascular sling, goiter), and loss of radial traction (e.g., emphysema). Table 33-1 lists the locations and mechanisms of the more common types of airway obstruction.

TABLE 33-1	Locations of various types of airway obstruction

Supraglottic Upper Airway
Pharyngeal abscess
Lingual and pharyngeal neoplasms
Obesity
Laryngocele
Laryngeal stenosis
Tonsilar hypertrophy
Angioedema

Glottic and Subglottic Extra Thoracic
Vocal cord dysfunction
Paraglottic neoplasms
Paraglottic hematoma
Laryngospasm
Foreign body aspiration
Laryngeal neoplasm
Subglottic stenosis
Tracheal neoplasm
Extrinsic compression from neck tumors and adenopathy
Extrinsic compression from great vessel vascular anomalies
Tracheomalacia
Goiter

Glottic and Subglottic Intra Thoracic
Tracheobronchial malacia
Infectious tracheobronchitis
Foreign body aspiration
Tracheobroncomegaly
Tracheobronchial neoplasms
Tracheobronchial granulomas
Tracheobronchial stenosis

Small Airways
Asthma
COPD
Bronchiolitis
Bronchiectasis
Pulmonary edema

Although asthma and chronic obstructive pulmonary disease (COPD) are the most common causes of airflow obstruction, many other conditions beginning in the mouth and affecting passage of air to the small airways (bronchioles 2 mm or less) may produce similar and sometimes confusing presentations. Typically, asthma is characterized by *intermittent* wheezing, chest tightness, and shortness of breath. In contrast, COPD typically presents with progressive chronic dyspnea, cough, and sputum production. Pulmonary specialists often are consulted by primary care providers to evaluate patients labeled with COPD or asthma who are unresponsive to traditional therapy. Although a lack of response may be due to suboptimal treatment, the patient's status may be due to incorrect diagnosis or unrecognized concomitant problems.

Spirometry should be the initial step in the evaluation of possible obstructive airways disease. A disproportionate reduction of FEV_1 as compared to FVC is characteristic of obstruction. Although "office spirometry" is increasingly popular, poorly performed spirometry may be deceptive and lead to over or under diagnosis of obstructive disease. For example, if exhalation is not performed vigorously, FEV_1 and FVC both appear diminished prompting misleading conclusions. It is crucial that patient demographics and clinical parameters are accurately accounted for when population based "normals" are used as a comparison. Spirometry of questionable quality or with clinically incongruous results should be repeated in a setting with properly trained technicians. The numerical values obtained with spirometry also may be misleading and a thorough visual review of flow-volume curves also is important in separating large from small airway obstruction. There are three classical appearances of a flow-volume loop that may alert clinicians to the presence of large airway obstruction and its probable location: (1) fixed obstruction, (2) variable extrathoracic obstruction, and (3) variable intrathoracic obstruction.

FIXED OBSTRUCTION

A truncation of both the inspiratory and expiratory limbs of the flow-volume loop should raise the suspicion of central airway occlusion. This can occur secondary to a variety of malignant and nonmalignant disorders causing either extrinsic or intrinsic narrowing of the central airway. Many patients with central airway obstruction from tumors or foreign bodies present acutely with obvious symptoms of impending respiratory failure. However, patients with slowly progressive disease may present with more insidious symptoms that can be misinterpreted as asthma or COPD unresponsive to treatment. In the absence of other associated pulmonary or cardiac pathology, dyspnea may be a late finding in these patients. In an adult, exertional symptoms typically indicate a tracheal diameter of less than 8 mm and rest dyspnea indicates a diameter of less than 5 mm. The suspicion for central airway obstruction may be raised if the history discloses a previous malignancy (which may recur in the central airway), prolonged mechanical ventilation (which may damage the tracheal wall), or inflammatory collagen vascular diseases (which may result in airway scarring). Although physical exam findings may be nonspecific, the presence of stridor, or unilateral wheezing, should always be taken seriously and prompt further investigation. In patients with evidence of obstruction, the absence of findings related to the small airways (prolonged exhalation, enhancement of wheezes during end exhalation, etc.) may also raise the suspicion for central airway obstruction.

Patients with acute and severe dyspnea should be assessed for impending respiratory failure from lack of a definitive airway. If airway control is compromised, it should be secured as quickly as possible. Paralyzing agents may lead to abrupt closure of a stenotic airway, and should be used only with extreme caution. Typically, intubation should be performed in consultation with either anesthesia or interventional pulmonology.

Plain chest radiographs are rarely diagnostic; therefore a computed tomography (CT) is the initial radiographic test of choice and should be performed with contrast to better define the lesion in relation to the surrounding mediastinal structures. A neck CT in addition to the standard chest radiograph should be considered to ensure adequate proximal localization of the obstructing lesion. Bronchoscopy plays a crucial role in the evaluation of central airway obstruction. It should be performed with caution, however, since contact with the stenotic airway may lead to tissue swelling and critical airway narrowing. In some cases, it is best performed after endotracheal intubation and definitive control of the airway, due to the potential for worsening airway compromise resulting from instrumentation and the use of sedative agents.

VARIABLE EXTRATHORACIC OBSTRUCTION

When truncation of the maximal inspiratory curve is seen, it should prompt suspicion for pathology in the trachea outside of the thorax. Although the expiratory limb should be normal in these disorders, the inability to take a full rapid inspiration before starting expiration can result in reduction in both peak expiratory flow and the FEV_1. There are multiple disorders which can result in this finding to include vocal cord paralysis/paresis (temporary loss of vocal cord function), malacia of the larynx or upper trachea, or functional vocal cord disorders.

Paralysis of the vocal cords can occur as a complication of prolonged intubation, surgery, or postradiation but can also be an indication of inflammatory disease such as rheumatoid arthritis or a neurological disorder such as Parkinson disease. This is in contrast to vocal cord dysfunction, which is a functional disorder that often mimics and sometimes coexists with asthma.

Inspiratory flow limitation is seen in about half of patients with vocal cord dysfunction, but spirometry is often normal. Direct laryngoscopy is essential for differentiating between true paralysis/paresis and inspiratory adduction as seen in vocal cord dysfunction. Patients with evidence of vocal cord injury or paralysis on laryngoscopy should be referred to an otolaryngologist promptly for further investigation. In regards to laryngoscopy for confirmation of vocal cord dysfunction, it is important to realize that paradoxical motion of the cords may only be present when the patient is experiencing symptoms. Exercise or voluntary hyperventilation may be required just prior to laryngoscopy in order to confirm this disorder. In patients with proven or suspected vocal cord dysfunction, triggers should be identified. Empiric treatment of gastroesophageal reflux disease, postnasal drip, and psychological evaluation are often helpful. Typically, a referral to speech therapy will provide significant benefit to patients with functional vocal cord disorders.

VARIABLE INTRATHORACIC OBSTRUCTION

When flow-volume loops show a sudden reduction of peak expiratory flow during the initial effort dependent portion of the forced expiratory maneuver, this indicates excessive central airway collapse. In normal individuals, the central airways will collapse partially on expiration, with bulging of the posterior membrane into the lumen. A greater than 50% collapse occurring during exhalation is, however, considered a pathologic degree of airway closure. Although excessive airway collapse can be asymptomatic, it often results in a characteristic barking cough, dyspnea, wheezing, and recurrent respiratory infections. There are two main causes of expiratory central airway collapse, which should be clinically differentiated. Tracheobronchomalacia is central airway collapse resulting from abnormal softening of the cartilaginous structures. It typically occurs in the setting of previous prolonged intubation, chronic compression from extraluminal masses, or cartilaginous disease such as relapsing polychondritis or chronic inflammation.

Excessive dynamic airway collapse, on the other hand, is excessive bulging of the posterior membrane in the presence of normal cartilaginous structural integrity. Excessive dynamic airway collapse normally occurs in patients with small airway obstruction such as COPD, and should not interfere with airflow which is predominantly limited by excessive resistance in the *small* airways. Differentiating between these two disorders can be difficult. Dynamic expiratory CT and bronchoscopy are both acceptable tools that can be used in a complimentary manner. Dynamic expiratory CT may quantify the degree of collapse and evaluate for associated extraluminal diseases. Typically, a greater than 50% collapse of the central airways is consistent with excessive airway collapse; however, there is some debate about this. A 2009 radiology study found that nearly 80% of normal individuals may collapse their central airways to this degree. On bronchoscopic examination, one can determine if the obstruction is confined to the posterior membrane (as would be expected in excessive dynamic airway collapse), or whether cartilaginous weakening of the anterior as well as lateral tracheal walls (suggestive of tracheomalacia) is present. In patients with excessive dynamic airway collapse, one should concentrate on treatment of the associated obstructive lung disease. In actual tracheomalacia or bronchiomalacia, noninvasive nocturnal ventilation may stent the airways open during exhalation. In patients with disease refractory to medical treatment, airway stents may provide symptomatic relief but are associated with significant complications. Symptomatic improvement after stent placement raises the possibility of permanent improvement with the more invasive, but potentially definitive, surgical tracheobronchoplasty.

Asthma and COPD are the most common disorders which result in increased resistance in the small airways (<2 mm). This occurs through a variety of mechanisms including destruction of alveolar support to the peripheral airways and narrowing of the lumen resulting from chronic inflammation. These, however, are not the only diseases which result in obstruction to flow in the small airways. There are numerous etiologies of small airway obstruction that can be uncovered by a thorough history and examination. The most common example is pulmonary edema in which bronchial edema narrows the airway lumina creating a "cardiac wheeze." A variety of less common disorders may cause inflammation and fibrosis of the bronchioles (bronchiolitis) and can mimic typical asthma or COPD. Obliterative bronchiolitis, most commonly associated with postlung transplant patients, can also occur after exposure to inhalational toxins (ammonia, toxic fires), industrial exposures (popcorn workers), in association with rheumatic disease, or can be idiopathic following viral infection. Another distinct entity called diffuse panbronchiolitis, which is an overlap syndrome between bronchiolitis and bronchiectasis has become increasingly recognized with associated sinus disease in patients of Asian descent. Bronchiolitis should be considered in middle-aged individuals without classic patterns of asthma or COPD who have rapidly declining, nonreversible reduction in FEV_1 and in younger individuals with toxic fume exposures presenting with new or progressive dyspnea. Since these disorders occur in the smallest airways that do not typically contribute to airflow resistance, spirometry can remain normal until the disease becomes advanced. Reduced average mid-expiratory flow rate (FEF_{25-75}) can be an early clue in the right clinical instance and should alert the practitioner to the possibility of these disorders, although this value alone is not sensitive or specific for small airway disease (see Chapter 3). In patients with normal spirometry and high suspicion for distal airway obstruction, forced oscillation testing can identify subtle increased resistance in the distal airway and may have a role in evaluation of symptomatic patients following industrial exposures. When small airway obstruction is being considered, end-expiratory high resolution CT may disclose mosaic attenuation. Often, the diagnosis is difficult to make solely with noninvasive testing and tissue biopsy is required. With the exception of postlung transplant bronchiolitis obliterans, transbronchial biopsy is rarely diagnostic and thoracoscopic lung biopsy is often needed to confirm the diagnosis of small airway obstruction.

FURTHER READING

1. Ernst A, Feller-Kopman D, Becker HD, et al. Central airway obstruction. *Am J Respir Crit Care Med.* 2004;169(12):1278–1297.

   This is an excellent review article for evaluation and management of central airway obstruction from prospective of the interventional pulmonologist. Included is a review of currently available bronchoscopic techniques. Included is a nice table summarizing the major clinical trials of airway stent placement for central airway obstruction as well as an algorithm for endoscopic management of central airway obstruction.

2. Murgu SD, Colt HG. Tracheobronchomalacia and excessive dynamic airway collapse. *Respirology.* 2006;11(4):388–406.

   This review coined the term "excessive dynamic airway collapse" and compares and contrasts this diagnosis to true tracheomalacia. Included is a section reviewing the pathophysiology of central airway flow limitation and a review of the currently available diagnostic and therapeutic treatments.

3. Miller RD, Hyatt RE. Obstructing lesions of the larynx and trachea: clinical and physiologic characteristics. *Mayo Clin Proc.* 1969;44(3):145–161.

   Original paper clarifying the three major patterns of central airway obstruction (fixed, variable intrathoracic, and variable extrathoracic).

4. Morris MJ, Christopher KL. Diagnostic criteria for the classification of vocal cord dysfunction. *Chest.* 2010;138(5):1213–1223.

   Detailed review of vocal cord dysfunction including potential etiologies clinical pearls followed by a proposed simple diagnostic criteria based on combination of clinical symptoms, laryngoscopy, and pulmonary function testing.

5. Maschka DA, Bauman NM, McCray PB Jr, et al. A classification scheme for paradoxical vocal cord motion. *Laryngoscope.* 1997;107(11, pt 1):1429–1435.

   An excellent review describing the organic as well as the nonorganic causes for paradoxical movement of the vocal cords.

6. Murgu SD, Colt HG. Complications of silicone stent insertion in patients with expiratory central airway collapse. *Ann Thorac Surg.* 2007;84(6):1870–1877.

   This report of 15 patients who underwent silicone stent placement for expiratory central airway collapse describes the immediate improvement in functional status as well as the typical stent-related complications that may result from the procedure.

7. Murgu SD, Colt HG. Expiratory central airway collapse: a concise review. *Egypt J Bronchol.* 2007;1(1):87–99.

    Provides a good review that contrasts excessive dynamic airway collapse (EDAC) with tracheobronchomalacia.

8. Boiselle PM, O'Donnell CR, Bankier AA, et al. Tracheal collapsibility in healthy volunteers during forced expiration: assessment with multidetector CT1. *Radiology.* 2009;252(1):255–262.

    Study looks at the wide variability of tracheal collapse in a normal subset of patients, and calls into question the criteria of 50% expiratory collapse which may lead to overdiagnosis of tracheomalacia.

9. Burgel PR. The role of small airways in obstructive airway diseases. *Eur Respir Rev.* 2011; 20(119):23–33.

    Reviews of the role of small airways in asthma and COPD. Reinforces our current limitations in knowledge in regard to the role of small airways in obstructive disease.

10. Oppenheimer BW, Golding RM, Herberg ME, et al. Distal airway function in symptomatic subjects with normal spirometry following World Trade Center dust exposure. *Chest.* 2007;132(4):1275–1282.

    This study looked at world trade center survivors with respiratory symptoms and found that impedance oscillometry (IOS) could detect reversible distal airway obstruction in many patients despite normal spirometry. This study reinforces the poor sensitivity of spirometry in ruling out small airway obstruction in patients with high pretest probability.

11. Allen TC. Pathology of small airways disease. *Arch Pathol Lab Med.* 2010;134(5):702–718.

    Provides an excellent review of the histopathology and classification of small airways disease.

12. Hogg JC, Chu F, Utokaparch S, et al. The nature of small-airway obstruction in chronic obstructive pulmonary disease. *N Engl J Med.* 2004;350(26):2645–2653.

    A review of pathologic specimens of small airways from patients with different stages of COPD.

34 Acute Hypercapnic Respiratory Failure

Timothy A. Morris

The principle function of the lungs is gas exchange; *hypercapnia* indicates severe compromise of this vital function. Although disease may substantially affect any of the functional elements of the respiratory system, the term *acute respiratory failure* is used only when gas exchange is so severely impaired that arterial hypoxemia or hypercapnia occurs. Hypoxemia may involve a multitude of respiratory and metabolic processes and may occur in the absence of hypercapnia. However, hypercapnia is more directly linked to inadequate gas exchange and dysfunction of one or more elements of the respiratory system (e.g., control of breathing, mechanical performance of the lungs, respiratory muscle function, lung parenchyma, and vasculature). Hypercapnic respiratory failure is often referred to as *alveolar hypoventilation* and nearly always involves some level of hypoxemia as well. Specific values of arterial Pco_2 ($Paco_2$) that indicate hypercapnic respiratory failure are not well defined, but most experts agree that a $Paco_2$ greater than 45 mmHg (in a previously eucapnic patient) reflects acute respiratory failure. In patients with chronic hypercapnic lung disease, a sudden increase of 5 mmHg or more of $Paco_2$ from a previously stable level represents acute hypercapnic respiratory failure superimposed on chronic respiratory failure.

DIAGNOSIS

The hallmark of acute hypercapnic respiratory failure is an elevated $Paco_2$. A rise in $Paco_2$ signals that pulmonary "clearance" of carbon dioxide is inadequate; that is, more carbon dioxide is being produced by body metabolism than what the respiratory apparatus can clear by ventilation. This relationship is defined by the equation:

$$Paco_2 = K \; \frac{\dot{V}co_2}{\dot{V}_A}$$

In this equation, $\dot{V}co_2$ represents carbon dioxide production; $\dot{V}_A$, alveolar ventilation; and K, a constant. An increase in $\dot{V}co_2$ secondary to elevated metabolic activity is almost never the primary cause of hypercapnia because the respiratory system usually can compensate for the higher ventilatory requirement. When other elements of the respiratory system impair alveolar ventilation, however, increases in $\dot{V}co_2$ (e.g., secondary to fever or sepsis) can contribute to hypercapnia. The central cause of hypercapnic respiratory failure remains inadequate alveolar ventilation.

Alveolar ventilation is a physiologic process described by the equation:

$$\dot{V}_E = \dot{V}_A + \dot{V}_D$$

$\dot{V}_E$ (the volume of gas expired per minute, or "minute ventilation") is a measurable quantity. The equation divides minute ventilation into two separate components: (1) alveolar ventilation ($\dot{V}_A$), which participates in gas exchange, and (2) dead space ventilation ($\dot{V}_D$), which does not. $\dot{V}_D$ also may be viewed as "wasted" ventilation, that is, ventilation that does not reach the gas-exchanging areas of the lung. Rearranging this equation,

$$\dot{V}_A = \dot{V}_E + \dot{V}_D$$

This way of considering alveolar ventilation makes it clear that hypercapnia may occur via two distinct mechanisms: (1) a reduction in minute ventilation itself (*absolute hypoventilation*), or (2) an increase in dead space ventilation (*relative hypoventilation*).

Although mixed forms of hypoventilation occur, the distinction between absolute and relative hypoventilation is useful in separating patients with hypercapnic respiratory failure into two major categories: those with normal lungs and those with intrinsic disease of the lungs. Patients with normal lungs manifest hypercapnia because of inadequate minute ventilation caused by abnormalities in respiratory control (induced by disease or drugs), neuromuscular disorders involving the respiratory nerves and muscles, or chest wall abnormalities. Lung function may be normal in this group. Patients with abnormal lungs manifest hypercapnia because of the increased dead space (wasted) ventilation associated with maldistribution of ventilation and perfusion. The net result of these derangements is inadequate carbon dioxide clearance, even though minute ventilation (and respiratory drive) is normal or increased.

Combined forms of hypercapnic respiratory failure occur occasionally, such as in a patient with chronic obstructive pulmonary disease (COPD) who receives sedatives or narcotics (e.g., for anxiety or sleeplessness, or because of a misdiagnosis of left ventricular failure). Similarly, excessive diuretic use or other circumstances may cause hypokalemia, hypomagnesemia, or hypocalcemia and impair diaphragmatic contractility. Somewhat controversial is the relationship of excessive amounts of supplemental oxygen to absolute and relative hypoventilation and acute deterioration of patients with chronic hypercapnia (discussed below).

Regardless of the pathogenesis, the consequences of hypercapnic respiratory failure are the same. All patients with acute hypercapnia have hypoxemia, acidosis, an increase in pulmonary vascular resistance, and dilatation of the cerebral vessels. Arterial hypoxemia is an inevitable consequence of hypercapnia because, as alveolar Pco_2 ($Paco_2$) rises, alveolar Po_2 (Pao_2) and therefore arterial Po_2 (Pao_2) must fall. The alveolar–arterial gradient ("A–a gradient") is a useful indicator of how much of a patient's hypoxemia is attributable to hypoventilation itself. The A–a gradient ($P(A a)O_2$) is calculated as

$$P(A-a)O_2 = PAO_2 - PaO_2$$
$$= \left[FIO_2 \times (\text{ambient pressure} - PAH_2O) - \frac{PACO_2}{0.8} \right] - PaO_2$$

At sea level, this equation becomes

$$P(A-a)O_2 = PAO_2 - PaO_2$$
$$= \left[FIO_2 \times (703) - \frac{PACO_2}{0.8} \right] - PaO_2$$

where PAO_2 is the alveolar oxygen pressure, PaO_2 is the arterial oxygen pressure, FIO_2 is the fraction of oxygen in inspired air, PAH_2O is the alveolar water vapor pressure (47 torr), and $PACO_2$ is the alveolar CO_2 pressure (which is equal to the $PaCO_2$). If hypercapnia alone is responsible for hypoxemia, the $P(A-a)O_2$ is not widened. If this difference is widened, hypoxemia is likely due to cardiopulmonary disease. For example, in acute respiratory failure induced purely by drug overdose, the $P(A-a)O_2$ might be normal, meaning that the hypoxemia might be fully explained by hypercapnia. However, if the patient has aspirated, zones of acute lung injury may create low ventilation–perfusion ($\dot{V}/\dot{Q}$) units leading to hypoxemia and an increased $P(A-a)O_2$.

ACIDOSIS

Acidosis is a direct consequence of hypercapnia, although patients with acute respiratory failure may have other reasons for acidosis. The severity of acidosis attributable to hypercapnia itself can be calculated using the equilibrium expression: CO

$$Ka = \frac{[H_2CO_3]}{[H^+][HCO_3^-]}$$

Rearranging the terms yields the Henderson-Hasselbalch equation:

$$pH = pKa + \log\left(\frac{[HCO_3^-]}{[H_2CO_3]} \right)$$

or

$$pH = 6.1 + \log\frac{[HCO_3^-]}{0.03} \times PaCO_2$$

The HCO_3^- concentration in this equation is the *actual* concentration in the blood, not the concentration reported in the typical chemistry panel, which is measured after all the CO_2 has left the serum. If the *actual* HCO_3^- concentration determined by the Henderson-Hasselbalch equation were normal, one could conclude that metabolic disorders are not contributing to the acid–base disorder. Although this might seem like a daunting mathematical task to perform at that bedside, a happy coincidence makes it quite easy. As it turns out, if the *actual* HCO_3^- concentration is normal, and the pH is between 7.0 and 7.5, the complicated Henderson-Hasselbalch equation comes very close to a straight line, with the formula:

$$\Delta pH = 0.008 \times \Delta PaCO_2$$

Within these limits, an acute change in $PaCO_2$ of 10 torr changes (in the opposite direction) the blood pH by 0.08. Changes in pH not predicted by this equation must be attributed to causes other than acute hypercapnia.

Regardless of the cause, alveolar hypercapnia, hypoxemia, and arteriovenous acidosis all contribute to constriction of pulmonary resistance vessels and an increased pulmonary arterial pressure. This can lead to a higher work requirement for the right ventricle and right ventricular failure. The same factors cause dilatation of cerebral resistance vessels and increases in intracranial pressure. For this reason, hypercapnic respiratory failure may manifest itself by symptoms such as disorientation, personality changes, coma, headache, papilledema, and asterixis.

MANAGEMENT

The primary goals of management in acute hypercapnic respiratory failure are to (1) prevent respiratory arrest in patients who are rapidly decompensating; (2) restore adequate gas exchange; and (3) treat the disorder(s) responsible for inducing respiratory failure. These goals can be pursued simultaneously.

Supplemental Oxygen

The development and worsening of hypercapnia strongly suggests that a patient's respiratory system is failing and dangerous degrees of hypoxemia are imminent. Under these circumstances, severe hypoxemia is the greatest danger to patient survival and requires immediate attention. In some cases of mild hypercapnic respiratory failure, supplemental oxygen alone may stabilize the patient. However, oxygen alone may not reverse the respiratory decompensation observed in many cases of severe hypercapnic failure. Furthermore, two potential risks are associated with the administration of high oxygen concentrations to patients with hypercapnic respiratory failure: respiratory depression and worsening of ventilation–perfusion mismatching.

The hazard of respiratory *depression* with oxygen delivery is confined to patients with hypercapnic respiratory failure in whom the normal stimuli to ventilation are compromised and in whom hypercapnia has been present for at least several days. In these patients, retention of bicarbonate leads to moderation of the acidosis that acute hypercapnia causes in both the arterial blood and cerebrospinal fluid—an acidosis that provides a strong drive to respiration. In acute hypercapnic respiratory failure, these drives are present and oxygen poses no depression hazard. In chronic hypercapnic states, however, particularly if the patient is obtunded or sedated, hypoxemia is the major residual drive to ventilation. Oxygen administration may blunt this drive; the patient ventilates less, and the $Paco_2$ rises.

More commonly in patients with COPD and other lung diseases, however, supplemental oxygen may cause the $Paco_2$ to rise even if the $\dot{V}_E$ stays the same or increases. The seemingly paradoxical decompensation during oxygen administration occurs because of worsened matching of ventilation and perfusion. Excessive supplemental oxygen raises the alveolar Po_2 in diseased areas of the lung that are normally not well perfused. In these areas, hypoxic vasoconstriction is a useful adaptation, which is reversed by the presence of supplemental oxygen. Blood flow to the diseased, poorly ventilated areas of the lung is increased. The increased perfusion to the diseased alveoli worsens ventilation–perfusion mismatching, leading to an apparent increase in $\dot{V}_D/\dot{V}_T$ and worsened hypercapnia.

Whatever the mechanisms, the fact remains that *excessive* oxygen administration to patients with chronic hypercapnia can induce hypercapnic coma and death. The problem can be worsened by sedatives, which should be used with extreme caution in patients with chronic hypercapnia. Although some oxygen therapy to relieve hypoxemia may be essential for patients with hypercapnic respiratory failure, it should be used judiciously in those with chronic hypercapnia. A reasonable goal of oxygen therapy in these patients is to obtain a Pao_2 in the 50- to 60-mmHg range, corresponding to an oxygen saturation of approximately 90%. In these cases, it is imperative to closely monitor the arterial Pao_2 and $Paco_2$ during therapy with oxygen.

Mechanical Ventilation

If supplemental oxygen fails to provide an adequate Pao_2 without inducing marked hypercapnia, or if clinical signs of respiratory decompensation are detected, the next step is use of a mechanical ventilator. This step is a major decision because it generally requires endotracheal intubation, may require sedation or paralysis, and makes patients totally dependent on a "closed system" and the personnel caring for them. Furthermore, this step exposes patients to new risks. Therefore, the decision to initiate mechanical ventilation should not be made until it is clear that simpler measures will not suffice. Despite intensive investigative efforts, no absolute criteria for intubation–ventilation exist. The decision still rests on an overall assessment of the individual patient, particularly the degree of hypoxemia and acidosis and, often, the response to a trial of nonventilator management.

A potential intermediate step to avoid intubation–ventilation in selected patients is the use of positive airway pressure through nasal masks or face masks, commonly termed "noninvasive mechanical ventilation." Noninvasive mechanical ventilation can be delivered as continuous positive airway pressure (CPAP), or it may provide different pressures during inhalation and exhalation (BiPAP). In selected patients, such as those with COPD and CHF, short-term use of noninvasive mechanical ventilation may avoid the need to control the airways with endotracheal intubation. Defining how often and in which patients noninvasive mechanical ventilation will be beneficial remains an investigative challenge.

Gas exchange aberrations pose an immediate risk to patient survival, and should be corrected. Prompt action must be taken to revert or avoid hazardous levels of hypoxemia, hypercapnia, and acidosis. Such levels must be defined rather arbitrarily, because coexistent conditions modify such definitions. For example, a degree of hypoxemia well tolerated by a young adult with a barbiturate overdose may be hazardous in a person who has recently sustained a myocardial infarction. In nearly all cases, however, Pao_2 below 40 mmHg is poorly tolerated by adults; these levels are commonly associated with cardiac arrhythmias and functional or anatomic abnormalities of the heart, brain, kidney, liver, and other organs. The dangerous effects of $Paco_2$ relate chiefly to the degree of associated acidosis. Thus, a chronically elevated $Paco_2$ of 60 mmHg with an essentially normal pH is not dangerous, whereas a sudden rise to 60 mmHg induces a potentially hazardous acidosis. In a patient with respiratory failure breathing without the assistance of a ventilator, a blood pH below 7.2 indicates imminent respiratory arrest, and available data indicate that the mortality risk rises with each decrement below 7.2. Once the risk of respiratory arrest has been minimized by intubation and mechanical ventilation, however, the levels at which hypercapnia and respiratory acidosis become harmful are more difficult to establish. Whereas acidosis itself potentiates the functional abnormalities induced by hypoxemia (such as pulmonary hypertension, cerebral vasodilatation, and depression of myocardial contractility), the level at which this occurs and the clinical consequences vary from patient to patient. For this reason, excessive attempts to lower $Paco_2$ in mechanically ventilated patients, by increasing minute ventilation at the cost of alveolar overdistention and lung damage, may not be necessary. To spare the lungs from trauma during mechanical ventilation, some experts use lower tidal volumes and respiratory rates, allowing the $Paco_2$ to rise to high (previously considered alarming!) levels. Within limits, this strategy of "permissive hypercapnia" is well tolerated by respiratory failure patients, provided that adequate blood oxygenation is ensured.

Underlying Causes

As the life-threatening alterations in gas exchange are being controlled, attention also is directed toward diagnosis and treatment of the disorder(s) that induced hypercapnic respiratory failure. In some instances, diagnosis of the precipitating disorder may determine decisions regarding institution of mechanical ventilation.

In patients with absolute hypoventilation (reduced $\dot{V}E$), the primary problem is usually readily identified and treated. For example, respiratory depression due to drug overdose may be treated with specific antagonists or by enhancing drug excretion using dialysis. Myasthenia gravis or myxedema can be treated with specific agents. In patients with Guillain-Barré syndrome, however, ventilatory support is required until the disorder runs its course.

Among patients with relative hypoventilation due to obstructive lung disease, therapy is directed toward the problems that caused acute deterioration in gas exchange. The most frequent reversible problems are accumulation of secretions, infection, and bronchospasm. As these abnormalities are resolved, the mechanical function of the lungs improves, ventilation–perfusion relationships return toward normal, and gas exchange is enhanced. In some patients, recovery depends on these factors alone. In others, the respiratory muscles may have become exhausted from hours or days of respiratory failure and mechanical ventilation may be necessary until they have adequately rested.

Symptomatic Treatment

Secretions are best removed by encouraging the patient to cough and by adequately hydrating the patient. There is little evidence that available "mucolytic" agents are of significant value. However, new agents with greater potency (e.g., DNase) need evaluation in this context. Hydration is best achieved by oral fluid intake; if this intake is not adequate, intravenous administration or aerosolization of water or both can be added. Sputum mobilization can be enhanced by chest percussion and vibration, and by instruction from a skilled respiratory or physical therapist. If necessary, catheters inserted by the nasal or oral route into the trachea can be used to suction secretions, or fiberoptic bronchoscopy can be performed.

The treatment of bronchospasm is an integral part of the management of most patients with hypercapnic respiratory failure associated with COPD because most patients have some degree of reversible bronchoconstriction (see Chapters 64 and 66).

Infection is a frequent cause and a common complication of hypercapnic respiratory failure in patients with COPD and other chronic lung diseases. Treatment with broad-spectrum antimicrobial drugs (ampicillin, tetracycline, trimethoprim-sulfamethoxazole, ciprofloxacin, and others) should be initiated on the presumption that infection is present. However, appropriate samples for smear and culture should be requested so that more specific therapy can be applied if indicated.

Corticosteroids are commonly given during the first few days of therapy, usually in high doses, to reverse airway inflammation and bronchospasm. Many clinicians initiate therapy with the equivalent of 100 to 125 mg of methylprednisolone on presentation, followed by about half this dose every 6 hours. Empiric trials suggest that such therapy has modest positive impact on the course of patients with hypercapnic respiratory failure. Unfortunately, large clinical trials comparing the effects of different corticosteroid doses are unavailable.

It is important to consider and search for other factors that may have induced hypercapnic respiratory failure, particularly left ventricular failure and pulmonary embolism, and attention to the patient's nutritional needs. Left ventricular failure may cause ventilation–perfusion aberrations due to alveolar edema as well as dysfunction of poorly perfused respiratory muscles. Cardiac ischemia is increasingly recognized as a reason for failure of some patients to wean from mechanical ventilation. Pulmonary embolism is common in patients with acute and chronic lung disease. In most patients who die with pulmonary embolism, clinicians had not suspected the diagnosis premortem, possibly because the characteristic signs and symptoms were attributed to other coexisting lung conditions (see Chapter 68). Many patients with COPD are malnourished; correction of nutritional depletion and avoidance of further depletion during a bout of acute respiratory failure may enhance recovery and forestall future episodes of acute respiratory failure (see Chapter 66).

The role of respiratory muscle performance and in respiratory control in the pathogenesis of hypercapnic respiratory failure has generated a great deal of research interest. Treatment for alterations of respiratory control is not yet available, but respiratory muscle performance may be improved by several proposed methods. Putting the respiratory muscles to rest may improve muscle performance in some patients with acute respiratory failure. Some patients have chronic respiratory muscle dysfunction and may benefit from pharmacologic therapy. Some physicians have advocated the use of theophylline preparations in this setting because these agents are known to modestly enhance diaphragmatic function.

COMPLICATIONS

Patients with hypercapnic respiratory failure are subject to complications associated with both respiratory failure and its treatment. Often such complications lead to acute deterioration in a previously stable or improving patient. Several common complications have been identified: (1) Cardiac arrhythmias of all types are common, relating to diverse factors including hypoxemia, wide swings in pH, electrolyte disturbances, and drugs that may be employed such as β-adrenergic agents, theophylline, and digoxin. (2) Gastrointestinal hemorrhage, chiefly from the stomach and duodenum, is frequent. Again, multiple factors may be involved, and the hemorrhage can be sudden and massive. (3) Pneumothorax occurs in a significant number of patients with respiratory failure, particularly among those who are mechanically ventilated. (4) Bronchial obstruction may occur due to thick, inspissated secretions or improper placement or obstruction of endotracheal tubes. Other complications include acute right or left ventricular failure (or both), pulmonary embolism, and convulsions from hypoxia or even alkalosis following sudden reversion of hypercapnia.

The patient with hypercapnic respiratory failure requires careful initial evaluation and close monitoring throughout management. Such patients are best cared for in a respiratory intensive care unit that is staffed by experienced personnel and properly equipped. In this environment, most patients can be stabilized promptly, decisions regarding the need to intubate and mechanically ventilate can be made properly, and therapy can be applied and monitored appropriately.

FURTHER READING

1. Dereune JP, Fleury B, Pariente R. Acute respiratory failure of chronic obstructive pulmonary disease. *Am Rev Respir Dis.* 1988;138:1006.

   An exhaustive review of the problem posed by acute respiratory failure in COPD, with more than 450 references.

2. West WW, Nagai A, Hodgkin JE, et al. The NIH intermittent positive pressure breathing trial: pathology studies, III: the diagnosis of emphysema. *Am Rev Respir Dis.* 1987;135:123.

   This large NIH trial has shed some light on the pathology of COPD and the value of certain interventions (including the nonvalue of intermittent positive pressure breathing).

3. Waldhorn RE. Nocturnal nasal intermittent positive pressure ventilation with bi-level positive airway pressure (Bi PAP) in respiratory failure. *Chest.* 1992;101:516.

4. Hill NS, Eveloff SE, Carlisle CC, et al. Efficacy of nocturnal nasal ventilation in patients with restrictive thoracic disease. *Am Rev Respir Dis.* 1992;145:365.

5. Strumpf DA, Millman RP, Carlisle CC, et al. Nocturnal positive-pressure ventilation via nasal mask in patients with severe chronic obstructive pulmonary disease. *Am Rev Respir Dis.* 1991;144:1234.

   References 3, 4, and 5 report on alternative approaches to intubation in patients with respiratory failure, employing other systems for enhancing ventilation.

6. Sassoon CS, Hassell KT, Mahuette CL. Hyperoxic-induced hypercapnia in stable chronic obstructive pulmonary disease. *Am Rev Respir Dis.* 1987;135:907.

7. Stadling JR. Hypercapnia during oxygen therapy in airway obstruction: a reappraisal. *Thorax.* 1986;41:897.

   These two papers emphasize that the mechanisms responsible for oxygen exacerbation of hypercapnia involve more than simple "blunting of hypoxic drive."

8. Aubier M, Murciano D, Lecocquic Y, et al. Effect of hypophosphatemia on diaphragmatic contractility in patients with acute respiratory failure. *N Engl J Med.* 1985;313:420.

   Hypophosphatemia is one of several electrolyte disturbances that may impair diaphragmatic function and lead to acute respiratory failure.

9. Wilson DO, Rogers M, Sanders MH, et al. Nutritional intervention in malnourished patients with emphysema. *Am Rev Respir Dis.* 1986;134:672.

10. Pingleton SK, Harmon GS. Nutritional management in acute respiratory failure. *JAMA.* 1987;257:3094.

    Two of many articles emphasizing that the nutritional status of COPD patients, in or out of acute respiratory failure, should not be neglected.

11. Frostell C, Fratacci MD, Wain JC, et al. Inhaled nitric oxide. *Circulation.* 1991;83:2038.

12. Rossaint R, Falke KJ, López F, et al. Inhaled nitric oxide for the adult respiratory distress syndrome. *N Engl J Med.* 1993;328:399.

    Inhalation of nitric oxide may improve ventilation–perfusion relationships by increasing blood flow to the best ventilated lung zones because of its pulmonary vasodilator activity. The potential clinical role of this new modality remains to be fully defined.

13. Anthonisen NR, Manfreda J, Warren CP, et al. Antibiotic therapy in exacerbations of chronic obstructive pulmonary disease. *Ann Intern Med.* 1986;106:196.

    New data dealing with an old question that indicates that antimicrobial therapy often helps. Sometimes "standard practice" is validated. But the controversy is not fully settled.

14. Bolder PM, Healy TE, Bolder AR, et al. The extra work of breathing through adult endotracheal tubes. *Anesth Analg.* 1986;65:853.

    One reason some patients do better when the tube is pulled.

15. Ishaaya AM, Nathan SD, Belman MJ. Work of breathing after extubation. *Chest.* 1995;107: 204–209.

    A well-performed series of physiologic experiments that suggests the opposite conclusion from the previous reference.

16. Albert RK, Martin TR, Lewis SW. Controlled clinical trial of methylprednisolone in patients with chronic bronchitis and acute respiratory insufficiency. *Ann Intern Med.* 1980;92:753.

    If you feel short-course steroids help, this paper validates your practice; if you do not, you will find fault with the paper.

17. Campbell EJ. The management of acute respiratory failure in chronic bronchitis and emphysema. *Am Rev Respir Dis.* 1967;96:626.

    Classic article emphasizing the rational administration of oxygen.

18. Rochester DF, Arora NS. Respiratory muscle failure. *Med Clin North Am.* 1983;67:573.

    An excellent review of the role respiratory muscles can play in hypercapnic respiratory failure and of strategies that may be useful in avoiding or moderating muscle fatigue.

19. Shapiro BA, Cane RD, Chomka CM, et al. Preliminary evaluation of intra-arterial blood gas system in dogs and humans. *Crit Care Med.* 1989;17:455.

20. Zimmerman JL, Dellinger LV. Initial evaluation of a new intra-arterial blood gas system in humans. *Crit Care Med.* 1993;21:495.

    References 20 and 21 review new approaches to monitoring of arterial blood gases with systems that do not require blood withdrawal.

21. Antonelli M, Conti G, Rocco M, et al. A comparison of noninvasive positive-pressure ventilation and conventional mechanical ventilation in patients with acute respiratory failure. *N Engl J Med.* 1998;339:429–435.

    Noninvasive ventilatory support may be a helpful adjunct to standard medical therapy in selected patients with respiratory failure due to exacerbations of COPD. However, the only COPD patients were entered into the trial, and patients appeared to require immediate intubation and mechanical ventilation were excluded.

22. Wysocki M, Tric L, Wolff MA, et al. Noninvasive pressure support ventilation in patients with acute respiratory failure. A randomized comparison with conventional therapy. *Chest.* 1995;107:761–768.

    Preliminary study suggesting that respiratory failure due to "non-COPD" causes was not as amenable to noninvasive ventilatory support.

Bronchiectasis
Kevin D. Shaw

Bronchiectasis is defined as an anatomic distortion of the normally tapering bronchi, characterized by persistent airway dilation, wall thickening, fibrosis, epithelial destruction, and failure to branch normally. The origin of the word comes from the Greek roots "bronkhos," referring to windpipe, and "ektasis," meaning a stretching out. Rene Laënnec, a French physician and father of the stethoscope, first characterized the condition in 1819. In 1950, Lynne Reid performed careful anatomic dissection in comparison to radiographic appearance of bronchiectasis on contrast bronchography, and described three separate but often overlapping morphologies. Since her work, bronchiectasis has generally been described as cylindrical, varicose, or saccular.

Bronchiectasis may best be considered an effect, rather than a cause, of pulmonary disease. It is almost always secondary to a state of chronic inflammation and repeated infections, which over time cause neutrophilic infiltration and subsequent destruction of the airway walls. A "vicious cycle" of bronchiectasis has been well recognized by many authors, and explains the persistence of symptoms and frequency of exacerbations: chronic airway infection leads to inflammation and airway wall damage with impaired mucociliary clearance, ultimately predisposing to further infection. Treatments for bronchiectasis are varied, and target each of these steps in the cycle.

Bronchiectasis is typically seen later in life, often in the fifth and sixth decades. Because bronchiectasis is a consequence of an underlying condition, investigation of the etiology should be performed.

PRESENTATION

Bronchiectasis can be identified in asymptomatic patients, and does not necessarily have a "classic" presentation. A patient may present with complaints of a chronic, wet cough, repeated episodes of chest congestion or infection, shortness of breath, wheezing, audible crackles, or hemoptysis. Physical examination may be notable for coarse crackles, occasional wheezing, a barrel chest, cachexia, and in severe cases, clubbing. Pulmonary function testing is frequently abnormal, with a mixture of obstructive and restrictive processes identified in mild cases. Severe bronchiectasis almost always presents with severe obstructive physiology.

Chest imaging is often diagnostic, but bronchiectasis may be missed on plain films. Contrast bronchography is no longer performed routinely, but had been used prior to computed tomography (CT) to define abnormal airway anatomy. Currently, high resolution CT scanning is the imaging modality of choice to identify and characterize bronchiectasis. Persistent airway dilation is the norm, often with surprisingly dilated airways seen near the periphery. On axial imaging, the "signet ring" sign is often appreciated: defined by an airway inner diameter exceeding that of the adjacent pulmonary artery, resembling a stone mounted on a ring. In addition, airway wall thickening, sometimes with adjacent fibrosis, may be found.

Radiographically, bronchiectasis can be divided into one of Reid's three categories. *Cylindrical* bronchiectasis is defined as persistent airway dilation in the medium-sized bronchi, and the absence of normal tapering that is expected as airways head toward the pleural surface. There are often near normal numbers of branching subdivisions of smaller airways when compared to controls. *Varicose* bronchiectasis is defined by its areas of airway outpouching and narrowing, similar to a varicose vein seen in cross section. *Saccular* bronchiectasis is characterized by large mucus-filled cysts, typically subpleural, which result from destruction and cavitation of normal bronchial anatomy. Although saccular bronchiectasis was originally thought to originate from the most distal bronchi, it is now recognized that the number of branching airway subdivisions in saccular disease is often markedly decreased, suggesting a proximal destructive process spreading into the distal parenchyma. Saccular bronchiectasis is typically associated with worsened symptoms, decreased lung function, worsened prognosis, and a higher incidence of *Pseudomonas aeruginosa* infection than the other two types of bronchiectasis.

The term *traction* bronchiectasis refers to the abnormally widened airways seen in the setting of parenchymal volume loss, as is often found in pulmonary fibrosis. Whether this is true bronchiectasis or pseudobronchiectasis is debatable, as these patients do not typically present with typical symptoms of chronic wet cough and do not exhibit similar airway pathology of chronic inflammation, repeated infection, and airway wall thickening. In acute pneumonia, similar volume loss secondary to consolidation can mimic bronchiectasis on chest imaging. This is also not true bronchiectasis, as it disappears with resolution of the pneumonia.

Microbes typically cultured from bronchiectatic patients include *Pseudomonas aeruginosa*, *Staphylococcus aureus*, *Haemophilus influenza*, *Moraxella catarrhalis*, mycobacteria (*avium/intracellulare* most commonly), and a variety of other Gram-negative organisms including *Escherichia coli*, *Klebsiella pneumoniae*, *Achromobacter xylosidans*, and *Stenotrophomonas maltophilia*. Fungi are also seen, most commonly *Aspergillus* species, *Scedosporium apiospermum*, or *Candida* species. It is important to differentiate bronchiectasis with colonizing fungus growth from allergic bronchopulmonary aspergillosis (ABPA), one of many potential etiologies of bronchiectasis. More recently, the virome of the bronchiectatic lung is being explored, with increasing importance placed on "top-down" suppression of bacterial growth by bacteriophage present in the airways.

Hemoptysis can be a particularly frightening complication of bronchiectasis for patients and practitioners alike. Patients may encounter flecks of blood only, or "massive hemoptysis" which is considered life threatening in nature. Because hemoptysis is difficult to accurately quantify, the definitions of "massive" often found in literature, ranging from 100 to 1,000 mL per 24 hours, are of limited utility. The source of bleeding is typically a bronchial artery, which has a higher mean arterial pressure compared with the pulmonary artery. In chronic or severe bronchiectasis, bronchial artery hypertrophy is often seen, which is a setup for more frequent and severe bleeding. Hemoptysis can occur while a patient is feeling otherwise well, but often presents in the setting of chest congestion, increased mucus production, and worsening dyspnea.

PATHOGENESIS

Bronchiectasis can be characterized as either diffuse or focal. Diffuse bronchiectasis is often the result of a systemic immunodeficiency, severe inhalation injury, or a congenital condition. Focal bronchiectasis may represent a sequela of prior infection or a singular insult. With focal disease, airway lesions such as tumor or foreign body may be considered, since bronchiectasis can occur in the setting of chronic infection distal to an obstruction.

The underlying mechanisms responsible for the development of bronchiectasis are similar amongst the recognized etiologies. Principal among them is the development of airway damage and inflammation, often resulting from an episode of airway infection. When an infection develops in the setting of obstruction, inflammatory airway debris cannot be efficiently cleared, predisposing to continued inflammation, epithelial damage, and repeated infections. Over time, this cycle of inflammation, obstruction, and infection leads to airway wall damage. Denuded airway epithelium, is often replaced by nonciliated, cuboidal, or squamous epithelium. Loss of basement membrane, smooth muscle, and cartilage integrity leads to tortuous, dilated airways, with thickened, fibrotic airway walls. Microabscesses may form within and alongside bronchial walls, causing further inflammatory and fibrotic damage, as well as airway obstruction. This abnormal airway anatomy with loss of ciliated epithelium predisposes to impaired sputum clearance and further cycles of infection.

The airway infections typically induce chronic *neutrophilic* infiltrates. The oxidative chemicals released during chronic neutrophil activation play a principle role in the subsequent airway wall trauma. Neutrophil chemotactic factors including interleukin-8, leukotriene B4, and tumor necrosis factor-alpha lead to increased neutrophil infiltration. Release of neutrophil-derived toxic products such as elastase and matrix metalloproteinases results in destruction of basement membrane collagen, elastin, and proteoglycan support molecules with subsequent loss of airway wall integrity. Bronchoalveolar lavage studies have demonstrated increased levels of these chemotactic and toxic factors. Sputum elastase concentration has been correlated with decreased lung function and increased cytokine expression.

A multitude of underlying etiologies have been identified. The most common cause of bronchiectasis is prior lung infection, historically attributed to tuberculosis, measles, or pertussis. These are typically childhood infections, with the ultimate development of bronchiectasis often recognized many years later. However, any necrotizing pneumonia, bacterial or viral, can result in bronchiectasis. Common responsible bacterial pathogens include *Streptococcus pneumoniae*, *Staphylococcus aureus*, *Klebsiella pneumoniae*, and *Pseudomonas aeruginosa*. Diffuse postinfectious bronchiectasis is typically related to repeated episodes of pneumonia, although may be due to a single, severe, multifocal episode.

Although bronchiectasis is often characterized as "idiopathic," a careful history may identify prior infections in many patients. In a study performed in Tyler, Texas, 70% of patients were able to identify a lung injury prior to development of bronchiectasis. Of these patients, greater than 50% identified a prior lung infection as the inciting event. In the older population, or those prone to dysphagia, chronic aspiration should be ruled out, especially if the bronchiectasis appears radiographically in the dependent portions of the lungs.

Granulomatous lung diseases, including mycobacterial disease, sarcoidosis, and fungal lung infections are frequent causes of bronchiectasis. Mycobacterial disease is often associated with predominantly right middle lobe and lingular bronchiectasis. In nonsmoking Caucasian women over age 50, there is a relatively increased incidence of right middle lobe or "Lady Windermere" syndrome, often attributed to the right middle lobe's "fish mouth" orifice and impaired drainage. Chest imaging often shows bronchiectasis with nodules and "tree-in-bud" opacities in these segments. Sarcoidosis and granulomatous fungal infections can involve airway walls, leading to focal areas of obstruction and impaired drainage, with resultant chronic infection and bronchiectasis.

Cystic fibrosis is the most commonly recognized genetic disease predisposing to bronchiectasis. These patients typically develop varicose and saccular changes in all lobes of the lung, but with an upper lobe predominance. Another associated genetic disease is primary ciliary dyskinesia, which may present as Kartagener syndrome (situs inversus, paranasal sinusitis, and bronchiectasis). Due to immotile cilia, these patients experience repeated sinus and pulmonary infections, leading to the subsequent cycle of inflammation and airway destruction. Alpha-1 antitrypsin deficiency may also lead to loss of airway wall integrity, chronic inflammation, and development of bronchiectasis. Other less commonly recognized genetic disorders associated with bronchiectasis include Mounier-Kuhn syndrome (tracheobronchomegaly), Williams-Campbell syndrome (cartilage malformation in distal bronchi), and Young syndrome (sinus and pulmonary infections with infertility).

Allergic bronchopulmonary aspergillosis is defined as a chronic, destructive type III immune complex reaction associated with airway colonization with *Aspergillus* species. Radiographically, patients typically have central bronchiectasis and fleeting infiltrates associated with episodes of exacerbation. Diagnosis is based on symptoms, consistent radiographs, Aspergillus-specific precipitating antibodies or a positive Aspergillus skin prick test, and an elevated IgE level. For reasons that are not clearly understood, the incidence of ABPA is elevated in the cystic fibrosis population.

Immunodeficiencies, whether congenital (severe combined immunodeficiency, X-linked agammaglobulinemia) or acquired (HIV, stem cell transplant), may lead to bronchiectasis. Patients with history of splenectomy are also at increased risk. Chronic immunosuppression associated with a variety of autoimmune and transplant recipient states may predispose to lung infection, including nontuberculous mycobacteria, with resultant bronchiectatic changes.

A less commonly recognized cause of bronchiectasis is inhalation injury, such as exposure to industrial fires, ethylene oxide (used in gas-sterilization), or other toxic fumes. Bronchiectasis is recognized in 40% of patients with Yellow Nail Syndrome, a condition marked by lymphedema, pleural effusion, and dystrophic yellow nails. Autoimmune conditions including rheumatoid arthritis, ulcerative colitis, Crohn disease, Sjögren syndrome, and systemic lupus erythematosus are all associated with bronchiectasis, independent of tumor necrosis factor inhibitor use.

DIAGNOSTIC TESTING

The diagnostic approach to bronchiectasis is dependent upon symptoms, prior history, and physical examination findings. The workup is 2-fold. The first step is to confirm the presence of bronchiectasis radiographically. The next step in the bronchiectasis workup is to determine the underlying etiology and inciting factors, which relies heavily on history and radiographic features.

Although the chest radiograph may be normal in up to 20% of patients with established bronchiectasis, typical abnormal findings may include ring shadows from thickened and fibrotic airway walls, reticular patterns of fibrosis, air-filled cystic structures, and vascular crowding. In mild or moderate bronchiectasis, these findings may not be specific. High-resolution CT is currently the most commonly used and reliable modality for detecting and characterizing bronchiectasis. This allows confirmation of the bronchiectatic changes themselves, and may also reveal associated findings such as parenchymal nodules, airway tumors, foreign bodies, lymphadenopathy, or strictures that may give clues to the underlying etiology. Although contrast bronchography is seldom performed in the age of computed tomography, it is possible to reconstruct the airways using three-dimensional computer modeling. The images can provide a detailed look into the tortuous nature of varicose and saccular disease.

Depending on the history provided, additional testing may include genetic screening for cystic fibrosis transmembrane conductance regulator (CFTR) mutations, sweat chloride measurement, quantitative analysis of immunoglobulin subclasses, rheumatologic workup, lung biopsy, colonoscopy, purified protein derivative (PPD), interferon release assay, sputum culture, swallow studies, nasal nitric oxide measurement, or nasal mucosal biopsy for electron micrography of ciliary structure. Focal bronchiectasis typically merits diagnostic bronchoscopy to rule out endobronchial obstructing lesions such as teeth, foreign bodies, tumors, or broncholiths.

TREATMENT

Medical Management

In the stable patient, typical management focuses on bronchial hygiene. Airway clearance therapies can reduce sputum load, which improves lung function and reduces the frequency of exacerbations. There is limited data in the noncystic fibrosis population, so many therapies mimic those used for typical cystic fibrosis patients. Mechanical devices such as a flutter valve, intrapulmonary percussive ventilator (IPV), percussion vest, manual percussion, postural drainage techniques, or exercise alone have all been evaluated in cystic fibrosis patients, with no single method showing superiority. Typically, patients find the method that is most useful and practical for them, which also improves compliance.

Azithromycin is beneficial in cystic fibrosis patients who grow *Pseudomonas*. There are several small studies suggesting that it also reduces exacerbations and improves lung function in noncystic fibrosis populations. Other macrolides have been investigated with equivocal to mildly positive results. Inhaled hypertonic saline and dornase alfa are beneficial for cystic fibrosis, but may not benefit noncystic fibrosis patients. Dornase alfa actually showed harm in a population of idiopathic bronchiectasis patients: it increased exacerbation frequency and caused a greater decline in lung function. Other therapies such as inhaled mannitol and *N*-acetyl cysteine have limited data; but they may ultimately play some role in bronchial hygiene.

FDA-approved inhaled antibiotics for cystic fibrosis patients with *Pseudomonas* colonization include tobramycin and aztreonam. For the noncystic fibrosis population, inhaled tobramycin leads to reduction in *Pseudomonas* sputum density, but has not shown clinical benefit. Tobramycin has also been associated with increased wheezing, dyspnea, and chest tightness. These agents, as well as inhaled fluoroquinolones, amikacin, gentamicin, colistin, and inhaled cephalosporins have shown varying degrees of success, or are currently being investigated. Inhaled corticosteroids may improve spirometry and sputum quantity at high doses, but do not reduce frequency of exacerbations or long-term outcomes.

In the setting of an acute exacerbation of bronchiectasis, the mainstay of therapy is reduction of bacterial burden via systemic antibiotics. Traditionally, the choice of therapy is based on recent sputum culture growth, including sensitivity to specific antibiotics. It has become apparent recently that organisms cultured in the laboratory represent only a small portion of the diversity of the lung ecosystem. A specific sputum sample may characterize the population of only one lung segment, or may represent species with robust growth in culture that do not play a dominant role *in vivo*. For this reason, effective antibiotic treatment tends to be broad spectrum, typically with Gram-negative and anaerobic coverage. With mild exacerbations, oral fluoroquinolones can often be effective in suppressing bacterial growth and resolving symptoms. For severe exacerbations, prolonged intravenous therapy is commonly necessary. Often multiple agents, working by differing mechanisms, are required. Typical examples include a broad-spectrum β-lactam agent, combined with an aminoglycoside or fluoroquinolone.

For severe disease with quality of life implications, pulmonary rehabilitation has been shown to improve quality of life measures, dyspnea scales, and 6-minute walk distance. Results are generally comparable to those seen in the chronic obstructive pulmonary disease (COPD) population.

Surgical Management

Surgical interventions are reserved for unique situations where symptoms cannot be adequately managed with medical therapy alone. Focal or lobar areas of destructive bronchiectasis may be surgically resected in certain situations in order to prevent the spread of infection to surrounding lung. This is sometimes employed with isolated lobar mycobacterial infections. It may also be performed in the setting of frequent bothersome exacerbations attributed to a single area, with the intention of surgical cure. Prior to any surgical procedure, the airways merit bronchoscopic evaluation to rule out endobronchial obstruction.

Hemoptysis is typically managed conservatively as part of a bronchiectasis exacerbation, but may require more invasive interventions. Angiography of the bronchial arteries with embolization is employed for massive hemoptysis. In the absence of ongoing detectable blood spillage, the angiographer searches for abnormal bronchial artery formations as the source of bleeding. With diffuse bronchiectasis, there may be numerous malformations within the bronchial arteries, making localization a challenge. Preangiogram computed tomography or bronchoscopy plays a role in defining an anatomic location for bleeding, and may guide the angiographer toward the problem area. Massive hemoptysis which is not amenable to arterial embolization may require urgent surgical intervention with lobar resection in life-threatening bleeds.

Lung transplantation remains an option in patients with suitable functional status and end-stage bronchiectasis. With exceedingly rare exceptions, these are performed bilaterally, due to concern that the new organ would become quickly infected by a native bronchiectatic lung. Cystic fibrosis patients are the most frequent recipients of bilateral transplantation, and are third most common population to receive lung transplants. They tend to have better outcomes than most lung transplant populations, with survival of 62% at 5 years in one recent UK cohort. This may be attributable to their overall younger age at time of surgery, or the higher incidence of bilateral transplantation. Although there is limited outcome data in the noncystic fibrosis bronchiectasis population, transplantation has proven to be a viable option for many patients.

CONCLUSIONS

Bronchiectasis encompasses a wide range of congenital and acquired diseases processes, with characteristic resultant lung destruction. Management of clinical disease is based on the underlying etiology, which makes the diagnostic workup important. Combination therapies including bronchial hygiene and suppressive antibiotics, as well as management of complications such as hemoptysis have improved overall outcomes in both the cystic fibrosis and noncystic fibrosis populations. For end-stage disease, appropriate patients may pursue lung transplantation.

FURTHER READING

1. Laënnec RTH. *De l'auscultation médiate, ou, Traité du diagnostic des maladies des poumons et du coeur: fondé principalement sur ce nouveau moyen d'exploration.* Paris: J-A. Brosson, et J-S. Chaudé; 1819.

   Initial description of bronchiectasis, included in his text describing the novel technique of auscultation with a stethoscope.

2. Reid L. Reduction in bronchial subdivision in bronchiectasis. *Thorax.* 1950;5(3):233–247.

   Classic study comparing bronchography with pathology specimens in bronchiectasis. Established the terms cylindrical, varicose, and saccular to describe morphology.

3. Bachman AL, Hewitt WR, Beekley HC. Bronchiectasis; a bronchographic study of sixty cases of pneumonia. *Arch Intern Med.* 1953;91(1):78–96.

   Bronchography performed in 60 consecutive patients with acute pneumonia, of whom 25 showed bronchial dilation suggestive of bronchiectasis. This resolved in 11/16 followed with serial bronchography. Coined the term "pseudo-bronchiectasis."

4. Cole PJ. Inflammation: a two-edged sword—the model of bronchiectasis. *Eur J Respir Dis Suppl.* 1986;147:6–15.

   Landmark paper describing the "vicious circle" hypothesis for bronchiectasis.

5. Currie DC, Cooke JC, Morgan AD, et al. Interpretation of bronchograms and chest radiographs in patients with chronic sputum production. *Thorax.* 1987;42(4):278–284.

   Historical interest, discussing bronchography for diagnosis of bronchiectasis. High degree of inter-radiologist disagreement noted.

6. Slutzker AD, Kinn R, Said SI. Bronchiectasis and progressive respiratory failure following smoke inhalation. *Chest.* 1989;95(6):1349–1350.

   Case report of bronchiectasis following many years after severe inhalational injury.

7. Currie DC, Peters AM, Garbett ND, et al. Indium-111 labelled granulocyte scanning to detect inflammation in the lungs of patients with chronic sputum expectoration. *Thorax.* 1990;45(7):541–544.

   Interesting use of indium to correlate degree of inflammation and expectorated sputum volume in bronchiectasis.

8. Ramsey BW, Dorkin HL, Eisenberg JD, et al. Efficacy of aerosolized tobramycin in patients with cystic fibrosis. *N Engl J Med.* 1993;328(24):1740–1746.

   Early trial demonstrating improved lung function and decreased exacerbations using inhaled tobramycin in CF patients.

9. Richman-Eisenstat JB, Jorens PG, Hébert CA, et al. Interleukin-8: an important chemoattractant in sputum of patients with chronic inflammatory airway diseases. *Am J Physiol.* 1993;264 (4, pt 1):L413–L418.

   Interleukin-8 is an important neutrophil chemoattractant in sputum from bronchiectasis patients.

10. Nicotra MB, Rivera M, Dale AM, et al. Clinical, pathophysiologic, and microbiologic characterization of bronchiectasis in an aging cohort. *Chest.* 1995;108(4):955–961.

    Oft-cited bronchiectasis cohort, describing clinical, spirometric, etiologic, and microbiologic findings.

11. Mikami M, Llewellyn-Jones CG, Bayley D, et al. The chemotactic activity of sputum from patients with bronchiectasis. *Am J Respir Crit Care Med.* 1998;157(3, pt 1):723–728.

    Interleukin-8 and leukotriene-B4 from bronchiectatic sputum have additive effects on neutrophil chemotaxis.

12. O'Donnell AE, Barker AF, Ilowite JS, et al; for the rhDNase Study Group. Treatment of idiopathic bronchiectasis with aerosolized recombinant human DNase I. *Chest.* 1998;113(5):1329–1334.

    Dornase alfa resulted in increased exacerbations and greater lung function decline in idiopathic bronchiectasis patients.

13. Tsang KW, Ho PL, Lam WK, et al. Inhaled fluticasone reduces sputum inflammatory indices in severe bronchiectasis. *Am J Respir Crit Care Med.* 1998;158(3):723–727.

    High dose inhaled fluticasone reduces sputum inflammatory cytokine concentration.

14. Lynch DA, Newell J, Hale V, et al. Correlation of CT findings with clinical evaluations in 261 patients with symptomatic bronchiectasis. *AJR Am J Roentgenol.* 1999;173(1):53–58.

    CT severity of bronchiectasis associated with physiologic impairment. Saccular bronchiectasis is associated with Pseudomonas *growth.*

15. Tsang KW, Ho PI, Chan KN, et al. A pilot study of low-dose erythromycin in bronchiectasis. *Eur Respir J.* 1999;13(2):361–364.

    Small trial suggesting erythromycin improves lung function in non-CF bronchiectasis.

16. Barker AF, Couch L, Fiel SB, et al. Tobramycin solution for inhalation reduces sputum *Pseudomonas aeruginosa* density in bronchiectasis. *Am J Respir Crit Care Med.* 2000;162(2, pt 1):481–485.

    One of many studies showing decreased Pseudomonas *sputum density, with increased adverse reactions.*

17. Mitchell TA, Hamilos DL, Lynch DA, et al. Distribution and severity of bronchiectasis in allergic bronchopulmonary aspergillosis (ABPA). *J Asthma.* 2000;37(1):65–72.

    Central varicose and cystic bronchiectasis is seen in most patients with clinical diagnosis of ABPA, and few with clinical diagnosis of asthma. CT can expedite diagnosis in patients with suspected ABPA.

18. Pasteur MC, Helliwell SM, Houghton SJ, et al. An investigation into causative factors in patients with bronchiectasis. *Am J Respir Crit Care Med.* 2000;162(4, pt 1):1277–1284.

    Exhaustive attempt to determine the etiology of bronchiectasis in 150 patients, in which 80 (53%) remained idiopathic.

19. Roberts HR, Wells AU, Milne DG, et al. Airflow obstruction in bronchiectasis: correlation between computed tomography features and pulmonary function tests. *Thorax.* 2000;55(3):198–204.

    Degree of airflow obstruction is associated with radiographic bronchial wall thickness and decreased expiratory attenuation, and not degree of overt bronchiectasis.

20. Shum DK, Chan SC, Ip MS. Neutrophil-mediated degradation of lung proteoglycans: stimulation by tumor necrosis factor-α in sputum of patients with bronchiectasis. *Am J Respir Crit Care Med.* 2000;162(5):1925–1931.

    Human bronchiectatic sputum stimulates neutrophil-mediated degradation of rat bronchoalveolar proteoglycans. This is stimulated by TNF-α, and attenuated by anti-TNF-α antibodies.

21. Tsang KW, Chan K, Ho P, et al. Sputum elastase in steady-state bronchiectasis. *Chest.* 2000;117(2): 420–426.

    24-Hour sputum elastase correlates with sputum volume, sputum inflammatory cytokine concentration, extent of bronchiectasis, and degree of spirometric impairment.

22. Couch LA. Treatment with tobramycin solution for inhalation in bronchiectasis patients with *Pseudomonas aeruginosa*. *Chest*. 2001;120(3)(suppl):114S–117S.

Randomized study in non-CF bronchiectasis with subjective end-points, and a trend toward worsened lung function.

23. Prieto D, Bernardo J, Matos MJ, et al. Surgery for bronchiectasis. *Eur J Cardiothorac Surg*. 2001;20(1):19–23, discussion 23–24.

Review of 119 surgical cases for bronchiectasis complications. Few complications reported, with similar post-op lung function.

24. Barker AF. Bronchiectasis. *N Engl J Med*. 2002;346(18):1383–1393.

Excellent, though dated, review article.

25. Equi A, Balfour-Lynn IM, Bush A, et al. Long term azithromycin in children with cystic fibrosis: a randomised, placebo-controlled crossover trial. *Lancet*. 2002;360(9338):978–984.

Azithromycin improves lung function in a pediatric CF population.

26. Wolter J, Seeney S, Bell S, et al. Effect of long term treatment with azithromycin on disease parameters in cystic fibrosis: a randomised trial. *Thorax*. 2002;57(3):212–216.

First large trial using azithromycin in CF.

27. Saiman L, Marshall BC, Mayer-Hamblett N, et al. Azithromycin in patients with cystic fibrosis chronically infected with *Pseudomonas aeruginosa*: a randomized controlled trial. *JAMA*. 2003;290(13):1749–1756.

Azithromycin in CF patients with Pseudomonas *improved lung function and decreased exacerbations over 6 months.*

28. Davies G, Wilson R. Prophylactic antibiotic treatment of bronchiectasis with azithromycin. *Thorax*. 2004;59(6):540–541.

Small study using azithromycin in non-CF bronchiectasis. Benefit seen in exacerbation frequency and intravenous antibiotic use.

29. Dupont M, Gacouin A, Lena H, et al. Survival of patients with bronchiectasis after the first ICU stay for respiratory failure. *Chest*. 2004;125(5):1815–1820.

Initial ICU admission for respiratory failure in non-CF bronchiectasis is associated with high ICU and 1-year mortality.

30. Speich R, Nicod LP, Aubert J-D, et al. Ten years of lung transplantation in Switzerland: results of the Swiss Lung Transplant Registry. *Swiss Med Wkly*. 2004;134(1–2):18–23.

Cystic fibrosis accounted for one-third of all lung transplantations in this cohort.

31. Cymbala AA, Edmonds LC, Bauer MA, et al. The disease-modifying effects of twice-weekly oral azithromycin in patients with bronchiectasis. *Treat Respir Med*. 2005;4(2):117–122.

Small, crossover study suggesting reduced exacerbation frequency with azithromycin in non-CF bronchiectasis.

32. Kellett F, Redfern J, Niven RM. Evaluation of nebulised hypertonic saline (7%) as an adjunct to physiotherapy in patients with stable bronchiectasis. *Respir Med*. 2005;99(1):27–31.

Hypertonic saline may augment sputum clearance prior to airway clearance therapy.

33. Newall C, Stockley RA, Hill SL. Exercise training and inspiratory muscle training in patients with bronchiectasis. *Thorax*. 2005;60(11):943–948.

Pulmonary rehabilitation is beneficial in bronchiectasis. Inspiratory muscle training may help extend benefit following rehabilitation.

34. Scheinberg P, Shore E. A pilot study of the safety and efficacy of tobramycin solution for inhalation in patients with severe bronchiectasis. *Chest*. 2005;127(4):1420–1426.

Unblinded pilot study in non-CF bronchiectasis. Some QoL benefit seen, at the expense of high adverse reaction rates.

35. Tillie-Leblond I, Tonnel A-B. Allergic bronchopulmonary aspergillosis. *Allergy*. 2005;60(8): 1004–1013.

Excellent clinical and pathophysiologic review of ABPA.

36. Tsang KW, Tan KC, Ho PL, et al. Inhaled fluticasone in bronchiectasis: a 12 month study. *Thorax*. 2005;60(3):239–243.

Essentially no benefit seen with high-dose fluticasone.

37. Elkins MR, Robinson M, Rose BR, et al. A controlled trial of long-term inhaled hypertonic saline in patients with cystic fibrosis. *N Engl J Med.* 2006;354(3):229–240.

   48-Week trial of hypertonic saline in CF patients, demonstrating sustained improvement in lung function, exacerbation frequency, antibiotic use, and absenteeism.

38. Martínez-García MA, Perpiñá-Tordera M, Román-Sánchez P, et al. Inhaled steroids improve quality of life in patients with steady-state bronchiectasis. *Respir Med.* 2006;100(9):1623–1632.

   Minimal benefit to very large doses of inhaled fluticasone in non-CF patients.

39. King PT, Holdsworth SR, Freezer NJ, et al. Microbiologic follow-up study in adult bronchiectasis. *Respir Med.* 2007;101(8):1633–1638.

   Prospective survey of sputum microbiology in non-CF bronchiectatics. Pseudomonas was associated with increased sputum volume, number, and severity of exacerbations, extent of disease, and decreased lung function.

40. Martínez-García MA, Soler-Cataluña J-J, Perpiñá-Tordera M, et al. Factors associated with lung function decline in adult patients with stable non-cystic fibrosis bronchiectasis. *Chest.* 2007;132(5):1565–1572.

   Pseudomonas colonization and severe exacerbations are associated with rapid decline in lung function in non-CF bronchiectasis.

41. Anwar GA, Bourke SC, Afolabi G, et al. Effects of long-term low-dose azithromycin in patients with non-CF bronchiectasis. *Respir Med.* 2008;102(10):1494–1496.

   Retrospective analysis of low-dose azithromycin in non-CF bronchiectasis, suggesting clinical benefit.

42. Meachery G, De Soyza A, Nicholson A, et al. Outcomes of lung transplantation for cystic fibrosis in a large UK cohort. *Thorax.* 2008;63(8):725–731.

   UK cohort of 176 CF lung transplant recipients, demonstrating 62% 5-year survival and 51% 10-year survival.

43. O'Donnell AE. Bronchiectasis. *Chest.* 2008;134(4):815–823.

   Excellent review of bronchiectasis by an expert in the field.

44. Quast TM, Self AR, Browning RF. Diagnostic evaluation of bronchiectasis. *Dis Mon.* 2008;54(8):527–539.

   Comprehensive guide to the workup of bronchiectasis, with etiology-specific recommendations.

45. Sidhu M, Wieseler K, Burdick TR, et al. Bronchial artery embolization for hemoptysis. *Semin Intervent Radiol.* 2008;25(3):310–318.

   Excellent review of arterial embolization for hemoptysis. Short-term success approaches 90%. Recurrence rates are high, but better for bronchiectasis patients than for neoplasm or aspergilloma.

46. Arya AK, Beer HL, Benton J, et al. Does Young's syndrome exist? *J Laryngol Otol.* 2009;123(5):477–481.

   Updated discussion on the declining recognition of Young syndrome.

47. Cantin L, Bankier AA, Eisenberg RL. Bronchiectasis. *AJR Am J Roentgenol.* 2009;193(3):W158–W171.

   Radiology review of bronchiectasis.

48. Javidan-Nejad C, Bhalla S. Bronchiectasis. *Radiol Clin North Am.* 2009;47(2):289–306.

   Brief review of bronchiectasis etiologies with excellent representative imaging.

49. Kapur N, Bell S, Kolbe J, et al. Inhaled steroids for bronchiectasis. *Cochrane Database Syst Rev.* 2009;(2):CD000996.

   Cochrane review, little evidence to support routine inhaled steroids for adults with bronchiectasis.

50. Lynch DA. Lung disease related to collagen vascular disease. *J Thorac Imaging.* 2009;24(4):299–309.

   Excellent summary of collagen vascular disease and associated radiographic abnormalities by an authority in the field.

51. Mohd Noor N, Mohd Shahrir MS, Shahid MS, et al. Clinical and high resolution computed tomography characteristics of patients with rheumatoid arthritis lung disease. *Int J Rheum Dis.* 2009;12(2):136–144.

   Description of chest radiographic abnormalities in a small cohort of rheumatoid arthritis patients. Bronchiectasis appreciated in 18/63 (29%) of patients.

52. Hayes D, Meyer KC. Lung transplantation for advanced bronchiectasis. *Semin Respir Crit Care Med.* 2010;31(2):123–138.

    Up-to-date review of bronchiectasis, including workup and management, with concentration on transplantation.

53. Stafler P, Carr SB. Non-cystic fibrosis bronchiectasis: its diagnosis and management. *Arch Dis Child Educ Pract Ed.* 2010;95(3):73–82.

    Excellent review of pediatric presentation, workup, and treatment for non-CF bronchiectasis.

54. Bilton D, Robinson P, Cooper P, et al. Inhaled dry powder mannitol in cystic fibrosis: an efficacy and safety study. *Eur Respir J.* 2011;38(5):1071–1080.

    Phase III clinical trial. Inhaled mannitol improves lung function in CF patients.

55. Ong H, Lee A, Hill C, et al. Effects of pulmonary rehabilitation in bronchiectasis: a retrospective study. *Chron Respir Dis.* 2011;8(1):21–30.

    Retrospective study suggesting pulmonary rehabilitation improves functional status and quality of life in bronchiectasis. Outcomes persist similar to COPD cohort.

56. Rolla M, D'Andrilli A, Rendina EA, et al. Cystic fibrosis and the thoracic surgeon. *Eur J Cardiothorac Surg.* 2011;39(5):716–725.

    Comments and historical summary of surgical approaches to CF pulmonary complications.

57. Serisier DJ, Martin ML. Long-term, low-dose erythromycin in bronchiectasis subjects with frequent infective exacerbations. *Respir Med.* 2011;105(6):946–949.

    Exploratory study. Uncontrolled cohort suggests reduced exacerbation frequency in non-CF bronchiectasis.

58. Teper A, Jaques A, Charlton B. Inhaled mannitol in patients with cystic fibrosis: a randomised open-label dose response trial. *J Cyst Fibros.* 2011;10(1):1–8.

    Dose-dependent effect of inhaled mannitol for CF patients.

36 The Difficult Airway

Erik B. Kistler and Jonathan L. Benumof

INTRODUCTION

Endotracheal intubation can be lifesaving for the patient in need of a definitive airway. An endotracheal tube (ETT) provides a secure respiratory conduit from the outside environment to the airway, enabling ventilation, oxygenation, relief of airway obstruction, control of respiratory acid-base status, and protection against aspiration. However, endotracheal intubation is a potentially dangerous intervention, especially when attempted emergently with inadequate preparation, and should not be undertaken lightly. A patient requiring out-of-operating room emergent intubation should be considered as having a potentially difficult airway and treated accordingly.

PREPARATION AND ENVIRONMENT

Arguably, the most important modifiable variable in securing a difficult airway is preparation. Personnel capable of securing the airway as well as ancillary staff (i.e., nursing, respiratory therapists) must be available and a definitive plan should be in place. The American Society of Anesthesiologists (ASA) Difficult Airway Algorithm (Fig. 36-1) is a widely used schema and is included at the end of the chapter as an exemplary guide. Finally, it is imperative that

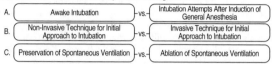

DIFFICULT AIRWAY ALGORITHM

1. Assess the likelihood and clinical impact of basic management problems:
    A. Difficult Ventilation
    B. Difficult Intubation
    C. Difficulty with Patient Cooperation or Consent
    D. Difficult Tracheostomy

2. Actively pursue opportunities to deliver supplemental oxygen throughout the process of difficult airway management

3. Consider the relative merits and feasibility of basic management choices:

    A. Awake Intubation — vs.— Intubation Attempts After Induction of General Anesthesia

    B. Non-Invasive Technique for Initial Approach to Intubation — vs.— Invasive Technique for Initial Approach to Intubation

    C. Preservation of Spontaneous Ventilation — vs.— Ablation of Spontaneous Ventilation

4. Develop primary and alternative strategies:

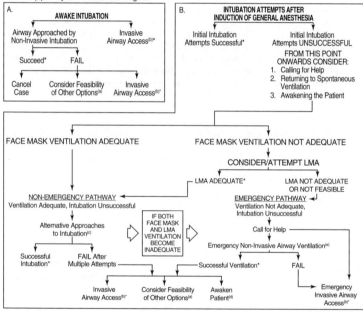

* Confirm ventilation, tracheal intubation, or LMA placement with exhaled CO_2

a. Other options include (but are not limited to): surgery utilizing face mask or LMA anesthesia, local anesthesia infiltration or regional nerve blockade. Pursuit of these options usually implies that mask ventilation will not be problematic. Therefore, these options may be of limited value if this step in the algorithm has been reached via the Emergency Pathway.

b. Invasive airway access includes surgical or percutaneous tracheostomy or cricothyrotomy.

c. Alternative non-invasive approaches to difficult intubation include (but are not limited to): use of different laryngoscope blades, LMA as an intubation conduit (with or without fiberoptic guidance), fiberoptic intubation, intubating stylet or tube changer, light wand, retrograde intubation, and blind oral or nasal intubation.

d. Consider re-preparation of the patient for awake intubation or canceling surgery.

e. Options for emergency non-invasive airway ventilation include (but are not limited to): rigid bronchoscope, esophageal-tracheal combitube ventilation, or transtracheal jet ventilation.

Figure 36-1. ASA Difficult Airway Algorithm. (From American Society of Anesthesiologists Task Force on Management of the Difficult Airway. Practice guidelines for management of the difficult airway: an updated report by the American Society of Anesthesiologists Task Force on Management of the Difficult Airway. *Anesthesiology.* 2003;98:1269–1277.)

equipment, including rescue options, be available for immediate use. A Difficult Airway cart that is stocked, accessible, and contains equipment familiar to the operator can be lifesaving.

RECOGNITION AND INTERVENTION IN THE DIFFICULT AIRWAY

Unlike scheduled operating room procedures where the patient's airway is carefully examined and comorbidities acknowledged and optimized, the patient with the difficult airway may present as a completely unknown entity, encountered for the first time in cardiopulmonary arrest. Therefore, it is not always possible to adequately assess the airway beforehand. Factors contributing to a difficult endotracheal intubation may be divided into anatomical and pathological categories. Anatomic factors are listed in Table 36-1. Pathologic factors such as an unstable cervical spine secured via halo stabilization devices or cervical collars, airway edema, blood, secretions and pus, and facial hair also contribute to the difficult airway. Every effort should be made to determine the presence of these risk factors as is clinically feasible. In general, earlier intervention should be considered if it is perceived that the airway may be difficult to manage.

The decision of when (and if) to intervene to secure the airway is often complex and involves a consideration of many different variables. These factors include but are not limited to patient oxygenation(SpO_2) in relation to the applied oxygen (FiO_2) as reflected by the difference in oxygen tension between the alveolus and arterial circulation (i.e., the A–a gradient), hypo- or hypercarbia ($PaCO_2$) in relation to minute ventilation and tidal volume, adventitious breath sounds, distended abdomen, fluid balance, use of accessory muscles of breathing, the patient's ability to speak in complete sentences, anxiety, and blood pressure and heart rate (as indices of Central Nervous System [CNS] activation). Sometimes it is the anticipated fate of other organ systems (brain, heart, liver, etc.) that determine when and if airway intervention is necessary.

TABLE 36-1	Components of the Airway Preoperative Physical Examination
Airway Examination Component	**Nonreassuring Findings**
1. Length of upper incisors	Relatively long
2. Relation of maxillary and mandibular incisors during normal jaw closure	Prominent "overbite" (maxillary incisors anterior to mandibular incisors)
3. Relation of maxillary and mandibular incisors during voluntary protrusion of cannot bring	Patient mandibular incisors anterior to (in mandible front of) maxillary incisors
4. Interincisor distance	Less than 3 cm
5. Visibility of uvula	Not visible when tongue is protruted with patient in sitting position (e.g., Mallambati class greater than II)
6. Shape of palate	Highly arched or very narrow
7. Compliance of mandibular space	Stiff, indurated, occupied by mass, or nonresilient
8. Thyromental distance	Less than three ordinary finger breadths
9. Length of neck	Short
10. Thickness of neck	Thick
11. Range of motion of head and neck	Patient cannot touch tip of chin to chest or cannot extend neck

This table displays some findings of the airway physical examination that may suggest the presence of a difficult intubation. The decision to examine some or all of the airway components shown in this table depends on the clinical context and judgment of the practitioner. The table is not intended as a mandatory or exhaustive list of the components of an airway examination. The order of presentation in this table follows the "line of sight" that occurs during conventional oral laryngoscopy.

(From American Society of Anesthesiologists Task Force on Management of the Difficult Airway. Practice guidelines for management of the difficult airway: an updated report by the American Society of Anesthesiologists Task Force on Management of the Difficult Airway. *Anesthesiology.* 2003;98:1269–1277.)

Depending on the etiology of the airway compromise, it may be beneficial and potentially lifesaving to attempt noninvasive techniques first. The patient should be optimally positioned, upright with the head-of-bed angled as high as possible, avoiding impingement of the belly on the lungs. This may require a less acute upright angle in obese patients (because of abdominal interference) compared to those of normal habitus. Supplemental oxygen and bronchodilator treatment are almost always indicated. "Noninvasive" mechanical ventilation modalities such as continuous positive airway pressure (CPAP) or bilevel positive airway pressure (BiPAP) can be effective in preventing respiratory failure in correctly selected patients. Hypercarbia and fluid-overload (i.e., CHF) are conditions most amenable to noninvasive airway interventions. However, if these interventions are ineffective, the airway should be secured without delay. Hypoxia, rarely resolves with noninvasive modalities, unless it is due to atelectasis alone. Diuretics and corticosteroids may have long-term benefit in preventing respiratory failure due to fluid overload and airway edema, respectively.

Proper Mask Ventilation Is the Bridge to Everything

An often neglected but vitally important airway skill is mask ventilation. Properly performed, mask ventilation can be lifesaving, requires only a mask, bag, and oxygen source, and may be continued indefinitely until a definitive airway is secured. Preoxygenation with effective mask ventilation provides a margin of safety for intubation. It is important that the jaw is brought to the mask rather than the mask crushed onto the face, and a seal maintained using the fingers of the left hand around the angle of the mandible and jaw. Oral and nasal airways may be invaluable in maintaining the patency of the naso- and oropharynx, especially in the edentulous and the obese. Straps around the head and attached to the mask can facilitate a seal around the face and be an invaluable adjunct. Occasionally two-man ventilation is required; in this case one operator maintains a two-hand patent seal of the airway and the other operator ventilates. When ventilating a spontaneously breathing patient, assisted breaths should be synchronized with those of the patient. In the nonbreathing patient, tidal volumes should be sufficient to provide chest excursion without overinflation and distention of the stomach. Ideally, each exhalation should result in an exhaled capnogram. (Capnography may be universally available in the future.)

Positioning for Optimal Outcomes

In addition to mask ventilation, correct positioning is another critical but often neglected aspect of airway management. Most patients presenting with respiratory compromise will be lying in a bed, which impedes optimal positioning. The patient's pillow should be removed and the head placed into a "sniffing" position with anterior flexion of the lower cervical spine and extension of the atlanto-occipital joint; placement of folded towels under the patient's head is probably the easiest and quickest way to accomplish this. Patients with cervical spine injuries require in-line stabilization without movement of the neck. For obese patients a ramp should be made under the patient that lifts the chest above the abdomen and the head above the chest, maintaining the sniffing position. Reverse-Trendelenburg positioning may be of help. The bed should be pushed away from the wall enabling personnel access to the head of the bed. Headboards and extraneous equipment (i.e., ortho bars) should be removed. If an awake fiberoptic intubation is considered, maintaining the patient as upright as possible is probably best.

Obtaining a Secure Airway

A secure airway is defined as a cuffed subglottic tube, either an ETT or a tracheostomy. Depending on the urgency of the situation, the definitive airway can be inserted while the patient is "awake" or "asleep." Both "awake" and "asleep" airways can be accomplished with direct laryngoscopy, fiberoptic intubation, or surgically. Techniques for these procedures are beyond the scope of this chapter.

The great advantage of securing the airway with the patient "awake" is that respiratory drive is preserved and the patient remains responsible for the vital function of respiration. The components of proper preparation for an awake intubation are patient psychological buy-in, drying of airway secretions (i.e., glycopyrrolate), topicalization (local anesthetic) and/or nerve block, and sedation. The importance of obtaining patient psychological buy-in to an awake intubation cannot be over emphasized, and it must be understood that adequate topicalization achieved by repetitive application of local anesthetic takes several minutes.

The awake intubation is usually accomplished fiberoptically. For fiberoptic intubation, the operator inserts a flexible fiberoptic bronchoscope loaded with an ETT into the patient's airway; proper topicalization is important in securing cooperation and optimizing intubating conditions. The "awake" patient also greatly aids the procedure by holding the airway open with "awake" competent pharyngeal muscles. Usually oral fiberoptic intubation is advocated because of the ability to place a larger ETT, and decreased risk of bleeding and infection in the upper airway compared to nasal fiberoptic intubation. Widely used conduits to the larynx include the pink Williams airway and the (intubating) laryngeal mask airway. Awake nasal fiberoptic intubation is an option in patients with limited mouth opening or otherwise nontypical oral structures. Nasal intubation may also be technically easier, as the ETT path from the nasal pharynx is fairly straight to the glottic opening. Note that the nasal passage will have to be adequately prepared with vasoconstrictors, local anesthetics, and dilating soft nasal trumpets. Nasal intubation is contraindicated in severe nasal or facial trauma and basilar skull fractures. Coagulation abnormalities represent a relative contraindication. Because psychological buy-in and topicalization cannot completely prepare the patient, some sedation is usually advocated in order to comfortably secure the airway for an awake fiberoptic intubation.

If "awake" intubation is absolutely contraindicated (e.g., outright refusal), or not indicated (e.g., airway assessed as "not difficult") the airway should then be obtained with the patient "asleep." Medications and dosing depend on the patient's hemodynamic stability, level of consciousness, and habitus (body mass), as well as the practitioner's experience. All drugs advocated for endotracheal intubation have benefits and drawbacks; among those most commonly used include etomidate, propofol, barbiturates, ketamine, narcotics, benzodiazepines, and dexmedetomidine. In addition to sedation, many practitioners advocate paralysis as well. This is the basis behind "rapid sequence intubation" (RSI), where a fast-acting neuromuscular drug is administered in conjunction with a sedation agent to achieve optimal intubating conditions in as short a time as possible. Classic RSI specifies the maintenance of cricoid pressure and holding ventilation until the ETT is secured in order to minimize the possibility of gastric reflux into the lungs. In practice, a modified RSI is often used, whereby cricoid pressure is held but the patient is gently mask ventilated until conditions are optimized. There are relative indications and contraindications (e.g., succinylcholine) to the use of particular paralytics; discussion of these is beyond the scope of this chapter. Chemical paralysis abolishes spontaneous respiration, making the patient dependent upon the operator for ventilation. Therefore, the practitioner must be able to effectively mask ventilate in order to assume this responsibility. Assuming ventilation via mask capability is at hand, it should be noted that successful intubation rates are higher in patients receiving paralytics in addition to sedation compared to those receiving sedation alone. An important caveat to the use of paralytics is that if direct laryngoscopy is unlikely to be successful, the patient should be intubated awake using fiberoptic intubation. If "asleep" fiberoptic intubation is to be performed, the Williams (pink) airway and laryngeal mask airway are excellent conduits to the larynx.

Once conditions are optimized, direct laryngoscopy is performed and the ETT is advanced through the vocal cords to secure the airway. Again, proper patient positioning in an optimal "sniff position" will facilitate this task. The "BURP" maneuver may improve visualization; this entails placement of pressure on the thyroid cartilage *B*ackwards (posterior), *U*pwards (cephalad), and to the *R*ight. Alternatively, guide devices such as the gum elastic bougie may be used.

ALTERNATIVE MODES OF SECURING THE AIRWAY

Direct laryngoscopy is not always successful in securing the airway, especially in the emergent situation. Therefore, an emergency backup plan should be formulated (as described in the ASA Difficult Airway Algorithm). Several alternative intubating techniques and devices are available; success depends on the operator's familiarity with them as well as their availability.

Among the many devices used to secure the failed airway, the laryngeal mask airway (LMA) is the most popular. It is easily placed and has a high success rate. However, the LMA is supraglottic and therefore does not protect the glottis nor the subglottic airway. For this reason, the LMA is not a truly secure airway. Also, the LMA is usually only sealed to approximately 20 cm H_2O; thus positive pressure ventilation may be difficult, especially in the morbidly obese or those with severely decreased pulmonary or chest wall compliance (i.e., severe pneumonia, acute respiratory distress syndrome [ARDS]). These limitations aside, the LMA can be lifesaving in the patient who otherwise cannot be intubated and is also an excellent conduit for fiberoptic intubation.

The video laryngoscope (e.g., GlideScope®) is a newer airway intervention modality that allows a view of the airway from the tip of the laryngoscope blade. These devices offer an excellent view of the anatomy and can be of immense benefit in the patient with a difficult airway. The learning curve is short (and intuitive), visualization is superior to the fiberoptic scope when the pharynx is filled with blood or secretions, and for those patients with decreased compliance and functional residual capacity (FRC) it may enable more rapid intubation than fiberoptic intubation. However, these devices are not a panacea for the patient with the difficult airway, and the novice should exercise particular care in depending upon them in the absence of a fundamental skill set.

Cricothyroidotomy is a measure of last resort when the airway is unable to be secured by other means. In order to be efficacious for the patient in need of a surgical airway, the surgeon must be called early, be fully gowned and gloved and the tracheostomy tray opened and functional. Percutaneous cricothyrotomy is a reasonable option if the operator has significant prior experience. In part because of the type of patient who presents with the failed difficult airway (large neck, anatomic abnormalities, etc.), an emergent cricothyroidotomy can be a high-risk, low-success procedure.

Verification of a Patent Airway

Except after fiberoptic intubation where the tube is directly visualized to be in the trachea upon withdrawal of the bronchoscope, indirect methods are used to verify correct ETT positioning. Although seemingly trivial, this step may be lifesaving, especially in the case of a difficult airway. In order to ensure successful endotracheal intubation, end-tidal CO_2 must be detected. While this is routine in the operating room, many ICUs are not equipped with end-tidal CO_2 monitors. However, portable CO_2 detectors (EZ Cap®) are widely available and should be used for all out-of-operating room intubations. Other methods to check for correct ETT placement include the esophageal bulb, fogging of the ETT upon expiration, and auscultation for bilateral breath sounds. These latter two methods are helpful in determining correct placement of the ETT but should not be relied on as sole indices of correct placement, and the practitioner should know the potential limitations of these techniques.

CONCLUSION

Endotracheal intubation can be lifesaving in the patient who requires a secure airway. However, out-of-operating room intubations are often difficult and can be fraught with peril. Successful airway management in a patient with a difficult airway demands preparation, prompt recognition of the difficult airway, optimal patient positioning, the ability to adequately mask ventilate, the proper use of "awake" and "asleep" conditions, alternative modes for securing the airway, and proper verification of the patent airway.

FURTHER READING

1. American Society of Anesthesiologists Task Force on Management of the Difficult Airway. Practice guidelines for management of the difficult airway: an updated report by the American Society of Anesthesiologists Task Force on Management of the Difficult Airway. *Anesthesiology.* 2003;98(5):1269–1277.

   This practice guideline is the cornerstone for difficult airway management. Although it may not be entirely applicable for out-of-operating-room airway management (awakening the patient is not usually feasible, for example), the ASA Guidelines present a framework for the decision-making process in the event of a difficult airway.

2. Schönhofer B, Kuhlen R, Neumann P, et al. Clinical practice guideline: non-invasive mechanical ventilation as treatment of acute respiratory failure. *Dtsch Arztebl Int.* 2008;105(24):424–433.

Deciding when to use noninvasive mechanical ventilation versus a secured airway in an emergent situation is one of the more difficult decisions a clinician can face. This article is an evidence-based practice guideline on when to choose one form of mechanical ventilation over another. As above, although not infallible, guidelines in this area provide an approach to optimal decision making practices.

3. Benumof JL. Preoxygenation: best method for both efficacy and efficiency. *Anesthesiology.* 1999;91(3):603–605.

A short and concise editorial that explains in detail the rationale and method for effective preoxygenation of the patient, and the amount of time available to the practitioner to secure the airway (the amount of time before the patient desaturates). A lot of valuable information in a short article.

4. McGee JP, Vender JS. Nonintubation management of the airway: mask ventilation. In: Hagburg CA, ed. *Benumof's Airway Management: Principles and Practice.* 2nd ed. Philadelphia, PA: Mosby; 2007:347.

A great resource in a classic reference; concise information included in the book, such as a table of the pros and cons of different supraglottic airway devices in this chapter, make this series a great resource for both in-depth research and as a quick reference guide. Wheeler et al.'s chapter on fiberoptic intubation is another standout in this book.

37 Occupational-Environmental Lung Disease

William G. Hughson

Occupational-environmental lung disease (OELD) describes a diverse group of conditions that are caused or aggravated by exposures in the workplace or environment; Table 37-1 lists some examples. Correct assessment of OELD requires systematic collection of data from multiple sources. Table 37-2 outlines the general approach to these patients, which begins with a careful review of the symptoms, with special emphasis on their relationship to patient activities. It is important to determine whether symptoms are worse at work and improve when away on weekends or holidays. Cigarette smoking and preexisting conditions such as asthma or allergies must be recorded. Nonrespiratory causes of dyspnea, including obesity or cardiac disease, should be evaluated as part of the general medical history.

A unique aspect of OELD is the crucial importance of the occupationalenvironmental history (Table 37-3); discovery of the correct diagnosis usually begins with sufficient attention to collecting and evaluating this information. It is essential to obtain a complete chronology of all jobs held by the patient. Many conditions (e.g., asbestosis) have a long latency between exposure and disease; enquiries limited to the current occupation may fail to identify the culpable exposures.

After a history is taken, a workplace or environmental cause may be suggested. Data are then collected to narrow the differential diagnosis. The physical examination should search for respiratory signs and for nonpulmonary causes of dyspnea such as heart disease and obesity. Chest radiographs are always important and can be central to the diagnosis of certain conditions (e.g., silicosis). However, the radiographs may be normal (e.g., in occupational asthma) or the findings may be nonspecific. For example, cigarette smoking increases the profusion of irregular densities in the parenchyma, confounding the diagnosis of asbestosis. Confusion can be avoided if the radiologist is a National Institute for Occupational Safety and Health-certified

TABLE 37-1	Examples of Occupational–Environmental Lung Disease		

Disorder	General Agent	Examples
Industrial bronchitis	Irritants	Gases
		Smoke
		Fumes
Occupational asthma	Chemicals	Isocyanates
	Animal proteins	Laboratory animals
Hypersensitivity pneumonitis actinomycetes	Biologic dusts	Thermophilic
Pneumoconiosis	Mineral dusts	Asbestos
		Coal
		Silica
Lung cancer	Mineral dusts	Asbestos
	Metal dusts	Arsenic
	Radiation	Radon

TABLE 37-2	General Approach to the Patient Suspected of Having Occupational–Environmental Lung Disease

Medical and respiratory history
    Symptoms (e.g., dyspnea, cough, sputum, wheezing)
    Smoking
    Past medical history (e.g., asthma, atopy, cardiorespiratory diseases)
Detailed occupational history (see Table 37-3)
    Physical examination
    Respiratory (e.g., wheezing, rales, rhonchi)
    Cardiac (e.g., coronary artery disease, congestive heart failure)
    Other (e.g., obesity, neuromusculoskeletal conditions, clubbing)
Laboratory data
    Chest radiographs (e.g., pneumoconiosis)
    Pulmonary function tests
    Special studies (e.g., serology, skin tests)
Industrial hygiene data
    Material safety data sheets
    Air sampling data
    Site visit
Research—literature review
Report preparation—disability evaluation
Prevention

TABLE 37-3	Essential Features of an Occupational–Environmental History
Chronologic list of all jobs, beginning with the first	
Job activities and materials used for each position	
Duration and intensity of exposure in each position	
Protective equipment (e.g., respirators, gloves, aprons)	
Adequacy of ventilation in workplace	
Activities and materials used by coworkers	
Health effects in coworkers	
Part-time jobs	
Domestic exposures (e.g., pets, hobbies)	
Chronology of disease in relationship to work or environmental exposures	

B reader experienced in OELD. Pulmonary function tests are used to determine the general pattern (e.g., restrictive or obstructive) and the degree of impairment. Exercise testing is often included to assess work capacity. Bronchial hyperreactivity can be identified using nonspecific agents (e.g., methacholine or histamine) or specific agents from the workplace. Special studies (e.g., skin tests, radioallergosorbent test assays) can be useful in identifying sensitization to workplace or environmental antigens. Invasive techniques (e.g., bronchoscopy, bronchoalveolar lavage, and open lung biopsy) may be necessary in selected cases.

After data have been collected from the patient, the focus shifts to the workplace and environment. Industrial hygiene information can be obtained from the employer. This includes material safety data sheets for all agents used by the patient. The employer is legally obligated to provide these safety data sheets, which describe each agent's chemical constituents and toxicity. In some cases, they can be supplemented with air testing data or results of previous inspections by government agencies. Often, the workers' compensation insurance company has information, including health effects in other workers. When possible, a site visit to the workplace can provide first-hand observation of workplace practices, ventilation, and personal protective equipment. Recommendations may then be made for additional air quality or other industrial hygiene testing. After exhausting all these sources, it is frequently necessary to perform a literature review concerning specific exposures and their known health effects. Consultation with experts such as industrial hygienists and toxicologists may be required.

Many cases of OELD involve litigation, and a formal report containing the clinician's opinions is needed for dispute resolution. The clinician may be asked to rate the pulmonary disability using systems such as the American Medical Association Guides to the Evaluation of Permanent Impairment or the Black Lung Benefits Act. It is important to become familiar with the relevant rating systems and to use appropriate terms when describing disability caused by OELD. Reports that are imprecise or do not contain the appropriate language cannot be used to provide benefits.

The issues of occupational exposure and subsequent disease in a particular patient may provide the basis for interventions or screening programs to prevent or identify OELD in others. Recognition of a specific risk factor for OELD has often begun with an unusual case report. If involved with patients with OELD, consider whether hazardous exposures or working conditions could be altered and make recommendations when appropriate.

FURTHER READING

1. Balmes JR. Occupational lung diseases. In: Ladou J, ed. *Current Occupational & Environmental Medicine.* 4th ed. New York, NY: McGraw-Hill; 2007:310–333.

   An excellent review chapter.

2. Cone JE, Ladou J. The occupational medical history. In: Ladou J, ed. *Current Occupational & Environmental Medicine.* 4th ed. New York, NY: McGraw-Hill; 2007:7–20.

   Includes websites for important databases such as Toxline and the EPA Integrated Risk Information System.

3. Greenberg GN. Internet resources for occupational and environmental health professionals. *Toxicology*. 2002;178:263.

   Gives Web sites for many important data bases providing information concerning hazardous exposures.

4. Guidotti TL, Abraham JL, Hughson WG, et al. Taking the occupational history. *Ann Intern Med*. 1983;99:641.

   Discusses how to take a detailed occupational history. Includes a one-page history form that can be completed by the patient.

5. Ling D, Menzies D. Occupation-related respiratory infections revisited. *Infect Dis Clin North approximately Am*. 2010;24:655–680.

   Comprehensive review of tuberculosis, SARS, and influenza in the healthcare setting.

6. Peden DB, Bush RK. Advances in environmental and occupational respiratory diseases in 2009. *J Allergy Clin Immunol*. 2010;125:559–562.

   Reviews recent data concerning allergens, approaches to immunotherapy, and methods to reduce risks for severe allergic disease.

7. Rom WN, Markovitz SB, eds. *Environmental and Occupational Medicine*. 4th ed. Philadelphia, PA: Lippincott Williams & Wilkins; 2007.

   Textbook that deals with all aspects of occupational medicine. Excellent chapters on occupational lung disease.

8. Sudhakar NJ, Godwin JD, Kanne JP. Occupational lung disease: a radiologic review. *Semin Roentgenol*. 2010;45:43–52.

   Comprehensive review article with excellent radiographic images.

9. Van Hee VC, Kaufman JD, Budinger GRS, et al. Update in environmental and occupational medicine 2009. *Am J Respir Crit Care Med*. 2010;181:1174–1180.

   Reviews recent data concerning air pollution and occupational lung diseases.

Solitary Pulmonary Nodule

Andrew D. Lerner and Samir S. Makani

A *solitary pulmonary nodule* (SPN) is a well-circumscribed spherical lesion completely surrounded by pulmonary parenchyma. SPNs may be distinguished from other focal lung opacities because (1) they are not associated with atelectasis, lymphadenopathy, or pneumonia; (2) they are not pleural or mediastinal based; and (3) they are less than 3 cm in diameter. Nodules larger than 3 cm are typically considered to be "masses," which are more likely than SPNs to be malignant.

Lung nodules commonly are diagnosed on chest radiographs and computed tomography (CT) scans. For example, up to half of smokers aged 50 or older may have pulmonary nodules on CT scan. More than 150,000 patients per year in the United States seek medical attention because of an incidental finding of a lung nodule on an imaging study. While many SPNs are benign, some may represent early stage (T1N0M0), bronchogenic carcinoma for which treatment has an excellent prognosis. Thus, it is important to determine which SPNs can be safely observed and which ones require diagnostic interventions or thoracotomy with resection. A comprehensive diagnostic approach is especially advantageous for patients at high risk for malignancy.

ETIOLOGIES OF SOLITARY PULMONARY NODULES

The two most common etiologies of SPNs are malignancy and granulomatous disease (e.g., tuberculosis, coccidioidomycosis, and histoplasmosis). SPN-associated malignancies are either primary lung cancer or metastatic disease. Bronchogenic carcinoma presents as an SPN in 10% to 20% of cases. Most malignant SPNs are adenocarcinomas, although squamous cell carcinoma, adenocarcinoma *in situ*, carcinoid tumors, and even small-cell carcinomas can present as SPNs. Approximately 5% of SPNs are metastatic lesions from other cancers such as colon, breast, kidney, testicular, sarcoma, or malignant melanoma. The possibility of discovering treatable cancer underlies the importance of prompt SPN evaluation and management, especially in patients with significant risk factors (e.g., smoking) or a previous history of cancer.

According to the large National Lung Cancer Screening Trial in 2011, 96.4% of SPNs identified in over 26,000 patients were false positive or benign. However, there is great variability in the rates of malignancy in patients with SPN, which depend on many clinical and radiologic factors. Benign nodules are typically infection-related granulomas, from tuberculous or fungal infections, or hamartomas. Less common causes include *Pneumocystis jirovecii* infection and viral infections (e.g., cytomegalovirus); both causes can appear nodular. Other less common causes include resolving pneumonia, lung abscess, pulmonary infarction, Kaposi sarcoma, pulmonary arteriovenous malformation, pulmonary contusion, pulmonary sequestration, Wegener granulomatosis, rheumatoid arthritis, mucoid impaction, dirofilariasis, and bronchogenic cysts.

CLINICAL AND RADIOGRAPHIC EVALUATION

Typically, an SPN is first detected as an incidental finding on chest imaging that was done for other reasons. The initial clinical approach is to identify risk factors that may help differentiate the presence of benign from a malignant nodule. A detailed history is an essential first step. It should include a smoking and occupational history, inquiry about previous cancer, and a detailed evaluation of the patient's home and travel environments (especially areas endemic for histoplasmosis or coccidioidomycosis). For example, nonsmoking, younger patients living in areas endemic for fungal disease are likely to have benign nodules associated with granulomatous disease.

A careful physical examination should focus on signs of other malignancies, such as melanoma, breast cancer, and testicular carcinoma. Unexplained hypoxemia may suggest arteriovenous malformation. Skin tests, interferon-gamma release assays, and serological tests for fungal infections can be helpful if tuberculosis or fungal diseases are suspected, especially in endemic areas.

Multiple imaging modalities may be used to evaluate SPNs, including posteroanterior (PA) and lateral chest radiographs, thoracic CT scans, and dynamic positron emission tomography (PET) scans. CT scans, especially thin-section studies, are cost effective and have become commonplace in the routine evaluation of SPNs. In fact, many SPNs are first detected and radiographically evaluated when patients undergo chest CT scanning for other purposes. Thoracic CT scans allow assessment of the nodule itself and of the mediastinum for potential lymphadenopathy. Inclusion of the upper abdomen allows the adrenals to be evaluated for metastases. Recent data also suggest the potential for use of serial CT imaging in high-risk patient populations for lung cancer screening (see Chapter 101).

Two radiographic features can be used with some degree of confidence to predict that a lesion will be benign: calcification and the absence of growth over time. An SPN is more likely benign if calcifications follow one of four distinct patterns: (1) central calcification; (2) ring or halo pattern; (3) diffusely speckled calcification; or (4) dense, irregular pattern termed *popcorn calcification*. It is noteworthy, however, that small, eccentric calcifications within an SPN can be due to malignancy that is embedded within scar tissue. Comparison of the SPN's size to the findings from prior images (if they are available) is an excellent way to estimate its growth characteristics.

Other radiographic features may be helpful as well. For example, clustering of multiple nodules in a single location tends to favor infection rather than malignancy. However, radiographic characteristics such as the shape, location, margins of the lesion, or presence of cavitation are unreliable for differentiating malignant from benign SPNs. Lobulation and larger size tend to be associated with malignancy, although these characteristics are not definitive.

PET imaging is a useful and noninvasive diagnostic modality for SPN evaluation. A pooled meta-analysis disclosed that the sensitivity and specificity of PET scanning for SPN-related malignancy are approximately 87% and 83%, respectively. Combination PET-CT is more sensitive for malignant nodules than CT or PET imaging alone. However, the sensitivity of PET scanning is low for nodules below 7 mm in diameter. In addition, false negatives may occur with tumors that have low metabolic activity, such as carcinoid tumors and adenocarcinomas *in situ* (historically called bronchioloalveolar carcinomas). This is due to the lack of a glucose-1 transporter, which leads to low fluorodeoxyglucose (FDG) uptake. On the other hand, false positives may occur with several nonmalignant etiologies such as active infections (e.g., tuberculosis and fungal etiologies) and inflammatory conditions (e.g., sarcoidosis and rheumatoid nodules). PET-CT findings cannot definitively confirm or rule out malignancy and should not be considered to be identical to a tissue diagnosis. Nevertheless, for low-risk patients with an SPN over 7 mm, a normal (no uptake) PET-CT has a high negative predictive value.

A special consideration is necessary when an SPN occurs in a patient with a history of malignancy. Tissue diagnosis may be a critical diagnostic step in those circumstances because conclusive evidence of metastatic disease may dictate further therapy. Pulmonary "metastatectomy" of the SPN may favorably influence survival, especially in patients with soft tissue sarcoma, melanoma, and colon cancer. On the other hand, an SPN can't be presumed to be metastatic in patients with a history of cancer, since there is a 50% likelihood that it will be either benign or a different, treatable primary malignancy. Metastatic disease is more likely if (1) the known primary tumor is an adenocarcinoma; (2) the lung lesion appears within 12 months after treatment of the primary tumor; (3) the patient is young and a nonsmoker; (4) the primary tumor was associated with metastatic lymphadenopathy; or (5) the location of the nodule is in the periphery or in the lower lobe. In the absence of known extrapulmonary malignancy, the SPN proves to be a metastasis in fewer than 5% of cases.

In summary, four clinical features are generally cited that suggest a benign etiology: (1) absence of growth of the nodule over a 2-year period; (2) absence of risk factors for cancer; (3) presence of calcium in characteristic patterns on imaging studies; and (4) age less than 35 years. Risks for malignancy increase with age, smoking history, and nodule size, although the probability for malignancy cannot be accurately based on any single characteristic.

MANAGEMENT
Surveillance Imaging

Management of patients with SPN includes balancing the goals of limiting the number of unnecessary lung resections for benign disease and expediting potential curative resections in patients with malignancy. This is especially important because of the relatively high survival rate of stage 1A non-small cell lung cancer compared with the high mortality of unresected cancer.

The clinical and radiologic factors described in the previous section help define the probability of cancer. The initial diagnostic and management decisions should be individualized based on the probability of cancer, as well as the patient's preferences, the patient's age, and other comorbid conditions. However, the 2005 Fleischner Society guidelines describe a useful standard management approach to SPNs in patients over 35 years of age. The guidelines recommend specific schedules for follow-up high-resolution CT scanning, and have helped decrease unnecessary imaging and radiation exposure. They were developed for SPNs that were discovered incidentally—not those that are associated with underlying disease or known malignancy. In those cases, follow-up is determined by two main factors: the nodule's size and the patient's risk for lung cancer. Risk for lung cancer is defined as low risk (minimal or absent history of smoking and of other known risk factors) or high risk (history of smoking or of other known risk factors). Size is determined by the widest diameter of the nodule. The recommendations are described in the Table 38-1.

Ground glass opacities (GGOs), although not technically classified as SPNs, warrant specific consideration. GGOs are CT findings of focal, noncalcified, veil-like opacifications of the lung, which do not obscure the vascular structures and do not yield air bronchograms. They are common nonspecific findings on CT scans, and represent a broad differential including pulmonary

TABLE 38-1	Guidelines for Follow-up of Lung Nodules
SPN Diameter and Clinical Risk of Cancer	**Recommended Follow-up**
≤4 mm nodule in a low-risk patient	No follow-up needed
≤4 mm nodule in a high-risk patient	Follow-up CT at 12 mo; if unchanged, no further follow-up
>4–6 mm in a low-risk patient	Follow-up CT at 12 mo; if unchanged, no further follow-up
>4–6 mm in a high-risk patient	Initial follow-up CT at 6–12 mo then at 18–24 mo if no change
>6–8 mm in a low-risk patient	Initial follow-up CT at 6–12 mo then at 18–24 mo if no change
>6–8 mm in a high-risk patient	Initial follow-up CT at 3–6 mo then at 9–12 and 24 mo if no change
>8 mm in a low-risk or high-risk patient	Follow-up CT at around 3, 9, and 24 mo, dynamic contrast-enhanced CT, PET, and/or biopsy
Nonsolid (ground-glass) or partly solid nodules	May require longer follow-up to exclude indolent adenocarcinoma or slow-growing carcinoid tumors

fibrotic disease, pulmonary edema, acute respiratory distress syndrome, and other pulmonary infections (i.e., *Pneumocystis jirovecii* and fungal pneumonias). Persistent GGO nodules, however, may represent malignancy, especially adenocarcinoma *in situ*. A recent retrospective study evaluated the management of GGO nodules with serial imaging and, in some cases, biopsy and resection. While approximately 90% of them resolved or do not grow during follow-up, those GGOs that grew in size or developed a solid component over time were highly associated with malignancy, specifically adenocarcinoma. Thus, surveillance imaging of persistent GGO nodules for up to 5 years may be necessary to evaluate them for the presence of slow-growing adenocarcinomas.

The decision to move from a "watchful waiting" approach with serial imaging to a more definite intervention is often based on changes in appearance or growth of the SPN. The growth rate of an SPN can be determined by measuring its doubling time (DT), which refers to doubling of the nodule's volume (not its diameter). DT is derived from the formula for a sphere: $V = 4r^3$, where V = volume and r = radius. For example, a 1-cm nodule that doubles in volume only increases 26% in diameter. A very slow (>2 years) or very fast (<7 days) DT suggests benignity, but this is not definitive.

INTERVENTION: BIOPSY AND EXCISION

SPNs greater than 8 mm found in patients with associated risk factors for malignancy, or nodules demonstrating interval growth, often require histopathologic evaluation. Diagnostic techniques include flexible bronchoscopy or percutaneous transthoracic needle aspiration. Occasionally, wedge resection is the initial procedure of choice for tissue sampling. The choice among the modalities is based upon several factors such as the nodule's size, location (central vs. peripheral), availability of the procedure, and local expertise.

Fiberoptic bronchoscopy can sample tissue by several different methods, such as standard bronchoscopy, navigational bronchoscopy, and radial endobronchial ultrasound (EBUS) bronchoscopy (see Chapter 7). Standard fiberoptic bronchoscopy is a useful approach for large, central lesions above 2 cm, with reported overall sensitivities reported up to 88%. Complications of standard bronchoscopy are infrequent and typically minor (major complication rate is <1%). Modalities used with bronchoscopy include forceps biopsy for visualized central lesions, washings, and brushings. Direct forceps biopsies provide the highest yields for visible endobronchial lesions (74%), followed by washings and brushings (48% and 59%, respectively).

The sensitivity of standard bronchoscopic approaches decreases with peripheral lesions and especially with smaller size nodules. Sensitivities of standard bronchoscopy for peripheral lesions less than 2 cm have ranged from 10% to 50% in various series. The performance of transbronchial biopsies under fluoroscopy increases the diagnostic sensitivity, as does increasing the number of biopsy passes. Current guidelines recommend obtaining up to six biopsy samples. Another feature that increases the yield of bronchoscopy is the finding of a *bronchus sign* on CT imaging (a bronchus extending to or contained within an SPN).

Adjunctive techniques to standard bronchoscopy include navigational bronchoscopy and radial EBUS. Navigational bronchoscopy uses an electromagnetic probe to help guide a catheter through the peripheral airways to the lesion. It is a valuable option for more peripheral lesions, but is performed only in specialized centers. Radial EBUS uses a small ultrasound probe at the end of a catheter that is inserted through a standard bronchoscope or extended working channel. EBUS allows for a 360° real-time ultrasound visualization of the peripheral airway and its surroundings. Navigational bronchoscopy and radial EBUS increase the positive diagnostic yield of peripheral lesions (up to 82%) with similar complication rates to standard bronchoscopy.

Transthoracic needle aspiration (TTNA), under fluoroscopic, ultrasound, or CT guidance, should be considered for peripheral nodules that are difficult to reach via bronchoscopy. The sensitivity of TTNA for peripheral lesions is higher than the sensitivity of bronchoscopy, with reports above 90%. The sensitivity depends on several factors, including the size and location of the nodule, the size of the needle, the number of needle passes, and the presence of on-site cytopathology examination. However, pneumothorax complicates TTNA more frequently than bronchoscopy. Minor pneumothoraces have been reported in approximately 25% of procedures and larger ones requiring chest tube drainage occur in approximately 5% of procedures. Risk factors that increase the risk of pneumothorax include underlying chronic obstructive pulmonary disease (COPD) and a long distance of the nodule from the pleura.

A nonspecific or nondiagnostic (normal) biopsy finding in a sample obtained by bronchoscopy or percutaneous TTNA requires careful clinical and radiographic follow-up. A "negative" finding does not preclude repeat biopsy or evaluation for surgical resection if there remains a high clinical suspicion for malignancy. If a malignancy is diagnosed by TTNA, bronchoscopy should be considered to evaluate the central airways.

Some experts have advocated thoracotomy, via open surgery or video-assisted thoracoscopic surgery (VATS) approach, as a first-line approach for obtaining tissue biopsies of SPNs. When compared with bronchoscopy or percutaneous needle aspiration, thoracoscopy is virtually 100% sensitive and 100% specific, offering an excellent, albeit expensive and invasive alternative. However, it also has a higher risk of complications than the less invasive sampling techniques. Smaller nodules or GGOs are occasionally difficult to palpate during surgery, and may require guidewire insertion or dye marking to assist in localization during resection.

Once the diagnosis is established, surgical resection remains the standard treatment for stage I non-small cell lung cancer. Resection can be accomplished via open thoracotomy or VATS. The typical practice currently is to perform a lobectomy for malignant SPNs. However, newer prospective studies suggest that segmentectomy with curative intent may be an alternative first-line therapy in specific patient populations.

For medically inoperable patients or those who refuse a surgical option, another therapeutic technique with curative intent is stereotactic body radiation therapy (SBRT). This procedure precisely targets radiation to a tumor while minimizing radiation to surrounding tissue, which limits the "collateral damage." This option is appealing for patients who are not good surgical candidates after confirmation of malignancy. It is also a potential option for empiric treatment in patients without established tissue diagnosis in whom underlying comorbidities make the performance of biopsy unsafe. Although there are no large randomized studies yet comparing SBRT to lobectomy for stage I disease, there are observational studies which suggest that SBRT may result in local control that is similar to surgical resection.

CONCLUSION

The overall goals in the management of SPNs are to delineate benign from malignant disease and to facilitate appropriate therapy. These goals require a comprehensive clinical evaluation of a patient's history, physical examination, and radiologic findings in order to estimate the likelihood of cancer. A patient's surgical risk and personal preferences also help determine the approach. Standard recommendations in surveillance CT imaging can help guide follow-up imaging. A decision to pursue tissue diagnosis is based on the clinical likelihood of cancer and on the changes in imaging characteristics over time. Standard bronchoscopy should be considered for larger central nodules. Navigational bronchoscopy and radial EBUS are two adjunctive bronchoscopic techniques that improve the diagnostic sensitivity for more peripheral lesions. TTNA has a high yield for peripheral SPNs, but carries a high risk of pneumothorax. Occasionally, surgical resection and radiation therapy remain good empiric treatment options for nodules highly suspicious for cancer in which prior confirmation of the diagnosis by other means was unobtainable.

FURTHER READING

1. MacMahon MB, Austin JH, Gamsu G, et al. Guidelines for management of small pulmonary nodules detected on CT scans: A statement from the Fleischer Society. *Radiology.* 2005;237(2):395.

   2005 Fleischner Society guidelines for the work up of solitary pulmonary nodules.

2. Patel VK, Naik SK, Naidich DP, et al. A practical algorithmic approach to the diagnosis and management of solitary pulmonary nodules. *Chest.* 2013;143(3):825–839.

   Good review of radiologic characteristics of nodules and imaging modalities.

3. National Lung Screening Trial Research Team; Aberle DR, Adams AM, et al. Reduced lung-cancer mortality with low-dose computed tomographic screening. *N Engl J Med.* 2011;365(5):395–409.

   Large NLST trial of over 50,000 patients evaluating the use of serial low-dose spiral CT in screening high-risk patients for lung cancer.

4. Baaklini WA, Reinoso MA, Gorin AB, et al. Diagnostic yield of fiberoptic bronchoscopy in evaluating solitary pulmonary nodules. *Chest.* 2000;117:1049–1054.

   Yield decreases with nodules of decreasing size.

5. Chang B, Hwang JH, Choi Y, et al. Natural history of pure ground-glass opacity lung nodules detected by low-dose CT scan. *Chest.* 2013;143(1):172–178.

   Recent trial on the screening of pure ground-glass opacity nodules.

6. Batra P, Brown K, Aberle DR, et al. Imaging techniques in the evaluation of pulmonary parenchymal neoplasms. *Chest.* 1992;101:239.

   A summary of the current roles of chest radiographs, CT scans, and magnetic resonance imaging in the evaluation of pulmonary opacities.

7. Collard JM, Reymond MA. Video-assisted thoracic surgery (VATS) for cancer: risk of parietal seeding and of early local recurrence. *Int Surg.* 1996;81:343.

   Special precautions should be used (such as enveloping specimens in an endobag) before removal through the intercostal tissues.

8. Cummings SR, Lillington GA, Richard RJ. Estimating the probability of malignancy in solitary pulmonary nodules: a Bayesian approach. *Am Rev Respir Dis.* 1986;134:449.

   Provides a table of likelihood ratios and a formula to determine the risk of cancer in an individual patient. This information may be useful in deciding on a conservative or aggressive approach to diagnosis.

9. Cummings SR, Lillington GA, Richard RJ, et al. Managing solitary pulmonary nodules: the choice of strategy is a "close call." *Am Rev Respir Dis.* 1986;134:453.

   Decision analysis is applied to the evaluation of SPNs, taking into consideration risks of procedure, treatment, and delayed treatment. The authors suggest that patients should play an active role in the decision-making process.

10. Goldberg SK, Walkenstein MD, Steinbach A, et al. The role of staging bronchoscopy and the preoperative assessment of a solitary pulmonary nodule. *Chest.* 1993;104:94.

    A retrospective review of 33 cases. No evidence of endobronchial disease was seen in 23 patients with malignant, asymptomatic SPNs. The authors advocate abandonment of routine staging fiberoptic bronchoscopy in patients with indeterminate SPNs.

11. Gould MK, Maclean CC, Kuschner WG, et al. Accuracy of positron emission tomography for diagnosis of pulmonary nodules and mass lesions. *JAMA*. 2001;285:914–924.

    Essential meta-analysis of data sources from 1966 to 200 using MEDLINE and CANCERLIT to estimate diagnostic accuracy of FDG-PET for malignant focal pulmonary nodules.

12. Gupta N, Gill H, Graeber G, et al. Dynamic positron emission tomography with F-18 fluorode-oxyglucose imaging in differentiation of benign from malignant lung/mediastinal lesions. *Chest*. 1998;114:1105.

    Distinct time–activity curve patterns were identified in malignant and benign lesions. Continued uptake is noted in malignant lesions, suggesting a role for PET scanning in patients with equivocal findings on other imaging studies.

13. Henschke CI, McCauley DJ, Yankelevitz DF, et al. Early lung cancer action project: overall design and findings from baseline screening. *Lancet*. 1999;354:99.

    Using helical CT scanning in a prospective study of 1,000 smokers, investigators detected noncalcified nodules in 233 (23%); 27 of these (12%) were subsequently found to have lung cancer. Only 7 of these 27 cancers were visible on chest radiographs.

14. Huston J III, Muhm JR. Solitary pulmonary nodules: evaluation with a CT reference phantom. *Radiology*. 1989;170:653.

    Describes techniques and use of reference phantoms.

15. Khan JH, McElhinney DB, Rahman SB, et al. Pulmonary metastases of endocrine origin: the role of surgery. *Chest*. 1998;114:526.

    Patients with carcinoid, thyroid, pheochromocytoma, and parathyroid tumors with pulmonary metastases should undergo surgical resection in cases of good control of the primary tumor, no evidence of extrathoracic disease, and satisfactory lung function.

16. Lewis RJ, Caccavale RJ, Sisler GE, et al. One hundred video-assisted thoracic surgical simultaneously stapled lobectomies without rib spreading. *Ann Thorac Surg*. 1997;63:1415.

    For lesions ranging from 1.5 to 8 cm, stapled lobectomy through VATS had results similar to those obtained from open surgical techniques. Hospitalization was less than 3 days on average.

17. Levine MS, Weiss JM, Harrell JH, et al. Transthoracic needle aspiration biopsy following negative fiberoptic bronchoscopy in solitary pulmonary nodules. *Chest*. 1988;93:1152.

    Authors suggest that nondiagnostic TTNA is more likely to occur with a benign rather than a malignant SPN and state that this procedure cannot be the decisive factor in opting for or against definitive resection.

18. Libby DM, Smith JP, Altorki NK, et al. Managing the small pulmonary nodule discovered by CT. *Chest*. 2004;125:1522–1529.

    Prospective, noncomparative study of smokers without prior malignancy also includes a review of the literature of CT screening and lung cancer.

19. Lillington GA. Management of solitary pulmonary nodules. *Dis Mon*. 1991;37:274.

    A careful review of SPNs, with a description of several decision analysis studies suggesting the importance of patients' wishes regarding management strategies.

20. O'Keefe ME Jr, Good CA, McDonald JR, et al. Calcification in solitary nodules of the lung. *AJR Am J Roentgenol*. 1957;77:1023.

    Benign patterns of calcification are described. Eccentric calcifications can occur in malignant lesions.

21. Mack MJ, Hazelrigg SR, Landreneau RJ, et al. Thoracoscopy for the diagnosis of the indeterminate solitary pulmonary nodule. *Ann Thorac Surg*. 1993;56:825.

    A multi-institutional review of 242 patients with SPNs undergoing thoracoscopic excisional biopsy as the primary diagnostic method. A definite diagnosis was obtained in all patients. A fine discussion follows the references, bringing to light several areas of controversy regarding this procedure.

22. McCormack PM, Ginsberg KB, Bains MS, et al. Accuracy of lung imaging in metastases with implications for the role of thoracoscopy. *Ann Thorac Surg*. 1993;56:863.

    A retrospective study in which CT scans differed from pathologic findings in 42% of patients (18 patients had more cancers than CT reported). Because thoracoscopy does not allow manual palpation of the lung to locate lesions not seen on the lung surface, the validity of using thoracoscopic resection as a definitive procedure is questioned.

23. Naidich DP, Sussman R, Kutcher WL, et al. Solitary pulmonary nodules: CT-bronchoscopic correlation. *Chest*. 1988;93:595.

A retrospective review of 65 patients undergoing thin-section CT scanning, which reports the value of a positive bronchus sign. Of the patients with positive bronchus sign, 60% were diagnosed bronchoscopically.

24. Swensen SJ. An integrated approach to evaluation of a solitary pulmonary nodule. *Mayo Clin Proc.* 1990;65:173.

    A fine review that also addresses TNM staging. Many references are provided.

25. Reichenberger F, Weber J, Tamm M, et al. The value of transbronchial needle aspiration in the diagnosis of peripheral pulmonary lesions. *Chest.* 1999;116:704.

    In this retrospective study of 172 patients (126 with malignant disease), transbronchial needle aspiration increased the diagnostic yield of bronchoscopy from 35% to 51%.

26. Tan BB, Flaherty KR, Kazerooni EA, et al. The solitary pulmonary nodule. *Chest.* 2003;123:89S–96S.

    Includes recommendations for imaging modalities and obtaining tissue preoperatively based on review of current literature.

27. Tschernko EM, Hofer S, Bieglmayes C, et al. Early postoperative stress: video assisted wedge resection/lobectomy vs conventional axillary thoracotomy. *Chest.* 1996;109:1636.

    In this study of 22 patients undergoing VATS and 25 undergoing axillary thoracotomy for pulmonary nodule, less postoperative pain and better oxygenation were noted in the VATS group.

28. Gould MK, Fletcher J, Iannettoni MD, et al. Evaluation of patients with pulmonary nodules: when is it lung cancer? ACCP evidence-based clinical practice guidelines (2nd edition). *Chest.* 2007;132:108S–130S.

    2007 ACCP guidelines of the diagnosis and management of lung cancer.

29. Rivera MP, Mehta AC. Initial diagnosis of lung cancer: ACCP evidence-based clinical practice guidelines (2nd edition). *Chest.* 2007;132:131S–148S.

    2007 ACCP guidelines of the diagnosis and management of lung cancer.

30. Geraghty PR, Kee ST, McFarlane G, et al. CT-guided transthoracic needle aspiration biopsy of pulmonary nodules: needle size and pneumothorax rate. *Radiology.* 2003;229(2):475–481.

    Complication rates and yields of TTNA.

31. Schuchert MJ, Abbas G, Awais O. Anatomic segmentectomy for the solitary pulmonary nodule and early-stage lung cancer. *Ann Thorac Surg.* 2012;93(6):1780–1785.

    Use of anatomic segmentectomy as therapy for malignant SPN.

32. Baumann P, Nyman J, Hoyer M, et al. Outcome in a prospective phase II trial of medically inoperable stage I non-small-cell lung cancer patients treated with stereotactic body radiotherapy. *J Clin Oncol.* 2009;27(20):3290–3296.

    Trial of SBRT in empiric therapy of SPN.

39 Mediastinal Masses

Timothy M. Fernandes

INTRODUCTION

The mediastinum is located in the central thorax and is bound by the thoracic inlet apically, the diaphragm caudally, and the sternum and spinal column in the anteriorposterior direction. The space may be divided into three anatomic compartments, knowledge of their normal contents helps narrow the differential diagnosis of masses that may arise in them. The *anterior compartment* is the area between the sternum and the anterior pericardium. Important structures contained in the anterior compartment include the trachea, ascending aorta, thymus gland, and numerous lymph nodes. The *middle compartment*, sometimes referred to as the visceral compartment, contains the pericardium and its contents along with the distal trachea, carina, main bronchi and their associated lymph nodes. The *posterior compartment* extends from the posterior pericardium to the vertebral column and the paravertebral gutters. This compartment includes the descending aorta, the esophagus, the sympathetic ganglion, and peripheral nerves.

CLINICAL PRESENTATION

Masses that arise in the mediastinum are extremely variable in the symptoms, or lack of symptoms, that are found at presentation. In adults, approximately half of all mediastinal masses are asymptomatic and are found incidentally on radiographic examination of the thorax. In children, however, the presentation may be subtle, with complaints such as cough or vague pain. The contents of the normal mediastinum may suffer specific effects when they are compressed by enlarging masses, which may give clues to trigger further investigation. In the anterior compartment, a mass may grow to compress the airways, causing recurrent pneumonia, wheezing, hemoptysis, or an intrathoracic obstruction seen on pulmonary function testing. Masses in the middle compartment also may cause airway compression. The recurrent laryngeal nerve is found in the middle compartment. Its usual course is to wrap under the left main bronchus; its disruption produces hoarseness and paralysis of the left vocal cord. The phrenic nerve arises from the cervical roots of the spinal cord and travels through the mediastinum to innervate the diaphragm; its disruption may lead to an elevated hemidiaphragm. The posterior mediastinum also contains the sympathetic chain ganglia which, if severed, can lead to Horner syndrome with the classic triad of ptosis (drooping of the upper eyelid), miosis (small pupils), and anhidrosis (lack of sweat production). Horner syndrome frequently is seen with masses that occur near the thoracic inlet and these may compress the superior vena cava leading to facial swelling and plethora (the superior vena cava syndrome).

Mediastinal masses (both malignant and benign) that originate from structures found within the mediastinum can cause associated symptoms, paraneoplastic syndromes, or other systemic diseases. Lymphomas in the mediastinum may present with "B symptoms" which include fevers, night sweats, and weight loss. Thymomas are found in the anterior mediastinum and are closely associated with myasthenia gravis, which may manifest as diplopia, muscle weakness, or easy fatigability. Other rare problems associated with thymomas include red cell aplastic anemia (5% of cases) and hypogammaglobinemia (5%–10% of cases). Parathyroid adenomas can present with hyperparathyroidism resulting in hypercalcemia and its associated features. Paraganglionomas may manifest clinically the features of pheochromocytoma, including intermittent flushing, headaches, and sweating. Intrathoracic goiters may occasionally be associated with thyrotoxicosis.

DIAGNOSIS

The evaluation of a mediastinal mass is directed by the differential diagnosis which, in part, is dictated by the anatomic location and the age of the patient. Routine chest radiographs should be carefully evaluated for abnormalities in the mediastinum. In the anteroposterior (AP) or posteroanterior (PA) views, subtle densities along the paratracheal stripe may hint at the presence of a mass but widening of the mediastinum is a more characteristic sign. A normal mediastinum should be less than 8 cm in transverse diameter in the PA view. The lateral film is useful in defining the compartments of the mediastinum. The retrosternal clear space, retrotracheal space, and the aortopulmonary window should all be carefully examined. Comparison with prior radiographs may aid in diagnosis of subtle abnormalities.

Chest computed tomography (CT) with intravenous contrast can be the first-line diagnostic imaging modality for mediastinal masses. Chest CT offers the ability to determine the exact location of a mass in relation to vessels or other structures of the thorax. The tissue attenuation also may suggest the etiology of the mass. Magnetic resonance imaging (MRI) is seldom needed to identify mediastinal masses themselves, although it may be useful for neurogenic masses and enteric foregut duplication cysts. In addition, MRI can provide information about vascular involvement, invasion of tissue planes, and can distinguish between cystic and solid masses. Other imaging modalities may be considered based on the suspected etiology of the mass. Radionucliotide scanning can be helpful for certain diagnoses. Thyroid ^{123}I scans (for thyroid masses and goiters), metaiodobenzylgnanidine (MIBG) scans (for suspected pheochromocytomas and paraganglionomas), and sestambi scans (for masses of parathyroid origin) all have utility based on clinical suspicion. Whole body position emission tomography-CT (PET-CT) is useful to rule out metastatic disease, especially for lymphomas, that may be easy to reach bronchoscopically for definitive tissue diagnosis. Laboratory testing may be helpful depending on the clinical context of the presentation. Germ cell tumors (GCT) should be suspected in a young male with an anterior mediastinal mass. Elevation of α-fetoprotein (AFP) and β-human chorionic gonadotropin (β-hCG) levels is found in nonseminomatous GCT. Other laboratory testing may be helpful, depending on the suspected etiology. Thyroid function tests may help diagnose a functioning goiter or intrathoracic thyroid. Serum calcium, phosphate, and parathyroid hormone levels are useful in parathyroid adenomas. In patients with paravertebral masses, paraganglionoma and pheochromocytoma may be suspected. These tumors commonly produce norepinepherine or epinephrine; serum free metanepherines are less sensitive than a 24-hour urine collection for metanepherines, urinary homovanillic acid, and vanillylmandelic acid in diagnosing these tumors.

Ultimately, tissue diagnosis is needed to determine a treatment plan for most suspected malignant mediastinal masses. In recent years, the use of minimally invasive techniques for obtaining biopsies of mediastinal masses have become more commonplace. Percutaneous needle biopsy under CT- or ultrasound-guidance, endobronchial ultrasound with transbronchial needle aspiration (EBUS-TBNA) or endoscopic ultrasound with fine needle aspiration (EUS-FNA) should be considered first line for amenable lesions. In a recent review of 140 patients with mediastinal masses of unclear etiology, the use of EBUS-TBNA proved diagnostic in 93% of all patients (88% of malignant lesions and 96% of benign lesions) and prevented more invasive procedures such as mediastinoscopy or thoracostomy in 80% of cases. With the use of flow cytometry, EBUS-TBNA has become extremely effective in diagnosing suspected lymphoma. One series from MD Anderson demonstrated EBUS-TBNA had a sensitivity of 91%, specificity of 100%, positive predictive value of 100%, and negative predictive value of 93% for the diagnosis of lymphoma. For duplication cysts of the middle mediastinum, needle drainage may provide both diagnosis and therapeutic benefit. For paraesophageal lesions in the posterior mediastinum, EUS-FNA can be valuable in obtaining tissue. An important exception to the needle biopsy approach is for suspected thymomas which have been reported to seed the biopsy needle's track. For metastatic disease, locally invasive disease, suspected lymphomas and malignancies presenting with bulky adenopathy, minimally invasive approaches to diagnosis should be first line since surgical resection is not part of the initial treatment algorithm. Additionally, GCT are typically treated with chemoradiation first followed by surgical resection, so minimally invasive approaches to diagnosis should be attempted upfront in this group as well. First-line mediastinoscopy should be reserved for lesions that are likely benign but are causing symptoms and for resection of suspected thymomas. Special caution should be used in the surgical planning of large anterior mediastinal masses given the risk of compression of the airway and great vessels once a recumbent patient is anesthetized. Awake, seated intubation followed by general anesthesia is sometimes the more prudent option.

ETIOLOGY

Overall, the frequency of malignant versus benign causes of mediastinal masses varies by age. In children, approximately half of mediastinal masses are malignant with tumors of neural origin representing about 33% of all lesions. Other malignancies that are common in childhood include lymphoma (14%) and teratomas (10%). The nonmalignant mediastinal masses that appear in childhood tend to be thymic hyperplasia or cystic remnants of embryologic development (such as bronchogenic cysts, enteric cyts, or pericardial cysts). Once adulthood is entered, the rates of both Hodgkin and non-Hodgkin lymphoma as well as GCT increases which makes it more likely that a mass found in a patient aged 20 to 40 will be malignant. Large series involving mostly adult patients report widely varying frequencies of different mediastinal lesions. By combining 13 reported studies involving 2,399 patients, the following mean (and range) percentage rates for mediastinal lesions are derived: neurogenic tumors, 20.7% (14%–36%); thymoma, 19.1% (10%–27%); cyst, 18.3% (0%–26%); lymphoma, 12.5% (5%–23%); germ cell tumor, 10.0% (5%–29%); endocrine tumor, 6.4% (0%–23%); mesenchymal tumor, 6.0% (0%–11%); primary carcinoma, 4.6% (0%–23%); and miscellaneous masses, 2.4% (1%–14%). Location within the mediastinum also affects the likelihood for malignancy. In one large retrospective review of 400 adult patients with mediastinal masses, the anterior, middle, and posterior compartments were found to harbor malignancy in 59%, 29%, and 16% of cases, respectively. Anterior mediastinal masses in children are less likely to be malignant than in adults whereas posterior mediastinal masses tend to have an increased risk of malignancy in the young.

Neurogenic tumors are one of the most common group of malignancies, representing 20% of adult and 35% of pediatric mediastinal masses. These lesions are the most common cause of masses in the posterior compartment. In the adult, approximately 90% of these lesions are benign and frequently are asymptomatic while, in children, over 50% of lesions are malignant. The neurogenic tumors are divided into those arising from peripheral nerves (such as schwannomas or neural sheath tumors) and those arising from ganglia (i.e., ganglioblastoma, neuroblastoma, and rarely parasympathetic ganglionoma). The neural sheath tumor is most common in adults and is benign whereas neuroblastoma is most common in children and is malignant. MRI is helpful in determining tissue planes for resection in these tumors, since the definitive treatment for any neural tumor is surgical resection. Malignant lesions should receive postsurgical radiation.

Thymomas are the most common anterior mediastinal mass and typically occur in the 40s to 60s with an equal frequency in men and women. More than 90% of thymomas are visible on the PA and lateral chest radiograph. Many thymomas are found after diagnosis of an associated paraneoplastic syndrome such as myasthenia gravis (present in one-third of thymoma cases, whereas 15% of myasthenia gravis patients have associated thymomas), red cell aplastic anemia (5% of thymoma cases), or hypogammaglobinemia (10% of thymoma cases). Approximately two-thirds of thymomas are contained in a thick capsule at the time of surgical resection; resection of thymomas without evidence of local invasion is considered curative. Invasive thymomas frequently involve the pleura or other intrathoracic structures. The mainstay of therapy remains local resection with postoperative radiation.

Other neoplasms may originate in the thymus but are histologically and clinically distinct from thymomas. Thymic carcinoma is an aggressive malignancy with early local invasion and distant metastases; this malignancy is frequently positive for Epstein-Barr virus and is treated by resection followed by a cisplatin-based chemotherapeutic regimen. Thymic carcinoid, thymolipoma, and thymic cysts are uncommon causes of anterior mediastinal masses.

GCT can be divided into benign teratomas, seminomas, and embryonal tumors which include nonseminomatous GCT. GCT are found predominantly in the anterior mediastinum and present in the third decade of life with a male predominance. Benign teratomas are derived from two of the three primitive germ cell layers and frequently contain tissue of ectodermal origin such as mature bone, teeth, or hair. These lesions are generally asymptomatic, but surgical resection is recommended as there is a rare risk for conversion to a malignant process such as rhabdomyosarcoma, adenocarcinoma, or anaplastic small cell carcinoma. Seminomas are found almost exclusively in males in their 20s and 30s. Seminomas tend to be especially responsive to cisplatin-based chemotherapy and radiation with surgical resection reserved for residual tumor; using this treatment algorithm, patients can expect an over 90% 5-year predicted survival. Nonseminomatous GCT include embryonal cell carcinomas, endodermal thymus tumors, choriocarcinomas, yolk sac tumors, and mixed GCT. Most patients have elevated AFP levels and a minority have elevations in β-hCG; high levels of both AFP and β-hCG are considered diagnostic for nonseminomatous GCT and may preclude the need for tissue diagnosis. Nonseminomatous GCT are aggressive lesions that are usually metastatic at the time of diagnosis. The standard approach to treatment includes frontline chemotherapy, usually with bleomycin, etoposide, and cisplatin followed by surgical resection for residual masses and salvage chemotherapy frequently using ifosfamide-based regimens. Despite this approach, the prognosis for nonseminomatous GCT remains poor with less than a 50% predicted 5-year survival.

Lymphomas, including both Hodgkin disease and non-Hodgkin lymphoma, are one of the more common malignancies on the mediastinum and can seen found in any of the three compartments. In total, Hodgkin disease is less prevalent than non-Hodgkin lymphoma (25% vs. 75%, respectively). However, in the mediastinum, Hodgkin disease represents upwards of 50% to 70% of all cases of lymphoma. Nodular sclerosing Hodgkin disease has a tendency to manifest in the lymph nodes of the anterior mediastinum and may involve the thymus. Of patients with lymphoma, only 5% to 10% present with primary mediastinal masses. Hodgkin disease occurs with a bimodal distribution, peaking in the early 20s and again in the 50s. The cure rates for Hodgkin disease, even with extensive disease above and below the diaphragm, have been upwards of 60% to 70% due to its responsiveness to combined chemotherapy and radiation. Bulky adenopathy and extension into adjacent lung tissue portend a worse prognosis.

The most common nonHodgkin lymphoma entities to involve the mediastinum are large B-cell lymphoma and lymphoblastic lymphoma; these also have a predilection for the anterior compartment. Non-Hodgkin lymphomas tend to present with advanced disease and frequently have extranodal involvement at diagnosis. The large B-cell subtype tends to affect primarily the mediastinal nodes and occurs in patients in their 20s with a female predominance. Lymphoblastic lymphoma is an aggressive, high-grade lymphoma that is closely linked to lymphoblastic leukemia and occurs most prevalently in male adolescents. Overall, non-Hodgkin lymphoma is associated with a poorer prognosis compared to Hodgkin disease, despite the use of aggressive chemotherapeutic regimens; bone marrow transplantation may be necessary.

Mediastinal developmental cysts are most commonly found in the middle compartment, are nearly always benign and, except in infants and young children, are usually asymptomatic at presentation. In a retrospective review of 105 cases of cysts at one institution in Osaka, Japan, 45% of cysts were bronchogenic in origin followed in prevalence by thymic cysts (29%), pericardial cysts (11%), pleural cysts (6%), and esophageal duplication cysts (4%). During embryogenesis, bronchogenic and esophageal cysts arise from an abnormal budding of the primitive foregut in the laryngotracheal groove; pericardial and pleural cysts are of mesothelial origin. Although the majority of bronchogenic cysts are asymptomatic, approximately 40% of patients may present with symptoms such as retrosternal chest pain or cough. In symptomatic patients, simple aspiration of the cyst usually leads to resolution; surgical resection is the definitive treatment but should be reserved for symptomatic lesions that fail aspiration given the invasiveness of the procedure and otherwise benign nature of the diagnosis. Cysts of mesothelial origin, including pericardial and pleural cysts, are asymptomatic in over 80% of cases and can be managed expectantly.

Other nonneoplastic mediastinal lesions to consider include *mediastinal infection, intrathoracic thyroid* (most commonly found in the middle compartment), *parathyroid adenomas* (commonly in the anterior mediastinum). and *sarcoidosis* (see Chapter 90). Mediastinal infections are most commonly found either after an intrathoracic procedure or in association with an esophageal perforation. These infections are usually mixed with aerobes and anaerobes including *Bacteroides*. Pneumomediastinum may be seen on chest radiography and barium swallow may help localize an esophageal perforation. Early treatment with broad-spectrum antibiotics and surgical drainage should be pursued.

FURTHER READING

1. Azizkhan RG, Dudgeon DL, Buck JR, et al. Life-threatening airway obstruction as a complication to the management of mediastinal masses in children. *J Pediatr Surg.* 1985;20:816.

    The risk of airway compression from mediastinal masses during anesthesia is discussed.

2. Besznyak I, Sebesteny M, Kurchar F. Primary mediastinal seminoma. *J Thorac Cardiovasc Surg.* 1973;65:930.

    A literature review of all mediastinal seminomas reported up to 1973.

3. Cohen AJ, Thompson L, Edwards FH, et al. Primary cysts and tumors of the mediastinum. *Ann Thorac Surg.* 1991;51:378.

   A large series over 45 years, emphasizes the change in preoperative evaluation and operative approach over that time.

4. Conkle DM, Adkins RB Jr. Primary malignant tumors of the mediastinum. *Ann Thorac Surg.* 1972;14:553.

   A single center's experience with malignant mediastinal masses; notes high incidence of symptoms and poor prognosis associated with malignant lesions.

5. Davis RD Jr, Oldham HN Jr, Sabiston DC Jr, et al. Primary cysts and neoplasms of the mediastinum: recent changes in clinical presentation, methods of diagnosis, management, and results. *Ann Thorac Surg.* 1987;44:229.

   A large series spanning 56 years. Emphasizes improved preoperative diagnosis of all lesions and improved survival in patients with Hodgkin disease and germ cell tumors in recent years.

6. Duwe BV, Sterman DH, Musani AI. Tumors of the mediastinum. *Chest.* 2005;128:2893–2909.

   Dr. Duwe, a former UCSD pulmonary fellow, presents a definitive review of the most common tumors of the mediastinum.

7. Ferguson MK, Lee E, Skinner DB, et al. Selective operative approach for diagnosis and treatment of anterior mediastinal masses. *Ann Thorac Surg.* 1987;44:583–586.

   Surgical options are discussed for anterior mediastinal masses of unclear etiology.

8. Marano R, Liguori C, Savino G, et al. Cardiac silhouette findings and mediastinal lines and stripes: radiograph and CT correlation. *Chest.* 2011;139(5):1186–1196.

   This article focuses on the normal margins of the mediastinum on chest X-rays then demonstrates how mediastinal masses may alter this normal borders; chest X-rays findings are further correlated with CT scans.

9. Kennedy MP, Jimenez CA, Bruzzi JF, et al. Endobronchial ultrasound-guided transbronchial needle aspiration in the diagnosis of lymphoma. *Thorax.* 2008;63:360–365.

   This article discusses the experience at MD Anderson with EBUS-TBNA for diagnosis of lymphoma.

10. Maggi G, Giaccone G, Donadio M, et al. Thymomas: a review of 169 cases, with particular reference to results of surgical treatment. *Cancer.* 1986;58:765.

    This large case series discusses tumor invasiveness and its effect on prognosis.

11. Ribet ME, Cardot GR. Neurogenic tumors of the thorax. *Ann Thorac Surg.* 1994;58:1091.

    Compared with adults, children more often are symptomatic at presentation, have nerve cell (vs nerve sheath) tumors, and have a higher incidence of malignancy.

12. Rubush JL, Gardner IR, Boyd WC, et al. Mediastinal tumors: review of 186 cases. *J Thorac Cardiovasc Surg.* 1973;65:216.

    A fine review of the distribution of mediastinal masses in a general hospital population. Excellent comparative tables review different series from the literature.

13. Strollo DC, Rosado de Christenson ML, Jett JR. Primary mediastinal tumors, part 1: tumors of the anterior mediastinum. *Chest.* 1997;112:511.

    The authors present an in-depth review of tumors of the anterior mediastinum in this two-part paper.

14. Strollo DC, Rosado de Christenson ML, Jett JR. Primary mediastinal tumors, part 2: tumors of the posterior mediastinum. *Chest.* 1997;112:1344.

    The second portion of this extensive review focuses on masses of the middle and posterior mediastinal compartments.

15. Suster S, Rosai J. Thymic carcinoma: a clinicopathologic study of 60 cases. *Cancer.* 1991;67:1025.

    The authors describe two distinct pathologic presenstations of thymic carcinoma; one group has a more favorable predicted outcome with over 50% 5-year survival while the other group demonstrates rapidly progressive and lethal disease.

16. Takeda S, Miyoshi S, Minami M, et al. Clinical spectrum of mediastinal cysts. *Chest.* 2003;124:125–132.

    One Japanese institution discusses their experience with mediastinal cysts and focus on features that defer between children and adults.

17. Weinreb JC, Naidich DP. Thoracic magnetic resonance imaging. *Clin Chest Med.* 1991;12:33.
    The authors discuss the limited utility of MRI in evaluating the mediastinum.
18. Whooley BP, Urschel JD, Antkowiak JG, et al. Primary tumors of the mediastinum. *J Surg Oncol.* 1999;70:95–99.
    The surgical oncologist perspective of primary malignancies of the mediastinum is provided.
19. Wychulis AR, Payne WS, Clagett OT, et al. Surgical treatment of mediastinal tumors: a 40-year experience. *J Thorac Cardiovasc Surg.* 1971;62:379.
    One center's experience with surgical management of mediastinal masses in the era before routine bronchoscopy is provided.
20. Yasufuku K, Nakajima T, Fujiwara T, et al. Utility of EBUS-TBNA in the diagnosis of mediastinal masses of unknown etiology. *Ann Thorac Surg.* 2011;91:831–836.
    The authors present their experience with EBUS in both establishing a diagnosis and avoiding further procedures for patient with a mediastinal mass of unclear etiology.

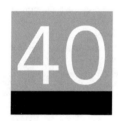

40 Eosinophilic Lung Disease

Timothy M. Fernandes

INTRODUCTION

The eosinophil plays a diverse role in human immunity from involvement with the allergic response to an antiparasitic function; when these functions go awry in the respiratory system, eosinophilic lung diseases may develop. Inherently, eosinophilic lungs diseases share a similar pathogenic cause: an over abundance of eosinophils in the lung. Eosinophilic cytokines, namely IL-5, IL-6, and IL-10, are present in abundance in bronchoalveolar lavage (BAL) samples from involved segments, consistent with an intense inflammatory response that draws more eosinophils to the area. Tissue eosinophilia is present on open lung biopsy of an involved lobe; peripheral eosinophilia or an eosinophilic predominant cell count in the bronchoalveolar wash may or may not be present as well. The eosinophilic pneumonias may be broadly classified as those of known and unknown etiology.

EOSINOPHILIC PNEUMONIAS OF KNOWN ETIOLOGY

Helminthic and Fungal Infection-Associated Eosinophilic Lung Disease

Worldwide, the most common cause of eosinophilic lung disease is transient infection with a parasitic organism. Wilhelm Löffler first described a series of patients with pulmonary infiltrates with high peripheral eosinophilia in 1932. In that series, all cases were associated with infection with one of four helminthes: either one of the roundworms (*Ascaris lumbricoides* or *Strongyloides stercoralis*) or one of the hookworms (*Ancylostoma duodenale* or *Necator americanus*). The term Löffler syndrome subsequently has been assigned to the constellation of transient and migratory interstitial infiltrates, peripheral eosinophilia, and mild pulmonary symptoms, such as cough and wheezing associated with the transpulmonary passage of larvae from a helminth infection. *Ascaris lumbricoides* remains the most common cause of Löffler syndrome worldwide. Patients typically present with low grade fever, nonproductive cough, and occasionally hemoptysis.

Ascaris and *Strongyloides* are found ubiquitously throughout the world. The human lifecycle begins with ingestion of ova from contaminated soil. The ova hatch in the small intestine and larvae enter the splanchnic circulation, eventually migrating to the pulmonary circulation. The larvae move into the alveoli and ascend into the large airways where they are swallowed to complete their life cycle by reproducing in the gastrointestinal tract. The pulmonary portion of the life cycle takes about 2 weeks to complete. Symptoms occur after the transpulmonary passage of the larvae, which may be seen in the sputum; peripheral eosinophilia peaks soon after. Frequently, stool examination for ova is negative until weeks after the respiratory symptoms have resolved. In general, these infections are self-limited but treatment with antihelminthic agents such as mebendazole may be warranted.

Other parasitic infections directly invade the lung parenchyma and may cause more profound and chronic pulmonary complications. Lung flukes, such as *Paragonimus,* are mainly found in central Africa or southeast Asia and infection is associated with undercooked or raw crab meat ingestion. This fluke invades the parenchyma and may cause pleural effusions and chocolate-colored sputum which may contain ova. Another more invasive organism is the cestode that causes echinococcosis. This tapeworm is usually found in dogs but may infect humans as well. Cystic lesions are commonly found in both the lungs and liver; patients are typically asymptomatic until compression of surrounding structures by the enlarging cysts. Therapy usually consists of a course of the antihelminthic agent, mebendazole, followed by surgical resection of the cystic cavity.

Tropical pulmonary eosinophilia is a separate entity which is seen after infection with the nematodes from the Filarioidea superfamily, *Wuchereria bancrofti* or *Brugia malayi*, which occupy the lymphatic system ("lymphatic filariae"). They are found in tropical regions of the world, with the highest prevalence in India, Southeast Asia, and parts of Africa. The filariae generate an intense eosinophil-mediated inflammatory response with elevated IgE levels and antifilarial antibodies. Patient present with wheezing, paroxysmal cough, and constitutional symptoms such as fevers and weight loss. The diagnosis of tropical eosinophilia due to filarial infection should be considered in all patients who have traveled to endemic regions and present with refractory asthma and a peripheral eosinophilia of greater than 3,000/mm^3. Establishing the prompt diagnosis of tropical eosinophilia is important as the symptoms usually resolve after a 21-day course of diethylcarbamazine and delay in diagnosis may lead to long-term complications such as pulmonary fibrosis or chronic bronchitis.

Other nonhelminthic infections also may cause peripheral and intrapulmonary eosinophilia. Coccidioidomycosis, discussed elsewhere in more detail, is common in the southwestern United States. It is frequently mistaken for an idiopathic eosinophilic pneumonia due to difficulty isolating the organism from tissue culture. Allergic bronchopulmonary aspergillosis (ABPA) represents a hypersensitivity reaction to the ubiquitous fungus, *Aspergillus fumigatus.* Patients frequently present with cough productive of brown sputum, central bronchiectasis, elevated IgE, and fevers. Pathologic examination of the lung in ABPA may demonstrate an eosinophilic interstitial infiltrate with bronchiolitis and mucus impaction.

Drug- and Toxin-Induced Eosinophilic Lung Disease

Drug and toxin exposure represent another common cause of eosinophilic lung disease and should be included in the differential diagnosis, since removal of the exposure usually leads to resolution of symptoms. There are many drugs that have been associated with pulmonary eosinophilia (Table 40-1), but nonsteroidal anti-inflammatory drugs (NSAIDS) and antibiotics such as daptomycin, sulfonamides, penicillins, and tetracyclines are some of the most common culprits. The website www.pneumotox.com is a good resource to query medications that have published case reports of an association with eosinophilic lung disease. Outside of pharmaceuticals, many toxins have been associated with pulmonary eosinophilia as well. Emergency relief workers at the World Trade Center have been documented to have an increased risk for eosinophilic lung disease. Over-the-counter supplements such as L-tryptophan and rapeseed oil contaminated with aniline have caused epidemics of eosinophilic pneumonias. Other exposures to screen for include inhaled cocaine and heroin, scorpion stings, aluminum dust exposure, fumes from rubber production, and sulfite exposure in grape workers.

TABLE 40-1	Drugs and Toxins Associated with Eosinophilic Lung Disease

Commonly Associated	Rarely Associated
NSAIDS	Sulfa-containing antibiotics
L-Tryptophan	Penicillamine
Pheyntoin	Minocycline
Methotrexate	Carbamazepine
Nitrofurantoin	GCSF
Amiodarone	Cocaine
Daptomycin	Angiotensin-converting enzyme inhibitors
Bleomycin	Sulfites
Iodonated contrast	

EOSINOPHILIC PNEUMONIAS OF UNKNOWN ETIOLOGY

Acute Eosinophilic Pneumonia

Idiopathic acute eosinophilic pneumonia often presents in a dramatic fashion with hypoxemic respiratory failure soon after symptom onset. Acute eosinophilic pneumonia was first described as a case series of four patients in 1989 and the authors' original definition has persisted. Patients must have (1) an acute febrile illness (>99.0 F), (2) severe hypoxemia (defined by partial pressure of arterial oxygen <60 mmHg, oxygen saturation of <90% on room air, or an A–a gradient of >40 mmHg), (3) diffuse pulmonary infiltrates, (4) greater than 25% eosinophils in BAL fluid or an eosinophilic predominant insterstital infiltrate on lung biopsy, and (5) the absence of an infectious or allergic nidus. Periphial eosinophilia is not common at the time of diagnosis. Acute eosinophilic pneumonia tends to occur in otherwise healthy, young patients with nearly an equal distribution between males and females and no previous history of asthma. In one case series of 22 patients with acute eosinophilic pneumonia, the average age at presentation was 29 years old (±15.8 years). While there has been no proven causative agent, many cases are associated with the recent start of cigarette smoking.

Radiographic findings on presentation require bilateral infiltrates, but pleural effusions are also commonly present. Early on, radiographs of acute eosinophilic pneumonia may disclose prominent interstitial marking that develop Kerley B lines and eventually pleural effusions. Several case series have been published that note a relatively high prevalence of pleural effusions on admission, between 50% and 60% in most series. This is in contrast to chronic eosinophilic pneumonia which rarely presents with effusions. The pleural fluid contains a high percentage of eosinophils and an elevated pH (>7.50). In acute eosinophilic pneumonia, pleural effusions are almost universally present at some point in the course and frequently are the last abnormality to resolve on chest radiographs.

Despite the dramatic clinical presentation of severe hypoxemic respiratory failure that may require mechanical ventilation, acute eosinophilic pneumonia patients tend to respond quickly to steroids with little risk of death . Initial therapy with intravenous methylprednisolone with a starting dose of about 1 mg/kg (in the range of 60–125 mg) every 6 hours is appropriate. Once enteral therapy can be tolerated, an oral prednisone taper can be initiated. The duration of steroids is dictated by the clinical response and radiographic disease resolution, but most patients require between 3 and 12 weeks of therapy. Data regarding the long-term follow-up of patients with acute eosinophilic pneumonia are lacking, but recurrence of acute eosinophilic pneumonia is rare. A small series of eight patients with acute eosinophilic pneumonia had pulmonary function testing done about 6 months after admission; of these eight, five patients had normal spirometry, one developed mild obstruction, and two patients developed new restrictive defects.

Chronic Eosinophilic Pneumonia

Unlike acute eosinophilic pneumonia, patients with chronic eosinophilic pneumonia tend to have a more indolent presentation, often with months of preceding cough, dyspnea, and fevers. The disease is more common in women and nonsmokers. Asthma is associated with over 50% of cases and may occur at any point in the presentation or after resolution. Peripheral eosinophilia is also more prevalent at diagnosis in chronic eosinophilic pneumonia but up to 20% of cases may lack peripheral eosinophilia. The initial chest radiograph frequently has pleural-based opacities that are often called "the photographic negative of pulmonary edema." To establish the diagnosis of chronic eosinophilic pneumonia, a bronchoscopy with BAL may demonstrate greater than 25% eosinophils. Often times, the BAL is nondiagnostic so lung biopsy is needed. Pathologic examination of the lung in chronic eosinophilic pneumonia will demonstrate interstitial and alveolar eosinophil invasion with evidence of bronchiolitis obliterans and organizing pneumonia. Fibrosis is rare in chronic eosinophilic pneumonia and close examination of the blood vessels should be undertaken. If eosinophilic vasculitis is present, the diagnosis of chronic eosinophilic pneumonia should be questioned in favor of Churg–Strauss syndrome.

The treatment of chronic eosinophilic pneumonia is characterized by prolonged courses of steroids. Typically, patients may require methylprednisolone (60–125 mg every 6 hours) intravenously for 3 to 5 days prior to transitioning to oral prednisone in a dose of 0.5 mg/kg/day. This high dose should be continued for weeks, then attempts should be made to taper the dose slowly. Relapses frequently occur during steroid tapers and may require dose escalation. The majority of patients require over 6 months of prednisone and about 40% will require prolonged use, i.e., greater than 12 months. These patients frequently encounter the complications of long-term steroid use including diabetes, weight gain, osteopenia, and Cushingoid features. Prophylaxis of *Pneumocystis* infection with trimethoprim and sulfamethoxazole may be helpful during steroid tapering. There have not been clinical trials to evaluate the use of steroid-sparing agents such as azathioprine in chronic eosinophilic pneumonia. Case reports suggest that the addition of an inhaled corticosteroid during dose tapering may help prevent relapses but inhaled corticosteroids should not be used as monotherapy.

Churg–Strauss Syndrome

Churg–Strauss syndrome is detailed elsewhere in this text. Briefly, Churg–Strauss syndrome is primarily an eosinophilic vasculitis that is associated with sinusitis and asthma, although other organs including the skin, heart, gastrointestinal tract and nervous system may be involved. Mononeuritis multiplex is common. Onset of Churg–Strauss syndrome has been associated with use of leukotriene antagonists, inhaled glucocorticoids, and cocaine. A positve p-antineutrophil cytoplasmic antibody (ANCA) can be seen in 60% of cases and is associated with renal involvement and peripheral neuropathy; "ANCA negative" cases of Churg–Strauss syndrome have more frequent cardiac involvement and fevers. The mainstay of therapy remains methylprednisolone with the addition of other immunosupression such as cyclophosphamide, azathioprine, or methotrexate based on the degree of systemic involvement of the vasculitis.

Idiopathic Hypereosinophilic Syndrome

The term idiopathic hypereosinophilic sydrome encompasses a variety of rare diagnoses that present with peripheral eosinophilia for over 6 months with associated eosinophil-mediated end-organ damage. These patients most commonly present with dermatologic manifestations first, including eczema, recurrent urticaria, and angioedema, but pulmonary complaints may be seen in up to half of these patients. The pulmonary manifestations can be varied and may include unexplained dyspnea, cough, or wheeze. Radiographs may demonstrate patchy parenchymal infiltrates with pleural effusions. In addition to peripheral eosinophilia, blood tests may reveal elevated levels of vitamin B_{12}, trypase, or IgE. Molecular testing for the FIP1L1/PDGFRA mutation helps establish a diagnosis of the myeloproliferative form of hypereosinophilic sydrome and portends a favorable response to imatinib. The T-cell lymphocytic variant of hypereosinophilic sydrome will demonstrate clonality on bone marrow biopsy with the most common phenotype being $CD3^-$ and $CD4^+$. Ultimately, treatment of hypereosinophilic sydrome centers on the use of steroids; the use of adjunctive therapy such as imatinib, hydroxyurea, or IGN-alpha depends on the variant of hypereosinophilic sydrome.

APPROACH TO DIAGNOSIS

As with all interstitial diseases, attention should be given to obtaining a detailed history with special focus on travel history, new mediations, and extrapulmonary symptoms. The duration of pulmonary symptoms and any evidence of preceding asthma should be elicited. A complete blood count with differential should be obtained to evaluate for peripheral eosinophilia, with the caveat that its absence does not exclude pulmonary eosinophilia. Additional laboratory testing may be indicated based on the history. Patients with recent travel to regions with endemic helminthic disease should have their stool examined for ova and parasites; further serologic testing may be necessary as well. Those who present with sinusitis and asthma as prominent features should have ANCA levels drawn to help establish a diagnosis of Churg–Strauss sydrome. IgE levels and erythrocyte sedimentation rates may be drawn as well, but these are nonspecific and may only be useful to follow as a marker of response to treatment.

Specific radiographic patterns may help yield a diagnosis. ABPA will demonstrate "fleeting" lung infiltrates and central bronchiectasis on computed tomography (CT); mucoid impaction in the central airways may appear as tubular opacities, the so-called "finger-in-glove" sign. Acute eosinophilic pneumonia may present with bilateral alveolar infiltrates in a pattern similar to acute respiratory distress syndrome (ARDS). Chronic eosinophilic penumonia can present with peripheral, subpleural consolidations in a "photographic negative of pulmonary edema pattern," but this pattern is only seen in about a third of chronic eosinophilic pneumonia cases. Churg–Strauss syndrome may present with centrilobular nodules, septal thickening or bronchial wall thickening. However, these signs are nonspecific.

FURTHER READING

1. Kita H, Sur R, Hunt LW, et al. Cytokine production at the site of disease in chronic eosinophilic pneumonia. *Am J Respir Crit Care Med.* 1996;153:1437–1441.

   This study compares the levels of cytokines found in bronchoalveolar lavage samples from both involved and uninvolved lobes of the lung from patients with chronic eosinophilic pneumonia. IL-5, IL-6, and IL-10, the eosinophil-active cytokines where increased in the involved lobes.

2. Ong RK, Doyle RL. Tropical pulmonary eosinophilia. *Chest.* 1998;113:1673–1679.

   A definitive review on filarial lung disease. The diagnosis should be considered in all patients with refractory asthma with eosinophilia greater than 3,000/mm³ who have traveled to endemic regions.

3. Allen JN, Pacht ER, Gadek JE, et al. Acute eosinophilic pneumonia as a reversible cause of noninfectious respiratory failure. *N Engl J Med.* 1989;321(9):569–574.

   A series of four patients presenting with hypoxemic respiratory failure and increased eosinophilic count on BAL (mean 42 percent) are described. This article represents the first description acute eosinophilic pneumonia in the literature.

4. Kunst H, Mack D, Kon OM, et al. Parasitic infections of the lung: a guide for the respiratory physician. *Thorax.* 2011;66(6):528–536.

   The authors provide an overview of many of the parasitic lung infections that can cause eosinophilia with a focus on radiographic changes that may hint at specific diagnoses.

5. Santivanez S, Garcia HH. Pulmonary cystic echinococcosis. *Curr Opin Pulm Med.* 2010;16(3): 257–261.

   The diagnosis of pulmonary cystic echinococcosis is made primarily by imaging and treatment involves premedicating with mebendazole, then surgical resection of cysts.

6. Philit F, Etienne-Mastroianni B, Parrot A, et al. Idiopathic acute eosinophilic pneumonia: a study of 22 patients. *Am J Respir Crit Care Med.* 2002;166:1235–1239.

   This article is a retrospective review of a French registry detailing the presentation of 22 patients with acute eosinophilic pneumonia and notes that pleural effusions are much more common in acute eosinophilic pneumonia than chronic eosinophilic pneumonia.

7. Pope-Harman AL, Davis WB, Allen ED, et al. Acute eosinophilic pneumonia: a summary of 15 cases and review of the literature. *Medicine.* 1996;75(6):334–342.

   A series of 15 cases of acute eosinophilic pneumonia in Columbus, Ohio is described. The authors present the only long-term follow-up data for acute eosinophilic pneumonia published to date.

8. Jeong YJ, Kim KI, Seo IJ, et al. Eosinophilic lung diseases: a clinical, radiographic and pathologic overview. *Radiographics.* 2007;27:617–637.

   Written from a radiologist perspective with multiple examples of chest radiographs and CT scans, this article focuses on the radiographic differences among the eosinophilic lung disease that can be used to help narrow the differential diagnosis.

9. Carrington CB, Addington WW, Goff AM, et al. Chronic eosinophilic pneumonia. *N Engl J Med.* 1969;280(15):787–798.

   The authors provide the first description of chronic eosinophilic pneumonia in nine women and coin the term "photographic negative of pulmonary edema" associated with the radiographic findings.

10. Minakuchi M, Niimi A, Matsumoto H, et al. Chronic eosinophilic pneumonia: treatment with inhaled corticosteroids. *Respiration.* 2002;70:362–366.

    Inhaled corticosteroids may be useful in addition to oral prednisone during tapers of the oral steroid but ICS should not be used as monotherapy.

11. Ogbogu PU, Bochner BS, Butterfield JH, et al. Hypereosinophilic syndrome: a multicenter, retrospective analysis of clinical characteristics and response to therapy. *J Allergy Clin Immunol.* 2009;124(6):1319–1325.

    The authors provide an overview of the most common manifestations of hypereosinophilic syndrome and suggest a treatment plan based on etiology.

12. Sable-Fourtassou R, Cohen P, Mahr A, et al. Antineutrophil cytoplasmic antibodies and the Churg-Strauss syndrome. *Ann Intern Med.* 2005;143(9):632.

    The presence or absence of p-ANCA in the Churg–Strauss syndrome predicts different clinical courses.

SECTION **III**

Diseases

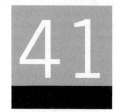

Pneumococcal Pneumonia

Julian P. Lichter

Pneumococcal pneumonia is the most common infection leading to hospitalization in the United States. It occurs in all age groups and is responsible for 500,000 cases of pneumonia and approximately 40,000 deaths annually. Pneumococcal pneumonia accounts for more than 50% of community-acquired pneumonias and 10% of nosocomial pneumonias. A resurgence of outbreaks of pneumococcal pneumonia has occurred, especially in chronic-care facilities where the strains are increasingly resistant to antibiotics. Although pneumococcal pneumonia can occur in any season, it is more common in winter and early spring.

The pneumococcus organism inhabits the nasopharynx of 40% to 50% of normal individuals for 4 to 6 weeks at a time. Disease is frequently caused by acquiring a serotype different from the colonizing serotype. The probability and severity of infection are influenced by host factors and by biologic properties of the bacterium itself. Patients who are most susceptible to pneumococcal infection include those with (1) disorders of swallowing and impairment of airway clearance mechanisms and mucociliary defenses, such as advanced age, seizure and other neurologic disorders, asthma, chronic bronchitis, and bronchiectasis; (2) alveolar fluid accumulation, such as congestive heart failure, burns, and acute respiratory distress syndrome; and (3) impaired phagocytosis and compromised humoral immunity, such as surgical or functional asplenia (e.g., sickle cell anemia, thalassemia, total irradiation), hypogammaglobulinemia, diabetes, HIV infection (50–100 times increase in invasive pneumococcal disease in HIV), multiple myeloma, lymphoma, cirrhosis, and transplant recipients (especially bone marrow). Such individuals are also susceptible to protracted or complicated pneumonias. Viral upper respiratory illness also seems to predispose patients to subsequent pneumococcal pneumonia. Viral disruption of respiratory epithelium increases expression of receptors for pneumococcal attachment and, thus, predisposes the patient to pneumococcal invasion. Other more recently described predisposing factors include alcohol abuse, smoking, pregnancy, homelessness, incarceration, and crack-cocaine use.

Of the more than 82 strains of pneumococci, only a few commonly cause pneumonia. The pathogenicity and virulence of particular strains are related to properties of the outer capsules and cell walls, as well as surface and cytoplasmic regulatory mechanisms. They may be identified in the laboratory by a characteristic capsular swelling (Quellung reaction) when incubated with a specific antibody. Current evidence suggests that the pneumococcal capsule protects the organism from phagocytosis and enhances its pathogenicity. Recent studies suggest that the development of type-specific, anticapsular antibody correlates with the resolution of fever and recovery in untreated patients.

Pneumococci are aerosolized from the nasopharynx to the alveolus, and then pass from alveolus to alveolus through the pores of Cohn, resulting in a mostly lobar distribution of consolidation. They invade alveolar type II cells, a process initiated through binding of bacterial surface choline to the receptor for platelet-activating factor (up-regulated on the alveolar cell surface, presumably by viral infection). Pathologically the consolidated lung evolves through well-described stages of alveolar engorgement followed by red hepatization and, after a few days, grey hepatization with alveoli packed with leukocytes. There is, however, little tissue destruction, and resolution occurs with minimal organization or permanent scarring. Dying pneumococci produce a potent cytotoxin, pneumolysin, which binds to cholesterol on the host's cell membranes, forming pores and killing the cells. Pneumolysin also promotes intra-alveolar bacterial replication, penetration from alveoli to interstitium, and dissemination into the bloodstream. Approximately 25% of cases of pneumococcal pneumonia were associated with bacteremia in the 1960s but recent studies report a much lower occurrence (as low as 1%–6%).

The clinical manifestations of classic pneumococcal pneumonia include high fever (100% in one series, although high fever may be absent in the elderly or in uremic patients), productive cough (98%), pleuritic chest pain (70%), and the abrupt onset of shaking chills (7%). The sputum is blood streaked or rusty (75%). Pleuritic pain may radiate into the abdomen, masquerading as an acute abdomen. Patients characteristically appear acutely ill, tachypneic, and demonstrate signs of consolidation on chest examination. A pleural rub is occasionally present. Herpes labialis is a relatively common finding. Older patients often present with confusion and delirium.

The chest roentgenogram usually reveals a lobar, alveolar-filling process, frequently with an ipsilateral pleural effusion. The roentgenographic presentations, however, are diverse and include a patchy bronchopneumonia, adult respiratory distress syndrome, and an interstitial appearance when occurring in an emphysematous lobe. The prevalence of these radiologic patterns may depend on the infecting serotype.

As with other bacterial pneumonias, the methods and criteria for establishing a diagnosis are controversial. Gram stain of expectorated sputum typically reveals numerous polymorphonuclear granulocytes and lancet-shaped Gram-positive diplococci. However, the predominant organism may not be obvious on some specimens because of heavy smear contamination with oropharyngeal flora. Sputum Gram stain and culture also can be misleading in patients who have received prior antibiotics and in patients with chronic obstructive pulmonary disease. Isolation of the organism in the sputum is not sensitive for the presence of infection; in fact, only 45% of patients with pneumonia and blood cultures positive for pneumococci grow the organism on sputum culture. For this reason, many culture-negative cases of pneumonia may be caused by the pneumococcus. Isolation of the organism from blood, pleural fluid, or other involved closed tissue space (e.g., joint, cerebrospinal fluid, pericardium) may be required for a firm diagnosis. A rapid urinary antigen test (Binax NOW) is available to detect pneumococcal pneumonia earlier in its course. The sensitivity is 60% to 70% (higher for bacteremic patients), whereas the specificity approaches 100%. Two recent studies have reported immunochromatographic tests capable of rapidly detecting streptococcus pneumonia antigen in sputum and pleural fluid. In the sputum study, the sensitivity was greater than the urinary antigen test and just as specific.

Much of our understanding of the natural history of pneumococcal pneumonia comes from experience during the preantibiotic era, when three clinical patterns were observed: (1) a 5- to 10-day course characterized by high fevers with defervescence and recovery occurring either gradually (lysis) or dramatically (crisis); (2) a protracted or recrudescent febrile course indicative of complications such as empyema, meningitis, endocarditis, and pericarditis; or (3) rapid respiratory deterioration and death. An initial leukocytosis exceeding 20,000 correlated with a good prognosis, whereas a normal or low leukocyte count implied a grave prognosis. An abrupt fall in leukocyte count often preceded resolution by crisis, but persistent leukocytosis frequently was a harbinger of complications such as empyema.

Although antibiotics have improved survival, pneumococcal pneumonia remains a serious disease. In the preantibiotic era, the overall mortality rate was 25% to 35%. In bacteremic patients, it exceeded 80%. Antibiotics have reduced the mortality rate to 5% and 20%, respectively most within the first week of illness. Of patients who die despite antibiotic therapy, 35% die within the first 24 hours of antibiotic treatment, underscoring the fulminant course this disease can pursue. Mortality in those who require mechanical ventilation remains high. Advanced age, presence of asthma or chronic obstructive pulmonary disease, and high acute physiology and chronic health evaluation (APACHE) scores are independent predictors of poor outcome in bacteremic pneumococcal disease. Inability to mount a fever and nosocomially-acquired pneumococcal pneumonia are additional risk factors for respiratory failure or death.

Penicillin G continues to be the drug of choice for sensitive pneumococcal pneumonia. It is effective either orally or intramuscularly in moderately to severely ill patients but should be administered intravenously in the critically ill and in those with empyema or extrapulmonary foci of infection. Penicillin-sensitive strains can also be treated with penicillin derivatives, and second and third-generation cephalosporins. First generation cephalosporins should not be used because poor penetration into the cerebrospinal fluid increases the risk of developing pneumococcal meningitis. Administration of at least one active antibiotic within 4 hours has been associated with reduced mortality and shortened length of stay especially in bacteremic patients. Therapy of uncomplicated pneumonia should be continued for 5 to 7 days or at least 3 to 5 days after defervescence of fever in more severe cases. Although monotherapy with a single effective antibiotic for pneumococcal pneumonia is standard, recent studies have shown a significant survival benefit for combination therapy in patients with bacteremic pneumococcal pneumonia who required intensive care unit admission. In one large study, mortality rate at 14 days was reduced from 55% to 14% with combination therapy.

Worldwide it is becoming more common to find pneumococcal strains that have developed intermediate or full resistance to penicillin, probably through alteration of cellular penicillin-binding proteins. Approximately 20% of pneumococcal strains in the United States show an intermediate resistance, indicated by a mean inhibitory concentration of 0.1 to 1.0 μg/mL. In this setting, increasing the penicillin dose to 12 to 18 million units per day may be effective, as would administration of cefotaxime, ceftriaxone, imipenem, or fluoroquinolones once sensitivities have been confirmed. Twenty percent of pneumococcal isolates are highly resistant (types 6, 9, 14, 19, and 23), with a mean inhibitory concentration of at least 2 μg/mL. Multiresistant strains (resistant to penicillin, trimethoprim–sulfamethoxazole, chloramphenicol, tetracycline, macrolides, and even second- and third-generation cephalosporins) have been isolated in the United States. Resistance to levofloxacin and moxifloxacin has been reported as well but rates remain low (<1%). Vancomycin, fluoroquinolones, or an alternative agent based on *in vitro* sensitivities should be used for strains with high-level penicillin resistance or resistance to multiple antibiotics. Drug-resistant infections have been observed in certain institutional settings, particularly daycare centers, hospitals, and nursing homes.

Interestingly, a number of studies have continued to show that antibiotic resistance to the pneumococcus is not necessarily associated with increased morbidity or mortality in patients with pneumococcal pneumonia with and without bacteremia. Treatment options, however, for meningitis and for infections treated with oral agents especially in children have been limited by resistance. A meta-analysis of 10 studies published in 2006 did find a significant difference in mortality rate (19.4% vs. 15.7%) between penicillin nonsusceptible and penicillin susceptible groups. It would seem that strategies to prevent or limit the development of resistance through appropriate antimicrobial use are to be encouraged by physicians and patients.

With regard to antibiotic response, in one large study of 358 patients, 71% were afebrile within 5 days of therapy. A slow clinical response is frequently associated with delayed radiographic resolution. In one series of bacteremic patients, only 13% had complete roentgenographic clearing within 2 weeks. Of the others, 61% cleared by 6 weeks, 78% cleared by 10 weeks, and 100% cleared by 18 weeks. Conversely, the chest roentgenogram can appear worse or unchanged, despite clinical improvement with antibiotics. Thus, slow radiographic resolutions do not indicate treatment failure in the face of clinical response.

Complications of pneumococcal pneumonia include necrotizing pneumonia, lung abscess, meningitis, endocarditis, septic arthritis, and pleural disease. Pleural complications are common, and most patients have pleuritic chest pain. A pleural friction rub has been reported in 17% of cases. Pleural effusions can be detected in nearly 60% of patients if repetitive lateral decubitus chest radiographs are obtained. Although the effusions usually are sterile (parapneumonic) exudates, the incidence of empyema is approximately 15%. Diagnostic thoracentesis is mandatory for all large effusions occurring with pneumococcal pneumonia. A pleural fluid pH less than 7.2 suggests that a complicated parapneumonic effusion or frank empyema is present and that chest tube drainage is indicated. Conservative treatment with antibiotics is usually successful if the pH is greater than 7.3. Both parapneumonic effusions and empyemas can accumulate during antibiotic therapy. Generally, the patient with empyema usually appears ill, with a persistent or recrudescent fever and leukocytosis. The degree of pleural disease correlates well with the extent of the initial pneumonia. Early therapy decreases the incidence of empyema.

Pneumococcal vaccines are an important weapon against the pneumococcus. For adults, the vaccine has evolved since 1983 to include 23 purified capsular polysaccharide antigens (the 23-valent vaccine) chosen to represent 90% of the serotypes that cause invasive disease in the United States. Pneumococcal infections have the highest mortality rate of any vaccine-preventable disease; about half of these deaths are felt to be preventable by the polysaccharide vaccine. Many trials have shown failure to protect against nonbacteremic community-acquired pneumonia, as well as those at the highest risk for pneumococcal pneumonia, but a large prospective study from Spain published in 2006 and involving 11,000 subjects, found that the 23-valent vaccine was very effective in preventing pneumococcal pneumonia with or without bacteremia and reducing hospitalization and mortality from pneumonia in adults greater than 65 years. This is consistent with an earlier Swedish study. A 2010 study involving 1,000 randomized nursing home residents showed reduced rates of pneumonia in the vaccinated subjects (12.5% vs. 20.6%) and reduced mortality from pneumococcal pneumonia (0% vs. 35%). There is recent evidence that HIV-infected adults who receive the vaccine have a lower rate of pneumonia, but there appears to be no benefit if the viral load is greater than 100,000 copies/mL at the time of vaccination. There is also consistent evidence that the polysaccharide vaccine significantly reduces the risk of pneumococcal bacteremia. A serotype prevalence study based on the Centers for Disease Control's pneumococcal surveillance system demonstrated a 57% overall protective effect of this vaccine against invasive disease. The reduction in pneumococcal bacteremia is felt to be reason enough to administer the vaccine. Pneumococcal vaccine can be administered concurrently with other vaccines. The antibody levels to most vaccine antigens remain elevated for at least 5 years in healthy adults. Vaccination is recommended for all persons older than age 65; those with chronic medical illnesses; patients who are immunosuppressed, especially by asplenia; and patients in chronic-care facilities. Routine revaccination of immunocompetent persons is not recommended. A single repeat vaccination is recommended for persons who are at highest risk for serious pneumococcal infection, provided that 5 years have elapsed since the first dose.

In February 2000, a promising new vaccine formulation was approved by the Food and Drug Administration (FDA) for use in children younger than age 2—the protein conjugate heptavalent vaccine (PCV-7). This vaccine links the capsular polysaccharide of seven serotypes to a protein carrier, thereby making it immunogenic in children younger than age 2. Studies have shown high efficacy (80%–100%) against invasive disease in children, modest efficacy against noninvasive vaccine type pneumococcal otitis media, and reduction in the carriage and transmission of nasopharyngeal pneumococcus including antibiotic-resistant isolates. One year after the licensing of the conjugate vaccine, a dramatic reduction in invasive disease was documented in children. At the end of 2004, all-cause pneumonia admission rates had declined by 39% in the United States for children younger than 2 years, the target population of the vaccination program. Between 2001 and 2007 there has also been a significant reduction in pneumococcal invasive disease rates and mortality in adults (HIV-infected as well), coupled with a reduction in nonsusceptible pneumococcal isolates. There has been a greater than 95% reduction in invasive pneumococcal disease caused by serotypes covered by the vaccine (types 4, 6B, 9, 14, 18C, 19F, 23F). Mortality in greater than greater than 65-year age group declined from 31% to 8% in Minnesota. Unfortunately although the disease caused by vaccine-containing serotypes has been reduced substantially, there has been a distinct unexpected increase in disease caused by nonvaccine "replacement" serotypes, especially serotypes 19A, 6 (non B), 11, 15, and 35. However, in a large prospective review of patients with pneumococcal bacteremia, there was no association between infection with invasive serotypes and mortality.

A 13-valent pneumococcal conjugate vaccine has been recently approved by the US FDA for children 6 weeks through 5 years for the prevention of invasive disease by the 13 strains of Streptococcal pneumoniae included in the vaccine. It has also been approved for adults 50 years and older for prevention of pneumococcal pneumonia and invasive disease caused by the 13 vaccine strains, on the basis of immune response to the vaccine. No controlled trial in adults, demonstrating a reduction in pneumococcal pneumonia or invasive disease following vaccination with the 13 valent vaccine, has yet been published. The Center for Disease Control and Prevention is awaiting the outcome of a large trial being conducted in Europe before deciding whether to recommend the vaccine for adults aged 50 or older.

FURTHER READING

1. Austrian R, Gold J. Pneumococcal bacteremia with special reference to bacteremic pneumococcal pneumonia. *Ann Intern Med.* 1964;60:759.

    A classic paper describing the natural history of pneumococcal pneumonia and the benefits (and limitations) of antibiotic therapy.

2. Austrian R. Pneumococcal pneumonia: diagnostic, epidemiologic, therapeutic, and prophylactic considerations. *Chest.* 1986;90:738.

    A general update from the previous paper.

3. Barret-Connor E. The nonvalue of sputum culture in the diagnosis of pneumococcal pneumonia. *Am Rev Respir Dis.* 1971;103:845.

    The isolation of pneumococci from sputum may be both difficult and misleading.

4. Bartlett JG, Mundy LM. Community-acquired pneumonia. *N Engl J Med.* 1995;333(24):1618.

    Pneumonia is the sixth leading cause of death in the United States. Prevention of influenza and pneumococcal pneumonia by vaccination should be assigned a high priority.

5. Davies D, Hodgson G, Whitby L. A study of pneumococcal pneumonia. *Lancet.* 1935;1:791.

    A clinical description of this disease in the preantibiotic era.

6. Waterer GW, Somes GW, Wunderink RG. Monotherapy may be suboptimal for severe bacteremic pneumococcal pneumonia. *Arch Intern Med.* 2001;161:1837–1842.

    Dual effective therapy reduces mortality compared with single effective therapy in bacteremic pneumococcal pneumonia.

7. Moroney JF, Fiore AE, Harrison LH, et al. Clinical outcomes of bacteremic pneumococcal pneumonia in the era of antibiotic resistance. *Clin Infect Dis.* 2001;33:797–805.

    Antimicrobial resistance in cases of invasive pneumococcal pneumonia appears to have no impact on mortality or need for ICU. Potential reasons discussed.

8. Doern GV. Antimicrobial resistance with *Streptococcus pneumoniae:* much ado about nothing? *Semin Respir Infect.* 2001;16:177–185.

   In vitro antibiotic resistance to S. pneumoniae *does not necessarily translate into diminished effectiveness in vivo.*

9. Aspa J, Rajas O, Rodriguez de Castro F, et al. Drug-resistant pneumococcal pneumonia: clinical relevance and related factors. *Clin Infect Dis.* 2004;38:787–798.

   Multicenter study of 638 cases of pneumococcal pneumonia in which high incidence of antibiotic resistance did not increase morbidity. Complications were, in fact, more common in penicillin-sensitive patients.

10. Marcos MA, Jimenez de Anta MT, de la Bellacasa JP, et al. Rapid urinary antigen test for diagnosis of pneumococcal community-acquired pneumonia in adults. *Eur Respir J.* 2003;21:209–214.

    The Binax NOW urinary antigen test is sensitive and specific for detecting pneumococcal pneumonia.

11. Lujan M, Gallego M, Fontanals D, et al. Prospective observational study of bacteremic pneumococcal pneumonia: effect of discordant therapy on mortality. *Crit Care Med.* 2004;32:625–631.

    Survival is improved if an antibiotic with in vitro activity against the isolated strain is administered within 24 hours.

12. Anderson KB, Tan JS, File TM Jr, et al. Emergence of levofloxacin-resistant pneumococci in immunocompromised adults after therapy for community-acquired pneumonia. *Clin Infect Dis.* 2003;37:376–381.

    Levofloxacin resistance is more likely in immunosuppressed patients after a recent prior course of levofloxacin.

13. O'Brien KL, Santosham M. Potential impact of conjugate pneumococcal vaccines on pediatric pneumococcal diseases. *AMJ Epidemiol.* 2004;159:634–644.

    Up-to-date review of the effectiveness of the new conjugated vaccine.

14. Drew WL. Value of sputum culture in diagnosis of pneumococcal pneumonia. *J Clin Microbiol.* 1977;6:62.

    Positive sputum cultures were obtained in 94% of bacteremic pneumococcal pneumonias. Poor culture yields may result from suboptimal technique.

15. Janoff EN, Breiman RF, Daley CL, et al. Pneumococcal disease during HIV infection: epidemiologic, clinical, and immunologic perspectives. *Ann Intern Med.* 1992;117:314.

    Streptococcus pneumoniae *is the leading cause of invasive bacterial respiratory disease in patients with HIV infection. Prompt diagnosis and treatment are associated with favorable outcome.*

16. Jay SJ, Johanson W, Pierce A. The radiographic resolution of *Streptococcus pneumoniae* pneumonia. *N Engl J Med.* 1975;293:798.

    A good study in bacteremic patients.

17. Ort S, Ryan JL, Barden G, et al. Pneumococcal pneumonia in hospitalized patients: clinical and radiologic presentations. *JAMA.* 1983;249:214.

    Atypical presentations are common.

18. Marfin AA, Sporrer J, Moore PS, et al. Risk factors for adverse outcome in persons with pneumococcal pneumonia. *Chest.* 1995;107:2.

    Risk factors identified at hospital admission can predict the outcome in persons with pneumococcal pneumonia and bacteremia.

19. Nuorti JP, Butler JC, Crutcher JM, et al. An outbreak of multidrug-resistant pneumococcal pneumonia and bacteremia among unvaccinated nursing home residents. *N Engl J Med.* 1998;338:1861.

    The first report in the United States of an epidemic outbreak of multidrug-resistant pneumococcal pneumonia in unvaccinated nursing home residents.

20. Taryle DA, Sahn SA. The incidence and clinical correlates of parapneumonic effusions in pneumococcal pneumonia. *Chest.* 1978;74:170.

    Effusions are common when looked for carefully. Their presence correlates with duration of symptoms before admission, bacteremia, and prolonged fever after therapy.

21. Tuomanen EI, Austrian R, Masure HRN. Pathogenesis of pneumococcal infection. *N Engl J Med.* 1995;332:1280.

    A review of some of the molecular details of the pathogenesis of pneumococcal infection in relation to the current understanding of the genesis of the clinical symptoms and signs.

22. Van Vetre T. Pneumococcal pneumonia treated with antibiotics: the prognostic significance of certain clinical findings. *N Engl J Med.* 1954;251:1048.

    Prognostic correlates in 358 cases.

23. Marrie TJ, Tuomanen EI. Pneumococcal pneumonia in adults. *UpToDate.* June 1, 2010.

    Comprehensive current review.

24. Sexton DJ, Jaggers LB. Invasive pneumococcal infections and bacteremia. *UpToDate.* May 13, 2010.

    Comprehensive current review.

25. Musher DM. Resistance of *Streptococcus pneumoniae* to beta-lactam antibiotics. *UpToDate.* June 4, 2009.

    Comprehensive current review.

26. Pletz MW, van der Linden M, von Baum H, et al; CAPNETZ study group. Low prevalence of fluoroquinolone resistant strains and resistance precursor strains in *Streptococcus pneumoniae* from patients with community-acquired pneumonia despite high fluoroquinolone usage. *Int J Med Microbiol.* 2011;301(1):53–57.

    Absence of resistance likely explained by high use of third-generation fluoroquinolones with enhanced activity against pneumococci.

27. Maruyama T, Taguchi O, Niederman MS. Efficacy of 23-valent pneumococcal vaccine in preventing pneumonia and improving survival in nursing home residents. *BMJ.* 2010;340: c1004.

    Pneumonia occurred in 12.5% of participants in the vaccine group and 20.6% in the placebo group. Mortality was 35% in placebo group and 0% in the vaccine group.

28. French N, Gordon SB, Mwalukomo T. A trial of a 7-valent pneumococcal conjugate vaccine in HIV-infected adults. *N Eng J Med.* 2010;362(9):812–822.

    The vaccine protected HIV-infected adults from recurrent pneumococcal infection caused by vaccine serotypes.

29. Garnacho-Montero J, Garcia-Cabrera E. Determinants of outcome in patients with bacteremic pneumococcal pneumonia: importance of early adequate treatment. *Scand J Infect Dis.* 2010;42(3):185–192.

    Adequate antibiotic therapy within 4 hours of arrival is a critical determinant of survival in bacteremic pneumococcal pneumonia.

30. Van der Poll T, Opal SM. Pathogenesis, treatment and prevention of pneumococcal pneumonia. *Lancet.* 2009;374(9700):1543–1556.

    Review of the versatility of the genome and virulence capability of the pneumococcus versus an array of host defenses shows that many vaccine antigens, antibiotic combinations, and immunoadjuvant therapies will be needed to control this microbe.

31. Juhn YJ, Kita H, Yawn BP, et al. Increased risk of serious pneumococcal disease in patients with asthma. *J Allergy Clin Immunol.* 2008;122(4):719–723.

    In this study, serious pneumococcal disease was associated with a history of asthma among all age groups, but especially adults.

32. Teshale EH, Hanson D, Flannery B, et al. Effectiveness of 23-valent polysaccharide pneumococcal vaccine on pneumonia in HIV-infected adults in the United States, 1998–2003. *Vaccine.* 2008;26(46):5830–5834.

    Vaccinated patients had lower rate of pneumonia, but no benefit when patients were vaccinated at HIV viral load greater than 100,000 copies/mL irrespective of CD4 count.

33. Jacobs MR. Antimicrobial-resistant *Streptococcus pneumoniae*: trends and management. *Expert Rev Anti Infect Ther.* 2008;6(5):619–635.

    Management of pneumococcal infections challenged by development of resistance, especially new resistant clones of serotypes following the introduction of the conjugate vaccine for children.

34. Ehara N, Fukushima K, Kakeya H, et al. A novel method for rapid detection of *Streptococcus pneumoniae* antigen in sputum and it's application in adult respiratory tract infections. *J Med Microbiol.* 2008;57(pt 7):820–866.

    Results suggest that this direct sputum detection kit may be more clinically useful than the urinary antigen detection kit in adult patients.

35. Berjohn CM, Fishman NO, Joffe MM, et al. Treatment and outcomes for patients with bacteremic pneumococcal pneumonia. *Medicine.* 2008;87(3):160–166.

    Overall in-hospital mortality was 10%. Receipt of at least one active antibiotic within 4 hours was associated with reduced mortality and shortened length of stay.

36. Brueggermann AB, Pai R, Crook DW, et al. Vaccine escape recombinants emerge after pneumococcal vaccine in the United States. *PLoS Pathog.* 2007;3(11):e168.

    Heptovalent conjugate vaccine introduced in the United States in 2000 has significantly reduced invasive pneumococcal disease. However, incidence of nonvaccine serotype invasive disease has increased. The study looks at the genetic events that may be giving rise to these novel serotypes.

37. Feldman C, Klugman KP, Yu VL, et al. Bacteremic pneumococcal pneumonia: impact of HIV on clinical presentation and outcome. *J Infect.* 2007;55(2):125–135.

    Multicenter prospective study showed that HIV patients with pneumococcal bacteremia have a significantly higher 14 day mortality especially if CD4 count was low as well.

38. Porcel JM, Ruiz-Gonzalez A, Falguera M, et al. Contribution of a pleural antigen assay (Binax NOW) to the diagnosis of pneumococcal pneumonia. *Chest.* 2007;131(5):1442–1447.

    The pleural antigen assay augments the standard diagnostic methods of blood and pleural fluid cultures and enhances the urinary antigen assay.

39. Mufson MA, Chan G, Stanek RJ. Penicillin resistance not a factor in outcome from invasive *Streptococcus pneumoniae* community-acquired pneumonia in adults when appropriate empiric therapy is started. *Am J Med Sci.* 2007;333(3):161–167.

    Combination antibiotic regimens effective in the treatment of invasive susceptible S. pneumonia are equally effective in the treatment of invasive resistant and of intermediate S. pneumoniae pneumonia.

40. Chiou CC, Yu VL. Severe pneumococcal pneumonia: new strategies for management. *Curr Opin Crit Care.* 2006;12(5):470–476.

    Parenteral penicillin remains the drug of choice to treat pneumococcal pneumonia regardless of in vitro resistance. Combination antimicrobial therapy will improve survival of critically ill patients with bacteremia.

41. Villa-Corcoles A, Ochoa-Gondar O, Hospital I, et al. Protective effects of the 23-valent pneumococcal polysaccharide vaccine in the elderly population: the EVAN-65 study. *Clin Infect Dis.* 2006;43(7):860–868.

    The 23-valent vaccine effectively prevented pneumococcal pneumonia (with or without bacteremia) and reduced hospitalization and mortality rates due to pneumonia in older (≥65 years) adults.

Staphylococcal and Streptococcal Pneumonias

Omar H. Mohamedaly and Laura E. Crotty Alexander

Staphylococcus and *Streptococcus* are Gram-positive cocci responsible for a broad spectrum of human disease and are common causes of pneumonia. Staphylococci typically grow in clusters, whereas streptococci occur in pairs and chains. Recovery of staphylococci from sputum culture is more reliable than for streptococci since antibiotics administered prior to obtaining culture specimens commonly inhibit streptococcal growth more than staphylococci.

Staphylococci secrete various catalases, which can be used to discriminate among species. *S. aureus,* a common pathogen in humans, is coagulase positive, which distinguishes it from the common contaminants *S. epidermidis* and *S. saprophyticus. S. aureus* is common in healthcare-associated pneumonia (HCAP). It is isolated in 15% to 23% of HCAP cases, compared to 3% to

9% of community-acquired pneumonia (CAP) cases. The incidence of *S. aureus* pneumonia continues to rise in both the HCAP and CAP settings. Risk factors for infection with *S. aureus* reflect impairment of host defenses, which include lung structure derangements (e.g., cystic fibrosis and bronchiectasis) as well as immunological defects (e.g., diabetes mellitus, alcoholism or postinfluenza).

S. aureus pneumonia commonly presents with fever, productive cough, and pleuritic chest pain. Radiographic patterns include extensive bilateral consolidation and cavitary lesions, especially early in the disease course. Pleural effusions are common. Empyema complicates about 20% of *S. aureus* pneumonias and the incidence appears to be rising; national registry data show a 3.3-fold increase in staphylococcal empyema between 1996 and 2008. Bacteremia may complicate as many as 60% of all *S. aureus* pneumonias.

Since it was first identified in 1961 on the basis of resistance to semisynthetic penicillins, methicillin-resistant *S. aureus* (MRSA) has come to represent a large proportion of staphylococcal diseases: over 60% of *S. aureus* isolates from US intensive care units are MRSA. Use of antibiotics, especially fluoroquinolones and cephalosporins, increases the risk of MRSA colonization and infection. Mortality is higher in invasive disease caused by MRSA as compared to methicillin-sensitive *S. aureus* (MSSA), with an odds ratio of 1.93.

MRSA more commonly causes HCAP than CAP (26.5% vs. 8.9% in one survey of 59 US hospitals covering 4,543 patients); however, the incidence is rising in the community setting. In particular, influenza patients who develop *S. aureus* super-infection most commonly have MRSA. The USA300 strain is a community-acquired MRSA that has rapidly spread across the world and is likely to continue increasing in prevalence and severity. It is characterized by the presence of the arginine catabolic mobile element (ACME) and production of Panton–Valentine leukocidin (PVL), a bicomponent pore-forming toxin responsible for neutrophil lysis, adhesion to mucous membranes, and an inflammatory response mediated by NF-κB. There are conflicting data on the morbidity and mortality attributable to PVL-positive strains. Another *S. aureus* virulence factor, α-hemolysin, might be more directly responsible for pneumonia-related mortality. Further investigation of other virulence factors implicates the superantigens responsible for staphylococcal toxic shock syndrome in the development of necrotizing pneumonias, for example, the small secreted protein SEIX, which is encoded by mobile genetic elements that are easily transmitted horizontally among strains.

The initial antimicrobial choice for *S. aureus* should be guided by local patterns of resistance and the degree of suspicion for MRSA. It can be tailored to culture and sensitivity results once they are available. Vancomycin remains the antimicrobial of choice for MRSA coverage. Though resistance is rare, minimum inhibitory concentration (MIC) creep is an increasing problem that has given rise to vancomycin-intermediate *S. aureus* (VISA), whichrequires higher doses to achieve sufficient MIC. High vancomycin doses, however, can be problematic in critically ill patients with renal failure. One emerging source of resistance is β-lactam-induced vancomycin resistance (BIVR), the clinical implications of which are not fully apparent at this point. Linezolid resistance has also been identified, but with stricter control of linezolid prescription practices, it has been kept from spreading. It is noteworthy the concentration of vancomycin in the alveolar epithelium is only 12% of the vancomycin plasma concentration, which is far less than the 415% noted with linezolid. Linezolid has the additional advantage that its volume of distribution is not affected by critical illness and volume shifts. However, a major clinical trial comparing vancomycin to linezolid for MRSA pneumonia treatment (ZEPHYR) did not demonstrate superiority of linezolid and had significant methodological flaws limiting its generalizability. The fifth-generation cephalosporins, ceftaroline and ceftobiprole, have some potential for MRSA treatment. They have been shown to be noninferior to the older cephalosporins and to linezolid.

Promising efforts are underway to develop vaccines against *S. aureus*. Several targets are being investigated, including PVL (despite the lack of a direct link to morbidity and mortality), cell surface proteins, and peptidoglycan cell wall components. Blockade of ADAM10 receptor binding by α-hemolysin has shown efficacy in protecting against lethal pneumonia in animal models. Multi-antigenic approaches to vaccination against *S. aureus* are likely to be developed in the future.

Although there are more streptococcal species than staphylococcal, only three, *S. pyogenes*, *S. agalactiae*, and *S. pneumoniae*, play a major role in human lung infection. Streptococci are classified by the pattern of hemolysis on blood agar culture media: α-hemolysis refers to partial or green hemolysis related to oxidation of iron in hemoglobin within red blood cells, β refers to complete hemolysis causing RBC rupture, γ refers to lack of hemolysis. β-hemolytic streptococci are further classified by Lancefield group: 20 serotypes named A to V (sans I and J), referring to the carbohydrate antigenic composition of their cell walls.

Group A streptococcus, *S. pyogenes,* is the etiologic organism of some of the most publicized diseases in medicine: streptococcal pharyngitis, necrotizing fasciitis (for which it earned the label "flesh-eating bacteria"), and toxic shock syndrome. It is also responsible for some of the most severe cases of CAP, although it fortunately remains a rare cause of CAP, accounting only for less than 1% of cases. Group A streptococcus outbreaks have occurred in nursing homes, in military recruitment facilities, and in families. Presenting symptoms include cough, fever, sore throat, pleuritic chest pain, and dyspnea. Group A streptococcal pneumonia is typically multilobar (59%). Parapneumonic effusion are more common in group A streptococcal pneumonia (23%) than in pneumonia caused by *S. pneumoniae* (16%). Infections can be complicated by development of toxic shock syndrome (6%), and treatment with clindamycin to restrain toxin production by group A streptococci may be helpful early in disease. Patients with group A streptococcal pneumonia tend to have longer duration of symptoms, longer hospitalizations, more morbidity, and higher mortality (38%) than those with pneumonia caused by *S. pneumoniae.*

Host genetic susceptibility to group A streptococcus plays a role in the susceptibility to infection. This is most apparent in outbreaks where family members have higher rates of infection (up to 42%) compared to unrelated military recruits (0.6%). Group A streptococcal infection should be suspected when multiple family members or persons living in close proximity present with symptoms of streptococcal disease. Antibiotic prophylaxis can be considered for individuals in close contact with infected patients, since their rate of infection is 200 times that of the general population (2.9 per 1,000 individuals). However assessment for group A streptococcus via throat culture prior to giving prophylaxis can decrease the number of contacts receiving unnecessary antibiotics.

Group B streptococcus, *S. agalactiae,* is a pathogen of neonates and the elderly (adults ≥65 years). It colonizes 25% of healthy elderly adults in the United States, a similar percentage to that of childbearing women. Just as in group A streptococcal disease, invasive group B streptococcal disease has increased 2- to 4-fold over the past two decades. Group B streptococcus most commonly causes pneumonia in the very young (due to transmission from mothers during childbirth) and in the elderly, with mortality rates of 4% and 14%, respectively. Pneumonia in the elderly accounts for over 50% of group B streptococcus-associated deaths. It often occurs as an HCAP, and presents with lobar or multilobar infiltrates, but no effusions. Presenting symptoms are similar to other bacterial pneumonias. No vaccine has been successfully developed against this major streptococcal pathogen, but much research is ongoing, particularly against group B streptococcal pili which are found on all 10 serotypes.

S. pneumoniae, also known as Pneumococcus, is an α-hemolytic streptococcus that grows as diplococci with a thick capsule. It is the major cause of CAP (30% of all cases) in all settings: outpatient, ward, and intensive care unit. Symptoms include fever, rigors, cough, pleuritic chest pain, and the classic "rust-colored sputum." Lobar consolidation is commonly seen on chest radiographs and can be associated with parapneumonic effusions and empyema. Cavitation is rare. Urinary pneumococcal antigen testing can aid in the diagnosis. It is sensitive, but by no means cost-effective. Pneumococcal pneumonia is accompanied by bacteremia in about 10% to 30% of cases. It most commonly affects children less than less than 2 years and adults greater than 65 years, but infects people of all ages in all settings, including HCAP and postinfluenza. The natural reservoir is the human nasopharynx. Impressively, 50% to 80% of children are colonized by 6 months of age. Despite advances in vaccination and treatment, pneumococcal mortality remains high, ranging from 6.4% to over 40%, depending on the setting.

Historically, penicillin was the antimicrobial treatment of choice for pneumococcal pneumonia. Resistance to penicillin has been on the rise since the first documentation in 1967, but it has not corresponded with an increase in mortality. Two large meta-analyses from the last decade came to conflicting conclusions on the impact of treatment failure on mortality. Regardless, third-generation cephalosporins such as ceftriaxone have become the standard antimicrobial for the empiric treatment of pneumococcal pneumonia, which is also reflected in the current guidelines for CAP treatment. Ceftaroline, the fifth-generation cephalosporin used in resistant MRSA cases, has activity against ceftriaxone-resistant Pneumococcus.

Macrolides, the other component of CAP treatment, have the advantage of immunomodulation in addition to their antimicrobial activity. It may be the former role that is of greater significance in the management of pneumococcal disease. The emergence of macrolide resistance without an increase in mortality bespeaks the immunomodulator theory. A recent small retrospective cohort study suggests that statin therapy might be more protective against pneumococcal mortality than macrolide use. It is noteworthy that greater than 80% of all penicillin and macrolide resistance worldwide is accounted for by only 6 of the 92 serotypes of *S. pneumoniae* (6A, 6B, 9V, 14, 19F, 23F). In the current era of continuous macrolide therapy for chronic obstructive pulmonary disease (COPD) and bronchiectasis, new resistance patterns and their effect on pneumonia prevalence and mortality may come to light.

Pneumococcal serotypes are relevant to the protection afforded by available vaccines and the controversy surrounding vaccine efficacy. As a combination of polysaccharide rather than protein antigens, the current 23-valent pneumococcal vaccine provides T-cell-independent immunity, thus eliciting no memory B cell formation and showing no anamnestic or booster response upon revaccination. In fact, hyporesponsiveness, the eliciting of an even weaker immune response upon revaccination, might be an issue despite current guidelines for revaccination after 5 years if the first dose was received under the age of 65 or the patient has a high risk for pneumococcal disease. A Cochrane review in 2008 disclosed a vaccine-related reduction in invasive pneumococcal disease with an OR of 0.26, though efficacy against all-cause pneumonia was unclear and there was no evidence of efficacy against all-cause mortality. A subsequent meta-analysis analyzing studies by methodological quality also failed to show the benefit of pneumococcal vaccination in reduction of pneumococcal pneumonia, all-cause pneumonia, or mortality. Nonetheless, observational studies suggest some benefit of vaccination, although it is limited to healthy adults, not elderly and immunocompromised patients that make up the population with the highest pneumococcal mortality. Specifically, there is no evidence of benefit in HIV patients despite vaccination recommendations for such patients. Most studies included in the aforementioned meta-analyses used the 14-valent rather than the 23-valent vaccine, thus further studies are needed to evaluate the efficacy of the 23-valent vaccine. A protein-conjugate vaccine, correcting the T-cell-independence of polysaccharide vaccines, is available for children. It offers coverage against fewer serotypes, but adults seem to benefit from the "herd immunity" effect conferred by childhood vaccination. Perhaps the most promise lies in investigation of protein-based vaccines, especially those targeting virulence factors conserved across different Pneumococcus serotypes, such as pneumolysin.

FURTHER READING

1. Kollef MH, Shorr A, Tabak YP, et al. Epidemiology and outcomes of healthcare-associated pneumonia. Results from a large US database of culture-positive pneumonia. *Chest.* 2005;128:3854–3862.

    4,543 patients with culture-positive peptide nucleic acid. Staphylococcus aureus *(SA, MSSA, and MRSA) was the most common pathogen in all groups, but higher prevalence in non-CAP. Non-CAP patients had higher mortality rates of 19% to 29%.*

2. Watkins RR, David MZ, Salata RA. Current concepts on the virulence mechanisms of methicillin-resistant *Staphylococcus aureus. J Med Microbiol.* 2012;61:1179–1193.

    A nice review of what is known and unknown about MRSA virulence factors, and where ongoing research efforts are focused.

3. Peyrani P, Allen M, Wiemken TL, et al. Severity of disease and clinical outcomes in patients with hospital-acquired pneumonia due to methicillin-resistant *Staphylococcus aureus* strains not influenced by the presence of the Panton-Valentine Leukocidin gene. *Clin Infect Dis.* 2011;53:766–771.

    Observational study of 109 cases of MRSA pneumonia, finding that expression of PVL has no impact on severity of disease or mortality, and thus is not a major virulence factor.

4. Ramirez P, Fernández-Barat L, Torres A. New therapy options for MRSA with respiratory infection/pneumonia. *Curr Opin Infect Dis.* 2012;25:159–165.

    A summary of what new MRSA treatments have been tried, and have failed! Vancomycin and linezolid remain the best, but telavancin may be used in patients without renal failure.

5. Holmes NE, Turnidge JD, Munckhof WJ, et al. Antibiotic choice may not explain poorer outcomes in patients with *Staphyloccus aureus* bacteremia and high vancomycin minimum inhibitory concentrations. *J Infect Dis.* 2011;204:340–347.

Interesting study demonstrating that patients whose MRSA or MSSA has a higher vancomycin MIC have higher mortality, and this is not related to what drug is used to treat them, consistent with the Vancomycin MIC being a surrogate marker for some other virulence factor present in these SA strains.

6. Conte JE Jr, Golden JA, Kipps J, et al. Intrapulmonary pharmacokinetics of linezolid. *Antimicrob Agents Chemother.* 2002;46:1475–1480.

A very nice study of how effectively linezolid penetrates the lung and gets into the epithelial lining fluid.

7. Stevens DL, Herr D, Lampiris H, et al. Linezolid versus vancomycin for the treatment of methicillin-resistant *Staphylococcus aureus* infections. *Clin Infect Dis.* 2002;34:1481–1490.

The first trial to show equivalence between linezolid and vancomycin in the treatment of MRSA pneumonia (as well as other sites of infection).

8. Blasi F, Mantero M, Santus P, et al. Understanding the burden of pneumococcal disease in adults. *Clin Microbiol Infect.* 2012;18:7–14.

Excellent summary of pneumococcal disease, vaccination, and treatment today.

9. Metlay JP. Antibacterial drug resistance: implications for the treatment of patients with community-acquired pneumonia. *Infect Dis Clin North Am.* 2004;18:777–790.

A discussion of antibiotic drug resistance trends and how changes in vaccination may change disease prevalence in the future.

10. Tleyjeh IM, Tlaygeh HM, Hejal R, et al. The impact of penicillin resistance on short-term mortality in hospitalized adults with pneumococcal pneumonia: a systematic review and meta-analysis. *Clin Infect Dis.* 2006;42:788–797.

Meta-analysis (10 studies) confirming that penicillin resistance is associated with a higher mortality rate in hospitalized patients with pneumococcal pneumonia.

11. Lynch JP III, Zhanel GG. Escalation of antimicrobial resistance among *Streptococcus pneumoniae*: implications for therapy. *Semin Respir Crit Care Med.* 2005;26:575–616.

A nice in-depth discussion of what antimicrobial resistance in S. pneumonia might mean.

12. Pfaller MA, Farrell DJ, Sader HS, et al. AWARE Ceftaroline Surveillance Program (2008-2010): trends in resistance patterns among *Streptococcus pneumoniae, Haemophilus influenzae,* and *Moraxella catarrhalis* in the United States. *Clin Infect Dis.* 2012;55(S3):S187–S193.

13. Huss A, Scott P, Stuck AE, et al. Efficacy of pneumococcal vaccination in adults: a meta-analysis. *CMAJ.* 2009;180:48–58.

Meta-analysis (22 trials) concluding that pneumococcal vaccination does not confer protection against pneumonia in general, and in the elderly and chronically ill in particular.

14. Moberley SA, Holden J, Tatham DP, et al. Vaccines for preventing pneumococcal infection in adults. *Cochrane Database Syst Rev* 2013;(1):CD000422.

Meta-analysis (25 studies) finding that pneumococcal vaccination does prevent pneumococcal pneumonia in adults (not as much in the chronically ill population though) especially in low-income countries.

15. Doshi SM, Kulkarni PA, Liao JM, et al. The impact of statin and macrolide use on early survival in patients with pneumococcal pneumonia. *Am J Med Sci.* 2013;345(3):173–177.

Interesting study which found that even though statin users had more chronic diseases and were sicker on admission than nonstatin users with pneumococcal pneumonia, the statin users had lower mortality at 7, 14, 20, and 30 days after admission. Treatment with a macrolide did not change survival.

16. Crum NF, Russell KL, Kaplan EL, et al. Pneumonia outbreak associated with group A *Streptococcus* species at a military training facility. *Clin Infect Dis.* 2005;40(4):511–518.

Case-control study of 56 Marine Corp personnel who developed group A Streptococcal pneumonia, and a finding that pharyngeal carriage rate of GAS was 16% at that time. This report confirmed the need for antibiotic prophylaxis in high-risk populations.

17. Edwards MS, Baker CJ. Group B Streptococcal infections in elderly adults. *Clin Infect Dis.* 2005;41(6):839–847.

18. Diep BA, Stone GG, Basuino L, et al. The arginine catabolic mobile element and staphylococcal chromosomal cassette mec linkage: convergence of virulence and resistance in the USA300 clone of methicillin-resistant *Staphylococcus aureus*. *J Infect Dis.* 2008;197(11):1523–1530.

ACME enhances growth and survival of MRSA strain USA300, while SCCmec protects against β-lactams.

Haemophilus influenzae Infections

Dennis E. Amundson and Jennifer M. Radin

Haemophilus influenzae are small, pleomorphic, nonmotile oxidative-positive, Gram-negative rods that occur in both encapsulated and nonencapsulated forms. The encapsulated forms (types A–F), and particularly *H. influenzae* type B, have increased virulence and are associated with invasive disease (e.g., meningitis, bacteremia, epiglottitis, pneumonia, and septic arthritis), primarily in children younger than age 5. In contrast, the genetically diverse unencapsulated (nontypeable) strains of *H. influenzae* commonly cause mucosal diseases such as community-acquired pneumonia in adults, sinusitis in children and adults, otitis media in children, and bronchitis in patients with chronic lung disease. All strains of *H. influenzae* are fastidious, tend to be overgrown by other bacteria in culture, and require special growth factors (X [hemin] and V [nicotinamide adenine dinucleotide]) to grow aerobically. These factors can be supplied with chocolate or supplemented agars. The six capsular forms are identified and differentiated from the heterogeneous nontypeable *H. influenzae* strains by a variety of serotyping methodologies (e.g., latex particle slide agglutination, countercurrent immunoelectrophoresis).

A dramatic shift has occurred in the epidemiology of *H. influenzae* infections in developed countries since the early 1990s because of the universal implementation of *H. influenzae* type B vaccines in infancy. *H. influenzae* type B is now only a small burden with an estimated incidence of 0.05/100,000 population in the United States. In contrast, all of the *H. influenzae* subtypes together have an estimated incidence of 1.63 of every 100,000 population in the United States and a case fatality rate of 15.3%, with most of the burden coming from the nontypeable strains. Concurrently, there has been increasing global recognition of the importance of nontypeable *H. influenzae* strains as causative agents for respiratory tract infections and for invasive disease. Nontypable strains cause 59% of invasive disease in children and 61% in adults.

Humans are the only known hosts for *H. influenzae*. The organisms, predominately the nontypeable strains, colonize the nasopharynx throughout life, beginning in infancy and can be cultured from 3% to 88% of asymptomatic individuals, depending on the population sampled. Higher rates, increased susceptibility, and more prolonged duration of carriage are observed in those with underlying lung disease (e.g., cystic fibrosis, chronic obstructive pulmonary disease [COPD]) as well as in the relatively immunosuppressed (e.g., chronic renal failure, myeloma, alcoholism, and diabetes). Colonization can be a very dynamic process, with coinfection and strain turnover within days to weeks. Unlike the nontypeable strains, *H. influenzae* type B and other encapsulated strains colonize only a few percentage of healthy individuals. The rate of carriage of *H. influenzae* type B has substantially declined in countries using the *H. influenzae* type B vaccine.

Bacterial transmission occurs through respiratory droplets or contact with secretions and fomites. Increased transmission occurs in closed settings, such as households, child day care centers, and nursing homes. *H. influenzae*, primarily nontypeable strains, cause approximately 20% of all otitis media infections in children and 20% to 25% of all sinus infections in adults. In addition, nontypeable *H. influenzae* strains are second only to *Streptococcus pneumoniae* as the causative agents in community-acquired pneumonia (12%–28% of cases) and are the most common cause of exacerbations of COPD and bronchiectasis. Infection with *H. influenzae* in bronchiectasis is particularly interesting in that the eradication of one strain of the bacteria is quickly followed by reacquisition of another. Additionally, the degree of bacterial load in bronchiectasis is associated with evidence of inflammatory infiltration of the airways and increased airway injury. Risk factors for *H. influenzae* pneumonia include (1) antecedent viral respiratory tract infection (especially influenza A); (2) chronic lung disease (e.g., COPD or bronchiectasis); (3) systemic diseases associated with immunosuppression (e.g., diabetes or cancer);

(4) environmental exposures (e.g., exposure to smoke); and, in some cases, (5) strain-specific virulence factors.

The pathogenesis of disease is very different between encapsulated and unencapsulated strains. The encapsulated strains are better able to survive in the bloodstream because the polysaccharide capsules confer virulence, as in the case of the polyribosylribitol phosphate moieties of *H. influenzae* type B. *H. influenzae* type B invades the nasopharyngeal vascular space; the ensuing bacteremia can result in sepsis, meningitis, epiglottitis, and other deep-seated infections. Other encapsulated serotypes (especially a and f) can cause invasive disease, especially in the immunocompromised population and in a small minority of immunocompetent individuals.

Pathogenesis of disease for the unencapsulated strains is by contiguous spread from a colonized nasopharynx, resulting in localized upper and lower respiratory tract infections. The oligoliposaccharide of *H. influenzae* plays a major role in microbe adherence and colonization. Historically, unencapsulated strains of *H. influenzae* rarely caused tissue invasion. Recent reports from both developing and developed countries suggest they are becoming more prevalent as causes of both invasive disease and pneumonia in healthy children and adults.

Nontypeable *H. influenzae* are common causes of pneumonia in adults and resemble other pneumonias in clinical presentation. Radiographically, multilobar involvement often occurs with patchy or lobar distribution of infiltrates. As with other bacterial pneumonias, bacteremia, parapneumonic effusions, and empyema can occur. Blood cultures and culture of other accessible specimens (e.g., parapneumonic pleural effusion) should be done, although the yield from blood cultures for nontypeable strains is low. Gram stain and culture of tracheobronchial secretions can be difficult to interpret, given the frequent colonization of the respiratory tract by *H. influenzae*. The diagnosis is supported if a predominance of Gram-negative bacilli and polymorphonuclear leukocytes are seen in a Gram stain of expectorated sputum (or transtracheal or bronchoscopic specimens). *H. influenzae*, however, may not be evident as the cause of pneumonia by either Gram stain or culture. Recent studies of real-time polymerase chain reaction (PCR) testing for *Haemophilus influenzae* suggest that it offers more sensitive and more specific results than other methods previously used. More invasive sampling (e.g., protected bronchial brush catheterization or needle aspiration of lung tissue) can increase the likelihood of a definitive diagnosis. These procedures, however, are not usually necessary in stable, immunocompetent individuals presenting with community-acquired pneumonia. Rather, most patients are treated with empiric antibiotic therapy that covers the more common causes of community-acquired pneumonia.

Nontypeable *H. influenzae* is also a common cause of acute bacterial exacerbation of COPD and bronchiectasis. Colonization with *H. influenzae* in "stable" COPD patients has been shown to increase total symptoms during exacerbations and to prolong the recovery of peak flow afterward. Additionally, bacteria isolated from patients with COPD subjected to molecular typing demonstrate that the acquisition of a new strain of *H. influenzae* is associated with a significantly increased risk of exacerbation. The clinical signs of an exacerbation can be subtle: low-grade fever; mild, increased shortness of breath; or a change in tracheobronchial secretions. Because of the ubiquity of the organism and the limitations of sputum Gram stain and culture (described above), empiric antibiotic therapy for COPD exacerbation should include coverage of nontypeable *H. influenzae*.

Acute epiglottis, as with the other clinical syndromes primarily associated with *H. influenzae* type B, is declining in incidence; however, it is a presentation that requires prompt recognition and management to circumvent progression to lethal airway obstruction. Acute epiglottitis is now more common in adults due to the *H. influenzae* type B vaccine in children. It should be suspected in the setting of a severe sore throat and painful swallowing. In later stages, the voice is often muffled and stridor is evident with rapid progression to severe upper airway obstruction. The epiglottis is bright red and edematous when visualized by indirect laryngoscopy; it is seen as an enlarged structure compromising the air column on lateral roentgenograms of the neck. In expert hands, laryngoscopic evaluation can be performed with relative safety and is diagnostically helpful. Establishing a patent airway is essential until the edema and inflammation subside. Although tracheostomy will bypass the obstruction, management of the airway by endotracheal intubation is increasingly used such that tracheostomy is not usually required. Importantly, as manipulation of swollen laryngeal tissues by attempts at visualization or intubation can result in more edema and obstruction, the provisions and expertise for tracheostomy should be immediately available. Management also includes appropriate antibiotics and may include systemic steroids, although the benefit of the latter has not been definitely established.

Serious infections with *H. influenzae* should be treated with parenteral antibiotics. Appropriate options include (1) selected second-generation cephalosporins (e.g., cefuroxime); (2) third-generation cephalosporins (e.g., ceftriaxone, cefotaxime); (3) fluoroquinolones (e.g., levo-, gati-, moxifloxacin); (4) monolactams (e.g., aztreonam); (5) extended-spectrum penicillins (e.g., piperacillin); and (6) imipenem-cilastatin. Less serious infections, including otitis media, sinusitis, bronchitis, and community-acquired pneumonia, may be treated with oral agents. A major consideration in selection of an oral agent is the occurrence of β-lactamase-producing *H. influenzae* strains, which were first reported in the 1970s. Both encapsulated and nontypeable strains can produce β-lactamase. Most recent national estimates suggest that approximately 26% of all isolates produce β-lactamase; however, the percentage appears to be decreasing (Heilmann, 2005). Thus, ampicillin or amoxicillin is only appropriate when the particular isolate has been shown to be sensitive. Reasonable options for either empiric oral therapy or therapy with a documented β-lactamase-producing strain include (1) trimethoprim-sulfamethoxazole (although resistance is approximately 24% in the United States) (Pfaller, 2012); (2) cefuroxime axetil; (3) amoxicillin-clavulanate; (4) doxycycline; (5) azithromycin; and (6) fluoroquinolones. Erythromycin, first-generation cephalosporins, clindamycin, and tetracycline have poor activity against *H. influenzae* and should not be prescribed empirically.

Currently, a number of licensed *H. influenzae* type B conjugate vaccines incorporate capsular polysaccharide into protein carriers and are highly immunogenic, even in infancy. The *H. influenzae* type B vaccines have been shown to be protective for invasive disease and to reduce carriage of *H. influenzae* type B, contributing to *herd immunity*. No cross-protection with other capsular strains or nontypeable *H. influenzae* strains exists. Since the addition of these vaccines in routine infant immunization schedules, follow-up surveillance has demonstrated significant reductions in the overall incidence of *H. influenzae* type B infections and the near elimination of invasive *H. influenzae* type B infection; however, strain replacement with serotype F and nontypeable strains has been noted in children below age 5 and the elderly (>60 years old) in some regions. These strain changes may be causing increases in disease of invasive *H. influenzae* among adults, especially the elderly, in some regions of the United States. However, overall rates in the United States in the greater-than-65-year age group appear stable. Research is ongoing to develop vaccines to prevent infections caused by nontypeable *H. influenzae*; however, the heterogeneity of the surface molecules of the various strains has made attempts challenging thus far. An oral monobacterial vaccine has shown some promise in small studies in reducing the frequency and severity of recurrent bronchitis exacerbations in adults, and a nasal vaccine used in mice was able to protect against middle ear and pulmonary infections. However, further work needs to be done.

In summary, *H. influenzae* is an important respiratory tract pathogen with a changing epidemiology and resistance pattern noted over the last decade. Encapsulated forms, predominately *H. influenzae* type B, and nontypeable strains are both pathogenic, but manifest different mechanisms of disease pathogenesis and outcomes. The introduction of *H. influenzae* type B immunization in infancy has sharply reduced the incidence of *H. influenzae* type B infections, which were predominately invasive infections of childhood. Nonencapsulated forms, which are common colonizers of the respiratory tract, primarily cause mucosal disease. Additionally, they are responsible for a significant proportion of otitis media in children, sinusitis and community-acquired pneumonia in adults, and lower respiratory tract infection in patients with chronic lung disease. Approximately 25% of both encapsulated and nontypeable strains produce β-lactamase, so empiric antibiotic therapy strategies should include agents with β-lactamase resistance. Research is in progress to develop an effective vaccine for nontypeable *H. influenzae*.

FURTHER READING

1. Adam HJ, Richardson SE, Jamieson FB, et al. Changing epidemiology of invasive *Haemophilus influenzae* in Ontario, Canada: evidence for herd effects and strain replacement due to Hib vaccination. *Vaccine.* 2010;28(24):4073–4078.

   The epidemiology of invasive Haemophilus influenzae *has changed in Ontario as a result of Hib vaccination introduced in the early 1990s. Now, older individuals frequently present with sepsis from nontypeable* H. influenzae *and strain replacement of Hib with serotype f and nontypeable strains has been seen in children under 5 years.*

2. Agrawal A, Murphy TF. *Haemophilus influenzae* infections in the *H. influenza* type b conjugate vaccine era. *J Clin Microbiol.* 2011;49(11):3728–3732.

   In places where Hib vaccination is widely used, invasive Hib disease has almost been eradicated. Currently, nontypeable strains are more commonly isolated than type b strains; however there is no evidence that incidence of non-type b strains are increasing.

3. Anevlavis S, Petroglou N, Tzavaras A, et al. A prospective study of the diagnostic utility of sputum Gram stain in pneumonia. *J Infect.* 2009;59(2):82–89.

   A sputum Gram stain has 0.79 sensitivity and 0.96 specificity for identifying Haemophilus influenzae *pneumonia when compared to a gold standard of blood and sputum cultures. Clinicians should take note of this uncertainty when diagnosing and treating patients.*

4. Dworkin M, Park L, Borchardt S. The changing epidemiology of invasive *Haemophilus influenzae* disease, especially in persons ≥65 years old. *Clin Infect Dis.* 2007;44(6):810–816.

   The incidence of invasive Haemophilus influenzae *increased from 1996 to 2004 in Illinois. Now* H. influenzae *it is most commonly seen in adults and caused by nontypeable strains, whereas before the vaccine, it was mostly seen in children and caused by serotype b.*

5. Garcia-Rodriguez JA, Martinez MJF. Dynamics of nasopharyngal colonization by potential respiratory pathogens. *J Antimicrob Chemother.* 2002;50(S2):59–73.

   This review summarizes factors involved in colonization of the nasopharynx with respiratory pathogens. Although, the factors are not entirely understood, adhesion to mucosal receptors, immune responses, bacterial properties, and colonization resistance dynamics play a role.

6. Guardiani E, Bliss M, Harley E. Supraglottitis in the era following widespread immunization against *Haemophilus influenzae* type B: evolving principles in diagnosis and management. *Laryngoscope.* 2010;120(11):2183–2188.

   After the start of widespread Hib vaccine use, patient demographics, presentation and course of supraglottitis have changed.

7. Heilmann KP, Rice CL, Miller AL, et al. Decreasing prevalence of β-lactamase production among respiratory tract isolates of *Haemophilus influenzae* in the United States. *Antimicrob Agents Chemother.* 2005;49(6):2561–2564.

   Isolates collected during the winter of 2002–2003 in the United States showed Haeomophilus influenzae *had decreased prevalence of β-lactamase production compared to national surveys before 1994.*

8. Kalies H, Siedler A, Gröndahl B, et al. Invasive *Haemophilus influenzae* infections in Germany: impact of non-type b serotypes in the post-vaccine era. *BMC Infect Dis.* 2009;9:45.

   This study using 8 years of postvaccination surveillance data from Germany and did not find an increase in non-type b invasive infections. They found a similar proportion of meningitis cases from capsulated non-type b compared to Hib infections and twice as many from noncapsulated Hi compared to Hib infections.

9. Ladhani S, Slack M, Heath PT. Invasive *Haemophilus influenzae* disease, Europe, 1996–2006. *Emerg Infect Dis.* 2010;16(3):455–463.

   A surveillance network of 14 countries in Europe from 1996 to 2006 found that the incidence of invasive non-type b H. influenzae *is higher than Hib and has a greater case fatality.*

10. Livorsi D, MacNeil J, Cohn A, et al. Invasive *Haemophilus influenzae* in the United States, 1999–2008: epidemiology and outcomes. *J Infect.* 2012;65:496–504.

    Increased risk of in-hospital death from H. influenzae *was associated with premature birth, older age, and several chronic diseases in adults. In the elderly, nontypeable* H. influenzae *was associated with higher mortality.*

11. MacNeil J, Cohn A, Farley M, et al. Current epidemiology and trends in invasive *Haemophilus influenzae* disease—United States, 1989–2008. *Clin Infect Dis.* 2011;53(12):1230–1236.

    After widespread use of Hib vaccines became established in the United States, the incidence of invasive H. influenzae *disease declined substantially. There is no evidence of replacement with non-b serotypes in young children.*

12. Nix EB, Hawdon N, Gravelle S, et al. Risk of invasive *Haemophilus influenzae* type B (Hib) disease in adults with secondary immunodeficiency in the post-Hib vaccine era. *Clin Vaccine Immunol.* 2012;19(5):766–771.

    Among patients with secondary immunodeficiency from severe disease, patients with multiple myeloma or chronic renal failure have an increased risk of invasive Hib disease. This study supports the benefit giving the pediatric Hib vaccine to some adults with secondary immunodeficiency.

13. Pfaller M, Farrell D, Sader H, et al. AWARE Ceftaroline Surveillance Program (2008–2010): trends in resistance patterns among *Streptococcus pneumonia, Haemophilus influenzae,* and *Moraxella catrrhalis* in the United States. *Clin Infect Dis.* 2012;55(suppl 3):S187–S193.

    Haemophilus influenzae *isolates collected for the AWARE Ceftaroline Surveillance Program from 2008 to 2010 were found to be very susceptible to ceftaroline regardless of β-lactamase production. However, increased rates of nonsusceptibility were seen for trimethoprim/sulfamethoxazole and azithromycin.*

14. Resman F, Ristovski M, Ahl J, et al. Invasive disease caused by *Haemophilis influenzae* in Sweden 1997–2009; evidence of increased clinical burden of non-type b strains. *Clin Microbiol Infect.* 2011;17(11):1638–1645.

    A retrospective study in Sweden between 1997 and 2009 found that there was a significant increase in the clinical burden from invasive nontypeable Haemophilus influenzae *and encapsulated strains type of* H. influenzae, *particularly in the elderly.*

15. Shah R, Roberson D, Jones D. Epiglottitis in the *Haemophilus influenzae* type B vaccine era: changing trends. *Laryngoscope.* 2004;114(3):557–560.

    Following Hib vaccination, the demographics, causative organisms, and natural history of epiglottitis have significantly changed.

16. Van Wessel K, Rodenburg G, Veenhoven R, et al. Nontypable *Haemophilus influenzae* invasive disease in the Netherlands: a retrospective surveillance study 2001–2008. *Clin Infect Dis.* 2011;53(1):1–7.

    A retrospective surveillance study in the Netherlands found that risk factors for invasive nontypeable Haemophilus influenzae *include premature birth, age greater than 65 years old, and a compromised immune system.*

17. Van den Bergh MR, Biesbroek G, Rossen J, et al. Associations between pathogens in the upper respiratory tract of young children: interplay between viruses and bacteria. *PLoS One.* 2012;7(10):e47711.

    This study summarizes the association of different bacterial and viral pathogens in the upper respiratory tract of young children. They found positive associations between Haemophilus influenzae *and rhinoviruses, respiratory syncitial viruses, and* S. pneumoniae *colonization.*

18. Wroblewski D, Halse T, Hayes J, et al. Utilization of a real-time PCR approach for *Haemophilus influenzae* serotype determination as an alternative to the slide agglutination test. *Mol Cell Probes.* 2013;27(2):86–89.

    This study found that a two-step real-time PCR approach was more sensitive than previously published PCR assays and was an easy alternative to the slide agglutination test.

Klebsiella Pneumonia

Steven J. Escobar

Klebsiella pneumoniae is a common nosocomial Gram-negative pathogen that has become an increasingly global concern due to its carbapenemase activity. Community-acquired pneumonia due to *K. pneumoniae* is rare in the United States and Europe but has been reported to be the second leading cause of severe pneumonia (following *Streptococcus pneumonia*) requiring hospitalization in Asia. A community-acquired *K. pneumoniae* primary bacteremic liver abscess syndrome with meningitis and/or endophthalmitis also has been described in Asia.

Klebsiella species are lactose-fermenting Gram-negative bacteria belonging to the Enterobacteriaceae family. *K. pneumoniae* has a very large polysaccharide capsule with antiphagocytic property, which contributes to its virulence. Encapsulated *K. pneumoniae* strains have a mucoid appearance in culture plates, and Gram stain demonstrates bipolar Gram positivity, as seen in other enteric organisms. *K. pneumoniae* may be suspected on Gram stain if there are clear zones around apparently Gram-negative bacteria.

K. pneumoniae carbapenemase (KPC) was first described from an isolate in North Carolina in 1996 and was infrequently isolated prior to several outbreaks in New York and New Jersey in 2001. KPC has now been reported in 42 states of the United States, Europe, South America, Middle East, and Asia. The rapid global spread has been attributed to international travel, patient-to-patient transmission, and interspecies transfer of KPC-producing organisms. KPC is an Ambler class A carbapenemase that through hydrolysis confers decreased susceptibility or resistance to virtually all β-lactams, including carbapenem. The transferable plasmid encoding KPC frequently contains genes encoding amnioglycoside, extended-spectrum β-lactamase (ESBL), and flouroquinolone resistance. These plasmids may be horizontally transmitted to other enterobacteriaceae and have been reported in *Pseudomonas aeruginosa* and *Acinetobacter baumannii*.

K. pneumoniae is a saprophyte which colonizes the gastrointestinal tract, nasopharynx, and, rarely, the skin. *K. pneumoniae* may be found in 5% to 38% of stool samples and has a 1% to 6% nasopharyngeal carrier rate among normal hosts in the community. However, the nasopharyngeal colonization rate has been found to be as high as 30% in ambulatory alcoholics. The carrier rate increases in the hospital environment in direct proportion to the length of stay, prior antibiotic use, comorbidities and invasive lines and tubes. In hospitalized patients, the gastrointestinal, nasopharyngeal, and skin carrier rates have been reported to be as high as 77%, 19%, and 42% respectively.

The classic presentation of community-acquired *K. pneumoniae* pneumonia (Friedlander pneumonia) is rare and consists of acute onset prostration, pleuritic chest pain, dyspnea, high fever, and productive cough with "currant jelly" (thick, bloody-appearing and mucoid-viscid) sputum. Physical examination discloses tachypnea and signs of lung consolidation. The posterior segment of the right upper lobe is the most often affected area of the lung. Patients may present with sepsis or septic shock, and blood cultures are positive in 25% of cases. Leukocyte counts can be high, normal, or low. Neutropenia indicates a worse prognosis. Respiratory distress or failure requiring endotracheal intubation and mechanical ventilation upon presentation is common. Lung abscess, cavitation, and pulmonary gangrene (a large cavity containing fragments of necrotic lung) may complicate the course of illness. Pleural effusion and empyema also are common. After recovery, unclosed cavities, residual fibrosis, and reduced lung volumes may be detected.

The presentation of hospital-acquired *K. pneumoniae* pneumonia is less severe and similar to other forms of ventilator-associated pneumonia or hospital-acquired pneumonia. Depending on the patient's underlying illness and ability to respond immunologically, localizing symptoms, physical findings, and radiographic appearances may be less apparent or less specific.

On chest radiograph, *K. pneumoniae* pneumonia has been described classically as a lobar consolidation with a "bulging" or "bowed" fissure sign more commonly affecting the upper lobes and on the right more often than the left. Pathologically, the "bulging" fissure sign is thought to result from the necrotizing pneumonia seen more often with *Klebsiella* pneumonia than pneumococcal pneumonia. Destruction of parenchyma within larger areas of consolidative lung is thought to lead to the loss of elastic recoil, and thus the "bulging" fissure sign. Subsequent reports have revealed that the "bulging" fissure sign is not specific to *Klebsiella* pneumonia and has been reported in *Haemophilus influenza* and *Streptococcus pneumoniae* pneumonia as well.

Challenging the classic description, a recent retrospective review from Japan of computer tomography findings in 198 patients with acute *K. pneumoniae* pneumonia demonstrated ground-glass attenuation (100%), consolidation (91.4%), and intralobular reticular opacities (85.9%), which were found in the periphery (96%) of both sides of the lungs (72.2%) and were often associated with pleural effusion (53%). Disease in the upper zones occurred in 13.1% compared to 55.6% in the lower zones and 31.3% with a random distribution.

The mortality rate for community-acquired *K. pneumoniae* pneumonia complicated by bacteremia is high despite adequate antimicrobial coverage. A recent study from Taiwan reported pneumonia mortality of 55% for bacteremic *Klebsiella* versus 27% for bacteremic *S. pneumoniae*. Nosocomial *K. pneumoniae* infections have similarly high mortality rates. Independent risk factors for death include older age, higher Acute Physiology and Chronic Health Evaluation (APACHE II) scores, and inappropriate antimicrobial coverage.

KPC may be difficult to detect with standard clinical microbiologic testing, since high-level carbapenem resistance may not be present due to a heterogeneously expressed enzyme. A slight increase in minimal inhibitory concentrations (MIC) (within the susceptible to intermediate range) may be the only laboratory manifestation. A phenotypic test is often required to detect KPC presence. The gold standard for detection is either spectrophotometry or polymerase chain reaction (PCR) of the bla$_{KPC}$ gene.

Treatment for community-acquired *K. pneumoniae* pneumonia should follow Infectious Diseases Society of America/American Thoracic Society (IDSA/ATS) guidelines. Treatment of resistant organisms can be tailored to susceptibility reports. For KPC-producing strains, tigecycline, colistin, aminoglycosides, and tetracycline have all demonstrated efficacy in case reports and small series, especially when used in combination therapy.

FURTHER READING

1. Korvick JA, Hackett AK, Yu VL, et al. Klebsiella pneumoniae in the modern era: clinicoradiographic correlations. *South Med J.* 1991;84:200.

   A prospective study of 15 patients with bacteremic Klebsiella pneumoniae *demonstrating the changes in clinical presentation and radiographic findings of this disease from the classic Gram-negative community-acquired pneumonia described by Friedlander to that of a predominantly hospital-acquired one affecting more immunocompromised hosts.*

2. Okada F, Ando Y, Honda K, et al. Clinical and pulmonary thin-section CT findings in acute *Klebsiella pneumoniae* pneumonia. *Eur Radiol.* 2009;19:809–815.

   Retrospective CT scan review of 198 patients with acute Klebsiella pneumoniae *pneumonia.*

3. Hoban DJ, Biedenbach DJ, Mutnick AH, et al. Pathogen of occurrence and susceptibility patterns associated with pneumonia in hospitalized patients in North America: results of the SENTRY Antimicrobial Surveillance Study (2000). *Diagn Microbiol Infect Dis.* 2003;45:279.

   Among patients hospitalized with pneumonia in North America, Klebsiella *spp. were isolated 7.5% of the time. Extended-spectrum beta-lactamases were detected at a rate of 5.4% among* Klebsiella *spp. They remain 100% susceptible to carbapenem (imipenem and meropenem).*

4. Hirsch EB, Tam VH. Detection and treatment options for *Klebsiella pneumoniae* carbapenemases (KPCs): an emerging cause of multidrug-resistant infection. *J Antimicrob Chemother.* 2010;65(6):1119–1125.

   Review of KPC's laboratory detection and antibiotic resistance patterns.

5. Zarkotou O, Pournaras S, Tselioti P, et al. Predictors of mortality in patients with bloodstream infections caused by KPC-producing *Klebsiella pneumoniae* and impact of appropriate antimicrobial treatment. *Clin Microbiol Infect.* 2011;17:1798–1803.

   Observational case-control study of 53 patients with KPC producing blood stream infections in a Greek hospital.

6. Nordmann P, Cuzon G, Naas T. The real threat of *Klebsiella pneumoniae* carbapenemase producing bacteria. *Lancet Infect Dis.* 2009;9:228–236.

   General review microbiology of KPC producing Klebsiella pneumoniae.

7. Tzouvelekis LS, Markogiannakis A, Psichogiou M, et al. Carbapenemases in *Klebsiella pneumoniae* and other *Enterobacteriaceae*: an evolving crisis of global dimensions. *Clin Microbiol Rev.* 2012;25(4):682.

   Review article on microbiology of KPCs.

8. Chen LF, Anderson DJ, Paterson DL. Overview of the epidemiology and the threat of *Klebsiella pneumoniae* carbapenemases (KPC) resistance. *Infect Drug Resist.* 2012;5:133–141.

   Review article on microbiology of KPCs.

9. Centers for Disease Control and Prevention. Carbapenemase-producing CRE in the United States. http://www.cdc.gov/hai/organisms/cre/TrackingCRE.html.

   Documents states with confirmed cases of KPC-producing bacteria.

10. Lin Y-T, Jeng Y-Y, Chen T-L, et al. Bacteremic community-acquired pneumonia due to *Klebsiella pneumoniae*: clinical and microbiological characteristics in Taiwan, 2001–2008. *BMC Infect Dis.* 2010;10:307.

    Retrospective review of 93 patients admitted to a Taiwanese hospital.

11. Kang C-I, Kim S-H, Bang J-W, et al. Community-acquired versus nosocomial *Klebsiella pneumoniae* bacteremia: clinical features, treatment outcomes, and clinical implication of antimicrobial resistance. *J Korean Med Sci.* 2006;21:816–822.

    Retrospective review of 377 patients with Klebsiella pneumoniae *bacteremia.*

12. Mandell LA, Wunderink RG, Anzueto A, et al. Infectious Diseases Society of America/American Thoracic Society Consensus Guidelines on the management of community-acquired pneumonia in adults. *Clin Infect Dis.* 2007;44(suppl 2):S27–S72.

Other Gram-Negative Pneumonias: *Pseudomonas aeruginosa, Escherichia coli, Proteus, Serratia, Enterobacter,* and *Acinetobacter*

James H. Williams, Jr.

BACKGROUND AND ETIOLOGY

The Gram-negative bacilli (GNB) *Pseudomonas aeruginosa, Escherichia coli,* and organisms of the *Proteus, Serratia, Enterobacter,* and *Acinetobacter* species are most commonly associated with nosocomial (hospital-acquired) pneumonia (HAP), including ventilator-associated pneumonia (VAP). GNB are associated with less than 20% of pneumonias among ambulatory patients with community-acquired pneumonia (CAP). However, these GNB are more commonly recovered from the airways of debilitated, institutionalized patients with pneumonia, who are included among those defined as health care–associated pneumonia (HCAP). GNB are associated with as many as half the deaths from bacterial pneumonia in these patients, and are common pathogens identified in the airways of hospitalized patients.

Predisposing factors for GNB pneumonia vary with the population at risk. In the community, chronic bronchitis, bronchiectasis, alcoholism, diabetes, altered mental status, and neutropenia appear to be the major risk factors. Prior antibiotic selection pressure contributes to the emergence of these organisms. In the hospital, GNB pneumonia most often occurs with prolonged intubation, including tracheostomy. Even without intubation, prolonged hospital stay (particularly in the ICU), recent thoracic or abdominal surgery, advanced age, and severe underlying illness all are risk factors. During acute and chronic illnesses, patients more often have relatively lower levels of some micronutrients (e.g., selenium, zinc), potentially resulting in altered host responses, while more frankly immune-compromised hosts are at particular risk for adverse outcomes from these infections.

Although contaminated respiratory equipment has caused occasional outbreaks, particularly those due to *Serratia* and *Pseudomonas* species, these outbreaks are uncommon with the use of disposable equipment and aseptic techniques. Medical staff can facilitate colonization of patients with potentially resistant organisms by careless hygiene, which can be diminished by careful cleansing of hands before and after patient contact and avoiding contact with commonly shared fomites (e.g., stethoscopes, door handles, bed controls, etc.) without cleansing. GNB pneumonias may result from bacteremia introduced by bladder catheters, intravenous catheters, or infections in the abdomen or elsewhere. However, GNB causing HCAP/HAP/VAP are more commonly delivered to the lungs via the airways.

Colonization of the upper airways, including the pharynx and nasal sinuses, by GNB generally precedes pneumonia. Nasal tubes increase retention of secretions in the nasal sinuses and drain into the posterior pharynx. Selection of GNB is encouraged in a hospital by a number of additional factors commonly encountered in the ICU, particularly antibiotic selection pressure, increased adherence of GNB to the airway epithelium, and retained secretions in seriously ill patients. Reflux of gastric contents into the posterior pharynx also can contribute, particularly in the supine position and with larger gastric volume. Suppression of gastric acidity selectively promotes GNB proliferation in the stomach, although the magnitude of this effect on the development of GNB HAP/VAP has been debated. Instillation of medications and nutrition via nasogastric tubes likely enhances the risk of aspiration, while passing feeding tubes beyond the stomach (postpyloric position) may reduce risk.

Access of nasopharyngeal flora to the lower airways is facilitated by a number of factors inherent to ICU patients, particularly intubation. Translaryngeal intubation mechanically holds open the epiglottis and vocal cords. Although cuffed endotracheal tubes (ETTs) diminish the rate at which large volumes can enter the lower airways, the reservoir of secretions above the cuff continue to ooze down around the cuff, which is kept at low pressure to avoid tracheal necrosis. Efforts to diminish the size of this subglottic secretion pool with specially designed ETTs have produced variable results, perhaps reflecting in part the tenacious character of and limited access to subglottic secretions. Bacteria adherent to the ETT provide an additional nidus for infection, and silver impregnated tubes may limit recovery of organisms in culture that would suggest VAP. However, these approaches have not been reliably demonstrated to translate into a reduction in overall mortality.

The normal reflex clearance of airway secretions is attenuated by many factors as well. Endotracheal and tracheostomy tubes create a smaller lumen through which to expectorate. The effectiveness of expectoration is also inhibited by CNS depression (e.g., narcotics, sedatives, metabolic instability, CNS lesions), local reflex depression (e.g., topical anesthetic, learned tolerance of foreign nasotracheal or nasogastric tubes), and pain (particularly chest and abdominal surgery). Mucociliary activity can be decreased (e.g., alcohol, chronic inflammation, metabolic disorders), and phagocytic activity can be impaired (e.g., immunocompromised patients, alcohol, overwhelmed reserves).

Tracheostomy has advantages for patients requiring prolonged intubation, including stabilization of airway access, patient comfort, and less physical interruption of airway closure during swallowing. However, tracheostomy also delays reestablishment of normal airway architecture during recovery. After weaning from ventilator support, clearance of secretions is still inhibited by diminished ability to generate a high positive pressure for cough and by flow limitations of the tube. Airway protection is also impaired by limiting the normally generated positive airway pressure during swallowing, by potentially hindering tracheal lift for closure of the epiglottis, and by applying pressure to the upper esophagus through the membranous posterior tracheal surface. These factors, along with the underlying problems of these patients, lead to a high incidence of recurrent pneumonia, often with GNB in this setting.

CLINICAL PRESENTATIONS

The clinical features of GNB infections are intertwined with the underlying diseases with which they are usually associated. The classic descriptions of GNB pneumonias focus on community-acquired cases, uncomplicated by adult respiratory distress syndrome (ARDS), heart failure, or fluid imbalance and, therefore, incompletely represent the spectrum of nosocomial GNB pneumonias. Regardless, they provide useful comparisons of pathologic responses in relatively fit individuals. In contrast, immunocompromised patients may exhibit relatively few signs or symptoms and less evidence of infiltrate on chest film. Even more difficult are patients with underlying acute or chronic lung injury who have similar signs and symptoms and areas of increased lung tissue density from prior injury. The presence of GNB organisms in such patients may reflect either colonization or acute infection, making diagnosis of acute GNB pneumonia more challenging.

P. aeruginosa frequently colonizes the skin or mucosa of patients as well as the hospital environment (soap, liquid media, and hospital staff). It can colonize or infect tracheostomy sites, burns, wounds, and the urinary tract as well as the lower airways of patients with chronic bronchitis/bronchiectasis. Mucoid strains often emerge in the airways of patients with cystic fibrosis. Pneumonia is usually acquired via the airway and tends to be more prominent in dependent lung zones, whereas hematogenous infections may lead to more widespread changes.

Pathologically, severe focal necrosis may be seen with nodular infarcts and vessel wall necrosis leading to hemorrhage and formation of small cavities. Purulent pleural effusions are more often found at autopsy. Clinically, patients often appear toxic, presenting with chills, fever, and dyspnea; sputum often is copious and can be blood-tinged. Pleuritic chest pain is less common. Ecthyma gangrenosum is an uncommon cutaneous maculopapular eruption representing infection and necrosis in vessel walls and may present as hemorrhagic bullae, ulcers, or nodular lesions. Though historically linked to bacteremia with these organisms, it can be seen with other infections. Radiographically, consolidation in dependent areas is most common and it is classically associated with abscesses varying in size from 2 to 11 cm. Small effusions also may be present. Bilateral patchy infiltrates or bilateral nodules are occasionally seen with hematogenous infection.

E. coli pneumonia may follow aspiration or hematogenous dissemination from urinary tract or gastrointestinal infections. Pathologically, a diffuse, hemorrhagic pneumonia is often present, but abscess formation is less common. Clinically, patients often appear toxic, with fever, dyspnea, productive cough, and, more often, pleuritic chest pain. Classically, one may see a relative bradycardia for the degree of temperature elevation and a paucity of signs of parenchymal consolidation. The chest roentgenogram usually demonstrates patchy bronchopneumonia, often in the lower lobes. Pleural effusion may be present.

Proteus species are less common causes of respiratory tract infection, frequently associated with altered consciousness, potentially leading to aspiration. Pathologically, the pneumonia is hemorrhagic and associated with small abscesses. Clinically, patients usually appear less toxic, although chills, fever, dyspnea, productive cough, and pleuritic chest pain may be present. The chest roentgenogram demonstrates dense infiltrates, more often in the dependent segments of the upper lobes and superior segment of the lower lobes, and volume contraction may be seen. Pleural effusion is less common.

Serratia species occasionally cause pneumonia. Clustered cases have been linked in the past to contaminated respiratory equipment. Pathologically, diffuse bronchopneumonia can occur with small (2–3 mm) abscesses. Patients typically are toxic, with fever, chills, and productive cough. Pseudohemoptysis, the production of sputum tainted with a red pigment produced by some strains, is classically described but is uncommon. The chest radiograph often demonstrates diffuse, patchy, bronchopneumonia similar to *Pseudomonas* pneumonia, although abscess formation has been reported less frequently. Pleural effusion and empyema may occur.

Enterobacter pneumonia is less well characterized than the other GNB pneumonias. In one small series, symptoms included fever, dyspnea, and cough productive of yellow sputum, but pleuritic pain was uncommon. Chest radiographs most often demonstrate bilateral bronchopneumonia, but abscesses and empyema formation are uncommon. The emergence of drug-resistant strains has increased the frequency and seriousness of infection from these organisms.

Acinetobacter species have emerged more recently as multidrug-resistant (MDR) organisms associated with HAP/VAP, likely in response to the prolific use of broad-spectrum antibiotics. Colonization of hospitalized patients with these organisms has been observed with increasing frequency. The presence of MDR *Acinetobacter* species in airway cultures of febrile intubated patients with pulmonary infiltrates presents diagnostic and therapeutic dilemmas. The chest roentgenogram may demonstrate multilobar infiltrates, occasionally with signs of necrosis (cavitation) or effusion.

DIAGNOSIS

The diagnosis of Gram-negative pneumonia by examination of airway secretions is problematic because of the frequency with which GNB colonize the airways of patients at risk, many of whom have infiltrates on chest radiographs for other reasons or infiltrates obscured behind the diaphragms and mediastinal shadows on portable anteroposterior (AP) films. Demonstration of numerous GNB and neutrophils on smears of airway secretions collected via expectoration or suctioning provides presumptive evidence of infection, particularly with intracellular organisms indicating evidence of a host response; however, this still may reflect bronchitis rather than pneumonia. Attempts to reach beyond the upper airway with bronchoscopic brushing or lavage are complicated by the fact that the upper airways are traversed in the process, contaminating the sampling channel during suctioning to maintain visualization. Fewer organisms sometimes recovered with these techniques may simply reflect a smaller or diluted sample. Therefore, while these samples provide a basis for a presumptive diagnosis, invasion by these organisms is more firmly supported by positive cultures from blood or pleural fluid. While routine use in this setting is debated, bronchoscopy can provide important access to samples in patients who cannot provide adequate lower airway samples and sometimes demonstrates organisms not reported in cultures of upper airway samples laden with other bacteria. Demonstrating a clear predominance of one organism increases confidence of its role in a respiratory infection, but recovery of multiple organisms does not preclude a role for one or more in an apparent pneumonia. Occasionally, if the patient is deteriorating while undergoing treatment, demonstration of tissue infection via lung biopsy may be warranted.

TREATMENT

Decisions about when and how to treat HCAP/HAP/VAP are sometimes difficult. Published guidelines provide useful direction, but clinical judgment is still required in individual cases. Issues related to diagnostic uncertainty complicate confidence in choosing antibiotics, and initiating antibiotics immediately adds selection pressure for emergence of drug-resistant strains. However, the high mortality associated with HAP/VAP with GNB is worsened by delay in starting antibiotics to which the organism is sensitive, particularly among those admitted to the ICU. This argues *for* aggressive, broad-spectrum empiric coverage initially, and *against* limited coverage while waiting for results of cultures, particularly among those who are critically ill.

The initial drug or drugs chosen should be based on current resistance patterns in the hospital and organisms likely to be present based on the patient's presentation and risk profile. For example, *Pseudomonas* is more likely among patients with VAP and those previously receiving antibiotics, particularly those with recurrent respiratory tract infections associated with bronchiectasis. To limit antibiotic selection pressure, current opinion favors a "de-escalation" strategy, starting with relatively broad coverage, particularly in critically ill patients, and then narrowing subsequent coverage based on the results of cultures. However, subsequent de-escalation can be worrisome when a patient is improving slowly on an initial regimen, particularly if there is uncertainty regarding sensitivity of cultures and in very sick patients with limited ability to tolerate deterioration. Recognizing that repetitive use of standardized regimens induces resistance, some rotate every few months the classes of drugs selected empirically. Underlying all such strategies is a desire to reserve certain classes of drugs for use with subsequent infections in both individuals and the institution and to reduce the emergence of multidrug-resistance profiles, although evidence of outcome benefit from specific approaches remains limited and continued investigation is needed.

When *Pseudomonas* species are demonstrated or suspected, two classes of drugs have been used simultaneously because drug resistance often emerges in these organisms. This may be particularly important with prior exposure to antipseudomonal antibiotics of the same class. Traditionally, a high dose semisynthetic penicillin (e.g., piperacillin) has been combined with an aminoglycoside (e.g., tobramycin, gentamycin, amikacin). In recent years, high doses of fluoroquinolones (e.g., ciprofloxacin, possibly levofloxacin) are often substituted for aminoglycosides, particularly among older, sicker patients at increased risk of ototoxicity and nephrotoxicity. Of note, while adding a β-lactamase inhibitor (e.g., piperacillin-tazobactam—pip/tazo) enhances piperacillin efficacy against many organisms, this is not true for *Pseudomonas* species. Therefore, the pip/tazo combination is usually recommended at higher doses (4.5 g every 6 hours) for *Pseudomonas* species. Several other β-lactam drugs can be substituted for semisynthetic penicillins, including some third- and fourth-generation cephalosporins (e.g., ceftazidime and cefepime, respectively). When severe allergy to β-lactam antibiotics makes use of cephalosporins and carbapenems a concern, monobactam aztreonam may be used, but it should be remembered that this choice sacrifices virtually any coverage of Gram positives. Carbapenems are often more effective when organisms with extended-spectrum beta-lactamase (ESBL) inhibitors have emerged. *Pseudomonas* species are usually sensitive to imipenem, meropenem, and doripenem, but not ertapenem. However, ertapenem is often effective against other GNB with ESBL resistance (e.g., *E. coli*), and does not induce resistance of emerging *Pseudomonas* species to the other carbapenems. Most worrisome is the continued emergence of MDR organisms, including *Acinetobacter* species, forcing consideration of colistin (polymyxin E) and polymyxin B, potentially more toxic agents. Of interest, recent data suggest that addition of rifampin to colistin may improve outcomes with some MDR strains.

While dual antibiotic therapy has been the standard for covering *Pseudomonas* species, a single broad-spectrum drug has been successful in the initial empiric treatment of patients with HCAP, pending results of cultures, unless there is reason for heightened concern for resistant organisms or for intolerance of the patient for clinical deterioration should subsequent culture results show resistance to that single drug. A growing list of orally active agents effective against GNB has facilitated outpatient management of persons with less severe illness, including very high doses of some quinolones (e.g., ciprofloxacin, levofloxacin) for pseudomonas coverage, or less broad spectrum cephalosporins and β-lactam inhibitor combinations (e.g., amoxicillin plus clavulanate) for other species. One might caution against the overuse of quinolones in hospitalized patients, where parenteral antibiotics are generally used, unless other options are unlikely to be effective or more likely to be toxic. Specific choice(s) should also take into account institutional sensitivity patterns.

Prior exposure to a class of antibiotics increases the probability of resistance, which argues for use of a different drug class with each new event. However, this must be weighed against the risk of broadening antibiotic selection pressure in the individual patient if recurrent infection is likely, a risk that may be shared with others in the health care environment as well. As such, the potential tolerance of the individual for a delay in appropriately targeted therapy should be considered in making the best decision for the patient, both short-term and long-term.

Delivery of antibiotics to infected regions of the lungs is inherently complicated by hypoxic vasoconstriction, and accumulated secretions may further diminish local concentrations. Bacteriocidal activity increases with higher local concentrations of aminoglycosides and quinolones, whereas activity of β-lactam drugs is not similarly enhanced by raising local concentrations above the bacteriocidal level. Therefore, although drug penetration is always an issue, it carries additional significance in comparing quinolones with aminoglycosides. Quinolones enjoy good tissue penetration and fairly good tolerance at relatively higher systemic doses, while aminoglycosides penetrate tissues more poorly and toxicity precludes systemic administration of higher doses. Of interest, airway instillation of aminoglycosides as an adjuvant to intravenous therapy more rapidly clears GNB from secretions, but direct instillation of less-than-usual systemic doses of aminoglycoside has little impact on the overall course of VAP when added to systemic administration. In contrast, repeated nebulization of very high doses of tobramycin (300 mg BID) alone has improved long-term outcomes in patients with cystic fibrosis and suppressed symptoms in other patients with bronchiectasis, with remarkably good tolerance. The role of nebulizing high doses of aminoglycosides as an adjunct to systemic therapy in HAP/VAP with GNB has not been well characterized. Aerosolization of other classes of antibiotics is also of interest, with some anecdotal successes with colistin for MDR infections, but data are not yet sufficient for specific recommendations regarding appropriate dosing or confidence in efficacy for treatment of HCAP/HAP/VAP.

The appropriate duration of antibiotic therapy varies with the severity of infection, comorbidities, overall severity of the clinical presentation, the organisms involved, the confidence in the diagnosis, and the characteristics of the antibiotic chosen, including sensitivity of the organisms, tissue penetration, and persistence at the targeted site. For example, among patients with CAP, which only infrequently is associated with GNB, a quinolone (levofloxacin) was found comparably effective orally at a high dose (750 mg daily) for 5 days when compared to a moderate dose (500 mg daily) for 10 days. Importantly, these regimens were not recommended for infections with pseudomonas. Among sicker patients with VAP, various regimens utilized for 8 days were found to be comparable to longer 15-day courses. This study was confirmed subsequently in patients studied earlier in the course of intubation. Limited data suggest that infusion of 3.375 g pip/tazo over 4 hours three times a day (TID) may be as effective as four times a day (QID) infusion over 30 minutes for HAP/VAP. However, a study of patients with VAP compared a 7-day course of similarly prolonged 4-hour infusion of 1 g of doripenem to a 10-day course of 1-hour infusion of 1 g imepenem-cilastatin, two carbapenems with broad spectrum activity in vitro, including pseudomonas, to which addition of amikacin was permitted if carbapenem resistance was suspected. Unexpectedly, mortality appeared greater with the shorter course of doripenem, particularly among those with *Pseudomonas* infections.

The 2005 American Thoracic Society/Infectious Diseases Society of America (ATS/IDSA) guidelines for HCAP/HAP/VAP recommend considering shorter courses (<8 days) for patients with rapid clinical response, but noted that longer courses are needed in some, perhaps most notably in those with *Pseudomonas* infections. Monitoring clinical responses helps determine appropriate duration of therapy. There is some evidence that declining levels of inflammatory markers (e.g., procalcitonin, C-reactive protein [CRP]) may be helpful. More prospective studies are needed to help guide duration of specific drug regimens and to differentiate between subsets of HCAP/HAP/VAP who are likely to respond differently.

The potential role of passive immunotherapy for treatment or prevention of GNB infections has been investigated much less than the use of new antibiotics. While passive immunization with antibodies induced in horse serum were useful prior to the development of effective antibiotics, results from more recent clinical trials of pharmacologic modulation of immune responses among patients with pneumonia have been variable and thus far disappointing. Examples of failed approaches include efforts to enhance apparently weak responses, and conversely to suppress potentially excessive host responses. Unfortunately, these interventions may dysregulate overall host response sufficiently to result in ineffective, or even harmful, overall effects. Commercially available agents include immunostimulants (e.g., granulocyte colony-stimulating factor [G-CSF], granulocyte-macrophage colony-stimulating factor [GM-CSF], interferons), and immunosuppressants (corticosteroids, tumor necrosis factor [TNF] antagonists). Although the value of these agents in most patients is unclear, severe neutropenia (<500/mm^3) is associated with very high risk and should usually be treated with bone marrow stimulants (G-CSF, GM-CSF). In contrast, patients with pneumonia who are in septic shock requiring vasopressors should receive at least a short course of corticosteroids to improve hemodynamic responses. Immunoglobulin supplements (intravenous immunoglobulin [IVIG]) should be administered to patients with severe immunoglobulin deficiencies, but a role for IVIG in treatment of others with HCAP/HAP/VAP has not as yet been established.

PROGNOSIS

Unfortunately, the mortality rate associated with GNB pneumonia remains high, although ranging widely from less than 20% to as high as 90% in an older report. Historic, observational data suggest mortality was higher with monotherapy relying on aminoglycosides compared to monotherapy with other, newer agents. However, mortality is largely determined by the severity of the underlying illness. Although bacteremia with GNB has not been reliably demonstrated to be associated with higher mortality in all patients, neutropenic patients with *P. aeruginosa* pneumonia and bacteremia may still suffer a mortality exceeding 80%. Supportive measures directed at treating underlying illnesses, and limiting multi-organ dysfunction in severe infections, likely impact overall outcome.

PREVENTION

A persistently high mortality rate from GNB pneumonia continues to stimulate interest in preventive therapy. Unfortunately, the need for intubation with respiratory failure, prior use of antibiotics for treatment of other apparent infections, and presence of other underlying serious illnesses in these patients significantly limit the impact of prevention efforts. Nevertheless, risk factors may be modified in some patients.

Avoidance of prolonged intubation can diminish HAP/VAP. Noninvasive (mask) ventilation (NIV) applied initially to patients with respiratory insufficiency may reduce HAP/VAP and associated mortality among patients with respiratory insufficiency, including those with neutropenia. However, the role of NIV after extubation for managing patients with recurrent respiratory failure is more complex. NIV can be helpful when applied routinely at the time of extubation of marginal patients, perhaps diminishing fatigue leading to recurrence of frank respiratory failure. However, outcomes appear worse when NIV is used to delay reintubation of patients already showing signs of frank respiratory failure after extubation.

If intubation is required, an oral, rather than nasal, route is recommended to avoid obstructing sinuses and, if feasible, an ETT with a dorsal lumen suction tube above the cuff for continuous or intermittent suction to reduce secretions in the subglottic space. At the time of extubation, careful attention to clearing these secretions is recommended to avoid larger volume aspiration. One practical approach is as follows: (1) temporarily increase positive pressure in the trachea by increasing positive end expiratory pressure (PEEP, about 8–10 cm H_2O), returning the ventilator mode to assist control (AC) with pressure control (PC, about 20–25 cm H_2O); (2) slowly deflate the cuff while capturing the few secretions that fall into the trachea with a suction catheter reaching to the tip of the ETT, hopefully hearing the bulk of secretions expelled into the pharynx above by the positive pressure; (3) reinflate the cuff; and then (4) clear the larger volume of secretions in the posterior pharynx with an oral suction device (e.g., Yankauer). After completing and possibly repeating this exercise, the volume of subglottic secretions should be minimized, and the patency of the upper airway confirmed by the audible air-leak with expulsion of secretions. Finally, (5) remove the ETT while continuously suctioning via a catheter extended to the tip of the ETT.

Among patients with a tracheostomy who no longer require ventilator support, but still need access for suctioning, deflation of the balloon and application of a one-way value (e.g., Passey valve) not only facilitates speech but also can reduce aspiration during swallowing. These valves permit inhalation via the tracheostomy tube and are generally more easily removed than locking tracheostomy tube caps when access is needed urgently. Among those who continue to require ventilator support, clearance of condensate in ventilator tubing is recommended, but frequent replacement of the tubing itself is not beneficial for patients who remain connected to the ventilator. Careful cleansing of hands and other contact surfaces is too often forgotten when moving from patient to patient.

Among high-risk patients, elevating the head of the bed 30° to 45° to avoid gastric reflux appears important, as does limiting gastric residua. However, protracted efforts to advance feeding tubes beyond the stomach are more costly, can delay onset of feedings, and have not demonstrated consistent benefit. Use of sucralfate for gastric protection from stress ulcerations, without alkalization, in ventilated patients has been studied repeatedly with some evidence of fewer VAP when compared to H_2 blockers, but less effective in preventing peptic ulcerations when compared to more potent acid inhibitors. Prophylactic administration of antibiotics intratracheally, intravenously, or by oral paste to achieve selective gut decontamination can reduce colonization with organisms susceptible to the agents and apparent respiratory infections, although there is no consistent reduction in mortality. Mortality benefit was demonstrated in a recent large study that combined oral decontamination with a 4-day course of intravenous cefotaxime, but concerns for inducing resistance over time remain. Use of tooth brushing does not reliably improve on the potential benefit of mouth wash with chlorhexidine.

The potential value of augmenting immune responses in high-risk patients continues to be explored both for prevention and treatment, including active immunization of high-risk individuals and passive enhancement of host responses in established infections. Dietary supplements to restore micronutrient deficiencies may enhance host immunity and epithelial repair and may reduce the risk of infection, although existing data regarding many selective nutrients remain inconsistent and insufficient for specific recommendations.

Continued research in this area holds promise of reducing the unacceptably high mortality rate caused by infection with GNB, but large randomized, controlled clinical trials are needed before recommending routine use of specific interventions. Because the importance of GNB recovered from the airways in these patients is often unclear, more valuable endpoints for such studies might include reduced mortality, shortened ICU and hospital stays, and reduced costs, not simply recovery of GNB organisms in the presence of an infiltrate on chest radiographs.

FURTHER READING

Recent General Reviews

1. Skrupky LP, McConnell K, Dallas J, et al. A comparison of ventilator-associated pneumonia rates as identified according to the National Healthcare Safety Network and American College of Chest Physicians criteria. *Crit Care Med.* 2012;40:281–284.
   Apparent incidence of VAP varies by criteria used.

2. Tablan OC, Anderson LJ, Besser R, et al. Guidelines for preventing health-care-associated pneumonia, 2003: recommendations of CDC and the Healthcare Infection Control Practices Advisory Committee. *MMWR Recomm Rep.* 2004;53:1–36.

   Prior review, listing 433 references, with specific recommendations that were carefully considered and generally not overstated.

3. American Thoracic Society, Infectious Diseases Society of America. Guidelines for the management of adults with hospital-acquired, ventilator-associated, and healthcare-associated pneumonia. *Am J Respir Crit Care Med.* 2005;171:388–416.

   Generally quoted ATS, IDSA guidelines.

4. Rotstein C, Evans G, Born A, et al. Clinical practice guidelines for hospital-acquired pneumonia and ventilator-associated pneumonia in adults. *Can J Infect Dis Med Microbiol.* 2008;19:19–53.

5. Woodhead M, Blasi F, Ewig S, et al. Guidelines for the management of adult lower respiratory tract infections. *Clin Microbiol Infect.* 2011;17(suppl 6):E1–E59.

   European Respiratory Society guidelines more recently updated.

6. Williams JH Jr. Fluoroquinolones for respiratory infections: too valuable to overuse. *Chest.* 2001;120:1771–1775.

   Editorial concern regarding emerging resistance to quinolones, bring only available oral antipseudomonal agents.

7. Florescu DF, Qiu F, McCartan MA, et al. What is the efficacy and safety of colistin for the treatment of ventilator-associated pneumonia? A systematic review and meta-regression. *Clin Infect Dis.* 2012;54:670–680.

   Review suggesting colisin (polymyxin E) therapy for multidrug resistant VAP, may be less toxic than generally believed.

8. Coffin SE, Klompas M, Classen D, et al. Strategies to prevent ventilator-associated pneumonia in acute care hospitals. *Infect Control Hosp Epidemiol.* 2008;29(suppl 1):S31–S40.

9. McClave SA, Martindale RG, Vanek VW, et al. Guidelines for the provision and assessment of nutritional support therapy in the adult critically ill patient. *JPEN J Parenter Enteral Nutr.* 2009;33:277–316.

10. Ho KM, Dobb GJ, Webb SA. A comparison of early gastric and post-pyloric feeding in critically ill patients: a meta-analysis. *Intensive Care Med.* 2006;32(5):639.

    Pneumonia not significantly reduced by efforts to pass feeding tube past pylorus, which can delay initiating feeding, and is not routinely beneficial in the absence of gastric emptying problems.

11. Afessa B, Shorr AF, Anzueto AR, et al. Association between a silver-coated endotracheal tube and reduced mortality in patients with ventilator-associated pneumonia. *Chest.* 2010;137(5):1015–1021.

    Secondary analysis of NASCENT study leaves impression that, while silver impregnation reduced mortality associated with apparent VAP, a larger increase in non-VIP associated mortality discounted desired benefit.

12. Bouadma L, Wolff M, Lucet JC. Ventilator-associated pneumonia and its prevention. *Curr Opin Infec Dis.* 2012;25:395–404.

    Reviews prevention efforts, continuing to support head elevation in most, and suggesting limited benefits of several independent measures, that may need to be bundled to show significant impact.

13. Brusselaers N, Labeau S, Vogelaers D, et al. Value of lower respiratory tract surveillance cultures to predict bacterial pathogens in ventilator-associated pneumonia: systematic review and diagnostic test accuracy meta-analysis. *Intensive Care Med.* 2013;39(3):365–375.

14. El-Solh AA, Pietrantoni C, Bhat A, et al. Microbiology of severe aspiration pneumonia in institutionalized elderly. *Am J Respir Crit Care Med.* 2003;167:1650–1654.

15. Gu WJ, Gong YZ, Pan L, et al. Impact of oral care with versus without toothbrushing on the prevention of ventilator-associated pneumonia: a systematic review and meta-analysis of randomized controlled trials. *Crit Care.* 2012;16:R190.

Recent Relevant Studies

16. de Smet AM, Kluytmans JA, Blok HE, et al. Selective digestive tract decontamination and selective oropharyngeal decontamination and antibiotic resistance in patients in intensive-care units: an open-label, clustered group-randomized, crossover study. *Lancet Infect Dis.* 2011;11(5):372–380.

17. El-Solh AA, Aquilina AT, Dhillon RS, et al. Impact of invasive strategy on management of antimicrobial treatment failure in institutionalized older people with severe pneumonia. *Am J Respir Crit Care Med.* 2002;166:1038–1043.

    Small study weakly supporting invasive diagnostic approach with failed outpatient Rx.

18. Esteban A, Frutos-Vivar F, Ferguson ND, et al. Noninvasive positive-pressure ventilation for respiratory failure after extubation. *N Engl J Med.* 2004;350:2452–2460.

    Multicenter trial of delaying reintubation with trial of NIV: outcome worse, including greater ICU mortality with NIV. Note: the results of this study contrast with others where NIV was applied before emergence of frank respiratory failure among marginal patients.

19. Burns KE, Adhikari NK, Keenan SP, et al. Noninvasive positive pressure ventilation as a weaning strategy for intubated adults with respiratory failure. *Cochrane Database Syst Rev.* 2010;(8):CD004127.

    Meta-analysis, mostly COPD patients, shows lower mortality and fewer pneumonia when NIV used to assist weaning from ventilator supports.

20. Freire AT, Melnyk V, Kim MJ, et al. Comparison of tigecycline with imipenem/cilastatin for the treatment of hospital-acquired pneumonia. *Diagn Microbiol Infect Dis.* 2010;68:140–151.

    Tigecycline was less effective than imipenem among patients with VAP.

21. Aydemir H, Akduman D, Piskin N, et al. Colistin vs. the combination of colistin and rifampicin for the treatment of carbapenem-resistant *Acinetobacter baumannii* ventilator-associated pneumonia. *Epidemiol Infect.* 2013;141(6):1214–1222.

    Suggests adding rifampin to colistin may enhance response with MDR organisms.

22. Chastre J, Wolff M, Fagon JY, et al. Comparison of 8 vs 15 days of antibiotic therapy for ventilator-associated pneumonia in adults: a randomized trial. *JAMA.* 2003;290:2888–2898.

    Seeking to reduce antibiotic selection pressure time, the shorter course unfortunately diminished efficacy for clearing nonfermenting, Gram-negative organisms.

23. Capellier G, Mockly H, Charpentier C, et al. Early-onset ventilator-associated pneumonia in adults randomized clinical trial: comparison of 8 versus 15 days of antibiotic treatment. *PLoS One.* 2012;7(8):e41290.

    A more recent study with similar results.

24. Fahimi F, Ghafari S, Jamaati H, et al. Continuous versus intermittent administration of piperacillin–tazobactam in intensive care unit patients with ventilator-associated pneumonia. *Indian J Crit Care Med.* 2012;16:141–147.

    Outcomes with VAP were similar using pip/tazo 3.375 g infused over 30 minutes every 6 hours, versus over 4 hours every 8 hours, with a relatively long duration of therapy (mean 19 days).

25. Kollef MH, Chastre J, Clavel M, et al. A randomized trial of 7-day doripenem versus 10-day imipenem-cilastatin for ventilator-associated pneumonia. *Crit Care.* 2012;16(6):R218.

    RCT stopped early as strong trend toward increased mortality with shorter 7 day course of doripenem, given as 4-hour infusions every 8 hours, particularly among those with pseudomonas infection, compared to longer 10 day imipenem treatment, given in more standard, shorter infusion times.

26. Short AE, Zadeiki N, Xiang JX, et al. A multicenter, randomized, double-blind, retrospective comparison of 5- and 10-day regimens of levofloxacin in a subgroup of patients aged >65 years with community-acquired pneumonia. *Clin Ther.* 2005;27:1251–1259.

27. Bouadma L, Luyt CE, Tubach F, et al. Use of procalcitonin to reduce patients' exposure to antibiotics in intensive care units (PRORATA trial): a multicentre randomised controlled trial. *Lancet.* 2010;375(9713):463–474.

    Monitoring acute inflammation marker allowed safe reduction in time on antibioitics in septic patients in ICU.

28. Gruson D, Hilbert G, Vargas F, et al. Strategy of antibiotic rotation: long-term effect on incidence and susceptibilities of Gram-negative bacilli responsible for ventilator-associated pneumonia. *Crit Care Med.* 2003;21:1908–1914.

    Unfortunate swing of late outcome data that eroded initially published enthusiasm for the approach.

29. Hamer DH. Treatment of nosocomial pneumonia and tracheobronchitis caused by multi-drug resistant *Pseudomonas aeruginosa* with aerosolized colistin. *Am J Respir Crit Care Med.* 2000;162:328–330.

    Three patients treated by nebulization of systemically toxic drug.

30. de Jonge E, Schultz MJ, Spanjaard L, et al. Effects of selective decontamination of digestive tract on mortality and acquisition of resistant bacteria in intensive care: a randomized, controlled trial. *Lancet.* 2003;362:1011–1016.

    A complex approach renews hope for a role of selective gut decontamination in reducing colonization with GNB, without increased resistance.

Historically Important References

31. Holzapfel L, Chastang C, Demingeon G, et al. A randomized study assessing the systematic search for maxillary sinusitis in nasotracheally mechanically ventilated patients: influence of nosocomial maxillary sinusitis on the occurrence of ventilator-associated pneumonia. *Am J Respir Crit Care Med.* 1999;159:695.

    Suggests early recognition and treatment of sinusitis reduces the incidence of nosocomial pneumonia in intubated patients

32. Reyes MP. The aerobic gram-negative bacillary pneumonias. *Med Clin North Am.* 1980;64:363.

    A readable review with many classic references.

33. Unger JD, Rose HD, Unger GF. Gram-negative pneumonia. *Radiology.* 1973;107:283.

    Discusses classic radiologic features.

34. Dorff GJ, Rytel MW, Scanlon G. Etiologies and characteristic features of pneumonia in a municipal hospital. *Am J Med Sci.* 1973;266:349.

    A study of 178 cases of pneumonia before the initiation of antibiotics.

35. Polednak AP. Postmortem bacteriology and pneumonia in a mentally retarded population. *Am J Clin Pathol.* 1977;67:190.

    Postmortem diagnosis that was most accurate!

36. Valdivieso M, Gil-Extremera B, Bodey GP. Gram-negative bacillary pneumonia in the compromised host. *Medicine (Baltimore).* 1977;55:214.

    A classic, large study of patients receiving tumor chemotherapy, with good discussions.

37. Zornoza J, Goldman AM, Bodey GP. Radiologic features of gram-negative pneumonias in the neutropenic patient. *AJR Am J Roentgenol.* 1976;127:989.

38. Andrews CP, Coalson JJ, Johanson WG. Diagnosis of nosocomial bacterial pneumonia in acute, diffuse lung injury. *Chest.* 1981;80:254.

    Gram-negative bacterial pneumonia is difficult to diagnose in adult respiratory distress syndrome.

39. Rose HD, Heckman MG, Unger JD. *Pseudomonas aeruginosa* pneumonia in adults. *Am Rev Respir Dis.* 1973;107:416.

    A classic description.

40. Fuchshuber PR, Lipman B, Kraybill WG, et al. *Ecthyma gangrenosum* secondary to *Escherichia coli* sepsis. *Infect Med.* 1998;15:798.

    The finding discussed is seen in infections other than Pseudomonas. This is a well-written case report of it in Escherichia coli *sepsis, with an illustrative description and thoroughly referenced list of the associated infectious agents.*

41. Jonas M, Cunha BA. Bacteremic *Escherichia coli* pneumonia. *Arch Intern Med.* 1982;142:2157.

    A good study and review.

42. Tillotson JR, Lerner MA. Characteristics of pneumonias caused by *Bacillus proteus*. *Ann Intern Med.* 1968;68:287.

    A classic study of outpatients.

43. Yu VL. *Serratia marcescens*: historical perspective and clinical review. *N Engl J Med.* 1979;300:887.

44. Hurley EJ, Viroslav J, Gray WR, et al. Pharyngeal aspiration in normal adults and patients with depressed consciousness. *Am J Med.* 1978;64:564.

    Aspiration is common, even in normals.

45. Torres A, Serra-Batlles J, Ros E, et al. Pulmonary aspiration of gastric contents in patients receiving mechanical ventilation: the effect of body position. *Ann Intern Med.* 1992;116:540.

    Emphasizes the importance of elevating the head of the bed after intubation, because the endotracheal tube only reduces acute aspiration volumes, not aspiration per se.

46. Mann HJ, Canafax DM, Cipolle RJ, et al. Increased dosage requirements of tobramycin and gentamicin for treating *Pseudomonas pneumonia* in patients with cystic fibrosis. *Pediatr Pulmonol.* 1985;1:238.

    Higher aminoglycoside doses were required to maintain levels in cystic fibrosis patients.

47. Johanson WG Jr, Seidenfeld JJ, Gomez P Jr, et al. Bacteriologic diagnosis of nosocomial pneumonia following prolonged mechanical ventilation. *Am Rev Respir Dis.* 1988;137:259.

    An important animal (baboon) study, suggesting bronchoalveolar lavage is more sensitive and correlates better with burden than protected brush and needle aspirates, although it is not more specific.

48. Brown RB, Kruse JA, Counts GW, et al. Double-blind study of endobronchial tobramycin in the treatment of gram-negative bacterial pneumonia. *Antimicrob Agents Chemother.* 1990;34:269.

    Added to intravenous therapy, aminoglycoside instillation accelerates bacterial clearance without a significant impact on overall hospital course.

49. Intravenous Immunoglobulin Collaborative Study Group. Prophylactic intravenous administration of standard immune globulin as compared to core-lipopolysaccharide immune globulin in patients at high risk of postsurgical infection. *N Engl J Med.* 1992;327:234.

    Nonimmune globulin inhibited GNB infections more effectively than specific immune globulin.

50. Hospital-acquired pneumonia in adults: diagnosis, assessment of severity, initial antimicrobial therapy, and preventive strategies: a consensus statement, American Thoracic Society, November 1995. *Am J Respir Crit Care Med.* 1996;153:1711–1725.

46 Anaerobic Lung Infections

Laura E. Crotty Alexander

Anaerobic bacteria aspirated into the lung can cause pneumonia, lung abscess, and empyema. Anaerobic lung infections typically smolder for weeks to months before a patient presents for medical care. Symptoms tend not to be as profound or specific as in other bacterial infections and include putrid sputum and breath, weight loss, and fever. Infection is caused by aspiration of multiple organisms normally residing in gingival crevices. Because anaerobes are not highly virulent organisms, they may require up to three or more concomitant bacterial species to establish infection in the lung via bacterial synergy. The concomitant species may be aerobic or anaerobic. Many times the concomitant bacteria will grow in culture, while the anaerobic bacteria do not. For this reason, the selective nature of diagnostic cultures may mask the true contribution of anaerobes to the infectious process. The top three anaerobic bacteria that cause lung infections are *Bacteroides melaninogenicus, Fusobacterium nucleatum,* and *Peptostreptococcus.*

Poor dentition and gingival disease in a patient with pulmonary symptoms should raise the suspicion for anaerobic infection, since these conditions are associated with higher amounts of bacteria in the oropharynx. Anaerobic bacteria infect the lung after large quantities are aspirated. For this reason, anaerobic lung infection is associated with conditions that lead to aspiration such as alcohol abuse, seizure, stroke or other neurologic disorders, dysphagia, and esophageal motility disorders. In addition, patients with nosocomial sinusitis have a high incidence of anaerobes as the etiologic organism. Sinusitis is commonly associated with pneumonia due to the same organism, presumably because of aspiration of the organisms from the nasopharyngeal space. Anaerobic infections also can occur in the setting of obstructing lung lesions, such as tumors or aspirated objects.

Patients with anaerobic lung infections tend to be less acutely ill than those with other community-acquired pneumonias. In one review of all ICU admissions over one year, not a single case was due to anaerobic lung infections or their sequelae. The onset of symptoms tends to be more insidious than in pneumonia due to more virulent bacteria. Patients with anaerobic empyema and lung abscess typically present after 14 to 15 days of symptoms. Twenty percent of patients who have aspirated anaerobic organisms will develop lung necrosis and abscesses in the following weeks. Some patients will develop empyema in 4 to 6 weeks. Because of the chronic nature of anaerobic infections, symptoms such as weight loss, anemia, and night sweats are common. However, in the hours following aspiration itself, patients may have symptoms of chemical pneumonitis, which symptomatically and radiographically should clear within 24 to 48 hours.

Radiographic findings of anaerobic lung infection include necrotic lesions, cavitations, and abscesses and complicated pleural effusions. Because aspiration is the primary process leading to infection, dependent lung segments in the recumbent position are most commonly involved, especially the superior segments of the lower lobes and the posterior segments of the upper lobes.

Diagnosis is almost entirely clinical but the presence of putrid sputum or empyema fluid is diagnostic because anaerobes are the only organisms to produce the short-chain volatile fatty acids that are associated with a distinctive odor and sour and foul taste. There have been no significant advancements in diagnosis in over 20 years. Methods that may be useful in making a diagosis include transtracheal lung sampling and protected brush specimens via bronchoscopy. However, neither method has become commonplace. Samples need to be rapidly processed under anaerobic conditions; any contamination with more robust bacterial species (*Staphylococcus*) can lead to overgrowth that masks the presence of anaerobes.

New methods might include polymerase chain reaction (PCR) detection of bacterial genomic markers in sputum and bronchoalveolar lavage (BAL) samples. However, because the bacteria that cause anaerobic infections are found normally in the oral cavity, contamination of expectorated specimens is common. One method of removing oral contaminations is to run tap water over sputum samples to remove any bacteria not embedded in the mucous and biofilm. Recovery of anaerobes from pleural fluid is the most convincing finding. However, even in the absence of culture data, any pleural fluid that smells putrid is strong evidence of anaerobic infection.

Antibiotic coverage for anaerobes is reasonable in the setting of out-of-hospital aspiration that results in pneumonia. Also, patients who appear to be nontoxic despite evidence of necrotizing pneumonia, lung abscess, or empyema should be treated for anaerobic lung infection. Many commonly used antibiotics have good anaerobic coverage, which may be the reason that anaerobic lung infections are often not diagnosed specifically and do not need additional coverage. For community-acquired pneumonia that may be related to aspiration, a fluoroquinolone plus clindamycin or a β-lactam/β-lactamase inhibitor is appropriate. If the clinical diagnosis is clearly aspiration pneumonia, single-drug therapy has been shown to be efficacious with clindamycin, β-lactam/β-lactamase inhibitor, and carbapenem. Nosocomial aspiration should be covered with imipenem, piperacillin-tazobactam (pip/tazo) or other Gram-negative bacteria coverage plus clindamycin. Clindamycin is one of the most commonly recommended antibiotics for anaerobic pneumonia, and is well supported by clinical research. However, monotherapy with ampicillin/sulbactam, amoxicillin-clavulanate, moxifloxacin, or carbapenems has resulted in outcomes comparable to clindamycin. Metronidazole is not as effective and is not recommended for single-drug treatment of anaerobes in the lung. If metronidazole is used, it must be combined with penicillin to provide coverage against streptococci.

Antibiotic treatment for anaerobic pneumonia should continue for 7 to 10 days. Aspiration pneumonitis is mostly chemical in nature and does not require antibiotic treatment if it occurred out of hospital. However, aspiration in hospitalized patients is associated with a 13% to 26% chance of bacterial superinfection. In those cases, coverage for Gram-negative and anaerobic species (e.g., a carbapenem or pip/tazo) would be prudent for 48 to 72 hours. It can be discontinued if lung infiltrates do not develop. Antibiotic treatment of several months may be necessary for lung abscesses, continuing until radiographic clearance (anywhere between 3 weeks to 8 months). Anaerobic empyemas require drainage and concomitant antibiotic treatment for

7 to 14 days beyond resolution of the empyema and defervescence. Pleural thickening, however, is a common residua, and its presence does not indicate a need to prolong antibiotic therapy.

Patients with aspiration-associated anaerobic pneumonia and lung abscess typically recover well. The Pneumonia Patient Outcomes Research Team (PORT) pneumonia severity index (PSI) score and CURB-65 scores (see Further Reading 23–25) can be used to predict short-term mortality and need for hospitalization, while the PSI score can also be used to predict long-term mortality. Outcomes for lung abscess depend greatly on the underlying condition of the patient. Relatively healthy patients, including alcoholics, have a 90% to 95% cure rate with antibiotics, while those who are immunocompromised or have cancer may have a mortality rate up to 75%.

FURTHER READING

1. Smith DT. Experimental aspiratory abscess. *Arch Surg.* 1927;14(1):231–239.

    The original discussion of why abscesses arise: embolic vs. aspiration.

2. Bartlett JG. Anaerobic bacterial infections of the lung and pleural space. *Clin Infect Dis.* 1993;(suppl 4):S248–S255.

    Dr. Bartlett is the world expert on anaerobic lung infections, and each of his papers and articles shine new light on the subject. This one is a thorough review of 193 cases, diagnosis, and treatment.

3. Wimberley NW, Bass JB Jr, Boyd BW, et al. Use of a bronchoscopic protected catheter brush for the diagnosis of pulmonary infections. *Chest.* 1982;81:556–562.

    Sixty-five patients in this study, and good microbiology data was acquired via protected brush, even in abscess patients (mixed aerobic and anaerobic bacteria recovered in these patients).

4. Bartlett JG. Anaerobic bacterial infections of the lung. *Chest.* 1987;91:901–909.

5. Le Moal G, Lemerre D, Grollier G, et al. Nosocomial sinusitis with isolation of anaerobic bacteria in ICU patients. *Intensive Care Med.* 1999;25:1066–1071.

    Culture of sinus contents is high-yield for obtaining bacteriologic data, and often correlates with organisms causing concomitant lung infection.

6. Mattison LE, Coppage L, Alderman DF, et al. Pleural effusions in the medical ICU: prevalence, causes, and clinical implications. *Chest.* 1997;111:1018–1023.

    Prospective observational study of pleural effusion prevalence and etiology in the MICU (only 1% due to empyema).

7. Bartlett JG. Anaerobic bacterial infection of the lung. *Anaerobe.* 2012;18:235–239.

8. Bartlett JG. How important are anaerobic bacteria in aspiration pneumonia: when should they be treated and what is optimal therapy. *Infect Dis Clin North Am.* 2013;27:149–155.

9. Kadowaki MY, Demura S, Mizuno D, et al. Reappraisal of clindamycin IV monotherapy for treatment of mild-to-moderate aspiration pneumonia in elderly patients. *Chest.* 2007;127:1276–1282.

    Clindamycin as a monotherapy is a valid treatment option in aspiration pneumonia, and has a lower incidence of posttreatment MRSA compared to penicillin and carbapenem therapies.

10. Levison ME, Mangura CT, Lorber E, et al. Clindamycin compared with penicillin for the treatment of anaerobic lung abscess. *Ann Intern Med.* 1983;98:466–471.

    Clindamycin is superior to penicillin as a monotherapy for lung abscess (no treatment failures and faster resolution of symptoms).

11. Gudiol F, Manresa F, Pallares R, et al. Clindamycin vs penicillin for anaerobic lung infections: high rate of penicillin failures associated with penicillin-resistant *Bacteroides melaninogenicus. Arch Intern Med.* 1990;150:2525–2529.

    Superiority of clindamycin over penicillin monotherapy in lung abscess and necrotizing pneumonia is frequently due to penicillin resistance in Bacteroides *(this trial successfully utilized transthoracic aspiration and protected brush via bronchoscopy to obtain culture data).*

12. Boyce JM, Walsh DA, Levison ME, et al. Anaerobic lung abscess: clindamycin or penicillin. *Ann Intern Med.* 1983;99:410.

13. Fernandez-Sabe N, Carratala J, Dorca J, et al. Efficacy and safety of sequential amoxicillin-clavulanate in the treatment of anaerobic lung infections. *Eur J Clin Microbiol Infect Dis.* 2003;22:185–187.

    IV followed by PO amoxicillin-clavulanate cured 35 sequential patients with lung abscess or necrotizing pneumonia.

14. Allewelt M. Aspiration pneumonia and primary lung abscess: diagnosis and therapy of an aerobic or an anaerobic infection. *Expert Rev Respir Med.* 2007;1:111–119.

    A nice review of anaerobic lung infections.

15. Ott SR, Allewelt M, Lorenz J, et al. Moxifloxacin vs ampicillin/sulbactam in aspiration pneumonia and primary lung abscess. *Infection.* 2008;36:23–30.

    Prospective, randomized trial with 139 patients demonstrated equivalence of moxifloxacin to amp/sulbactam in aspiration pneumonia and lung abscess.

16. Tokuyasu H, Harada T, Watanabe E, et al. Effectiveness of meropenem for the treatment of aspiration pneumonia in elderly patients. *Intern Med.* 2008;48:129–135.

    Prospective study of 62 elderly patients with aspiration pneumonia demonstrated that anaerobes can be detected by bronchoscopy (in 20% of cases), meropenem is effective as a monotherapy, and mortality is 10% in this population.

17. Sanders CV, Hanna BJ, Lewis AC. Metronidazole in the treatment of anaerobic infections. *Am Rev Respir Dis.* 1979;120:337–343.

    The first study to demonstrate that metronidazole should not be used as a monotherapy to treat anaerobic pleuropulmonary infections (38%–61% failure rate).

18. Perlino CA. Metronidazole vs clindamycin treatment of anerobic pulmonary infection: failure of metronidazole therapy. *Arch Intern Med.* 1981;141:1424–1427.

19. Mandell LA, Wunderink RG, Anzueto A, et al. Infectious Diseases Society of America/American Thoracic Society consensus guidelines on the management of community-acquired pneumonia in adults. *Clin Infect Dis.* 2007;44(suppl 2):S27–S72.

    Consensus guidelines from ATS and the ID Society of America, covering management of all types of CAP, incuding aspiration pneumonia.

20. Bynum LJ, Pierce AK. Pulmonary aspiration of gastric contents. *Am Rev Respir Dis.* 1976;114:1129–1136.

    Beautiful description of the natural history of aspiration: 62% aspiration pneumonitis that clears quickly, 26% developed aspiration pneumonia and 60% of those died, and 12% died shortly after the initial aspiration event. And a description of patients who aspirate.

21. Cameron JL, Mitchell WH, Zuidema GD. Aspiration pneumonia: clinical outcome following documented aspiration. *Arch Surg.* 1973;106:49–52.

    Forty-seven cases of aspiration were reviewed and a mortality rate of 62% was found, 90% if two or more lung lobes were involved.

22. Dines DE, Titus JL, Sessler AD. Aspiration pneumonitis. *Mayo Clin Proc.* 1970;45:347–360.

23. Aujesky D, Auble TE, Yealy DM, et al. Prospective comparison of three validated prediction rules for prognosis in community-acquired pneumonia. *Am J Med.* 2005;118:384–392.

    Prospectively followed 3,181 patients with CAP and found that the Pneumonia Severity Index (PSI) was more powerful than CURB and CURB-65 for predicting short-term mortality and defining low-risk patients.

24. Johnstone JD, Eurich T, Majumdar SR, et al. Long-term morbidity and mortality after hospitalization with community-acquired pneumonia: a population-based cohort study. *Medicine (Baltimore).* 2008;87:329–334.

    Prospective study of 3,415 subjects with CAP which found that initial PSI class predicted not only short-term mortality, but also long-term postdischarge morbidity and mortality.

25. Fine MJ, Auble TE, Yealy DM, et al. A prediction rule to identify low-risk patients with community-acquired pneumonia. *N Engl J Med.* 1997;336:243–250.

    The original PORT score, which identifies patients at low-risk of death from CAP.

26. Bartlett JG. *Lung abscess and necrotizing pneumonia.* Philadelphia, PA: WB Saunders; 1992.

    Informative book chapter.

27. Pohlson EC, McNamara JJ, Char C, et al. Lung abscess: a changing pattern of the disease. *Am J Surg.* 1985;150:97–101.

    Description of patients with lung abscess admitted to a community hospital, which found a 9% mortality rate contributable to lung abscess.

47 Atypical Pneumonias: *Mycoplasma, Chlamydophila* (Chlamydia), Q Fever, and *Legionella*

Maida V. Soghikian

Historically, the term *atypical pneumonia* was applied to pulmonary infections that were without identifiable causative organisms on routine culture and did not respond to standard antimicrobial therapy. They had unusual clinical and radiographic presentations compared with classic bacterial pneumonias. Subsequently, a variety of causative organisms were identified that are often considered synonymous with the term atypical pneumonia, including *Mycoplasma pneumoniae, Chlamydophila psittaci* (psittacosis), *Chlamydophila pneumoniae* (formerly *C. psittaci*, strain TWAR), *Coxiella burnetii* (Q fever), *Legionella* species, and various viruses. This group of organisms is responsible for at least 25% of all community-acquired pneumonias (CAP) worldwide. The illnesses caused by these organisms differ in their epidemiology and natural history, but they are all thought to be transmitted via particle or droplet inhalation and all are resistant to beta lactam antibiotics. CAP empiric therapy guidelines specifically address atypical pathogens, and some scoring systems have been developed in an attempt to differentiate typical from atypical CAP. Because laboratory identification of these infections remains difficult, much effort has gone into developing newer diagnostic techniques such as polymerase chain reaction (PCR). Mortality with these pathogens is characteristically less than with other common causes of CAP and many, including *Legionella*, are frequently managed as outpatients. The enhanced ability to identify these infectious agents and their relative frequency leads some to argue that atypical is now a misnomer.

M. pneumoniae is a free-living organism without a cell wall that readily attaches to mucosal surfaces. It was first described in 1938, and at that time it was believed to be caused by a nonfilterable virus. It was later found to be associated with a rise in cold agglutinins and to be a bacterial infection. It is the most common cause of atypical pneumonia, accounting for 10% to 30% of pneumonias in ambulatory patients (some reports suggest even higher). It had previously been called "walking pneumonia" due to the discordance between radiographic infiltrates and relative paucity of symptoms. *M. pneumoniae* is the most common cause of pneumonia in young adults and teenagers, though the frequency is also increased in the elderly. Hospitalization is rarely required except in individuals who are chronically ill or develop complications. *M. pneumoniae* has an incubation period averaging 2 to 3 weeks. The infection is usually endemic, occurring most frequently in the fall and winter months. The rate of infection is greatest in areas of close personal contact (e.g., military bases, households). *M. pneumoniae* infection most commonly presents as tracheobronchitis with intractable cough and low-grade fever. Relatively few infected persons develop frank pneumonia (3%–6%). Pulmonary exam may be normal but often demonstrates diffuse inspiratory rales that correspond to unilateral or bilateral infiltrates on radiographs. Lobar consolidation is rare. Small pleural effusions occur in up to 25% of patients. Leucocytosis is often absent. In addition to respiratory illness, *M. pneumoniae* can cause a myriad of extrapulmonary illnesses either by direct invasion or by immune mechanisms, such as nonexudative pharyngitis, bullous myringitis, diarrhea, and erythema multiforme. Rarely, patients may present with central nervous system (CNS) manifestations (meningoencephalitis, transverse myelitis) or cardiac manifestations (pericarditis, myocarditis). A potentially serious extrapulmonary manifestation is cold agglutinin-induced hemolysis, which results from IgM antibodies that cross-react with the erythrocyte I antigen. A nonspecific elevation in cold agglutinin titers occurs in 75% of patients by the first to second week of the illness, but may be mild and without associated complications. Diagnosis by a 4-fold rise in antibody titers by enzyme-linked immunosorbent assay (EIA) is both sensitive and specific. PCR is not yet standardized or available for routine use. It is recommended to treat empirically, while using paired EIA serology and rapid PCR assays if available. *M. pneumoniae* infection is self-limited in most cases; in one large series, it represented only 5% of patients hospitalized with pneumonia. The overall mortality rate is extremely low and generally attributed to neurologic and cardiac sequelae. *M. pneumoniae* can be treated with azithromycin 500 mg initially followed by 250 QD mg daily for 4 days or with doxycycline 200 mg initially, then 100 mg Q12H for 10 to 14 days, although macrolide resistance is an increasing problem. The respiratory fluoroquinolones, moxifloxacin or levofloxacin, are effective alternatives and given for 5 days.

The *Chlamydophila* species are obligate intracellular bacteria and include two species associated with human pneumonia in adults: *C. psittaci* and *C. pneumoniae*. *Chlamydia trachomatis* causes conjunctivitis and pneumonia in newborn infants but has not been implicated as a cause of adult respiratory disease. *C. psittaci* is primarily an avian pathogen but also causes infection in humans (psittacosis) after contaminated droppings from diseased birds are inhaled. Parrots and parakeets (psittacine birds) are the most common sources of human infection, but domestic (chickens, ducks, and turkeys) and urban (pigeons) fowl also have been described as a source of infection. Infected birds are commonly asymptomatic but can develop an illness of ruffled feathers, respiratory symptoms, conjunctivitis, or diarrhea. Psittacosis occurs sporadically but frequently is seen in association with avian outbreaks. It is a serious occupational hazard in poultry-processing plants, with turkeys being the most commonly involved bird in the United States and ducks in Europe. After the organism gains access to the upper respiratory tract, it spreads hematogenously to the lungs and to the reticuloendothelial system. The incubation period is 5 to 21 days. Human-to-human transmission is unusual, although infection of healthcare workers by patients has been described. The reported incidence is 0.01/100,000 in the United States, but this is likely an underrepresentation since clinical disease is often mild and likely underdiagnosed. Psittacosis is responsible for less than 5% of hospitalized pneumonia cases. It can affect any age, but is more common in young and middle-aged adults. The clinical spectrum of psittacosis is protean and ranges from a mild, flulike illness with fever, dry cough, and headache (the majority) to fulminant sepsis with multiorgan failure. Pneumonia, although generally mild, can present as a severe, multilobar, consolidative process associated with splenomegaly and relative bradycardia. Many extrapulmonary manifestations have been described, including severe headache, photophobia, myalgias, arthralgias, nausea and vomiting, lymphadenopathy, hepatosplenomegaly, and thyroiditis. Serious manifestations such as meningoencephalitis, endocarditis, myocarditis, and nephritis can be seen. Dermatologic manifestations include erythema nodosum, erythema marginatum, and a pink, roselike, macular rash (Horder spots). The chest radiograph is abnormal in 80% of patients, most often with lobar consolidation. Labs are nonspecific. Fulminant psittacosis is an infrequent but important complication manifested by hypoxic respiratory failure, septic shock, impaired cognition, and renal, hepatic, and hematologic failure. Poor prognostic signs include increased age, confusion, leukopenia, severe hypoxemia, and renal and multilobar pulmonary involvement. The mortality rate was 20% in the preantibiotic era and now is about 1% with appropriate treatment.

C. pneumoniae occurs most commonly in elderly. In contrast to *C. psittaci*, no animal vector (other than humans) has been discovered. Transmission is likely from person to person through respiratory secretions. Serologic evidence indicates that infection is common throughout the world. About 5% to 15% of community-acquired pneumonia is attributed to this organism, although serologic tests used to make such estimates have suffered from poor specificity. Repeated infection and persistent infection can occur. Dual infections in combination with *Streptococcus pneumoniae* or *M. pneumoniae* have been reported. Often the patient has a brief prodrome of headache and myalgias and then high fever and shaking chills, but they may be asymptomatic. Cough and pharyngitis are frequently present. Other clinical manifestations include sinusitis and delirium. Extrapulmonary signs and symptoms are less common but can include arthritis, myocarditis, Guillian-Barre syndrome, and meningoencephalitis. In addition to causing pneumonia, *C. pneumoniae* has been identified as an etiologic factor in acute exacerbations of chronic obstructive pulmonary disease and coronary artery disease. Laboratory data are not specific, and radiographs generally have patchy subsegmental infiltrates. Diagnosis is most commonly made by demonstrating a 4-fold rise in complement fixation (CF) titers drawn 2 weeks apart. The clinical utility of serial titer measurement is limited by lack of specificity (with significant cross-reactivity between *C. psittaci* and *C. pneumoniae*) and by the delay incurred while waiting for a second sample. Microimmunofluorescence (MIF) is a specific assay that can be positive on the basis of a single IgM titer of 16 or greater; however, it is less readily available than other tests. PCR of sputum and bronchoalveolar lavage (BAL) samples is a rapid and specific diagnostic test, but it is not routinely available outside of reference laboratories. Cell culture techniques are not generally available except in specialized labs (*C. psittaci* is classified as a dangerous pathogen).

The antibiotic of choice for *Chlamydophila* pneumonias is doxycycline for 10 to 14 days for *C. pneumoniae* and 14 days for *C. psittaci*. Tigecycline and fluoroquinolones have in vitro activity, but clinical treatment data are limited. Newer macrolides have in vitro activity against *Chlamydophila* species and are an appropriate choice in pregnancy and childhood. Birds infected with *C. psittaci* should be treated with doxycycline to cure or at least suppress any major ongoing exposure risk.

Q fever is a zoonosis, named "Query fever" in 1936 following an outbreak in Australia of a febrile illness characterized by headache, malaise, anorexia, and myalgia in abattoir workers. *Coxiella burnetii*, the etiologic agent of Q fever, is an obligate intracellular bacterium with a large natural reservoir that includes rodents, cattle, sheep, and goats. In nature, a tick vector maintains the disease. *C. burnetii* is a reportable disease in the United States and a Centers for Disease Control and Prevention (CDC) category B bioterrorism agent, meaning it has the potential for large-scale dissemination but generally causes less illness and death than category A agents. Humans acquire the disease through contact with infected milk, feces, urine, or placentas of farm animals. Human-to-human spread, although theoretically possible, has never been documented. The incubation period averages 2 to 3 weeks. Outbreaks have been reported in stockyard and meat packinghouse employees, dairy workers, animal hair processors, and medical school employees (in research facilities using contaminated sheep placentas). Infection can result in acute or chronic illness and induces a range of immunomodulatory responses in the host from immunosuppression in those with chronic Q fever to nonspecific stimulation after vaccination that results in autoantibody induction, especially to smooth muscle and cardiac muscle. There was an average of 51 cases per year in the United States from 2000 to 2004. It remains more common in Australia and is endemic in many European countries. Acute Q fever can be present as a nonspecific febrile illness, pneumonia, or hepatitis, the clinical presentation being influenced by geography. Q fever pneumonia patients present with some combination of fevers, severe headache, cough, pleuritic chest pain, digestive symptoms, and arthromyalgia, though other nonspecific symptoms may occur. Other more severe extrapulmonary manifestations include endocarditis, myocarditis, pericarditis, glomerulonephritis, and meningoencephalitis. Hematologic and dermatologic complications can occur, not unlike other atypical pathogens. Chronic Q fever, defined as lasting over 6 months, occurs in 1% to 5% of infected patients. It presents as endocarditis, osteomyelitis, and hepatitis and can complicate pregnancy. History often provides the most important clue of exposure. Exam may reveal hepatosplenomegaly and nonspecific rales. Liver function abnormalities occur in the majority of patients and both thrombocytopenia and autoantibodies are commonly seen. Radiographic manifestations are not specific though multiple rounded opacities are not infrequently found. Diagnosis of Q fever is most commonly by immunofluorescence antibody testing. Persistence or reappearance of high levels of antibodies may indicate chronic infection. PCR has been used in cell cultures and clinical samples; however, isolation must be done in a biosafety containment facility because of its extreme infectivity. The treatment of choice for Q fever pneumonia is doxycycline for 10 days. There is heterogeneous susceptibility to macrolides, and fluoroquinolone resistance has been reported. Pregnant patients should be treated with cotrimoxazole for the duration of pregnancy. Q fever pneumonia is usually a self-limited illness with an excellent prognosis though symptoms can last for weeks. Patients with cardiac valvular lesions who develop Q fever are at risk for endocarditis months or years later and should be followed serologically or treated prophylactically for 1 year. Vaccines have been developed for use in high-risk populations.

Legionella is an obligate aerobic Gram-negative nonfermenting bacillus that was first recognized during the 1976 outbreak at American Legion Convention in Philadelphia. It is now known to be a common cause of both CAP and nosocomial pneumonia. Legionellosis refers to the two clinical syndromes caused by *Legionella* species: Legionnaires' disease, the most common acute pneumonic syndrome, and Pontiac fever, a nonpneumonic acute syndrome manifested by a febrile, self-limited, flulike illness. The family Legionellae consists of more than 70 serogroups. *L. pneumophila*, serogroups 1 to 6 account for most human infections (90% are serogroup 1), but other *Legionella* species are known to cause similar human disease. *Legionella* organisms are predominantly intracellular, infecting mononuclear cells (e.g., alveolar macrophages) in the lung. The natural habitat of *Legionella* species is fresh water sources, such as cooling towers, evaporative condensers, humidifiers, and nebulizers, as well as potable water systems. There is a seasonal peak of *Legionella* CAP in the late summer and early fall. Sporadic cases and outbreaks (including nosocomial outbreaks) are often related to exposure to colonized water sources. Superheating and hyperchlorination can eradicate the organism.

Legionella is often an opportunistic pathogen. Smokers, the elderly, patients with chronic illnesses, those on corticosteroids, and those with impairment in cellular immunity are particularly susceptible. There was an unexplained increase in Legionnaires' disease during the H1N1 influenza pandemic.

The greater severity of illness seen with *Legionella*, frequently requiring hospitalization and intensive care, distinguishes it from the other atypical pneumonias. The incubation period ranges from 2 to 18 days. *Legionella* may present subacutely, but commonly presents acutely with severe illness, manifested by a high fever, rigors, and significant hypoxemia. Gastrointestinal symptoms are a prominent feature. Radiographic studies are nonspecific, but rapidly progressive asymmetrical patchy infiltrates are characteristic. Although uncommon, Legionnaires' disease is associated with many extrapulmonary findings. Some features more consistent with Legionnaires' disease are temperature greater than 39, confusion, relative bradycardia (pulse temperature deficit), mild transaminitis, loose watery stool, microscopic hematuria, hypophosphatemia, hyponatremia, markedly elevated ferritin, relative lymphopenia, and absence of dermatologic or upper respiratory tract symptomatology.

Diagnosis is made by culture of respiratory secretions on selective media. Monoclonal DFA of respiratory secretions is diagnostic, but positivity decreases rapidly with anti-*Legionella* therapy. The urinary antigen for *L. pneumophila* serogroups 1 to 6 is commonly used. It may be negative early, but positivity lasts for several days and the results can be available in hours. The newer ICT (immunochromatographic membrane) assay for urinary antigen reports a sensitivity of 80% and specificity of 97% to 100%. PCR-based tests are available but currently not routinely used nor recommended by CDC. The mainstays of *Legionella* therapy are fluoroquinolones, which are highly active against *Legionella* and penetrate well into alveolar macrophages, concentrating intracellularly to supraserum concentrations. Tigecycline is also active and concentrates well in lung tissue and alveolar macrophages. Use is recommended if intolerant of fluoroquinolones. Prior to fluoroquinolones, doxycycline was the treatment of choice. Macrolides, considered the drug of choice for empiric treatment of atypical pneumonia, have variable effectiveness. Duration of therapy is 2 weeks unless the patient has severely limited cardiopulmonary function, which may require longer therapy. Prognosis is dependent on host cardiopulmonary function, cellular immune function, innoculum size, and promptness of therapy. Legionnaires' disease can be fatal, but with early diagnosis and appropriate therapy mortality is less than 5% in immunocompetent patients.

Although important differences in severity and outcome exist, the clinical manifestations of *M. pneumoniae, C. pneumoniae,* psittacosis, Q fever, and Legionnaires' disease can be similar and nonspecific. These pneumonic illnesses characteristically have unimpressive physical findings, nonspecific routine laboratory tests and chest radiographs, absence of bacterial pathogens on Gram stain and routine culture of clinical samples. Clues to the etiologic agents, however, can often be discerned from medical history, including environmental and occupational exposures coupled with patterns of organ involvement. Specific antigens, PCR, and serologic tests exist, but there is no widely accepted gold standard that can be routinely recommended for all pneumonia patients, though multiplex PCRs being tested show promise for the future. Standardized, reliable tests will help not only in diagnosing individual patients but also in establishing accurate incidence and prevalence of these elusive organisms. As is the case with other types of pneumonia, a decision to treat must be made before laboratory confirmation of a specific diagnosis is made. Single empiric antibiotic options for outpatient therapy that will cover atypical pathogens include the macrolides, the respiratory fluoroquinolones, and the tetracyclines. The Infectious Diseases Society of America has developed useful guidelines for empiric treatment of these and other community-acquired pneumonia

FURTHER READING

1. Murdoc DR, Chambers ST. Atypical Pneumonia-time to breathe new life into a useful term? *Lancet Infect Dis.* 2009;9:512–519.

   Reviews the history and terminology of atypical pneumonia suggesting that we should reevaluate what we call an atypical pneumonia or perhaps abolish using the term altogether.

2. Casey KR. Atypical pneumonia and environmental factors: where have you been and what have you done? *Clin Chest Med.* 1991;12:285.

   Underscores the importance of obtaining a thorough occupational, environmental, travel, and social history in patients with atypical pneumonias. Clues obtained from the history are crucial in trying to identify a specific cause of acute pneumonitis, whether it be infectious or noninfectious.

3. Cunha CB. The first atypical pneumonia: the history of the discovery of *Mycoplasma pneumoniae*. *Infect Dis Clin North Am.* 2010;24:1–5.

   The history of primary atypical pneumonia, a sporadic pneumonia occurring predominantly in younger individuals associated with cold agglutinins and an elusive organism called the Eaton agent which was subsequently classified as Mycoplasma pneumoniae.

4. Cunha BA, Pherez FM. *Mycoplasma pneumoniae* community-acquired pneumonia (CAP) in the elderly: diagnostic significance of acute thrombocytosis. *Heart Lung.* 2009;38:444–449.

   Review of Mycoplasma pneumoniae *and some distinguishing features between other atypical pathogens. Use these characteristics to evaluate an elderly patient with CAP and thrombocytosis.*

5. Stewardson AJ, Grayson ML. Psittacosis. *Infect Dis Clin North Am.* 2010;24:7–25.

   Review of microbiology, epidemiology and spectrum of disease of Chlamydophila psittacosis.

6. Monno R, De Vito D, Losito G, et al. *Chlamydia pneumoniae* in community-acquired pneumonia: seven years of experience. *J Infect.* 2002;45:135.

   Of 311 patients with CAP, 39 (12.5%) met diagnostic criteria of acute Chlamydia pneumoniae *infection. Four had coinfection with other organisms. Incidence was greater in the winter and early spring. Macrolides and levofloxacin were effective for treatment. Of 250 patients hospitalized for acute exacerbations of chronic obstructive pulmonary disease, 73 (33%) met serologic criteria for the diagnosis of* C. pneumoniae *infection.*

7. File TM Jr, Plouffe JF Jr, Breiman RF, et al. Clinical characteristics of *Chlamydia pneumoniae* infection as the sole cause of community-acquired pneumonia. *Clin Infect Dis.* 1999;29: 426–428.

   Description of clinical characteristics of C. pneumoniae *based on 26 patients diagnosed with community-acquired pneumonia caused by the organism.*

8. Kumar S, Hammerschlag MR. Acute respiratory infection due to *Chlamydia pneumoniae*: current status of diagnostic methods. *Clin Infect Dis.* 2007;44:568–576.

   Review of diagnostic methods for diagnosing pneumoniae and the ongoing challenges in adopting standardized diagnostic methods to obtain valid and reliable results.

9. Miyashita N, Fukano H, Yoshida K, et al. Is it possible to distinguish between atypical pneumonia and bacterial pneumonia?: evaluation of the guideline for community-acquired pneumonia in Japan. *Respir Med.* 2004;98:952–960.

   Evaluates the utility of the 9 point Japanese Respiratory Society (JRS) scoring system to differentiate typical (S. pneumoniae *and* H. influenzae) *from atypical pneumonias* (M. pneumoniae *and* C. pneumoniae), *noting that it is better for single etiologic agent* M. pneumoniae *than for* C. pneumoniae.

10. Thurman KA, Warner AK, Coawrt KC, et al. Detection of *Mycoplasma pneumoniae, Chlamydia pneumoniae,* and *Legionella* spp. in clinical specimens using a single-tube multiplex real-time PCR assay. *Diagn Microbiol Infect Dis.* 2011;70:1–9.

    Development of a multiplex real-time PCR assay that can detect three leading causes of CAP (M. pneumoniae, C. pneumoniae, L. pneumophila) *with high sensitivity.*

11. Cillóniz C, Ewig S, Polverino E, et al. Microbial aetiology of community-acquired pneumonia and its relation to severity. *Thorax*. 2011;66:340–346.

Etiology and severity of CAP in 3,523 patients (85% inpatient, 15% outpatient). Forty-two percent had etiology established with 36% outpatients and 16% of inpatients having atypical pathogens (L. pneumophila, M. pneumoniae, C. pneumoniae, C. burnetii). The frequency of atypical pathogens decreased as the severity scores (CURB-65 and PSI) of the patients increased. All of these pathogens were low risk and/or treated as outpatients with the exception of Legionella that was equally distributed across all settings and severity scores.

12. Lui G, Ip M, Lee N, et al. Role of "atypical pathogens" among adult hospitalized patients with community-acquired pneumonia. *Respirology*. 2009;14:1098–1105.

Assessed clinical significance and outcome of atypical pathogens (M. pneumoniae and C. pneumoniae) infection in adults hospitalized with CAP. A constructed clinical prediction rule was unable to distinguish between CAP due to these atypical pathogens from other organisms.

13. Smith LG. *Mycoplasma* pneumonia and its complications. *Infect Dis Clin North Am*. 2010;24:57–60.

Review of Mycoplasma *pneumonia history, clinical features, diagnostic strategies and management.*

14. Te Witt R, van Leeuwen WB, van Belkum A. Specific diagnostic tests for atypical respiratory tract pathogens. *Infect Dis Clin North Am*. 2010;24:229–248.

Diagnostic improvement in laboratory techniques used in establishing the diagnosis of Mycoplasma, Legionella, Chlamydia *pneumonia.*

15. Marrie TJ. Q fever pneumonia. *Infect Dis Clin North Am*. 2010;24:27–41.

Concise review of Q fever microbiology, epidemiology, presentation and treatment.

16. Okimotoe N, Asaoka N, Osaki K, et al. Clinical features of Q fever pneumonia. *Respirology*. 2004;9:278–282.

Review of clinical features of Q fever in Japan and four case reports, suggesting that two types of pneumonia occur; one with the usual features of atypical pneumonia and the other presenting with features of typical bacterial pneumonia in the elderly due to mixed bacterial infection.

17. Marrie TJ, Peeling RW, Fine MJ, et al. Ambulatory patients with community-acquired pneumonia: the frequency of atypical agents and clinical course. *Am J Med*. 1996;101(5):508–515.

Prospective cohort of 149 patients with CAP presenting to ED in Nova Scotia evaluated for etiology and prospectively followed and evaluated at 30 days for outcome. 49.7% of patients had identifiable etiologic agent (M. pneumoniae 22.8%, C. pneumoniae 10.7%, C. burnetii 2.7%, H. influenza A 2.7%, dual infection 3.4%, conventional bacteria 2%, other 7.4%). 48.3% had no identified etiology. Outcomes were similar in atypical and undetermined etiology patients.

18. Sampere M, Font B, Font J, et al. Q fever in adults: review of 66 clinical cases. *Eur J Clin Microbiol Infect Dis*. 2003;22:108.

The most common clinical presentation was pneumonia (56%); eight patients had hypoxia and five developed respiratory failure. Over 70% of patients received empiric macrolides as opposed to tetracyclines to cover for the organisms that most frequently cause atypical pneumonia in the region. Outcomes were favorable, although the use of macrolides in Q fever was noted to be controversial

19. Fraser DW, Tsai TR, Orenstein W, et al. Legionnaires' disease: description of an epidemic pneumonia. *N Engl J Med*. 1977;297(22):1189–1197.

Description and epidemiologic analysis of the Philadelphia American Legion convention outbreak of a previously unrecognized bacterium in 182 people including 29 fatalities.

20. Cunha BA. Legionnaires' disease: clinical differentiation from typical and other atypical pneumonias. *Infect Dis Clin North Am*. 2010;24:73–105.

Excellent review of history and characteristic features of Legionnaires' disease as compared to other typical and atypical etiologies of community-acquired pneumonia.

21. Gacouin A, Le Tulzo Y, Lavoue S, et al. Severe pneumonia due to *Legionella pneumophila*: prognostic factors, impact of delayed appropriate antimicrobial therapy. *Intensive Care Med*. 2002;28:686.

This study examined patients with severe Legionella *pneumonia admitted to an ICU. Delays in admission to the ICU and the need for intubation were associated with increased mortality. Starting a fluoroquinolone within 8 hours of ICU admission significantly reduced mortality*

22. Mykietiuk A, Carratali J, Fernandez-Sabi N, et al. Clinical outcomes for hospitalized patients with *Legionella* pneumonia in the antigenuria era: the influence of levofloxacin therapy. *Clin Infect Dis.* 2005;40(6):794–799.

    Prospective observational review of 1,934 cases of Legionella pneumophila *pneumonia analyzed for outcome with respect to antibiotic treatment. The early and overall case fatality rates were 2.9% and 5%. 86.3% received appropriate initial antimicrobial therapy with levofloxacin gradually replacing macrolides. Patients receiving levofloxacin had faster defervescence and shorter length of stay but no difference in complications or mortality.*

23. Dominguez J, Gali N, Matas L, et al. Evaluation of a rapid immunochromatographic assay for the detection of *Legionella* antigen in urine samples. *Eur J Clin Microbiol Infect Dis.* 1999;18(12):896.

    Evaluation of a new urinary antigen test was compared to Binax EIA antigen test with 98.1% agreement. Sensitivity for L. pneumophila *serogroup 1 was 97.2% in concentrated urine.*

24. Lindsay DSJ, Abraham WH, Findlay W, et al. Laboratory diagnosis of Legionnaires' disease due to *Legionella pneumophila* serogroup 1: comparison of phenotypic and genotypic methods. *J Med Microbiol.* 2004;53:183.

    Both the urine antigen test and PCR were found to be sensitive and specific for the diagnosis of Legionnaires' disease.

25. Bruin JP, Peeters MF, Ijzerman EP, et al. Evaluation of *Legionella* V-Test for the detection of *Legionella pneumophila* antigen in urine samples. *Eur J Clin Microbiol Infect Dis.* 2010;29(7):899–900.

    Evaluated sensitivity and specificity of new urinary antigen tests for Legionella pneumophila *serogroup 1.*

26. Zarogoulidis P, Alexandropoulou I, Romanidou G, et al. Community-acquired pneumonia due to *Legionella pneumophila*, the utility of PCR, and a review of the antibiotics used. *Int J Gen Med.* 2010;4:15–19.

    Case of Legionnaires' disease and discussion of how newer diagnostic and therapeutic strategies have improved outcomes.

27. Mandell LA, Wunderink RG, Anzueto A, et al. Infectious Diseases Society of America/American Thoracic Society consensus guidelines on the management of community-acquired pneumonia in adults. *Clin Infect Dis.* 2007;44(suppl 2):S27.

    Background and discussion of community-acquired pneumonia in adults with expert guidelines for empiric therapy.

Viral Pneumonia

Bao Q. Luu

Viruses are recognized increasingly as a primary cause of pneumonia and also as coinfection with bacterial pneumonia. Interest in viral pneumonia has increased in recent years because of several factors: (a) the increasing number of immunosuppressed patients resulting from hematologic stem cell and solid organ transplants; (b) the availability of new molecular diagnostic techniques such as nucleic acid amplification (i.e., polymerase chain reaction [PCR]); and (c) the development of new, effective antiviral therapies as well as preventive measures (i.e., immunization as well as chemoprophylaxis). In addition, interest has been heightened by recent epidemics of respiratory illness caused by novel strains of viruses such as severe acute respiratory syndrome (SARS) in 2003, avian flu (H5N1) from 2006 to 2008, swine flu (H1N1) in 2009, and, most recently, the H7N9 reassortment of influenza A causing severe flu with high mortality rate among rural Chinese exposed to infected poultry.

This chapter reviews several of the most common viral pneumonias in *immune-competent* hosts. In such individuals, most viral respiratory infections have similar clinical presentations. Diagnosis, therefore, depends heavily on a high index of suspicion based on the epidemiologic context and confirmation by diagnostic tools such as serologic and immunohistochemical data as well as molecular diagnostic techniques such as PCR.

Influenza viruses remain the most common cause of pulmonary viral infections. These are RNA-containing viruses in the myxovirus family. They are divided into three groups (A, B, and C) on the basis of internal membrane (M) and nucleoprotein (NP) antigens. Group A is further divided into a variety of antigenic subtypes based on two distinct surface glycoproteins: hemagglutinin (H) and neuraminidase (N). Hemagglutinin is necessary for binding and penetrating the host cell membrane. Neuraminidase aids in the release and spread of replicated viral particles. Influenza A viruses can mutate spontaneously, producing new strains with changes in the H and N glycoproteins. The complete nomenclature of a strain of influenza virus includes the viral type (A, B, or C), geographic location of discovery, strain number, year, and H and N numbers (e.g., A/California/7/2009[H1N1]). All three types (A, B, and C) can undergo minor structural changes; however, only type A produces serologically distinct strains designated by numerical subscripts in the H and N loci. Immunity to influenza infection depends on the host's production of antibodies to these glycoproteins. When a small antigenic change (*antigenic drift*) occurs, the effect on immunity is relatively minor. However, with a major antigenic change (*antigenic shift*) most people are not immune to the new (e.g., novel) virus resulting in a pandemic. The swine flu (H1N1) virus responsible for the 2009 pandemic is an example of such an antigenic shift. The WHO estimated that 16,226 deaths were attributed to H1N1 from April 2009 to January 2010. A growing body of literature supports the theory that aquatic birds and other animals (e.g., pigs) serve as important reservoirs of influenza virus, allowing genetic recombination leading to new, antigenically distinct, and, thus, more virulent strains of virus.

Influenza A is the most virulent subtype and the cause of the annual epidemics. Influenza B usually causes disease in populations confined to closed spaces such as daycare centers and boarding schools. Influenza C is the least virulent and found in sporadic cases. Typically, patients present with fever, cough, myalgia, headache, conjunctivitis, and prostration. Significant gastrointestinal symptoms, rhinorrhea, and pharyngitis are uncommon. Infections often exacerbate chronic illnesses such as chronic obstructive pulmonary disease (COPD), asthma, cystic fibrosis, and congestive heart failure. Chest radiographs are often negative. However, in cases of pneumonia, infiltrates are usually patchy and bilateral. Infiltrates are generally self-limited and resolve within 3 weeks. Occasionally, influenza pneumonia evolves into diffuse pneumonia with bilateral infiltrates, severe hypoxemia, and acute respiratory distress syndrome (ARDS).

Coinfection with bacteria such as *Staphylococcus aureus, Streptococcus pneumoniae,* and *Haemophilus influenza* can occur within days and up to 2 weeks of influenza infection. Bacterial coinfection is a significant factor in the high mortality rate seen during epidemics and pandemics. The clinical course is determined in part by the specific bacterial pneumonia. However, complications such as abscess formation (especially with *S. aureus*), septic shock, empyema, and Reye syndrome are common.

Neurological sequelae of influenza, including Guillan-Barre syndrome, seizures, and transverse myelitis, have been reported. Severe myositis with elevated serum creatinine and phosphokinase levels also have been reported. Other rare complications include myoglobinuria, thrombocytopenia, renal failure, myocarditis, and disseminated intravascular coagulation.

Vaccination remains the most important preventive measure against the epidemic of influenza A. The Centers for Disease Control and Prevention (CDC) recommends that vaccination efforts be directed toward at-risk populations including children aged 6 months to 4 years; adults aged 50 and older; persons with chronic pulmonary, cardiovascular (except hypertension alone), renal, hepatic, neurologic, hematologic, or metabolic disorders (including diabetes mellitus); and immunosuppressed patients, and women who are pregnant or will be pregnant during the influenza season. Vaccination is also recommended for residents of nursing homes and chronic care facilities, healthcare workers, household contacts, caregivers of children younger than 5 years and adults 50 years and older, and household contacts and caregivers of persons with medical conditions that put them at higher risk for severe complications from influenza.

Amantadine and rimantadine have been approved for prevention and treatment of influenza A but are not effective against influenza B. However, many influenza A strains are now resistant to these drugs; thus, they are no longer recommended for empiric single-drug therapy.

Oseltamivir and zanamivir are drugs that block the surface protein neuraminidase and trap the virus within the infected respiratory epithelium preventing its dissemination. They should be administered, preferably within 48 hours of the onset of symptoms. They are active against both influenza A and B. In cases of severe pneumonia, medication should be provided even after 48 hours of symptom onset.

In cases of severe hypoxemic respiratory failure with ARDS as seen in the H1N1 pandemic, rescue maneuvers such as prone ventilation and extracorporeal membrane oxygenation (ECMO) may be instituted in addition to antiviral therapy.

Respiratory syncytial virus (RSV) is part of the *Paramyviridae* family and is an important cause of croup, bronchiolitis, and pneumonia in infants and young children. It has also now been recognized as an important cause of pneumonia in adults, especially the elderly. It is highly contagious, spreading through droplets and fomites, leading to a few outbreaks in nursing homes. Treatment is mainly supportive. However, ribavirin is currently available as antiviral therapy effective against RSV and is recommended for severe cases and those at high risk of complications from RSV. Intravenous immunoglobulin specific for RSV (palivizumab) can also be used in combination with ribavirin in critically ill patients and those at high risk for complications, especially bone marrow transplant recipients.

Parainfluenza, a paramyxovirus classified into four subtypes (1, 2, 3, and 4), is a common cause of viral respiratory infections in children and a recognized cause of pneumonia in adults. However, severe cases of pneumonia are usually seen only in immunocompromised adults. In immunocompetent hosts, it commonly leads to exacerbation of chronic diseases and rarely causes severe pneumonia.

Adenovirus causes a particularly aggressive form of pneumonia in neonates, triggering necrotizing bronchiolitis and alveolitis. In large closed quartered populations, such as military recruits, it can cause viral pneumonia similar to other atypical pneumonias. In the general population, however, adenovirus pneumonia is seen rarely, but is a common cause of pharyngitis, tracheobronchitis, and conjunctivitis. Treatment is supportive, although in severe cases and in immunocompromised hosts antiviral therapy with cidofovir and ribavirin has been used.

During 2002 and 2003, a coronavirus (SARS-coV) caused SARS, a severe respiratory infection in more than 8,000 people, leading to 774 deaths. Up to a third of those infected became critically ill. Pneumonia with lung injury was noted in 16% of all infected individuals and 80% of critically ill patients. In contrast to other viral infections, adults were affected more than children.

More recently, in September 2012, a novel coronavirus (initially termed HCoV-EMC, now designated as Middle East respiratory syndrome coronavirus, MERS-CoV) was discovered to have caused severe pneumonia and renal failure in a healthy 60-year-old man with a fatal outcome. According to the WHO, up to February of 2013, there have been 13 laboratory-confirmed cases, 6 of which were fatal. It was hypothesized that these cases were secondary to zoonotic events, possibly contact with bats as the reservoir host.

Rhinovirus is most commonly recognized as the cause of the common cold. Although controversial, some studies have found this virus in up to 30% of cases of severe pneumonia requiring hospitalization with ICU admission.

Varicella-zoster virus (VZV) causes varicella, a highly contagious childhood exanthema with variable systemic syndrome. In adults, some form of pulmonary involvement complicates about 5% to 15% of instances of adult chickenpox. Risk factors for progression to pneumonia include pregnancy, smoking, older age, chronic pulmonary disease, and immunosuppression. In addition to the typical polymorphic rash with vesciles, pustules, and crusty lesions, patients with VZV pneumonia have chest X-rays with diffuse nodules which may resolve into miliary calcified densities. High resolution CT scan of the thorax often shows numerous ill-defined centrilobular nodules, randomly distributed in both lungs with surrounding ground-glass opacities. Treatment is with acyclovir and supportive care. Most healthy adults have a favorable outcome with complete recovery. However, in immunocompromised patients, mortality can reach 50% despite aggressive treatment.

Measles (rubeola) is another highly contagious systemic viral illness of childhood that can cause serious pneumonia in susceptible adults. With effective vaccination using the inactivated virus, measles pneumonia is now seen rarely.

Cytomegalovirus (CMV) is highly prevalent in the general population. In immunocompromised hosts such as bone marrow and organ transplant recipients, it can cause severe, life-threatening pneumonia leading to respiratory failure. In immunocompetent hosts, CMV can cause community-acquired viral pneumonia; however, the incidence is quite low. Patients present with typical viral syndrome with symptoms of fever, chills, cough, and malaise. Chest X-rays may show patchy infiltrates or a reticular pattern. Thoracic CT scan typically demonstrates ground-glass infiltrates, but a reticular pattern and consolidation have also been described. The diagnosis can be made by viral culture of respiratory secretions or bronchoalveolar lavage fluid or cytology showing typical viral inclusions. Serologic diagnosis is based on elevated CMV IgM or on increasing titer of IgG over time. More recently, CMV PCR has allowed for both more rapid diagnosis and close follow-up by quantitative PCR. Of note, blood CMV PCR can be negative in immunocompetent hosts with primary CMV pneumonia. Treatment is with ganciclovir or valganciclovir. In immunocompetent hosts, prognosis is usually favorable.

Herpes simplex virus (HSV) type I is transmitted via close contacts through saliva or vesicular fluid and is typically associated with gingivostomatitis. It can also cause vesicular-ulcerative lesions on the mucosa of the lower respiratory tract. Commonly, HSV-I causes tracheobronchitis in predisposed patients such as those with severe burns, malignancies, AIDS, and bone marrow and organ transplants. Occasionally, HSV-I can be found in immunocompetent patients with a recent myocardial infarction or COPD exacerbation, and also in elderly patients. Pneumonia is uncommon, except for predisposed patients in whom the spectrum ranges from an innocent bystander to fulminant disease leading to ARDS. HSV-II rarely causes pulmonary disease except in cases of hematogenous dissemination. Definitive diagnosis of HSV pneumonia is often difficult and requires lung biopsy. Treatment is with acyclovir with foscarnet as an alternative for acyclovir-resistant HSV.

The *hantavirus pulmonary syndrome* (HPS) is caused by the *Sin Nombre virus* (SNV). *Sin Nombre* means "no name" in Spanish. Humans become infected through contact with hantavirus-infected rodents or their urine and droppings. Infection can lead to severe illness with fever, severe myalgia, cough, headache, and malaise. Rhinorrhea and sore throat are seen rarely. Disease can progress to hemorrhagic fever and renal failure. Patients with HPS can develop rapid respiratory failure from noncardiogenic pulmonary edema cause by massive pulmonary capillary leak. Routine laboratory findings are nonspecific, but frequently leukocytosis with bandemia and metamyelocytes are found in the peripheral blood. Thrombocytopenia and erythrocytosis are common. Chemistry panels show low albumin, elevated lactate dehydrogenase (LDH), and elevated aspartate aminotransferase (AST) and alanine aminotransferase (ALT). As critical illness progresses, respiratory failure and cardiac failure develop. In contrast to septic shock, shock seen in HPS is characterized by low cardiac output.

HPS was first recognized in 1993, when a cluster of deaths occurred in residents of the Four Corners area of the southwestern United States. It is now known that SNV infects the common deer mouse, *Peromyscus maniculatus*. Zoonotic transmission occurs when humans come in contact with urine or droppings of infected mice. More recently, in the summer of 2012, another outbreak occurred at Curry Village in Yosemite National Park where 10 people were infected, supposedly when campers came in contact with infected mice droppings or urine in their tents. Two of these cases were fatal. Diagnosis should be suspected in the appropriate context. Acute infection can be confirmed by enzyme-linked immunosorbent assay (ELISA) to detect IgM antibodies to SNV. Four-fold rise in IgG between acute and convalescent titer or the presence of IgM in the acute phase is diagnostic. Reverse-transcriptase PCR is also available as a diagnostic tool. Immunohistochemistry is usually used in postmortem or retrospective analyses.

Treatment entails aggressive early ICU support with inotropic agents, mechanical ventilation, and renal replacement therapy. No specific antiviral agent is effective, although ribavirin has been tried. Mortality in HPS remains quite high, up to 76%. Rodent control is the most effective preventive measure.

FURTHER READING

1. Ruuskanen O, Lahti E, Jennings L, et al. Viral pneumonia. *Lancet.* 2011;377:1264–1275.

   An excellent seminar on viral pneumonia including review of recent SARS, Avian flu and Swine flu pandemic of 2009.

2. Neto OG, Leite RF, Baldi BG. Update on viral community-acquired pneumonia. *Rev Assoc Med Bras.* 2013;59(1):78–84.

   A brief review of the most common viruses causing respiratory illnesses including community-acquired pneumonia.

3. Marcos MA, Esperatti M, Torres A. Viral pneumonia. *Curr Opin Infect Dis.* 2009;22:143–147.

   Another review raising the question of viral-bacterial co-infection.

4. Falsey AR, Wash E. Viral pneumonia in older adults. *Clin Infect Dis.* 2006;42:518–524.

   A review with special attention to viral pneumonia in geriatric population.

5. Huijskens EGW, van Erkel AJM, Palmen FMH, et al. Viral and bacterial aetiology of community-acquired pneumonia in adults. *Influenza Other Respir Viruses.* 2013;7(4):567–573.

   A comprehensive study of the etiologies of community-acquired pneumonia from the Netherlands from April 2008 to April 2009. Interestingly, during this period there was an outbreak of Coxiella burnetti.

6. Johnstone J, Majumdar SR, Fox J, et al. Viral infection in adults hospitalized with community acquired pneumonia. *Chest.* 2008;134(6):1141–1148.

   This studies include patients admitted to five Canadian hospitals with community-acquired pneumonia from 2004 to 2006. Etiologic pathogen was found in 39% of patients, 15% was viral, 30% was bacterial, and 4% was mixed.

7. Wiemken T, Peyrani P, Bryant K, et al. Incidence of respiratory viruses in patients with community-acquired pneumonia admitted to the intensive care unit: results from the Severe Influenza Pneumonia Surveillance (SIPS) project. *Eur J Clin Microbiol Infect Dis.* 2013;32:705–710.

   In this population 23% of adults and 19% of pediatric patients admitted to ICU with CAP were found to have viral etiologies. Influenza remains the most common virus found.

8. Choi SH, Hong SB, Ko GB, et al. Viral infection in patients with severe pneumonia requiring intensive care unit admission. *Am J Respir Crit Care Med.* 2012;186(4):325–332.

   Korean studies included CAP as well as HCAP using BAL as well as nasopharyngeal swabs and RT-PCR to look for viral pathogen contributing to pneumonia.

9. Rello J, Chastre J. Update in pulmonary infections 2012. *Am J Respir Crit Care Med.* 2013; 187(10):1061–1066.

   Concise update on old and emergent causes of pulmonary infection, viral respiratory infection included.

10. Ananthanarayanan V, Mueller J, Taxy J, et al. Unexpected fatal pneumonia in an immunocompetent adult: a tale of a father and a son. *J Clin Microbiol.* 2012;50(10):3151, 3414.

    A case of fatal adenovirus causing pneumonia in an adult.

11. Zaki AM, van Boheemen S, Bestebroer T, et al. Isolation of a novel coronavirus from a man with pneumonia in Saudi Arabia. *N Engl J Med.* 2012;367:1814–1820.

    First description of HCoV-EMC, a novel coronavirus causing fatal pneumonia and renal failure. The author hypothesized that this was a zoonotic event with bats being the reservoir.

12. Grilli E, Galati V, Bordi L, et al. *Cytomegalovirus* pneumonia in immunocompetent host: case report and literature review. *J Clin Virol.* 2012;55(4):356–359.

    CMV pneumonitis in a healthy man treated with ganciclovir.

13. Voore N, Lai R. Varicella pneumonia in a immunocompetent adult. *CMAJ.* 2012;184(17):1924.

    A case of VZV pneumonia in a 30-year-old woman treated and recovered uneventfully with acyclovir.

14. Schomacker H, Schaap-Nutt A, Collins P, et al. Pathogenesis of acute respiratory illness cause by human parainfluenza viruses. *Curr Opin Virol.* 2012;2(3):294–299.

    A brief review of parainfluenza respiratory infections.

49 Tuberculosis: Epidemiology, Diagnosis, and Treatment of Latent Infection

Philip A. LoBue

Tuberculosis is a pulmonary and systemic infectious disease caused by *Mycobacterium tuberculosis*. It is spread from person to person by airborne transmission of droplet nuclei 1 to 5 μm in diameter. Several factors determine the probability of transmission: (1) infectiousness of the source patient—a positive sputum smear for acid-fast bacilli or a cavity on chest radiograph being strongly associated with infectiousness; (2) host susceptibility of the contact; (3) duration of exposure of the contact to the source patient; and (4) the environment in which the exposure takes place: a small, poorly ventilated space providing the highest risk. Even among household contacts of active tuberculosis patients, the risk of infection is surprisingly low; the United States Public Health Service (USPHS) reported an approximate 28% incidence of infection in household contacts. In addition, animal and human studies have demonstrated that tuberculosis transmission may dramatically decrease within days to weeks of instituting effective treatment.

Despite this relatively low transmission rate, tuberculosis remains a major global public health problem. There are almost 9 million new tuberculosis cases per year throughout the world and about 1.4 million people die of the disease annually. The human immunodeficiency virus (HIV) epidemic has dramatically altered tuberculosis epidemiology and is driving much of the global epidemic, especially in Africa. Nearly one quarter of worldwide HIV deaths are tuberculosis-related. The current epidemic has been accompanied by a rise in drug-resistant tuberculosis. Currently, it is estimated that each year there are almost 500,000 new cases of multidrug-resistant (MDR) tuberculosis (resistant to isoniazid and rifampin) globally, of which approximately 10% are extensively drug-resistant (MDR plus resistance to a fluorquinolone and any second-line injectable drug [amikacin, kanamycin, and capreomycin]).

In the United States, there had been a steady 4% to 7% annual decline in the case rate until 1984. Between 1985 and 1992, however, the annual incidence of tuberculosis increased by 20%. This increase was concentrated in young (predominantly aged 25–44), urban (especially New York, New Jersey, and California), racial, and ethnic minority populations. Tuberculosis also was found to be prevalent among the homeless, injection and noninjection drug users, and inmates of correctional facilities. In many of these groups, the rise in tuberculosis was linked to high rates of HIV infection. A second epidemiologic trend emerged with increased immigration to the United States of persons from countries where tuberculosis is prevalent (especially Latin America, South and Southeast Asia, Africa, and Eastern Europe). Before 1986, foreign-born persons accounted for 22% of tuberculosis cases. By 1997, this number had increased to 39% and in 2009 it reached 59%. In some locations, this phenomenon is even more pronounced. In California, for example, more than 75% of tuberculosis cases occur in persons born outside the United States. Because of extensive national, state, and local control efforts, the annual incidence of tuberculosis has been on the decline again since 1992, falling 57% between 1992 and 2011 (from 26,673 cases to 10,528 cases). Despite this welcome decline, the associations of tuberculosis with conditions such as HIV infection, homelessness, injection drug use, and foreign birth remain. Approximately 1% of US tuberculosis cases are MDR.

The tuberculin skin test (TST) is a major tool for investigating tuberculosis infection. It can be used diagnostically in the individual patient and epidemiologically in the general population. The TST (Mantoux method) is performed by the intracutaneous injection of a standardized, stabilized dose of 5 TU of purified protein derivative (PPD). The extent of induration is measured 48 to 72 hours later. Multiple puncture techniques (e.g., tine test) are not recommended. The interpretation of the TST is based on an individual's epidemiologic risk factors for tuberculosis infection. The 2000 American Thoracic Society (ATS) guidelines for interpretation of TST results are as follows: (a) 5-mm induration is considered positive for (i) individuals with HIV infection or other comparable immunosuppression (equivalent to receiving 15 mg or greater of prednisone for 1 month or more), (ii) close contacts to an active tuberculosis case, or (iii) patients with a chest radiograph suggestive of prior tuberculosis (e.g., fibronodular) disease (also termed inactive disease); (b) 10-mm induration is considered positive for (i) recent immigrants (within the last 5 years) from high-incidence countries; (ii) injection drug users; (iii) residents and employees of high-risk congregate facilities, such as nursing homes, homeless shelters, or prisons; (iv) mycobacterial laboratory personnel; (v) persons with underlying medical conditions, such as diabetes, silicosis, end-stage renal disease, certain malignancies, and low body weight (loss of at least 10% of ideal body weight); or (vi) children younger than age 4 and infants, children, or adolescents exposed to adults at high risk; and (c) 15-mm induration is considered positive for all others.

A positive TST result is considered to indicate the presence of infection with *M. tuberculosis*. In the United States, it is recommended that persons who test positive receive treatment for latent tuberculosis to prevent progression to disease. Thus, an intent to test for latent tuberculosis should indicate an intent to treat for latent tuberculosis if it is found. Consequently, testing should be reserved for persons at high risk for latent infection or at high risk to progress to disease based on their epidemiologic profile.

In a number of situations, the TST is neither sensitive nor specific for tuberculosis infection. A positive TST result is a manifestation of type IV delayed hypersensitivity. Certain biologic conditions, such as viral illnesses (including HIV infection), malignancies, other debilitating illness (including advanced active tuberculosis) and certain medications will suppress the type IV response and T-lymphocyte function. In addition, proper application of the TST requires careful attention to technique and interpretation. TST should be performed by well-trained, experienced operators. False-positive test findings can occur for a number of reasons, including cross-reactions caused by nontuberculous (atypical) mycobacterial infection bacillus Calmette-Guérin (BCG) vaccination.

In 2001, a new test, the QuantiFERON-TB test (QFT), was approved by the FDA for the diagnosis of latent tuberculosis infection. This test, which measures interferon-γ response to PPD in whole blood, was found to have good agreement with the TST in a number of populations. Subsequently, newer versions of interferon-gamma release assays (IGRAs) were developed that substituted synthetic peptides mimicking *M. tuberculosis* antigens, such as ESAT-6 and CFP-10, for PPD. Because these antigens are not found in BCG or most nontuberculosis mycobacteria, IGRAs are much less subject to false-positive reactions due to cross-reactivity. Per current CDC guidelines, IGRAs are recommended to be used in any situation in which the TST is used. Furthermore, IGRAs are preferred in persons who have received BCG vaccination or for groups that historically have had low rates of return for TST reading (e.g., homeless persons). Because of limited data about the performance of IGRAs in young children at present, the TST is preferred in children less than 5 years of age.

Two methods have been used for tuberculosis prevention: BCG vaccination and isoniazid therapy for latent infection. BCG is a live, attenuated bacterial vaccine that has been evaluated extensively. The World Health Organization recommends administering BCG once at birth in endemic countries. Except for occasional local reactions, its toxicity is minimal. In controlled trials, the efficacy of case reduction has varied from 0% to 80%. In most trials, the incidence of miliary and meningeal tuberculosis in children has been greatly reduced. Variations in the efficacy of case reduction have been explained by differences in vaccine potency. A large trial conducted in India using a very potent BCG vaccine failed to show a protective effect against tuberculosis in adults, however, suggesting that vaccine potency is not the only factor determining efficacy. BCG is best used in the noninfected (TST-negative) population. The vaccine generally converts an individual's TST to positive, at least in the short term. However, the TST response has been somewhat variable with different vaccines and in different individuals, and it correlates poorly with vaccine effectiveness. BCG may, therefore, limit the diagnostic value of the TST in certain circumstances. BCG has not been used in the United States because of the low incidence of tuberculosis. It has been most useful in areas of the world where the case rate and new infection rate remain high.

The principal preventive tool in the United States has been treatment of latent infection with isoniazid. In the 1950s, when isoniazid became available as an inexpensive, bactericidal, and relatively nontoxic drug for the treatment of active tuberculosis disease, controlled trials were instituted to determine its efficacy for the treatment of latent infection. In more than 70,000 patients, the USPHS and others consistently demonstrated a 60% to 70% case reduction rate attributable to isoniazid therapy. Follow-up for as long as 15 years confirmed the long-term protection isoniazid provides against progression to disease.

Concern regarding toxicity, especially hepatotoxicity, and the need for adherence to a prolonged course of therapy have limited isoniazid therapy's effectiveness as a public health intervention. Older studies revealed that isoniazid-associated liver injury occurred in about 1% of patients, and deaths secondary to isoniazid-induced liver injury were reported. More recently, however, public health clinics in Seattle and San Diego reported incidences of hepatotoxicity of 0.1 and 0.3%, respectively, among more than 14,000 patients treated. There were no deaths reported and only one hospitalization. Despite the low incidence of liver injury, completion rates for 6 months of therapy were below 65% in both reports.

ATS and CDC recommend that all persons with latent tuberculosis infection receive treatment. Clinical monitoring, on a monthly basis at minimum, is recommended for all patients receiving isoniazid. Routine transaminase monitoring should be reserved for individuals at particular risk for hepatotoxicity, including those who are pregnant or in the immediate postpartum period (first 3 months) or those with HIV infection, a history of liver disease, a history of excess alcohol use, or other risks for liver disease. The preferred duration of isoniazid therapy is 9 months for all groups of patients, including those with HIV infection, those with a chest radiograph suggestive of prior tuberculosis disease (inactive tuberculosis), and children. Six months of treatment is considered an acceptable alternative for immunocompetent adults without evidence of prior tuberculosis on chest radiograph, but this shorter duration is felt to be less effective based on existing data.

Initial studies done in HIV-infected patients suggested that the combination of daily rifampin and pyrazinamide for 2 months was equally efficacious and safe for the treatment of latent tuberculosis when compared with 6 or 12 months of isoniazid. Subsequently, as this regimen came in to general use, multiple hospitalizations and deaths resulting from hepatotoxicity associated with this regimen were reported. ATS and CDC now recommend that the combination of rifampin and pyrazinamide should generally not be offered to persons with latent tuberculosis infection for either HIV-negative or HIV-infected persons.

A 12-dose regimen of isoniazid and rifapentine (once weekly for 12 weeks) has been evaluated as a possible short-course substitute for 9 months of isoniazid. An initial study from Brazil showed this regimen was well tolerated and appeared to be effective. A much larger clinical trial that randomized more than 8,000 patients, mainly in the United States, to either 9 months of isoniazid or 12 weekly doses of isoniazid and rifapentine found that 12 weekly doses of isoniazid and rifapentine was as good as 9 months of isoniazid. CDC subsequently recommended use of isoniazid and rifapentine-using directly observed therapy for otherwise healthy patients aged greater than or equal to 12 years who have latent tuberculosis infection and factors that are predictive of tuberculosis developing (e.g., recent exposure to contagious tuberculosis).

For contacts exposed to isoniazid-resistant, rifampin-susceptible tuberculosis patients, rifampin (4 months duration) can be used. It is important to note that rifampin and a closely related medication, rifabutin, interact with protease inhibitors and nonnucleoside reverse transcriptase inhibitors used to treat HIV. Consultation with an expert familiar with both HIV and tuberculosis treatment is recommended in this situation. For MDR tuberculosis exposures, some have suggested the use of a fluoroquinolone alone or in combination with either pyrazinamide or ethambutol if the source-case *M. tuberculosis* isolate is susceptible to these drugs. Two-drug combinations, especially those including pyrazinamide, tend not to be well tolerated, and completion rates are very low. Data on the efficacy of these regimens are not available.

FURTHER READING

1. World Health Organization. *Global Tuberculosis Control, 2012.* Geneva, Switzerland: World Health Organization; 2012.

   WHO annual report on global TB control. It includes data on case notifications and treatment outcomes from all national TB control programs that have reported to WHO.

2. World Health Organization. *Anti-tuberculosis Drug Resistance in the World: Fourth Report.* Geneva, Switzerland: World Health Organization; 2008.

   Fourth WHO anti-tuberculosis drug resistance survey estimated that greater than 489,000 MDR cases emerged in 2006, and that the global proportion of resistance among all cases was 4.8%.

3. Centers for Disease Control and Prevention. *Reported Tuberculosis in the United States, 2011.* Atlanta, GA: US Department of Health and Human Services, CDC; 2012.

   Report of tuberculosis morbidity and trends in the United States.

4. American Thoracic Society, Centers for Disease Control and Prevention. Targeted tuberculin testing and treatment of latent tuberculosis infection. *Am J Respir Crit Care Med.* 2000;161:S221–S247.

   Comprehensive guidelines for tuberculin skin testing and treatment of latent tuberculosis. These guidelines included the use of rifampin and pyrazinamide as a recommended treatment regimen. However, after multiple reports of severe liver injury associated with this combination, an amendment was published recommending that this regimen not be used for treatment of latent tuberculosis.

5. Pai M, Zwerling A, Menzies D. Systematic review: T-cell-based assays for the diagnosis of latent tuberculosis infection: an update. *Ann Intern Med.* 2008;149:177–184.

   Systematic review of performance of IGRAs for diagnosing latent tuberculosis infection.

6. Mazurek GH, Jereb J, Vernon A, et al. Updated guidelines for using Interferon Gamma Release Assays to detect *Mycobacterium tuberculosis* infection—United States, 2010. *MMWR Recomm Rep.* 2010;59(RR-5):1–25.

   Guidelines for use of IGRAs published by the CDC.

7. LoBue P, Menzies D. Treatment of latent tuberculosis infection: an update. *Respirology.* 2010;15:603–622.

   A comprehensive review of latent tuberculosis infection treatment.

8. Schechter M, Zajdenverg R, Falco G, et al. Weekly rifapentine/isoniazid or daily rifampin/pyrazinamide for latent tuberculosis in household contacts. *Am J Respir Crit Care Med.* 2006;173:922–926.

   A study of latent tuberculosis infection treatment among household contacts in Brazil using a 12-dose regimen of isoniazid and rifapentine.

9. Sterling TR, Villarino ME, Borisov AS, et al; TB Trials Consortium PREVENT TB Study Team. Three months of rifapentine and isoniazid for latent tuberculosis infection. *N Engl J Med.* 2011;365:2155–2166.

   Large, randomized clinical trial demonstrating 12 weekly doses of isoniazid and rifapentine is noninferior to 9 months of isoniazid.

10. Centers for Disease Control and Prevention (CDC). Recommendations for use of an isoniazid-rifapentine regimen with direct observation to treat latent *Mycobacterium tuberculosis* infection. *MMWR Morb Mortal Wkly Rep.* 2011;60:1650–1653.

    The combination regimen of isoniazid and rifapentine given as 12 weekly directly observed doses is recommended in otherwise healthy patients aged greater than or equal to 12 years who have a predictive factor for greater likelihood of tuberculosis developing, which includes recent exposure to contagious tuberculosis, conversion from negative to positive on an indirect test for infection, and radiographic findings of healed pulmonary tuberculosis.

11. Brewer TF. Preventing tuberculosis with bacillus Calmette-Guérin vaccine: a meta-analysis of the literature. *Clin Infect Dis.* 2000;31(suppl 3):S64–S67.

    Meta-analysis of effectiveness of BCG vaccination in prevention of tuberculosis.

50 Tuberculosis: Clinical Manifestations and Diagnosis of Disease

Philip A. LoBue

TB has a wide array of pulmonary and extrapulmonary clinical manifestations. Inhaled droplet nuclei of *Mycobacterium tuberculosis* initially lodge in the middle or lower lung zones where regional ventilation is greatest, resulting in a local inflammatory reaction with spread to regional lymph nodes and subsequent hematogenous dissemination. Distant organs, especially the kidneys, bone, CNS, as well as the lung apices, are seeded, but overt clinical disease of these areas does not usually ensue. A low-grade fever and symptoms of an upper respiratory illness also may be present. The chest radiograph may show a small area of pneumonitis and often hilar and paratracheal lymphadenopathy. Prominent hilar adenopathy is frequent in children; it is found less commonly in adults.

This initial infection, termed *primary TB*, resolves spontaneously in most individuals. Healed lesions appear on chest radiograph as calcified parenchymal nodules and are often associated with calcified hilar lymph nodes. In a small percentage of individuals, the initial infection progresses and can manifest as (1) rupture of subpleural infectious foci into the pleural space resulting in tuberculous pleuritis; (2) extensive caseous pneumonia; (3) enlargement of tuberculous lymph nodes causing bronchial obstruction (collapse–consolidation lesion); (4) rupture of a tuberculous focus into a bronchus leading to extensive endobronchial spread throughout one or both lungs; or (5) rupture of a tuberculous focus into a pulmonary blood vessel with hematogenous spread leading to acute disseminated disease.

TB can reactivate months to years after containment of the primary infection. The factors causing reactivation lesions are poorly understood. Certain conditions increase the likelihood of progression from latent TB infection to disease, including malnutrition, alcoholism, poorly controlled diabetes mellitus, silicosis, immunosuppression (by disease processes or drugs), gastrectomy, chronic hemodialysis, and jejunoileal bypass surgery. In most patients, however, no predisposing factor can be identified.

Radiographically, reactivation or postprimary pulmonary TB usually presents as an infiltrate in the apical and posterior segments of the upper lobes. The patient can be entirely asymptomatic or have nonspecific symptoms of chronic respiratory infection (e.g., fever, weight loss, productive cough, and hemoptysis). The chest radiograph may reveal a somewhat nondescript fibronodular or fluffy alveolar filling process in the upper lung fields but frequently shows cavity formation, fibrosis with volume loss, or both. The process occasionally heals spontaneously but more frequently progresses locally in the absence of drug therapy. Advanced disease can be associated with rupture of a hypertrophied pulmonary artery (Rasmussen aneurysm) into a cavity, resulting in massive hemoptysis, although this is exceedingly uncommon in the era of effective therapy. Rapid progression of pulmonary disease with severe ventilation–perfusion disturbances presenting as the adult respiratory distress syndrome is also seen in rare instances. New hematogenous dissemination and extrapulmonary disease may follow pulmonary reactivation.

Routine laboratory studies in pulmonary TB are nonspecific. Hematologic studies often reveal a mild anemia, leukopenia, or a monocytosis, but more profound pancytopenia or leukocytosis has been reported. Hyponatremia, usually attributable to the syndrome of inappropriate antidiuretic hormone production, occurs in more than 10% of patients with pulmonary TB. Addison disease is a very rare cause of hyponatremia in patients with TB.

The definitive diagnosis of pulmonary TB depends on obtaining a positive culture from infected secretions or tissue. If cultures are negative or obtaining a culture is not possible, a presumptive diagnosis can be made from clinical inference and therapeutic trial. The tuberculin skin test (TST) and interferon-gamma release assays (IGRAs) provide information as to whether a tuberculous infection is present, but do not distinguish between disease and latent infection. False-negative TST and IGRA results may occur in immunosuppressed patients (advanced TB, itself, being sufficiently immunosuppressive). A typical chest radiograph is helpful but non-specific: a variety of nontuberculous processes can have a similar appearance. Spontaneous or aerosol-induced sputum sampling (at least three specimens) is the initial method of choice for bacteriologic assessment. Initially, the specimens are stained by the Ziehl-Neelsen or fluorescent techniques for acid-fast bacilli (AFB). When sputum analyses are unrevealing, bronchoscopy with lavage, brushings, transbronchial biopsy, or needle aspiration may be considered. Broncho-scopic sampling can enhance both the speed and likelihood of making a diagnosis for an indi-vidual patient. Recent systematic studies have not found bronchoscopy to provide an aggregate diagnostic yield superior to aerosol-induced sputum sampling, however. All sputum, lavage, and tissue specimens should be cultured for mycobacteria. Cultures are essential, because (1) smears alone will miss up to 50% of active TB cases, (2) mycobacteria other than *Mycobacterium tuber-culosis* can produce positive smears, and (3) cultures are necessary for drug susceptibility testing. Special culture media are required, and the laboratory should have proficiency in mycobacterial techniques.

One of the major limitations of mycobacterial culture in the past was that 6 to 8 weeks were required to obtain results. Newer laboratory diagnostic techniques significantly reduced culture times. With broth-based culture methods, mycobacterial growth can be detected in as few as 5 to 8 days, although on average it takes 2 to 3 weeks. DNA probe technology can provide a very rapid (within hours) method of differentiating *Mycobacterium tuberculosis* complex from non-tuberculous mycobacteria in growing cultures. This technique has proved to be highly specific and sensitive.

Nucleic acid amplification (NAA) tests performed on direct specimens (i.e., without the need for a growing culture) for the diagnosis of TB have been available since the 1990s. Two commercially available NAA tests have been approved by the FDA for use on AFB smear-positive respiratory specimens: the polymerase chain reaction (PCR) and transcription-mediated amplification. Transcription-mediated amplification has also been FDA-approved for use on AFB smear-negative specimens. NAA tests can be performed in several hours. The combination of a positive AFB smear and positive NAA test is essentially diagnostic of active TB. A negative NAA test in the face of a positive AFB smear suggests that the patient has infection with non-tuberculous mycobacteria. NAA tests are also approximately 25% more sensitive than the AFB smear and can be of use when the smear is negative and the clinical suspicion for TB remains moderate or high. Based on these findings, current Centers for Disease Control and Prevention (CDC) guidelines recommend that NAA testing should be performed on at least one respiratory specimen from each patient with signs and symptoms of pulmonary TB for whom a diagnosis of TB is being considered but has not yet been established, and for whom the test result would alter case management or TB control activities. There is less experience with the use of NAA tests for nonrespiratory specimens. Several studies suggest they can be useful for the diagnosis of extrapul-monary TB, especially for meningitis. The finding of a positive NAA test does not obviate the need for cultures, as FDA-approved NAA tests do not give any information about drug suscep-tibilities. Rapid molecular assays that can detect both *Mycobacterium tuberculosis* and mutations associated with resistance to certain anti-TB drugs, such as rifampin, have been developed, and initial studies suggest they are highly accurate. However, commercial versions of these tests have not yet been approved by FDA and therefore are not currently available in the United States.

Extrapulmonary TB can occur with or without concurrent active pulmonary TB. Most fre-quently, the pathogenesis is that of recrudescence of a previously quiescent hematogenous lesion. However, upper airway and laryngeal disease, lymphatic TB, and pleural or pericardial TB com-monly arise by extension from contiguous structures. Gastrointestinal TB can follow ingestion of expectorated infectious sputum or of unpasteurized dairy products from cattle infected with *Mycobacterium bovis* (a rare cause of human TB).

Large airway (endobronchial) and laryngeal TB can be present with a normal chest radiograph but is usually associated with extensive cavitary pulmonary disease. Hoarseness is a common pre-senting symptom. Classically, laryngeal TB has been considered extremely infectious; however, it may be that the often-associated extensive pulmonary disease, rather than the laryngeal disease per se, is responsible for the increased contagiousness.

Pleural TB usually presents as a unilateral, exudative, predominantly lymphocytic, pleural effusion often associated with ipsilateral pulmonary TB. Symptomatic improvement frequently occurs spontaneously. With thoracentesis and pleural biopsy, the diagnosis can be made in 80% to 90% of cases. High levels of adenosine deaminase and interferon-γ in the pleural fluid have been associated with pleural TB in numerous studies, and these tests should be considered if available. Younger patients with an idiopathic pleural effusion and a positive TST reaction are often treated for pleural TB solely on clinical grounds. However, multiple closed pleural biopsies or thoracoscopic or surgical exploration should be strongly considered when resolution of the effusion is not prompt.

Pericardial TB can present with clinical features of tamponade or chronic constrictive pericarditis. Pericardial involvement should be considered in all TB patients with cardiomegaly, unexplained heart failure, or arrhythmias. A calcified pericardium on chest radiograph strongly suggests the diagnosis. Echocardiography may demonstrate the presence of pericardial fluid; however, pericardiocentesis and possibly pericardiectomy are necessary to confirm the diagnosis in the absence of confirmation of disease from another anatomic site. Cultures of pericardial fluid are positive in only 50% of cases.

Miliary TB refers to widespread dissemination of *Mycobacterium tuberculosis* from a previously established focus. It is seen more commonly in primary TB or in association with immunosuppression (HIV, organ transplantation, tumor necrosis factor α antagonists). Sputum AFB smears and cultures are positive in 30% to 60% of patients. Culture material should be obtained from a transbronchial biopsy or extrapulmonary sources (e.g., liver biopsy, bone marrow biopsy, and urine) if the diagnosis is being considered and sputum specimens are not diagnostic.

Tuberculous meningitis usually results from acute hematogenous spread and is present in up to 33% of cases of miliary disease. Rarely, it can result from breakdown in a silent granuloma or residua from remote hematogenous dissemination and, in children, by direct spread from a tuberculous otitis. Meningitis can present insidiously with lethargy, confusion, and headache. The cerebrospinal fluid (CSF) often shows a lymphocytic pleocytosis, a glucose level less than 20 mg/dL, and a significantly elevated protein level. The CSF smear is positive in only 10% to 20% of cases, whereas cultures are positive in 45% to 70%. Pathologically, an occlusive cranial arteritis can lead to infarction, cranial nerve palsies, and hydrocephalus.

Genitourinary TB classically presents as painless hematuria and sterile pyuria, but dysuria and secondary bacterial infection are not infrequent. Of all TB patients, 5% to 7% may have positive urine cultures for *Mycobacterium tuberculosis*, despite the absence of urinary symptoms and normal urinalyses. The renal parenchyma, caliceal system, ureters, bladder, and reproductive organs all can be affected. If renal TB is suspected, early-morning urine cultures, an intravenous pyelogram, renal ultrasound, or cystoscopy may be indicated.

Bone and joint TB can be difficult to diagnose in the early stages of disease. Pain and joint swelling can occur, and there may be paraosseus (cold) abscesses and sinus tract formation. The weight-bearing bones and joints are most commonly affected, especially the spine (Pott disease), hips, and knees. Early diagnosis by joint aspiration or biopsy is essential to prevent significant disability and to avoid the need for surgery.

TB in HIV-infected patients often presents differently than it does in immunocompetent patients. Atypical features of TB found in HIV patients include (1) higher frequency of negative TSTs (61% vs. 10%); (2) higher frequency of extrapulmonary sites (60% vs. 28%); (3) higher frequency of diffuse or miliary infiltrates (60% vs. 32%); (4) higher frequency of hilar adenopathy (20% vs. <5%); (5) higher frequency of normal chest radiographs with pulmonary involvement (15% vs. <1%); (6) lower frequency of focal infiltrates (35% vs. 68%); and (7) lower frequency of cavities (18% vs. 67%). Atypical clinical and radiographic features of TB in HIV patients are more likely to be seen in those patients with lower CD4 counts, especially below 200. Patients infected with HIV are much more likely to develop rapidly progressive, sometimes fatal, disease.

FURTHER READING

1. Jeong YJ, Lee KS. Pulmonary tuberculosis: up-to-date imaging and management. *AJR Am J Roentgenol*. 2008;191:834–844.

   Reviews chest radiographic findings in pulmonary tuberculosis including information on CT and PET imaging.

2. Jones BE, Young SM, Antoniskis D. Relationship of the manifestations of tuberculosis to CD4 cell counts in patients with human immunodeficiency virus. *Am Rev Respir Dis*. 1993;148:1292–1297.

   Extrapulmonary tuberculosis and atypical chest radiographic abnormalities are associated with lower CD4 counts in patients with HIV.

3. Greco S, Girardi E, Navarra A, et al. Current evidence on diagnostic accuracy of commercially based nucleic acid amplification tests for the diagnosis of pulmonary tuberculosis. *Thorax*. 2006;61:783–790.

   Commercial NAA tests can be confidently used to exclude TB in patients with smear positive samples in which environmental mycobacteria infection is suspected and to confirm TB in a proportion of smear negative cases.

4. Centers for Disease Control and Prevention (CDC). Updated guidelines for the use of nucleic acid amplification tests in the diagnosis of tuberculosis. *MMWR Morb Mortal Wkly Rep*. 2009;58:7–10.

   CDC guidelines for use of NAA tests for diagnosis of pulmonary tuberculosis.

5. Boehme CC, Nabeta P, Hillemann D, et al. Rapid molecular detection of tuberculosis and rifampin resistance. *N Engl J Med*. 2010;363:1005–1015.

   A rapid molecular test was shown to be sensitive for detection of tuberculosis and rifampin resistance directly from untreated sputum in less than 2 hours with minimal hands-on time.

6. Conde MB, Soares SL, Mello FC, et al. Comparison of sputum induction with fiberoptic bronchoscopy in the diagnosis of tuberculosis: experience at an acquired immune deficiency syndrome reference center in Rio de Janeiro, Brazil. *Am J Respir Crit Care Med*. 2000;162:2238–2240.

   Aerosol-induced sputum sampling and bronchoscopy were found to have similar diagnostic yields in HIV-positive patients.

7. Liang QL, Shi HZ, Wang K, et al. Diagnostic accuracy of adenosine deaminase in tuberculous pleurisy: a meta-analysis. *Respir Med*. 2008;102:744–754.

   ADA determination is a relatively sensitive and specific test for the diagnosis of tuberculous pleurisy.

8. Fontanilla JM, Barnes A, von Reyn CF. Current diagnosis and management of peripheral tuberculous lymphadenitis. *Clin Infect Dis*. 2011;53:555–562.

   Definitive diagnosis is by culture or nucleic amplification of Mycobacterium tuberculosis; *demonstration of acid fast bacilli and granulomatous inflammation may be helpful. Excisional biopsy has the highest sensitivity at 80%, but fine-needle aspiration is less invasive and may be useful, especially in immunocompromised hosts and in resource-limited settings.*

9. Brancusi F, Farrar J, Heemskerk D. Tuberculous meningitis in adults: a review of a decade of developments focusing on prognostic factors for outcome. *Future Microbiol*. 2012;7:1101–1116.

   Reviews epidemiology, clinical and laboratory presentation, management and prognostic factors for outcomes of tuberculous meningitis.

10. Syed FF, Mayosi BM. A modern approach to tuberculous pericarditis. *Prog Cardiovasc Dis*. 2007;50:218–236.

    Tuberculous pericarditis has a high mortality (17% to 40%). Early diagnosis and institution of appropriate therapy are critical. Definitive diagnosis is made by detection of tubercle bacilli in pericardial fluid or on tissue biopsies of the pericardium. A presumptive diagnosis can be made if tuberculosis is found at another anatomic site in the presence of otherwise unexplained pericarditis, pericardial fluid sampling reveals a lymphocytic pericardial exudate with chemical markers of tuberculous infection, and/or there is a response to a trial of antituberculosis therapy.

11. Trecarichi EM, Di Meco E, Mazzotta V, et al. Tuberculous spondylodiscitis: epidemiology, clinical features, treatment, and outcome. *Eur Rev Med Pharmacol Sci*. 2012;16(suppl 2):58–72.

    Review of all aspects spinal tuberculosis and covers roles of chemotherapy and surgery in its management.

12. Gardam M, Lim S. Mycobacterial osteomyelitis and arthritis. *Infect Dis Clin North Am.* 2005;19:819–830.

    Reviews bone and joint disease caused by Mycobacterium tuberculosis *and nontuberculous mycobacteria.*

13. Abbara A, Davidson RN. Etiology and management of genitourinary tuberculosis. *Nat Rev Urol.* 2011;8:678–688.

    In genitourinary tuberculosis, the kidneys are the most commonly infected sites (through hematogenous spread of the bacilli), with subsequent spread through the renal and genital tract. Diagnosis is often delayed because signs, symptoms, and laboratory findings are not specific; therefore, a high degree of suspicion and a systematic approach to diagnosis are necessary.

14. Rasheed S, Zinicola R, Watson D, et al. Intra-abdominal and gastrointestinal tuberculosis. *Colorectal Dis.* 2007;9:773–783.

    As with other forms of extrapulmonary tuberculosis, the diagnosis of gastrointestinal and peritoneal tuberculosis can be a challenge because of nonspecific presentation and rare occurrence in industrialized countries. Tuberculosis can affect all portions of the gastrointestinal tract, but ileocecal region is most common site.

15. Sharma SK, Mohan A, Sharma A, et al. Miliary tuberculosis: new insights into an old disease. *Lancet Infect Dis.* 2005;5:415–430.

    Miliary tuberculosis is a potentially lethal form of tuberculosis that is more common in young children and immunocompromised adults. Although response to first-line antituberculosis drugs is usually good, there is uncertainty around optimal duration of treatment and the role of adjunctive corticosteroids.

51

Tuberculosis: Treatment of Disease

Philip A. LoBue

Although the principles of effective antituberculous chemotherapy are reasonably straightforward, even well-trained physicians may treat tuberculosis patients inappropriately. The problem likely reflects the relatively limited experience many physicians have with this disease. As a consequence, local health departments have assumed a greater role in the management of patients with tuberculosis. Whether care is being managed primarily by a private physician or by the health department, the medical provider has two major responsibilities: (1) to prescribe a treatment regimen with appropriate drugs, dosages, and duration, and (2) to ensure adherence to the regimen until the treatment is complete. When non–health department providers assume a primary patient-management role, they should work in partnership with the health department to ensure these responsibilities are met.

Drugs used to treat tuberculosis can be divided into first- and second-line agents. The first-line (i.e., most effective and least toxic) drugs consist of isoniazid, rifampin, pyrazinamide, and ethambutol. Isoniazid and rifampin are very effective bactericidal drugs. Isoniazid's major adverse reactions include hepatitis and neuritis. The major adverse effects of rifampin are hepatotoxicity and hypersensitivity reactions. Some evidence suggests that the combination of rifampin and isoniazid can be associated with a greater incidence of liver injury than with either drug alone. Hypersensitivity reactions, including a flulike syndrome, thrombocytopenia, and, rarely, acute renal failure, have been reported, usually with intermittent rifampin therapy. Rifampin increases hepatic metabolism of some drugs, causing important drug interactions. Oral contraceptives can be ineffective at normal doses because their hepatic metabolism is increased.

In addition, rifampin can induce methadone withdrawal. Pyrazinamide is used for the first 2 months in many treatment regimens. Its principal side effects are hepatotoxicity and hyperuricemia, with the latter rarely leading to gout or renal failure. Ethambutol is a bacteriostatic agent that has been in general use for over three decades. Retrobulbar optic neuritis has occasionally complicated therapy with doses in excess of 20 mg/kg for prolonged periods, but is almost never seen when using 15 mg/kg.

Second-line medications are generally reserved for therapy of drug-resistant disease or for patients intolerant of first-line medications. Fluoroquinolones are among the latest additions to the array of antituberculous drugs. They are generally well-tolerated and several have good in vitro activity against *Mycobacterium tuberculosis*. Levofloxacin has in vitro activity superior to older fluoroquinolones and a good safety profile with long-term use. The newer fluoroquinolones, such as moxifloxacin, have better in vitro activity, but there is less clinical experience with their use for tuberculosis treatment. Rare gastrointestinal side effects, such as nausea and bloating, and neurologic side effects, including dizziness, insomnia, tremulousness, and headache, may occur with fluoroquinolones. Several second-line medications require intramuscular or intravenous administration. Streptomycin, the first drug available for tuberculosis therapy, is still used occasionally; however, its value is limited by dose-related renal and eighth cranial nerve toxicities and an increasing incidence of drug resistance. Other injectable agents, such as capreomycin, kanamycin, and amikacin, have similar toxicities and may be slightly less effective. *p*-Aminosalicylic acid (PAS), ethionamide, and cycloserine are oral preparations that are usually used only in multidrug-resistant (MDR) tuberculosis. PAS and ethionamide can cause severe gastrointestinal distress, whereas cycloserine is associated with personality changes, depression, frank psychoses, and, in high doses, seizures. Linezolid, clofazimine, imipenem, macrolides, and amoxicillin/clavulanate are sometimes used as "third-line" drugs in patients with disease-resistant to first- and second-line medications.

Since the development of streptomycin in the 1940s, the treatment of tuberculosis has changed considerably. Although individual patients or situations can require tailored regimens, the combination of isoniazid, rifampin, and pyrazinamide is currently the mainstay of treatment for patients with susceptible organisms. Other drugs, especially ethambutol, fluoroquinolones, and injectable agents have important roles in certain contexts.

For patients with isoniazid- and rifampin-susceptible pulmonary tuberculosis, standard treatment is divided into an initial phase of 2 months (8 weeks) followed by a continuation phase of 4 months (18 weeks). Because of the relatively high rate of isoniazid resistance found in adults, their initial-phase treatment should consist of isoniazid, rifampin, pyrazinamide, and ethambutol pending availability of drug-susceptibility test results. For children, ethambutol usually is not needed, unless there is particular concern for isoniazid resistance or the child has a clinical pattern usually seen in adults (i.e., upper lobe infiltration, cavity formation). Once susceptibility results become available, ethambutol may be discontinued (or omitted if drug susceptibility results are known before treatment is started) if the organism is susceptible to isoniazid and rifampin. The initial phase may be given daily throughout, daily for 2 weeks and then twice weekly for 6 weeks, or three times weekly throughout. Twice-weekly therapy is never recommended for human immunodeficiency virus (HIV)-infected patients with CD4 counts less than 100 in the initial or continuation phases of tuberculosis treatment (see below).

The standard continuation-phase therapy for drug-susceptible tuberculosis consists of isoniazid and rifampin. Treatment may be given daily, two times weekly (except if HIV-infected and CD4 count below 100), or three times weekly. For HIV-negative patients with non–cavitary pulmonary tuberculosis and negative sputum smear results at the completion of 2 months of treatment, an alternative continuation-phase treatment is isoniazid and rifapentine (a long-acting analog of rifampin) given once weekly. The duration of the continuation phase is 4 months (6 months total treatment) for most patients with drug-susceptible tuberculosis. Patients with positive sputum cultures after 2 months of therapy and cavities on chest radiograph are more likely to fail treatment or relapse. Therefore, such patients should have their continuation phase extended to 7 months (9 months total treatment), as should patients being treated with once-weekly isoniazid and rifapentine with positive sputum cultures after 2 months of treatment, regardless of chest radiographic findings.

Since the 1990s, use of directly observed therapy (DOT) by local health departments has become a major tool in tuberculosis control. With DOT, some or all doses of medication are taken in the presence of a health professional (e.g., nurse) or a trained outreach worker. This can be done by having the patient come to the clinic or by sending an outreach worker to the patient's home or other mutually agreed upon site. Use of DOT minimizes the risk of treatment failure and acquired drug resistance due to nonadherence. DOT is a core management strategy for patients with tuberculosis. It is considered especially important when using intermittent (i.e., other than daily) therapy. Because DOT is resource-intensive, some health departments may not be able to provide it to all patients. Priority for DOT is given to children, individuals with drug-resistant disease, and those who are likely to be nonadherent (e.g., injection and non–injection drug users, persons with psychiatric disorders, homeless persons).

Completion of treatment is defined not just by the duration of therapy, but by the number of doses taken. For example, a patient receiving daily standard treatment for drug-susceptible disease should take 56 doses (over 8 weeks) of medication in the initial phase and 126 doses (over 18 weeks) in the continuation phase. This should be kept in mind when deciding when to discontinue therapy.

To monitor response to therapy, sputum cultures should be collected every month until cultures are negative for 2 consecutive months. Since more than 90% of patients have negative sputum cultures after 3 months of treatment, any individual with a positive sputum culture at this point should be carefully evaluated to try to identify the etiology of this delayed response to therapy. A patient with a positive sputum culture after 4 months of treatment is considered a treatment failure. Possible reasons for treatment failure include nonadherence and medication malabsorption. In addition to addressing the reasons for treatment failure, repeat susceptibility testing should be performed to assess for acquired drug resistance. If the treatment regimen is going to be modified, at least three new drugs to which the patient's organism would be expected to be susceptible should be added. A cardinal rule of tuberculosis therapy is that a single drug should never be added to a failing regimen.

Patients infected with organisms that are resistant to isoniazid, rifampin, or both require modifications in their drug regimens. For tuberculosis that is isoniazid-resistant (but rifampin-susceptible), the recommended regimen is daily rifampin, ethambutol, and pyrazinamide for 6 to 9 months. A fluoroquinolone may be added to strengthen this regimen in patients with extensive disease. For tuberculosis resistant to rifampin (but isoniazid-susceptible), the recommended therapy is isoniazid, ethambutol, and a fluoroquinolone for 12 to 18 months with pyrazinamide added for the first 2 months. Tuberculosis that is resistant to at least isoniazid and rifampin is termed MDR. Treatment of MDR tuberculosis is often complex and should be done with the consultation of a tuberculosis expert. MDR tuberculosis should be treated with four to six medications to which the organism is susceptible. Therapy should continue for 18 to 24 months. MDR tuberculosis that is also resistant to a fluoroquinolone and any second-line injectable agent is called extensively drug-resistant (XDR) tuberculosis is very difficult to treat, and outcomes in some studies have been comparable to those found in the preantibiotic era. Surgical resection of heavily diseased areas of the lung is sometimes used as an adjunctive therapy for MDR tuberculosis and should be considered in suitable candidates.

Chemotherapy for extrapulmonary tuberculosis does not differ in principle from that for pulmonary tuberculosis. Duration of therapy is the same as for pulmonary disease, with the exceptions of (1) meningitis, for which 9 to 12 months of treatment is recommended, and (2) bone and joint disease, for which some experts recommend extending treatment to 9 months. Corticosteroids should be used routinely in the treatment of central nervous system tuberculosis, including meningitis and pericarditis, but are not recommended as an adjunct for treatment of other forms of tuberculosis.

Tuberculosis treatment of HIV-infected patients is similar to that of HIV-negative patients, although there are several differences. The combination of once-weekly isoniazid and rifapentine should never be used in HIV-infected individuals, as this has resulted in high rates of treatment failure and relapse associated with acquired rifampin resistance. Biweekly therapy should not be used in HIV-infected patients with CD4 counts below 100 for the same reason. The preferred approach to HIV/tuberculosis treatment is combining efavirenz-based antiretroviral therapy (i.e., efavirenz plus two nucleoside analogs) with a standard rifampin-based tuberculosis regimen. For patients unable to take efavirenz, antiretroviral therapy should consist of a protease inhibitor with two nucleoside analogs and tuberculosis treatment should substitute rifabutin for rifampin. Because of the complex interactions between antiretroviral and tuberculosis medications, it is strongly recommended that tuberculosis management of HIV-infected patients be carried out in consultation with a clinical HIV expert.

Temporary exacerbation of tuberculosis symptoms and lesions can occur in patients with HIV who are taking antiretroviral therapy. This phenomenon, known as the immune reconstitution inflammatory syndrome (IRIS) or paradoxical reaction, has been attributed to recovery of the delayed hypersensitivity response in these patients and increased exposure to tuberculosis antigens after the initiation of bactericidal antituberculous therapy and/or antiretroviral therapy for HIV. In general, modifications of tuberculosis therapy and antiretroviral therapy are not necessary, and a short course of corticosteroids may ameliorate symptoms associated with this reaction if it is severe.

Tuberculosis in children is treated similarly to adult disease. In the past, concern was expressed about the use of ethambutol in very young children because of the difficulty in screening for retrobulbar neuritis. More recent data, however, suggest that ethambutol is safe in this population.

Isoniazid, ethambutol, and rifampin have been used successfully and safely in pregnancy. Pyrazinamide has not been shown to be teratogenic, but there is insufficient experience with this drug in pregnancy to assure its safety; its use during pregnancy is not generally recommended. Streptomycin causes eighth cranial nerve damage to the fetus and should not be used. All other second-line drugs, with the possible exception of PAS, either have known teratogenic effects or are lacking sufficient safety data to endorse their use in pregnancy.

Adverse drug reactions can occur at any time during treatment. Often difficult to diagnose, they can be confused with manifestations of tuberculosis or other concurrent illnesses. Sometimes, drug reactions are relatively mild so that stopping therapy is not warranted. Specific reactions can be handled by discontinuing the suspect drug. Often drugs have overlapping toxicity and reactions are nonspecific (e.g., fever, rash, jaundice). In such cases, all drugs should be stopped for a brief period (e.g., 1 week) and then reintroduced singly, the least likely offender first. Some clinicians reinitiate drugs at low doses, whereas others resume full-dose therapy. If a reaction appears a second time, then another drug may need to be substituted. (One drug can be added to a successful regimen as long as the entire regimen is adequate.)

All patients being treated for tuberculosis should be counseled and tested for HIV infection. Patients with risk factors for hepatitis B or C should be tested for these viruses. Baseline serum transaminase, bilirubin, alkaline phosphatase, and creatinine levels and a platelet count should be measured for all adults. Visual acuity and color testing should be performed for all patients receiving ethambutol. Routine follow-up measurements of liver or renal function or platelet count are not necessary unless there were abnormalities at baseline or there are clinical indications for additional blood tests. Patients who have stable abnormalities of hepatic or renal function at initial testing should have repeat measurements early in the course of treatment, then less frequently to ensure that there is no deterioration. At minimum, patients receiving ethambutol should be questioned regarding visual disturbances at monthly intervals; however, formal monthly repeat testing of visual acuity and color vision is often done routinely and is strongly recommended for individuals receiving more than 15 mg/kg or for those taking the medication for more than 2 months. Monitoring tests for individual second-line drugs can be found in the American Thoracic Society/Centers for Disease Control and Prevention/Infectious Diseases Society of America 2003 Treatment of Tuberculosis statement.

Surgery is rarely necessary except in selected cases of MDR tuberculosis and for complications of tuberculosis such as (1) emergency treatment of massive hemoptysis, (2) therapy of bronchopleural fistulas, (3) drainage of true (purulent) tuberculous empyemas (not free flowing, nonpurulent effusions, which are much more common), or (4) relief of mechanical problems in skeletal tuberculosis, such as spinal stabilization procedures in selected individuals with Pott disease.

FURTHER READING

1. American Thoracic Society, Centers for Disease Control and Prevention, Infectious Diseases Society of America. Treatment of tuberculosis. *MMWR Recomm Rep.* 2003;52(RR-11):1–77.

   National guidelines for the treatment of active tuberculosis. Also gives background information on various tuberculosis medications and guidelines for special situations, such as children, pregnancy, and drug resistance.

2. Combs DL, O'Brien RJ, Geiter LJ. USPHS Tuberculosis Short-Course Chemotherapy Trial 21: effectiveness, toxicity, and acceptability. The report of final results. *Ann Intern Med.* 1990;112:397–406.

   A 6-month regimen, beginning with isoniazid, rifampin, and pyrazinamide for 2 months, followed by isoniazid and rifampin for 4 months, is similar in effectiveness and toxicity to the 9-month regimen.

3. Chan ED, Laurel V, Strand MJ, et al. Treatment and outcome analysis of 205 patients with multidrug-resistant tuberculosis. *Am J Respir Crit Care Med.* 2004;169:1103–1109.

   Compared to a prior cohort of MDR patients, this group had more favorable initial treatment responses and long-term outcomes. Use of fluoroquinolones and adjunctive surgery was associated with improved clinical and microbiologic outcomes.

4. Centers for Disease Control and Prevention. Managing drug interactions in the treatment of HIV-related tuberculosis [online]. 2007. Available from http://www.cdc.gov/tb/TB_HIV_Drugs/default.htm.

   Reviews tuberculosis treatment in HIV-infected patients and drug interactions between tuberculosis medications and antiretrovirals.

5. Narita M, Ashkin D, Hollender ES, et al. Paradoxical worsening of tuberculosis following antiretroviral therapy in patients with AIDS. *Am J Respir Crit Care Med.* 1998;158:157–161.

   Describes the paradoxical reaction which can occur in patients being treated for HIV and tuberculosis.

6. Weis SE, Slocum PC, Blais FX, et al. The effect of directly observed therapy on the rates of drug resistance and relapse in tuberculosis. *N Engl J Med.* 1994;330:1179–1184.

   Use of DOT results in decreased rates of relapse, acquired drug resistance, and primary drug resistance in the community.

7. Yee D, Valiquette C, Pelletier M, et al. Incidence of serious side effects from first-line antituberculosis drugs among patients treated for active tuberculosis. *Am J Respir Crit Care Med.* 2003;167:1472–1477.

   Among 430 patients, the incidence of all major adverse effects was 1.48 per 100 person-months of exposure. The incidence of pyrazinamide-induced hepatotoxicity and rash during treatment for active TB was substantially higher than with the other first-line anti-TB drugs, and higher than previously recognized.

8. Patel AM, McKeon J. Avoidance and management of adverse reactions to antituberculous drugs. *Drug Saf.* 1995;12:1–25.

   Comprehensive review of adverse effects of medications used to treat tuberculosis, including sections on prevention, monitoring, and management.

9. Francis J. Curry National Tuberculosis Center and California Department of Public Health. *Drug-resistant tuberculosis: a survival guide for clinicians*, 2nd ed, San Francisco, CA: Francis J. Curry National Tuberculosis Center; 2008.

   Excellent, comprehensive guide on management of drug-resistant tuberculosis.

10. LoBue P. Extensively drug-resistant tuberculosis. *Curr Opin Infect Dis.* 2009;22:167–173.

    XDR TB is an emerging global health threat. The disease is difficult and expensive to diagnose and treat, and outcomes are frequently poor.

52 Nontuberculous Mycobacterial Pulmonary Infections

Marisa Magaña and Antonino Catanzaro

INTRODUCTION

Nontuberculous mycobacterial (NTM) infections encompass a variety of acid-fast bacilli that are biologically distinct from *Mycobacterium tuberculosis* and *M. leprae*. They had long been considered saprophytes or culture contaminants. More recently, they have been recognized as significant, although uncommon, human pathogens. Rates of NTM infection have increased due in part to the rising frequency of infection encountered in patients with chronic lung disease and the AIDS epidemic, where disseminated *M. avium-intracellulare* (MAC) can be life-threatening. Although the rates of tuberculosis (TB) are declining in many industrialized countries, the prevalence of pulmonary disease caused by NTM appears to be increasing.

While over 100 species of NTM have been identified, only a few species account for the majority of human infections. NTM diseases occur in most industrialized countries with an incidence of approximately 3 per 100,000 persons. Pulmonary disease caused by *M. avium* complex is the most common NTM infection in most areas. There are some regional differences in the prevalence of certain other species. For example, *M. abscessus* is the second most common in the United States and Korea, whereas *M. kansasii* is the second most common NTM in Canada. Unlike the *M. tuberculosis* complex, NTM are widely dispersed in the environment and commonly isolated from soil, drinking water, rivers, hospital instruments (i.e., bronchoscopes), and municipal water sources. Unlike tuberculosis, there is no person-to-person transmission.

DIAGNOSIS

Diagnosis of pulmonary disease caused by NTM may be difficult, as the organisms are commonly isolated from environmental sources, and therefore, many isolates are in fact contaminants. The American Thoracic Society has published guidelines outlining specific diagnostic criteria for pulmonary disease caused by NTMs. Broadly, these guidelines require the presence of a compatible clinical and radiographic presentation, supporting microbiological data, and the exclusion of other potential etiologies. These criteria are based on experience with common and well-described respiratory pathogens, such as MAC and *M. abscessus*. However, there is little experience with most of the other NTM to know if these criteria are uniformly applicable. Because NTM are ubiquitous, the ATS has recommended specific microbiologic criteria which attempt to differentiate between a contaminant and a true pathogen. The microbiologic criteria may be any one of the following: a positive culture from at least two expectorated sputum samples, a positive culture from at least one bronchial wash, a biopsy with mycobacterial histopathologic features and positive culture, or a biopsy with mycobacterial histopathologic features and one or more sputum/bronchial washings that are culture-positive for NTM. Once a microbiologic confirmation of disease has been made, the guidelines require that the patient display symptoms as well as radiographic evidence of disease before establishing a diagnosis of pulmonary disease due to the NTM. Most series have demonstrated that only 25% to 50% of patients with an NTM isolate will meet the 2007 ATS criteria for infection. The decision to treat a patient is a decision that requires further consideration of various factors that will be discussed later in this chapter.

MICROBIOLOGY

Several recent advances have enabled laboratories to detect and identify mycobacteria more rapidly and accurately. The use of liquid-based culture media such as BACTEC (Becton Dickinson, Sparks, Maryland) has greatly reduced the time in which results are available; many NTM can now be recovered in days rather than weeks. In addition, the increased use of liquid culture is also likely a factor in the increase in isolation of some of these organisms. High-performance liquid chromatography (HPLC) can be used to identify species based on interpretation of the mycolic acid pattern they display. The differentiation between *M. tuberculosis* and NTM is reliable using this method as is the differentiation of many other mycobacterium species or groups. Chemi-luminescent DNA probes (such as AccuProbe, GeneProbe Inc., San Diego, California) are now being used as confirmatory tests to identify some of the more common families. These probes are reported to be nearly 100% sensitive and specific and have become the most commonly used method of rapid mycobacterial identification.

While many mycobacterial species can now be detected more rapidly because of the advent of liquid media and molecular testing, the old growth characteristics are still used as part of the classification system. The rapidly growing mycobacteria or RGM are characterized by visible growth on solid media within 7 days. *M. abscessus* complex accounts for 65% to 80% of lung disease caused by RGM and will be discussed in detail later in this chapter, as it has become a common cause of NTM lung disease.

The approach to management of pulmonary disease due to NTM depends primarily on the causative species. Therefore, treatment for some of the more common NTMs will be discussed in this chapter by species.

M. avium Complex

Pulmonary infection with NTM is most often caused by MAC. There are at least two species within this complex, *M. avium* and *M. intracellulare*, and they may sometimes be referred to as MAC or MAI. *M. avium* appears to be more linked with disseminated disease, while *M. intracellulare* is more often found as an isolated respiratory pathogen. At present, there does not appear to be any prognostic advantage to differentiating these two species, and therefore, this is not routinely done.

In HIV-negative patients with pulmonary disease caused by MAC, two main types of radio-graphic presentation, are currently recognized. The first is an apical fibrocavitary disease, resembling findings seen in TB patients. This tends to occur in males aged 40 to 50 with a history of tobacco and alcohol use. This type of presentation tends to progress, leading to lung destruction and loss of lung function, without treatment. The second type of pulmonary MAC disease is a nodular and bronchiectatic presentation that tends to occur in patients without any underlying lung disease. Most often, these radiographic changes are present in the lingula and right-middle lobes. This presentation tends to be slowly progressive and occurs mostly in postmenopausal, tall, thin and nonsmoking women. This second type of presentation is sometimes called the "Lady Windermere syndrome." Lady Windermere syndrome was first described in 1892 after the character in Oscar Wilde's play *Lady Windermere's Fan*.

In addition to its occurrence in the above-mentioned at-risk patient populations, pulmonary disease due to MAC is increasingly being recognized as a pathogen in patients with cystic fibrosis. One potentially important discovery is the presence of CFTR mutations (the gene responsible for cystic fibrosis) in patients without cystic fibrosis who have a diagnosis of bronchiectasis, pulmonary NTM, or both. The significance of this is unclear. When MAC is recovered from patients with cystic fibrosis, it is often difficult to determine whether the radiographic changes are due to MAC, the underlying cystic fibrosis or nonmycobacterial pathogens such as pseudomonas. It is recommended that all potential nonmycobacterial pathogens be aggressively treated prior to initiation of MAC therapy in patients with cystic fibrosis. In recent years, there has been increasing use of the macrolides in cystic fibrosis patients for their anti-inflammatory effects. This phenomenon could potentially lead to the development of macrolide resistant strains of NTM. It is recommended that cystic fibrosis patients undergo evaluation for NTM disease prior to initiation of macrolide monotherapy.

M. avium Complex—Treatment

Treatment of MAC can be difficult, especially due to the fact that with the exception of the macrolides (azithromycin and clarithromycin), the in vitro susceptibilities do not predict clinical outcomes. Based on the available literature, the ATS has recommended that treatment regimens contain a macrolide (clarithromycin 1,000 mg/day or azithromycin 250 mg/day), ethambutol (15 mg/kg/day), and rifampin (10 mg/kg/day, 600 mg/day max.). If there is severe disease or previous treatment, then an IV aminoglycoside (streptomycin or amikacin) should be added for the first 2 to 3 months. Three times weekly treatment can be considered in patients with less-severe nodular, bronchiectatic disease who are treatment naive. There are some patients in whom a microbiological cure will not be possible because of the potential side effects or drug interactions. In these patients, the MAC infection may be viewed as a noncurable, chronic, indolent infection, and other treatment regimens may be more appropriate for suppressive-type therapy.

Bronchial hygiene is an important, often overlooked adjunctive therapy for those patients with preexisting lung disease. Routine drug susceptibility testing is not recommended as the organism shows in vitro resistance to most antituberculous drugs. However, in vitro sensitivities should be obtained for those patients who are failing therapy or experiencing a relapse after prior treatment. Sputum should be sampled monthly to document negative conversion, and blood tests should be monitored routinely while on treatment as the potential for drug toxicity is high.

Treatment should continue for 12 months after the first documented negative sputum culture. One study using 12 months of negative sputum cultures as an endpoint observed no relapses with a mean follow-up period of 18 months. Of note, early relapses were observed if 10 months of culture negativity was used as a therapy endpoint. Others recommend 24 months of therapy, although the extended treatment benefits have not been clearly proven. In addition, some advocate stopping therapy all together for those patients who have difficulty tolerating the medications or who do not show clear improvement after 6 months or more of treatment. In general, patients on a macrolide-containing regimen should show clinical improvement in 3 to 6 months and should continue treatment for at least 12 months after culture conversion. When anatomically feasible, early surgical intervention (under chemotherapeutic coverage) is recommended by some but should only be undertaken by very experienced surgeons. Bacteriologic conversion rates varying from 40% to 90% have been achieved with such combined medical and surgical therapy.

To improve the tolerability of a regimen, it is recommended that the drugs be introduced gradually with escalating dosages. In addition, one drug should be initiated at a time with medications added at 1- to 2-week intervals to avoid side effects. When amikacin is used, baseline audiometry with repeat interval testing should be performed. In addition, patients receiving amikacin should be specifically warned about the signs and symptoms of toxicity, including unsteady gait, tinnitus, and diminished hearing. Similarly, patients receiving ethambutol should be instructed to report visual changes in addition to undergoing periodic visual acuity and color discrimination testing as optic neuritis is a potential side effect. Rifampin commonly causes discoloration of body secretions and tissues, and patients should be warned about this. Liver function tests only need to be monitored if patients are at high risk of hepatitis, otherwise only if clinically suspected based on symptoms.

Disseminated *M. avium* Complex Infection and AIDS

In HIV-positive patients, MAC infection often presents with disseminated disease, in contrast to the presentation in patients who are immunocompetent. There was a striking increase in the incidence of disseminated MAC during the 1980s with the HIV/AIDS epidemic. Subsequently, with the introduction of antiretroviral therapy, the incidence of disseminated MAC has markedly decreased over the past three decades. Disseminated MAC carries a high mortality and should be aggressively treated. Treatment consists of antimicrobial therapy as well as immune reconstitution with antiretroviral therapy. Clarithromycin appears to clear bacteremia quicker than azithromycin and is therefore the preferred antibiotic. Ethambutol and typically rifabutin (rather than rifampin because reduced interactions with the antiretroviral medications) are added. Treatment is generally lifelong or until the CD4 count is greater than 100 cells/μl for at least 12 months. Primary prevention of disseminated MAC with azithromycin 1,200 mg once weekly is recommended for patients with CD4 count less than 50 cells/μl.

M. abscessus

M. abscessus is the second most common NTM causing lung disease after MAC. It occurs more commonly in young women, often with no underlying lung disease. Although many have bronchiectasis, it is unclear if this is a result, rather than the cause, of the *M. abscessus* infection. *M. abscessus* has become an increasingly common cause of NTM lung disease in patients with cystic fibrosis. On HRCT, the radiographic pattern is similar to that of the nodular bronchiectatic

MAC infection. In most patients who do not have underlying lung disease, infection with *M. abscessus* follows a very indolent course. However, a subset of patients may have rapidly progressive and destructive disease that requires aggressive treatment.

Treatment outcomes of *M. abscessus* has historically been very poor; however, there have been very few studies published on the topic. Recent data suggests that treatment outcomes correlate with macrolide in vitro sensitivities, much like for MAC lung disease. ATS–IDSA guidelines do not recommend any particular drug regimen for treatment of *M. abscessus* because of the lack of reliable cure with any one particular drug regimen. These guidelines do however recommend that a macrolide and parenteral therapy with amikacin, cefoxitin, or imipenem be used if surgery is not a viable option. A recent study reviewing treatment outcomes in 65 patients in Korea demonstrated maintenance of negative sputum cultures in 58% of patients treated with the following regimen: oral clarithromycin (1,000 mg/day), ciprofloxacin (1,000 mg/day), and doxycycline (200 mg/day) along with an initial 4 weeks of IV amikacin (15 mg/kg/day in two divided doses) and cefoxitin (200 mg/kg/day, max 12 mg/day in three divided doses). In vitro susceptibilities to the macrolides were the only sensitivities that correlated with clinical outcomes. Sputum conversion rates were significantly lower in patients whose isolates were resistant to macrolides when compared with patients whose isolates demonstrated in vitro macrolide sensitivity/intermediate sensitivity 17% versus 64%. In general, treatment should probably continue for 12 months after sputum culture conversion.

M. abscessus complex has been shown to comprise three closely related species: *M. abscessus, M. massiliense,* and *M. bolletti*. Recent data suggests that species distinction is important because antibiotic susceptibilities and treatment outcomes vary by subspecies. Patients with *M. abscessus* infection compared with patients with *M. massiliense* have poorer clinical outcomes defined as culture conversion, symptom, and imaging resolution as well as relapse rates. The reason for this difference is thought to occur because of a clarithromycin inducible resistant gene that *M. abscessus* has but *M. massiliense* does not. Presently, most laboratories do not differentiate between these subspecies; however, it may be useful to do so in the future if these data are confirmed.

M. kansasii

M. kansasii is another common NTM that causes pulmonary disease. Of all the NTM, *M. kansasii* most closely parallels the clinical course of *M. tuberculosis*, with up to 90% of HIV-negative patients presenting with cavitary infiltrates. Like the other NTM, it is not transmissible from person to person. Risk factors for developing pulmonary disease by *M. kansasii* include pneumoconiosis, chronic obstructive pulmonary disease, previous mycobacterial disease, malignancy, and alcoholism. This NTM primarily affects middle-aged white men. *M. kansasii* also produces pulmonary disease in HIV-infected patients who usually have the same symptoms as immunocompetent patients. Radiographically, interstitial infiltrates and hilar adenopathy are more commonly seen with HIV-infected patients than cavities. *M. kansasii* can also cause disseminated disease, particularly in severely immunocompromised patients, such as those with advanced AIDS and those who have undergone organ transplantation. In the appropriate clinical setting, a single culture-positive specimen for *M. kansasii* is sufficient to make a diagnosis and initiate therapy as this NTM is considered to be the most virulent.

M. kansasii responds well to chemotherapy. Similar to the other NTMs, in vitro susceptibility studies do not necessarily correlate with in vivo drug efficacy. The initial regimen should include isoniazid, ethambutol, and, most importantly, rifampin. Rarely, regimens including four or five drugs may be necessary to achieve a bacteriologic cure. Treatment should be continued for at least 18 months; shorter courses have not been studied extensively and appear to have a higher relapse rate. More than 90% success has been achieved with drug therapy alone. Adjunctive surgery is rarely indicated, except in well-localized disease that has responded poorly to adequate chemotherapy.

NONPULMONARY DISEASE CAUSED BY NTM SPECIES

Well-documented infections involving bone, joints, urinary tract, skin, soft tissues, lymph nodes, liver, kidney, and meninges have been reported with a variety of the NTM. Widely disseminated disease may occur, especially in immunosuppressed individuals and those with hematologic abnormalities. Guidelines regarding treatment of these conditions and some of the less-common NTM organisms is beyond the scope of this chapter; however, readers are referred to the 2007 ATS/IDSA Statement on the Diagnosis, Treatment and Prevention of Nontuberculous Mycobacterial Diseases for more information.

FURTHER READING

1. Griffith DE, Aksamit T, Brown-Elliott BA, et al. An official ATS/IDSA statement: diagnosis, treatment, and prevention of nontuberculous mycobacterial disease. *Am J Respir Crit Care Med.* 2007;175:367–416.

    This official statement covers diagnostic criteria for the most common nontuberculous mycobacterium. In addition, it proposes diagnostic criteria and treatment regimens for each of the NTMs.

2. Daley CL, Griffith DE. Pulmonary non-tuberculous mycobacterial infections. *Int J Tuberc Lung Dis.* 2010;14(6):665–671.

    An excellent review on the epidemiology, diagnosis and treatment of common NTM pulmonary infections.

3. French AL, Benator DA, Gordin FM. Nontuberculous mycobacterial infections. *Med Clin North Am.* 1997;81:361–379.

    An excellent review article covering MAC, Mycobacterium kansasii, and other nontuberculous mycobacteria, with special emphasis on infection in AIDS patients.

4. Kim RD, Greenberg DE, Ehrmantraut MR, et al. Pulmonary nontuberculous mycobacterial disease: prospective study of a distinct preexisting syndrome. *Am J Respir Crit Care Med.* 2008;178:1066–1074.

    Prospective evaluation of 63 patients with pulmonary NTM infection. These patients were taller and thinner than control patients. In addition, there was a high incidence of scoliosis, pectus excavatum and mitral valve prolapse in patients with pulmonary NTM infection.

5. Tanaka E, Kimotot T, Tsuyuguchi K, et al. Effect of clarithromycin regimen for *Mycobacterium avium* complex pulmonary disease. *Am J Respir Crit Care Med.* 1999;160:866–872.

    The authors examined the efficacy of a four-drug regimen for MAC that contained clarithromycin. They found that the regimen benefited newly treated patients, but problems remained for retreated patients, such as adverse side effects and low sputum conversion rates.

6. Corpe RF. Surgical management of pulmonary disease due to *Mycobacterium avium-intracellulare.* *Rev Infect Dis.* 1981;3:1064.

    Of 131 patients with pulmonary infections due to MAC, 124 had excisional surgery plus chemotherapy; and 7 had definitive thoracoplasties.

7. Van Ingen J, Verhagen AFTM, Dekhuijzen PNR, et al. Surgical treatment of non-tuberculous mycobacterial lung disease: strike in time. *Int J Tuberc Lung Dis.* 2010;14:99–105.

    Retrospective review of one center's experience with surgical intervention for pulmonary NTM disease.

8. Reich JM, Johnson RE. *Mycobacterium avium* complex pulmonary disease. *Am Rev Respir Dis.* 1991;143:1381.

    The experience with pulmonary disease caused by MAC was examined during a 12-year period in a nonreferral setting.

9. Reich JM, Johnson RE. *Mycobacterium avium* complex pulmonary disease presenting as an isolated lingular or middle lobe pattern: the Lady Windermere syndrome. *Chest.* 1992;101:1605.

    This case series describes the syndrome and its occurrence predominantly in elderly women and hypothesizes that voluntary cough suppression may lead to its development.

10. Swensen SJ, Hartman TE, Williams DE. Computed tomographic diagnosis of *Mycobacterium avium-intracellulare* complex in patients with bronchiectasis. *Chest.* 1994;105:49.

    Evaluated the usefulness of bronchiectasis and multiple nodules on CT imaging for predicting MAC infection. These CT findings had a sensitivity of 80%, and a specificity of 87% for MAC infection.

11. Jeon K, Kwon OJ, Lee NY, et al. Antibiotic treatment of *Mycobacterium abscessus* lung disease. *Am J Respir Crit Care Med.* 2009;180:896.

    Retrospective review of clinical outcomes in 65 patients with M. abscessus treated with the following regimen: oral clarithromycin, ciprofloxacin and doxycycline along with an initial 4 weeks of IV amikacin and cofoxitin in Korea.

12. Koh W, Jeon K, Lee NY, et al. Clinical significance of differentiation of *Mycobacterium massiliense* from *Mycobacterium abscessus*. *Am J Respir Crit Care Med.* 2011;183:405.

Retrospective review that examined the outcomes of disease based on species. Data suggests that patients with M. abscessus do much worse clinically and that this is because of inducible macrolide resistance.

13. Mitchison DA, Ellard GA, Grosset J. New antibacterial drugs for the treatment of mycobacterial disease in man. *Br Med Bull.* 1988;44:757.

A nice review of the mechanism of action of drugs used to treat mycobacterial diseases.

14. O'Brien RJ, Geiter LJ, Snider DE Jr. The epidemiology of nontuberculous mycobacterial diseases in the United States: results from a national survey. *Am Rev Respir Dis.* 1987;135:1007.

The data suggested a changing epidemiologic picture of nontuberculous mycobacterial disease due perhaps to the decreased incidence of tuberculosis, the increased prevalence of chronic lung disease, and increased culturing of diagnostic specimens, as well as possibly a change in the ecology of these organisms.

15. Cassidy PM, Hedberg K, Saulson A, et al. Nontuberculous mycobacterial disease prevalence and risk factors: changing epidemiology. *Clin Infect Dis.* 2009;49:e124–e129.

Evaluated the prevalence of NTM disease using the ATS/IDSA 2007 microbiologic criteria alone to estimate disease prevalence. Disease prevalence was higher in women than in men.

16. Kotloff RM. Infection caused by nontuberculous mycobacteria: clinical aspects. *Semin Roentgenol.* 1993;28:131.

A discussion of the differential diagnosis of nontuberculous mycobacterial disease from the perspective of a radiologist.

17. MacDonell KB, Glassroth J. *Mycobacterium avium* complex and other nontuberculous mycobacteria in patients with HIV infection. *Semin Respir Infect.* 1989;4:123.

Initiation of drug therapy for MAC may decrease the severity of disease symptoms in some HIV-infected patients.

18. Nightingale SD, Cameron DW, Gordin FM, et al. Two controlled trials of rifabutin prophylaxis against *Mycobacterium avium* complex infection in AIDS. *N Engl J Med.* 1993;329:828.

MAC infection develops in most patients with AIDS. Two randomized, double-blind, multicenter trials of daily prophylactic treatment with either rifabutin (300 mg) or placebo were conducted. Untreated disseminated disease carries a very poor prognosis with only a 13% one year survival rate.

19. O'Brien RJ. The epidemiology of nontuberculous mycobacterial disease. *Clin Chest Med.* 1989;10:407.

The most common forms of disease are chronic pulmonary disease resembling tuberculosis, benign cervical adenopathy in children, skin and soft tissue infection, and disseminated disease in immunocompromised persons.

20. Kirschner RA Jr, Parker BC, Falkinham JO. Epidemiology of infection by nontuberculous mycobacteria. *Am Rev Respir Dis.* 1992;145:271.

M. avium, M. intracellulare, *and* M. scrofulaceum *in acid, brown-water swamps of the southeastern United States and their association with environmental variables.*

21. Wallace RJ, Brown BA, Griffith DE, et al. Clarithromycin regimens for pulmonary *Mycobacterium avium* complex: the first 50 patients. *Am J Respir Crit Care Med.* 1996;153:1766–1772.

22. Heifets L. Mycobacterial infections caused by nontuberculous mycobacteria. *Semin Respir Crit Care Med.* 2004;25:283–295.

A relatively concise review on the topic of NTM with excellent references and a focus on pulmonary disease.

23. Phillips MS, von Reyn CF. Nosocomial infections due to nontuberculous mycobacteria. *Clin Infect Dis.* 2001;33:1363–1374.

A review of the spectrum of potential nosocomial infections due to NTM.

24. Griffith DE, Brown-Elliott BA, Wallace RJ. Diagnosing nontuberculous mycobacterial lung disease: a process in evolution. *Infect Dis Clin North Am.* 2002;16:235–239.

A discussion of the ongoing controversies in diagnosing NTM pulmonary disease.

25. Chemlal K, Portaels F. Molecular diagnosis of nontuberculous mycobacteria. *Curr Opin Infect Dis.* 2003;16:77–83.

    A review of the various molecular diagnostic tools available to diagnose NTM.

26. Brown-Elliott BA, Griffith DE, Wallace RJ. Diagnosis of nontuberculous mycobacterial infections. *Clin Lab Med.* 2002;22:911–925.

    This article reviews the methods of laboratory diagnosis of NTM.

Coccidioidomycosis

Robert Bercovitch and Antonino Catanzaro

INTRODUCTION

Coccidioidomycosis is an infection caused by the fungus *Coccidioides*. Inhalation is the main route of infection. Coccidioidomycosis causes a wide spectrum of pulmonary disease, including acute and chronic pneumonia, pulmonary nodules, and cavitary disease. Dissemination via the bloodstream can occur to any organ, including the lungs, but the most common sites of dissemination are skin and bone. Infection is common in endemic areas, and travelers to these areas are at risk for infection. Healthcare providers in endemic and nonendemic areas should be aware of the clinical manifestations, diagnosis, and management of coccidioidomycosis.

MICROBIOLOGY

In addition to *Coccidioides immitis,* a second species, *Coccidioides posadii,* has been identified. Although the two organisms are genetically distinct and geographically separated, there are no known differences in terms of the immune response or clinical disease. *Coccidioides* is a dimorphic fungus. It proliferates in the mycelial form during the rainy season and forms arthroconidia, the infectious spore, when the climate becomes hot and dry. Wind or soil disruption causes the arthroconidia to become airborne, and infection is caused when they are inhaled. Once inhaled, the arthroconidia undergoes transformation into a spherule. The spherule undergoes internal division, forming numerous endospores. With rupture of the spherule, endospores are released, each able to mature into a spherule. The findings of spherules and endospores on histology is characteristic of coccidioidomycosis.

EPIDEMIOLOGY

Coccidioides grows in the soil in endemic areas, including the lower Sonoran life zone (southern California, Arizona, Nevada, New Mexico, and Texas), and in northern Mexico and parts of Central and South America. Infection has been reported in nonendemic areas returning travelers or persons exposed to objects containing dust sent from an endemic area. Coccidioidomycosis outbreaks can follow natural disasters such as earthquakes, which can vigorously disturb soil and cause the release of arthroconidia. Construction can also disrupt soil and contribute to outbreaks.

CLINICAL PRESENTATION

The primary coccidioidal infection is asymptomatic in 60% of individuals; the remainder have a similar presentation to other causes of community-acquired pneumonia (CAP) with fever, chills, malaise, cough, dyspnea, chest pain, arthralgias, pharyngitis, and rash. In endemic areas, coccidioidomycosis is a common cause of CAP, with evidence of infection in up to 29% of patients presenting for evaluation of lower respiratory tract symptoms.

In general, physical findings in primary coccidioidomycosis are nonspecific. Signs of pulmonary parenchymal consolidation may be present and often are very localized and transient; pleural rubs are unusual. San Joaquin Valley Fever represents a characteristic symptom complex of primary coccidioidomycosis and classically includes erythema nodosum (with or without erythema multiforme), arthralgias, malaise, and fever. Skin manifestations are common in primary infection, occurring in approximately 5% of men and 25% of women. A fine erythematous maculopapular exanthem, toxic cutaneous erythema, is said to be very common but is an extremely evanescent, early event.

The chest X-ray is often abnormal, even in asymptomatic individuals, and infiltrates are observed in 80% of patients requiring hospitalization. The infiltrates vary widely in size, location, character, and duration. Hilar adenopathy occurs in 20% of cases and does not influence the prognosis unless it is persistent and accompanied by rising serologic titers. Pleural effusion is seen in less than 10% of symptomatic individuals; in most patients, the effusion is small (<1 L). Pleural effusions in coccidioidomycosis can be eosinophilic exudates.

Coccidioidomycosis is considered chronic or progressive when symptoms or signs of pulmonary involvement are present or increasing beyond 6 to 8 weeks. Manifestations of chronic pulmonary coccidioidomycosis may include acute progressive pneumonia that is usually symptomatic, chronic progressive pneumonia, pulmonary nodule or nodules, and pulmonary cavities. Coccidioidomas represent isolated residua of active pulmonary disease, and organisms have been cultured from lesions that remained unchanged for decades. Cavities may be thin-walled and often represent the initial radiographic manifestation of infection. The thin-walled cavities have a tendency to expand. Most coccidioidal cavities are clinically silent, but hemorrhage and rupture leading to bronchopleural fistulas can occur, although this is typically limited to the initial phase of the disease and related to necrotizing pneumonia. Occasionally, secondary bacterial infection of cavities can occur. Empyema may result and be either bacterial or fungal in etiology. In persistent pulmonary coccidioidomycosis, serologic evidence of activity (e.g., elevated complement fixation [CF] titers) may be absent but, when present, should raise the possibility of intrapulmonary dissemination.

A worse prognosis and an increased risk of dissemination may be indicated by the findings of (1) elevated CF titers, (2) pulmonary infiltrates or hilar or paratracheal adenopathy that persists more than 6 weeks, and (3) significant weight loss. Extrapulmonary dissemination is estimated to occur in less than 5% of symptomatic infections. The risk of dissemination is increased in patients with depressed cell-mediated immune (CMI) responses. Certain individuals appear predisposed to severe, prolonged, or disseminated infections. These include immunocompromised individuals, most notably those with AIDS; patients taking immunosuppressive drugs, particularly prednisone and tumor necrosis factor (TNF) antagonists; individuals of Black, Filipino, or American Indian extraction; and those in the last trimester of pregnancy. Age older than 55 carries a greater risk of continuing illness even after 1 year of treatment. Recently, mutations in the IL-12/IL-23/IFN pathway have been identified in certain individuals with disseminated coccidioidomycosis, but it is not known whether genetic polymorphisms in this axis underlie the ethnic differences in disseminated disease that have been observed.

The most frequent sites of dissemination are the skin, bones, soft tissues, and meninges; however, single- or multiple-mass lesions or abscesses may occur in any organ. Typical miliary lesions occur in 4% of cases. Cutaneous fistula formation from deep-seated lesions is common. Meningitis is the most ominous form of dissemination because of anatomic disruption that can lead to hydrocephalus, and because of the difficulty in getting drugs to the site of infection. There is some evidence that patients with facial lesions due to coccidioidomycosis have a greater risk for developing meningitis than patients who had lesions only on the body. This association may allow for earlier detection and treatment of coccidioidomycosis meningitis. If dissemination has occurred or is suspected, a careful evaluation of its extent should be undertaken, including analysis of the cerebrospinal fluid (CSF) for CF titer. CSF may be negative in 25% of cases on an initial examination. If clinical suspicion is high, a spinal tap should be repeated in 1 or 2 weeks. Bone scans are very useful in the search for subclinical sites of dissemination.

DIAGNOSIS

Coccidioidomycosis can be diagnosed by culture, histology, or serology. In addition, the presence of tissue eosinophilia, while nonspecific, should raise suspicion for coccidioidomycosis in the correct clinical context. Skin testing was performed frequently in the past to determine cellular immunity to *Coccidioides*. Unfortunately, the skin test reagent has been unavailable for a number of years, but it may be reintroduced.

The finding of spherules containing endospores on direct microscopy is considered pathognomonic for coccidioidomycosis. The organism can be detected on histopathology using standard hematoxylin–eosin (H&E), periodic acid Schiff (PAS), or Grocott methenamine silver (GMS) stains, with the GMS stain considered the most sensitive. Sputum samples can be prepared with potassium hydroxide (KOH) or calcofluour white (CFW), although these methods lack sensitivity.

Coccidioides can be cultured on a wide variety of culture media, including some bacterial media. Visible growth is usually evident by 4 to 5 days. Identification is usually by direct microscopy of the specimen, but a nucleic acid probe for rapid identification is also commercially available. In vitro drug susceptibility testing has not been shown to correlate with clinical response and is not routinely performed in clinical labs. Culture of *Coccidioides* represents a potential risk to lab personnel as arthroconidia in culture specimens may become airborne and are highly infectious. Accidental lab exposure can be prevented with proper handling. Recently, real-time polymerase chain reaction (PCR) has been shown to be highly sensitive and specific for detecting *Coccidioides* without the need for culture, but is not yet commercially available.

Several serological tests have been used to detect coccidioidomycosis, including the tube precipitin, immunodiffusion, latex agglutination, CF, and enzyme immunoassay (EIA) tests. Precipitin tests become positive early in the course of infection (1–3 weeks), whereas CF and immunodiffusion tests are more delayed in their conversion to positive. The latex agglutination test is problematic. It detects both immunoglobulins G and M (IgG, IgM) antibodies; unfortunately, it is positive in up to 10% of normals and negative in 30% of confirmed cases of coccidioidomycosis. For these reasons, it is usually necessary to confirm the results of latex agglutination. The EIA test also detects IgG and IgM and is highly sensitive, but is not very specific and is often used as a screening test. The CF and immunodiffusion tests are important, because titers tend to correlate with the extent of infection and are useful with respect to prognosis and management. CF titers are greater than 1:32 or 1:64 in 90% of disseminated disease; however, a high titer is not always present in disseminated disease. That notwithstanding, a high titer by itself is not sufficient evidence to diagnose dissemination. The coccidioidal CF test may give some reaction in other fungal infections, most notably in patients with histoplasmosis. CF tests using spherulin antigen are even more nonspecific. The immunodiffusion test is ideally suited to demonstrate antigenic cross-reactivity. A new enzyme-linked immunosorbent assay (ELISA) for coccidioidal antigens has become available. This test has very good sensitivity and is technically much easier to automate and more widely available than the older tests. At this point in time, it may be best to confirm positive ELISA test results with one of the other serologic tests described above. This is particularly the case for following the patient, as it is sometimes difficult to correlate the results of this test with benchmarks established for CF antibody levels.

TREATMENT

Treatment considerations are largely influenced by the specifics of the case, such as the extent of disease, the immune response, and risk factors such as age, gender, and ethnicity. It is necessary to establish the extent of disease, particularly involvement of the central nervous system or bones, as well as the immune response of the host to the infection in terms of cell-mediated immunity and antibody response. These steps will allow a better estimation of the prognosis, as well as establish a baseline that is necessary to monitor treatment.

Amphotericin B was the first antifungal that showed efficacy in the treatment of coccidioidomycosis and, for many years, was the drug of choice for this and many other fungal infections. Amphotericin B is not absorbed orally, tissue distribution is poor, and it is highly toxic. For these reasons, it is not considered the drug of choice in many situations.

Many experts now consider the triazoles, fluconazole and itraconazole, to be first-line drugs to treat coccidioidomycosis. They have been demonstrated to be efficacious in open trials. Each should be started at 400 mg/day. Fluconazole can be given intravenously or at higher doses as needed. Fluconazole or itraconazole at a dose of 400 mg/day is effective in more than half the cases. Itraconazole is more toxic, particularly at higher doses, and interacts with many drugs. Itraconazole is not available in a parenteral formulation and has unacceptable toxicities at dosages of more than 600 mg/day. A liquid formulation is available and, while more costly, does result in higher blood levels. Fluconazole is less toxic and can be given at much higher doses in those cases that do not respond to conventional doses. In refractory cases, as much as 2 g/day can be given without toxicity. In these cases, the dose can be lowered when control of the disease is established. Treatment with a 400 mg/day dose of fluconazole is well-tolerated and fairly effective for the treatment of chronic coccidioidomycosis. However, alopecia is a side effect associated with higher doses (400 mg/day) or long-term use. Alopecia is usually reversed when therapy is stopped. Although ketoconazole is active against *Coccidioides*, the safety margin is small, and at the effective dose, 200 to 600 mg/day, it may cause gastrointestinal irritation, hepatitis, and adrenal and testicular dysfunction. The newer extended-spectrum azole antifungals, voriconazole and posaconazole, have activity against coccidioidomycosis and have been shown to be effective in cases refractory to treatment with standard therapy, however have not been studied in systematic trials. Relapse is a risk when treatment with any antifungal is completed. Relapses are seen in 50% of cases treated with ketoconazole and 25% to 30% of patients treated with fluconazole or itraconazole. Oldfield et al. confirmed a long-held clinical suspicion that negative skin tests and a titer of greater than or equal to 1:256 were associated with increased risk of coccidioidomycosis relapse.

With the advent of the azoles, amphotericin B has been moved to a niche drug. Reduction in kidney function is a nearly universal side effect of this drug. This complication can be highly problematic, particularly in diabetic patients. Liposomal formulations of amphotericin are clearly less nephrotoxic. In addition, they alter the distribution of the drug, which can be a distinct advantage. Amphotericin B or its liposomal formulations are very useful, but only for special situations, for example, patients who are pregnant, those who are critically ill, and those who have failed therapy with azoles.

Coccidioidal meningitis is usually treated with fluconazole, which has good penetration into the CSF. The best study reported the results of treatment with 400 mg/day; however, since the response is suboptimal, most clinicians start at 800 to 1,000 mg/day. Unfortunately, when the drug is stopped, meningitis is likely to recur. Occasionally, meningitis continues even with azole treatment. In these cases, amphotericin must be used. Amphotericin B is probably best considered as second-line therapy for meningitis. It does not cross the blood–brain barrier in concentrations needed to treat coccidioidal meningitis, so it must be administered intrathecally. Lumbar injections are easiest to deliver amphotericin to the CSF, but almost always result in chemical arachnoiditis. Cisternal injections may reduce the incidence of chemical arachnoiditis, but must be performed by a specially trained practitioner. An intraventricular catheter with an Ommaya reservoir circumvents some problems, but if outflow of fluid from the ventricles becomes obstructed, the drug may not get to the site of the infection.

In general, coccidioidomycosis is not a surgical disease. However, surgery is critical in several situations, specifically in establishing the diagnosis in difficult cases, for draining pus; in treating certain problems, such as life-threatening hemoptysis; or as an adjunct to medical treatment of tenosynovitis.

CONTROL AND PREVENTION

Control of coccidioidomycosis can be improved by early diagnosis, through careful clinical evaluation (including a thorough travel history) and specific testing, as well as individualized case management, including a multidisciplinary approach. Further progress is possible through scientific research efforts and intelligent institutional policies. Several promising vaccine candidates have been tested in animals, but an effective vaccine for humans is not yet available.

FURTHER READING

1. Galgiani JN, Ampel NM, Catanzaro A, et al; for the Infectious Diseases Society of America. Practice guideline for the treatment of coccidioidomycosis. *Clin Infect Dis.* 2000;30:658–661.

   Guidelines for management of patients diagnosed with coccidioidomycosis, covering the most common clinical manifestations of the disease.

2. Catanzaro A, Galgiani JN, Levine BE, et al; for NIAID Mycoses Study Group. Fluconazole in the treatment of chronic pulmonary and nonmeningeal disseminated coccidioidomycosis. *Am J Med.* 1995;98:249–256.

   Open-label study of fluconazole 200 or 400 mg/day for treatment of coccidioidomycosis. This study demonstrated the effectiveness of fluconazole, but relapses were high after discontinuation of therapy.

3. Oldfield EC, Bone WD, Martin CR, et al. Prediction of relapse after treatment of coccidioidomycosis. *Clin Infect Dis.* 1997;25:1205–1210.

   The authors report on their findings of a retrospective cohort study designed to determine factors associated with relapse after successful treatment of coccidioidomycosis. A peak CF titer greater than 1:256 and negative serial skin testing were associated with an increased risk of relapse.

4. Arsura EL, Kilgore WB, Caldwell JW, et al. Association between facial cutaneous coccidioidomycosis and meningitis. *West J Med.* 1998;169:13–16.

   Through a retrospective review, the authors determined that patients are more likely to develop meningitis if they have facial lesions than those with lesions on the body only.

5. Einstein HE, Johnson RH. Coccidioidomycosis: new aspects of epidemiology and therapy. *Clin Infect Dis.* 1993;16:349.

   A good summary of the extent of the epidemic of coccidioidomycosis in 1992 to 1994 and some of the clinical experiences arising from the epidemic confirming many presumed risk factors for poor outcomes.

6. Richardson HB Jr, Anderson JA, McKay BM. Acute pulmonary coccidioidomycosis in children. *J Pediatr.* 1967;70:376.

   Excellent description of coccidioidomycosis in the pediatric population.

7. Greendyke WH, Resnick DL, Harvey WC. The varied roentgen manifestations of primary coccidioidomycosis. *Am J Roentgenol Radium Ther Nucl Med.* 1970;109:491.

   Categorizes roentgenographic abnormalities. The article states that 46% demonstrated segmental pneumonias, 27% had minimal infiltrates, and 19% each had hilar lymphadenopathy or pleural effusions.

8. Wack EE, Ampel NM, Galgiani JN, et al. Coccidioidomycosis during pregnancy: an analysis of ten cases among 47,120 pregnancies. *Chest.* 1988;94:376.

   Ten cases of coccidioidomycosis during pregnancy are described. Three of these cases were diagnosed during the third trimester, two of which developed disseminated disease.

9. DiTomasso JP, Ampel NM, Sobonya RE, et al. Bronchoscopic diagnosis of pulmonary coccidioidomycosis: comparison of cytology, culture, and transbronchial biopsy. *Diagn Microbiol Infect Dis.* 1994;18(2):83–87.

   A retrospective review of bronchoscopic techniques for diagnosis of coccidioidomycosis. BAL cytology was only diagnostic in 42% of HIV-infected patients and 31% of patients without HIV. Culture was more sensitive.

10. Jaroszewski DE, Halabi WJ, Blair JE, et al. Surgery for pulmonary coccidioidomycosis: a 10-year experience. *Ann Thorac Surg.* 2009;88(6):1765–1772.

    A retrospective review of 86 cases of surgery for pulmonary coccidioidomycosis. The main indicatios for surgery was disease symptoms or progression despite antifungal therapy. Higher morbidity was seen after surgery for cavitary disease, with prolonged air leak and bronchopleural fistula as the most common complications.

11. Johnson RH, Einstein HE. Coccidioidal meningitis. *Clin Infect Dis.* 2006;42(1):103–107.

    An excellent review of diagnosis and management of coccidioidal meningitis.

12. Vincent T, Galgiani JN, Huppert M, et al. The natural history of coccidioidal meningitis: VA-Armed Forces cooperative studies, 1955–1958. *Clin Infect Dis.* 1993;16:247.

This new analysis of old cases of meningitis reviews the clinical course of 25 patients who had coccidioidal meningitis before the advent of effective antifungal therapy. Surprisingly, cerebrospinal fluid white blood cell count markedly decreased over time even without therapy.

13. Pappagianis D, Zimmer BL. Serology of coccidioidomycosis. *Clin Microbiol Rev.* 1990;3:247.

    A very nice review of the use of serology in the diagnosis of this disease.

14. Como JA, Dismukes WE. Oral azole drugs as systemic antifungal therapy. *N Engl J Med.* 1994; 330:263.

    An excellent general review of the antifungal agents available and their indications for certain mycoses.

15. Graybill JR, Stevens DA, Galgiani JN, et al. Itraconazole treatment of coccidioidomycosis. NA- IAD Mycoses Study Group. *Am J Med.* 1990;89:282.

    Open-label study of itraconazole (100–400 mg/day) for 51 patients with nonmeningeal coccidioidomycosis were considered for treatment with itraconazole. Of the patients treated, 57% achieved remission.

16. Masannat FY, Ampel NM. Coccidioidomycosis in patients with HIV-1 infection in the era of potent antiretroviral therapy. *Clin Infect Dis.* 2010;50(1):1–7.

    Immunosuppression from HIV has been recognized as a risk factor for severe coccidioidomycosis. In the era of potent antiretroviral therapy, the authors find that the incidence of symptomatic infection has decreased. Coccidioidomycosis infection was associated with lower CD4 counts.

17. Arsura EL, Bellinghausen PL, Kilgore WB, et al. Septic shock in coccidioidomycosis. *Crit Care Med.* 1998;26:62–65.

    Report of eight patients with septic shock from coccidioidomycosis. Infection was not diagnosed until after the onset of septic shock in five patients. Despite treatment with amphotericin B, there was 100% mortality in this series.

18. Bergstrom L, Yocum DE, Ampel NM, et al. Increased risk of coccidioidomycosis in patients treated with tumor necrosis factor alpha antagonists. *Arthritis Rheum.* 2004;50:1959–1966.

    Report of 13 cases of documented coccidioidomycosis were associated with TNF-α antagonist therapy.

19. Dewsnup DH, Galgiani JN, Graybill JR, et al. Is it ever safe to stop azole therapy for *Coccidioides immitis* meningitis? *Ann Intern Med.* 1996;124:305–310.

    Fourteen of 18 patients with coccidioidal meningitis had relapse with disseminated disease after discontinuation of therapy. Relapse occurred both soon and after therapy was discontinued. Relapse had serious consequences in some patients; three died.

20. Galgiani JN, Catanzaro A, Cloud GA, et al; for the Mycoses Study Group. Comparison of oral fluconazole and itraconazole for progressive, nonmeningeal coccidioidomycosis: a randomized, double-blind trial. *Ann Intern Med.* 2000;133:676–686.

    Comparison of oral fluconazole, 400 mg/day, or itraconazole, 200 mg twice daily, for progressive, nonmeningeal coccidioidomycosis. Overall response was higher with itraconazole (63% vs. 50%). Patients with skeletal infections responded twice as frequently to itraconazole as to fluconazole. Relapse rates after discontinuation of therapy did not differ significantly between drugs. Both drugs were well tolerated.

21. Kushwaha VP, Shaw BA, Gerardi JA, et al. Musculoskeletal coccidioidomycosis: a review of 25 cases. *Clin Orthop.* 1996;(332):190–199.

    A case series of 25 patients with musculoskeletal coccidioidomycosis. Only seven patients had a history of overt pneumonia. Delay in diagnosis was common. Surgical debridement was performed in all but one patient.

22. Stevens DA, Rendon A, Gaona-Flores V, et al. Posaconazole therapy for chronic refractory coccidioidomycosis. *Chest.* 2007;132(3):952–958.

    Open label study of posaconazole (800 mg/day in divided doses) for chronic coccidioidomycosis that was refractory to treatment with amphotericin B with or without an azole antifungal. Complete or partial response was achieved in 73%, suggesting that posaconazole should be considered for cases of chronic refractory coccidioidomycosis.

23. Schneider E, Hajjeh RA, Spiegel RA, et al. A coccidioidomycosis outbreak following the North- ridge, Calif, earthquake. *JAMA.* 1997;277:904–908.

    Report of an outbreak of coccidioidomycosis following a large earthquake.

Histoplasmosis
Omar Saeed and J. Jonas Carmichael

The term *histoplasmosis* refers to any one of a variety of disorders resulting from infection with the thermal dimorphic fungus *Histoplasma capsulatum*. Pulmonary histoplasmosis is an important cause of morbidity in the United States and Latin America. Up to 50 million people in the United States have been infected by *H. capsulatum* and up to 500,000 new infections occur each year.

Infections with *H. capsulatum* are ubiquitous within the major endemic ranges of the Ohio, St. Lawrence, and Mississippi river valleys. The distribution pattern reflects conditions favorable to the organism, such as humidity, moderate climate and soil components. *H. capsulatum* is fertilized by nitrogen-rich guano from birds or bats. Particularly high guano concentrations occur in areas such as old chicken coops, decayed trees, starling roosts, river or creek banks, and caves with bat colonies. Activities that disturb these sites cause aerosolization of spores and mycelial fragments that can be inhaled. Air currents can carry conidia for miles, exposing distant hosts. Although most cases represent isolated events, numerous epidemics have been traced to activities associated with high-risk exposures creating occupational hazards such as earth moving activities at landfills, construction sites, bird coops, or in caves.

PATHOPHYSIOLOGY

Inhaled spores convert to yeast forms and multiply within airspaces at body temperature. After an ineffective neutrophil response, alveolar macrophages phagocytize the yeast and spread the infection to hilar and mediastinal lymph nodes. The infection spreads hematogeneously and involves distant organs, as evidenced by the calcified granulomas found in the liver and spleen. The severity of the illness depends on the inoculum size as well as the immune status and underlying lung architecture of the host.

Acute Pulmonary Histoplasmosis

The clinical manifestations range from asymptomatic to life-threatening respiratory failure secondary to severe pneumonia. The majority of patients experience an influenza-like syndrome 1 to 2 weeks after infection. Acute pulmonary histoplasmosis is a self-limited condition associated with localized, diffuse or multinodular pulmonary infiltrates. Symptoms usually include fever, chills, headaches, and myalgias. However, if the patient is exposed to a large inoculum (e.g., a closed exposure to a high concentration of bird guano), bilateral infiltrates can progress to respiratory failure requiring mechanical ventilation.

Subacute pulmonary histoplasmosis is characterized by symptomatic illness persisting for more than 1 month, with focal infiltrates and hilar and/or mediastinal lymphadenopathy. Patients develop inflammatory manifestations such as pericarditis, erythema nodosum (in female patients), pleuritis, polyarthritis, and cystic coalescence of mediastinal lymph nodes known as *mediastinal granuloma*.

Chronic Pulmonary Histoplasmosis

Infection of distorted lung architecture in an emphysematous lung can cause chronic pulmonary histoplasmosis. Patients have a prolonged duration of symptoms lasting greater than 3 months with cavitary and/or reticulonodular apical infiltrates. Clinical and radiological findings can resemble reactivation tuberculosis with weight loss, dyspnea, productive cough, and hemoptysis.

Progressive Disseminated Histoplasmosis

Acute pulmonary histoplasmosis can be complicated by disseminated infection in patients who have cellular immunodeficiency due to human immunodeficiency virus (HIV) infection, malignancy, immunosuppressive therapy, or advanced age. Besides interstitial pneumonitis, the clinical manifestations are secondary to involvement of spleen, liver, bone marrow, lymph nodes, gastrointestinal tract, adrenal gland, integument, meninges, or heart valves, particularly the aortic valves. Patients often develop hepatosplenomegaly, and 5% to 20% of cases present with focal brain lesions or chronic meningitis.

Other Manifestations

Sites of *H. capsulatum* infection that heal and condense leading to nodule formation are called *histoplasmomas*. Typical central and concentric calcification does occur. The time required for a nodule to calcify is unpredictable, which may pose a problem in distinguishing it from malignant growth. Diagnosis can be challenging as some lesions might never calcify and biopsy samples rarely stain positive for the organism. *Broncholithiasis* occurs when calcified lymph nodes erode into the airway, causing respiratory symptoms. *Fibrosing mediastinitis* is a reactive, calcified fibrosis which can lead to compression of central vessels and airways. It is considered a late but serious complication of histoplasmosis, especially if it involves both lungs. Approximately 1 in 100,000 infected patients develops this condition, 20% of which will involve both lungs.

IMMUNOCOMPROMISED PATIENTS

Patients with an immunocompromised state, especially T-cell immune deficiencies, are particularly susceptible to histoplasmosis. In its endemic range, histoplasmosis is one of the most prevalent AIDS-defining illnesses. Those coinfected often have untreated severe AIDS with CD4 counts less than 100 cells/μL and high HIV RNA levels. HIV patients not on antiretroviral treatment are much more likely to be symptomatic with primary *H. capsulatum* infection, and the majority of those patients are found to have progressive disseminated histoplasmosis. Pulmonary involvement without dissemination is uncommon; however, 40% to 50% of patients with progressive disseminated histoplasmosis have pulmonary manifestations. HIV patients with progressive disseminated histoplasmosis manifest the fevers, night sweats, malaise, dyspnea, hepatosplenomegaly, adenopathy, and skin lesions seen in immunocompetent patients but often lack the focal infiltrate seen in acute pulmonary histoplasmosis. Bilateral, diffuse interstitial, or reticulonodular opacities are present in more than half of patients with progressive disseminated histoplasmosis, though the initial imaging may be normal. Other clues of progressive disseminated histoplasmosis include thrombocytopenia, anemia, leukopenia, hepatic enzyme elevation, and adrenal insufficiency. Advanced age, renal insufficiency, fungemia, aspartate aminotransferase (AST) levels greater than 2.5 times the upper limit of normal, and decreased platelet counts have been associated with increased mortality. Severe disease can progress to multiorgan failure or meningitis that carries a mortality approaching 50% even with appropriate antimicrobials.

Cell-mediated immunity is necessary for control of an infection with *H. capsulatum*. Histoplasmosis is a serious cause of infection in patients taking TNF-α antagonists and has complicated that therapy more than any other endemic mycosis. In a series of 19 patients from an endemic area on TNF-α antagonists who developed histoplasmosis, 17 (89%) patients presented clinically with progressive disseminated histoplasmosis and 15 (79%) had pulmonary involvement. In contrast to HIV patients, radiographic evidence of focal pneumonitis, nodules, or mediastinal lymphadenopathy may predominate, although diffuse, bilateral reticulonodular or military disease is associated with dissemination. The radiographic hallmarks of prior histoplasmosis such as calcified nodules, nodes, or splenic lesions do not portend an increased risk of acute pulmonary histoplasmosis or progressive disseminated histoplasmosis. Etanercept, perhaps by its limited effect on the full array of TNF forms and reduced induction of complement-mediated cell lysis, has been associated with fewer cases of histoplasmosis than infliximab and adalimumab. An immune reconstitution inflammatory syndrome (IRIS) can occur with cessation of TNF-α antagonists following a documented histoplasmosis infection. Although 42% of such patients in one series developed IRIS symptoms, all recovered with antifungals.

Solid organ transplant recipients rarely develop histoplasmosis, even patients with positive pretransplant *Histoplasma* serologies. A study of transplant recipients performed in an endemic area found no cases of histoplasmosis over 3 years of observation. A previous retrospective study also found it rare in these patients (1 case per 1,000 transplant-person years). If it does occur, unfortunately, it is typically manifested as progressive disseminated histoplasmosis. Cases develop late in comparison to other posttransplant infections, which suggests that the infections are primary rather than reactivation histoplasmosis.

DIAGNOSIS

The diagnosis of histoplasmosis is dependent not only on the characteristics of the infection (location, duration, severity) but also on other factors such as the patient's prior exposures, sampling, and the experience of the pathologist. An understanding of the limitations of the various tests is necessary to develop a testing strategy for each of the histoplasmosis clinical syndromes. A combination of studies that may include histopathology, cultures, antigen detection, and serologic tests are often needed to establish a diagnosis.

Serum and/or urine antigen and antibody testing has a higher sensitivity in patients presenting with acute, diffuse pulmonary disease (in which the fungal burden is presumably highest) than in localized or subacute disease. In progressive disseminated histoplasmosis or acute pulmonary histoplasmosis, *H. capsulatum* galactomannan antigen testing sensitivity is in the range of 83% to 92% and is highest if both serum and urine samples are tested. It is most sensitive in AIDS and in more severe disease. Complement fixation methods display a greater sensitivity than immunodiffusion testing (95% vs. 90%), though fixation lacks specificity and low titers can occur in patients with active disease. Unfortunately, these tests may be falsely negative early in the course of the infection or in the immunocompromised. They may be falsely positive from a prior illness or cross react with other fungal organisms that cause granulomatous diseases. In patients with a high clinical suspicion of histoplasmosis but negative testing, repeat antigen and antibody testing, bronchoscopy, and/or biopsy may be necessary. The utility of *Histoplasma* antigen detection in bronchoalveolar lavage specimens was supported in a study identifying antigens in 29 of 31 patients with mostly diffuse pulmonary histoplasmosis. The utility of polymerase chain reaction in lavage specimens is unclear. Though it is often positive in chronic pulmonary histoplasmosis, cultures and histologic specimens may be positive in only 40% of acute histoplasmosis cases.

When it is isolated in culture, *H. capsulatum* should never be regarded as an airway colonizer. Culture specimens are placed on Sabouraud dextrose agar incubated at 25°C for up to 6 weeks and diagnosis is confirmed by a highly specific DNA probe. Histologic specimens generally display caseating granulomas with mononuclear cell infiltrates and lymphohistiocytic aggregates. The small, ovoid, yeast-phase of *H. capsulatum* displays narrow-based budding on Gomori methenamine silver or periodic acid Schiff stains and is often confused with *Pneumocystis jirovecii*, *Candida glabrata*, or *Cryptococcus neoformans*. Patients presenting with reactive mediastinal fibrosis and histoplasmomas may have *H. capsulatum* identified on biopsy and evidence of prior infection with low grade antibody titers but rarely have positive cultures or antigen detection.

TREATMENT

Guidelines for the treatment of histoplasmosis have been developed by the Infectious Disease Society of America (IDSA) and the American Thoracic Society (ATS) based largely on nonrandomized trials, cohort studies, and expert opinion. Therapy should be managed by a provider comfortable with the administration, interactions, and monitoring of levels and toxicities of the necessary antifungals. Patients presenting with severe acute pulmonary histoplasmosis or progressive disseminated histoplasmosis should be treated with the lipid formulation of amphotericin B (3–5 mg/kg IV daily for 1–2 weeks) then transitioned to intraconazole (200 mg three times daily for 3 days, then 200 mg twice daily) for a total of 12 weeks in acute pulmonary histoplasmosis or 12 months in progressive disseminated histoplasmosis. HIV and AIDS patients are often continued on protracted intraconazole maintenance therapy at least until CD4 counts are greater than 200 cells/μL. Methylprednisolone or prednisone (40–60 mg/day or equivalent) can be used in patients with severe respiratory compromise or IRIS, but its use is controversial. Adrenal insufficiency from adrenal involvement by histoplasmosis should be considered in patients failing to respond to therapy and can be another indication for steroids. For mild or moderate acute pulmonary histoplasmosis, treatment is held until the symptoms progress or persists for greater than 1 month at which time initiation of intraconazole is recommended (200 mg three times daily for 3 days, then 200 mg once or twice daily for 6–12 weeks). Though resistance may emerge during treatment, fluconazole has been used as an alternative to intraconazole. With its reasonable side-effect profile, posaconazole shows promise in murine models of histoplasmosis and case reports of salvage therapy. Chronic pulmonary histoplasmosis treatment is similar to symptomatic acute pulmonary histoplasmosis but continued for at least 1 year with ongoing monitoring for relapse. Antifungal treatment is generally not recommended in mediastinal fibrosis or culture-negative histoplasmomas, though patients with vascular stenosis or airway involvement may require stenting. Other than excluding malignancy in at-risk patients or the removal of a complicated mediastinal granuloma, there is generally no role of surgery either in the removal of histoplasmomas or for mediastinal disease.

FURTHER READING

1. Ajello L, Chick W, Furculow MF, eds. *Histoplasmosis*. Springfield, IL: Charles C Thomas; 1971.
   Described the emergence of Histoplasmosis as a prevalent clinical entity over tuberculosis.

2. Kauffman CA, Pappas PG, Dismukes WE, eds. *Essentials of Clinical Mycology*. New York, NY: Oxford University Press; 2011.
   Brief review in focused text on mycology.

3. Cano M, Hajjen RA. The epidemiology of histoplasmosis: a review. *Semin Respir Infect.* 2001;16:109–118.
   Describes the history and groundwork to establish the epidemiology and ecologic features of histoplasmosis.

4. McKinsey DS, Smith DL, Driks MR, et al. Histoplasmosis in Missouri: historical review and current clinical concepts. *Mo Med.* 1994;91(1):27–32.

5. Chamany S, Mirza SA, Fleming JW, et al. A large histoplasmosis outbreak among high school students in Indiana, 2001. *Pediatr Infect Dis J.* 2004;23(10):909–914.

6. Furculow ML, Tosh FE, Larsh HW, et al. The emerging pattern of urban histoplasmosis: studies on an epidemic in Mexico, Missouri. *N Engl J Med.* 1961;164:1226–1230.

7. Huhn GD, Austin C, Carr M, et al. Two outbreaks of occupationally acquired histoplasmosis: more than workers at risk. *Environ Health Perspect.* 2005;113(5):585–589.
   Interesting description highlighting the occupational hazards of acute histoplasmosis in two outbreaks in Illinois among laborers at a landfill in 2001 and at a bridge reconstruction site in 2003.

8. Kauffman CA. Histoplasmosis: a clinical and laboratory update. *Clin Microbiol Rev.* 2007; 20(1):115–132.
   Comprehensive journal review with good discussion on diagnostic modalities.

9. McKinsey DS, McKinsey JP. Pulmonary histoplasmosis. *Semin Respir Crit Care Med.* 2011; 32(6):735–744.
   Exemplary review briefly but critically covering all aspects of histoplasmosis management.

10. Wheat LJ, Conces D, Allen SD, et al. Pulmonary histoplasmosis syndromes: recognition, diagnosis, and management. *Semin Respir Crit Care Med.* 2004;25(2):129–144.
    Review with good description on differentiating clinical presentations and appropriate evaluation and treatment.

11. Wynne JW, Olsen GN. Acute histoplasmosis presenting as the adult respiratory distress syndrome. *Chest.* 1974;66(2):158–161.
    Reference article of fulminant, acute histoplasmosis.

12. Baum GL, Schwarz J. Chronic pulmonary histoplasmosis. *Am J Med.* 1962;33:873–879.
    Reference article describing chronic pulmonary histoplasmosis.

13. Hage CA, Wheat LJ. Diagnosis of pulmonary histoplasmosis using antigen detection in the bronchoalveolar lavage. *Expert Rev Respir Med.* 2010;4:427–429.
    Critical review of the utility of BAL antigen detection for histoplasmosis diagnosis.

14. Wheat LJ, Wass J, Norton J, et al. Cavitary histoplasmosis occurring during two large urban outbreaks: analysis of clinical, epidemiologic, roentgenographic, and laboratory features. *Medicine (Baltimore).* 1984;63:201–209.
    Study reviewing the contrasting clinical characteristics of patients with cavitary histoplasmosis versus other forms of histoplasmosis.

15. Goodwin RA Jr, Shapiro JL, Thurman GH, et al. Disseminated histoplasmosis: clinical and pathological correlations. *Medicine (Baltimore).* 1980;59:1–33.
    Early description of the manifestations of disseminated histoplasmosis.

16. Hage CA, Ribes JA, Wengenack NL, et al. A multicenter evaluation of tests for diagnosis of histoplasmosis. *Clin Infect Dis.* 2011;53:448–454.

Study performed in 218 patients with different categories of histoplasmosis determining antigen detection in disseminated histoplasmosis is higher in immunocompromised patients than in immunocompetent patients and in patients with more severe illness.

17. Croft DR, Trapp J, Kernstine K, et al. FDG-PET imaging and the diagnosis of non–small cell lung cancer in a region of high histoplasmosis prevalence. *Lung Cancer.* 2002;36:297–301.

Study of 90 patients with FDG-PET imaging for pulmonary nodules in a region with a high prevalence of pulmonary fungal infection revealing a low specificity and NPV for identifying NSCLC.

18. Goodwin RA Jr, Snell JD Jr. The enlarging histoplasmoma: concept of a tumor-like phenomenon encompassing the tuberculoma and coccidioidoma. *Am Rev Respir Dis.* 1969;100:1–12.

19. Menivale F, Deslee G, Vallerand H, et al. Therapeutic management of broncholithiasis. *Ann Thorac Surg.* 2005;79:1774–1776.

20. Goodwin RA Jr, Nickell JA, Des Prez RM. Mediastinal fibrosis complicating healed primary histoplasmosis and tuberculosis. *Medicine.* 1972;51:227–246.

21. Lloyd JE, Tillman BF, Atkinson JB, et al. Mediastinal fibrosis complicating histoplasmosis. *Medicine.* 1988;67:295–310.

22. Baddley JW, Sankara IR, Rodriquez JM, et al. Histoplasmosis in HIV-infected patients in a southern regional medical center: poor prognosis in the era of highly active antiretroviral therapy. *Diagn Microbiol Infect Dis.* 2008;62(2):151–156.

Cohort of 46 HIV-infected patients with related histoplasmosis defining the increased poor outcomes and mortality associated with fungemia, renal insufficiency, and older age.

23. Wheat LJ, Connolly-Stringfield PA, Baker RL, et al. Disseminated histoplasmosis in the acquired immune deficiency syndrome: clinical findings, diagnosis and treatment, and review of the literature. *Medicine.* 1990;69(6):361.

Early review describing the clinical characteristics of disseminated histoplasmosis in a pre-highly active antiretroviral therapy era.

24. Conces DJ, Stockberger SM, Tarver RD, et al. Disseminated histoplasmosis in AIDS: findings on chest radiographs. *AJR Am J Roentgenol.* 1993;160(1):15–19.

25. de Francesco Daher E, de Sousa Barros FA, da Silva Junior GB, et al. Risk factors for death in acquired immunodeficiency syndrome-associated disseminated histoplasmosis. *Am J Trop Med Hyg.* 2006;74(4):600–603.

Retrospective study of 164 HIV-infected patients with disseminated histoplasmosis identifying low hemoglobin levels, increased serum AST levels, acute renal failure, and respiratory insufficiency as independent risk factors for death.

26. Couppié P, Aznar C, Carme B, et al. American histoplasmosis in developing countries with a special focus on patients with HIV: diagnosis, treatment, and prognosis. *Curr Opin Infect Dis.* 2006;19(5):443–449.

Review describing the variable presentation, diagnosis, and management difficulties in resource-poor countries.

27. McKinsey DS, Spiegel RA, Hutwagner L, et al. Prospective study of histoplasmosis in patients infected with human immunodeficiency virus: incidence, risk factors, and pathophysiology. *Clin Infect Dis.* 1997;24(6):1195–1203.

Cohort of 304 HIV-infected patients with histoplasmosis describing the incidence (4.7%), characteristics, symptoms, and risk factors for infection (exposure to coops, positive baseline serology, and CD4 lymphocyte count <150).

28. Hage CA, Bowyer S, Tarvin SE, et al. Recognition, diagnosis, and treatment of histoplasmosis complicating tumor necrosis factor blocker therapy. *Clin Infect Dis.* 2010;50(1):85–92.

General review of the reported cases of histoplasmosis presenting during TNF blocker therapy providing a methodical discussion of diagnosis, treatment, immune reconstitution, and prevention in the emerging group of patients.

29. Olson TC, Bongartz T, Crowson CS, et al. Histoplasmosis infection in patients with rheumatoid arthritis, 1998–2009. *BMC Infect Dis.* 2011;11(1):145.

Single center review of the presentation and treatment of 26 patients with rheumatoid arthritis describing longstanding arthritis and multiple immunomodulatory agents, specifically anti-TNF treatment as risk factors for infection.

30. Vail G, Young R, Wheat L, et al. Incidence of histoplasmosis following allogeneic bone marrow transplant or solid organ transplant in a hyperendemic area. *Transpl Infect Dis.* 2002;4(3):148–151.

    Retrospective review of 137 allogenic bone marrow and 449 solid organ transplant patients performed in an endemic area with no histoplasmosis identified over a mean of 16 months follow-up.

31. Cuellar-Rodriguez J, Avery R, Lard M, et al. Histoplasmosis in solid organ transplant recipients: 10 years of experience at a large transplant center in an endemic area. *Clin Infect Dis.* 2009;49(5):710–716.

    Large retrospective study of 3,436 solid organ transplant patients identifying the potential utility of prophylactic treatment and low incidence (1 case per 1,000 transplant-person-years) of posttransplant histoplasmosis.

32. Wheat LJ, Slama TG, Norton JA, et al. Risk factors for disseminated or fatal histoplasmosis: analysis of a large urban outbreak. *Ann Intern Med.* 1982;96(2):159.

    Classic description of an outbreak of 488 histoplasmosis infections in an endemic area identifying age greater than 54 years and immunosuppression as the only risk factors for disseminated or fatal infection.

33. Hage CA, Davis TE, Fuller D, et al. Diagnosis of histoplasmosis by antigen detection in BAL fluid. *Chest.* 2010;137(3):623–628.

    Study determining the diagnostic performance of the quantitative antigen detection assay in comparison with serum and urine antigen detection.

34. Wheat LJ, Freifeld AG, Kleiman MB, et al. Clinical practice guidelines for the management of patients with histoplasmosis: 2007 update by the Infectious Diseases Society of America. *Clin Infect Dis.* 2007;45(7):807–825.

    Recent IDSA management guidelines.

35. Limper AH, Knox KS, Sarosi GA, et al. An official American Thoracic Society statement: treatment of fungal infections in adult pulmonary and critical care patients. *Am J Respir Crit Care Med.* 2011;183(1):96–128.

    Recent ATS treatment guidelines.

36. La Hoz RM, Loyd JE, Wheat LJ, et al. How I treat histoplasmosis. *Curr Fungal Infect Rep.* 2012:1–8.

    Current review of the pharmacologic management of the different manifestations of histoplasmosis.

Blastomycosis
David Wayne Dockweiler

Blastomycosis is a relatively uncommon disease caused by the dimorphic fungus *Blastomyces dermatitidis*. After inhalation of fungal spores by the host, the organism may give rise to a spectrum of clinical syndromes ranging from an acute, self-limited, flulike illness to rapidly progressive, widely disseminated, fatal disease. The primary reservoir for human infection is soil that is moist and rich in organic debris.

The vast majority of cases have been described in North America in endemic areas that include the southeastern and south-central United States and the region around the Great Lakes; thus, the disease also has been known as North American blastomycosis. With the demonstration of cases in Europe, Africa, South America, and the Middle East, this term is clearly no longer appropriate.

Blastomycosis most often is a disease of young to middle-aged men, although cases have been described in both sexes and in ages ranging from newborn to the elderly. A significant number of patients have a history of outdoor activities, especially hunting. Interestingly, canine blasto-mycosis, a condition similar to human disease, is more commonly seen in animals that are used in hunting, pointing to exposure of both humans and animals from a common outdoor source. Blastomycosis is not considered an opportunistic infection, per se, and has not been identified in immunocompromised patients to the same degree as other fungal pathogens, such as histoplas-mosis or cryptococcosis; however, cases have occurred in patients with renal transplants, chronic steroid use, and AIDS. Not surprisingly, disseminated disease and an increased incidence of central nervous system (CNS) involvement are seen in such individuals.

Primary infection with *B. dermatitidis* almost always results from inhalation of fungal spores. Far less commonly, the disease is sexually transmitted through prostatic secretions or spread by maternal–fetal transmission. A laboratory accident associated with percutaneous inoculation has resulted in disease. Person-to-person transmission by aerosol has never been documented.

After deposition of the spores in the alveoli, an inflammatory response is initiated that consists of polymorphonuclear leukocytes, monocytes, and alveolar macrophages. Granuloma formation follows in most cases. Several clinical courses may ensue, depending on factors such as host resistance and the inhaled dose. First, there may be spontaneous resolution of mild or clinically silent pulmonary involvement that, in a presumably small number of cases, may disseminate. Second, there may be the development of acute pneumonitis with nonspecific symptoms, such as fever, cough, purulent sputum, chills, myalgias, pleuritic chest pain, and occasionally, erythema nodosum. Third, patients may present with a severe progressive pulmonary process leading to hypoxemia, respiratory failure, and prostration. Fourth, the infection may present as a chronic pulmonary infiltrate, easily confused with other fungal diseases or tuberculosis. Patients with this chronic form of blastomycosis often present with a long history of constitutional complaints, such as malaise, weight loss, chronic cough, fever, and blood-tinged sputum. Significant hemop-tysis is rare. Dissemination is said to take place in up to 70% of patients with chronic pulmonary blastomycosis, and multiple-organ involvement is the rule. Lastly, there may be disseminated disease, which may occur with the previously mentioned patterns of pulmonary involvement or in isolation, representing reactivation of the disease long after the primary focus of infection has resolved.

Although disseminated blastomycosis may present anywhere, the skin, as the organism's name suggests, is by far the most commonly involved organ. The skin lesions typically begin as small subcutaneous nodules or pustules that may grow rapidly and ulcerate to form large verru-cous ulcers with heaped-up edges. Although skin lesions may occur at any site, the face and trunk are favored. Bony lesions, typically osteolytic, are next in frequency. Areas commonly involved include the vertebral bodies, skull, ribs, long bones, and pelvis. Overlying soft tissue may be in-volved, joint spaces may be infected by direct extension, and vertebral body disease may give rise to paraspinous abscesses. The male genital tract (epididymis, testes, prostate) has been estimated to be involved in about 10% to 30% of patients with disseminated disease. Infected prostatic se-cretions have been documented and presumably explain sexual transmission of the disease. Less often, laryngeal involvement is seen and may be difficult to distinguish grossly from carcinoma. Adrenal involvement with adrenal insufficiency has been reported. Meningeal blastomycosis is rare in immunocompetent hosts but occurs more frequently in patients with AIDS.

Roentgenographic findings are variable and correlate only moderately well with the clini-cal presentation. In patients with acute disease, the chest radiograph and computed tomogram (CT) are more likely to demonstrate pneumonic, consolidative, nodular, or interstitial infiltrates that are segmental or nonsegmental. Multiple lobes may be involved, though upper lobe in-volvement appears to be more common. Despite the relatively common occurrence of pleurisy, pleural effusions are unusual. Cavitary changes are unusual, seen only in up to 10% of cases. Chronic forms of blastomycosis are somewhat more likely to present as central mass lesions and may closely mimic bronchogenic carcinoma. Hilar and mediastinal adenopathy appear to be infrequent, even on CT examination. Lymph node calcification, common in histoplasmosis, is rare in blastomycosis.

Standard laboratory studies are nondiagnostic. Hematologic abnormalities (e.g., anemia, leukocytosis) are variable and rarely significant. Serum chemistries are usually normal. Skin testing for blastomycosis is not useful. Serologic tests are similarly unhelpful. An antigen test is available for use with urine, cerebrospinal fluid (CSF), and bronchoalveolar lavage fluid, and while sensitive, false positives occur in patients with histoplasmosis or paracoccidioidomycosis.

Definitive diagnosis of the disease requires the demonstration of the fungus in the tissues, either microscopically or by culture. *B. dermatitidis* is often found in sputum smears (potassium hydroxide [KOH] or Papanicolaou), bronchoscopy washings, pleural fluid, urine (especially after prostate massage), or tissue biopsy specimens. The organism is best demonstrated with methenamine silver or para-aminosalicylic acid (PAS) stains. Culture of the organism from all the above sources has a very high diagnostic yield, but growth may require up to 30 days, a problematic delay in the acutely ill patient. Once cultured, the yeast form of the fungus is relatively easy to identify microscopically, as *B. dermatitidis* grows in mycelial form when cultured at 25°C and as a single budding yeast with a characteristically thick refractive cell wall at 37°C. Because tissue colonization with blastomycosis does not occur, finding the organism provides a definitive diagnosis.

Although most experts agree that the majority of cases of blastomycosis are probably self-limited, treatment is now recommended for all recognized cases of both acute and chronic pulmonary blastomycosis.

In cases of mild to moderate pulmonary or disseminated disease, itraconazole at a dosage of 200 to 400 mg/day for 6 to 12 months is recommended. Like the other oral azoles, itraconazole is fungistatic and does not cross the blood–brain barrier; therefore, its use as monotherapy should be limited to treating immunocompetent individuals with nonmeningeal, non–life-threatening disease.

For moderately severe to severe pulmonary disease, disseminated disease, and in immunosuppressed patients where the CNS is not involved, an initial course of amphotericin B for 1 to 2 weeks is recommended. This should be followed by itraconazole for an additional 6 to 12 months with pulmonary disease, and 12 months with disseminated disease or in the immunosuppressed. In cases with CNS involvement, amphotericin B should be given for 4 to 6 weeks, followed by either itraconazole or voriconazole for at least a year. Pregnant patients should receive only amphotericin B as systemic azoles are contraindicated in pregnancy.

Corticosteroids may be helpful in treating refractory hypoxemia when acute respiratory distress syndrome (ARDS) is secondary to blastomycosis.

FURTHER READING

1. Bariola JR, Perry P, Pappas PG, et al. Blastomycosis of the central nervous system: a multicenter review of diagnosis and treatment in the modern era. *Clin Infect Dis.* 2010;50(6):797–804.

   Retrospective review of 22 patients with CNS blastomycosis leads authors to recommend voriconazole following initial course of amphotericin B.

2. Brown LR, Swensen SJ, Van Scoy RE, et al. Roentgenologic features of pulmonary blastomycosis. *Mayo Clin Proc.* 1991;66:29.

   In 35 cases of pulmonary blastomycosis, consolidation (26%) and mass lesion (31%) were the most common findings. Hilar adenopathy, pleural effusion, and calcification were uncommon.

3. Chapman SW, Dismukes WE, Proia LA, et al. Clinical practice guidelines for the management of blastomycosis: 2008 update by the Infectious Diseases Society of America. *Clin Infect Dis.* 2008;46(12):1801–1812.

   Recent treatment guidelines for blastomycosis.

4. Farber ER, Leahy MS, Meadows TR. Endometrial blastomycosis acquired by sexual contact. *Obstet Gynecol.* 1968;32:195.

   First well-documented case of sexually transmitted blastomycosis.

5. Hussein R, Khan S, Levy F, et al. Blastomycosis in the mountainous region of northeast Tennessee. *Chest.* 2009;135(4):1019–1023.

   Mass-type pulmonary lesions have become more common in this endemic region, and itraconazole has emerged as the therapy of choice.

6. Klein BS, Vergeront JM, Weeks RJ, et al. Isolation of *Blastomyces dermatitidis* in soil associated with a large outbreak of blastomycosis in Wisconsin. *N Engl J Med.* 1986;314:529.

First convincing demonstration of soil as the reservoir for the organism.

7. Kravitz GR, Davies SF, Eckman MR, et al. Chronic blastomycotic meningitis. *Am J Med.* 1981; 71:501.

    All three cases presented as a chronic meningitis and obstructive hydrocephalus developed. Cerebrospinal fluid cultures from lumbar taps were not diagnostic, but ventricular taps were.

8. Lahm T, Neese S, Thornburg AT, et al. Corticosteroids for blastomycosis-induced ARDS: a report of two patients and review of the literature. *Chest.* 2008;133(6):1478–1480.

    Refractory hypoxemia improved dramatically in two previously healthy men with ARDS secondary to blastomycosis after treatment with corticosteroids.

9. Martynowicz MA, Prakash UBS. Pulmonary blastomycosis: an appraisal of diagnostic techniques. *Chest.* 2002;121:768–773.

    Noninvasive specimens were positive on culture in 86%, compared with a 92% yield from specimens obtained by bronchoscopy.

10. Pappas PG. Blastomycosis in the immunocompromised patient. *Semin Respir Infect.* 1997; 12:343–351.

    Clinical disease in this patient population is much more likely to disseminate and involve multiple organs, especially the central nervous system.

11. Patel RG, Patel B, Petrini MF, et al. Clinical presentation, radiographic findings, and diagnostic methods of pulmonary blastomycosis: a review of 100 consecutive cases. *South Med J.* 1999;92:289–295.

    Clinical presentation was found to correlate with findings on chest radiograph in about 60% to 70% of cases. Diagnosis was made in most cases with sputum examination, culture, or cytology.

12. Saccente M, Woods GL. Clinical and laboratory update on blastomycosis. *Clin Microbiol Rev.* 2010;23(2):367–381.

    An excellent recent review.

13. Watts EA, Gard PD, Tuthill SW. First reported case of intrauterine transmission of blastomycosis. *Pediatr Infect Dis.* 1983;2:308.

    A case of maternal-to-fetal transmission of blastomycosis is described.

14. Winer-Muram HT, Beals DH, Cole FH. Blastomycosis of the lung: CT features. *Radiology.* 1992;182:829.

    CT scans of 16 patients with blastomycosis found a low incidence of pleural effusion and hilar and mediastinal adenopathy.

Aspergillus Lung Disease

Judd W. Landsberg

Aspergillus species are responsible for a diverse spectrum of human pulmonary diseases, ranging from hypersensitivity reactions to necrotizing angioinvasive infection. Overall, the incidence of *Aspergillus* lung disease is on the rise, largely as a result of increased numbers of immunosuppressed patients. Worldwide, *Aspergillus* is the most common cause of invasive mold infection. Although the host immune status influences disease susceptibility (e.g., allergic reaction with atopy vs. invasive aspergillosis with neutropenia), the notion that invasive disease is seen exclusively in neutropenic individuals is incorrect. Only 31% of patients with invasive pulmonary aspergillosis (IPA) are neutropenic when diagnosed. Increasingly, IPA has been recognized to occur in solid organ transplant patients, HIV infected individuals, and those receiving systemic glucocorticoid therapy for chronic inflammatory disease.

There are more than 200 species of *Aspergillus*, but *Aspergillus fumigatus* is responsible for more than 90% of human disease; the remainder is mostly caused by *A. flavus* (5%–10%), *A. terreus* (2%–5%), or *A. niger* (1%–2%). *Aspergillus* is ubiquitous and found worldwide in organic debris and soil. It commonly contaminates sputum and laboratory specimens exposed to unfiltered air. *Aspergillus* can be isolated from sputum in 1% to 6% of healthy individuals; higher rates of asymptomatic colonization are found in cigarette smokers and patients with chronic lung disease or HIV infection.

In the environment, the fungi produce small spores that are routinely inhaled and rapidly cleared from the normal host. However, inhalation in patients with underlying lung disease, immunologic sensitization, or immunocompromised status, may result in saprophytic colonization, hypersensitivity, or invasive disease. Person-to-person transmission has not been reported, but clustered mini-outbreaks of aspergillosis in immunocompromised patients have been reported from environmental exposure.

Aspergillus can cause at least seven distinct pulmonary syndromes, depending on host susceptibility and immune response, leading to colonization, allergy, or invasive disease. Patients with parenchymal lung disease are susceptible to (1) aspergilloma and (2) chronic pulmonary aspergillosis (CPA). Individuals with immune sensitization are vulnerable to (3) immunoglobulin E (IgE)-mediated asthma, (4) hypersensitivity pneumonitis (HP), and (5) allergic bronchopulmonary aspergillosis (ABPA). Patients with even minor degrees of immune suppression are at risk of (6) IPA ranging from bronchopneumonia to vessel invasive disseminated disease and, less commonly, (7) tracheobronchial aspergillosis. Although each syndrome has a unique pathogenesis, there is significant overlap between these syndromes in individual patients (e.g., an individual with ABPA developing tracheobronchial aspergillosis after high-dose prednisone therapy for a systemic inflammatory disease).

ASPERGILLOMA AND CHRONIC PULMONARY ASPERGILLOSIS

Aspergilloma (*mycetoma or fungus ball*) refers to a mass of fungal mycelia, inflammatory cells, and tissue debris, typically occurring in a preexisting, poorly draining lung cavity. Cavities occur most commonly in association with tuberculosis (TB), emphysematous bullae, treated lung cancer, ABPA-associated bronchiectasis, sarcoidosis, endemic fungal infection, chronic *Pneumocystis carinii* (PCP) infection (in HIV disease), and bronchial cysts.

An aspergilloma may be discovered on routine chest imaging in asymptomatic individuals or may be associated with recurrent mild hemoptysis. Most aspergillomas remain stable and up to 10% regress spontaneously. Typical imaging reveals an upper-lobe cavity with an intraluminal irregularity. Fluoroscopy may demonstrate mobility of the irregularity with positional changes. Sputum culture for *Aspergillus* may be negative in 50% of cases. Serum IgG *Aspergillus*-specific antibodies are present in over 90% of patients with associated cavitation and fibrosis, but may be falsely negative in patients on systemic corticosteroids, or in patients infected with non-*Aspergillus* species. *Aspergillus* skin testing is uniformly negative in patients with aspergilloma. Lesions tend to be solitary, but bilateral disease occurs in 5% to 10%. Asymptomatic patients with stable chest imaging require no antifungal therapy.

Simple aspergillomas and asthmatics with ABPA may progress to CPA. Classically called chronic invasive aspergillosis or chronic necrotizing aspergillosis, CPA encompasses a spectrum of indolent *Aspergillus* infections occurring in patients with underlying lung disease and often mild degrees of immunosuppression in which saprophytic colonization of abnormal parenchyma progresses to local invasion, often in a fibrocavitary pattern. CPA typically occurs in middle-aged and elderly patients with chronic obstructive pulmonary disease (COPD), late-stage ABPA, prior granulomatous disease (both mycobacterial and fungal), cystic fibrosis (CF), and other diseases involving parenchymal distortion. Patients may be immunocompetent but typically have varying degrees of mild immunosuppression secondary to diabetes mellitus, low-dose oral glucocorticoid therapy, alcoholism, poor nutrition, or connective tissue disease. Some patients with CPA appear to have an immune predisposition involving both a poor antibody response to polysaccharide antigens and a failure to produce interferon-γ (IFN-γ) (a recent therapeutic target). Clinically, patients complain of weight loss (94%), dry cough (78%), recurrent hemoptysis (58%), and dyspnea (50%). Fever and sputum production are less common and should prompt consideration for bacterial infection. Imaging typically demonstrates multiple upper-lobe, often confluent thick-walled, cavities with intraluminal irregularities, associated fibrosis, and adjacent pleural thickening. Up to 70% of these patients do not have a clearly discernible fungus ball. Given the presence of underlying lung disease, old imaging studies are essential to look for subtle changes surrounding preexisting areas of parenchymal scar, cavity, or aspergilloma. The presence of a significant air fluid level suggests bacterial superinfection more than CPA.

Biopsy is the diagnostic gold standard. However, given the poor yield from transbronchial biopsy and complications associated with transthoracic, thoracoscopic or open-lung biopsy in patients with severe underlying lung disease, diagnosis is usually made on clinical grounds. Diagnostic criteria include (1) compatible clinical and radiographic features; (2) isolation of *Aspergillus* species in sputum or bronchoalveolar lavage (BAL) fluid. If cultures are negative but suspicion is high, the presence of a positive galactomannan test (BAL more sensitive than serum) and/or IgG-specific *Aspergillus* antibodies can further suggest the diagnosis; and (3) exclusion of other conditions with similar presentations (e.g., active TB, atypical mycobacterial infection, bacterial superinfection, endemic fungal infection, and lung cancer), often through combined BAL, serology results, and close clinical and radiographic follow-up. Patients with ongoing parenchymal destruction (increased cavity size, wall thickness, and fibrosis) are at risk of worsening lung function, recurrent bacterial superinfection, and massive hemoptysis.

Bronchial artery embolization is an appropriate initial step in the management of massive, life-threatening, hemoptysis, though recurrent bleeding from collateral blood vessels is very common. Although surgical resection of the cavity provides definitive treatment, mortality (7%) and morbidity (23%) can be very high in the presence of coexisting lung disease. Younger patients without significant underlying lung disease have significantly lower rates of morbidity (18%) and mortality (1.5%). In general, surgery is reserved for patients with massive hemoptysis who have adequate pulmonary reserve and fail embolization.

Clinically symptomatic and or radiographically progressive CPA requires antifungal therapy. Immunocompetent patients, with subacute disease can typically be treated with oral itraconazole (more data) or voriconazole (better absorption and tissue penetration). The duration of therapy ranges from 6 months to lifelong chronic suppressive therapy for patients with substantial immunosuppression. Imaging improves gradually with cavity walls thinning and intraluminal irregularities resolving. Surgical resection is rarely an option, reserved for the young patient with focal disease and good pulmonary reserve. Treatment failures should prompt consideration for drug-level testing and possible IV therapy as well as the possibility of common disease mimics (e.g., bacterial superinfection or lung cancer). The long-term prognosis for patients with CPA has not been well studied, but 2-year survival is reported to be 70%, with the majority of deaths attributed to underlying lung disease or comorbidities, rather than *Aspergillus* infection.

IgE-MEDIATED ASTHMA

Patients with severe extrinsic IgE-mediated asthma attributable to environmental *Aspergillus* antigens (a.k.a. severe asthma with fungal sensitization) must be differentiated from those with asthma and ABPA. Immediate skin test reactivity to *Aspergillus* is present in as many as 25% to 40% of patients in asthma clinics. The absence of bronchiectasis, mucus plugging, and elevated IgE levels (<2,400 ng/mL or <1,000 IU/mL) argues against ABPA in this group. As in all allergic asthma, both avoidance of antigen (e.g., gardening, moldy environments) and anti-inflammatory therapy are mainstays.

HYPERSENSITIVITY PNEUMONITIS

Inhalation of organic matter contaminated with *Aspergillus* species has been associated with HP. *Aspergillus* antigens are associated with malt worker's lung, paper mill worker's lung, and, more recently, a cluster of hypersensitivity pneumonitis cases in plaster workers exposed to *Aspergillus*-contaminated esparto fibers.

ALLERGIC BRONCHOPULMONARY ASPERGILLOSIS

ABPA refers to a clinical syndrome involving a hypersensitivity to *A. fumigatus* which compli-cates asthma and CF. It is characterized by episodic chest radiograph infiltrates, IgE elevations, and poorly controlled asthma (20% of the time, asthma is well controlled on medications). The peak incidence is in the fourth to fifth decades. The clinical course is characterized by a cough productive of golden-brown sputum plugs (containing *Aspergillus* hyphae), hemoptysis, intermittent fever, chest pain, and recurrent pneumonias. Often, there is a discrepancy between significant chest radiograph consolidation and muted clinical findings. During disease flares, serum IgE levels are typically elevated greater than 1,000 ng/mL. After disease is established, exacerbations may be clinically silent, requiring vigilant chest radiograph and serum IgE surveil-lance. While ABPA may remain quiescent for many years, it rarely (if ever) resolves.

The pathogenesis of ABPA involves both failures in innate and adaptive immunity which al-low persistence of *Aspergillus* spores in the tracheobronchial tree, which in turn germinate leading to hyphal growth. In the predisposed (HLA DR2/DR5) hyphal antigen, presentation leads to a Th2 predominant phenotype and increased total IgE, *Aspergillus*-specific IgE, pulmonary eo-sinophilic inflammation, and tissue damage. Radiographic findings include fleeting upper-lobe infiltrates, branching homogeneous (gloved finger) shadows of mucoid impaction, and tramline and ring shadows indicative of thickened bronchial walls. Computed tomographic (CT) scans may identify central bronchiectasis (medial two-thirds of the chest) that classically terminates abruptly, leaving distal airways uninvolved. More recent imaging series suggest ABPA bronchiec-tasis may involve distal airways up to 40% of the time. Recurrent episodes of ABPA with mucus plugging and airway inflammation can lead to end-stage bronchiectasis, mixed obstructive–re-strictive lung disease, and respiratory failure. ABPA has been historically classified by the pres-ence or absence of bronchiectasis and clinically staged according to disease activity. Recently, the International Society of Human and Animal Mycology (ISHAM) convened a working group of experts entitled "ABPA in asthmatics" to refine the classification and staging of ABPA. Though not yet widely adopted, the refinements address some the most significant misconceptions and vagaries in the previous classification and staging scheme, and thus will be discussed here. Ad-ditionally, they suggest the concept that central bronchiectasis is a *sine qua non* for the diagnosis of ABPA should be replaced by the CT finding of high attenuation mucus (HAM) impaction, a finding purported to be pathognomonic for ABPA, as well as predicting relapsing progressive dis-ease. Typical mucus impaction is low attenuation. In general, treatment focuses on both control of inflammation with steroids and decreasing organism burden with antifungals.

Traditionally, the essential features required for the diagnosis of ABPA are (1) asthma, (2) immediate cutaneous reactivity to *Aspergillus* and, in patients not on systemic glucocorticoids, (3) total serum (IgE) greater than 1,000 ng/mL, (4) elevated serum IgE-Af, and/or (5) IgG-Af specific to *Aspergillus*. Common, but not required features include (6) episodic chest radiograph infiltrates and (7) peripheral eosinophilia. During flares, sputum stains may be positive for fungal elements and cultures positive for *Aspergillus*. To improve diagnostic accuracy, ISHAM experts recommend that a diagnosis of ABPA requires *all* of the following characteristics: (1) predisposing condition (asthma or CF), (2) type I allergic response to *Aspergillus* (positive serum IgE-Af or skin test), and (3) total IgE elevation greater than 2,400 ng/mL (1,000 IU/mL) during a flare (this is higher than the current accepted cutoff of 1,000 ng/mL). Individuals then need two of the following three: (1) positive IgG-Af specific to *Aspergillus*, (2) radiographic findings consistent with ABPA, and/or (3) total eosinophil count greater than 500 cells/μL during a flare. Patients meeting some but not all of the criteria are deemed "at-risk" for ABPA and should be followed expectantly. The differential diagnosis of ABPA includes allergic bronchopulmonary mycosis, IgE-mediated asthma, pulmo-nary infiltration with eosinophilia syndromes, helminthic lung disease, and other types of HP.

Patients with ABPA are divided into five clinical stages (without necessary progression): (1) acute, (2) remission, (3) exacerbation, (4) corticosteroid-dependent asthma, and (5) fibrotic. Stage 1 (acute) describes patients who initially present with classic ABPA. Most patients achieve stage 2 (remission), defined as no recurrence for at least 6 months after corticosteroid therapy is discontin-ued. Remissions can be sustained, but relapses have occurred as long as 7 years after initial remis-sion. Patients in remission should be followed with IgE levels every 3 to 6 months for the first year,

Stage 3 (exacerbation) occurs in 25% to 50% and may be clinically silent, consisting of only as-ymptomatic infiltrate or an increase in IgE levels (doubling from baseline is the generally accepted criterion for exacerbation, but 10-fold increases are common). As many as 45% become stage 4 (corticosteroid-dependent asthma). Infiltrates may or may not recur, and IgE levels are only variably elevated. Occasionally, the diagnosis of ABPA will be made at stage 4 during evaluation of a patient with long-standing steroid-dependent asthma. In this situation, serology is less useful. The presence of proximal bronchiectasis and/or HAM impaction on chest CT scan is very suggestive, as are previ-ous chest radiographs revealing fleeting upper-lobe infiltrates. Stage 5 (fibrotic) refers to patients with ABPA who develop mixed obstructive–restrictive lung disease with pulmonary fibrosis, often compli-cated by hypoxia, cor pulmonale, bacterial superinfection, and respiratory failure.

Treatment of ABPA should produce rapid improvement with resolution of infiltrates by 4 weeks, improved asthma, reduced sputum with clearing of *Aspergillus*, decreased peripheral blood eosinophilia, and decreased total serum IgE (by at least 35% in 6 weeks). Standard treat-ment for stages 1 (acute) and 3 (exacerbation) is prednisone 40 mg (about 0.5 mg/kg) daily for at least 2 weeks, followed by every other day dosing for 2 months. Prednisone can then be tapered rapidly and stopped unless infiltrates, clinical symptoms, or a rise in total serum IgE recurs.

Antifungals should be used if patients cannot be tapered off of prednisone or if patients suf-fer an exacerbation. A randomized clinical trial of itraconazole for patients with stage 4 ABPA (cannot be tapered) showed a 29% increase in clinical response rate over prednisone alone (with no significant adverse events). Another randomized trial demonstrated that itraconazole (400 mg/day) over 16 weeks resulted in fewer exacerbations requiring oral glucocorticoid therapy, reduced eosinophilic airway inflammation, and reduced IgE levels in patients with stage 2 (remission). Anecdotal evidence suggests itraconazole also may be used as a steroid-sparing agent for stage 5 (fibrotic) disease. The role of itraconazole and newer azoles in the treatment of stages 1 and 3 disease remains to be defined. A randomized controlled trial comparing itraconazole monotherapy to prednisone for stage 1 disease (MIPA) is currently underway.

Therapeutic bronchoscopy should be considered if proximal airway mucus impaction and collapse are not relieved with chest physiotherapy. Persistent proximal mucus impaction (>3 weeks) increases the risk of irreversible airway malacia. With adequate management, the prognosis for ABPA is good and long remissions are often achieved.

INVASIVE PULMONARY ASPERGILLOSIS

IPA represents a spectrum of acute invasive pulmonary *Aspergillus* infections occurring primarily in patients with prolonged neutropenia, but also in patients with only modest degrees of im-mune suppression. Although the majority of IPA occurs in patients with underlying hematologic malignancies (28%) or allogeneic hematopoietic stem cell transplants (HSCT) (25%), up to 9% of cases occur in patients with chronic lung disease and only modest degrees of immunosup-pression. Solid organ transplant (9%), AIDS (8%), autologous HSCT (6%), and other immune deficiencies (6%) account for the rest. Up to 2% of cases are reported in patients with no under-lying disease; therefore, the diagnosis of IPA should be considered in immunocompetent patients in the proper scenario. Individuals with chronic granulomatous disease and mannose-binding lectin deficiency are uniquely susceptible to invasive disease. The clinical radiographic pattern of aspergillosis varies dramatically based on the host's immune status. Patients with persistent neutropenia often have a fulminant course with rapid progression to vessel invasion, thrombo-sis, massive hemoptysis, lung infarction, and acute cardiopulmonary death. Individuals with milder degrees of immunosuppression more commonly present as typical or atypical bacterial bronchopneumonia, which if inadequately treated may progress to disseminated angioinvasive catastrophic disease. Reported mortality rates vary, and may be as high as 90% or as low as 16%, depending on the host's immune status, speed of diagnosis, and aggressiveness of therapy. While biopsy with culture remains the gold standard, CT scan, BAL, and galactomannan testing are the mainstays of diagnosis. Therapy is often started empirically based on clinical and radiographic features. Voriconazole is first-line therapy for IPA, and echinocandins are available for salvage therapy. Amphotericin B is typically reserved for salvage therapy, but may be used as a first-line agent if the diagnosis is uncertain and a significant concern for mucormycosis exists.

Invasive aspergillosis has become a leading cause of death in allogeneic HSCT recipients, in addition to being the most common cause of community-acquired pneumonia in those with graft-versus-host disease (GVHD). The epidemiology of IPA in allogeneic HSCT recipients reveals three periods of vulnerability: (1) after the first neutropenia during the conditioning phase, (2) associated with acute GVHD (<100 days posttransplant), and (3) associated with chronic GVHD (>100 days posttransplant). In fact, IPA occurs more commonly in allogeneic HSCT patients suffering from GVHD than in neutropenia patients. The clinical presentation of IPA is variable. Early in the disease, up to 30% of neutropenic patients may be asymptomatic. Initial symptoms will include fever, dry cough, pleurisy, and, occasionally, hemoptysis. If untreated, the disease will progress rapidly. Physical examination is nonspecific but may reveal a pleural rub.

CT is a significant tool in the early diagnosis of IPA in allogeneic HSCT recipients. The most common CT finding is multiple small nodules (<1 cm) seen in 43% followed by consolidation in 26%, large nodules and masses in 21%, and peribronchial infiltrates in 9%. Other less common findings include tracheobronchial thickening, pleural invasion, and hilar or mediastinal masses. The halo sign, a circumferential low attenuation ground-glass opacity surrounding a nodule (resulting from hemorrhage) occurs in up to 95% of patients at the time of diagnosis but is present in only 19% at 2 weeks. Conversely, the air crescent sign (necrosis of the nodule after neutrophils and inflammation return) is absent at diagnosis but present 63% after 2 weeks. Serial CT imaging should not be used to assess early response to therapy. Despite response, the volume of lesions typically increases 4-fold from the first week and then remains stable between days 7 and 14. The differential diagnosis includes pneumonia from other typical and atypical pathogens capable of causing multiple small nodules and/or necrotic consolidations in the immunosupressed (e.g., *Pseudomonas, Staphylococcus, Klebsiella, Nocardia,* viruses, mycobacteria, and other fungi), as well as neoplasm and pneumonitis from radiation or chemotherapy.

Invasive aspergillosis also threatens solid organ transplant recipients, especially lung and liver, often with a late onset (>3 months posttransplant). Cases have also been reported in individuals receiving every intensity of immunosuppressive therapy as well as immunocompetent critically ill patients. These nonneutropenic patients may present as a typical pneumonia with focal consolidations, ground-glass, and often nodular infiltrates being the predominant imaging findings. Cough and fever are typical but may be absent.

A definitive diagnosis of IPA requires lung biopsy, demonstrating septate hyphae with acute-angle branching in tissue (best seen with silver stain), and simultaneous growth of the organism in culture. Unfortunately, both transbronchial biopsy and sputum culture have a high false-negative rate. Thoracoscopic or open-lung biopsy may delay diagnosis and carry significant bleeding risk in the thrombocytopenic patient. For most patients at high risk for IPA, a less invasive diagnosis can be made by combining clinical, radiographic suspicion with the results of microbiologic and galactomannan testing.

Growing *Aspergillus* in sputum or BAL has a positive predictive value of 80% to 90% in very high-risk patients. Additionally, identifying branching hyphae on BAL cytology defines invasion in the right clinical setting. That said, other filamentous fungi have a similar appearance (e.g., *Scedosporium, Fusarium*). More recent data suggests the overall positive predictive value of growing *Aspergillus* in lower respiratory tract specimens is 72% for neutropenic patients and 58% for solid organ transplant recipients. Up to 50% of patients with invasive aspergillosis have negative cultures. Traditional *Aspergillus* serology (IgG-Af and IgE-Af) is not helpful in the determination of invasive disease.

Galactomannan is a polysaccharide produced during hyphal growth, detectable by an enzyme-linked immunosorbent assay (ELISA) Food and Drug Administration (FDA)-approved for the diagnosis of invasive aspergillosis. The FDA has licensed an OD index cutoff value of greater than or equal to 0.5 to represent a positive result. A meta-analysis of 27 studies with 4,000 patients found its overall sensitivity to be 71% and its specificity to be 89%. Sensitivity and specificity vary widely based on the prevalence of the disease in the tested population. In BAL specimens, using the same cutoff of greater than or equal to 0.5, the sensitivity is 93% and the specificity 87%. In lung transplant patients, the specificity of a positive BAL galactomannan has been reported as high as 95%. False positives occur most commonly in the first 100 days after HSCT possibly due to the combination of dietary intake of galactomannan and poor bowel wall integrity. False positives are also well documented to occur with piperacillin-tazobactam administration. False negatives commonly occur when treatment has begun.

The Infectious Disease Society of America (IDSA) and the American Thoracic Society (ATS) have published guidelines regarding therapy for invasive aspergillosis. Voriconazole is first-line. Herbrecht et al. found that after 12 weeks of therapy patients treated with voriconazole had improved survival (71% vs. 58%) and fewer severe side effects compared with amphotericin B. Voriconazole should be dosed at 6 mg/kg intravenously (IV) twice daily on the first day and then 4 mg/kg IV twice daily. For those who are unable to take voriconazole, liposomal amphotericin B, dosed at 3 to 5 mg/kg IV daily, is second-line. Caspofungin, an echinocandin, is a fungistatic peptide that inhibits the synthesis of fungal cell wall glucan and is approved for salvage therapy. It is often used in combination with voriconazole in this capacity (in lieu of compelling data). Caspofungin is dosed 70 mg IV daily for the first day and then 50 mg IV daily thereafter.

The optimal duration of therapy is unknown and must be weighed against the extent of infection, degree and rate of immune reconstitution, and degree of radiographic resolution. Practice guidelines suggest induction therapy with IV medication should be continued until the infection stabilizes, followed by oral maintenance therapy until complete resolution of radiographic findings or immune reconstitution occurs. The role of surgical resection remains controversial. Patients most likely to benefit from surgery are those with focal residual disease, often threatening a great vessel, and those who will be significantly immunosuppressed again in the future. The roles of granulocyte colony–stimulating factor (GCSF), IFN-γ, and other immune-based therapies are currently emerging.

TRACHEOBRONCHIAL ASPERGILLOSIS

Beyond the mucoid impaction seen in ABPA, *Aspergillus* causes a range of invasive tracheobronchial diseases in immunosuppressed patients. Tracheobronchial aspergillosis represents a unique presentation of IPA in which large airway mucosal invasion leads to thick, adherent, nodular plaques that cause endobronchial narrowing, obstruction, and significant distal plugging. The manifestations of tracheobronchial aspergillosis vary from obstructing tracheobronchitis to ulcerative tracheobronchitis, to an extensive pseudomembranous tracheobronchitis. Symptoms include cough, dyspnea, fixed wheeze, and radiographic evidence of atelectasis. Diagnosis is made by bronchoscopy with biopsy and culture. If the condition is not promptly diagnosed and treated, respiratory failure may result from airway obstruction, progression to frank IPA, or rarely perforation of the trachea or bronchi.

Beyond the obvious risk factors of hematologic malignancy and HIV infection, cases of fulminant tracheobronchitis have been reported in patients with only modest immunosuppression. Individuals with HIV infection and lung transplant recipients have a predilection for tracheobronchial aspergillosis.

In the 6 months after lung transplant, the bronchial anastomosis (BA) is uniquely vulnerable to saprophytic *Aspergillus* colonization and subsequent invasion, given its poor perfusion. The reported incidence of posttransplant *Aspergillus* colonization is approximately 30%, with isolated tracheobronchial aspergillosis occurring 5% to 25% of the time. The median time of diagnosis is 35 days posttransplant. Prognosis is good with a more than 80% response rate to combined antifungal therapy and bronchoscopic debridement. Mortality ranges from 1% to 5%. Residual airway complications after BA *Aspergillus* infection occur about 20% of the time, consisting mainly of bronchial stenosis and less frequently bronchomalacia. Routine, posttransplant surveillance bronchoscopy is recommended. Treatment consists of antifungal therapy for invasive aspergillosis and bronchoscopic debridement.

FURTHER READING

1. Agarwal R, Chakrabarti A, Shah A, et al; ABPA complicating asthma ISHAM working group. Allergic bronchopulmonary aspergillosis: review of literature and proposal of new diagnostic and classification criteria. *Clin Exp Allergy*. 2013;43:850–873.

An excellent review of the literature with an emphasis on genetic susceptibility as well as refined guidelines involving the diagnosis, staging, and management of the disease, written by the experts in the field.

2. Baron O, Guillaume B, Moreau P, et al. Aggressive surgical management in localized pulmonary mycotic and nonmycotic infections for neutropenic patients with acute leukemia: report of eighteen cases. *J Thorac Cardiovasc Surg.* 1998;115:63.

   Eighteen patients with hematologic diseases diagnosed with localized invasive pulmonary aspergillosis were treated with aggressive surgical resection. No perioperative deaths or complications occurred. Sixty-six percent of patients were alive after a mean follow-up of 29.1 months. No statistically significant difference was found between the invasive and the noninvasive pulmonary aspergillosis groups.

3. Binder RE, Faling LJ, Pugatch RD, et al. Chronic necrotizing pulmonary aspergillosis: a discrete clinical entity. *Medicine (Baltimore).* 1982;61:109–124.

   Original description of chronic necrotizing pulmonary aspergillosis as a clinical entity.

4. Buchheidt D, Weiss A, Reiter S, et al. Pseudomembranous tracheobronchial aspergillosis: a rare manifestation of invasive aspergillosis in a non-neutropenic patient with Hodgkin's disease. *Mycoses.* 2003;46:51–55.

   Case report of pseudomembranous tracheobronchial aspergillosis occurring in a patient with recurrent Hodgkin's disease.

5. Cornet M, Mallat H, Somme D, et al. Fulminant invasive pulmonary aspergillosis in immuno-competent patients—a two-case report. *Clin Microbiol Infect.* 2003;9:1224–1227.

   Report describing two cases of fulminant invasive pulmonary aspergillosis in immunocompetent patients with chronic lung disease treated with a short course of systemic corticosteroids.

6. Davies SF, Sarosi GA. Fungal pulmonary complications. *Clin Chest Med.* 1996;17:725.

   An excellent general review.

7. Denning DW, Riniotis K, Dobrashian R, et al. Chronic cavitary and fibrosing pulmonary and pleural aspergillosis: case series, proposed nomenclature change, and review. *Clin Infect Dis.* 2003; 37:265–280.

   An excellent review and case series of chronic pulmonary Aspergillus infection. This is the first detailed description of chronic cavitary and chronic fibrosing Aspergillus infection.

8. Herbrecht R, Denning DW, Patterson TF, et al. Voriconazole versus amphotericin B for primary therapy of invasive aspergillosis. *N Engl J Med.* 2002;347:408–415.

   Prospective randomized trial of 277 patients with invasive aspergillosis, 144 in the voriconazole group and 133 in the amphotericin B group. The survival rate at 12 weeks was 70.8% in the voriconazole group compared with 57.9% in the amphotericin B group, changing the standard of care for invasive pulmonary aspergillosis to voriconazole.

9. Husain S, Kwak EJ, Obman A, et al. Prospective assessment of Platelia *Aspergillus* galactomannan antigen for the diagnosis of invasive aspergillosis in lung transplant recipients. *Am J Transplant.* 2004;4:796–802.

   Prospective clinical trial investigating the utility of the Platelia Aspergillus galactomannan antigen test for the early diagnosis of invasive aspergillosis, in 70 lung transplant recipients. Although the specificity of the test was 95%, the sensitivity was only 30%.

10. Kahn FW, Jones JM, England DM. The role of bronchoalveolar lavage in the diagnosis of invasive pulmonary aspergillosis. *Am J Clin Pathol.* 1986;86:518.

    Demonstrated was 97% specificity, but only 53% sensitivity, of bronchoalveolar lavage in patients suspected of having invasive aspergillosis pneumonia.

11. Limper AH, Knox KS, Sarosi GA, et al; for the American Thoracic Society Fungal Working Group. An official American Thoracic Society statement: treatment of fungal infections in adult pulmonary and critical care patients. *Am J Respir Crit Care Med.* 2011;183:96–128.

    Diagnosis and treatment recommendations from the American Thoracic Society Fungal Working Group.

12. McCarthy DS, Pepys J. Pulmonary aspergilloma: clinical immunology. *Clin Allergy.* 1973;3:57.

    Serology findings in patients with aspergilloma.

13. McCarthy DS, Simon G, Hargreave FD. The radiological appearances in allergic bronchopulmonary aspergillosis. *Clin Radiol.* 1970;21:366.

    A classic description.

14. Mehrad B, Paciocco G, Martinez FJ, et al. Spectrum of *Aspergillus* infection in lung transplant recipients: case series and review of the literature. *Chest*. 2001;119:169–175.

   Retrospective review of 133 transplantations demonstrating airway colonization, isolated tracheobronchitis, and invasive pneumonia due to Aspergillus *species occurred in 29%, 5%, and 8%, respectively.*

15. Mennink-Kersten MA, Donnelly JP, Verweij PE. Detection of circulating galactomannan for the diagnosis and management of invasive aspergillosis. *Lancet Infect Dis*. 2004;4:349–357.

   Review reporting that in all studies thus far the specificity of the galactomannan assay was greater than 85%; however, the sensitivity of the assay varied considerably between 29% and 100%. Reasons for variable performance are discussed in detail.

16. Moreno-Ancillo A, Dominguez-Noche C, Carmen Gil-Adrados A, et al. Familial presentation of occupational hypersensitivity pneumonitis caused by *Aspergillus*-contaminated esparto dust. *Allergol Immunopathol*. 2003;31:294–296.

   Case report of a cluster of HP cases in plaster workers exposed to Aspergillus-*contaminated esparto fibers.*

17. Munoz P, Alcala L, Sanchez Conde M, et al. The isolation of *Aspergillus fumigatus* from respiratory tract specimens in heart transplant recipients is highly predictive of invasive aspergillosis. *Transplantation*. 2003;75:326–329.

   Study demonstrating that the isolation of Aspergillus *from the respiratory tract of heart transplant recipients is highly predictive of invasive aspergillosis.*

18. Nunley DR, Gal AA, Vega JD, et al. Saprophytic fungal infections and complications involving the bronchial anastomosis following human lung transplantation. *Chest*. 2002;122:1185–1191.

   Review of 61 lung transplant recipients who underwent surveillance bronchoscopy demonstrating saprophytic fungal infection of the bronchial anastomosis (80% Aspergillus, *20%* Candida) *in 24.6%. Infection was associated with bronchial stenosis nearly 20% of the time.*

19. Pfeiffer CD, Fine JP, Safdar N. Diagnosis of invasive aspergillosis using a galactomannan assay: a meta-analysis. *Clin Infect Dis*. 2006;42:1417–1427.

   A meta-analysis of 27 studies with 4,000 patients showing the overall sensitivity to be 71% and the specificity to be 89%.

20. Rello J, Esandi ME, Mariscal D, et al. Invasive pulmonary aspergillosis in patients with chronic obstructive pulmonary disease: report of eight cases. *Clin Infect Dis*. 1998;26:1473.

   A seminal description of hospital-acquired Aspergillus *disease.*

21. Robinson LA, Reed EC, Galbraith TA, et al. Pulmonary resection for invasive *Aspergillus* infections in immunocompromised patients. *J Thorac Cardiovasc Surg*. 1995;109:1182.

   In immunocompromised patients with hematologic diseases or liver transplantation with invasive pulmonary aspergillosis, early pulmonary resection should be strongly considered.

22. Rosenberg M, Patterson R, Roberts M, et al. The assessment of immunologic and clinical changes occurring during corticosteroid therapy for allergic bronchopulmonary aspergillosis. *Am J Med*. 1978;64:599.

   Serum IgE levels, both specific and nonspecific for Aspergillus, *are elevated in individuals with ABPA and mirror disease activity. Elevated IgE levels generally precede clinical exacerbations and fall toward normal in response to steroid therapy.*

23. Safirstein BH, D'Souza MF, Simon G, et al. Five-year follow-up of allergic bronchopulmonary aspergillosis. *Am Rev Respir Dis*. 1973;108:450.

   Oral corticosteroids may be important in prevention of long-term sequelae.

24. Salez F, Brichet A, Desurmont S, et al. Effects of itraconazole therapy in allergic bronchopulmonary aspergillosis. *Chest*. 1999;116:1665.

   An interesting report on the efficacy of itraconazole in long-standing ABPA in reducing steroid requirements and improving lung function.

25. Segal BH. Aspergillosis. *N Engl J Med*. 2009;360:1870–1884.

   Thorough, up-to-date review with an emphasis on the immunopathology.

26. Stevens DA, Schwartz HJ, Lee JY, et al. A randomized trial of itraconazole in allergic bronchopulmonary aspergillosis. *N Engl J Med*. 2000;342:756–762.

Randomized, double-blind, placebo-controlled trial of 16 weeks of itraconazole treatment in 28 patients with ABPA and corticosteroid-dependent allergic asthma, demonstrating a 46% response rate with no significant adverse events.

27. Wark PA, Hensley MJ, Saltos N, et al. Anti-inflammatory effect of itraconazole in stable allergic bronchopulmonary aspergillosis: a randomized controlled trial. *J Allergy Clin Immunol.* 2003;111:952–957.

A randomized, double-blind, placebo-controlled trial of itraconazole in 29 stable subjects with ABPA showing reduced eosinophilic airway inflammation, systemic immune activation, and exacerbations requiring glucocorticoid therapy.

Nocardiosis and Actinomycosis

Wael ElMaraachli and Antonino Catanzaro

INTRODUCTION

Nocardiosis and Actinomycosis are caused by bacteria in the genus *Nocardia* and the genus *Actinomyces*, respectively. These two organisms masquerade as fungi due to characteristic filamentous branching structures. They cause similar clinical syndromes that are nonspecific and diverse, and there is an inherent difficulty in cultivating either organisms; hence, their common presentations as masqueraders. Both organisms belong to the order Actinomycetales, but *Nocardia* is aerobic while *Actinomyces* is anaerobic.

NOCARDIOSIS
Microbiology and Epidemiology

Nocardia can be identified on Gram stain, with a typical appearance of delicate, Gram-positive, irregularly staining, beaded, branching filaments (hence, its previous misclassification as a fungus). It must be identified under oil immersion because of the extremely fine nocardial filaments (0.5–1.0 μm in diameter). The filaments can fragment easily into nondescript, coccobacillary forms. The organism is partially acid-fast due to the mycolic acid content of the wall.

Nocardia asteroides was formerly thought to be the most common species associated with human disease, but the group pathogenic to humans has been redefined as a complex that includes *N. asteroides, N. farcinica, N. nova,* and *N. transvalensis. N. farcinica* is more virulent than the others and more resistant to antimicrobials. It typically requires third-generation cephalosporins and tobramycin.

Nocardia species are not found in normal human flora. They are soil saprophytes, found worldwide in soil, decaying vegetable matter, and aquatic environments. They can become airborne, and inhalation is thought to be the most common mode of entry as evidenced by the observation that most infections involve the lung. Other modes of entry include ingestion and direct inoculation into the skin. There have been some reports of nosocomial transmission, but person-to-person transmission is generally not thought to occur.

The majority of patients with nocardial infection are immunocompromised (64% in one review). The most common causes of immunocompromise associated with nocardial infection are glucocorticoid therapy, malignancy, organ and hematopoietic stem cell transplantation, and

HIV infection (especially when CD4 cell count is below 100 cells/μL). Chronic lung disease and alcoholism are also risk factors.

Clinical Manifestations

The sites of infection in nocardiosis, in decreasing frequency, are pulmonary, systemic (≥2 sites involved), central nervous system (CNS), and cutaneous. Unlike actinomycosis, pulmonary disease is the primary manifestation of nocardiosis in the majority of cases. Pulmonary infection can be acute, subacute, or a chronic suppurative infection with periods of remission and exacerbation. The most common symptoms are cough, purulent (occasionally bloody) sputum, chest pain, weight loss, high fever, chills, and night sweats.

Acute nocardial infection can appear as an isolated lung abscess or a bronchopneumonia that may lead to a lung abscess. Consolidation and large irregular nodules are common, and they may be cavitary. Masses and interstitial patterns also occur. Pleural involvement ranges from simple, uncomplicated effusion to empyema. Lymph nodes can be enlarged. Spread to other parts of the lung or chest wall rarely happens; however, sinus tracts and perforation of the chest wall can occur.

Chronic infection can appear as small abscesses or chronic fibronodular disease. The lesions may be confined to a small portion of the lungs or scattered throughout the lungs. The later presentation may mimic miliary tuberculosis.

Extrapulmonary clinical manifestations depend on the site of infection. *Nocardia* frequently disseminates hematogenously and commonly spreads to the CNS, causing meningitis or brain abscesses. For this reason, it is prudent for all patients with nocardiosis to have diagnostic brain imaging (unless they are immunocompetent and the infection is confined to the skin).

Chest imaging can demonstrate single or multiple nodules, lung masses (sometimes with cavitation), reticulonodular infiltrates, lobar consolidations, and pleural effusions.

Diagnosis

Diagnosis requires direct visualization or culture of *Nocardia* in clinical specimens. However, the organism can be difficult to detect. The yield is much higher when the specimens are obtained through invasive means (bronchoscopy, percutaneous lung aspiration, and open lung biopsy) than in expectorated specimens. Gram stain shows the typical delicate, Gram-positive, irregularly staining, beaded, branching filaments that may have fragmented into nondescript, coccobacillary forms. The organism is partially acid-fast and must be identified under oil immersion because of the extremely fine nocardial filaments (0.5–1.0 μm in diameter). It does not stain on hematoxylin–eosin and will be missed on typical tissue biopsies unless special stains are performed. In routine culture media, 5 to 21 days are required for growth, so the microbiology laboratory must be informed and a request made to keep the culture plates longer if *Nocardia* is suspected. Polymerase chain reaction testing on samples appears to be sensitive and specific but is not clinically available at most centers.

Treatment

Successful treatment of nocardiosis includes the use of appropriate antibiotics and, if necessary, surgical drainage. Trimethoprim–sulfamethoxazole (TMP-SMX) is still the treatment of choice for nocardiosis infection. However, variable susceptibilities are now being reported. As a result, in severe disease (some cases of pulmonary disease, and any cases of disseminated or CNS disease), it may be best to begin with intravenous therapy with TMP-SMX and another agent such as amikacin for disease outside the CNS, imipenem for CNS disease, and both amikacin and imipenem for disease that occurs in the CNS and in other organs. After 3 to 6 weeks of therapy, switching to oral therapy may be considered, based on susceptibility. Several potential alternative treatments have been used, such as minocycline, clarithromycin, amikacin, imipenem, meropenem, linezolid, third-generation cephalosporins such as ceftriaxone and cefotaxime, fluoroquinolones, and amoxicillin–clavulanate. Species identification and susceptibility testing are useful in choosing a successful alternative treatment. The duration of therapy is uncertain, but 6 to 12 months is usually necessary to prevent dissemination or recurrence. Immunosuppressed patients should be treated for a minimum of 12 months, and an ongoing suppressive regimen should be considered.

ACTINOMYCOSIS

Actinomycosis is most often caused by *Actinomyces israelii*, and less often by *A. naeslundii/viscosus* complex, *A. odontolyticus*, *A. meyeri*, and *A. gerencseriae*. These organisms are filamentous, branching, Gram-positive, non–acid-fast anaerobic bacteria that were considered to be fungi in the past. However, responsiveness to antibiotics and a cell-wall composition established these organisms as true bacteria. They are normal inhabitants of the oropharynx, gastrointestinal tract, and female genital tract in humans. Men develop infection more often than women, but there is no occupational or environmental predisposition. In humans, the organism may cause disease in the cervicofacial, abdominopelvic, and thoracic area (in decreasing frequency). However, any site in the body can be affected. There is no person-to-person transmission, and infection usually occurs in immunocompetent individuals. Pulmonary infection is commonly caused by aspiration of organisms residing around carious teeth. The incidence appears to be greatest between ages 11 and 20, and 35 and 50, corresponding to the time when infection is most common in tonsils and teeth.

Thoracic actinomycosis can involve the lung parenchyma, pleura, mediastinum, or chest wall. There are several possible routes of infection, including aspiration of oropharyngeal secretions or gastric contents, direct extension of cervicofacial infection, transdiaphragmatic or retroperitoneal spread from the abdomen, or, rarely, hematogenous dissemination. Pathologically, infection results in a chronic granulomatous infiltrate, often with abscess formation. The organism is usually obvious on hematoxylin–eosin stain, forming a mass of filamentous hyphae staining densely with hematoxylin.

Clinically, pulmonary actinomycosis may present with cough that is often productive of purulent or blood-tinged sputum, as well as chest pain, weight loss, and fever that may mimic tuberculosis or malignancy. Chest-wall swelling may occur, although cutaneous abscesses or frank broncho-cutaneous fistulas rarely develop. Pleural extension with resultant empyema is a frequent complication of primary pulmonary actinomycosis; rarely, secondary bacterial infection may complicate empyema.

Examination may reveal rales, digital clubbing, and signs of consolidation or pleural effusion. Roentgenographically, actinomycosis may appear acutely as a diffuse alveolar-filling process typical of other acute bacterial pneumoniae. Alternatively, chronic infection may appear as a large mass, resembling bronchogenic carcinoma. This mass may extend across fissures or into the pleural space or chest wall, creating a soft-tissue mass or causing rib destruction. Extensive pulmonary fibrosis has been noted in a few patients with chronic infection. Extrapulmonary extension to the pericardium, mediastinum, pulmonary arteries, and beneath the diaphragm is a recognized complication to pulmonary infection. Hematogenous dissemination is rare.

The diagnosis of actinomycosis is based on demonstration of the organisms in tissue or pleural fluid, although this remains a difficult task. Advancements in both tissue sampling and radiographic techniques have improved our diagnostic abilities. In a retrospective review, a ring-like peripheral rim enhancement was seen on contrast computed tomography (CT) in 77% of patients with histopathologically proven thoracic actinomycosis. The presence of sulfur granules (white or yellow, 1- to 2-mm clumps of mycelia) in sputum or in drainage from a sinus tract is highly suggestive of the diagnosis; however, cultural confirmation is required.

Penicillin in large doses and for long duration is the treatment of choice. Administration should be intravenous for the first 4 to 6 weeks, followed by oral administration for 6 to 12 months. However, recent data suggest that short courses of treatment can be used, and that treatment can be tailored based on the initial burden of disease, whether surgical resection is performed, and response to therapy. Other effective alternatives are tetracycline, chloramphenicol, erythromycin, and clindamycin. One case report documents the successful use of a third-generation cephalosporin. There is also a small series of patients who were successfully treated with imipenem–cilastatin. A shorter duration of penicillin therapy was recently used successfully in two patients with esophageal and cervicofacial actinomycosis. To date, however, there are little data to support an abbreviated course in patients with thoracic disease. Suppurative lesions (empyema) should be excised or drained, or both. Surgical debridement of soft-tissue lesions is believed by some to be of critical importance. Appropriate therapy yields an approximate 80% recovery rate.

FURTHER READING
Nocardiosis

1. Sullivan DC, Chapman SW. Bacteria that masquerade as fungi: actinomycosis/*Nocardia*. *Proc Am Thorac Soc.* 2010;7:216–221.

   Excellent review of nocardiosis and actinomycosis that additionally compares and contrasts these two morphologically similar, but phylogenetically distinct, organisms.

2. Conant EF, Wechsler RJ. Actinomycosis and nocardiosis of the lung. *J Thorac Imaging.* 1992; 7(4):75–84.

   Another review of the two infections.

3. Menendez R, Cordero PJ, Santos M, et al. Pulmonary infection with *Nocardia* species: a report of 10 cases and review. *Eur Respir J.* 1997;10:1542.

   Reviews the clinical features and prognostic factors of 10 cases of pulmonary infection by Nocardia *species.*

4. Saubolle MA, Sussland D. Nocardiosis: review of clinical and laboratory experience. *J Clin Microbiol.* 2003;41(10):4497–4501.

   Review of nocardiosis with emphasis on the species isolate and, spectrum of disease in a series of infections in Arizona.

5. Uhde KB, Pathak S, McCullum I, et al. Antimicrobial-resistant *Nocardia* isolates, United States, 1995–2004. *Clin Infect Dis.* 2010;51(12):1445–1448.

   A 10-year retrospective evaluation of Nocardia *isolates submitted to the Centers for Disease Control and Prevention for susceptibility testing.*

6. Peleg AY, Husain S, Qureshi ZA, et al. Risk factors, clinical characteristics, and outcome of *Nocardia* infection in organ transplant recipients: a matched case-control study. *Clin Infect Dis.* 2007;44:1307–1314.

   Greater than 5,000 organ transplant recipients were followed, 35 of whom were identified as having Nocardia *infection. Independent risk factors for infection were assessed.*

7. Jinno S, Jirakulaporn T, Bankowski M, et al. Rare case of *Nocardia asteroides* pericarditis in a human immunodeficiency virus-infected patient. *J Clin Microbiol.* 2007;45(7):2330–2333.

8. Munoz J, Mirelis B, Aragon LM, et al. Clinical and microbiological features of nocardiosis 1997–2003. *J Med Microbiol.* 2007;56:545–550.

   Nocardia *isolates over a 7-year period were retrospectively reviewed to assess species distribution, pathogenecity, and antimicrobial susceptibility.*

9. Oszoyoglu AA, Kirsch J, Mohammed TL. Pulmonary nocardiosis after lung transplantation: CT findings in 7 patients and review of the literature. *J Thorac Imaging.* 2007;22(2):143–148.

10. Moylett EH, Pacheco SE, Brown-Elliott BA, et al. Clinical experience with linezolid for the treatment of *Nocardia* infection. *Clin Infect Dis.* 2003;36:313–318.

    Six clinical cases of nocardial infection (four had disseminated disease, two of these had brain abscesses) were successfully treated with linezolid, either as a monotherapy, or as part of a combination regimen.

11. Rivero A, Garcia-Lazaro M, Perez-Camacho I, et al. Successful long-term treatment with linezolid for disseminated infection with multiresistant *Nocardia farcinica. Infection.* 2008;36:389–391.

    The authors describe a patient with pulmonary and CNS nocardiosis. After discontinuing initial therapy for various reasons, linezolid was used and was continued for 17 months with resolution of the infection.

12. Khan BA, Duncan M, Reynolds J, et al. *Nocardia* infection in lung transplant recipients. *Clin Transplant.* 2008;22:562–566.

    A chart review of 410 lung transplant recipients was performed to better define the incidence of nocardial infection. The species isolated, their susceptibility patterns and clinical courses are described.

13. Naik S, Mateo-Bibeau R, Shinnar M, et al. Successful treatment of *Nocardia nova* bacteremia and multilobar pneumonia with clarithromycin in a heart transplant patient. *Transplant Proc.* 2007; 39:1720–1722.

In this patient, TMP-SMX had to be discontinued because of side-effects. Clarithromycin was used successfully.

14. Palmer SM Jr, Kanj SS, Davis RD, et al. A case of disseminated infection with *Nocardia brasiliensis* in a lung transplant recipient. *Transplantation.* 1997;63:1189.

A discussion of a patient's course with the unusual presentation of N. brasiliensis after lung transplant.

15. Yoon HK, Im JG, Ahn JM, et al. Pulmonary nocardiosis: CT findings. *J Comput Assist Tomogr.* 1995;19:52.

Discusses the computed tomographic (CT) results of five immunocompromised patients and recommends that nocardiosis should be included in the differential diagnosis with certain findings.

16. de Vivo F, Pond GD, Rhenman B, et al. Transtracheal aspiration and fine needle aspiration biopsy for the diagnosis of pulmonary infection in heart transplant patients. *J Thorac Cardiovasc Surg.* 1988;96:696.

17. Rodriguez JL, Barrio JL, Pitchenik AE. Pulmonary nocardiosis in the acquired immunodeficiency syndrome: diagnosis with bronchoalveolar lavage and treatment with non-sulphur containing drugs. *Chest.* 1986;90:912.

18. Garlando F, Bodmer T, Lee C, et al. Successful treatment of disseminated nocardiosis complicated by cerebral abscess with ceftriaxone and amikacin: case report. *Clin Infect Dis.* 1992;15:1039.

Actinomycosis

19. Brook I. Actinomycosis: diagnosis and management. *South Med J.* 2008;101(10):1019–1023.

Excellent review.

20. Mabeza GF, Macfarlane J. Pulmonary actinomycosis. *Eur Respir J.* 2003;21:545–551.

Excellent review.

21. Choi J, Koh WJ, Kim TS, et al. Optimal duration of IV and oral antibiotics in the treatment of thoracic actinomycosis. *Chest.* 2005;128:2211–2217.

A retrospective review of 28 patients with thoracic disease was performed in order to evaluate the duration of treatment.

22. Sudhaker SS, Ross JJ. Short term treatment of thoracic actinomycosis: two cases and a review. *Clin Infect Dis.* 2004;38:444–447.

Describes cases of esophageal and cervicofacial disease successfully treated with short-term antibiotic therapy.

23. Cheon JE, Im JG, Kim MY, et al. Thoracic actinomycosis: CT findings. *Radiology.* 1998;209: 229–233.

Discusses CT findings of 22 immunocompetent patients from a retrospective review.

24. Hsu WH, Chiang CD, Chen CY, et al. Ultrasound-guided fine needle aspiration biopsy in the diagnosis of chronic pulmonary infection. *Respiration.* 1997;64:319–325.

After studying 14 patients with abnormal chest X-rays, the authors found that ultrasound-guided fine needle aspiration biopsy was useful for pinpointing the diagnosis of chronic pulmonary infections.

25. Hamed KA. Successful treatment of primary *Actinomyces viscosus* endocarditis with third-generation cephalosporins. *Clin Infect Dis.* 1998;26:211–212.

A case review of a patient with endocarditis caused by Actinomyces species who was allergic to penicillin and treated successfully with third-generation cephalosporins.

26. Yew WW, Wong PC, Lee J, et al. Report of eight cases of pulmonary actinomycosis and their treatment with imipenem-cilastatin. *Monaldi Arch Chest Dis.* 1999;54:126–129.

A prospective study of eight patients explored the efficacy of treatment with imipenem–cilastatin. The study showed that this treatment alternative strategy shows promise.

27. Brown JR. Human actinomycosis: a study of 181 subjects. *Hum Pathol.* 1973;4:319.

Concise clinical review. Thoracic (lung or chest wall) involvement was present in 24%.

28. Frank P, Strickland B. Pulmonary actinomycosis. *Br J Radiol.* 1974;47:373.

   Most frequent alternative diagnosis is bronchogenic carcinoma. There is often a history of oral trauma, loss of consciousness, epileptic episodes, or dental caries.

29. Newsom BD, Hardy JD. Pulmonary fungal infection: survey of 159 cases with surgical implications. *J Thorac Cardiovasc Surg.* 1982;83:218.

   One hundred fifty-nine cases of pulmonary fungal disease treated at the hospital of the University of Mississippi are presented. This clinical review describes the presentation of the various fungal infections as well as the results of treatment regimens used at that hospital.

30. Smith R, Heaton CL. Actinomycosis presenting as Wegener's granulomatosis. *JAMA.* 1978; 240:247.

   Sulfur granules were absent in biopsied lesions. Ultimate diagnosis confirmed by an aerobic growth in thioglycolate broth.

31. Merdler C, Greif J, Burke M, et al. Primary actinomycotic empyema. *South Med J.* 1983;76:411.

   The clinical findings of this entity are described, along with a response to treatment with cefazolin and pleural drainage.

32. Smego RA, Foglia G. Actinomycosis. *Clin Infect Dis.* 1998;26:1255.

   An excellent concise review of the spectrum of disease, diagnosis, and treatment.

33. Sudhakar SS, Ross JJ. Short-term treatment of actinomycosis: two cases and a review. *Clin Infect Dis.* 2004;38:444.

   Two case reports of successful shorter durations of treatment for esophageal and cervicofacial actinomycosis.

Cryptococcosis

58

Wael ElMaraachli and Antonino Catanzaro

MICROBIOLOGY AND EPIDEMIOLOGY

Cryptococcosis is an invasive fungal infection caused by *Cryptococcus neoformans* or *C. gattii*. Meningoencephalitis is the most frequent manifestation of disease, but pulmonary disease is frequently seen as well. *Cryptococcus* is a single-budding yeast and has a thick polysaccharide capsule that is responsible for its characteristic visualization by India ink. *C. neoformans* has been categorized into four serotypes, A, B, C, and D, based on the immunologic properties of their capsular polysaccharide. Serotypes B and C are now considered a separate species called *C. gattii*. Infection due to the two species (*C. neoformans* and *C. gattii*) is generally indistinguishable, although there may be some important distinctive features in the type of host (*C. gattii* has more of a propensity to infect healthy hosts), and in the prognosis of intracranial infection in HIV-negative hosts.

   C. neoformans has been found in soil samples around the world in areas frequented by birds, especially chickens and pigeons, making cryptococcosis a mostly urban disease. However, human infection usually occurs without a history of direct contact with birds. *C. gattii*, generally occurs in the tropics and subtropics and is found in decaying vegetation, particularly the river red gum (eucalyptus) trees. An outbreak of *C. gattii* infections on Vancouver Island and surrounding areas of Canada and the Northwest United States was linked to the importation of eucalyptus trees from Australia. Most patients with cryptococcosis due to *C. neoformans* have underlying conditions that compromise cell-mediated immunity, such as HIV infection (dramatic increase in risk with CD4 cell counts below 100 cells/µL), lymphoproliferative disorders, corticosteroid therapy, organ transplantation, rheumatologic disorders, sarcoidosis, chronic liver diseases, and the use of tumor necrosis factor-α antagonists.

Widespread use of highly active antiretroviral therapy (HAART) has lowered the incidence of cryptococcosis in medically developed countries; however, it is the fourth most common opportunistic infection in AIDS. It is estimated that 1 million cases of cryptococcosis occur worldwide each year, with the largest burden in Africa. Prognosis in pulmonary cryptococcosis depends on the host's immune status. Immunocompetent patients usually recover without sequelae. In HIV patients, however, prognosis depends on the presence and severity of acute meningoencephalitis. Despite the availability of HAART and appropriate treatment, the 3-month mortality approximates 20%.

PATHOGENESIS AND CLINICAL MANIFESTATIONS

Cryptococcus is a basidiomycetous yeast that survives environmentally in the sexual form, producing hyphae with terminal basidiospores (chains of unbudded yeast). However, it is the asexual form (encapsulated yeast), which is found in clinical specimens. The portal of entry of the organism is the respiratory tract. Basidiospores may break off from the hyphae, become aerosolized, and are small enough to deposit in the alveoli. After inhalation, the yeast comes into contact with alveolar macrophages, and more inflammatory cells are recruited through chemokine release. In immunocompetent individuals, the yeasts can remain dormant in hilar lymph nodes or pulmonary foci asymptomatically for years and then disseminate outside these complexes if local immunity becomes suppressed. In cases of severely suppressed cell-mediated immunity, the yeasts reactivate and disseminate to other sites.

Several virulence factors aid in infection. These include an antiphagocytic polysaccharide capsule, and an enzyme that catalyzes the conversion of diphenolic compounds (such as dopamine) to melanin, which may have a biologic role in protecting the yeast from oxidative stress (hence the proposed propensity of the organism for the central nervous system [CNS], where there is an abundance of dopamine). In addition, its ability to grow at 37°C adds to its virulence.

Clinical manifestations of pulmonary infection range from an asymptomatic pulmonary nodule on radiograph to subclinical, mild, and self-limited symptoms (in an immunocompetent host) up to life-threatening fungal pneumonia. Symptoms include fever, productive cough, chest pain, weight loss, and respiratory distress (with the more severe symptoms occurring in immunocompromised persons). Roentgenographic abnormalities include pulmonary nodules or masses (solitary or multiple), airspace consolidations, reticular patterns, and ground-glass attenuation. Nodules can be single or multiple, and consolidations can be uni- or multi-focal. Cavitation occurs more frequently in immunocompromised hosts. Other associated findings can include lymphadenopathy, pleural effusion, and, rarely, endobronchial lesions causing collapse.

Dissemination from lungs to CNS occurs in 65% to 94% of cases of HIV-associated pulmonary cryptococcosis. In fact, most immunocompromised patients present with CNS rather than pulmonary symptoms in a clinical syndrome of subacute meningoencephalitis.

C. gattii infections have been recognized in immunocompetent hosts, producing pulmonary or CNS cryptococcosis. In certain areas of the world, *C. gattii* tends to cause cerebral cryptococcomas and hydrocephalus with or without large pulmonary lesions in immunocompetent hosts. Other organs that may be involved include skin, prostate, eyes, bone, and blood.

DIAGNOSIS

Several methods are used for the diagnosis of cryptococcosis, including direct examination of body fluids, histopathology of infected tissues, serologic studies, and culture.

Direct examination using India ink staining on cerebrospinal fluid (CSF) can be performed, showing a halo around the organism representing the polysaccharide capsule. This has a sensitivity of 30% to 50% in non–AIDS-related cryptococcal meningitis and 80% in AIDS-related cryptococcal meningitis. Specificity can be an issue if the ink becomes contaminated. *Cryptococcus* also can be identified by histologic stains of tissues from affected organs (e.g., fine needle aspiration [FNA] of a lung nodule) showing the budding yeast. Testing for the cryptococcal polysaccharide antigen (CRAG) with latex agglutination is the primary tool used for diagnosis. Serum CRAG has a sensitivity and specificity of 93% to 100%, and 93% to 98% in disseminated cryptococcosis. The test is not as sensitive when there is no other extrapulmonary involvement. Serum CRAG is often used as a screening test; however, false-negative rates of up to 48% have been reported in non–HIV-infected individuals with only pulmonary involvement (with single pulmonary nodules having the lowest rate of antigen positivity than all other radiographic presentations). On the other hand, a positive serum CRAG in a patient with suspected pulmonary cryptococcosis appears to reflect extrapulmonary, or disseminated, disease. It is recommended that a lumbar puncture should be performed to evaluate for meningitis in all patients with suspected pulmonary cryptococcosis (even without CNS symptoms), except those who are immunocompetent and in whom there is no suspicion of extrapulmonary disease. Bronchoscopic sampling (washings and bronchoalveolar lavage) is often diagnostic when the specimens are properly stained. However, there does not appear to be added benefit from transbronchial biopsy. Direct CRAG measurements can also be performed on bronchoscopic lavage and transthoracic needle aspirates of infiltrates and have a higher sensitivity for pulmonary cryptococcosis (without dissemination) than serum measurements of the antigen. As alluded to earlier, if cryptococci are recovered from respiratory samples, the CSF should be examined in most, if not all, cases.

MANAGEMENT

The recommendations for the treatment of cryptococcal infection differ depending on the host risk factors, severity of the disease, and organ(s) infected. The recommendations are based on the 2010 IDSA update of the clinical practice guidelines for the management of cryptococcal disease. Treatment of pulmonary disease without dissemination has not been studied with modern treatments. Therefore, the treatment recommendations for the most common syndrome in the immunocompromised, meningoencephalitis, will be outlined as there is frequently overlap with pulmonary cryptococcosis. In addition, the recommendation is to treat severe pulmonary disease the same as CNS disease. Some of the alternative treatment regimens will be outlined below; however, this is not a comprehensive list.

In cryptococcal meningoencephalitis in HIV-infected individuals, induction and consolidation consists of amphotericin B (0.7–1.0 mg/kg/day IV) and flucytosine (100 mg/kg/day PO in four divided doses) for at least 2 weeks, followed by fluconazole 400 mg PO daily for at least 8 weeks. Lipid formulations of amphotericin B can be substituted for amphotericin B in patients with or predisposed to renal dysfunction. The consolidation portion can be extended to 4 to 6 weeks in cases of treatment failure or high disease burden. In cases in which flucytosine or amphotericin cannot be used, the following alternative regimens can be used: amphotericin B (same dose) plus fluconazole (800 mg daily) for 2 weeks followed by fluconazole (800 mg daily) for at least 8 weeks, or fluconazole (1,200 mg daily) plus flucytosine (100 mg/kg daily) for 6 weeks. Maintenance (suppressive) therapy consists of fluconazole 200 mg/day orally for at least one year. Itraconazole 200 mg twice a day orally is a less effective alternative. Discontinuation of suppressive therapy can be considered (after at least 1 year) if patients are on HAART and have a CD4 cell count greater than 100 cells/μL and an undetectable or very low viral load for greater than or equal to months. In organ transplant recipients, lipid formulations of amphotericin B should be used because of the higher risk of renal toxicity in combination with the calcineurin inhibitors. There are several complications that may need to be addressed during treatment, including, but not limited to, persistence, relapse, elevated CSF pressure, immune reconstitution inflammatory syndrome (IRIS), and cerebral cryptococcomas.

Pulmonary cryptococcosis (isolated pulmonary disease) must first be ascertained in immunosuppressed patients in whom bronchoalveolar lavage or sputum culture results are positive for *Cryptococcus*. This is done with blood and CSF cultures and cryptococcal antigen measurements.

Pneumonia associated with CNS disease or documented dissemination and/or severe pneumonia is treated like CNS disease. Steroids may be considered in acute respiratory distress syndrome (ARDS) in the context of the IRIS. For mild to moderate symptoms, absence of pulmonary infiltrates, absence of severe immunosuppression, and absence of evidence for dissemination, fluconazole (400 mg/day orally) for 6 to 12 months should be used. In addition, based on sporadic experience some experts recommend voriconazole or posaconazole in patients who are treatment failures or unable to tolerate standard therapy.

C. gattii infection has a greater propensity to form pulmonary cryptococcomas. This may be explained by the greater containment of the foci of infection by the healthy immune response. Single cryptococcomas should be treated with fluconazole (400 mg/day orally). For very large and multiple cryptococcomas, consider a combination of amphotericin B and flucytosine for 4 to 6 weeks, followed by fluconazole for 6 to 18 months, depending on whether surgery was performed (this should be considered in the context of failure to reduce the size of the cryptococcomas after 4 weeks of therapy).

FURTHER READING

1. Speed B, Dunt D. Clinical and host differences between infections with the two varieties of *Cryptococcus neoformans*. *Clin Infect Dis*. 1995;21:28–34.

2. Perfect JR, Dismukes WE, Dromer F. Clinical practice guidelines for the management of cryptococcal disease: 2010 update by the Infectious Diseases Society of America. *Clin Infect Dis*. 2010;50:291–322.

   Updated practice guidelines for the management of cryptococcal disease, built on the previous guidelines published in 2000.

3. Garcia-Hermoso D, Janbon G, Dromer F. Epidemiological evidence for dormant *Cryptococcus neoformans* infection. *J Clin Microbiol*. 1999;37:3204.

   A genetic analysis of isolates from nine African expatriates diagnosed with cryptococcosis while living in France, a median of 110 months and without contact with an African environment for as long as 13 years. These isolates were significantly different than those isolates recovered from 17 European patients and were more similar to those isolates known to be from Africa.

4. Chang W, Tzao C, Hsu H, et al. Pulmonary cryptococcosis: comparison of clinical and radiographic characteristics in immunocompetent and immunocompromised patients. *Chest*. 2006; 129(2):333–340.

   Clinical characteristics and imaging findings were compared between immunocompetent and immunocompromised patients diagnosed with pulmonary cryptococcosis. They were followed for one year to better define the role of serum cryptococcal antigen and radiographs for follow up.

5. Chayakulkeeree M, Perfect JR. Cryptococcosis. In: Hospenthal DR, Rinaldi MG, eds. *Infectious Disease: Diagnosis and Treatment of Human Mycoses*. 1st ed. Totowa, NJ: Humana Press; 2008.

   Excellent review of cryptococcosis.

6. Chechani V, Kamholz SL. Pulmonary manifestations of disseminated cryptococcosis in patients with AIDS. *Chest*. 1990;98:1060–1066.

   A retrospective review of 48 AIDS patients with disseminated cryptococcosis was conducted to study pulmonary manifestations. Symptoms and roentgenographic manifestations were described.

7. Zinck SE, Leung AN, Frost M, et al. Pulmonary cryptococcosis: CT and pathologic findings. *J Comput Assist Tomogr*. 2002;26(3):330–334.

   CT scans and pathologic findings (from specimens obtained by open lung biopsy and transbronchial biopsy) in a series of patients are described.

8. Murayama S, Shuji S, Soeda H. Pulmonary cryptococcosis in immunocompetent patients HRCT characteristics. *Clin Imaging*. 2004;28(3):191–195.

   The CT characteristics of 13 immunocompetent patients diagnosed with pulmonary cryptococcosis were analyzed, with special emphasis on the differentiation from tuberculosis. The conclusion of the study is that pulmonary cryptococcosis mimics TB (hypothesized to be due to their shared mechanism of granulomatous inflammation) except for the absence of tree-in-bud abnormalities in crypto.

9. Baddley JW, Perfect JR, Oster RA, et al. Pulmonary cryptococcosis in patients without HIV infection: factors associated with disseminated disease. *Eur J Clin Microbiol Infect Dis*. 2008;27:937–943.

   A retrospective chart review of 15 medical centers was performed on 166 HIV-negative patients who were diagnosed with pulmonary cryptococcosis. Multiple factors were evaluated to differentiate those who had additional extrapulmonary disease.

10. Baughman RP, Rhodes JC, Dohn MN, et al. Detection of cryptococcal antigen in bronchoalveolar lavage fluid: a prospective study of diagnostic utility. *Am Rev Respir Dis.* 1992;145:1226.

A prospective study in 220 immunocompromised patients (188 with HIV infection, 32 with other causes of immunosuppression) undergoing BAL for fever and pulmonary symptoms led to the eventual diagnosis of cryptococcal pneumonia in 8 patients. All eight patients had a cryptococcal antigen titer greater than or equal to 1:8. There were four patients without cryptococcal pneumonia who had cryptococcal antigen titers of 1:8; none had higher titers. For a cryptococcal antigen titer of 1:8 or higher, there was 100% sensitivity, 98% specificity, a positive predictive value of 67%, and a negative predictive value of 100%. The measurement of cryptococcal antigen in the bronchoalveolar lavage can be a rapid, simple way to make a diagnosis of cryptococcal pneumonia in immunosuppressed patients with pneumonia.

11. Mahida P, Morar R, Mahomed AG, et al. Cryptococcosis: an unusual case of endobronchial obstruction. *Eur Respir J.* 1996;9:837–839.

Case report of a 43-year-old immunocompetent patient who presented with right middle and lower lobe collapse due to an endobronchial lesion, sampling of which showed cryptococcal organisms.

12. Singh N, Alexander BD, Lortholery O, et al. Pulmonary cryptococcosis in solid organ transplant recipients: clinical relevance of serum cryptococcal antigen. *Clin Infect Dis.* 2008;46:e12–e18.

A prospective study was conducted on 48 patients with pulmonary cryptococcosis. The factors influencing antigen positivity were evaluated.

13. Malabonga VM, Basti J, Kamholz SL. Utility of bronchoscopic sampling techniques for cryptococcal disease in AIDS. *Chest.* 1991;99:370–372.

Eleven AIDS patients over a 32-month period who were admitted with a clinical syndrome of pneumonia and diagnosed with cryptococcal pneumonia were studied. The goal of the study was to assess the sensitivity of nonbiopsy bronchoscopic sampling techniques (washings and lavage) compared with transbronchial biopsy.

14. Liaw YS, Yang PC, Yu CJ, et al. Direct determination of cryptococcal antigen in transthoracic needle aspirate for diagnosis of pulmonary cryptococcosis. *J Clin Microbiol.* 1995;33(6):1588–1591.

A prospective study was conducted on patients suspected of having cryptococcal pneumonia to assess the value of direct determination of cryptococcal antigen in lung aspirate for diagnosis of pulmonary cryptococcosis.

15. Brouwer AE, Rajanuwong A, Chierakul W, et al. Combination antifungal therapies for HIV-associated cryptococcal meningitis: a randomised trial. *Lancet.* 2004;363:1764–1767.

Sixty-four patients with a first episode of HIV-associated cryptococcal meningitis were randomised to initial treatment with: amphotericin B (0.7 mg/kg daily); amphotericin B plus flucytosine (100 mg/kg daily); amphotericin B plus fluconazole (400 mg daily); or triple therapy with amphotericin B, flucytosine, and fluconazole to assess which is the most fungicidal regimen.

16. Saag MS, Powderly WG, Cloud GA, et al; for The NIAID Mycoses Study Group and the AIDS Clinical Trials Group. Comparison of amphotericin B with fluconazole in the treatment of acute AIDS-associated cryptococcal meningitis. *N Engl J Med.* 1992;326:83–89.

A randomized trial was performed to compare the use of amphotericin with fluconazole during the induction regimen of AIDS-associated cryptococcal meningitis.

17. van der Horst CM, Saag MS, Cloud GA, et al; for the National Institute of Allergy and Infectious Diseases Mycoses Study Group and AIDS Clinical Trials Group. Treatment of cryptococcal meningitis associated with the acquired immunodeficiency syndrome. *N Engl J Med.* 1997; 337(1):15–21.

In a double-blind multicenter trial, patients with a first episode of AIDS-associated cryptococcal meningitis were assigned to treatment with higher-dose amphotericin B with or without flucytosine for 2 weeks (step 1), followed by 8 weeks of treatment with itraconazole or fluconazole (step 2). Treatment was considered successful if cerebrospinal fluid cultures were negative at 2 and 10 weeks or if the patient was clinically stable at 2 weeks and asymptomatic at 10 weeks.

18. Milefchik E, Leal MA, Haubrich R, et al. Fluconazole alone or combined with flucytosine for the treatment of AIDS-associated cryptococcal meningitis. *Med Mycol.* 2008;46:393–395.

An all oral consolidation treatment for cryptococcal meningitis was studied. Fluconazole at varying doses alone for 10 weeks or with flucytosine for 4 weeks were the regimens tried, and survival and time to culture conversion was analyzed.

19. de Gans J, Portegies P, Tiessens G, et al. Itraconazole compared with amphotericin B plus flucyto-sine in AIDS patients with cryptococcal meningitis. *AIDS.* 1992;6:185–190.

    A comparison of itraconazole versus amphotericin B plus flucytosine for the initial treatment of crypto-coccal meningitis was studied.

20. Bozzette SA, Larsen RA, Chiu J, et al; for the California Collaborative Treatment Group. A placebo-controlled trial of maintenance therapy with fluconazole after treatment of cryptococ-cal meningitis in the acquired immunodeficiency syndrome. California Collaborative Treatment Group. *N Engl J Med.* 1991;324:580–584.

    A controlled, double-blinded trial was performed to compare fluconazole versus placebo for maintenance therapy of cryptococcal meningitis.

21. Saag MS, Cloud GA, Graybill JR, et al; for the National Institute of Allergy and Infectious Diseases Mycoses Study Group. A comparison of itraconazole versus fluconazole as maintenance therapy for AIDS-associated cryptococcal meningitis. *Clin Infect Dis.* 1999;28:291–296.

    This study was designed to compare the effectiveness of fluconazole versus itraconazole as maintenance therapy for AIDS-associated cryptococcal meningitis.

22. Singh N, Lortholary O, Alexander BD, et al. Antifungal management practices and evolution of infection in organ transplant recipients with *Cryptococcus neoformans* infection. *Transplantation.* 2005;80:1033–1039.

    Antifungal treatment practices were assessed for cryptococcosis in a cohort of prospectively followed organ transplant recipients with respect to the choice of antifungal and duration of treatment.

23. Pappas PG, Perfect JR, Cloud GA, et al. Cryptococcosis in human immunodeficiency virus-nega-tive patients in the era of effective azole therapy. *Clin Infect Dis.* 2001;33:690.

    A case study of HIV-negative patients with cryptococcosis that further highlights the demographics, therapies, and prognostic factors associated with this disease.

24. Chen S, Sorrell T, Nimmo G, et al; for the Australasian Cryptococcal Study Group. Epidemiol-ogy and host- and variety-dependent characteristics of infection due to *Cryptococcus neoformans* in Australia and New Zealand. *Clin Infect Dis.* 2000;31:499–508.

    A prospective population-based study was conducted in Australia and New Zealand during 1994 to 1997 to elucidate the epidemiology of cryptococcosis due to Cryptococcus neoformans *var.* neofor-mans *(CNVN) and* C. neoformans *var.* gattii *(CNVG) and to relate clinical manifestations to host immune status and cryptococcal variety.*

25. Raad II, Graybill JR, Bustamante AB, et al. Safety of long-term oral posaconazole use in the treat-ment of refractory invasive fungal infections. *Clin Infect Dis.* 2006;42(12):1726–1734.

    In this study, 428 patients with fungal infections refractory to other treatments were treated with posaconazole. Forty-six of these patients had crypto. Here, the safety profile of the treatment was evalu-ated and found to be acceptable, leading to the author's recommendations to consider use of posaconazole in salvage treatment.

26. Perfect JR, Marr KA, Walsh TJ, et al. Voriconazole treatment for less-common, emerging, or refractory fungal infections. *Clin Infect Dis.* 2003;36(9):1122–1131.

    Patients with a variety of fungal infections who were refractory to, or not tolerating treatment, were treated with voriconazole. Patients with crypto showed around 40% efficacy rate.

59 Nematode and Trematode Diseases of the Lung

Konrad L. Davis

Helminthic (worm-related) pulmonary infections are caused by either roundworms (nematodes) or flatworms, which include flukes (trematodes) and tapeworms (cestodes). Although helminthic infection is ubiquitous in nature, human helminthic lung disease is relatively infrequent in North America. The diagnosis is usually considered in travelers returning from endemic regions. The parasites reach the lungs by hematogenous spread or direct migration, and disease is caused by either the parasites themselves or by the host's immune response to helminthic antigens. Pulmonary manifestations vary from asymptomatic to catastrophic. Nearly all helminthic life cycles require a phase of growth externalized to their host. The four modes of transmission to a human host include fecal–oral, transdermal, vector-borne, and predator–prey.

The principal pathologic nematodes include *Ascaris*, hookworm species (*Ancylostoma duodenale* and *Necator americanus*), *Strongyloides,* and *Filaria*. *Ascaris lumbricoides* is among the most common intestinal nematodes in the world, infecting approximately 25% of the global population. Though found predominately in the tropics, it also infects up to 4 million people living in the southern United States, especially in rural areas. Humans are infected by ingestion of contaminated soil or food that contains the *Ascaris* egg, which then hatches in the gastrointestinal tract. The larvae subsequently migrate through the venous system to the lungs, where they enter the alveoli and ascend the tracheobronchial tree. The worms are then swallowed, where they are returned to the intestine to mature into adult worms capable of reproduction just 2 to 3 months after initial ingestion.

Pulmonary disease results from a hypersensitivity response to migrating larvae. The manifestations are usually limited to transient pulmonary infiltrates and peripheral eosinophilia. A few patients develop the stigmata of Löffler syndrome (mild fever, cough, dyspnea, wheezing, sternal pain, and mild hemoptysis associated with migratory pulmonary infiltrates and peripheral eosinophilia). This typically occurs 1 to 2 weeks after egg ingestion. Secondary bacterial pneumonia is common, and mechanical airway obstruction has been described in the presence of a high worm burden.

Eosinophilia and elevated serum immunoglobulin E (IgE) levels are common. Chest radiographs may show patchy consolidation or diffuse miliary infiltrates. Sputum is rich in eosinophils and in crystallized protein from fragmented eosinophils (Charcot–Leyden crystals). Eggs are rarely found in the sputum but may be recovered from gastric aspirates. The diagnosis can be made by demonstration of *Ascaris* eggs in the stool within 3 months of a self-limited eosinophilic pneumonitis. Serum serologies are available, but their use is mainly as a research tool in endemic areas. Preferred treatment includes albendazole (400 mg single oral dose) or mebendazole (100 mg twice daily for 3 days).

The hookworms, *Ancylostoma duodenale* and *N. americanus,* infect humans through direct penetration of skin by larvae found in moist contaminated soil. The geographic distribution is worldwide and includes the southeastern Unites States (*N. americanus*). As with *Ascaris,* the hookworm larvae migrate to the lung through the venous system and can produce a self-limited Löffler syndrome (see above) before they inhabit the small intestine. Also similar to ascariasis, the stool examination may not be positive for up to 2 months after the pulmonary symptoms develop. Symptoms are usually self-limited, and treatment for pulmonary complaints is generally not necessary, but inhaled bronchodilators may provide symptomatic relief. Eradication of the parasite can be achieved with mebendazole (100 mg two times a day for 3 days or a 500-mg single dose) or albendazole (400-mg single oral dose).

Strongyloides stercoralis is endemic in tropical and subtropical areas and in the southeastern United States. A relatively unique feature of *Strongyloides stercoralis* is its ability to complete its life cycle entirely within the human (termed "autoinfection"), potentially leading to a substantial worm burden. Although the acute and chronic stages generally produce only mild symptoms in normal hosts, in immunocompromised conditions (AIDS, corticosteroids, and malignancy), it can be devastating. Strongyloides migrate hematogenously to the lungs after the larvae penetrate the skin. From here, they ascend the tracheobronchial tree and are swallowed. In the duodenum, they mature and produce larvae, some of which can penetrate the colonic mucosa or perianal skin, resulting in autoinfection.

The initial skin penetration by strongyloides may lead to local inflammation, edema, and a serpiginous erythematous track that rarely comes to medical attention. The gastrointestinal manifestations include duodenitis, abdominal pain, and malabsorption that can be seen with high worm burdens. The pulmonary manifestations in the immunocompetent patient include cough, wheezing, and a recurrent pneumonitis. Peripheral blood eosinophilia is not necessarily present. Asthma induced by chronic strongyloidosis will paradoxically worsen with corticosteroid administration.

In the immunocompromised host (e.g., those using corticosteroids), the colonic penetration of filariform larvae occurs unchecked and can widely disseminate to lungs, liver, central nervous system, and other organs. This so-called *hyperinfection syndrome* carries an extremely high mortality (>90%). The pulmonary manifestations at this stage include adult respiratory distress syndrome (ARDS) or secondary bacterial infections caused by enteric Gram-negative bacilli translocating with the worms.

The diagnosis of *Strongyloides* infection is often made by examination of multiple stool specimens (as a single stool sample has a low sensitivity, roughly 25%). Enzyme-linked immunosorbent assays (ELISA) are about 90% sensitive and have a negative predictive value of 95% in some populations. In hyperinfection syndrome, strongyloidosis has been diagnosed by examination of sputum or cerebrospinal fluid. Ivermectin (200 μg/kg/day for 2 days) is preferred over albendazole (400 mg twice daily for 3 days) for treatment.

Filariasis is caused by a nematode infection of the lymphatics and subcutaneous tissue. The most common filarial species include *Wuchereria bancrofti, Brugia malayi,* and *Brugia timori.* Humans are the definitive host of these mosquito-borne infections. Infection of the lungs may cause an immune hyperresponsiveness reaction called "tropical pulmonary eosinophilia." Tropical pulmonary eosinophilia is most common in India, Southeast Asia, and Sri Lanka, and is more prevalent in men. In the acute phase, tropical pulmonary eosinophilia causes paroxysmal nonproductive cough and wheeze, which are typically worse at night. Physical examination may reveal hepatomegaly and generalized lymphadenopathy. Laboratory evaluation typically reveals significant peripheral eosinophilia, elevated IgE, and eosinophilic alveolar exudates. Filarial antibodies are usually present, but microfilariae are not seen. The chest radiograph shows fluffy reticulonodular opacities in the mid and lower lung zones. A miliary pattern also has been described. Up to 20% of patients may have normal radiographs. Some patients develop chronic tropical pulmonary eosinophilia, manifested by a restrictive fibrotic pulmonary process without peripheral or alveolar eosinophilia. Most patients with acute tropical pulmonary eosinophilia respond to diethylcarbamazine (6 mg/kg/day in three doses for 12–21 days), but relapse (or reinfection) and chronically unresponsive disease are well described. Corticosteroids may be useful. The clinical response is poor in chronic disease.

Dirofilaria immitis (dog heartworm) can be transmitted to the human by a mosquito vector and has been reported increasingly in the United States. In dogs, coyotes, and cats, the larvae develop into sexually mature worms that travel to the right ventricle. In the human host, larvae cannot mature and subsequently die but are passively transported to the lung through the venous system, where they may cause thrombosis, infarction, and a granulomatous reaction. The infection generally manifests itself as an asymptomatic pulmonary nodule but can present with cough, chest pain, and hemoptysis. Because of its radiographic similarities to lung cancer, *D. immitis* manifested as a pulmonary nodule is often diagnosed by surgical resection.

Toxocariasis (visceral larvae migrans) is caused by human infection with a dog or cat ascarid. Endemic to North America, England, and Mexico, *Toxocara canis* and *Toxocara cutis* eggs are ingested from contaminated soil and food. As is the case with dog heartworm, the human is an imperfect host and maturation of the larvae cannot occur. The eggs hatch in the gut and the larvae migrate through host tissue, including the liver and lungs. This migration causes an inflammatory granulomatous response that is considered the source of the clinical manifestations of the disease. Serum and bronchoalveolar lavage (BAL) show increased IgE, as well as an increased eosinophil count. Pulmonary involvement is present in 20% to 80% of cases. Severity of symptoms is related to the worm burden. Visceral larva migrans is generally asymptomatic but can have a fulminant course with central nervous system involvement, hepatitis, acute pneumonia, or severe asthma.

Infection is most common in children (especially those with pica) and can be associated with cough, wheezing, and pulmonary infiltrates. Peripheral eosinophilia is significant and hepato-splenomegaly may be present. A definitive diagnosis depends on the demonstration of larvae in tissue; however, ELISA (using antitoxocara antibodies) and specific larva-related IgE tests are useful. Stool examination is not helpful, as the ascarid cannot reproduce in human hosts.

Generally, the disease is self-limited and treatment is generally not indicated; however, albendazole (400 mg orally twice daily for 5 days) is recommended if drug treatment is necessary. In cases of severe respiratory, myocardial, or neurologic involvement, concomitant prednisone (0.5 to 1 mg/kg for adults) should be considered.

The most common trematodes (flatworms) that cause human infection include *Schistosoma* and *Paragonimus*. Schistosomiasis is caused by a digenetic parasitic trematode that infects an estimated 200 million people worldwide. Several species can cause human disease: (1) *Schistosoma japonicum,* found in Japan, China, and the Philippines; (2) *Schistosoma mansoni,* found in Africa, Arabia, and South America; (3) *Schistosoma haematobium,* found in Africa and the Middle East; and (4) *Schistosoma intercalatum,* found in western Africa. Infection occurs through contact with fresh water that contains infective cercariae released from snails. The cercariae penetrate the intact skin of the definitive mammalian host and undergo transformation into migrating larvae. These larvae migrate via the hemolymphatic system, through the lungs, to the portal circulation of the liver where they mature into sexually active adults. Mature adults then localize in mesenteric (*Schistosoma mansoni* and *Schistosoma japonicum*) or bladder vesicle venules (*Schistosoma haematobium*) and produce eggs that are excreted in the urine and stool. Eggs are also carried in the venous system to the pulmonary vascular beds.

Pulmonary manifestations of schistosomiasis occur in acute and chronic forms. Acute pulmonary schistosomiasis occurs in nonendemic patients, typically manifests 3 to 8 weeks after schistosome penetration, and is characterized by shortness of breath, wheezing, and dry cough. Symptoms may be temporally related to a well-described febrile illness (Katayama fever), but respiratory complaints often persist well after resolution of the fever. Eosinophilia (30%–40% of total leukocytes) with mild leukocytosis, elevated IgE, and abnormal liver function tests are common. Radiographic abnormalities (ill-defined nodules, increased interstitial markings, hilar prominence) may be absent or may only appear after antischistosomal therapy is instituted. It is thought that these manifestations are immunologically related and are seen after release of schistosomal antigens. Transbronchial biopsy and BAL typically reveals only eosinophils. The sensitivity of stool and urine for detecting ova is low because of sporadic passage of eggs and the low worm burden. Serologies are currently used as a research tool.

Chronic pulmonary schistosomiasis is a syndrome of endemic individuals consisting of chest pain, dyspnea, fatigue, and cough. Cor pulmonale and right-sided congestive heart failure may be present. The syndrome results from an inflammatory reaction to eggs in the circulatory system, which lodge in the distal pulmonary vasculature and cause granulomatous inflammation. Serologies are not helpful, nor are transbronchial biopsies, because of the sporadic nature of the pathology. Lesions are typically fibrotic and thus respond poorly to therapy. However, because of the relative safety of praziquantel, a course of therapy may be warranted if the disease is strongly suspected.

Paragonimiasis is a disease with a widespread geographic range that is caused by the trematode *Paragonimus*. The best known species (also having the widest distribution) is *Paragonimus westermani*, which is prevalent in Asia, India, Latin America, and Africa. Humans become definitive hosts by consuming uncooked crustaceans that harbor the larvae of this lung fluke. Infection may also result from eating undercooked pork that carries the larvae. Once ingested, the larvae penetrate into the peritoneal cavity and migrate through the diaphragm and pleura into the lung. Once in the lungs, the larvae become encysted and produce eggs that are either expectorated or swallowed. Unlike most other helminths, pulmonary involvement is essential in this fluke's development. Clinically, this stage of infection can last for several years and carry few symptoms. Rupture of the cysts will cause blood-streaked sputum containing parasite eggs, necrotic tissue, and Charcot–Leyden crystals. Radiographically, small cavitary nodules, ring shadows, and masslike lesions may be present in addition to unilateral, eosinophilic, exudative pleural effusions. A peripheral eosinophilia is generally present in the acute setting, although the total leukocyte count may be normal. Eosinophilia is more common in patients who complain of pleurisy and less common with parenchymal disease. In the absence of eosinophilia, the clinical picture may be confused with tuberculosis, fungal infection, or cancer. The worms may also infest other organs than the lungs. The adult worms may produce 20,000 eggs per day, and live within humans for up to 20 years.

The diagnosis is established by demonstrating parasite eggs in sputum, feces, pleural fluid, or tissue. A single sputum examination has a sensitivity of 30% to 45%, and the yield is increased with multiple collections. BAL samples have a sensitivity of 60% to 70%. Stool examination is generally less sensitive than sputum or pleural fluid analysis. ELISA and immunoblotting assay techniques can help make the diagnosis also. An intradermal test is available but used only in highly endemic areas and in research studies. The first-line therapy is praziquantel (25 mg/kg three times a day for 3 days), with cure rates approaching 100%.

In summary, pulmonary helminthic infections may present with a broad array of signs and symptoms. A high index of suspicion should be maintained in patients with a pertinent travel history, underlying immune deficiency, or both. Diagnosis and therapy should be tailored to the specific infective agent. The Centers for Disease Control and Prevention (CDC) maintains a Web site at www.cdc.gov/travel/diseases.htm, which provides helpful information for travelers and physicians.

FURTHER READING

1. Allen JN, Davis WB. Eosinophilic lung diseases. *Am J Respir Crit Care Med.* 1994;150:1423–1438.

   Excellent overview of the PIE (pulmonary infiltrates with eosinophilia) syndromes to include helminthic infections.

2. Concha R, Harrington W, Rogers AI. Intestinal strongyloidiasis. *J Clin Gastroenterol.* 2005;39:203–211.

   Succinct yet thorough review of the manifestations, management, and prognostic variables associated with intestinal strongyloidiasis.

3. Drugs for parasitic infections. *Med Lett Drugs Ther.* 1998;40:1–12.

   An overview of the available antiparasitic drugs with side effects, dosing schedules, and availability.

4. Flieder DB, Moran CA. Pulmonary dirofilariasis: a clinicopathologic study of 41 lesions in 39 patients. *Hum Pathol.* 1999;30:251–256.

   Good clinical and pathologic information on dirofilariasis with excellent photomicrographs and a detailed description of their lifecycle.

5. Kagawa FT. Pulmonary paragonimiasis. *Semin Respir Infect.* 1997;12:149–158.

   Broad overview of paragonimiasis with epidemiologic, pathophysiologic, diagnostic, and therapeutic information for this lung fluke.

6. Lane MA, Barsanti MC, Santos CA, et al. Human paragonimiasis in North America following ingestion of raw crayfish. *Clin Infect Dis.* 2009;49:e55–e61.

   Well written case-based review of North American paragonimiasis infections.

7. Morris W, Knauer CM. Cardiopulmonary manifestations of schistosomiasis. *Semin Respir Infect.* 1997;12:159–170.

   Detailed description of pulmonary manifestations of schistosomiasis. This entire text has valuable information on a variety of helminthic infections.

8. Ong RK, Doyle RL. Tropical pulmonary eosinophilia. *Chest.* 1998;11:1673.

   A good review of this uncommon cause of eosinophilia and pulmonary infiltrates, with information on how to obtain recommended antifilarial medications.

9. Pavlin BI, Kozarsky P, Cetron MS. Acute pulmonary schistosomiasis in travelers: case report and a review of the literature. *Travel Med Infect Dis.* 2012;10:209–219.

   Excellent review of pulmonary shistosomiasis, with color photos of cercarial dermatitis and a nicely organized table detailing the wide array of potential symptoms (along with additional references for each of them).

10. Perez-Arellano JL, Andrade MA, Lopez-Aban J, et al. Helminths and the respiratory system. *Arch Bronconeumol.* 2006;42(2):81–91.

    Broad and introductory review of pulmonary helminthic infections, including comparative tables of their epidemiology, clinical syndromes, methods of diagnosis, and treatment.

11. Ryan ET. Health advice and immunizations for travelers. *N Engl J Med.* 2000;342:1716–1725.

    A nice resource for both patients and providers, with information on recommended immunizations, preventative therapy, and endemic diseases.

12. Sarinas PS, Chitkara RK. Ascariasis and hookworm. *Semin Respir Infect.* 1997;12:130–137.

    This series has comprehensive information on nematode infections.

13. Schwartz E. Pulmonary schistosomiasis. *Clin Chest Med.* 2002;23:433–443.

    This Clinics on tropical lung diseases has many valuable sections including this one on schistosomiasis, reviews the lifecycle and epidemiology, as well as diagnosis and therapy.

14. Shah MK. Human pulmonary dirofilariasis: review of the literature. *South Med J.* 1999;92:276–279.

    Comprehensive look at pulmonary manifestations of Dirofilaria.

15. Siddiqui AA, Berk SL. Diagnosis of *Strongyloides stercoralis* infection. *Clin Infect Dis.* 2001;33:1040–1047.

    Current opinion and review of the different testing options for diagnosis of this blood fluke.

16. Udwadia FE. Tropical eosinophilia: a review. *Respir Med.* 1993;87:17.

    A classic description of this pulmonary helminthic disease.

17. Velez ID, Ortega JE, Velasquez LE. Paragonimiasis: a view from Columbia. *Clin Chest Med.* 2002;23:421–431, ix–x.

    Up-to-date review of paragonimiasis including some atypical presentations.

18. Zaha O, Hirata T, Kinjo F. Strongyloidiasis: progress in diagnosis and treatment. *Intern Med.* 2000;39:695–700.

    Includes information on therapeutic interventions, as well as a review of common and specialized tests for the diagnosis of Strongyloides.

Amebiasis and Echinococcal Diseases of the Lung

William L. Ring

AMEBIASIS

Amebiasis is caused by the protozoan *Entamoeba histolytica* and is most common in tropical and subtropical regions. *E. histolytica* is morphologically identical to the nonpathogenic species *E. dispar* and *E. moshkovskii*. In the United States, infection is observed most commonly in (1) travelers and immigrants exposed in endemic areas, (2) patients in mental health institutions, and (3) HIV-positive patients. The organism is usually confined to the colon, producing either no symptoms or amebic dysentery. The disease is usually contracted by ingestion of food or water contaminated by feces or by fecal–oral contact.

Rarely, mature organisms (trophozoites) penetrate the bowel wall and migrate to the liver by the hepatic veins, where an abscess may form. This invasive form of amebiasis is 3 to 10 times more common in men, is associated with alcohol abuse, and is more common in individuals who are malnourished or immunosuppressed. Most patients with invasive disease present with several weeks of right upper quadrant abdominal pain and fevers. By the time a hepatic abscess forms, no dysenteric symptoms are present in up to two-thirds of patients, and most patients do not have parasites detectable in their stool.

Thoracic involvement occurs in 13% to 35% of patients with hepatic amebiasis. The usual route of pleuropulmonary infection is by extension from a hepatic or subdiaphragmatic abscess. Less commonly, direct parasitic migration occurs into the thorax. In addition, hematogenous spread to the lung rarely occurs by hemorrhoidal veins or lymphatics. All modes of spread can result in empyema or lung abscess. Pleuropulmonary disease can also occur without actual parasitic invasion in the form of lower-lobe infiltrates and exudative effusions; the mechanism for this is not clear, but it is presumably a response to subdiaphragmatic infection.

Amebic pleuropulmonary disease is 10 to 15 times more common in men than in women, with a peak incidence between ages 20 and 40. Patients usually have a history of amebic dysentery and may complain of right upper quadrant pain, weight loss, and cough. Rarely, the cough is productive of thick, dark *chocolate sauce* or *anchovy paste* sputum or even bile (biliptysis), indicating hepatobronchial and bronchobiliary fistulas, respectively. Fever and signs of empyema or consolidation may also be present. Chest roentgenogram typically reveals a right-sided effusion or right lower-lobe lung abscess. In addition, areas of consolidation may be seen in the right lower lobe, middle lobe, or both. The right hemidiaphragm may be elevated and have decreased motility. In cases involving the left lobe of the liver, changes can occur in the left lung. Computerized tomography will show the liver abscess. Magnetic resonance imaging can directly visualize the secondary diaphragmatic rupture. Thoracentesis usually reveals a sterile exudate; however, organisms are rarely present.

Routine laboratory examination may show a mild leukocytosis and eosinophilia. Cysts are rarely found in the sputum or the pleural fluid; however, when present, they confirm the diagnosis. A serum hemagglutination test for antibodies to amebae is positive in up to 95% of invasive infections, and will remain positive for years after the infection. Fecal antigen detection tests for amebae are rapid, highly specific, and widely available.

It is reasonable to initiate therapy in the presence of an appropriate clinical presentation. The generally recommended medications for extraintestinal amebiasis are metronidazole (750 mg tid) orally for 10 days followed by a luminal agent such as iodoquinol (650 mg tid for 20 days), paromomycin (25–35 mg/kg/day in three divided doses for 7 days), or diloxanide furoate (500 mg tid for 10 days). Failure to respond to treatment should call into question the diagnosis or suggest the possibility of a secondary bacterial infection. The rare patient with invasive amebiasis who does not respond to this regimen should be treated with chloroquine and percutaneous drainage of the liver abscess and any pleural fluid. Surgery is rarely indicated.

ECHINOCOCCAL DISEASE

Echinococcosis or hydatid disease is caused by the postlarval metacestode stage of the tapeworm *Echinococcus*. Humans are an intermediate host for this parasite. After ingestion of contaminated food, water, or soil, the oncosphere penetrates the intestine and migrates into the systemic circulation, whereby it is ultimately deposited within an organ, especially the liver or lungs. Once in an organ, cellular differentiation occurs, resulting in the development of a *hydatid cyst*. The mature cyst consists of an inner germinal layer, the endocyst; an outer chitinous layer, the exocyst; and a peripheral fibrous layer caused by host reaction, the pericyst.

Four species of *Echinococcus* cause human disease. *E. granulosus* is the most common because of its wide distribution and its high prevalence in sheep; it involves the lung 60% of the times and often has a protracted and relatively benign course. *E. granulosus* causes cystic echinococcosis, the classic hydatid disease, with often large, unilocular cysts. *E. multilocularis* is less common. It is primarily a liver disease with occasional involvement of the lung and typically has an aggressive, malignant course. *E. multilocularis* causes alveolar echinococcosis, with somewhat smaller, multilocular cysts, which at pathology appear to have an alveolar appearance. *E. vogeli* and *E. oligarthus* are restricted to parts of Central and South America and only rarely cause human disease. They cause polycystic echinococcosis.

E. granulosus is endemic in pastoral regions of the Mediterranean, Eastern Europe and Russia, the Near and Middle East, Central Asia, Australia, and parts of South America and East Africa. In North America, it has been reported in both Canada and the United States, particularly in the Mississippi River Valley and Alaska. Dogs and other carnivores serve as the definitive hosts, whereas humans, sheep, and cattle are intermediate hosts. Infection is prevalent in areas where dogs are used to care for herds.

Pulmonary hydatid cysts are typically 1 to 10 cm in diameter, but can grow much larger. The cysts usually grow at a rate of less than 1 cm per year in diameter, but growth rates of up to 5 cm per year have been reported. The cysts are usually located in the lower lobes and are twice as frequent on the right. When multiple (20%–30%), they are most often unilateral (80%). A cyst can rupture into the bronchial tree, in which case the fluid is replaced with air, or into the pleural space. Pulmonary cysts often (10%–60%) coexist with hepatic cysts. Clinically, most patients are asymptomatic. Hydatid cysts are discovered most frequently on routine chest radiographs. Cough, hemoptysis, and chest pain occur uncommonly. Mediastinal cysts can erode into adjacent structures, causing bone pain, hemorrhage, or airflow obstruction. Uncommonly, rupture of a cyst, either spontaneously or during surgery, can result in an acute hypersensitivity reaction. Roentgenographically, the cyst(s) appears as a dense, well-circumscribed oval or spherical mass that can reach enormous dimensions and fill an entire hemithorax. Debris within the fluid of the cyst, which is called *hydatid sand*, has typical characteristics. If bronchial communication has occurred, air between the pericyst and exocyst can produce the appearance of a thin layer around the cyst—the meniscus or moon skin sign. Air penetrating the interior of the cyst may outline the inner surface of the exocyst, producing parallel arches of air—Cumbo sign. As air fills the space, the endocyst and the exocyst may detach, showing an irregular air–fluid layer, with the collapsed membranes floating on the fluid surface; this is known as the water lily, lotus on water, or camelot sign. Calcification of the cyst is rare. Eosinophilia, usually not prominent, is found in less than 50% of patients. A skin test (Casoni) for delayed hypersensitivity to cyst material is generally positive but does not correlate with disease activity.

A number of sensitive, serologic tests are available and are used to support the clinical diagnosis. Cysts in the lung, however, are less likely to elicit antibody response than cysts in the liver, and, regardless of localization, antibody detection tests are least sensitive in patients with intact hyaline cysts. In a highly suggestive presentation, a negative serological workup does not rule out echinococcal disease. Fiberoptic bronchoscopy may reveal whitish–yellow gelatinous material in the bronchi. Conclusive diagnosis can be made if components of the hydatid cysts, including possibly scolexes or degenerated hooklets, are identified in bronchoalveolar lavage fluid, pleural fluid, or sputum. Although some risk has been observed with percutaneous aspiration of a cyst, some studies have suggested that this can be done safely. Traditionally, the treatment of choice has been close monitoring in asymptomatic patients and surgical resection in symptomatic patients. Some studies have suggested that medical treatment alone with a benzimidazole (albendazole or mebendazole) can be a safe, initial strategy.

E. multilocularis may cause the more dangerous condition of alveolar echinococcosis. *E. multilocularis* is endemic in an area extending from the White Sea to the Bering Straits, including the former Soviet Union, the European alpine countries, southern and central Canada, northeastern United States, Alaska, Japan, and China. The red fox, Arctic foxes, coyotes, and wolves are the definitive hosts, and certain wild rodents are intermediate hosts. The infection originates from larval penetration through the duodenal wall and transit through the portal vein. Most are trapped in the hepatic sinusoids, but alveolar echinococcosis occurs when some larvae pass through and are subsequently trapped in the alveolar capillaries. Cysts can form in the liver, the lung, or in both organs. Progressive larval invasion to contiguous regions, as well as occasional metastases to distant sites, leads to massive tissue destruction. When the lung is involved by direct invasion from the diseased liver, typically only the right lower-lung field is abnormal, often appearing roentgenographically as an abscess. With hematogenous spread, multiple small cysts can form diffusely in the lung. Typically, pulmonary symptoms are overshadowed by hepatic dysfunction.

Serologic testing, particularly the Em2-enzyme-linked immunosorbent assay (ELISA), is both sensitive and specific and useful to both assist in the diagnosis of the disease and monitor for recurrence. Alveolar echinococcosis is frequently fatal if not treated. Surgical resection remains the treatment of choice. In cases with limited disease, radical resection can lead to cure. Prolonged drug therapy with mebendazole or albendazole has a significant impact on disease progression.

FURTHER READING

1. Pritt BS, Clark CG. Amebiasis. *Mayo Clin Proc.* 2008;83:1154.

   A concise, overall review of amebiasis.

2. Shamsuzzaman SM, Hashiguchi Y. Thoracic amebiasis. *Clin Chest Med.* 2002;23:479.

   A detailed, overall review of thoracic amebiasis.

3. Fotedar R, Stark D, Beebe N, et al. Laboratory diagnostic techniques for *Entamoeba* species. *Clin Microbiol Rev.* 2007;20:511.

   An overview of amebiasis with a detail discussion of laboratory diagnostic strategies.

4. Stephen SJ, Uragoda CG. Pleuro-pulmonary amoebiasis: a review of 40 cases. *Br J Dis Chest.* 1970;64:96.

   A classic review from Ceylon of pleuropulmonary amebiasis.

5. Cameron EW. The treatment of pleuropulmonary amebiasis with metronidazole. *Chest.* 1978;73:647.

   Describes the management of 140 cases classified by chest radiographic findings; revised the indications for surgical intervention in view of the efficacy of metronidazole.

6. Landay MJ, Setiawan H, Hirsch G, et al. Hepatic and thoracic amebiasis. *AJR Am J Roentgenol.* 1980;135:449.

   Reviews sonographic and radiographic findings in 27 cases of hepatic amebiasis; half had nonspecific findings on chest radiographs, including elevated right hemidiaphragm, basilar infiltrates, and pleural effusions.

7. Lichtenstein A, Kondo AT, Visvesvara GS, et al. Pulmonary amebiasis presenting as superior vena cave syndrome. *Thorax.* 2005;60:350.

   A case report of amebiasis without hepatic involvement presenting with the development of superior vena cava syndrome.

8. Deshmukh H, Prasad S, Patankar T, et al. Percutaneous management of a bronchobiliary fistula complicating ruptured amebic liver abscess. *Am J Gastroenterol.* 1999;94:289.

   A case report of external biliary diversion as part of the treatment of a bronchobiliary fistula.

9. McManus DP, Zhang W, Li J, et al. Echinococcosis. *Lancet.* 2003;362:1295.

   A concise review of this disease.

10. Brunetti E, Kern P, Vuitton DA. Expert consensus for the diagnosis and treatment of cystic and alveolar echinococcosis in humans. *Acta Trop.* 2010;114:1–16.

    An extensive, detailed review of echinococcosis from the World Health Organization.

11. Santivanez S, Garcia HH. Pulmonary cystic echinococcosis. *Curr Opin Pulm Med.* 2010;16:577.

    A detailed review of pulmonary echinococcosis.

12. Amir-Jahed AK, Fardin R, Farzad A, et al. Clinical echinococcosis. *Ann Surg.* 1975;182:541.

    A retrospective study of 221 patients in Iran with hydatid disease who were treated before benzimidazoles were available.

13. Sarsam A. Surgery of pulmonary hydatid cysts: review of 155 cases. *J Thorac Cardiovasc Surg.* 1971;62:663.

    A review of the various surgical approaches to treating cystic echinococcosis.

14. Lewal DB. Hydatid disease: biology, pathology, imaging and classification. *Clin Radiol.* 1998;53:863.

    A review of the radiology of hydatid disease, including the nomenclature and sequelae of ruptured cysts.

15. Oztek I, Baloglu H, Demirel D, et al. Cytologic diagnosis of complicated pulmonary unilocular cystic hydatidosis: a study of 131 cases. *Acta Cytol.* 1997;41:1159.

   Reports on the cytology of E. granulosus *pulmonary cysts.*

16. Voros D, Katsarellias D, Polymeneas G, et al. Treatment of hydatid liver disease. *Surg Infect.* 2007;6:621.

   Review of one major echinococcal treatment center's treatment strategies, including complete surgical resection, laparoscopic surgery, percutaneous drainage, and chemotherapy.

17. Franchi C, Di Vico B, Teggi A. Long-term evaluation of patients with hydatidosis treated with benzimidazole carbamates. *Clin Infect Dis.* 1999;29:304.

   A prospective study of 448 patients with 929 E. granulosus *hydatid cysts (195 cysts in the lung), treated with mebendazole or albendazole and followed up for up to 15 years; 74% responded to treatment, but 25% of those relapsed; however, more than 90% of the relapsed cases responded to additional medical treatment.*

18. Bulman W, Coyle CM, Brentijens TE, et al. Severe pulmonary hypertension due to chronic echinococcal pulmonary emboli treated with targeted pulmonary vascular therapy and hepatic resection. *Chest.* 2007;132:1356.

   Reports on a rare complication of echinococcal disease: echinococcal pulmonary embolleading to severe pulmonary hypertension, generally felt to be a fatal disease. In this case, the patient was treated with bosentan and epoprostenol followed by hepatic resection, with a good response.

19. Topuzlar M, Eken C, Ozkurt B, et al. Possible anaphylactic reaction due to pulmonary hydatid cyst rupture following blunt chest trauma: a case report and review of the literature. *Wilderness Environ Med.* 2008;19:119.

   Anaphylactic reaction is a rare presentation of pulmonary hydatid cyst disease, but can occur after rupture of a pulmonary cyst.

20. Kern P. Clinical features and treatment of alveolar echinococcosis. *Curr Opin Infect Dis.* 2010;23:505.

   A detailed review of E. multilocularis.

Pulmonary Infections and Complications in HIV-Infected Patients

Jennifer Blanchard

Patients infected with HIV are predisposed to a variety of infectious, inflammatory, and neoplastic pulmonary diseases. Over the past decade, significant changes in the spectrum of HIV-related pulmonary complications have been observed after the introduction of highly active antiretroviral therapy (HAART—a combination of protease inhibitors taken with reverse transcriptase inhibitors) and the widespread use of effective prophylaxis against opportunistic infection. Moreover, the population characteristics and risk factors associated with HIV infection have evolved; AIDS is observed increasingly in women, children, and intravenous drug abusers. Homosexual and bisexual men still represent the majority of cases of HIV, but their percentage is decreasing in the United States.

The most prevalent opportunistic infection in patients infected with HIV is *Pneumocystis* pneumonia, which is an AIDS-defining illness. It has been officially renamed *P. jirovecii* pneumonia, but is still called PCP (for "*PneumoCystis* pneumonia") in the infectious disease community. Since the advent of HAART, the incidence has declined. The mode of transmission is not entirely known. Person-to-person airborne transmission is possible, but an environmental exposure is the most likely mode of transmission. Respiratory isolation of PCP-infected patients is not necessary. The risk of infection with PCP in HIV-infected patients increases sharply once the CD4 count drops below 200 cells/mm or there is a history of oropharyngeal candidiasis. In addition, the annual risk of recurrence after an episode of PCP is greater than 60%. For these reasons, HIV-infected patients with CD4 counts less than 200 or with a prior history of PCP should receive chemoprophylaxis. Primary or secondary prophylaxis can be discontinued in patients who have a response to HAART vigorous enough to raise the CD4 count to more than 200 for a period of 3 or more months. However, prophylaxis should be reinstituted if the CD4 cell count drops to less than 200. Drugs recommended for the prophylaxis are listed in Table 61-1.

The presentation of PCP in AIDS patients is usually indolent, with the onset of a nonproductive cough, progressive dyspnea, and fever over days to weeks. This is in contrast to the abrupt onset of symptoms typically observed in cancer patients. The physical examination is dominated by tachypnea and tachycardia; auscultatory findings can range from none to diffuse rales and rhonchi. Symptoms of local inflammation are distinctly absent (i.e., pleurisy, productive cough), and the presence of these should raise the possibility of an alternative diagnosis. Symptoms may be mild and permit outpatient management with oral therapy; however, severe hypoxemia mandates hospital admission and intravenous therapy.

Laboratory abnormalities often are nonspecific, revealing lymphopenia and anemia. Serum lactate dehydrogenase (LDH) is almost always elevated, although it probably reflects the inflammation of the lung parenchyma and is not a specific marker for PCP. The serum LDH, while nonspecific, is useful as a prognostic indicator, that is, a higher LDH signals a higher burden of disease. The chest radiograph is abnormal in 80% to 90% of cases and typically displays bilateral perihilar interstitial infiltrates that can progress to diffuse and homogenous opacities. Less common radiographic findings include solitary or multiple nodules, upper-lobe infiltrates in patients receiving inhaled pentamidine, pneumatoceles, and pneumothorax. Although the chest radiograph may be normal in 5% to 10% of patients, high-resolution computed tomography (HRCT) commonly discloses extensive ground-glass attenuation or cystic lesions. An HRCT with normal findings essentially rules out the diagnosis of PCP. Pleural effusions and thoracic lymphadenopathy are suggestive of other (or coexisting) diagnoses such as bacterial pneumonia, mycobacterial disease, or malignancy.

The arterial Po_2 is abnormal in most cases and is a key prognostic indicator. Patients presenting with near-normal oxygenation generally do well with treatment. An abnormal carbon

TABLE 61-1	Medications for PCP Prophylaxis	
Drug	**Dose**	**Comments**
TMP-SMX	One double-strength tablet daily or One single-strength tablet daily or One double-strength tablet three times per week	Most effective and most widely recommended Short-term intolerance is common and prophylaxis can frequently be continued
Pentamidine	300 mg monthly	Given by inhalation
Dapsone	100 mg daily	Ensure patient does not have G6PD deficiency
Atovaquone	1,500 mg daily	Give with meals to improve absorption

monoxide diffusing capacity, oxygen desaturation during exercise, and an abnormal gallium lung scan are sensitive but nonspecific for PCP infection.

Because the organism cannot be cultured, microscopic examination of an appropriate specimen is required to make the diagnosis. Patients with AIDS and PCP have significantly more organisms in their lungs than PCP patients without AIDS. Because of the higher organism burden, induced sputum has a diagnostic yield of 50% to 90% in AIDS patients and should be the initial diagnostic procedure if PCP is suspected. If induced sputum is either negative or not available, bronchoalveolar lavage (BAL) fluid obtained by fiberoptic bronchoscopy has a 90% to 95% sensitivity for PCP in the AIDS population. Transbronchial or open-lung biopsy is seldom needed. However, with an atypical presentation (e.g., focal disease), other diseases become more likely and transbronchial biopsy should be considered. The clinician should be aware that the (presumably dead) *P. jirovecii* cysts can persist for weeks to months after successful treatment, so a positive result on repeat testing does not necessarily indicate relapse.

Trophic forms of *Pneumocystis* can be detected with modified Papanicolaou or Wright–Giemsa stain. The cysts can be stained with Gomori methenamine silver, toluidine blue O, or calcofluor white. Immunohistochemical stains detect both the trophic forms and cysts and have higher sensitivity and specificity in induced sputum samples than conventional tinctorial stains. However, BAL fluid usually contains such a high density of organisms that immunohistochemistry is unnecessary.

Nucleic acid amplification using polymerase chain reaction (PCR) on respiratory specimens has greater sensitivity and specificity for the diagnosis of PCP than conventional staining. In patients with a positive PCR but a negative smear, treatment is recommended if the patient is immunosuppressed. PCR testing of serum samples has not yet been shown to be useful.

Those with mild cases of PCP can be treated as outpatients with close follow-up. Hospitalization is usually indicated when the alveolar–arterial oxygen gradient ($P[A–a]o_2$) is greater than 35 mmHg or the chest radiograph is clearly abnormal. Trimethoprim-sulfamethoxazole (TMP-SMX) is the preferred form of therapy. In moderate to severe disease, parenteral therapy initially is preferred. Drugs used in the treatment of PCP are listed in Table 61-2.

Administration of adjunctive corticosteroids is indicated in patients with a $Pao_2 < 70$ mmHg or $P(A–a)o_2 > 35$ mmHg. A recommended treatment regimen is prednisone given orally at a dose of 40 mg twice daily for 5 days, then 40 mg daily on days 6 through 11, and then 20 mg daily on days 12 through 21.

TABLE 61-2 Medications Used in the Treatment of PCP

Medication	Dose	Route	Common Adverse Reactions	Comments
TMP-SMX	15–20 mg/ kg of the trimethoprim component	Oral or intravenous	Rash, fever, transaminase elevations, pancytopenia, and hyperkalemia	First choice of therapy
Pentamidine	4 mg/kg daily	Intravenous	Nephrotoxicity, pancreatitis, leukopenia, arrhythmias, and dysglycemia	Switching to pentamidine after failure of TMP-SMX does not improve prognosis
Primaquine plus clindamycin	30 mg daily + 600 mg three times a day	Oral	Abdominal pain, anemia, fever, and hemolysis	Screen for G6PD deficiency
Atovaquone	750 mg twice daily	Oral	Abdominal pain, nausea, anemia, and neutropenia	Should take with meals

With the widespread use of sulfa drugs for prophylaxis and treatment of PCP, there is some concern about mutations in the dihydropteroate synthase (DHPS) gene of *P. carinii*. Some investigators have reported a correlation between prior sulfa prophylaxis and the occurrence of this mutation; however, the clinical significance of this mutation is still poorly understood. Failure of sulfa-based treatment is considered so rare that patients with sulfa allergies failing alternative therapies are desensitized to sulfa and treated with high-dose TMP-SMX at our institution.

Pneumothoraces in the setting of PCP can lead to prolonged air leaks and long-term morbidity. Conservative management is associated with high failure rates and prolonged hospitalization. Needle drainage, tube thoracostomy, Heimlich valve drainage, pleurodesis, pleurectomy, video-assisted thoracoscopic surgery, and thoracotomy may be needed. The reported success rates of tube thoracostomy in the evacuation of pneumothorax are variable. Heimlich valve drainage has been shown to facilitate earlier discharge from acute-care facilities. Surgery is needed if tube thoracostomy does not resolve the pneumothorax. The reported recurrence rates of spontaneous pneumothorax in AIDS are high (11%–60%), with pneumothorax in PCP being an independent predictor of mortality.

The introduction of HAART in patients may be complicated by the Immune Reconstitution Inflammatory Syndrome (IRIS). This syndrome, first described in patients with tuberculosis, has been reported with every opportunistic infection as well as hepatitis B and C. For example, patients with PCP can develop a pneumonic syndrome after effective PCP treatment and subsequent HAART initiation. No pathogens are identified on bronchoscopy, and the BAL CD4/CD8 ratio is much higher than in the initial illness. The evidence suggests that an influx of CD4 cells may be responsible for the syndrome. It can become severe enough to cause respiratory failure requiring mechanical ventilation.

Bacterial pneumonia remains a common complication of HIV infection. *Streptococcus pneumonia* and *Haemophilus influenzae* are the most frequent causes of community-acquired pneumonia in HIV-infected patients. "Atypical" organisms are found in approximately 3% of cases, usually with another organism. Nosocomial organisms are usually associated with advanced disease, recent hospitalization, and prior antibiotic exposure. Although the clinical presentation of community-acquired pneumonia is similar between HIV-infected and non–HIV-infected patients, bacteremia occurs more frequently in the presence of HIV, and the incidence and severity increases with worsening immunodeficiency. In HIV-infected patients, the yield from routine sputum cultures in the diagnosis of community-acquired pneumonia equals that of other, more invasive diagnostic procedures. Treatment of bacterial pneumonia in patients infected with HIV is no different than in immunocompetent patients, although mortality may be higher. Pneumococcal vaccination is recommended for HIV-infected patients.

Mycobacterium tuberculosis (see Chapters 49–51) is a serious threat to patients with HIV. Patients with HIV infection and a positive tuberculin skin test have an 8% to 10% risk per year of developing clinical tuberculosis. For this reason, tuberculin skin testing or use of an interferon-γ release assay, and appropriate tuberculosis prophylaxis are essential in the care of those with HIV infection. In this patient group, 5-mm induration should be considered to represent a positive tuberculin skin test and justify prophylaxis with isoniazid monotherapy. Because of an increased risk for fatal or severe hepatotoxicity, a 2-month regimen of daily rifampin and pyrazinamide is not recommended for latent tuberculosis infection treatment regardless of HIV status. Results from a randomized clinical trial comparing isoniazid daily therapy for 9 months with 12 doses of once-weekly isoniazid-rifapentine in HIV+ patients are pending.

Tuberculosis can occur as a primary infection, or as reactivation of a prior infection. It tends to present earlier in the course of HIV-related disease than most other infectious complications.

Chest radiographic findings depend on the degree of immunosuppression. Typical upper-lobe infiltrates are most common among patients with normal or mildly diminished CD4 cell counts. With advancing HIV infection, cavitation becomes rare, and nonapical or diffuse infiltrates predominate. Miliary pattern is seen in advanced disease. The approach to the diagnosis and treatment of tuberculosis in the HIV-infected patient is similar to that in patients without AIDS. There is, however, some concern that shorter regimens (24 weeks) may be associated with a higher rate of recurrence or relapse in patients infected with HIV.

In patients in whom HAART is initiated during the treatment of tuberculosis, temporary worsening of tuberculosis signs and symptoms can occur secondary to the IRIS. This phenomenon, also known as the paradoxical response, is seen in as many as 30% of patients. The diagnosis can be made after a thorough evaluation to rule out other etiologies such as infection with multidrug-resistant tuberculosis, or inadequate drug levels due to interactions with HAART or malabsorption. In many patients, no change in therapy is required. However, a short course of corticosteroids may be required for those in whom the inflammatory response is exaggerated. The IRIS usually occurs within the first 45 days after initiation of HAART but can occur from weeks to months later. Another form of the syndrome is the development of symptoms due to untreated occult disease that has been "unmasked" by the newly reconstituted immune system.

The optimal timing of initiation of HAART in AIDS patients with tuberculosis who are not already on HAART is not clear. Options include simultaneous tuberculosis treatment and HAART or treatment of tuberculosis first with delay of HAART by several weeks to months. A positive aspect of starting both regimens simultaneously is the possible prevention of progressive HIV disease and reduction in morbidity or mortality associated with tuberculosis or other opportunistic infections. A downside to the approach is the possibility of overlapping toxicities, drug interactions, a high pill burden, and the possibility of developing the IRIS or a paradoxical reaction. These factors must be weighed carefully when choosing the best time to start HAART in individual patients. Due to drug interactions with HAART, rifabutin is usually substituted for rifampin. Dose adjustments of rifabutin may be necessary, depending on the exact medications in the patient's HAART regimen. Consultation with an infectious disease or HIV/AIDS expert is recommended.

Although infection resulting from *M. avium* complex is common in advanced HIV disease (and is commonly cultured from pulmonary secretions), it is a rare cause of pulmonary signs and symptoms. On the other hand, *M. kansasii, M. xenopi,* and *M. gordonae* can all cause pulmonary disease. Both antimycobacterial therapy and surgical resection have been described in the treatment of *M. xenopi.*

Fungal pneumonia is well described in advanced HIV disease. Commonly reported organisms are *Cryptococcus neoformans, Histoplasma capsulatum, Coccidioides immitis,* and *Blastomycosis dermatitidis.* Disseminated infection is often part of the clinical presentation, and the radiographic findings are extremely varied.

The presentation of aspergillosis in the HIV-infected host is varied. In HIV-infected patients with pulmonary mycetoma, the clinical course differs in several ways from that seen in the immunocompetent host. HIV-infected patients are less likely to have hemoptysis but have a greater risk of disease progression. Invasive aspergillosis is associated with an extremely high mortality rate. However, combination therapy with antiretroviral and antifungal therapy has been reported to improve the outcome in these patients.

Although rarely reported, cryptogenic organizing pneumonia (COP) should be considered in the differential diagnosis of bilateral patchy infiltrates in a patient with AIDS. The clinical presentation is nonspecific, with fever, cough, dyspnea, and night sweats reported most commonly. The diagnosis can be made with open or thoracoscopic lung biopsy and the response to corticosteroids is generally good. Therapy is the same as what is used in the immunocompetent host.

Kaposi sarcoma is the most common HIV-related malignancy involving the lungs and (outside of sub-Saharan Africa) occurs almost exclusively in homosexual or bisexual men. Mucocutaneous manifestations are seen in the majority of patients with pulmonary disease. Fever and dyspnea are the most common symptoms at presentation. The chest radiograph may show patchy perihilar infiltrates with or without pleural effusions. Although lymphadenopathy may be seen, bulky disease suggests an alternative (or coexisting) diagnosis.

The visualization on bronchoscopy of characteristic reddish, flat, or raised endobronchial lesions is typically diagnostic. Biopsy of these lesions is usually not performed owing to the risk of bleeding and poor diagnostic yield from the small amount of tissue obtained. In the absence of endobronchial disease, open-lung biopsy may be necessary for diagnosis.

Before the introduction of HAART, Kaposi sarcoma carried a very poor prognosis. Even in those who responded to chemotherapy, the median survival was less than 12 months. The administration of HAART to patients receiving chemotherapy for Kaposi sarcoma significantly improves survival.

Bronchogenic carcinoma occurs more frequently in HIV-infected patients in the post-HAART era than it did in prior years. Unfortunately, the outcome remains poor despite HAART. HIV-infected patients are also at risk of developing B-cell lymphoma, in which pulmonary involvement is common.

HIV-related pulmonary hypertension is a complication of HIV infection that has become recognized with increased frequency over the past few years. HIV-infected patients have a 2,500-fold increased risk of developing pulmonary arterial hypertension (PAH) over the general population. The etiology remains unclear. There are several antiretroviral medications with minimal drug interactions; therefore, HAART should not preclude the treatment of pulmonary hypertension, nor vice versa.

FURTHER READING

1. Abdool Karim SS, Naidoo K, Grobler A, et al. Timing of initiation of antiretroviral drugs during tuberculosis therapy. *N Engl J Med.* 2010;362(8):697–706.

   Integrated HAART vs. sequential HAART during tuberculosis therapy is associated with improved survival.

2. CDC. Guidelines for prevention and treatment of opportunistic infections in HIV-infected adults and adolescents: Recommendations from CDC, the National Institutes of Health, and the HIV Medicine Association of the Infectious Diseases Society of America. MMWR 2009;58(No. RR-4);1–198.

   Comprehensive, up-to-date, evidence-based recommendations for prophylaxis of HIV-related infections.

3. Barry SM, Lipman MC, Deery AR, et al. Immune reconstitution pneumonitis following *Pneumocystis carinii* pneumonia in HIV-infected subjects. *HIV Med.* 2002;3:207–211.

   Indolent infection with P. carinii may lead to inflammatory pneumonitis after the institution of HAART.

4. Bower M, Powles T, Nelson M, et al. HIV-related lung cancer in the era of highly active antiretroviral therapy. *AIDS.* 2003;17:371–375.

   A description of the incidence of lung cancer in HIV-infected patients during the HAART era.

5. Bozzette SA, Sattler FR, Chiu J, et al; for the California Collaborative Treatment Group. A controlled trial of early adjunctive treatment with corticosteroids for *Pneumocystis carinii* pneumonia in the acquired immunodeficiency syndrome. *N Engl J Med.* 1990;323:1451.

   In 251 patients, early adjunctive steroids reduced the risk of oxygenation failure from 30% to 14% and of death from 23% to 11%.

6. Cicalini S, Chinello P, Petrosillo N. HIV infection and pulmonary arterial hypertension. *Expert Rev Respir Med.* 2011;5(2):257–266.

   HIV-infected patients have a 2,500-fold increased risk of developing PAH.

7. Cool CD, Rai PR, Yeager ME, et al. Expression of human herpes virus 8 in pulmonary hypertension. *N Engl J Med.* 2003;349:1113–1122.

8. Cordero E, Pachon J, Rivero A, et al. Usefulness of sputum culture for diagnosis of bacterial pneumonia in HIV-infected patients. *Eur J Clin Microbiol Infect Dis.* 2002;21:362–367.

   Routine sputum cultures have a diagnostic yield comparable to other standard, more invasive diagnostic methods.

9. DeLorenzo LJ, Huang CT, Maguire GP, et al. Roentgenographic patterns of *Pneumocystis carinii* pneumonia in 104 patients with AIDS. *Chest.* 1987;91:323.

   Bilateral interstitial infiltrates occurred in 75%, but alveolar infiltrates (25%), cysts (7%), unilateral infiltrates (5%), and other atypical features were not rare.

10. Franke MF, Robins JM, Mugabo J, et al. Effectiveness of early antiretroviral therapy initiation to improve survival among HIV-infected adults with tuberculosis: a retrospective cohort study. *PLoS Med.* 2011;8(5):e1001029.

    Initiation of HAART at day 15 of tuberculosis therapy is associated with a survival benefit compared to later initiation.

11. Greenberg AK, Knapp J, Rom WN, et al. Clinical presentation of pulmonary mycetoma in HIV-infected patients. *Chest.* 2002;122:886–892.

    Presentation and outcome of aspergillosis in HIV-infected patients.

12. Gordin FM, Simon GL, Wofsy CB, et al. Adverse reactions to trimethoprim-sulfamethoxazole in patients with the acquired immunodeficiency syndrome. *Ann Intern Med.* 1984;100:495.

    Adverse reactions, including rash, fever, neutropenia, and transaminase elevation, occurred in 29 of 35 patients (79%) and was dose limiting in 19 (54%).

13. Huang L, Hecht FM, Stansell JD, et al. Suspected *Pneumocystis carinii* pneumonia with a negative induced sputum examination: is early bronchoscopy useful? *Am J Respir Crit Care Med.* 1995;151:1866.

    Large series of patients with suspected PCP and negative induced sputum in a center where the yield of induced sputum is more than 90%. Even then, bronchoscopy had a high yield for PCP and other pathogens.

14. Huang L, Schnapp LM, Gruden JF, et al. Presentation of AIDS-related pulmonary Kaposi's sarcoma diagnosed by bronchoscopy. *Am J Respir Crit Care Med.* 1996;153:1385.

    The largest case series published. Chest radiograph and serum lactate dehydrogenase, not clinical presentation, distinguished those with and without concomitant infection.

15. Johnson JL, Okwera A, Hom DL, et al. Duration of efficacy of treatment of latent tuberculosis infection in HIV-infected adults. *AIDS.* 2001;33:1762–1769.

    Six months of isoniazid for latent tuberculosis infection is initially protective, but efficacy is lost within a year of therapy.

16. Kagawa FT, Kirsch CM, Yenokida GG, et al. Serum lactate dehydrogenase activity in patients with AIDS and *Pneumocystis carinii* pneumonia. *Chest.* 1988;94:1031.

    Findings in all 30 patients were abnormal.

17. Khater FJ, Moorman JP, Myers JW, et al. Bronchiolitis obliterans organizing pneumonia as a manifestation of AIDS: case report and literature review. *J Infect.* 2004;49:159–164.

    Description of presentation, diagnosis, and treatment of BOOP in the HIV-infected patient.

18. Kovacs JA, Ng VL, Masur H, et al. Diagnosis of *Pneumocystis carinii* pneumonia: improved detection in sputum with use of monoclonal antibodies. *N Engl J Med.* 1988;318:589.

    Immunofluorescent staining was 92% sensitive, compared with 80% for the best tinctorial stain, toluidine blue O.

19. Kovacs JA, Gill VJ, Meshnick S, et al. New insights into transmission, diagnosis and drug treatment of *Pneumocystis carinii* pneumonia. *JAMA.* 2001;286:2450–2460.

    Gene mutations provide evidence for person-to-person transmission of P. carinii.

20. Koval CE, Gigliotti F, Nevins D, et al. Immune reconstitution syndrome after successful treatment of *Pneumocystis carinii* pneumonia in a man with human immunodeficiency virus type 1 infection. *Clin Infect Dis.* 2002;35:491–493.

    Pneumonitis following improvement in immune function.

21. Leoung GS, Feigal DW Jr, Montgomery AB, et al. Aerosolized pentamidine for prophylaxis against *Pneumocystis carinii* pneumonia: the San Francisco community prophylaxis trial. *N Engl J Med.* 1990;323:769.

    Aerosolized pentamidine was 50% to 75% effective.

22. Lopez-Palomo C, Martin-Zamorano M, Benitez E, et al. Pneumonia in HIV-infected patients in the HAART era: incidence, risk, and impact of the pneumococcal vaccination. *Med Virol.* 2004;72:517–524.

    Evaluates the efficacy of pneumococcal vaccination in HIV-infected patients.

23. Magnenat JL, Nicod LP, Auckenthaler R, et al. Mode of presentation and diagnosis of bacterial pneumonia in human immunodeficiency virus-infected patients. *Am Rev Respir Dis.* 1991;144:917.

    Half of the patients taken to bronchoscopy for undiagnosed HIV-related pneumonia had an atypical presentation of bacterial infection.

24. Masur H, Ognibene FP, Yarchoan R, et al. CD4 counts as predictors of opportunistic pneumonias in human immunodeficiency virus (HIV) infection. *Ann Intern Med.* 1989;111:223.

CD4 counts obtained within 60 days were less than 200 in 46 of 49 episodes and less than 250 in 48 of 49 episodes. Patients with higher counts had other diseases.

25. Metersky ML, Colt HG, Olson LK, et al. AIDS-related spontaneous pneumothorax: risk factors and treatment. *Chest.* 1995;108:946.

A large case series with multivariate analysis. Pneumatoceles and prophylactic aerosolized pentamidine predicted risk of pneumothorax. Surgical and chemical pleurodesis prevented recurrence.

26. Miller RF, Foley NM, Kessel D, et al. Community-acquired lobar pneumonia in patients with HIV infection and AIDS. *Thorax.* 1994;49:367.

The most common pathogens were S. pneumoniae, S. aureus, P. carinii, H. influenzae, and P. aeruginosa.

27. Narita M, Ashkin D, Hollender ES, et al. Paradoxical worsening of tuberculosis following antiretroviral therapy in patients with AIDS. *Am J Respir Crit Care Med.* 1998;158:157.

Combination retroviral therapy initiated during treatment for tuberculosis-induced temporary worsening of signs and symptoms in one-third of patients, although usually not severe enough to warrant discontinuation of therapy. The phenomenon was associated with the return of a positive purified protein derivative (PPD) skin test and likely represented enhanced immune response to infection with tuberculosis.

28. Sattler FR, Frame P, Davis R, et al. Comparison of trimetrexate with leucovorin versus trimethoprim-sulfamethoxazole for moderate-severe episodes of *Pneumocystis carinii* pneumonia in patients with AIDS. *J Infect Dis.* 1994;170:165.

Trimethoprim-sulfamethoxazole therapy was superior to trimetrexate with leucovorin for patients presenting with $P(A-a)O_2$ greater than 30 mmHg, although trimetrexate was better tolerated.

29. Schneider MM, Hoepelman AI, Eeftinck Schattenkerk JK, et al. A controlled trial of aerosolized pentamidine or trimethoprim-sulfamethoxazole as primary prophylaxis against *Pneumocystis carinii* pneumonia in patients with human immunodeficiency virus infection. *N Engl J Med.* 1992;327:1836.

Of patients on monthly aerosolized pentamidine and patients on once or twice daily trimethoprim-sulfamethoxazole, 11% and 0%, respectively, developed first-episode Pneumocystis *pneumonia.*

30. Selwyn PA, Pumerantz AS, Durante A, et al. Clinical predictors of *Pneumocystis carinii* pneumonia, bacterial pneumonia and tuberculosis in HIV-infected patients. *AIDS.* 1998;12:885.

At admission, simple clinical variables differentiate tuberculosis, PCP, and bacterial pneumonia.

31. Shafer RW, Kim DS, Weiss JP, et al. Extrapulmonary tuberculosis in patients with human immunodeficiency virus infection. *Medicine (Baltimore).* 1991;70:384.

Diagnosis was often delayed because of decreased PPD reactivity and usually negative sputum smears (despite 90% of sputum eventually growing Mycobacterium tuberculosis*). Aspirates of lymph nodes, bone marrow, and the liver had the highest immediate yield.*

32. Staikowsky F, Lafon B, Guidet B, et al. Mechanical ventilation for *Pneumocystis carinii* pneumonia in patients with the acquired immunodeficiency syndrome: is the prognosis really improved? *Chest.* 1993;104:756.

Mortality rate was 50% if respiratory failure developed within 5 days of initial medical therapy and 95% if it developed after 5 days.

33. Toma E, Fournier S, Dumont M, et al. Clindamycin/primaquine versus trimethoprim-sulfamethoxazole as primary therapy for *Pneumocystis carinii* pneumonia in AIDS: a randomized, double-blind pilot trial. *Clin Infect Dis.* 1993;17:178.

Combination clindamycin-primaquine with trimethoprim-sulfamethoxazole as primary treatment for mild to moderately severe PCP. Efficacy of both regimens was equal, with no significant difference in toxicity, survival, or rate of relapse.

34. Thomas CF, Limper AH. *Pneumocystis* pneumonia. *N Engl J Med.* 2004;350:2487–2498.

Comprehensive review of Pneumocystis *pneumonia, clinical presentation, diagnosis, treatment, and biology of the disease.*

35. Visconti E, Ortona E, Mencarini P, et al. Mutations in dihydropteroate synthase gene of *Pneumocystis carinii* in HIV patients with *Pneumocystis carinii* pneumonia. *Int J Antimicrob Agents.* 2001;18:547–551.

Genetic mutations in P. carinii *occur as a result of selective pressure from sulfa therapy. Such mutations may not translate into worse outcome or nonresponse to therapy.*

36. Weverling GJ, Mocroft A, Ledergerber B, et al. Discontinuation of *Pneumocystis carinii* pneumonia prophylaxis after start of highly active antiretroviral therapy in HIV-1 infection. *Lancet.* 1999;353:1293.

   During 247 person-years of follow-up after discontinuation of prophylaxis at median CD4 count of 270, no cases of PCP developed. Almost all had been receiving primary prophylaxis.

37. White DA, Stover DE. Pulmonary complication of HIV infection. *Clin Chest Med.* 1996;17:621.

   A review of essentially all major clinical issues relating to HIV-related lung disease. Some of the chapters: P. carinii; Mycobacterial complications of HIV infection; Approach to the patient with pulmonary disease.

38. Woldehanna S, Volmink J. Treatment of latent tuberculosis infection in HIV-infected persons. *Cochrane Database Syst Rev.* 2004;(1):CD000171.

   Review of the treatment of latent tuberculosis infection.

39. Wolff AJ, O'Donnell AE. HIV-related pulmonary infections: a review of the recent literature. *Curr Opin Pulm Med.* 2003;9:210–214.

   The authors review some of the more recent literature pertaining to HIV-related pulmonary infections.

40. Zuper JP, Calmy A, Evison JM, et al. Pulmonary arterial hypertension related to HIV infection: improved hemodynamics and survival associated with antiretroviral therapy. *Clin Infect Dis.* 2004;38:1178–1185.

   Antiretroviral therapy improved survival in HIV-infected patients with pulmonary hypertension.

Hospital-Acquired Pneumonia

Kim M. Kerr

Hospital-acquired pneumonia (HAP) is defined as pneumonia occurring 48 hours or more after hospital admission. The definition excludes pulmonary infection that may be incubating at the time of admission. Pneumonia is the second most common hospital-acquired infection, and is associated with the highest mortality rate of all nosocomial diseases. Between 5 and 10 cases of HAP occur per 1,000 hospital admissions, but the incidence is 6 to 20 times higher in mechanically ventilated patients. In this group, the development of pneumonia (ventilator-associated pneumonia [VAP]) is associated with significant morbidity and higher mortality and substantially increases the cost of patient care.

In the immunocompetent host, HAP can be divided into early onset and late-onset infections. Early pneumonia occurs during the first 4 days of hospitalization and is often caused by community-acquired pathogens such as *Streptococcus pneumoniae,* methicillin-sensitive *Staphylococcus aureus,* and *Haemophilus influenzae.* Specific risk factors can alter the likely pathogens. For instance, if a patient has a witnessed aspiration, anaerobes, enteric Gram-negative bacilli, *S. aureus* should be considered. Recent thoraco-abdominal surgery and the presence of an obstructing foreign body are both additional risk factors for anaerobic pneumonias. Patients with coma, head injury, recent influenza, recent intravenous drug use, diabetes mellitus, or chronic renal failure are at increased risk for *S. aureus* pneumonias. Corticosteroids predispose patients to pneumonias from fungi, *Pseudomonas aeruginosa,* and, in some regions of the country, *Legionella* species.

Late-onset HAP, occurring 4 days or more after admission, is more commonly caused by, *S. aureus, P. aeruginosa,* or *Acinetobacter* or *Enterobacter* species. Resistant organisms such as methicillin-resistant *S. aureus* (MRSA), *P. aeruginosa,* and *Acinetobacter baumannii* tend to emerge after prolonged mechanical ventilation (>7 days), prior antibiotic use, and the use of broad-spectrum antibiotics (third-generation cephalosporins, fluoroquinolones, or carbapenems).

Understanding the pathogenesis of HAP may help in developing mechanisms of prevention. In the normal nonsmoking host, the upper respiratory tract is colonized with aerobic and anaerobic bacteria, whereas the respiratory tract below the vocal cords is sterile. Changes in host defenses can lead to inoculation of the lower respiratory tract with potentially pathogenic bacteria. Colonization and potentially fatal infection can follow inoculation.

Although pathogens can gain access to the lung by inhalation, hematogenous seeding, and contiguous spread, aspiration is the major route of bacterial access in patients with and without endotracheal tubes. Organisms such as *P. aeruginosa* can be inoculated directly into the endotracheal tube of intubated patients, whereas *Enterobacteriaceae* usually colonize the oropharynx before the trachea. Studies of oral care in the intensive care unit (ICU) show that chlorhexidine significantly decreases the risk of VAP. Subgroup analysis suggests that favorable effects were most pronounced in patients who were treated with 2% chlorhexidine and in cardiosurgical patients.

Mechanical ventilation almost always requires the presence of an artificial airway (endotracheal tube or tracheostomy tube). However, the presence of such an airway reduces the effectiveness of the cough reflex, compromises mucociliary clearance, can cause direct injury to the tracheal epithelial surface, and provides a direct pathway for pathogens from the ICU environment to the lower respiratory tract. A biofilm of bacteria-laden accretions on the luminal surface of the endotracheal tube also can contribute to the development of VAP if accretions dislodge into distal airways. Novel solutions to the biofilm problem include the development of less-adhesive polymers to prevent accumulation of infected material in the lumen of the tube or coating the tube with antimicrobial agents. Aspiration around the cuff of the endotracheal tube is another mechanism by which bacteria can access the lower respiratory tract. To reduce the amount of secretions pooling on top of the endotracheal tube cuff, a specific endotracheal tube was designed with a separate lumen that allows drainage of secretions from the subglottic space above the tube. Randomized trials have shown a reduction in the incidence of VAP with the use of this technique. Problems with the use of this device are the additional cost and the need to have these endotracheal tubes available when patients undergo endotracheal intubation in a variety of settings (e.g., emergency rooms, operating rooms, ICUs, and hospital wards).

Noninvasive ventilation has been shown to reduce the need for endotracheal intubation and decrease the likelihood of pneumonia. It should be considered in appropriate patients. The risk of developing VAP is approximately 3% per day for the first 5 days of intubation, 2% per day from days 6 to 10, and 1% per day after that. Some studies suggest that a daily routine of interruption of continuous sedation and assessment of readiness to wean may shorten the duration of mechanical ventilation. Theoretically, shortening the duration of intubation should reduce the incidence of VAP, but these protocols have yet to demonstrate a reduction in VAP.

Nasogastric feeding tubes have been implicated as a risk factor for pneumonia, presumably because of an associated increased incidence of gastroesophageal reflux and aspiration. The supine head position also is a risk factor for the development of VAP, since it has been linked to an increased incidence of aspiration and bacterial colonization of the lower airways in ventilated patients. Clinical data suggest that the simple maneuver of elevating the head of the bed, especially for patients with feeding tubes, may be a safe and inexpensive means of lowering the incidence of VAP.

The role of gastric colonization in facilitating VAP is controversial and has generated multiple clinical trials yielding conflicting data. Central to the controversy is the relationship between VAP, gastric colonization, and stress ulcer prophylaxis. The acidic environment of the gastric lumen prevents bacterial growth under normal physiologic circumstances. However, gastric acidity can be reduced by critical illness, advanced age, and administration of antacids or H_2 antagonists. The cytoprotective agent, sucralfate, may prevent stress ulcers without altering gastric acidity. There have been multiple analyses of more than 20 randomized, controlled clinical trials trying to settle the issue of the effect of stress ulcer prophylaxis on the development of VAP with mixed results: sucralfate decreased gastric colonization and VAP versus H_2 antagonists in some but not all studies. Given its relatively low cost and safe pharmacologic profile, sucralfate is an appealing way of providing stress-related upper gastrointestinal (GI) bleeding prophylaxis. However, sucralfate is not as effective as H_2 antagonists in preventing upper GI bleeding and one must weigh the benefit of the potential decreased risk of VAP against the potential decreased protection against GI bleeding. Whether proton pump inhibitors are more effective than H_2 antagonists in preventing significant upper GI bleeding associated with stress ulcers remains unclear. Limited data suggests the incidence of VAP is similar in those patients who receive H_2 antagonists or proton pump inhibitors for stress ulcer prophylaxis. In summary, the optimal agent that minimizes the risk of both stress ulcers and VAP has yet to be determined.

Although the role of gastric colonization in VAP is uncertain, the evidence is convincing that colonization of the oropharynx often precedes colonization of the trachea and subsequent development of VAP. Selective decontamination of the digestive tract is a strategy designed to prevent oropharyngeal and gastric colonization with aerobic Gram-negative bacilli and *Candida* species without altering the anaerobic flora of the gut. Some proposed regimens use a combination of nonabsorbable antibiotics applied as a paste to the oropharynx or given through the nasogastric tube, whereas others also include a short course of a systemic antibiotic. Some clinical trials have demonstrated a decrease in the rates of lower respiratory tract infections with selective decontamination of the digestive tract; others, however, have found no difference in the incidence of VAP. Because of concerns about the emergence of antibiotic-resistant organisms with these regimens, the routine use of selective decontamination of the digestive tract to prevent VAP is not recommended at present.

Despite some convincing evidence to support specific interventions to prevent VAP, studies have shown that many critical care nurses and physicians do not follow published recommendations. To facilitate guideline implementation, many facilities have adopted "care bundles," a small set of interventions derived from evidence-based guidelines that are expected to improve patient outcomes when they are performed together. The Institute for Healthcare Improvement (IHI) has proposed a "ventilator bundle" with four components (elevation of the head of the bed 30°–45°, daily sedation vacation and daily assessment of readiness to extubate, peptic ulcer disease prophylaxis, and deep venous thrombosis prophylaxis). While the science supporting the individual components of this bundle recently have been challenged, institutions adopting this ventilator bundle have reported decreased incidences of VAP.

The diagnosis of HAP, and in particular VAP, has been the subject of numerous studies and heated debates. It is generally accepted that reliance solely on clinical criteria (e.g., fever, leukocytosis, purulent tracheal secretions, and a new or progressive infiltrate on chest radiographs) often can be misleading. What is yet to be agreed upon is the role of "blind" and bronchoscopically guided culture techniques in the diagnosis of VAP. At issue for all microbiologic techniques are (1) the accuracy and reproducibility of the collection methods used, (2) the appropriate bacteriologic thresholds to define pneumonia, (3) the costs and risks associated with each procedure, and (4) the effect of the techniques on overall clinical outcomes. One problem in assessing the various diagnostic maneuvers is that no true gold standard for accuracy exists with which to compare diagnostic techniques, such as quantitative tracheal aspirates, quantitative bronchoalveolar lavage (BAL), or protected brush specimens. Even when open-lung biopsy has been performed, significant interobserver variability has been noted among pathologists when making the diagnosis of pneumonia on the basis of histologic criteria.

Given the subjectivity involved in the previous definitions of VAP, the Center for Disease Control has proposed a new surveillance definition of VAP that requires objective evidence of worsening oxygenation (need for increased supplemental oxygen or positive end–expiratory pressure); objective evidence of infection (fever, hypothermia, leukocytosis, or leukopenia); and purulent secretions and/or positive microbiologic results that are treated by the clinician. These criteria will likely change measured VAP rates, but they are intended to be used only for surveillance and not to guide clinical care.

Because of the significant questions regarding the sensitivity, specificity, and reproducibility of invasive diagnostic techniques for the diagnosis of HAP, a conservative approach seems warranted. When nosocomial pneumonia is suspected, a sputum or tracheal aspirate specimen should be obtained for Gram stain and culture. The Gram stain allows for the evaluation of the quality of the respiratory sample. Finding more than 10 squamous epithelial cells per low-powered field in an expectorated sputum specimen suggests oropharyngeal contamination; culture results from those samples will likely be unreliable. In addition, if the sample demonstrates fewer than 10 neutrophils per low-powered field, a diagnosis other than pneumonia should be suspected. However, the absence of neutrophils does not conclusively exclude an infectious process, because factors such as sampling errors and leukopenia can make this finding misleading. In the intubated patient, contamination of oropharyngeal specimens is less of a concern, but colonization of the endotracheal tube lumen itself can confound the interpretation of microbiologic studies. Cultures of tracheal aspirates are sensitive for detecting the organism responsible for the pneumonia, but they are not specific. Differentiating organisms that are colonizers from those that are true pathogens is extremely difficult. Semiquantitative cultures can provide information regarding the relative number of pathogenic bacteria in the specimen, but will not necessarily distinguish between colonizing and infecting bacteria. In addition, semiquantitative cultures are not available at all institutions, and many patients who develop HAP are already receiving antibiotics that may alter the results of this technique. Blood cultures should be obtained in the evaluation of suspected HAP, as should pleural fluid analysis in patients with pleural effusion. Isolation of organisms from these normally sterile fluids is typically diagnostic of the underlying pneumonia.

Treatment of nosocomial pneumonia should be initiated promptly and should not await the results of microbiologic tests. Early use of appropriate antibiotic therapy, before obtaining culture results, appears to have the greatest likelihood of improving patient outcome. The American Thoracic Society (ATS) published recommendations that, along with local (hospital/ICU) resistance patterns, may help in selecting appropriate antibiotics for empiric treatment of HAP. Consideration of previous antibiotics the patient may have received is also necessary when selecting empiric coverage for HAP. Inadequate initial empiric antibiotic therapy most frequently results from omission of treatment for MRSA or Gram-negative bacteria (*P. aeruginosa, Acinetobacter* species, *Klebsiella pneumoniae,* and *Enterobacter* species), or with resistance to previously used antibiotics. It is associated with a high mortality.

Of particular relevance to the choice of empiric antibiotic regimens for HAP are (1) the presence or absence of underlying medical conditions; (2) the time during the hospital course that the patient developed HAP (early <4 days, or late >4 days); and (3) the presence of specific risk factors for infection with particular organisms. The ATS and Infectious Disease Society of America (IDSA) guidelines state that previously healthy patients who develop early onset HAP can usually be treated with a nonpseudomonal third-generation cephalosporin or ampicillin/sulbactam or a quinolone (levofloxacin, moxifloxacin, or ciprofloxacin) or ertapenem. Those who develop late-onset HAP, are critically ill, or have risk factors for multidrug-resistant pathogens should receive broader antibiotic coverage to include resistant and virulent organisms such as *P. aeruginosa, Acinetobacter* species, *K. pneumoniae* (ESBL), *Enterobacter* species, and MRSA. Empiric therapy in these circumstances commonly includes two synergistic antipseudomonal agents as well as vancomycin or linezolid. If patients develop HAP during or shortly after antibiotic treatment for a different infection, use of the same class of antibiotics should be avoided in selecting initial empiric therapy. Knowledge of the antibiotic susceptibility patterns of local flora within a particular unit and hospital is essential in selecting appropriate initial empiric therapy. Frequently, the spectrum of antibiotic coverage can be narrowed 2 to 3 days into the treatment course, based on culture and sensitivity results and on the patient's response. Tailoring of antibiotic treatment as soon as possible is important to minimize the development of resistant organisms and to avoid the cost and adverse effects of unnecessary medications. Treatment of specific organisms is addressed elsewhere in this book. The duration of therapy is usually 7 to 14 days, based on the severity of illness, the infecting pathogen, and the rapidity of clinical response.

FURTHER READING

1. American Thoracic Society and Infectious Diseases Society of America. Guidelines for the management of adults with hospital-acquired, ventilator-associated, and healthcare-associated pneumonia. *Am J Respir Crit Care Med.* 2005;717:388 416.

   Extensive review of the epidemiology, pathogenesis, diagnostic strategies, and treatment of hospital-acquired pneumonia. Supported by 294 references.

2. Bonten MJ, Gaillard CA, de Leeuw PW, et al. Role of colonization of the upper intestinal tract in the pathogenesis of ventilator-associated pneumonia. *Clin Infect Dis.* 1997;24:309–319.

3. Bouadma L, Wolff M, Lucet JC. Ventilator-associated pneumonia and its prevention. *Curr Opin Infect Dis.* 2012;25:395–404.

   An excellent critical review of the recent literature focusing on measures to prevent ventilator-associated pneumonia.

4. Chastre J, Wolff M, Fagon J, et al. Comparison of 8 vs 15 days of antibiotic therapy for ventilator-associated pneumonia in adults. *JAMA.* 2003;290:2588–2598.

   Four hundred and one patients with VAP were randomized to 8 or 15 days of antibiotics. There was no difference in mortality, recurrent infection, duration of mechanical ventilation, or length of ICU stay between the two groups. Those with VAP caused by nonfermenting Gram-negative bacilli, who were treated with 8 days had a higher pulmonary infection recurrence than those who received 15 days of antibiotics.

5. Corley DE, Kirtland SH, Winterbauer RH, et al. Reproducibility of the histologic diagnosis of pneumonia among a panel of four pathologists: analysis of the gold standard. *Chest.* 1997;112:458.

   This study challenges histology as a gold standard in the diagnosis of VAP. Recognition of histologic pneumonia varies among pathologists.

6. Fagon JY, Maillet JM, Novara A. Hospital-acquired pneumonia: methicillin resistance and intensive care unit admission. *Am J Med.* 1998;104:17S.

7. Gerbeaux P, Ledoray V, Boussuges A, et al. Diagnosis of nosocomial pneumonia in mechanically ventilated patients. *Am J Respir Crit Care Med.* 1998;157:76.

   Results using BAL are reasonably reproducible in the absence of pneumonia, but in the presence of pneumonia, BAL is not repeatable.

8. Grgurich PE, Hudcova J, Lei Y, et al. Diagnosis of ventilator-associated pneumonia: controversies and working toward a gold standard. *Curr Opin Infect Dis.* 2013;26(2):140–150.

   A review of the literature and associated controversies and dilemmas in the diagnosis of VAP for clinical and surveillance purposes.

9. Hess DR. Noninvasive positive-pressure ventilation and ventilator-associated pneumonia. *Respir Care.* 2005;50:924–929.

   A review of 12 randomized trials comparing the incidence of pneumonia in patients treated with noninvasive positive-pressure ventilation (NPPV), compared to those treated with tracheal intubation and mechanical ventilation. All but one trial demonstrated a significant reduction in the incidence of pneumonia in patients randomized to NPPV.

10. Ibrahim EH, Tracy L, Hill C, et al. The occurrence of ventilator-associated pneumonia in a community hospital: risk factors and clinical outcomes. *Chest.* 2001;120:555–561.

    Prospective study of a medical and a surgical ICU in a community hospital. VAP developed in 15% of the 880 mechanically ventilated patients. Logistic regression analysis demonstrated that tracheostomy, multiple central venous lines, reintubation, and the use of antacids were independently associated with the development of VAP.

11. Iregui M, Ward S, Sherman G, et al. Clinical importance of delays in the initiation of appropriate antibiotic treatment for ventilator-associated pneumonia. *Chest.* 2002;122:262–268.

    Delay in appropriate antibiotic treatment occurred in 30.8% patients with VAP and was associated with a higher mortality (odds ratio [OR] 7.68). The most common reason for the delay in appropriate therapy was a delay in writing the antibiotic orders.

12. Kirtland SH, Corley DE, Winterbauer RH, et al. The diagnosis of ventilator-associated pneumonia: a comparison of histologic, microbiologic, and clinical criteria. *Chest.* 1997;112:445–457.

    No combination of clinical criteria correlated with the presence or absence of histologic pneumonia. Quantitative cultures (protected specimen brushing [PSB], BAL) did not accurately separate the histologic pneumonia and nonpneumonia groups. Tracheal aspirate had a sensitivity of 87% in recognizing bacterial species simultaneously present in lung parenchyma.

13. Kollef MH, Ward S. The influence of mini-BAL cultures on patient outcomes: implications for the antibiotic management of ventilator-associated pneumonia. *Chest.* 1998;113:412–420.

    Selection of appropriate initial antibiotic therapy improves the mortality rate in patients with suspected VAP. The most common organisms not appropriately covered with initial therapy were Gram-negative bacteria resistant to a prescribed third-generation cephalosporin.

14. Kress JP, Pohlman AS, O'Connor MF, et al. Daily interruption of sedative infusions in critically ill patients undergoing mechanical ventilation. *N Eng J Med*. 2000;342:1471–1477.

15. Labeau SO, Van de Vyver K, Brusselaers N, et al. Prevention of ventilator-associated pneumonia with oral antiseptics: a systematic review and meta-analysis. *Lancet Infect Dis*. 2011;11:845–854.

16. Liberati A, D'Amico R, Pifferi S, et al. Antibiotic prophylaxis to reduce respiratory tract infections and mortality in adults receiving intensive care. *Cochrane Database Syst Rev*. 2009;(4):CD000022.

    A review of 36 trials comparing prophylactic antibiotics in the prevention of respiratory tract infections in ICU patients. Trials using a combination of systemic and topical antibiotics demonstrated a significant reduction in respiratory tract infections and mortality in the treated group. In trials, comparing topical antimicrobials alone there was a significant reduction in respiratory tract infections, but not total mortality.

17. Luna CM, Vujacich P, Niederman MS, et al. Impact of BAL data on the therapy and outcome of ventilator-associated pneumonia. *Chest*. 1997;111:676–685.

    Delay of adequate therapy until bronchoscopy is performed or until BAL results are known, results in increased mortality in patients with suspected VAP.

18. Mehta S, Burry L, Cook D, et al. Daily sedation interruption in mechanically ventilated critically ill patients cared for with a sedation protocol: a randomized controlled trial. *JAMA*. 2012;308:1985–1982.

19. Muscedere J, Rewa O, McKechnie K, et al. Subglottic secretion drainage for the prevention of ventilator-associated pneumonia: a systematic review and meta-analysis. *Crit Care Med*. 2011;39:1985–1991.

    A review of 13 randomized clinical trials of comparing the effectiveness of standard endotracheal tubes to those with subglottic secretion drainage in the prevention of ventilator-associated pneumonia. Twelve studies reported a reduction in VAP and in meta-analysis, the use of subglottic secretion drainage was associated with an overall risk ratio for VAP of 0.55 (95% confidence interval, 0.46–0.66, P < .00001).

20. Pilkington KB, Wagstaff MJ, Greenwood JE. Prevention of gastrointestinal bleeding due to stress ulceration: a review of current literature. *Anaesth Intensive Care*. 2012;40:253–259.

21. Pinciroli R, Mietto C, Berra L. Respiratory therapy device modifications to prevent ventilator-associated pneumonia. *Curr Opin Infect Dis*. 2013;26(2):175–183.

    A thorough review of newer technologies, such as subglottic secretion drainage, antimicrobial coatings, endotracheal cuff materials, and pressure control in the prevention of VAP.

22. Rello J, Olendorf D, Oster G, et al. Epidemiology and outcomes of ventilator-associated pneumonia in a large US database. *Chest*. 2002;122:2115–2121.

    US study with 842 VAP patients and 2,243 control subjects. The incidence of VAP was 9.3%; the mean interval between intubation and development of VAP was 3.3 ± 6.6 days. VAP resulted in an increase in ICU/hospital stay, duration of mechanical ventilation, and hospital charges.

23. Rello J, Torres A, Ricart M, et al. Ventilator-associated pneumonia by *Staphylococcus aureus*: comparison of methicillin-resistant and methicillin-sensitive episodes. *Am J Respir Crit Care Med*. 1994;150:1545–1549.

    Risk factors for developing methicillin-resistant S. aureus ventilator-associated pneumonia (MRSA VAP) include previous antibiotic therapy, therapy with steroids, mechanical ventilation more than 6 days, age older than 25 years, and preceding chronic obstructive pulmonary disease. MRSA VAP had a greater bacteremic rate and a worse outcome than MSSA VAP.

24. Trouillet JL, Chastre J, Vuagnat A, et al. Ventilator-associated pneumonia caused by potentially drug-resistant bacteria. *Am J Respir Crit Care Med*. 1998;157:531–539.

    Using logistic regression analysis, three variables were identified as risk factors for the development of VAP with potentially drug-resistant bacteria: mechanical ventilation more than 7 days, prior antibiotic use, and prior use of broad-spectrum antibiotics.

63 Asthma

Timothy D. Bigby and Patricia W. Finn

Asthma is characterized clinically by reversible airway obstruction in association with symptoms of dyspnea, cough, and sputum production. Asthma is defined in pathophysiological terms by emphasizing the physiologic finding of airway hyperresponsiveness and the pathologic finding of airway inflammation.

Asthma is a common disorder worldwide. The World Health Organization recently stated that approximately 300 million people have asthma. Asthma is not distributed equally throughout the world: industrialized, Western countries have a higher incidence. In the United States, asthma afflicts 25 million people, including more than 7 million children. Asthma is the most common chronic disease of childhood. In the United States, asthma is more common in urban than in rural populations, and the incidence is higher among minority populations. Epidemiologic studies indicate that most asthma begins in early childhood, although it can develop at any age. At least one half of children who develop asthma will have remission as adults, but adult-onset asthma rarely abates. The prevalence, severity, and mortality rates associated with asthma have increased over the last 40 years. The explanation is unclear, but urban living conditions, exposure to oxidant pollutants, diet, nutrition, passive smoking, obesity, and even current therapies have been implicated. More recent concerns have been raised about relationships to the modernization of Western culture, including a decreased incidence of common childhood infectious diseases, widespread antibiotic use, declining physical fitness in children, and rising incidence of obesity beginning in childhood. Although many of these issues have been related to affluence, the greatest rise in asthma in the United States has occurred in inner-city, African-American children (prevalence of 17% in 2009, a 50% rise over the decade).

The hallmark of airway pathology in asthma is mixed inflammatory cell infiltration; eosinophils are the most striking feature, but the infiltrates also include large numbers of less easily recognized mast cells, neutrophils, lymphocytes, and macrophages. The inflammatory changes are also associated with denudation of airway epithelium and mucous gland hypertrophy. Long-standing asthma can be associated with subepithelial fibrosis and smooth muscle hypertrophy. Severe asthma is often associated with inflammation having a neutrophil predominance.

The etiology of asthma remains enigmatic. It does not appear to be a single disease, but a syndrome. An older hypothesis suggested that so-called *intrinsic asthma* (i.e., asthma in individuals without identifiable triggers) might be neurally mediated. However, a distinct abnormality of the sympathetic, parasympathetic, or peptidergic nervous systems has not been found in asthmatics. Mutations of the β_2-adrenergic receptor have now been described, but these mutations may be more important in dictating response to treatment than in the etiology of the disease itself. Substantial data support an allergic pathogenesis mediated predominantly by both inhaled and systemic antigens. Allergy appears to play a central role in sustained wheezing in early childhood that can be characterized clinically as asthma. Cytokines released by T-helper (T_H)2 lymphocytes are increasingly recognized as important in allergic and, possibly, all asthma. Pivotal cytokines include interleukins 13, 4, 5, and 9. Adaptive, allergic dependent immunity has been shown to play pivotal roles in asthma pathogens. Recent studies suggest that the interface between adaptive and innate new antigen-dependant immunity is also crucial. This interface has been suggested to play a role in the increase in asthma prevalence. An attempt to link the increase in asthma in the industrialized world to improved healthcare and decreased childhood infections has been termed the *hygiene hypothesis*. If hygiene does play a role in the development of asthma; it may do so through the interface between innate and adaptive immunity.

Multiple studies have demonstrated that airway inflammation precedes the development of hyperresponsiveness. In some models, hyperresponsiveness does not develop if this inflammatory cell influx is blocked. Most investigators now believe that, despite multiple triggers for the inflammatory cell influx, airway inflammation is the common pathway by which airway hyperresponsiveness is induced. Inflammatory cells also appear to be the source of mediators that induce acute bronchoconstriction, mucus hypersecretion, airway edema, and further inflammatory cell influx. The inflammatory milieu is complex, and a single inflammatory cell or inflammatory mediator is unlikely to explain all the clinical features of asthma. Although a genetic component of asthma clearly exists, it is not explained by a single gene, but instead is a complex genetic disorder. Thus, asthma appears to be polygenic, and the phenotypic expression of involved genes is significantly influenced by environmental factors. A variety of candidate genes in asthma are currently under investigation. Some very large genome-wide association studies have shown strong associations between asthma and eosinophilia with single nucleotide polymorphisms in genes encoding for IL-1RL1, the receptor for IL-33, and IL-33 gene. These studies suggest an important and perhaps central role for this cytokine and its receptor. However, the true significance of these associations is unknown.

Intermittent reversible airway obstruction is a clinical hallmark of asthma. However, symptoms improve or can fully remit between episodes. During episodes, symptoms can vary from mild to severe, with profound limitation of activity and symptoms at rest. Patients may not notice symptoms of obstruction until their acute exacerbation is of moderate to severe intensity. A detailed history of factors that precipitate acute symptoms is critical in subsequent management.

The 2007 National Asthma Education and Prevention Program (NAEPP), Expert Panel Report III, and the 2010 Global Initiative for Asthma (GINA) stratify severity of disease into levels that can be used to determine the appropriate step of therapy (a *step-care* approach). These guidelines have been well received by pulmonary and allergy clinicians. The current NAEPP and GINA guidelines differ from prior reports in that they have included 6 and 5 steps, respectively. The stratification includes mild intermittent (step 1), mild persistent (step 2), moderate persistent (steps 3 and 4), and severe persistent disease (step 5). Patients with mild intermittent asthma have only occasional symptoms (two or fewer times per week), normal pulmonary function, use intermittent inhaled β_2-agonists no more than twice per week, and modest variability in peak expiratory flow (PEF), a measure of airflow obstruction that can be obtained by patients themselves. Patients with mild persistent asthma have symptoms more than twice per week but less than once per day, normal pulmonary function between exacerbations, and more significant variability in PEF with exacerbations. Patients with moderate persistent asthma have daily symptoms that interfere with activity, require daily use of a β_2-agonist for quick relief, and have abnormal baseline pulmonary function with more severe variability of PEF. Patients with severe, persistent asthma have continuous symptoms that significantly impair their lives, limit physical activity, and are associated with frequent exacerbations. Baseline pulmonary function is abnormal, and there is more dramatic variability of PEF.

Historical details, such as age of onset, frequency and severity of episodes, requirements for medications, hospitalizations, and prior need for mechanical ventilation, are important to document. Daily fluctuations in symptoms also are important. Some patients have predominantly nocturnal symptoms, which can be associated with uncontrolled reflux esophagitis, sinusitis, or pharyngeal dysfunction. Daily fluctuations also can be precipitated by exertion or exposure to a variety of environmental agents, including cold, dry air, oxidant pollutants, tobacco smoke, perfumes, dust, or provocative agents in the workplace. Symptoms that increase throughout the workday or work week and tend to improve with days off from work suggest the possibility of occupational asthma. A history of allergy, atopy, eczema, allergic rhinitis, or nasal polyps may be elicited. Medication allergies or symptoms associated with the use of nonsteroidal antiinflammatory drugs (NSAIDs) also can be associated with asthma. The syndrome of sensitivity to NSAIDs, nasal polyps, and asthma has been termed *triad asthma* or Samter syndrome. Patients with asthma should be instructed to avoid these drugs, and those with sensitivity to them should be advised to strictly avoid them.

Occasionally, cough is the only symptom of asthma, thus underscoring the importance of considering asthma in the differential diagnosis of this symptom. Cough associated with asthma may be dry, but it is often productive of thick, tenacious sputum that may contain mucous plugs. The sputum may become purulent as symptoms worsen. This may represent secondary bacterial infection but more often is caused by inflammatory cell infiltration without viral or bacterial superinfection. This purulent sputum most often contains numerous eosinophils, but severe exacerbations may be associated with neutrophils in sputum.

Physical findings in asthma correlate poorly with more objective measures of airway obstruction, such as pulmonary function tests, that are obtained in a laboratory setting. Nevertheless, the findings are clinically useful. In an asymptomatic asthmatic patient, physical findings may be absent; however, wheezing may be elicited by forced expiration. Mild bronchospasm, in general, is associated with wheezing only during expiration. With greater degrees of obstruction, wheezing is heard in both the inspiratory and expiratory phases, with prolongation of the expiratory phase. With profound obstruction, wheezes may be heard only during the inspiratory phase or even may be absent with profoundly diminished air movement. When wheezing is correlated with other physical examination findings, a more reliable assessment can be made of the severity of obstruction. Normally, the inspiratory-to-expiratory ratio is less than 1:2, but this ratio increases in a graded fashion to 1:3 or more with increasing degrees of airway obstruction. Patients also begin to use accessory muscles of respiration with moderate to severe acute bronchospasm and may have active rather than passive expiration. With significant obstruction, evidence also may be seen of hyperinflation with low diaphragms and an increased anteroposterior diameter. Pulsus paradoxus is a term used to describe an indirect measure of fluctuations in transpulmonary pressure that occur with severe obstruction. Rather than truly paradoxical, pulsus paradoxus is an exaggerated decline in blood pressure with inspiration. The degree of obstruction correlates crudely with pulsus paradoxus. A pulsus greater than 10 mmHg is abnormal, and greater than 20 mmHg suggests profound obstruction. However, this measure has been supplanted and should not substitute for direct measures of the degree of obstruction by bedside or home PEF measurements. Measurement of forced expiratory volume in 1 second (FEV_1) is the gold standard, but is obtainable in a pulmonary function laboratory and is thus less readily available. With severely labored respirations, the patient can become diaphoretic, anxious, and unable to speak in full sentences. A respiratory rate greater than 30 breaths per minute and a heart rate of 120 beats per minute or more suggest severe bronchospasm. Agitation, confusion, somnolence, and cyanosis are foreboding findings and suggest impending respiratory failure. Unilateral loss of breath sounds can be consistent with mucous plugging and secondary atelectasis, but these findings also must raise the possibility of pneumothorax.

The clinical laboratory examination of asthmatics is often of limited value. Peripheral blood eosinophilia is frequently present but rarely exceeds 25%. Serum immunoglobulin E (IgE) is often elevated in asthmatics, and in allergic asthmatics specific antibodies can be detected. Very high serum IgE should raise the question of allergic bronchopulmonary aspergillosis. Likewise, examination of sputum or nasal mucus can often reveal the presence of increased numbers of eosinophils.

During bronchospasm, pulmonary function tests, including spirometry, reveal obstruction with a decrease in FEV_1 and decreased mid-expiratory flows. The ratio of FEV_1 to forced vital capacity (FVC) also is reduced. With more severe obstruction, hyperinflation is evident, with an increased residual volume and functional residual capacity more than total lung capacity. The flow-volume loop reveals evidence of obstruction with diminished flows and coving inward of the expiratory limb. One of the hallmarks of asthma is partial or complete reversal of airway obstruction after the administration of a bronchodilator. This response also can be used to gauge the adequacy of treatment. However, the lack of response to a one-time dose of a bronchodilator does not preclude a reversible component to the patient's obstruction. Moreover, it is now recognized that asthma is often associated with a progressive decline in lung function over years; presumably, this decline is caused by fixed airway obstruction associated with airway remodeling. The diffusing capacity of the lung for carbon monoxide is often increased in asthmatics who do not smoke. The exact mechanism of this increase is unknown, but it is thought to represent an increase in pulmonary capillary blood volume associated with obstruction. PEF measurements, which are inexpensive, simple measurements that patients can assess and interpret, are also reduced during bronchospasm.

Bronchial challenge testing can establish the presence of airway hyperresponsiveness. Nonspecific bronchial hyperresponsiveness is demonstrated by exaggerated bronchoconstriction to inhaled histamine or methacholine. Nonspecific bronchial challenge is most useful in the evaluation of cough or to establish the diagnosis of asthma when the history is compatible, but physical examination and pulmonary function evidence of obstruction are lacking. However, bronchial challenge can be hazardous and should not be performed when significant airway obstruction is present. Bronchial challenge with specific provocative agents has utility in selected cases. The most commonly used specific bronchial challenges are exercise or cold air. Specific airway challenges with other agents (e.g., antigen) should only be performed in specialized centers having experience with these procedures.

Assessment of arterial blood gases usually is not necessary in the management of mild to moderate asthma. However, pulse oximetry may be of value during moderately severe exacerbations, and arterial blood gas assessment may be indicated during severe exacerbations. Hypoxemia is a frequent finding in this setting, and the arterial Pco_2 is usually decreased. During prolonged and severe episodes of airway obstruction, the patient can develop respiratory muscle fatigue, and the Pco_2 may normalize or become elevated. A normal or elevated Pco_2 during a severe exacerbation is an ominous sign, suggesting impending respiratory failure.

In the setting of chronic asthma and in the absence of another underlying condition, chest radiographic findings are usually normal. During an exacerbation, chest radiographs are not required unless fever, sputum production, chest pain, leukocytosis, or physical evidence of barotrauma are present. Hyperinflation of the lung can be present during severe exacerbations.

The diagnosis of asthma is made principally on clinical grounds; laboratory data are used in a supplementary or confirmatory fashion. A history of episodic wheezing in a nonsmoking patient, with findings of wheezing on physical examination, is strongly suggestive of asthma. Other causes of wheezing should be excluded. The diagnosis is confirmed with spirometry, which demonstrates obstruction (a FEV_1/FVC ratio of less than 70% with or without a significant reduction of FEV_1) that normalizes or significantly improves with use of a bronchodilator. If spirometry is normal, it should be repeated after a forced expiratory maneuver, which usually induces a fall in FEV_1 in asthmatics. If spirometry still remains normal, bronchial challenge testing should be considered. Alternatively, the patient can be followed over time with serial spirograms (or PEF monitoring) to demonstrate variable obstruction.

Not all patients who wheeze have asthma. Additional diagnoses should be sought in both acute and chronic settings. Upper airway obstruction, tracheomalacia, and tracheal or bronchial masses can all masquerade as asthma. These disorders are usually distinguished by the presence of stridor or focal wheezing on physical examination with flow limitation on a flow-volume loop. Laryngeal (vocal-cord) dysfunction can be clinically indistinguishable from asthma. This disorder is caused by inappropriate apposition of the vocal cords during the respiratory cycle, which can be successfully treated by speech therapy. Laryngeal dysfunctions are often misdiagnosed and, when severe, can be treated with systemic corticosteroids for presumed severe asthma. Flow-volume loops demonstrate normal or near-normal expiratory flow with a flow-limited inspiratory limb. Vocal-cord dysfunction is confirmed by direct laryngoscopy.

Patients with chronic fixed airway obstruction (e.g., emphysema or chronic bronchitis) can have acute wheezing episodes, most often associated with exacerbations of their disease. These patients often have airway hyperresponsiveness that is present or enhanced during their exacerbation. In the past, these patients were labeled as having *asthmatic bronchitis*. A history of smoking, poor response to aggressive bronchodilator therapy, and spirometric findings of obstruction that do not reverse over time differentiate them from asthmatics. Acute bronchitis can also be associated with the development of airway hyperresponsiveness, most commonly after a viral respiratory tract infection. Most patients have transient symptoms that resolve spontaneously, but a small subgroup may develop sustained clinical asthma. Similarly, other respiratory tract infections are associated with wheezing, and some patients may develop sustained asthma. Left-ventricular failure, pulmonary embolus, hypersensitivity pneumonitis, sarcoidosis, lymphangiomyomatosis, and pulmonary helminth infections should also be considered. Eosinophilic vasculitis (Churg–Strauss syndrome) can also masquerade as asthma, with the symptoms or signs of vasculitis masked by the use of corticosteroids, but these patients have very high eosinophil counts ($>10,000/\mu l$).

The goals of asthma management in the NAEPP 2007 guidelines changed to focus on impairment and risk. Impairment is prevented by (1) preventing symptoms, (2) reducing the need for short-acting medications, (3) maintaining pulmonary function as close to normal as possible, (4) maintaining normal activity levels, and (5) meeting the patients' expectations of care. The additional goal of reducing risk includes (1) preventing exacerbations and the need for urgent care, (2) avoiding the loss of lung function, and (3) avoiding adverse effects of medications through optimal pharmacotherapy. The key components of asthma care as identified in the 2010 GINA Guidelines are (1) develop a patient/doctor partnership; (2) identify and reduce exposure to risk factors; (3) assess, treat, and monitor; and (4) manage exacerbations.

Development of the patient/doctor partnership is critical to attain optimal asthma care. Therefore, patient education is the most important nonpharmacologic intervention. A comprehensive understanding of asthma and its treatment allows the patient to participate actively in the care program, recognize potential problems, obtain early treatment, and avoid exacerbations that might lead to hospitalization. The correct use of metered-dose inhalers (MDIs) and the value of "spacers" (simple devices that connect to MDIs and improve the efficiency of aerosol delivery to the distal lung) should be emphasized. Inexpensive and portable peak flow meters may be of great value for patients with moderate to severe persistent asthma. Daily monitoring of PEF provides a simple, quantitative, and reproducible index of airflow obstruction and can detect early changes in airway function and disease status. Spirometry is indicated at baseline and after stabilization to document a patient's personal best function and should be repeated every 1 to 2 years to assess airway function. Optimal asthma management is best facilitated by a written action plan describing the steps a patient should take based on symptoms and PEF. Forms for written action plans and examples of detailed plans are available on multiple Web sites and are critical to effective prevention and early management of exacerbations.

Successful long-term management of asthma can be challenging. Reducing risk involves identifying and reducing exposure to inhaled allergens, occupational precipitants, and irritants. The patient should be asked about exposure to pets, house-dust mites, cockroaches, indoor molds, and outdoor allergens. Patients with an allergic component should avoid, or at least reduce, exposure to specific allergens. Patients with persistent asthma with an inconclusive allergic history may undergo skin testing. If a clear relationship between an allergen and symptoms is detected, immunotherapy may be considered if allergen avoidance and conventional pharmacotherapy fail to control symptoms. All asthmatics should abstain from smoking and avoid exposure to second-hand smoke. Children are particularly vulnerable to smoke exposure. Patients with severe persistent asthma, nasal polyps, or a history of sensitivity to aspirin or other nonsteroidal anti-inflammatory drugs should obviously avoid these agents, as fatal exacerbations have occurred. However, subclinical sensitivity to these agents is more common, suggesting that asthmatics should avoid these agents whenever possible. Patients should also avoid nonselective β-blockers, including topical ophthalmologic preparations, as these agents may surreptitiously cause exacerbations. Patients with persistent asthma should receive yearly influenza vaccine. Pneumococcal vaccine is currently recommended by the Center for Disease Control for adult asthmatics. Careful evaluation and treatment of concomitant conditions (e.g., chronic rhinitis, chronic sinusitis, vocal-cord dysfunction, and gastroesophageal reflux disease) may alleviate particularly difficult-to-control asthmatic symptoms.

Asthma medications are classified as *quick-relief* (rescue) and *long-term* (control) medications. Quick-relief medications, taken to promptly reverse airflow obstruction and relieve symptoms, include short-acting β_2-agonists, anticholinergics, and systemic corticosteroids (the earliest effect of corticosteroids is the upregulation of β_2-receptors within 8 hours). Long-term medications, taken daily to maintain control of persistent asthma, include corticosteroids, long-acting β_2-agonists (LABAs), leukotriene modifiers, theophylline, nedocromil, and cromolyn. The use of anti-IgE therapy can be beneficial in patients who do not achieve control with less costly and more convenient therapies. The role of anticholinergics in the treatment of asthma is currently being reevaluated with studies examining long-acting inhaled anticholinergics.

Current guidelines recommend stepping pharmacological care up or down depending on each patient's current impairment and future risk. Although the NAEPP 2007 guidelines identified six steps to reflect changes in the doses of inhaled corticosteroids (low, medium, and high) and an indication for anti-IgE antibody in severe disease, the GINA 2010 guidelines have consolidated these somewhat into five.

For mild intermittent asthma, the mainstay of pharmacologic therapy is an inhaled, short-acting β_2-agonist, taken as needed for symptoms without the use of daily, long-term control medication. Patients whose asthma is not adequately controlled with this medication alone are considered to have persistent disease. Mild persistent asthma is defined, in part, as asthma requiring inhaled β_2-agonists more than twice per week for relief of symptoms (GINA, December 2010). Patients with persistent disease require long-term control medication in addition to a short-acting β_2-agonist, which is used only when the patient is symptomatic. The control agent of choice is low-dose inhaled corticosteroids (equivalent to 8–10 puffs of beclomethasone per day). Numerous studies have suggested that inhaled corticosteroids can have clinically relevant long-term side effects, including dysphonia, posterior subcapsular cataracts, and osteoperosis. The use of a spacer device, followed by rinsing the mouth after inhalation, decreases local side effects and systemic absorption. A dose-dependent reduction in bone-mineral content probably occurs with long-term inhaled corticosteroids. For this reason, physicians should consider calcium and vitamin D supplementation for postmenopausal women. For patients who cannot or will not take inhaled corticosteroids, alternatives can include leukotriene modifiers or theophylline. The cromone drugs, cromolyn and nedocromil, have limited usefulness. These agents are less effective than inhaled corticosteroids as first-line control therapy except in specific circumstances (see below). The Federal Drug Administration has warned that LABAs should not be considered as a substitute for inhaled corticosteroids or prescribed in the absence of inhaled corticosteroids because of the risk of worsening disease. A rare but measurable increase in mortality has been observed with LABAs.

New recommendations for treatment of patients with moderate persistent asthma (GINA step 3) are daily low-dose inhaled corticosteroids in combination with long-acting inhaled β_2-agonists. This is based on scientific evidence from research studies in moderate asthmatic children older than age 12 and adults that indicate these patients benefit most from combination controller therapy. This approach is superior to increasing the dose of inhaled corticosteroid. Alternatively, medium-dose inhaled corticosteroids can be used as monotherapy, but this approach is clinically inferior (NAEPP, 2007; GINA, 2010). For patients with symptoms that remain uncontrolled (GINA step 4), the inhaled corticosteroid can be increased to medium (equivalent to 16 puffs of beclomethasone per day) or high doses (equivalent to 24 puffs of beclomethasone per day). This is probably the most economical, but additional add-on therapies may be more effective than increasing corticosteroids alone. The anti-IgE antibody, omalizumab, can also be considered in these patients.

Patients with severe, persistent asthma not adequately controlled with high-dose inhaled corticosteroids along with other long-term controller therapies may require oral corticosteroids for control, but because of serious long-term consequences of chronic systemic corticosteroids, every attempt should be made to improve the management of these patients with environmental control and attempts to taper systemic corticosteroids to the lowest dose possible. Patients receiving chronic oral corticosteroids should be treated no more frequently than once per day, except in rare circumstances; alternate-day therapy is preferred whenever possible. They should also be monitored closely for adverse medication effects. All patients at steps 4 and 5 should be referred to an asthma specialist. Occasionally, patients with severe persistent asthma may not be adequately controlled despite daily systemic corticosteroids. After careful reevaluation and maximal adjustment of medications, these patients may be considered for cytotoxic or immunosuppressive therapy. This should be considered only by a specialist who is experienced in the use of such medications.

Written self-management plans, especially for patients with moderate or severe persistent asthma with good fundamental understanding of their disease, are useful both for chronic management and during acute exacerbations. The usual initial plan during an exacerbation is to increase the dose and shorten the interval of short-acting inhaled β_2-agonists. Ipratropium bromide used with a short-acting β_2-agonist may provide additional bronchodilation. Purulent sputum with fever requires early medical attention and evaluation for possible concomitant pneumonia. However, purulent secretions are common during exacerbations and often are due to inflammatory influx into the airways unassociated with infection. Antibiotics are not recommended for the treatment of acute asthma exacerbations, except as needed for comorbid or exacerbating infectious conditions, such as bacterial pneumonia or suspected bacterial sinusitis. When symptoms do not remit with more aggressive use of inhaled β_2-agonists, early intervention with systemic corticosteroids is pivotal and should always precipitate contact with a physician. A typical schedule would begin with 40 to 60 mg/day of prednisone, tapered over 10 to 14 days. The dosage can be tapered rapidly and discontinued if the total course is less than 14 days. However, patients with more severe or more frequent exacerbations or those with prior use of corticosteroids may require more gradual tapering to avoid treatment failure and readmission. When the dose of oral corticosteroid has been reduced to approximately 20 mg/day of prednisone, or equivalent, reinstitution of inhaled corticosteroids is appropriate. Usually, inhaled corticosteroids are discontinued during acute exacerbations because of the tendency for some of these preparations to exacerbate bronchospasm through irritant effects. This is most common for inhaled corticosteroids supplied as a suspension rather than a solution. This issue has been reevaluated in recent years; some inhaled corticosteroids can provide therapeutic benefit during exacerbations. The physiologic abnormalities associated with exacerbation may persist well after symptomatic improvement, and, therefore, intensive therapy and close follow-up should be continued for an extended period after resolution of symptoms.

Status asthmaticus is life-threatening asthma characterized by sustained, severe airway obstruction refractory to treatment. These patients should always seek emergent medical care. Initial treatment should include oxygen, higher and more frequent doses of inhaled β_2-agonists, and early institution of systemic corticosteroids because of the delay in the observed clinical response (i.e., 6–8 hours). Small-volume nebulizers, MDIs, and continuous administration by a nebulizer are all effective methods for delivering β_2-agonists; however, numerous studies indicate that an MDI with a spacer is both as effective and more cost-effective than a nebulizer. Spacers are particularly important when an MDI is used for adults who are unable to coordinate their inspiratory effort with activation of the MDI. β-Agonists have been administered by the subcutaneous route in the past; however, this results in greater toxicity and has no greater benefit over the aerosol route. A commonly used corticosteroid is methylprednisolone in a dose of approximately 60 mg every 6 hours. These high doses are not benign; potential complications include hypokalemia, hyperglycemia, acute central nervous symptom alterations, hypertension, and peripheral edema. Use of parenteral theophylline in this setting is not recommended; many studies have shown no added bronchodilator effect and substantial increases in toxicity. The value of one or two doses of intravenous magnesium sulfate in the treatment of status asthmaticus is modest, but can buy time for other therapies and in turn help avoid intubation. Inhaled helium delivered as a helium–oxygen mixture has similarly been effective as a temporizing measure because of its favorable rheologic properties that decreased the work of breathing.

During severe exacerbations, respiratory failure can develop despite maximal therapy. Hypercapnia alone does not necessitate intubation and can be effectively managed in some cases with noninvasive mechanical ventilation by face mask. The goal is to allow time to optimize pharmacologic management. The presence of peak flows (<150 L/min), pulsus paradoxus (>20 mmHg), thoracoabdominal paradox, hypoxemia despite oxygen therapy, or an increasing $Paco_2$ signals the potential for progression to respiratory failure requiring intubation and mechanical ventilation.

For patients requiring intubation and mechanical ventilation, normal saline should be infused to attenuate hypotension that is frequently observed after the institution of positive pressure ventilation. Sodium thiopental, etomidate, narcotics, ketamine, and benzodiazepines have all been used safely for sedation or anesthesia at the time of intubation in the acute asthmatic patient. Paralysis may be required to intubate the patient safely and can be accomplished with succinylcholine; however, acidemic patients should be monitored carefully because of the potential for hyperkalemia. Concomitant use of nondepolarizing, neuromuscular blocking agents with systemic corticosteroids has been associated with myopathy and severe peripheral muscle weakness; thus, they should be used with caution.

Once the patient is intubated, careful attention to tidal volumes, peak flows, and inspiration to expiration ratios is necessary to minimize barotrauma and dynamic hyperinflation, which are significant risks in this setting. Sedation with opioids, benzodiazepines, or propofol is required to facilitate ventilator synchrony. To minimize intrinsic positive end-expiratory pressure (PEEPi), the time available for expiration should be maximized by increasing the inspiratory flow rate and reducing the respiratory frequency. It also may be necessary to reduce the tidal volume to increase expiratory time. In turn, permissive hypercapnia in some patients may help to avoid dramatically elevated airway pressures. Intravenous bicarbonate can be used with permissive hypercapnia to partially compensate for the resulting respiratory acidosis, but it must be used judiciously to maintain arterial pH greater than 7.20. Often, higher doses of inhaled β_2-agonists and ipratropium bromide are required through in-line MDI treatments at more frequent intervals because of the severe bronchospasm and the decreased efficiency of aerosol delivery through the ventilator circuit. Monitoring of peak-to-plateau airway pressure gradients and auto-PEEP may help in assessing the severity of bronchospasm and response to therapy. These patients should receive an extended course of oral corticosteroids (at least 4–6 weeks) and should not be tapered below 20 mg/day until seen by a physician, preferably an asthma specialist, in follow-up.

Some specific circumstances warrant special considerations in asthma. Exercise-induced asthma is common, especially in young asthmatics. Symptoms are often controlled by use of short-acting, inhaled β_2-agonists before exercise. For more persistent symptoms, regularly scheduled LABAs or leukotriene modifier should be considered. Persistent nocturnal symptoms despite inhaled corticosteroids require addition of long-term control therapy with LABAs, leukotriene modifiers, or theophylline. Patients with aspirin-sensitive asthma usually have moderate to severe symptoms that can be difficult to control. Leukotrienes are thought to play a particularly important role; thus, leukotriene modifiers should be strongly considered in these patients.

Asthma is the most common potentially serious medical condition complicating pregnancy. Uncontrolled asthma during pregnancy can produce complications in both the mother and the fetus. A recent report by the Working Group on Asthma and Pregnancy found that undertreatment, principally attributable to unfounded fears of fetal effects of medication, is the major problem in asthma management during pregnancy. The greatest experience in the pregnant patient is with inhaled β_2-agonists and theophylline; however, corticosteroids and anticholinergics have all been used safely. Thus, asthma should be treated as aggressively in pregnant as in nonpregnant women. A recent large study of pregnant women has raised concern about use of oral corticosteroids and theophylline. In this population, an increased risk of preterm delivery has been observed. Special emphasis should also be placed on nonpharmacologic measures to avoid asthma triggers, including first- and second-hand smoking, which is harmful for both mother and fetus. Asthma care should include monitoring of fetal growth, maternal symptoms, and maternal lung function. All pregnant asthmatics should be tested with spirometry; the single best index of severity is the FEV_1, which is not significantly altered by pregnancy. Patients with moderate or severe asthma should be monitored with twice-daily measurements of PEF rate and should report the values to the physician at each prenatal visit. After the first trimester, patients should receive influenza vaccine.

The basic management of asthma during pregnancy is very similar to that in nonpregnant patients and is based on asthma severity classification. If the patient's asthma is more than mild intermittent, anti-inflammatory therapy is recommended. If inhaled corticosteroids are used, beclomethasone is preferred. The immediate goals of therapy of severe asthma exacerbation in pregnancy are to correct hypoxemia, alleviate bronchospasm, avoid maternal exhaustion or respiratory failure, and prevent fetal morbidity and mortality. The management of acute exacerbation includes oxygen to maintain a minimum PaO_2 (>60 mmHg; oxygen saturation >95%), inhaled β_2-agonists, and a short course of systemic corticosteroids. During labor and delivery, patients who have required long-term systemic corticosteroids should be given hydrocortisone because of the risk of maternal adrenal suppression.

Asthmatics are at risk for respiratory complications during and after surgery, including acute bronchospasm triggered by intubation and hypoxemia. Therefore, patients with asthma should be evaluated before surgery, including a review of symptoms and medications, measurement of pulmonary function, and attempts made to optimize lung function. A short course of corticosteroids may be necessary. It is recommended that patients who have received systemic corticosteroids for more than 2 weeks during the past 6 months be given hydrocortisone (100 mg every 8 hours) intravenously on the day of surgery, with a rapid reduction of the dose within 24 hours after surgery.

Asthma specialists should particularly be involved in the care of patients with severe persistent asthma, and possibly those with moderate persistent asthma, as well as those who have had a life-threatening asthma exacerbation.

FURTHER READING

1. National Asthma Education and Prevention Program. *Expert Panel Report 3: Guidelines for the Diagnosis and Management of Asthma.* Bethesda, MD: National Institutes of Health, National Heart, Lung, and Blood Institute; 2007. http://www.nhlbi.nih.gov/guidelines/asthma/asthgdln.htm. Updated 2007. Accessed August 6, 2011.

   This is the current NIH guideline for the diagnosis and management of asthma. It is well-done, but long. A more abbreviated version is available.

2. Global Initiative for Asthma. *Global Strategy for Asthma Management and Prevention.* 2010. http://www.ginasthma.org/guidelines-gina-report-global-strategy-for-asthma.html. Updated 2010. Accessed August 6, 2011.

   This is the current World Health Organization guideline that updates many features of the NIH guidelines, but is a collaborative effort with the NIH. It is shorter and more practical.

3. Blake KV, Hoppe M, Harman E, et al. Relative amount of albuterol delivered to lung receptors from a metered-dose inhaler and nebulizer solution: bioassay by histamine bronchoprovocation. *Chest.* 1992;101(2):309–315.

   A study addressing the question of the effectiveness of MDI versus nebulizer delivery of β_2-agonists. These authors used histamine bronchoprovocation to evaluate the delivery systems. They found 10 puffs of the MDI to be equivalent to 2.5 mg of nebulized solution. This study suggests the need to use higher doses of MDIs during the treatment of acute asthma exacerbation. (Old, but the value is unchanged.)

4. Busse WW, Lemanske RF Jr, Gern JE. Role of viral respiratory infections in asthma and asthma exacerbations. *Lancet.* 2010;376(9743):826–834. PMCID: 2972660.

   An authoritative and clinically relevant review of viruses in asthma.

5. Busse WW, Morgan WJ, Gergen PJ, et al. Randomized trial of omalizumab (Anti-IgE) for asthma in inner-city children. *N Engl J Med.* 2011;364(11):1005–1015.

   A current view of the use of anti-IgE therapy in children in an area that has significantly evolved.

6. Chapman KR, Verbeek PR, White JG, et al. Effect of a short course of prednisone in the prevention of early relapse after the emergency room treatment of acute asthma. *N Engl J Med.* 1991;324(12):788–794.

   Classic paper that describes the use of the value of oral corticosteroids in preventing relapse of exacerbations requiring emergency care.

7. Corren J, Lemanske RF, Hanania NA, et al. Lebrikizumab treatment in adults with asthma. *N Engl J Med.* 2011;365(12):1088–1098.

   An initial report examining the potential value of an anti-IL-33 antibody in the treatment of adults with asthma.

8. Ege MJ, Mayer M, Normand AC, et al. Exposure to environmental microorganisms and childhood asthma. *N Engl J Med.* 2011;364(8):701–709.

   A definitive report on exposure to multiple microorganisms on a farm, early in childhood reduces asthma in children.

9. Finkelman FD, Hogan SP, Hershey GK, et al. Importance of cytokines in murine allergic airway disease and human asthma. *J Immunol.* 2010;184(4):1663–1674.

   A careful review of animal research on cytokines in asthma and its validation in studies in people.

10. Gold DR. Environmental tobacco smoke, indoor allergens, and childhood asthma. *Environ Health Perspect.* 2000;108(suppl 4):643–651. PMCID: 1637671.

    A review of the significant impact of tobacco smoke on the development of asthma.

11. Grainge CL, Lau LC, Ward JA, et al. Effect of bronchoconstriction on airway remodeling in asthma. *N Engl J Med.* 2011;364(21):2006–2015.

    A provocative study implicating mechanical forces in the development of airway remodeling in asthma.

12. Idris AH, McDermott MF, Raucci JC, et al. Emergency department treatment of severe asthma: metered-dose inhaler plus holding chamber is equivalent in effectiveness to nebulizer. *Chest*. 1993;103(3):665–672.

    This classic paper was an early one demonstrating that metered dose inhalers with spacers were effective in the treatment of acute exacerbations and they also addressed dose equivalency.

13. Kim HY, DeKruyff RH, Umetsu DT. The many paths to asthma: phenotype shaped by innate and adaptive immunity. *Nat Immunol*. 2010;11(7):577–584. PMCID: 3114595.

    A scholarly review of the interface between innate and adaptive immunity and its importance in allergic asthma.

14. Lange P, Parner J, Vestbo J, et al. A 15-year follow-up study of ventilatory function in adults with asthma. *N Engl J Med*. 1998;339(17):1194–1200.

    A landmark study demonstrating the accelerated loss of lung function in asthma.

15. Lazarus SC. Clinical practice: emergency treatment of asthma. *N Engl J Med*. 2010;363(8):755–764.

    An excellent state-of-the-art review of emergent care of asthma exacerbations.

16. Lemanske RF Jr, Mauger DT, Sorkness CA, et al. Step-up therapy for children with uncontrolled asthma receiving inhaled corticosteroids. *N Engl J Med*. 2010;362(11):975–985. PMCID: 2989902.

    A careful study demonstrating that step-up therapy in children can be complex and alternatives to long-acting β-agonists need to be carefully considered.

17. Lin RY, Pesola GR, Bakalchuk L, et al. Superiority of ipratropium plus albuterol over albuterol alone in the emergency department management of adult asthma: a randomized clinical trial. *Ann Emerg Med*. 1998;31(2):208–213.

    An important early study demonstrating the value of anticholinergics in the treatment of asthma exacerbations.

18. Littenberg B, Gluck EH. A controlled trial of methylprednisolone in the emergency treatment of acute asthma. *N Engl J Med*. 1986;314(3):150–152.

    A landmark study demonstrating the value of early intervention with systemic corticosteroids in emergent care of asthma exacerbations.

19. Mapp CE, Boschetto P, Maestrelli P, et al. Occupational asthma. *Am J Respir Crit Care Med*. 2005;172(3):280–305.

    An excellent state-of-the-art review of occupational asthma.

20. Martinez FD. The origins of asthma and chronic obstructive pulmonary disease in early life. *Proc Am Thorac Soc*. 2009;6(3):272–277. PMCID: 2677402.

    A review of data indicating that the development of asthma is the consequence of genetics and early life events. The author also reviews data that asthma leads to irreversible airway obstruction later in life. Early intervention is suggested to prevent this.

21. Morris MJ, Christopher KL. Diagnostic criteria for the classification of vocal cord dysfunction. *Chest*. 2010;138(5):1213–1223.

    An up-to-date review of vocal cord dysfunction by the one of the authors of the first report.

22. Murphy VE, Gibson PG. Asthma in pregnancy. *Clin Chest Med*. 2011;32(1):93–110, ix.

    A common, important topic that is under-discussed. Read it.

23. Peters SP, Kunselman SJ, Icitovic N, et al. Tiotropium bromide step-up therapy for adults with uncontrolled asthma. *N Engl J Med*. 2010;363(18):1715–1726.

    A provocative paper that provides data that we may have alternative step-up therapies already in our midst.

24. Price D, Musgrave SD, Shepstone L, et al. Leukotriene antagonists as first-line or add-on asthma-controller therapy. *N Engl J Med*. 2011;364:1695–1707.

    A potential new indication for a class of drugs that has been on the market since the 1990s.

25. Reddel HK, Barnes DJ. Pharmacological strategies for self-management of asthma exacerbations. *Eur Respir J*. 2006;28(1):182–199.

    Self-management strategies are underutilized. This paper provides a solid review of the topic and why physicians should make more use of this.

26. Rodrigo GJ, Neffen H, Castro-Rodriguez JA. Efficacy and safety of subcutaneous omalizumab vs placebo as add-on therapy to corticosteroids for children and adults with asthma: a systematic review. *Chest.* 2011;139:28–35.

    This study addresses an expanded indication for anti-IgE therapy. The cost as well as clinical efficacy must be a consideration.

27. Sleiman PM, Flory J, Imielinski M, et al. Variants of DENND1B associated with asthma in children. *N Engl J Med.* 2010;362(1):36–44.

    Another potential asthma gene detected in a genome-wide association study that appears to have significance for individuals of African decent.

28. Stevenson DD, Szczeklik A. Clinical and pathologic perspectives on aspirin sensitivity and asthma. *J Allergy Clin Immunol.* 2006;118(4):773–786; quiz 87–88.

    A review of aspirin-sensitive asthma by two of the world's experts.

29. Ververeli K, Chipps B. Oral corticosteroid-sparing effects of inhaled corticosteroids in the treatment of persistent and acute asthma. *Ann Allergy Asthma Immunol.* 2004;92(5):512–522.

    An important reminder about the many values of inhaled corticosteroids.

30. Woodcock A, Forster L, Matthews E, et al. Control of exposure to mite allergen and allergen-impermeable bed covers for adults with asthma. *N Engl J Med.* 2003;349(3):225–236.

    A well-done study that indicates that environmental control in allergic asthma is not as effective as we might of thought and this may be in part due to the difficulty of accomplishing it.

Chronic Obstructive Pulmonary Disease: Definition and Epidemiology

Andrew L. Ries

Chronic obstructive pulmonary disease (COPD) refers to a group of disorders that have in common the presence of persistent and progressive airflow obstruction that is not fully reversible. The airflow limitation is usually progressive and is associated with an abnormal inflammatory response of the lung to noxious particles or gases, primarily caused by cigarette smoking.

From the viewpoint of the pathologist, chronic bronchitis and emphysema are distinct processes, the former limited to the airways and the latter to the pulmonary parenchyma. From the viewpoint of the clinician, such a distinction is difficult for several reasons: (1) some degree of each may coexist in the same patient; *pure* forms of chronic bronchitis and emphysema are exceptions rather than the rule; (2) both are characterized by expiratory flow obstruction on simple spirometric testing; (3) patients with both processes often present with the same symptom—dyspnea on exertion; and (4) the presence of airway hyperreactivity (*asthma,* acutely reversible airways disease) in many patients with chronic bronchitis or emphysema further complicates the distinction. Faced with such complexities, it is understandable that the clinician often lumps together patients with chronic expiratory obstruction under the label COPD.

Nevertheless, distinct advantages are found in attempting to distinguish chronic bronchitis from emphysema, or at least to define the relative extent of each in a given patient. Such advantages relate particularly to the selection of therapy and to the natural history of these disorders, which is reflected in the individual patient's prognosis. For example, recent studies have indicated that mucous gland hypertrophy and mucus hypersecretion—both hallmarks of chronic bronchitis—are not major factors in causing airflow obstruction. Attempts at distinction also are essential to determine the pathogenetic differences between chronic bronchitis and emphysema, although the dominant role of cigarette smoking in both is clear.

The confusion between chronic bronchitis and emphysema has been compounded by the manner in which they have been defined by various scientific societies, in different studies, and in different nations. In defining chronic bronchitis and emphysema, three options are available: pathologic, clinical, and physiologic. In fact, all three options have been used. This is not surprising because pathologic evidence is rarely sought (or advisable) while the patient is alive; the physiologic techniques that allow distinction are still not generally applied; and attempts to provide clinical definitions were useful when neither pathologic nor physiologic criteria were available.

Chronic bronchitis has long been defined in clinical terms. The most widely used definition is that of the American Thoracic Society, which defines chronic bronchitis as "a clinical disorder characterized by excessive mucous secretion … manifested by chronic or recurrent productive cough … on most days for a minimum of three months in the year and for not less than two successive years." This clinical definition is now known to have serious deficits. First, other disorders with similar manifestations must be excluded, such as bronchiectasis, tuberculosis, and lung abscess. Furthermore, patients with predominant asthma or emphysema may fit this definition. Finally, many patients with pathologic or physiologic hallmarks of chronic bronchitis may not qualify under this definition (i.e., they do not cough).

If pathologic findings were used to define chronic bronchitis, the task would be relatively easy. Pathologically, the hallmark of chronic bronchitis is the hyperplastic and hypertrophied mucous glands found in the submucosa of large cartilaginous bronchi. The ratio of bronchial gland thickness to bronchial wall thickness (Reid index) is increased. The small airways (noncartilaginous bronchioles <2 mm in diameter) may also be involved, demonstrating mucous plugging, mural fibrosis and narrowing, goblet-cell hyperplasia, and inflammatory cell infiltrates. Thus, in the absence of parenchymal change, these findings in the airways would characterize *pure* chronic bronchitis.

Because such pathologic evidence is not conveniently available, much effort has been devoted to correlating pathologic data with physiologic tests. By physiologic testing, the pure chronic bronchitis patient should demonstrate

1. Relatively normal total lung capacity (TLC) with modest elevation of the residual volume (RV) and functional residual capacity (FRC)
2. Some degree of expiratory and inspiratory flow obstruction (both flows are abnormal because the airway lumen is narrowed)
3. Flow obstruction not acutely improved by bronchodilator administration
4. Significant disturbances of gas exchange producing hypoxemia because of ventilation–perfusion imbalance. Hypercapnia can develop with more severe disease
5. Normal diffusing capacity for carbon monoxide.

In contrast with the clinical description of chronic bronchitis, emphysema has long been defined in anatomic–pathologic terms. The widely used American Thoracic Society definition states that emphysema is present when there is "an anatomical alteration of the lung characterized by an abnormal enlargement of the airspaces distal to the nonrespiratory bronchioles, accompanied by destructive changes of the alveolar walls." Thus, pure emphysema is a parenchymal (airspace) disease in which the bronchi are not involved. In recent years, high-resolution computed tomography has been used to detect emphysema based on anatomic changes in the lung parenchyma.

Pathologically, emphysema is characterized by disruption of the alveolar walls at some location within the acinus, which is the lung division distal to the terminal bronchiole that includes the respiratory bronchioles, alveolar ducts, and terminal alveoli. Depending on the dominant site of involvement, emphysema is defined pathologically as centrilobular (proximal acinar), in which the proximal part of the acinus is involved, or as panacinar, in which the whole acinar structure is involved.

A clinical definition of emphysema is lacking; if one did exist, it would be dominated by the historic finding of effort dyspnea.

Physiologically, patients with pure emphysema demonstrate distinct features:

1. The lung volumes show evidence of hyperinflation, namely, an elevated FRC, RV, and RV:TLC ratio. Often, TLC is increased. Early in the course of disease, vital capacity (VC) may be preserved (i.e., concomitant elevation in RV and TLC). With more severe disease, VC may be reduced in proportion to the elevation in RV when further elevation in TLC is limited by the chest wall. Such measurements are best made in a body plethysmograph, because the lung volume measured by gas dilution techniques (e.g., helium dilution, nitrogen washout) may underestimate the lung volume in emphysema due to airspaces that communicate poorly with the airways.

2. Significant expiratory flow obstruction is present with preservation of inspiratory flows. This observation is most dramatically demonstrated by flow–volume curves that show normal flow rates during inspiration but severely reduced flow rates on expiration.

3. Expiratory obstruction is not immediately improved by bronchodilator administration.

4. Elastic recoil is low (i.e., low pleural pressures exist at TLC and other specified lung volumes) and compliance is increased (i.e., small pleural pressure changes are associated with large increases in lung volume). These findings are the physiologic correlates of alveolar disruption and are the hallmarks of emphysema.

5. Gas exchange is well preserved in the stable state, despite advanced spirometric abnormalities.

6. The diffusing capacity for carbon monoxide is reduced.

Therefore, to the extent that chronic bronchitis and emphysema exist in pure forms, they can be distinguished from each other and from asthma by physiologic tests that reflect the pathology involved. In practical terms, as already noted, mixed forms are the rule. This is particularly true when advanced disease is present.

Controversy exists about whether asthma itself is part of the spectrum of COPD. Nonspecific airway hyperresponsiveness has been proposed as a risk factor that predisposes smokers to developing COPD (the Dutch hypothesis). Asthmatic bronchitis is one of the recognized epidemiologic patterns of COPD. Asthma can result in chronic airflow obstruction and should probably be included within the clinical spectrum of COPD.

COPD is a major cause of death and disability. Because COPD is insidious, with a long latency period before clinical recognition, official statistics underestimate morbidity and mortality. As of 1990, COPD had moved up to the fourth leading cause of death in the United States. In 2008, COPD was listed as the underlying cause of more than 141,000 deaths. From 1980 to 2000, the COPD death rate among women increased dramatically from 20.1 to 56.7/100,000, whereas for men there was a more modest increase from 73.0 to 82.6/100,000. Also, in 2000, for the first time, the number of women dying from COPD surpassed the number of men. It should be noted that mortality rates for COPD significantly underestimate the magnitude of the problem because many decedents with COPD have their deaths attributed to other causes. In 1998, only 45% of death certificates mentioning COPD listed COPD as the underlying cause of death, even though people with COPD listed on their death certificate typically have severe disease. Thus, COPD is likely a more important contributor to death than generally recognized.

In the United States, the overall prevalence of COPD is approximately 6% in adults aged 25 and older based on self-reports of chronic bronchitis or emphysema. Using extensive questionnaires and physical examination, including spirometry testing, the Third National Health and Nutrition Examination Survey (NHANES III) reported a 14% prevalence of airway obstruction in a representative sample of US adults surveyed from 1988 to 1994. Similar results have been reported in international studies. COPD is also being recognized increasingly as a significant public health problem in developing countries.

The impact of COPD on morbidity is even greater than on mortality. In 2000, COPD was responsible for 8 million physician office or hospital outpatient visits, 1.5 million emergency department visits, and 726,000 hospitalizations. As a cause of disability-adjusted life-years (DALYs), in 1996 COPD was estimated to be the eighth among men and seventh among women. Worldwide, COPD is expected to move up from the 12th leading cause of DALYs in 1990 to 5th in 2020.

Epidemiologic studies have identified two main syndromes, with different risk factors and natural histories. The usual emphysematous form is associated closely with cigarette smoking. Patients develop airflow obstruction insidiously over many years, with minimal symptoms, followed by clinical disease in later years, with progressive symptoms and high morbidity and mortality. The second form of COPD, chronic asthmatic bronchitis, is associated with risk factors of atopy, high serum immunoglobulin E (IgE), and bronchial hyperreactivity. Patients develop chronic airflow obstruction independent of smoking, although smoking can add risk. Asthmatic bronchitis is more amenable to medical therapy and has a better prognosis and survival than the emphysematous type.

Cigarette smoking is the major risk factor, accounting for the majority of COPD cases. However, it is now recognized that more than one quarter of COPD occurs in individuals who never smoked. Compared with nonsmokers, current smokers have approximately 10 times the relative risk of developing COPD. The risk is equal for men and women. Previously, COPD was more common in men because of their higher smoking rates; however, the disease now exhibits more gender equality, reflecting similar smoking rates for men and women.

Significant individual variation in susceptibility is seen, and host factors play an important role. Only 10% to 15% of smokers develop significant obstructive lung disease. In susceptible persons, smoking is associated with an accelerated decline in lung function over many years that is related to the amount of smoking. Because of the large reserve in healthy lungs, disease is not typically recognized until later in life.

Besides cigarette smoking, other risk factors include environmental exposure to dusts, gases, and biomass smoke, malnutrition, early life infections, and asthma and airway hyperreactivity. Exposure of nonsmokers to the smoke of others in an indoor environment (second-hand smoke) is associated with an increase in respiratory infections and lung disease in children and with modest changes in lung function in adults. However, it has not been clearly established that passive smoke exposure leads to clinically significant obstructive lung disease.

One credible theory about the pathogenesis of emphysema is that the disease results from an imbalance between lung proteases and antiproteases, enzymes that, respectively, promote injury and protect the lung against injury. Human neutrophil elastase is released from granules of the neutrophil during phagocytosis and after stimulation, chemotaxis, and cell death. Cigarette smoke components appear to promote the release of (1) neutrophil chemotactic factors from alveolar macrophages and (2) human neutrophil elastase from neutrophils. The activity of human neutrophil elastase is mitigated by a serum protein, α_1-antiprotease, which is synthesized by the liver and migrates freely into alveoli. Formulation of the protease/antiprotease theory of emphysema was catalyzed by the discovery that emphysema is common among individuals who are severely deficient in α_1-antiprotease, a globulin that is a potent inhibitor of several enzymes, including trypsin and elastase. It is postulated that elastase, which is found in polymorphonuclear leukocytes and in alveolar macrophages, is normally released from these cells; larger quantities may be released in response to lower respiratory tract infections. When α_1-antiprotease is present, elastase is inhibited; in its absence, released elastase is free to digest the lung.

The gene for α_1-antiprotease deficiency is inherited in an autosomal recessive pattern—Pi MM is the normal phenotype, Pi ZZ the most common phenotype of homozygous deficiency. Although heterozygous persons have reduced levels of α_1-antiprotease, they do not have a clearly increased risk for developing disease. In congenital emphysema, anatomic changes predominate at the lung bases rather than in the upper lung fields. Less than 1 of 2,000 individuals is severely deficient in α_1-antiprotease. More than 90% of the population—and the vast majority of patients with emphysema—are of the normal (MM) phenotype and have normal serum levels of α_1-antiprotease. Nevertheless, the same concept of enzyme–inhibitor balance may apply to other patients with emphysema. This possibility is supported by animal experiments in which emphysema-like disorders have been induced by intrapulmonary instillation of papain, elastase, and leukocyte homogenates. Evidence that a protease–antiprotease imbalance exists in the alveoli of patients deficient in α_1-antiprotease, and that this balance can be restored by intravenous administration of α_1-antiprotease, adds further weight to this hypothesis, as does the demonstration that certain oxidants (including components of cigarette smoke) can inactivate α_1-antiprotease, rendering it unable to inhibit elastase and other proteolytic enzymes.

It should be noted that the term *emphysema* is also applied to several conditions in which lung hyperinflation occurs without alveolar destruction. Among these conditions is congenital lobar emphysema, in which overinflation of a lobe (usually the left upper lobe) occurs, which can be life-threatening. Pathologically, overdistention of single or multiple lobes is seen. *Compensatory emphysema* is a term applied to overinflation of the remaining lung in the face of collapse, destruction, or resection of other lung zones. Partial obstruction of a major bronchus does not cause tissue destruction characteristic of emphysema, although it does result in overdistention of alveoli. *Senile emphysema* is a term applied to the normal modest overinflation of the lung that occurs with aging and is reflected in an increase in RV:TLC ratio, and is better referred to as the *aging lung*.

FURTHER READING

1. Celli BR, MacNee W; committee members of ATS/ERS Task Force. Standards for the diagnosis and treatment of patients with COPD: a summary of the ATS/ERS position paper. *Eur Respir J.* 2004;23:932–946.

   Official statement published jointly by the American Thoracic Society and European Respiratory Society that updates official practice guidelines for the diagnosis and treatment of COPD. An online version of the document is available at www.thoracic.org/copd.

2. Rabe KF, Anzueto A, Barnes PJ, et al. Global strategy for the diagnosis, management, and prevention of chronic obstructive pulmonary disease: GOLD executive summary. *Am J Respir Crit Care Med.* 2007;176:532–555.

   International evidence-based review cosponsored by NHLBI and World Health Organization (WHO) providing guidelines for diagnosis and management. Major initiative to raise awareness about the global epidemic of COPD. Full online resources available at www.goldcopd.com.

3. Similowski T, Whitelaw WA, Derenne J-P, eds. *Clinical Management of Chronic Obstructive Pulmonary Disease.* New York, NY: Marcel Dekker; 2002.

   Excellent reference and resource in the Lung Biology in Health and Disease series. Comprehensive reviews of many topics related to pathogenesis, diagnosis, and management of COPD.

4. Snider GL. Nosology for our day: its application to chronic obstructive pulmonary disease. *Am J Respir Crit Care Med.* 2003;167:678–683.

   Excellent summary of terminology and definitions for COPD.

5. Snider GL. Emphysema: the first two centuries—and beyond. A historical overview, with suggestions for future research: Part 1. *Am Rev Respir Dis.* 1992;146(5, pt 1):1334–1344.

   Distinguished J. Burns Amberson's lecture, with an excellent review of the history and pathogenesis of emphysema.

6. Snider GL. Emphysema: the first two centuries—and beyond. A historical overview, with suggestions for future research: Part 2. *Am Rev Respir Dis.* 1992;146(6):1615–1622.

   Distinguished J. Burns Amberson's lecture, with an excellent review of the history and pathogenesis of emphysema.

7. Fishman AP. One hundred years of chronic obstructive pulmonary disease. *Am J Respir Crit Care Med.* 2005;171:941–948.

   Excellent review of the history of COPD.

8. Fletcher CM, Peto R. The natural history of chronic airflow obstruction. *Br Med J.* 1977;1:1645–1648.

   Classic epidemiologic study of London working men, demonstrating the gradual decline in forced expiratory volume in 1 second (FEV_1) in nonsmokers and an accelerated decline in susceptible smokers.

9. Burrows B. Epidemiologic evidence for different types of chronic airflow obstruction. *Am Rev Respir Dis.* 1991;143:1452.

   Report from the Tucson Epidemiologic Study of Obstructive Airway Diseases of a population sample of 1,467 in 1971 to 1972. Suggests at least two different types of COPD: chronic asthmatic bronchitis and the usual form of emphysematous COPD.

10. Mannino DM. The epidemiology and economics of chronic obstructive pulmonary disease. *Proc Am Thorac Soc.* 2007;4:502–506.

    Recent summary of the epidemiology, morbidity, mortality, and costs associated with COPD.

11. Mannino DM, Buist SA. Global burden of COPD: risk factors, prevalence, and future trends. *Lancet.* 2007;370:765–773.

    Discussion of global impact of COPD and increasing future trends.

12. Centers for Disease Control and Prevention. Chronic obstructive pulmonary disease surveillance—United States, 1971–2000. *MMWR Surveill Summ.* 2002;51(SS06):1–16.

    Centers for Disease Control and Prevention (CDC) report of trends in COPD over the past 30 years.

13. Centers for Disease Control and Prevention. Deaths: preliminary data for 2008. *Natl Vital Stat Rep.* 2010;59:1–71.

    Recent CDC mortality data.

14. Lamprecht B, McBurnie MA, Vollmer WM, et al. COPD in never smokers: results from the population-based burden of obstructive lung disease study. *Chest.* 2011;139:752–763.

    Results from the 14 country, population based BOLD study reporting that approximately 6% of never smokers had irreversible airway obstruction and that greater than 25% of COPD occurs in individuals who never smoked.

15. Fang X, Wang X, Bai C. COPD in China: the burden and importance of proper management. *Chest.* 2011;139:920–929.

    Review of known information about prevalence, mortality, disease burden, risk factors, diagnosis, and management of COPD in China. Reported COPD prevalence ranged from 5% to 13%. COPD ranked as the fourth leading cause of death in urban areas, third in rural areas.

16. Eriksson S. Pulmonary emphysema and alpha-1-antitrypsin deficiency. *Acta Med Scand.* 1964;17:197.

17. Eriksson S. A 30-year perspective on α1-antitrypsin deficiency. *Chest.* 1996;110:237S.

    Original description of syndrome (11) and a recent perspective (12) from the discoverer of the α_1-antitrypsin deficiency syndrome.

18. American Thoracic Society. Guidelines for the approach to the patient with severe hereditary α_1-antitrypsin deficiency. *Am Rev Respir Dis.* 1989;140:1494–1497.

    Official statement of the American Thoracic Society, describing the background, diagnosis, and treatment of patients with α_1-antitrypsin deficiency.

19. DeMeo DL, Silverman EK. Genetics of chronic obstructive pulmonary disease. *Semin Respir Crit Care Med.* 2003;24:151–159.

    Succinct summary of current knowledge about genetics of COPD, emphasizing variability in susceptibility and heterogeneity. Deficiency of α_1-antitrypsin is the only proven genetic risk to date.

Chronic Obstructive Pulmonary Disease: Clinical and Laboratory Manifestations, Pathophysiology, and Prognosis

Andrew L. Ries

Chronic obstructive pulmonary disease (COPD) typically appears later in life. Although characterized primarily by airway obstruction and reduced expiratory airflow, COPD is increasingly recognized as a systemic disease with significant extrapulmonary manifestations as well resulting from systemic inflammation.

Dyspnea is the hallmark symptom that brings the patient to medical attention and leads to a diagnosis. A careful history of the insidious onset of breathlessness on exertion, with or without a history of cough, sputum, or frequent lung infections, often provides the clue to diagnosis.

Because of the slow, progressive course of disease and the large reserve in lung function, a long preclinical period typically elapses during which the person who has smoked for years "without a problem" begins to note breathlessness with physical activities previously accomplished without difficulty. This may be attributed to "getting older" or "being out of shape." Reduced expiratory flow rates may be detected at this stage. Later, the patient may come to medical attention after a critical event, such as a winter cold from which recovery has been slow. Disease onset is often attributed to this time; in reality, however, this event just pushed the patient over the clinical edge of recognition, much like a rope weakened by progressive fraying breaks when *only* a small weight is attached.

Cough is a frequent symptom, often attributed as a "smoker's cough" early in disease. It is usually productive; sputum is described as mucoid. Often, there is a history of frequent respiratory infections associated with increased cough, purulent sputum, and breathlessness. The patient may note that it takes longer than usual to recover from these infections.

Some patients with COPD develop abnormal gas exchange with hypoxemia or hypercapnia. Hypoxemia can be associated with cognitive or personality changes, polycythemia, and cyanosis. Chronic hypercapnia can cause headache, particularly on arising, and increased somnolence. During exercise, the arterial Po_2 may change significantly and unpredictably from the resting level. In many patients, the Pao_2 decreases with physical activity; in others, it does not change or may actually increase.

On physical examination, decreased maximal expiratory flow may be apparent even in early disease. Therefore, it is important to assess maximal expiratory flow in persons at high risk (e.g., smokers). In early disease, the examination may be normal, but later, prolonged expiration or wheezing can be detected on forced exhalation. This can be assessed easily with the forced expiratory time, a useful screening test for expiratory obstruction. In this maneuver, the patient exhales with maximal effort through an open mouth after a full inspiration. The examiner listens with the bell of the stethoscope over the trachea in the suprasternal notch and records the time in seconds until airflow ceases. Normal persons can exhale completely within 4 seconds. A forced expiratory time greater than 6 seconds signifies significant expiratory obstruction.

Other physical signs of COPD often are not present until the disease becomes moderate to severe. Overinflation of the lungs can result in an increased anteroposterior diameter of the thorax and a low, flat diaphragm with reduced respiratory excursion. The flattened diaphragm contributes less to inspiration, placing more burden on the accessory breathing muscles (neck and intercostals) and producing greater respiratory movement in the upper chest. With severe hyperinflation, the diaphragm can even become inverted and move paradoxically—up on inspiration, down on expiration. This can be detected best with the patient supine, noting the inward movement of the lower rib cage and abdomen during inspiration. With advanced emphysema, the breath sounds are diminished because of reduced flow and increased lung inflation. Signs of pulmonary hypertension and right-sided heart failure (e.g., peripheral edema and hepatic congestion) are not usually detected until an advanced stage of disease.

The central diagnostic feature of COPD is reduced expiratory airflow, resulting from increased airway resistance due to airway narrowing. Spirometry is the standard pulmonary function test for measuring maximal airflow and is relatively simple, reliable, and reproducible. It is useful for detecting airflow obstruction, staging severity, and following the disease course. A reduction in the forced expiratory volume in 1 second (FEV_1) in relation to the forced vital capacity (FVC)—the FEV_1:FVC ratio—is a standard measure of obstruction. The FEV_1 is the best measure of disease severity; it correlates with exercise tolerance and survival. Other measures of expiratory airflow can also be helpful.

Measures of lung volumes reveal hyperinflation with an increase in residual volume, functional residual capacity, and, sometimes, total lung capacity. These tests can help to confirm the diagnosis suggested from spirometry. Emphysema causes a greater increase in total lung capacity than other obstructive diseases, as well as a reduced carbon monoxide diffusing capacity (D_{LCO}), primarily because of the loss of alveolar–capillary surface area. However, D_{LCO} is neither specific nor sensitive for emphysema.

Chest radiographs have limited usefulness in diagnosing or staging COPD; early in disease, they may be normal. Their main use is in detecting other parenchymal lung or cardiovascular diseases that can present with similar symptoms. With advanced emphysema, the chest radiograph may reveal overinflation of the lungs with a low, flat diaphragm and an increase in the retrosternal airspace (anterior to the heart) on the lateral film. The emphysematous lungs also may appear radiolucent because of bullous changes and a paucity of vascular shadows. High-resolution computed tomography may be useful in documenting pathologic evidence of emphysema and characterizing its distribution.

Arterial blood gas analysis may reveal hypoxemia and hypercapnia, particularly in advanced disease. The relationship between gas exchange abnormalities and other measures of lung function is poor. Hypoxemia can worsen with exercise, sleep, or changes in body position.

The electrocardiogram is usually normal early in disease; later, signs may appear of right-sided heart strain, including right-axis shift, increased R waves over the right precordial leads (V_1 and V_2), and peaked P waves (P pulmonale). These changes do not correlate well with the level of pulmonary hypertension.

Two characteristic clinical patterns of COPD were originally described by Dornholst: the *pink puffer* (type A or emphysematous type) and the *blue bloater* (type B or bronchitic type). Type A patients typically have severe dyspnea, with little cough and sputum. They are usually thin with a hyperinflated chest. Arterial blood gases reveal mild, if any, hypoxemia (i.e., *pink* without cyanosis) and normal to low arterial P_{CO_2} (i.e., *puffing* with increased breathing effort). Type B patients typically have a history of chronic bronchitis with cough, sputum, and recurrent exacerbations with respiratory tract infections. Dyspnea on exertion is a prominent symptom, but is often episodic. On examination, they tend to be overweight and cyanotic (*blue*) and have dependent edema, dilated neck veins, and hepatomegaly because of right-ventricular failure (*bloated*). Auscultation of the lungs reveals diffuse expiratory and inspiratory rhonchi. Arterial blood gases demonstrate severe hypoxemia and hypercapnia with CO_2 retention (reflecting low ventilation). These differences may reflect variations in ventilation–perfusion mismatching and central respiratory drive.

In clinical practice, most patients with COPD have a mixture of type A and type B disease and fall between these two extremes. In addition, many patients with COPD have an element of asthma (i.e., reversible airways obstruction with bronchospasm). As discussed in the previous chapter, epidemiologic studies of COPD have identified two main syndromes with different risk factors and prognosis: emphysematous form and chronic asthmatic bronchitis.

The pathophysiologic basis of emphysema is a consequence of slowly progressive alveolar fragmentation, loss of lung elasticity, and mechanically related expiratory airflow obstruction. If acute problems (e.g., infection, anesthesia, sedation, left-ventricular failure) do not occur, the patient slowly becomes more breathless, inactive, and wasted. This decline can extend over a period of many years. The development of acute respiratory failure is usually an ominous sign, because it occurs near the end stage (i.e., when very advanced parenchymal destruction is present).

On the other hand, the patient with more predominant bronchitis and asthmatic components of disease tends to have a more episodic course punctuated with exacerbations and reactive airway disease. Such patients tend to respond more to medical therapy and have a better prognosis.

Periodic exacerbations are an important aspect of COPD and have an important effect upon the natural history and disease progression. These episodes of periodic worsening are typically defined by a combination of symptoms of increasing dyspnea, cough, and sputum production. Repeated exacerbations may accelerate the progressive loss of lung function over time. Recovery from exacerbations is slow, and patients frequently do not return to the same level of baseline function.

FURTHER READING

1. Anthonisen NR, Wright FC, Hodgkin JE. Prognosis in chronic obstructive pulmonary disease. *Am Rev Respir Dis.* 1986;133:14–20.

A 3-year follow-up of 985 patients with COPD in the National Institutes of Health—Intermittent Positive Pressure Breathing trial. Age and FEV$_1$ were best predictors of mortality.

2. Bates DV. The fate of the chronic bronchitic: a report of the ten-year follow-up in the Canadian Department of Veterans' Affairs coordinated study of chronic bronchitis. *Am Rev Respir Dis.* 1963;108:1043.

   In approximately 10% of men who smoke, pulmonary function deteriorates faster than the normal rate of decline. This accelerated deterioration can occur in the absence of chest infections.

3. Burrows B, Bloom JW, Traver GA, et al. The course and prognosis of different forms of chronic airways obstruction in a sample from the general population. *N Engl J Med.* 1987;317:1309.

   The 10-year mortality rate among nonatopic smokers without a history of asthma was close to 60% versus 15% among atopic subjects or nonsmokers with known asthma. The mean rate of decline in FEV₁ was 70 mL/year in the former group and less than 5 mL/year in the latter group.

4. Postma DS, Burema J, Gimeno F, et al. Prognosis in severe chronic obstructive pulmonary disease. *Am Rev Respir Dis.* 1979;119:357.

   Five-year and 10-year cumulative survival rates in 129 patients (initial FEV₁ < 1,000 mL) were 69% and 40%, respectively. Best indicators of survival were a decrease in FEV₁/year and an increase in FEV₁ after inhaled bronchodilator.

5. Renzetti AD, McClement JH, Citt BD. The VA cooperative study of pulmonary function, III: mortality in relation to respiratory function in chronic obstructive lung disease. *Am J Med.* 1968;44:115.

   Excellent correlation found between degree of physiologic abnormality and mortality rate. A higher mortality rate was also noted in the patient group at moderately elevated altitude.

6. Peto R, Speizer FE, Cochrane AL, et al. The relevance in adults of airflow obstruction, but not of mucus hypersecretion, to mortality from chronic lung disease. *Am Rev Respir Dis.* 1983;128:491.

   A study of 2,718 British men. Death rates were not significantly related to initial mucus hypersecretion among men with similar initial airflow obstruction.

7. Fletcher C, Peto R, Tinker C, et al. *The Natural History of Chronic Bronchitis and Emphysema.* London, England: Oxford University Press; 1976.

   An important prospective study of nearly 800 working men. The authors emphasize that COPD and mucus hypersecretion are two independent consequences of smoking.

8. Nussbaumer-Ochsner Y, Rabe KF. Systemic manifestations of COPD. *Chest.* 2011;139:165–173.

   Overview of changing perspective about COPD from a purely pulmonary to a systemic disease process.

9. Celli BR, Cote CG, Marin JM, et al. The body-mass index, airflow obstruction, dyspnea, and exercise capacity index in chronic obstructive pulmonary disease. *N Engl J Med.* 2004;350:1005–1012.

   Description and development of the BODE index, a simple grading system that was found to be better than the FEV₁ in predicting risk of death from COPD.

10. Murphy TF, Sethi S. Bacterial infection in chronic obstructive pulmonary disease. *Am Rev Respir Dis.* 1992;146:1067.

    A comprehensive review of the role of bacterial infection as a risk factor, cause of acute exacerbation, and promoter of lung damage in COPD.

11. O'Connor GT, Sparrow D, Weiss ST. The role of allergy and nonspecific airway hyperresponsiveness in the pathogenesis of chronic obstructive pulmonary disease. *Am Rev Respir Dis.* 1989;140:225.

    An excellent review of allergy and airway hyperresponsiveness as risk factors for the development of COPD and as influences on the response to therapy and prognosis in patients with COPD.

12. Parker DR, O'Connor GT, Sparrow D, et al. The relationship of nonspecific airway responsiveness and atopy to the rate of decline of lung function. *Am Rev Respir Dis.* 1990;141:589.

    Among 790 men 40 to 79 years of age, airway responsiveness, as measured by methacholine challenge, was associated with a more rapid decline in FEV₁. This relationship was stronger among skin test-negative cigarette smokers and does not support a relationship between atopy and decline in FEV₁.

13. MacNee W. Pathophysiology of cor pulmonale in chronic obstructive pulmonary disease. *Am J Respir Crit Care Med.* 1994;150:833, 1158.

    A two-part state-of-the-art review of the pathogenesis of right ventricle failure in COPD, including a discussion of techniques used to assess cardiovascular function and management.

14. Washko GR. Diagnostic imaging in COPD. *Semin Respir Crit Care Med.* 2010;31:276–285.
    Review of role of radiographic imaging in COPD.

15. Hogg JC, Macklem PT, Thurlbeck WM. Site and nature of obstruction in chronic obstructive lung disease. *N Engl J Med.* 1968;278:1355.
    A major site of obstruction is in small airways.

16. Niewoehner DE. The impact of severe exacerbations on quality of life and the clinical course of chronic obstructive pulmonary disease. *Am J Med.* 2006;119:S38–S45.

17. Wedzicha JA, Seemungal TAR. COPD exacerbations: defining their cause and prevention. *Lancet.* 2007;370:786–796.

References 16 and 17 review the importance of exacerbations on the progression and natural history of COPD.

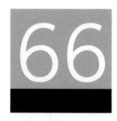

Chronic Obstructive Pulmonary Disease: Management

Andrew L. Ries

Chronic obstructive pulmonary disease (COPD) is a chronic, progressive, and largely irreversible disease, so the primary goals of management should be directed toward preventive health strategies to slow progression and reduce complications. Secondary goals are to improve symptoms and function and treat reversible components. Optimal management depends on the stage of disease. For patients with mild to moderate disease, early detection and diagnosis and counseling regarding appropriate preventive health strategies are important. For patients with moderate to severe disease, symptomatic treatment is also indicated.

According to the current international guidelines of the Global Initiative for Chronic Obstructive Lung Disease (GOLD), staging, and consequently treatment, should be based on a combination of both spirometric evidence of expiratory flow obstruction (i.e., GOLD grades 1 to 4 based on percent of predicted forced expiratory volume in 1 second [FEV_1]) as well as assessment of symptoms with standard questionnaires. Additional therapy should be considered for more symptomatic patients within the same GOLD grade according to spirometry.

Teaching the patient and family members how to participate in the patient's management as active partners with the physician is a key goal that affects all other goals. Patients who are adequately informed and motivated can work with the physician and maintain a level of function that the uninformed, poorly motivated, *passive* patient cannot.

Most patients with COPD are former or current cigarette smokers. Controlling smoking behavior is essential, regardless of the stage of disease. Smoking cessation will slow the rate of decline in FEV_1 and decrease coughing and sputum production. Naturally, the more advanced the functional loss, the less the impact will be. Therefore, early detection of COPD, particularly in smokers who are at high risk, and smoking cessation should be emphasized. Physicians play an important role by setting a smoke-free example in their lives and workplace. Physician advice is important and effective in inducing smokers to quit and maintain abstinence. Several studies have demonstrated that a physician who spends a few minutes inquiring about smoking status and providing advice to quit can achieve abstinence rates of up to 10% to 20% at 1 year. The use of additional modalities such as a comprehensive smoking cessation program, nicotine replacement therapy (gum, dermal patches, nasal spray, or oral inhaler), bupropion, or clonidine (oral or patches) can lead to long-term cessation rates of as high as 50% in motivated patients.

Pulmonary infection is the most common complication in COPD. Prophylactic influenza vaccination should be administered annually, preferably in the early fall. Pneumococcal vaccination, with the expanded version (containing the capsular polysaccharide of 23 serotypes), should be administered once or twice (if <65 years of age when first vaccinated). As effective antiviral agents become available (e.g., amantadine), consider their use for the patient with COPD, particularly during epidemics of influenza A.

Another preventive approach is to assess patient exposure to occupational–environmental air pollutants and, if possible, eliminate or reduce that exposure. A final method used to prevent complications is to avoid therapies and drugs that can compromise patient function. Patients with COPD tend to become victims of polypharmacy. To avoid this problem, carefully consider the risk-to-benefit characteristics of each therapy (drug, oxygen, or mechanical device) before it is instituted. Constantly review the treatment regimen, deleting elements that have been of no benefit, particularly if they can induce long-term toxicity.

For patients with recognized COPD, pharmacotherapy is directed toward the reversible component of airway obstruction and control of secretions. Bronchodilators used to improve symptoms and increase airway caliber include sympathomimetic β-agonists, anticholinergics, and (less commonly) the methylxanthine, theophylline. The decision to treat a patient with a bronchodilator should not depend on demonstrating an acute response, as many patients who do not demonstrate an acute response during testing do respond to long-term regular therapy. Airway hyperreactivity is common in patients with COPD, and long-term therapy with bronchodilators can serve to prevent airways constriction caused by inhaled irritants. Also, these medications may have effects beyond just bronchodilation. If a long-acting bronchodilator is used for maintenance therapy, then a short-acting agent is also needed for rescue therapy.

Sympathomimetic bronchodilators are used commonly. Newer β_2 agents are more selective and longer-acting and have fewer side effects than older, nonselective drugs. In addition to bronchodilation, β-agonists can also reduce airway hyperresponsiveness and enhance mucociliary clearance. The most common side effects are tachycardia and skeletal muscle tremor.

Anticholinergics have recently gained prominence in the treatment of COPD. Although their bronchodilating effects have been known for many years, the selectivity and reduced side effects of newer agents have increased their usefulness. Bronchodilation is thought to be caused by inhibition of cholinergic-mediated bronchomotor tone. The drugs are reported to be more effective in larger airways, making them particularly useful for patients with COPD. They can be used concomitantly with β_2-agonists. Both short- and long-acting agents are now available.

The preferred method of administration for both β-agonists and anticholinergics is by inhalation, usually with a metered-dose inhaler (MDI). This produces more bronchodilation with fewer side effects than oral or other systemic routes. Used properly, an MDI is equally effective and less expensive than a liquid nebulizer and can be used in acute and emergency department settings. Extensions or spacers may help persons who have difficulty coordinating the MDI, particularly children and older adults. The key to MDI use is proper technique. All patients should be instructed and observed in following several key steps in using MDIs: (1) shake inhaler, remove cap, and hold upright; (2) exhale to functional residual capacity or below; (3) place inhaler 2 to 4 cm in front of open mouth; (4) activate inhaler just after the start of a slow, deep inhalation; (5) hold breath for 5 to 10 seconds; (6) exhale slowly; and (7) wait at least 1 minute before next puff.

Theophylline preparations have been used in treating patients with COPD for many years, but their use has decreased because of a narrow toxic–therapeutic margin, frequent problems with toxicity, and the advent of newer, more selective bronchodilating agents. The mechanism of bronchodilation from theophylline is still not clearly defined. Theophylline has other potentially beneficial effects, such as improved diaphragmatic function, reduced dyspnea, increased mucociliary clearance, and stimulation of respiratory drive. Because of individual variability in metabolism and the many factors that can alter metabolism (e.g., drugs such as cimetidine, erythromycin, and ciprofloxacin), blood levels must be monitored with chronic therapy. The target therapeutic level is typically 10 to 20 μg/mL. Minor side effects such as tremor, insomnia, irritability, and gastrointestinal upset can occur with levels well below 20 μg/mL. More serious side effects, including vomiting, dysrhythmias, hypotension, and seizures, generally develop at higher blood levels. Older patients are particularly susceptible to toxicity.

Corticosteroids can be beneficial for some patients with COPD. The complications of long-term use are well-known, and chronic use of systemic corticosteroids should be avoided, if possible. A meta-analysis of 16 clinical trials of oral steroid therapy for stable patients found that a 20% improvement in FEV_1 occurred in approximately 10% more patients on steroids than on placebo. Many patients on corticosteroids report subjective symptom improvement, but long-term steroid use is associated with many serious side effects. A limited trial of corticosteroids is probably justified in patients who cannot be managed with standard bronchodilators alone. A single morning dose of prednisone (20–40 mg) for 5 to 7 days is a typical starting point. Treatment beyond a few weeks should be continued only with a significant improvement in pulmonary function and symptoms. For long-term therapy, the dose should be kept as low as possible to minimize side effects.

Inhaled steroids, best used through a spacer device to minimize oral deposition, are safer than systemic steroids, but their effectiveness in COPD has not been clearly established. Several multicenter clinical trials have evaluated the role of inhaled corticosteroids in the management of COPD. There is some evidence that inhaled corticosteroids may be associated with clinical benefits, such as reduced exacerbations and hospitalizations, even without documented improvement in lung function. Dysphonia and upper airway thrush are the most common adverse consequences of inhaled corticosteroids. However, prolonged use of these agents, particularly at high doses, may also produce systemic side effects (e.g., subcapsular cataracts and decreased bone-mineral density).

For patients with chronic cough and sputum, techniques to control secretions are important. Patients should be encouraged to drink several glasses of fluid per day, but excessive hydration is not warranted. They should also be taught the technique of controlled coughing, which involves a deep inspiration, breath-holding for a few seconds, and then coughing two or three times. Postural drainage is effective in patients with heavy sputum production. The use of mucolytic agents to thin secretions and promote clearance is controversial. Theoretically, therapy with drugs such as oral iodinated glycerol, nebulized acetylcysteine, or, more recently, recombinant human deoxyribonuclease works best in thinning secretions that are thick, mucoid, and heavy. Whether this produces physiologic or symptomatic improvement is unclear. Cough suppressant therapy is generally not recommended, as cough is an essential protective mechanism.

Exacerbations of COPD result in adverse effects and may cause permanent further loss of lung function. Most are thought to be due to infection, but sputum cultures and smears are not generally helpful since a specific bacterial pathogen cannot usually be identified. Because of impaired mucociliary clearance and less-effective cough, secretions can pool in dependent portions of the lung and be difficult to clear. For acute exacerbations, when sputum changes color and increases in volume, treatment with antibiotics is typically indicated. In many cases of acute bronchitis, it is appropriate to institute a course (7–10 days) of antibiotics empirically without a sputum culture. Oral antibiotics are commonly chosen to cover pathogens colonizing the respiratory tract, including *Haemophilus influenzae, Streptococcus pneumoniae,* and *Moraxella catarrhalis.* Most studies demonstrating benefits from antibiotics in exacerbations have been conducted with older antibiotics, such as trimethoprim–sulfamethoxazole, ampicillin, amoxicillin–clavulanate, tetracycline, or erythromycin. It is not clear whether newer drugs, such as macrolides and fluoroquinolones, are more effective. Short courses (up to 14 days) of systemic corticosteroids are also used commonly to treat acute exacerbations.

In the severely hypoxemic patient, oxygen therapy has been shown to improve survival and reduce morbidity from consequences such as right-ventricular failure, polycythemia, and psychologic–mental dysfunction. Less clearly defined are the possible benefits of supplemental oxygen for nonhypoxemic patients or for patients with hypoxemia only under certain conditions (e.g., exercise, sleep). The results of two multicenter clinical trials (one in Great Britain, the other in the United States) justify long-term oxygen therapy for patients with significant resting hypoxemia (arterial $Po_2 \leq 55$ mmHg or oxygen saturation $[So_2] \leq 88\%$). For patients with an arterial Po_2 between 56 and 59 mmHg, oxygen is indicated in cases of erythrocytosis (hematocrit 55 or more) or cor pulmonale. The decision for long-term therapy should be made only in stable patients on optimal treatment for at least 30 days. Patients recovering from an acute illness should be reevaluated after a period of stability before committing to this expensive treatment. Several options exist for long-term oxygen therapy. Home care providers, respiratory therapy personnel, and pulmonary rehabilitation professionals are excellent sources of information about available options, including gas sources (e.g., liquid, compressed gas, concentrators) and delivery devices (e.g., nasal, transtracheal, or conserving catheters and inspiratory demand regulators). Hypoxemic patients living at high altitude may benefit by moving to sea level, where the ambient oxygen tension is higher. If air travel is contemplated, arrangements may be necessary for supplemental oxygen because commercial aircraft cabins are pressurized at 5,000 to 8,000 feet.

Surgery may play a role in a few patients with COPD. Bullectomy may benefit selected patients with large space-occupying bullae. Lung transplantation for COPD is feasible and has been performed in many centers; criteria for selection and long-term follow-up are still evolving. In selected subgroups of patients with severe emphysema, lung-volume reduction surgery has been found to result in improved survival, exercise tolerance, symptoms, and quality of life compared with medically treated patients. The benefits were most evident in patients with a predominance of upper-lobe distribution of emphysema and very low exercise tolerance.

Pulmonary rehabilitation is an established preventive health strategy that enhances standard therapy for persons with chronic lung disease to control and alleviate symptoms, optimize function, and reduce the medical and economic burdens of disease (see Chapter 10). Multidisciplinary programs include education, respiratory and chest physiotherapy instruction, psychosocial support, and exercise training. As with other rehabilitation programs, the primary goal is to restore the patient to the highest possible level of independent function. This can be accomplished by helping patients become more knowledgeable about their disease, more actively involved in their own healthcare, more independent in daily care activities, and less dependent on family, friends, and health professionals and other expensive medical resources. Benefits of pulmonary rehabilitation include improved exercise tolerance and symptoms and reduced hospitalizations and use of expensive medical resources. Patients report improved quality of life with a reduction in respiratory symptoms, an increase in exercise tolerance and ability to perform physical activities of daily living, and improved psychological function, with less anxiety and depression and increased feelings of hope, control, and self-esteem.

Breathing retraining techniques include instruction in pursed-lip breathing and breathing patterns. Pursed-lip breathing imparts a subjective relief of dyspnea in some individuals. In theory, it prevents airway collapse during expiration. Pursed-lip breathing is often accompanied by an instantaneous diminution in activity of the accessory muscles of respiration. Slow, deep breathing often provides a subjective sense of improved respiratory control. The increased tidal volume can serve to reduce wasted ventilation.

Formal rehabilitation programs have obvious advantages for both patients and physicians. But, however achieved, patient education is essential. Patients who understand their disease, medications, and the other elements of their regimen are likely to avoid hospitalization and a variety of other untoward events.

FURTHER READING

1. Celli BR, MacNee W; committee members of ATS/ERS Task Force. Standards for the diagnosis and treatment of patients with COPD: a summary of the ATS/ERS position paper. *Eur Respir J.* 2004;23:982–994.

   Official statement published jointly by the American Thoracic Society and European Respiratory Society that updates official practice guidelines for the diagnosis and treatment of COPD. An online version of the document is available at www.thoracic.org/copd.

2. The Global Initiative for Chronic Obstructive Lung Disease (GOLD). Update 2011. Full online resources available at www.goldcopd.com.

   International evidence-based review cosponsored by NHLBI and WHO providing guidelines for diagnosis and management. Major initiative to raise awareness about the global epidemic of COPD.

3. Niewoehner DE. Outpatient management of severe COPD. *N Engl J Med.* 2010;362:1407.

   Excellent, succinct summary of recommendations for management of COPD.

4. Anthonisen NR, Connett JE, Kiley JP, et al. Effects of smoking intervention and the use of an inhaled anticholinergic bronchodilator on the rate of decline of FEV_1: the Lung Health Study. *JAMA.* 1994;272:1497.

   Results of the Lung Health Study, a multicenter, randomized trial of smoking cessation and inhaled anticholinergic bronchodilator therapy in 5,887 smokers with early COPD. Over 5 years of follow-up, smoking cessation significantly reduced the age-related decline in FEV_1. Anticholinergic therapy led to a small improvement in FEV_1 but did not influence long-term decline.

5. The Smoking Cessation Clinical Practice Guideline panel and staff. The Agency for Health Care Policy and Research Smoking Cessation Clinical Practice Guideline. *JAMA.* 1996;275:1270.

   Consensus panel recommendations about smoking cessation techniques for primary care clinicians, smoking cessation specialists, and healthcare administrators. Emphasizes the need for systematic practices and a multipronged attack to identify smokers and encourage smoking cessation practices.

6. Tashkin DP, Altose MD, Bleecker ER, et al. The Lung Health Study: airway responsiveness to inhaled methacholine in smokers with mild to moderate airflow limitation. *Am Rev Respir Dis.* 1992;145:301.

   Airway hyperresponsiveness was found in 85% of female and 59% of male smokers with mild to moderate COPD. Emphasizes the importance of airway reactivity in these patients.

7. Advisory Committee on Immunization Practices. Recommended adult immunization schedule. *Ann Intern Med.* 2009;150:40.

   Current US recommendations for influenza and pneumococcal vaccination.

8. Sin DD, McAlister FA, Man SFP, et al. Contemporary management of chronic obstructive pulmonary disease: scientific review. *JAMA.* 2003;290:2301.

   Systematic review of long-acting bronchodilators, inhaled corticosteroids, nocturnal noninvasive mechanical ventilation, pulmonary rehabilitation, domiciliary oxygen therapy, and disease management programs in COPD. Concluded that long-acting bronchodilators and inhaled corticosteroids reduced exacerbations, oxygen therapy improved survival in patients with resting hypoxemia, and pulmonary rehabilitation improved health status. Noninvasive ventilation and disease management programs have not been shown to improve outcomes.

9. Tashkin DP, Celli B, Senn S, et al. A 4-year trial of tiotropium in chronic obstructive pulmonary disease. *N Engl J Med.* 2008;359:1543.

10. Vogelmeier C, Hederer B, Glaab T, et al. Tiotropium versus salmeterol for the prevention of exacerbations of COPD. *N Engl J Med.* 2011;364:1093.

    References 9 and 10 describe recent large multicenter trials evaluating the benefits of long acting anticholinergic therapy in COPD.

11. Callahan CM, Dittus RS, Katz BP. Oral corticosteroid therapy for patients with stable chronic obstructive pulmonary disease: a meta-analysis. *Ann Intern Med.* 1991;114:216.

    A meta-analysis of published studies of oral corticosteroids in patients with stable COPD. Overall, a more than 20% improvement in FEV_1 was seen 10% more often in patients on steroid therapy compared with controls.

12. Niewoehner DE, Erbland ML, Deupree RH, et al. Effect of systemic glucocorticoids on exacerbations of chronic obstructive pulmonary disease. *N Engl J Med.* 1999;25:1941.

    A randomized clinical trial of systemic corticosteroids in 271 patients hospitalized for exacerbation of COPD in which steroid therapy was associated with improved clinical outcomes.

13. Alsaeedi A, Sin DD, McAlister FA. The effects of inhaled corticosteroids in chronic obstructive pulmonary disease: a systematic review of randomized placebo-controlled trials. *Am J Med.* 2002;113:59–65.

    Summary and systematic review of randomized clinical trials of inhaled corticosteroids in COPD. Concludes that there is a beneficial effect on reducing COPD exacerbations. Modest survival benefit was not statistically significant.

14. Highland KB, Strange C, Heffner JE. Long-term effects of inhaled corticosteroids on FEV_1 in patients with chronic obstructive pulmonary disease: a meta-analysis. *Ann Intern Med.* 2003;138:969–973.

    Meta-analysis of randomized clinical trials that did not find a significant relationship between the use of inhaled corticosteroids and the rate of decline in FEV_1 in COPD.

15. Rennard S. New approaches to COPD therapy. *Adv Stud Med.* 2003;3:S408–S415.

    Succinct review of newer classes of agents being evaluated for treatment of COPD, such as phosphodiesterase 4 inhibitors and other anti-inflammatory agents, retinoids, long-acting anticholinergics, and anabolic steroids.

16. Murphy TF, Sethi S. Bacterial infection in chronic obstructive pulmonary disease. *Am Rev Respir Dis.* 1992;146:1067.

    A state-of-the-art review of bacterial infection in COPD, including a discussion of its role in exacerbations, microbiology, and treatment. A treatment algorithm emphasizes use of Gram stain without sputum culture and empiric choice of antibiotics.

17. Saint S, Bent S, Vittinghoff E, et al. Antibiotics in chronic obstructive pulmonary disease exacerbations: a meta-analysis. *JAMA.* 1995;273:957.

    A meta-analysis summarizing published randomized trials on the effectiveness of antibiotics in treating COPD exacerbations. Results suggest a small but statistically significant improvement.

18. Kirilloff LH, Owens GR, Rogers RM, et al. Does chest physical therapy work? *Chest.* 1985;88:436.

19. Rochester DF, Goldberg SK. Techniques of respiratory physical therapy. *Am Rev Respir Dis.* 1980;122:133.

    References 18 and 19 review the rationale for and use of chest physiotherapy and breathing retraining techniques in patients with chronic lung diseases.

20. Petty TL. The National Mucolytic Study: results of a randomized, double-blind, placebo-controlled study of iodinated glycerol in chronic obstructive bronchitis. *Chest.* 1990;97:75.

    A randomized, double-blind, placebo-controlled multicenter study demonstrating efficacy of iodinated-glycerol (60 mg four times daily) given as an adjunctive therapy. Although dyspnea showed a "trend toward improvement," the physicians' global evaluation did not differ between the two groups. The test agent improved chest symptoms and patient well-being.

21. American Thoracic Society/European Respiratory Society. ATS/ERS statement on pulmonary rehabilitation. *Am J Respir Crit Care Med.* 2006;173:1390.

22. Ries AL, Bauldoff GS, Carlin BW, et al. Pulmonary rehabilitation: joint ACCP/AACVPR evidence-based clinical practice guidelines. *Chest.* 2007;131(suppl 5):4S.

    An updated statement (reference 21) and evidence-based practice guideline (reference 22) about pulmonary rehabilitation from major respiratory organizations.

23. Medical Research Council Working Party. Long-term domiciliary oxygen therapy in chronic hypoxic cor pulmonale complicating chronic bronchitis and emphysema. *Lancet.* 1981;1:681.

24. Nocturnal Oxygen Therapy Trial Group. Continuous or nocturnal oxygen therapy in hypoxemic chronic obstructive lung disease: a clinical trial. *Ann Intern Med.* 1980;93:391.

    References 23 and 24 are classic multicenter clinical trials conducted in Great Britain and the United States that demonstrated improved survival from oxygen therapy in hypoxemic patients with COPD.

25. Crockett AJ, Cranston JM, Moss JR, et al. A review of long-term oxygen therapy for chronic obstructive pulmonary disease. *Respir Med.* 2001;95:437–443.

    Systematic review evidence for use of long-term oxygen therapy in COPD.

26. National Emphysema Treatment Trial Research Group. A randomized trial comparing lung-volume reduction surgery with medical therapy for severe emphysema. *N Engl J Med.* 2003;348:2059–2073.

27. National Emphysema Treatment Trial Research Group. Cost effectiveness of lung-volume reduction surgery for patients with severe emphysema. *N Engl J Med.* 2003;348:2092–2102.

    These two references report primary outcomes of the National Emphysema Treatment Trial, a landmark study sponsored by NHLBI, CMS, and AHRQ to evaluate lung volume reduction surgery. Ideal patients were those with predominant upper lobe distribution of emphysema and lowest exercise tolerance. Emphasizes the poor prognosis of medically treated patients.

28. Orens JB, Martinez FJ. Lung and heart-lung transplantation: indications, timing, and results. *Semin Respir Crit Care Med.* 2001;22:477–587.

    Compendium of eight articles related to lung and heart-lung transplant.

The Acute Respiratory Distress Syndrome

Robert M. Smith

A marked increase in the permeability of the alveolar–capillary membrane to water, solutes, and plasma proteins is the defining characteristic of the acute respiratory distress syndrome (ARDS); clinically, it is associated with diffuse lung infiltrates, respiratory distress, and respiratory failure. A prospective study using the 1994 American-European Consensus Conference (AECC) definitions of ARDS and acute lung injury (ALI) suggested that the age-adjusted incidence was 86.2 per 100,000 person-years. The incidence increased with age, reaching 306 per 100,000 person-years for those aged 75 to 84 years. On the basis of these statistics, it is estimated that more than 190,000 cases occur annually in the Unites States and that these cases are associated with 74,500 deaths. Although there is some suggestion that the incidence has decreased somewhat over time, ARDS remains a frequent and dreaded problem in modern intensive care units.

ETIOLOGY

Events that have preceded and appear to act as precipitants to ARDS are remarkably diverse (Table 67-1), although sepsis and trauma are the most common associated clinical settings. The wisdom of grouping patients with such disparate precipitating factors together under the umbrella of ARDS has been debated frequently. However, because the biochemical and cellular pathways that lead to ARDS are not understood and because patients have a number of apparent physiologic and histologic features in common, it has proven useful to consider them together.

TABLE 67-1	Clinical Settings Associated with the Development of ARDS
Clinical Processes Where ARDS Occurs in More Than 1% of Patients at Risk	
Aspiration of gastric contents	
Pneumonia requiring intensive care unit	
Severe sepsis	
Multiple trauma	
Disseminated intravascular coagulation (usually associated with other events)	
Other Clinical Processes Associated with ARDS	
Near drowning	
Smoke inhalation	
Inhalation of irritant or toxic gases	
Fat or air embolism	
Pancreatitis	
Hypertransfusion	
Thermal burn	
Cardiopulmonary bypass	
Narcotic administration	

The probability of developing ARDS increases with multiple risk factors, but it is not known whether different precipitants act independently or via some common pathway that leads to lung injury.

The processes responsible for tissue injury in ARDS remain obscure. The lung is diffusely inflamed, and inflammatory cells (particularly neutrophils and their granular products) have been implicated in the pathogenesis of ARDS in animal models. Similarly, the production of highly reactive oxygen radical species by neutrophils or by resident lung macrophages may contribute to ARDS either by direct tissue injury or by modification of proteins, lipids, or DNA leading to inactivation (e.g., α_1-proteinase inhibitor) or abnormal function. A number of factors may lead to neutrophil accumulation in the lung. Cytokines, elaborated systemically or locally in the lung following sepsis or trauma, may act as chemotactic factors (e.g., interleukin [IL]-8) or can cause up-regulation of endothelial and leukocyte adhesion molecules (e.g., IL-1). Preliminary studies suggested that elevated levels of IL-8 in alveolar lavage fluid of patients at risk for ARDS may predict the subsequent development of the full-blown syndrome. However, this finding has not been confirmed in larger studies, and the complex interplay between the various cytokines is not yet well understood. The occurrence of ARDS in severely neutropenic patients and the lack of neutrophil participation in some animal models of ARDS suggest that neutrophil-independent mechanisms of tissue injury also are important. Loss of surfactant activity in lung lavage specimens is seen early in ARDS and is a potential explanation for many of the physiologic abnormalities. The loss of surfactant activity is caused in part by alterations in surfactant production by type II pneumocytes and in part by inhibition of surfactant activity by the ingress of plasma proteins.

Over the last two decades it has become increasingly clear that the ways in which mechanical ventilatory support is applied may influence the progress and potentially the development of ARDS. In animal models, positive-pressure ventilation alone can initiate diffuse lung injury with radiographic and histologic features indistinguishable from ARDS. This injury occurs in animals with even modest levels of positive pressure (e.g., sustained peak airway pressures of 30 cm H_2O for 24 hours). Data suggest that injury may be a result of cyclic opening and closing of alveoli or overdistension and stretching of the alveolar capillary membrane at peak inflation. Injury is diminished in these models by limiting maximal ventilatory excursion or by the application of positive end-expiratory pressure (PEEP). Further studies have demonstrated the elaboration of proinflammatory cytokines and the alteration of surfactant structure and function in the lungs of animals as a result of positive-pressure ventilation. Although these studies do not shed light on the etiologic events initiating ARDS, they do support the hypothesis that the ventilatory support necessary to preserve gas exchange may worsen or modify the course of the underlying lung injury.

PATHOPHYSIOLOGY

There are no specific physical or laboratory findings that identify patients with ARDS. Prior to the development of frank respiratory failure, respirations are rapid and shallow, and the patient may be cyanotic. Auscultation usually reveals bronchial breath sounds; rales are often absent. Serum chemistries and blood-cell counts tend to reflect the underlying diseases, rather than ARDS itself. The chest radiograph shows rapidly progressing widespread infiltrates, often with characteristics suggesting alveolar filling. Occasionally, there is a brief early period during which an interstitial infiltrate predominates. Particularly in the early stages, the infiltrates may look patchy or appear to spare some parts of the lung, leading to a mistaken diagnosis of pneumonia. Arterial blood gas analyses typically show markedly reduced Pao_2 with a normal or reduced $Paco_2$.

The 1994 AECC definition of ARDS utilized the level of hypoxemia to stage the severity. In that definition, a Pao_2/Fio_2 ratio between 200 and 300 corresponded to a diagnosis of ALI, while a Pao_2/Fio_2 ratio of less than 200 corresponded to full-blown ARDS. Despite its overall success and broad use as a research tool, the AECC definition had a number of limitations (such as the absence of a specification for PEEP). An expert panel (the ARDS Definition Task Force) has proposed an expanded definition (Table 67-2) that corrects these deficiencies. In the presence of PEEP or continuous positive airway pressure (CPAP) levels greater than or equal to 5 cm H_2O, Pao_2 levels between 200 and 300 mmHg correspond to mild

TABLE 67-2	The "Berlin" Definition of Acute Respiratory Distress Syndrome
Timing	Within 1 wk of a known clinical insult or new or worsening respiratory symptoms
Chest imaging[a]	Bilateral opacities—not fully explained by effusions, lobar/lung collapse, or nodules
Origin of edema	Respiratory failure not fully explained by cardiac failure or fluid overload
	Need objective assessment (e.g., echocardiography) to exclude hydrostatic edema if no risk factor present
Oxygenation[b]	
Mild	200 mmHg < Pao_2/Fio_2 ≤ 300 mmHg with PEEP or CPAP ≥ 5 cm H_2O[c]
Moderate	100 mmHg < Pao_2/Fio_2 ≤ 200 mmHg with PEEP ≥ 5 cm H_2O
Severe	Pao_2/Fio_2 ≤ 100 mmHg with PEEP ≥ 5 cm H_2O

Abbreviations: CPAP, continuous positive airway pressure; Fio_2, fraction of inspired oxygen; Pao_2, partial pressure of arterial oxygen; PEEP, positive end-expiratory pressure.
[a]Chest radiograph or computed tomography scan.
[b]If altitude is higher than 1,000 m, the correction factor should be calculated as follows: (Pao_2/Fio_2 * [barometric pressure/760]).
[c]This may be delivered noninvasively in the mild ARDS group. Adapted from The ARDS Definition Task Force. Acute respiratory distress syndrome: the Berlin definition. *JAMA.* 2012;307(23):2526–2533.

ARDS, between 100 and 200 mmHg correspond to moderate ARDS, and those less than or equal to 100 mmHg define severe ARDS. When applied retrospectively, this consensus definition appeared to correlate with mortality and duration of need for mechanical ventilation.

Clinically, physiologically, and pathologically, ARDS typically progresses through successive stages. After exposure to the triggering event, there is often an interval of apparently normal lung function lasting hours to days. With the onset of symptoms, there is rapidly worsening gas exchange with decreasing lung compliance and functional residual capacity over 1 to 3 days. Subsequently, lung compliance decreases further, and increases occur in the proportion of the total ventilation going to unperfused "dead space" lung regions ($\dot{V}_D/\dot{V}_T$) and in pulmonary vascular resistance. Multiple organ system failure, which may include renal dysfunction, hepatic dysfunction, and biventricular cardiac dysfunction, often becomes apparent at this point, although it may occur at any time. It is not known whether impairment in these organ systems is caused by the same process precipitating ARDS (e.g., sepsis) or to distinct pathologic processes. In addition, the interventions used to support gas exchange, such as mechanical ventilation or PEEP, may also have deleterious effects on the function of extrapulmonary organs. From 10 to 30 days after the onset of symptoms, the patient may enter a more chronic stage in which pulmonary function has stabilized, although persistent functional impairment remains. If the patient survives the acute events long enough to enter the chronic stage, there is usually a gradual improvement in lung function over weeks to months. The risk of mortality at this stage is more often related to nonpulmonary causes.

Histologic examination of pulmonary tissue supports the differentiation of ARDS into acute and chronic stages. In the early stages, termed the *exudative phase,* alveolar type I epithelial cells are focally destroyed, and endothelial cells may appear swollen. Neutrophils clog the capillaries and extravasate into the interstitium. Interstitial edema is found, with cuffs of more intense edema around bronchioles and vessels. The alveoli are filled with proteinaceous exudate containing red blood cells, neutrophils, macrophages, and cell fragments. Increased numbers of cells are recovered in bronchoalveolar lavage fluid. Polymorphonuclear neutrophil leukocytes, which normally make up less than 2% of recovered cells, predominate in the lavage fluid of ARDS.

A more chronic stage of ALI, termed the *fibroproliferative phase,* is apparent after 1 to 2 weeks. Plasma cells, histiocytes, and lymphocytes are seen in the interstitium and are accompanied by proliferation of pericytes and fibroblasts. Intravascular microthrombi are common. Cuboidal epithelial cells cover the surfaces of alveoli and alveolar ducts, and the acinar architecture of the lung is progressively replaced by thick bands of fibrotic tissue.

MANAGEMENT

Initial management of the patient with ARDS focuses on supporting the patient while identifying and treating potentially reversible processes that may exacerbate or mimic ARDS. An aggressive diagnostic approach is warranted in the patient with known or suspected immunocompromise. In particular, bronchoscopy with lavage and brushings may be useful to determine the presence of *Pneumocystis carinii* pneumonia for patients suspected of having AIDS. Transbronchial biopsy may be considered, but it should be used with caution in light of the risk of complications during mechanical ventilation. Open-lung biopsy may be helpful for those patients in whom no specific diagnosis can be made with less invasive techniques.

Oxygenation of the arterial blood and delivery of oxygen to peripheral tissues are the primary goals of supportive therapy in ARDS. These goals must be balanced with the equally important goal of limiting further lung injury from ventilatory support. Initially, supplemental oxygen via facemask or nasal cannula may be adequate. However, tracheal intubation and positive-pressure ventilation are usually needed and should be instituted as soon as it is apparent that an acceptable Pao_2 cannot be maintained with supplemental oxygen alone. The optimal method of supplying ventilatory support remains controversial. However, the National Institutes of Health-sponsored ARDS net trial of low-stretch ventilation (low tidal volume) compared with high-stretch ventilation (high tidal volume) demonstrated marked reduction in ARDS mortality when the low-stretch, "lung-protective" strategy was followed. In this study, patients ventilated with 6 mL/kg tidal volumes had a 30% mortality compared to the 40% mortality experienced by patients subjected to "standard" 12 mL/kg tidal volume ventilation. Although this study used a volume-controlled method of mechanical ventilation, end-inspiratory plateau pressures were limited to 25 and 45 cm H_2O in the low- and high-stretch arms, respectively. It is likely that other ventilatory strategies that limit end-inspiratory pressure to a similar level of 25 cm H_2O (such as pressure-cycled ventilation) would be equally successful.

Ventilation strategies that achieve low tidal volumes often result in hypoventilation with resulting increases in Pco_2 and falls in arterial pH. It is generally accepted that it is safe to allow the pH to fall to 7.20 during mechanical ventilation, and this strategy of "permissive hypercapnia" is typically well tolerated. Sedation is frequently needed to optimize patient comfort during this technique.

PEEP at levels from 10 to 15 cm H_2O should be applied when volume-limited positive-pressure ventilation cannot maintain a Pao_2 greater than 55 to 60 mmHg using an Fio_2 of 0.6 or less. The physiologic effects of PEEP are thought to result from (1) redistribution of capillary blood flow, resulting in improved ventilation–perfusion matching, and (2) the recruitment of previously collapsed alveoli and prevention of their collapse during exhalation. The net effect of these changes is an improvement in Pao_2, which then allows a reduction in Fio_2. The improvement in lung function due to PEEP may require 30 to 60 minutes to become apparent, but is lost more rapidly if PEEP is removed. PEEP also may have significant deleterious consequences. As end-expiratory pressure is increased, mean thoracic pressure may also increase, compromising venous return. In addition, PEEP may directly impact cardiac function by restricting the filling of the atria or ventricles during diastole. On the plus side, the application of PEEP appears to limit alveolar excursion during positive-pressure ventilation and protects from ventilation-associated lung injury in animal models. Although PEEP is essential for the support of patients at nontoxic Fio_2, early "prophylactic" PEEP is ineffective in preventing ARDS.

It is vital to recognize the deleterious effects of ventilatory support techniques and balance them against their benefits. Improvements in Pao_2 brought about by the incremental application of PEEP must be weighed against any decrement in cardiac output that may in fact decrease oxygen delivery. To achieve this balance, it may be helpful to monitor the variables that determine cardiac function (pulmonary artery and pulmonary artery wedge pressures), as well as those that measure total arterial oxygen delivery (arterial oxygen saturation, hemoglobin, and cardiac output). Measurements of the mixed venous oxygen tension (Pvo_2) and the difference between arterial and mixed venous oxygen contents ($C[a-v]o_2$) may be useful to monitor as well. The optimum level of PEEP is usually the lowest level, allowing a Pao_2 between 55 and 60 mmHg with an acceptable cardiac output. Further increases of PEEP may improve Pao_2, but may significantly increase the risk of barotraumatic injury and impaired cardiac function.

Alternative methods of ventilatory support have been explored with only limited success. High-frequency jet ventilation and high-frequency oscillation coupled with positive-pressure ventilation may improve gas exchange in certain patients. Similarly, the use of pressure-cycled inverse ratio ventilation (i.e., inspiratory time greater than expiratory time) may occasionally provide benefit, as may ventilation of patients in the prone position or using airway pressure-release ventilation. Application of extracorporeal bypass with membrane oxygenation or extracorporeal carbon dioxide removal through a venovenous bypass circuit may preserve function in selected patients where other approaches fail. Although each of these approaches have their adherents and have pathophysiologic rationale, none have had efficacy demonstrated in a robust controlled clinical trial. Inhalation of nitric oxide improves Pao_2 acutely, but has similarly not had a measurable impact on survival in a number of well-controlled trials.

Ongoing management of the patient with ARDS requires meticulous attention to detail and careful surveillance for possible complications. As for any critically ill patient, appropriate early attention must be paid both to nutritional support and to prevention of venous thrombosis. For patients with severely compromised lung function, sedation and muscle paralysis may be required to prevent struggling against the ventilator and increased oxygen utilization. Any sudden deterioration in hemodynamic status, increase in peak airway pressure, or drop in Pao_2 should suggest the possibility of a tension pneumothorax and prompt immediate action. Daily chest films and frequent examination of the chest for asymmetric breath sounds should be performed to survey for slowly developing air leaks.

In selected patients, pharmacologic agents (e.g., inotropic agents, vasodilators, or both) may be useful if cardiac output cannot be preserved with acceptable low left-ventricular filling pressures. Optimization of cardiac function as a physiologic goal, however, is another topic of ongoing debate, since it may conflict with other therapeutic strategies. For example, maximizing filling pressures to prevent a drop in cardiac output with PEEP conflicts with the strategy of reducing filling pressures to decrease the leak of fluid across the alveolar–capillary membrane. In general, strategies that aim toward reducing lung edema by limiting filling pressures appear more successful, although each situation warrants an individual decision. There does not appear to be any survival advantage conferred by elevating cardiac output and tissue oxygen delivery to supranormal levels.

Low tidal ventilation, the management strategy that has the greatest demonstrated effectiveness, remains inconsistently implemented even in otherwise high-performing intensive care units. The reasons for poor adherence are multifactorial. However, despite barriers to implementation, accumulated data to date suggest that implementation of lung-protective ventilation should become a part of routine critical care practice.

Specific therapy for ARDS is not yet available. Attempts to block elements of the inflammatory cascade (e.g., cyclooxygenase inhibitors or protease inhibitors) or attempts to manipulate cytokine cascades (e.g., anti–tumor necrosis factor or IL-1 receptor antagonists) have been unsuccessful clinically. Similarly, despite encouraging results in animal models, instillation of surfactant products into the airways early in ARDS has not shown benefit. Manipulation of dietary lipids or administration of glutathione precursors may be useful as part of the support of patients with lung injury.

Corticosteroid therapy in ARDS remains controversial. Earlier studies demonstrated that high-dose corticosteroid therapy did not prevent the development of ARDS or alter its eventual outcome. More recent studies suggested that moderate-dose corticosteroid therapy (0.5 to 2.5 mg/kg/day of methylprednisolone or its equivalent) administered during the early fibroproliferative phase of ARDS reduces mortality and increases ventilator-free days. Unfortunately, the methodologies used in the different studies varied substantially and the strength of the conclusions has been debated. However, those studies did demonstrate that moderate doses of corticosteroids have an acceptable side-effect profile. Given the high mortality that continues to be demonstrated in ARDS, the use of moderate doses of corticosteroids at day 5 to 10 of unresolving ARDS may be warranted on an individualized basis. If so, the steroids are typically used for no more than 7 to 10 days and tapered over that time. There is little evidence to support prolonged corticosteroid therapy or therapy in later-stage disease.

PROGNOSIS

The mortality of patients who develop moderate or severe ARDS remains distressingly high (~30%–40%), although estimate is an improvement over the 90% mortality reported in the initial studies of ARDS. Mortality appears to be age-related: the rates are 24% in those aged 15 to 19 but 60% in those 85 years and older. In general, mortality in ARDS correlates more with the presence of multiple organ failure and with other coexisting or preexisting disease than with the severity of pulmonary impairment. The long-term outlook for survivors of ARDS is relatively good in spite of the severe physiologic impairment and pathologic changes present during and immediately following hospitalization. Lung volumes and compliance often return to predicted levels within 6 to 18 months, and there is often only minimal impairment in exercise capacity compared to premorbid levels. Dyspnea persisting months after recovery should prompt a search for causes other than residual fibrosis from ARDS (e.g., tracheal stenosis). Unfortunately, however, patients with the most severe derangement of function during their acute illness are more likely to have persistent derangement of pulmonary function and have a persistent decrease in health-related quality of life.

FURTHER READING

1. The Acute Respiratory Distress Syndrome Network. Ventilation with lower tidal volumes as compared with traditional tidal volumes for acute lung injury and the acute respiratory distress syndrome. *N Engl J Med.* 2000;342:1301.

   In this randomized trial of "standard" 12 mL/kg tidal volumes compared to lower (6 mL/kg lean body weight, 5.2 mL/kg total body weight) tidal volumes, the use of lower tidal volumes and reduced respiratory system pressures was associated with a reduction in overall mortality from 40% to 30%.

2. The ARDS Definition Task Force. Acute respiratory distress syndrome: the Berlin definition. *JAMA.* 2012;307(23):2526–2533.

   An expert panel convened in 2011 under the auspices of the European Society of Intensive Care Medicine, the American Thoracic Society, and the Society of Critical Care Medicine proposed a definition of ARDS requiring development within 1 week of a known clinical insult, bilateral chest imaging opacities, and with respiratory failure not explained by cardiac failure or fluid overload. The level of injury was further stratified by oxygenation criteria as mild, moderate, or severe. When applied retrospectively the definition appeared to predict mortality and duration of mechanical ventilation.

3. Bachofen M, Weibel ER. Alterations of the gas exchange apparatus in adult respiratory insufficiency associated with septicemia. *Am Rev Respir Dis.* 1977;116:589.

   A classic description of the electron microscopic findings seen at various stages of ARDS. The authors showed that neutrophil infiltration and interstitial edema occurred before endothelial changes were found.

4. Bernard GR, Luce JM, Sprung CL, et al. High-dose corticosteroids in patients with the adult respiratory distress syndrome. *N Engl J Med.* 1987;317:1565.

   Methylprednisolone (30 mg/kg q6h for four doses) was administered in a double-blind, randomized trial to patients with ARDS (defined as refractory hypoxemia and bilateral infiltrates). Patients had received mechanical ventilation for an average of 3 days prior to steroid administration. The authors found no significant difference in mortality or in rates of disease remission or infectious complications.

5. Bernard GR, Artigas A, Brigham KL, et al. The American-European Consensus Conference on ARDS. Definitions, mechanisms, relevant outcomes, and clinical trial coordination. *Am J Respir Crit Care Med.* 1994;149:818.

   The initial consensus conference defining ARDS and acute lung injury, and recommending standards for future usage.

6. Briel M, Meade M, Mercat A, et al. Higher vs lower positive end-expiratory pressure in patients with acute lung injury and acute respiratory distress syndrome: systematic review and meta-analysis. *JAMA*. 2010;303(9):865–873.

   Meta-analysis of 2,299 individual patients in three trials suggested that treatment with higher levels of PEEP was associated with improved survival for patients with ARDS but not those with ALI.

7. Dreyfuss D, Basset G, Soler P, et al. Intermittent positive-pressure hyperventilation with high inflation pressures produces pulmonary microvascular injury in rats. *Am Rev Respir Dis*. 1985;132:880–884.

   Classic study showing that positive pressure ventilation resulted in lung injury in an animal model and demonstrated the protective effect of PEEP in the same model.

8. Gobien RP, Reines HD, Schabel SI. Localized tension pneumothorax: unrecognized form of barotrauma in adult respiratory distress syndrome. *Radiology*. 1982;142:15.

   With severe ARDS, the lung often does not collapse as expected in the presence of a pneumothorax. The radiographic features of pulmonary barotrauma are often subtle.

9. Herridge MS, Tansey CM, Matté A, et al. Functional disability 5 years after acute respiratory distress syndrome. *N Engl J Med*. 2011;364:1293–1304.

   Although pulmonary function returned to normal or near-normal level, exercise limitation, decreased quality of life, and increased use of health care resources persist after survival from ARDS. Younger patients had a greater rate of recovery than older.

10. Lewis JF, Jobe AH. Surfactant and the adult respiratory distress syndrome. *Am Rev Respir Dis*. 1993;147:218.

    A comprehensive review of the current knowledge of the role played by surfactant in the pathophysiology of ARDS (181 references).

11. Meduri GU, Headley AS, Golden E, et al. Effect of prolonged methylprednisolone therapy in unresolving acute respiratory distress syndrome: a randomized controlled trial. *JAMA*. 1998;280:159.

    The administration of methylprednisolone (2 mg/kg/day, n = 16) was compared to placebo (n = 8) in patients with unresolving ARDS. Steroid therapy was associated with improved lung injury score and mortality in a small scale trial.

12. Michael JR, Barton RG, Saffle JR, et al. Inhaled nitric oxide versus conventional therapy: effect on oxygenation in ARDS. *Am J Respir Crit Care Med*. 1998;157:1372.

    Nitric oxide therapy resulted in short-term improvement in PaO_2, but failed to improve mortality in ARDS. Similar results were reported by a European multicenter trial in the same volume.

13. The National Heart, Lung, and Blood Institute ARDS Clinical Trial Network. Higher versus lower positive end-expiratory pressures in patients with the acute respiratory distress syndrome. *N Engl J Med*. 2004;351:327.

    When patients were ventilated with 6 mL/kg tidal volume ventilation, the routine application of higher levels of PEEP did not improve or impair outcomes when compared with lower levels.

14. Needham DM, Colantuoni E, Mendez-Tellez PA, et al. Lung protective mechanical ventilation and two year survival in patients with acute lung injury: prospective cohort study *BMJ*. 2012;344:e2124.

    Among 485 patients with acute lung injury at academic hospitals only 41% had ventilation management adhering to lung-protective strategies. Increased adherence was associated with improvement in mortality.

15. Pepe PE, Hudson LD, Carrico CJ. Early application of positive end-expiratory pressure in patients at risk for the adult respiratory distress syndrome. *N Engl J Med*. 1984;311:281.

    The authors performed a randomized trial of the application of 8 cm H_2O of PEEP for 72 hours to patients at risk for ARDS. There was no reduction in the subsequent development of ARDS.

16. Rubenfeld GD, Caldwell E, Peabody E, et al. Incidence and outcomes of acute lung injury. *N Engl J Med*. 2005;353(16):1685–1693.

    Prospective application of the AECC definitions of ARDS and ALI found an age-adjusted incidence of 86.2 per 100,000 person years and in in-hospital mortality of 38.5%.

17. Spragg RG, Lewis JF, Walmrath HD, et al. Effect of recombinant surfactant protein C-based surfactant on the acute respiratory distress syndrome. *N Engl J Med*. 2004;351:884.

In a randomized blinded study of 448 patients with ARDS, the instillation of a synthetic surfactant containing recombinant surfactant protein C improved hypoxemia during the treatment period, but did not change overall mortality.

18. Tang BM, Craig JC, Eslick GD, et al. Use of corticosteroids in acute lung injury and acute respiratory distress syndrome: a systematic review and meta-analysis. *Crit Care Med.* 2009;37:1594–1603.

    Meta-analysis of four randomized and five cohort studies of steroid use in ALI and ARDS. While the authors concluded that low dose (0.5 to 2.5 mg/kg/day) of methylprednisolone or equivalent was associated with reduction in mortality, the studies varied significantly in the initiation and duration of corticosteroid use.

19. Tsuno K, Miura K, Takeya M, et al. Histopathologic pulmonary changes from mechanical ventilation at high peak airway pressures. *Am Rev Respir Dis.* 1991;143:1115.

    A description of the histologic and gas exchange abnormalities found in sheep subjected to positive pressure ventilation with peak airway pressure of 30 cm H₂O for 24 to 96 hours.

Thromboembolic Disease: Epidemiology, Natural History, and Diagnosis

Timothy A. Morris

Venous thromboembolism (VTE) can be entirely preventable or treatable. Yet, it is a persistent and prevalent cause of significant morbidity and mortality in the United States and is responsible for an estimated 50,000 deaths and 500,000 nonfatal episodes each year. Despite important diagnostic and therapeutic developments, medical science is only scratching the surface at understanding VTE, and clinical strategies have only partially impacted disability and death following VTE.

Venous thromboembolism, by definition, originates in systemic venous thrombosis, and is pathologically distinct from arterial thrombosis. Conditions that favor thrombosis fall into three categories (as predicted by Virchow over a century ago): (1) venous stasis, (2) injury to the venous intima, and (3) alterations in the coagulation–fibrinolytic system. The potential role of all three factors has been demonstrated in a variety of situations. Venous stasis occurs during bed rest and is associated with deep venous thrombosis (DVT); using intermittent compression stockings to restore venous flow reduces the risk for DVT. Injury to the venous wall is the most likely mechanism of the large number of lower extremity DVTs observed in proximity to sites of trauma and major orthopedic surgery. Coagulation abnormalities that occur alone or in concert with other conditions can promote clinical venous thrombosis. For example, there is an increased risk for VTE associated with mutations in factor V (factor V_Lieden) and in the untranslated region of the gene encoding prothrombin (although the procoagulant mechanism of the later mutation is still under investigation). Other less prevalent, but probably more potent, "thrombophilias" include deficiencies of antithrombin III, protein C, and protein S; aberrations in the thrombolytic system; and the presence of the doubly misnamed "lupus anticoagulant." Clinical conditions that involve combinations of these fundamental risk factors are associated with a higher risk of thrombosis.

Many large studies have identified the major risk factors for DVT of the lower extremities. These include: (1) surgery involving general anesthesia for more than 30 minutes, (2) injury or surgery involving the lower extremities or pelvis, (3) congestive heart failure, (4) prolonged immobility from any cause, and (5) pregnancy, particularly during the postpartum period. Other conditions that increase risk are cancer, obesity, advancing age, varicose veins, a prior episode of DVT, use of estrogen-containing compounds, and dehydration. Predictably, these risk factors are cumulative.

The deep veins of the lower extremities are the dominant source of clinically significant pulmonary emboli—an important epidemiologic, diagnostic, and therapeutic consideration. Less commonly, thrombi can arise in superficial veins or in prostatic, uterine, renal, and other veins. They also can occur in the right cardiac chambers in patients with right ventricular failure. However, more than 95% of clinically significant pulmonary emboli arise from DVT in the lower extremities (whether or not such DVT is clinically detectable).

The events initiating venous thrombosis are not fully understood. The valves of the lower extremity veins, especially in the calves, are common sites for the initial event. The development of a small nidus leads to the elaboration of clot-potentiating materials that trigger prolongation of the thrombus with red blood cells (RBCs), fibrin and, to a lesser degree, platelets. Once formed, the thrombus grows by accumulating additional RBC, fibrin, and platelet "layers," seen pathologically as the lines of Zahn.

Even as thrombosis is occurring, the process of resolution is beginning. The thrombi resolve by one or both of two mechanisms: fibrinolysis and organization. *Fibrinolysis* refers to actual dissolution of the thrombus by plasma enzymes. It is a relatively rapid process, proceeding over a period of hours to several days. If fibrinolysis is not totally successful, organization finishes the job of resolution. Reparative cells infiltrate the residual thrombus and replace the "thrombotic components" with connective tissue. The fibrotic residuum is then incorporated into the venous wall and re-endothelialized. Organization usually thickens the venous wall, which may provide loci for further thrombus formation. The thickening may also incorporate one or more venous valves, rendering them incompetent. Whatever the fate of a given thrombus, available data indicate that the sequence of resolution is complete within 7 to 10 days. By that time, the initial thrombus is gone or has been incorporated into the venous wall. In the latter case, the pathology is more accurately termed a *venous scar* than an *old clot*.

At any time during the process of resolution, pulmonary embolism (PE) can occur. It is important to recognize that embolism is not a new disorder; it is a serious complication of DVT. Because thrombi are most friable early in their development, embolic risk is highest during the first few days after thrombus formation. Thereafter, dissolution or organization sharply limits embolic risk (as long as no new thrombotic material has been laid down in the interval).

When emboli arise and lodge in one or more pulmonary arteries, hemodynamic and respiratory consequences occur. The hemodynamic consequences include a decrease in the available cross-sectional area of the pulmonary arterial system through both mechanical obstruction and release of vasoconstrictive thrombus metabolites directly into the vascular bed. The pulmonary vascular resistance rises, causing an increased pulmonary arterial pressure, and therefore an increased right ventricular workload. If these consequences are severe, the right ventricle may not tolerate the workload and the cardiac output will fall. Respiratory consequences include: (1) altered ventilation–perfusion relationships, which (combined with a fall in cardiac output and resulting lowered venous oxygen concentration) may lead to arterial hypoxemia, (2) development of one or more zones of alveolar dead space (zones that are ventilated but not perfused), (3) transient pneumoconstriction of these same zones, (4) hyperventilation (the reasons for which are debated), and (5) loss of surfactant in the underperfused zones. The first four events occur immediately; the fifth requires approximately 24 hours of total occlusion before alveolar surfactant is depleted. The two major consequences of surfactant depletion are atelectasis and an increase in permeability of the alveolar–capillary membrane, causing further problems with gas exchange.

Pulmonary infarction is a rare consequence of embolism; fewer than 10% of emboli lead to infarction. Therefore, embolism is by no means synonymous with infarction.

An important clinical question concerns the hemodynamic deterioration observed in some patients with PE in the first few days after embolization. Although PE can be immediately fatal, a large number of patients who eventually succumb, do so one or more days after presentation. It stands to reason that these "late fatalities" are caused by either progressively deteriorating myocardial fatigue (right ventricular infarction or other myocyte injury) or by increases in workload because of factors such as recurrent emboli, embolus propagation, or further release of vasoactive mediators from the embolus.

The phenomenon of embolic fragments entrapped in the right atrium and ventricle has been recognized in experimental embolism for some time; as cardiac echocardiography is more extensively utilized, this phenomenon has become more widely recognized in human disease as well. The clinical significance of these sessile cardiac thrombi has not been studied in a controlled fashion. However, it is likely that these thrombi may embolize; therefore, larger cardiac thrombi may warrant emergent surgical removal, especially in the presence of preexisting hemodynamic compromise.

Beyond these acute events, emboli (like venous thrombi) tend to resolve if prevented from propagating by anticoagulants. Precise data on the speed of resolution in humans are not available. The earliest reported time of total embolic resolution is about 2 days; most resolve substantially or completely within a few weeks. A very small number fail to dissolve, for unknown reasons, and form permanent vascular scars within the pulmonary arteries, causing chronic thromboembolic pulmonary hypertension (see Chapter 67).

Signs and symptoms of DVT are inconsistent and are essentially manifestations of its two consequences: inflammation of the venous wall and venous obstruction. The former may lead to local pain, tenderness (tenderness along the vessel wall is particularly suggestive), redness, and warmth; the latter may lead to edema in the leg zones drained by the vein(s) involved. Unfortunately, studies have demonstrated that fewer than half of patients with DVT have signs or symptoms at all and few have sufficient inflammation or edema to allow a clinical diagnosis to be made. Therefore, reliable and early detection requires that laboratory tests be used to supplement history and physical examination.

Three well-validated diagnostic procedures are generally available to diagnose and follow the course of DVT: compression ultrasound, impedance plethysmography, and contrast venography. Radiolabeled fibrinogen, a previously invaluable investigative tool for detecting thrombus presence and propagation, is no longer available. Other tests such as serologic markers of thrombosis/thrombolysis, magnetic resonance imaging (MRI) and, radiolabeled thrombus-specific agents are under development, but have not been completely validated for clinical use.

Compression ultrasonography involves the use of ultrasound visualization and Doppler analysis to distinguish between solid (thrombus) and fluid (blood) contents of the proximal deep veins of the leg. Failure to compress visualized veins suggests that at least part of the lumen is filled with solid material and is the only reliable criterion for DVT diagnosis. Findings such as "echogenic densities" or Doppler blood flow velocity measurements have not proved reliable in clinical studies and should not be used to make the diagnosis. The technique is not reliable in detecting thrombi limited to the calf or iliac veins. In addition, the vessel wall thickening from prior DVTs causes wall thickening in nearly half of the cases, which can cause non-compressibility on ultrasound. Even the most rigorously controlled clinical trials, using complex algorithms to compare old and new studies side by side, distinguished new thrombi from old scars only with great difficulty. In its current state, compression ultrasonography should not be used to diagnose recurrent DVT at the site of prior thrombosis.

Impedance plethysmography (IPG), which measures the rate of venous drainage from the leg, is positive when there is substantial obstruction to venous outflow at any point from the popliteal vein to the inferior vena cava. It is sensitive to above-the-knee thrombi, especially when unilaterally positive. The test has been well-validated in clinical studies and is a relatively inexpensive, standardized method to detect DVT. A great deal of work has been performed comparing the accuracy of IPG to that of compression ultrasound. As a group, these studies show compression ultrasound to be more accurate, although it is more expensive and highly operator-dependent. Unlike ultrasound, IPG has the benefit of returning to normal within weeks of an acute DVT, making it useful for diagnosing DVT recurrence. It should be noted that neither of these noninvasive tests reliably detects calf thrombi or asymptomatic proximal vein thrombi.

Contrast venography is an invasive test in which radiopaque contrast is injected into the leg veins, yielding a very complete image of leg DVTs on radiographs, even in the calves. However, it has substantial drawbacks, including expense and discomfort. At the present time, contrast venography is usually reserved for special situations, such as patients suspected of having recurrent DVT, those with equivocal results on IPG or ultrasound testing, or in whom those tests cannot be done (e.g., those with extensive lower extremity trauma or casts).

Among the promising newer techniques for DVT diagnosis are serologic tests of thrombosis (fibrinopeptide A and B, prothrombin fragment F1.2, thrombin–antithrombin complexes, and soluble fibrin monomer) and/or thrombolysis (D-dimer). A potential advantage of these blood tests is that their results may correlate with the presence of both DVT and PE. The D-dimer assay is the only one that has been extensively evaluated clinically; however, it suffers from two drawbacks. The first is practical; only carefully performed, precise methods to measure D-dimers can distinguish normal controls from VTE patients, who may have only modestly elevated plasma levels. Furthermore, even when D-dimers are measured using sophisticated enzyme-linked immunoassays, the plasma elevations are so common in medical illnesses that relatively few hospitalized patients have normal values for this assay.

MRI has been explored as a diagnostic tool for DVT. The results of initial studies performed by investigators at specialized centers have been encouraging and suggest that the technique can be used to diagnose DVT and PE, and perhaps even distinguish new DVTs from old venous scars. These reports, however, are preliminary and must be interpreted with caution. Large trials comparing MRI results to standard venography have not been performed. Outcome studies have not verified the safety of managing patients based on MRI results. Another consideration is that the interpretative performance of the expert readers who are pioneering this new technology may not be easily matched in general practice.

Radiolabeled thrombus-specific agents, such as antibodies targeted at components of fibrin and platelets, are under investigation. When these agents are systemically injected, they bind to acute thrombi and localize them as "hot spots" on nuclear medicine scans. Like MRI, these scans have the potential for diagnosing both PE and DVT simultaneously. Furthermore, because they are specific for the biochemical components of acute thrombi, they do not bind to venous scars and may distinguish them from recurrent DVTs. Finally, agents specific for propagating thrombi may foster unique insights about the ability of different anticoagulant drugs to "extinguish" active clotting.

As is true for DVT, clinical data are not sufficient to confirm or exclude the diagnosis of PE. This fact notwithstanding, the recognition of signs and symptoms suggestive of PE is the single most important factor in preventing death from this disease. This point is highlighted by the rather chilling observation that, in the vast majority of patients who die with PE, the condition was not diagnosed or even suspected ante mortem. Furthermore, although few patients who succumb to pulmonary emboli manifest all of the "textbook" clinical clues, almost all manifested at least one of them. The clinical impact of sophisticated diagnostic technology in reducing fatality from PE pales in comparison to the role of the astute clinician who maintains a low threshold for suspicion.

Signs and symptoms (even nonspecific ones) unexplained by other pathologies should raise the possibility of PE and trigger a workup. Dyspnea of sudden onset is a nonspecific, but common symptom. Pleuritic chest pain and hemoptysis, which indicate infarction, occur in a minority of patients. Other individual symptoms, such as syncope and substernal chest pain, are even less common and suggest myocardial damage or strain. In addition, specific physical findings are usually few. Tachycardia of variable duration is also nonspecific, but observed in the majority of patients. Other cardiac findings (e.g., increased pulmonic valve closure sound, right ventricular S3, right ventricular tap) can be subtle and typically occur only in the (fortunately) rare cases of massive embolism. Examination of the lungs rarely discloses a pleural friction rub or evidence of pleural effusion (because these require infarction). Scattered rales or focal wheezing may be heard but are hardly diagnostic.

Clinical clues are crucial for suggesting the diagnosis of PE, but as is true for DVT, objective testing is necessary to confirm or exclude it. Unfortunately, "routine" tests cannot offer such confirmation. The arterial Po_2 is variable and a low value is commonly observed in other respiratory disorders. The chest x-ray is most often either normal or discloses nonspecific findings such as small pleural effusions. The ECG commonly shows only sinus tachycardia. Although such tests may be highly suggestive and are useful in ruling out other diagnoses (e.g., pneumothorax, myocardial infarction), a definitive diagnosis can be arrived at only through a limited number of specific tests.

The currently available diagnostic techniques include: (1) ventilation and perfusion scinti-photography, (2) computer-assisted tomography (computed tomographic [CT] scanning and MRI) and DVT studies, and (3) pulmonary angiography. All have potential roles in the workup of a potential PE. Each test has, in turn, been declared the "optimal study"; however, they all have specific values and limitations. It is better to individualize the choice and interpretation of these complimentary imaging studies to the particular clinical situation. Unfortunately, blood tests are not yet capable of diagnosing PE in clinical practice.

The pulmonary perfusion scan is highly sensitive, but nonspecific and is recommended as the first test for most patients suspected of PE. A negative scan is invaluable because it excludes the diagnosis as reliably as a pulmonary angiogram; however, a positive scan may be caused by many disorders other than embolism. Combining perfusion lung scans with ventilation scans and/or chest x-rays enhances the specificity of the procedure. There is some evidence to suggest that the accuracy of scintigraphic ventilation/perfusion (V/Q) scans can be enhanced when the patients are scanned with single photon emission computerized tomography (SPECT), rather than with planar scans. Embolism can also be diagnosed when there are segmental or larger perfusion defects in the presence of a clear chest x-ray (indicating normally ventilated lungs). Defects anatomically "matched" by radiographic opacities or ventilation defects should be regarded as nondiagnostic and should prompt further workup. Smaller perfusion defects occur less commonly with PE, but these scan findings, regardless of ventilation results, should be regarded as nondiagnostic.

Cross-sectional tomographic imaging of the thorax with CT or, less commonly, MRI, is a popular diagnostic tool for PE. Both CT and MRI use intravascular contrast to fill the lumen of the pulmonary arteries. (Unfortunately, the initial optimism that non-contrast MR imaging would distinguish thromboemboli based on their specific signal characteristics did not come to fruition.) Currently, CT scanning has the advantages over MRI of higher special resolution, wider availability, and larger clinical series demonstrating its value. Both technologies are constantly advancing and the diagnostic value of each test is likely to improve. In both types of scans, emboli are detected as focal defects in pulmonary artery filling.

There is a great deal of evidence that CT, when performed and interpreted correctly, is capable of identifying emboli in the segmental or larger pulmonary arteries. However, certain areas, such as the hila, are prone to false positives. Reading emboli in these areas should be done with special care. Perhaps more importantly, CT scans have variable accuracy in imaging emboli in subsegmental pulmonary arteries. There are insufficient data to support the notion that thromboembolic disease invisible to thoracic tomography does not require treatment. At the present time, a negative thoracic CT scan I (or MRI) does not necessarily indicate that emboli are absent. In some cases, such as where severely limited cardiopulmonary reserve may make undetected emboli (or recurrent emboli) particularly dangerous, nondiagnostic CT scans should be followed up with further testing.

If the diagnosis of PE is in doubt after noninvasive testing, searching for DVT is a sensible strategy. Because the two diagnoses are manifestations of the same disease, the treatments are largely the same. The yield of noninvasive testing for DVT is low (<10%) in PE suspects without leg symptoms. However, the potential benefits of making the diagnosis without further thoracic imaging justifies the performance of noninvasive leg testing, even in patients without leg symptoms.

If other tests fail to confirm or refute the suspicion of PE, angiography may be indicated. Although it is used less commonly, pulmonary angiography is a valuable tool because it can demonstrate the embolus itself, even in subsegmental pulmonary arteries. The procedure is invasive, but can be performed with little risk in most situations, if special care is exercised. The most common serious complications arise from the use of contrast dye: the same amount of contrast dye used for helical CT scanning. The decision to perform angiography in patients with equivocal results from noninvasive studies must be based on the specific clinical situation.

New procedures to diagnose PE are generally the same as those discussed for DVT, including the use of radiolabeled monoclonal antibodies directed against other thromboembolic components and MRI. These agents are still under investigation and their diagnostic value remains to be defined.

Regardless of the imaging techniques employed, there are circumstances when the clinician must make the decision to withhold treatment or to treat on the basis of nondiagnostic test results, or to continue the work-up. The decision should be guided by careful consideration of the consequences of an incorrect choice: unnecessary long-term anticoagulation or, conversely, complications of untreated thromboembolism. The fundamental rule is that the greater the risk involved in making a therapeutic decision, the higher the degree of diagnostic certainty required.

FURTHER READING

1. Bell WR, Simon TL, DeMets DL. The clinical features of submassive and massive pulmonary emboli. *Am J Med.* 1997;62:355.

   A breakdown of the clinical features of the participants in the urokinase–streptokinase trials. Pleuritic chest pain and hemoptysis were more common in submassive than in massive emboli.

2. Dalen J, Mathur VS, Evans H, et al. Pulmonary angiography in experimental pulmonary embolism. *Am Heart J.* 1966;72:509.

   An excellent review of criteria to be used in angiographic diagnosis of PE.

3. De Nardo G, Goodwin DA, Ravasini R, et al. The ventilatory lung scan in the diagnosis of pulmonary embolism. *N Engl J Med.* 1970;282:1334.

   A classic study indicating the enhanced diagnostic specificity achieved by combining ventilation with perfusion scanning in patients with PE.

4. Heijboer H, Beuller HR, Lensing AW, et al. A comparison of real time compression ultrasonography with impedance plethysmography for the diagnosis of deep-vein thrombosis in symptomatic outpatients. *N Engl J Med.* 1993;329:1365–1369. See comments.

   Ultrasound had a slightly higher sensitivity and specificity for symptomatic proximal DVT than did IPG. However, both of their sensitivities depend on the serial performance of the tests when the first result is negative. Also, the IPG in this trial performed much worse than it had in a previous clinical trial on a similar patient population performed by the same investigators.

5. Hull R, Hirsh J, Carter CJ, et al. Pulmonary angiography, ventilation lung scanning, and venography for clinically suspected pulmonary embolism in the abnormal perfusion scan. *Ann Intern Med.* 1983;98:891.

   A prospective study showing that emboli are present in 86% of patients with segmental or larger Q defects, normal ventilation, and a clear chest X-ray. Other scan patterns are much less commonly associated with emboli; venous studies are important in the initial evaluation.

6. The PIOPED Investigators. The value of the ventilation/perfusion scan in acute pulmonary embolism. *JAMA.* 1990;263:2753.

   A complex scheme for interpreting lung scans was developed by the teams of investigators involved in this study.

7. Hull RD, Raskob GE. Low-probability lung scan findings: a need for change. *Ann Intern Med.* 1991;114:142.

   This report indicates that "low probability" scan interpretations are best deleted from the scan-reporting vocabulary because they confuse rather than clarify.

8. Karwinski ES. Comparison of clinical and postmortem diagnosis of pulmonary embolism. *J Clin Pathol.* 1989;42:135–139.

   A university hospital in Norway with a 75% to 80% autopsy rate (!) did a retrospective analysis of 21,529 cases. In patients who died from PE, the diagnosis was made before death in only 10% to 20% of cases. In addition, the rates of ante mortem diagnosis got worse over the 20-year span of the study.

9. Kearon C, Julian JA, Newman TE, et al. Noninvasive diagnosis of deep venous thrombosis. McMaster Diagnostic Imaging Practice Guidelines Initiative. *Ann Intern Med.* 1998;128:663–677. See comments.

   A well-written review of previous clinical studies. Although both tests are accurate enough to use as management tools, CUS has a slightly higher accuracy than IPG. However, either test can be in error and should be confirmed with venography if the results are discordant with clinical suspicion.

10. Kakkar V, Howe CT, Flanc C, et al. Natural history of post-operative deep vein thrombosis. *Lancet.* 1969;2:230.

   One of the early studies with radiolabeled fibrinogen, indicating that clinical detection of DVT is unreliable.

11. Kipper MS, Moser KM, Kortman KE, et al. Long-term follow-up of patients with suspected pulmonary embolism and a normal lung scan. *Chest.* 1982;82:411.

   Study indicating that a normal perfusion scan has the same value as a normal pulmonary angiogram in ruling out embolism (and the need for anticoagulant therapy).

12. Moser KM, Fedullo PF. Venous thromboembolism. Three simple decisions (Part 1). *Chest.* 1983;83(1):117–21.

13. Moser KM, Fedullo PF. Venous thromboembolism. Three simple decisions (Part 2). *Chest.* 1983;83(2):256–60.

14. Moser KM, Guisan M, Bartimmo EE, et al. In vivo and postmortem dissolution rates of pulmonary emboli and venous thrombi in the dog. *Circulation.* 1973;48:170.

   A study that demonstrates the speed with which fresh venous thrombi and pulmonary emboli can resolve in the dog.

15. Quinn PA, Thompson BT, Terrin ML, et al. A prospective investigation of pulmonary embolism in women and men. *JAMA.* 1992;268:1689.

   Women in the PIOPED study had a somewhat lower frequency of embolism than men but had the same risk factors—except that those on oral contraceptives had a higher postsurgical risk.

16. Stein PD, Henry JW. Prevalence of acute pulmonary embolism among patients in a general hospital and at autopsy. *Chest.* 1995;108:978–981.

   Even during a time when the investigators were recruiting patients for a multicenter trial for PE diagnosis (the PIOPED study), 70% of patients who died with PE had the disease unsuspected premortem.

17. Hoellerich VL, Wigton RS. Diagnosing pulmonary embolism using clinical findings. *Arch Intern Med.* 1986;146:1699.

   The authors indicate that a battery of 92 clinical items, including lung scans, disclosed no one variable of significant power in predicting the diagnosis of embolism by angiography. However, a battery of eight items (including the lung scan) had reasonable diagnostic power.

18. Hull RD, Raskob GE, Carter CJ, et al. Pulmonary embolism in outpatients with pleuritic chest pain. *Arch Intern Med.* 1988;148:838.

   Pulmonary embolism was present in only 21% of patients presenting in an emergency room with pleuritic chest pain. Clinical variables were not very sensitive (85%) or specific (36%). They conclude that objective tests (scan, angiogram) were necessary for diagnosis.

19. Huisman MV, Büller HR, ten Cate JW, et al. Serial impedance plethysmography for suspected deep venous thrombosis in outpatients. *N Engl J Med.* 1986;314:823.

   Careful study demonstrating excellent outcomes in outpatients with suspected venous thrombosis who had negative serial IPG tests and were not treated.

20. Huisman MV, Büller HR, ten Cate JW. Utility of impedance plethysmography in the diagnosis of recurrent deep-vein thrombosis. *Arch Intern Med.* 1988;148:881.

   Initially positive IPGs in patients with acute above-knee DVT return to normal in 95% over 12 months. Serial testing at 3-month intervals may allow detection of recurrence if an IPG that has returned to normal again becomes positive.

21. Davidson BI, Elliott CG, Lensing AW. Low accuracy of color Doppler ultrasound in the detection of proximal leg vein thrombosis in asymptomatic high-risk patients. *Ann Intern Med.* 1992;117:735.

   Color Doppler ultrasound was found to be insensitive to proximal DVT in asymptomatic high-risk patients.

22. Lensing AW, Prandoni P, Brandjes D, et al. Detection of deep vein thrombosis by real-time B-mode ultrasonography. *N Engl J Med.* 1989;320:342.

   A careful study of this technique. Using strict diagnostic criteria (ability to compress popliteal and femoral veins), ultrasound had same diagnostic value as IPG in symptomatic patients. Echogenicity was not a useful criterion; calf thrombi were poorly detected. Serial studies, as with IPG, were necessary to rule out thrombus extension.

A careful study of this technique. Diagnostic criteria need to be refined and other populations require acute and long-term study before the technique can be fully validated. Currently, as with IPG, detection of calf-limited thrombosis is poor (36%).

23. Anderson DR, Lensing AW, Wells PS, et al. Limitations of impedance plethysmography in diagnosis of clinically-suspected deep-vein thrombosis. *Ann Intern Med.* 1993;118:25.

    Questions the sensitivity and specificity of IPG versus ultrasound. The following two references point out serious methodologic problems with this study that place its conclusions in question.

24. Raskob GE. Impedance plethysmography and DVT diagnosis [letter to editor]. *Ann Intern Med.* 1993;119:247.

25. Wheeler HB, Anderson FA Jr. Impedance plethysmography and DVT diagnosis [letter to editor]. *Ann Intern Med.* 1993;119:246.

26. Rubinstein I, Murray D, Hoffstein V. Fatal pulmonary emboli in hospitalized patients. *Arch Intern Med.* 1988;148:1425.

    The authors conclude from this autopsy study that embolism is still underdiagnosed. Only 31% of this series with embolism at autopsy had the diagnosis suspected prior to death.

27. Pond GD, Ovitt TW, Capp MP. Comparison of conventional pulmonary angiography with intravenous digital subtraction angiography for pulmonary embolic disease. *Radiology.* 1983;147:345.

    Motion limits diagnostic sensitivity of the technique in embolism beyond the main pulmonary arteries, but its application in selected patients is useful. Technologic advances may improve the results further.

28. Prandoni P, Lensing AWA, Büller HR, et al. Deep vein thrombosis and the incidence of subsequent symptomatic cancer. *N Engl J Med.* 1992;327:1128.

    An old question, much debated, is revisited. These authors conclude that patients with idiopathic DVT, especially those with recurrences, have an increased incidence of cancer during long-term follow-up (7.6% in idiopathic DVT versus 1.9% in those with clear risk factors). A randomized trial is suggested to determine whether the cost and discomfort of excluding cancer in such patients are worthwhile.

29. Ginsberg JS, Liang MH, Newcomer L, et al. Anticardiolipin antibodies and the risk for ischemic stroke and venous thrombosis. *Ann Intern Med.* 1992;117:997.

    Anticardiolipin antibodies are a definite risk factor for venous thrombosis.

30. Bounameaux H, Schneider PA, Reber G, et al. Measurement of plasma D-dimer for the diagnosis of deep venous thrombosis. *Am J Clin Pathol.* 1989;91:82.

31. Heijboer H, Ginsberg JS, Büller HR, et al. The use of the D-dimer test in combination with non-invasive testing versus serial non-invasive testing alone for the diagnosis of deep vein thrombosis. *Thromb Haemost.* 1992;67:510.

32. Bounameaux H, Cirafici P, de Moerloose P, et al. Measurement of D-dimer in plasma as diagnostic aid in suspected pulmonary embolism. *Lancet.* 1991;337:196.

    The previous three references discuss the potential value of D-dimer assays in diagnosis of DVT and PE. The value of this assay to "rule out" these diagnoses remains unsettled.

33. Morris TA, Marsh JJ, Chiles PG, et al. Single photon emission computed tomography of pulmonary emboli and venous thrombi using anti–D-dimer. *Am J Respir Crit Care Med.* 2004;169:987–993.

    New approach to the diagnosis of VTE. Further study is needed to determine the value of these and similar "thrombus-targeted" methods.

Thromboembolic Disease: Prophylaxis

Timothy M. Fernandes and Timothy A. Morris

The most effective means to reduce the morbidity and mortality from venous thromboembolism (VTE) is by preventing the occurrence in the first place. The risk for VTE is especially high in patients hospitalized for medical illness with as many as 14.9% of patients having sonographic evidence of deep veins thrombosis (DVT) within 2 weeks of admission. When performed properly, the risks of VTE prophylaxis are small and are outweighed by a reduction in VTE. However, the decision regarding whether to offer pharmacologic prophylaxis must be made on a patient-to-patient basis, weighing the individualized risks of both bleeding and thrombosis. When the benefits favor provision of pharmacologic prophylaxis, the physician has several options and can be guided by costs and ease of reversibility.

RISK ASSESSMENT

The risk for hospital-acquired VTE varies among patients; several risk assessment models exist to help identify those at highest risk. While none of these risk assessment models have been prospectively validated, there are several important known factors that increase the risk of VTE: increasing age, active malignancy, and prior VTE are almost universally included in available risk assessment models. Also, the patient's mobility and predicted length of stay should be taken into account. For example, prophylaxis should be seriously considered for patients over 40 years of age who are admitted with expected periods of bed rest or immobilization for greater than 3 days. All patients admitted to the intensive care unit (ICU) are at high risk for VTE and more aggressive prophylaxis should be considered in this group.

The risk of bleeding must also be considered in the decision to provide thromboprophylaxis. Unfortunately, there are few data to guide this assessment directly. Only one risk model, developed using the IMPROVE registry but never externally validated, has been published. While some of the factors that increase bleeding risk are obvious, such as active gastroduodenal ulcer, hepatic failure, or thrombocytopenia, many of the same risk factors that predispose to thrombosis also predispose to bleeding. These include increasing age, ICU admission, and active cancer.

Ultimately, the risk factors for both thrombosis and bleeding are cumulative and the total clinical picture should determine whether prophylaxis is used and the aggressiveness of the methods to be employed. Patients who are deemed to be at high risk of developing VTE and low risk for bleeding, such as those undergoing extensive lower extremity orthopedic surgeries, require aggressive mechanical as well as moderate-dose anticoagulant prophylaxis. Patients at low risk of VTE (e.g., young patients admitted for short stays and who are not immobilized) may not require either mechanical or pharmacologic prophylaxis. In between these two groups lies a spectrum of patients in whom the proper course of action is less clear. The clinician's best judgment and the patient's personal preferences must be employed to guide this decision.

NATURAL HISTORY OF VTE

Strategies to prevent VTE should address the mechanisms by which venous thrombi are formed and progress to clinically significant disease. The basic science underlying the pathogenesis and natural history of VTE is only partially understood, a fact that is reflected in our inability to completely prevent this disease. Hospitalization appears to affect all three aspects of Virchow Triad: stasis due to immobility, endothelial injury related to the reason for hospitalization, and hypercoagulability related to comorbid conditions such as cancer. In addition, clinical studies to evaluate prophylactic methods suffer from an incomplete understanding of how best to define and detect "clinically significant VTE." Nevertheless, the prophylactic methods developed and validated have had a tremendous impact on the incidence of this disease.

When considering prophylaxis, DVT and pulmonary embolism (PE) should be considered as different manifestations of VTE, rather than as separate disorders. The vast majority (>95%) of clinically significant pulmonary emboli arise from deep veins of the lower extremities. Thus the prevention of PE, for the most part, is really the prevention of lower extremity DVT.

Substantial data suggest that only lower extremity DVTs extending into the proximal deep veins (popliteal and above) cause clinically apparent emboli; thrombi that remain confined to calf veins pose no significant embolic risk. It is not known whether this observation reflects the fact that thrombi restricted to the calf veins do not embolize or that such emboli are so small that clinical disease does not result, although the latter is more likely. Whatever the case, it is now evident that the key to preventing PE is the prevention of lower extremity DVT or, failing this, prevention of the extension of calf vein thrombosis into the more proximal venous system.

PHARMACOLOGIC PROPHYLAXIS

The weight of available evidence favors providing some form of pharmacologic prophylaxis in the vast majority of hospitalized medical patients. With anticoagulation, the risk of both DVT and nonfatal PE are reduced by about half. Several anticoagulation options have been validated in prospective randomized clinical trials for the prevention of VTE in hospitalized medical patients. These options range from the inexpensive yet effective unfractionated heparin (UFH) to the comparably effective yet tremendously expensive rivaroxaban. The decision as to which of the myriad of available options to provide may be influenced by cost, the local formulary, and ease of reversibility.

Of all the available options, subcutaneous UFH has been studied the most widely and has the most clinical experience behind it. Doses of 5,000 to 7,500 U subcutaneously every 8 to 12 hours have proved safe and effective in preventing VTE in most populations. Direct comparisons have not demonstrated any significant difference in VTE prevention or bleeding between t.i.d. and b.i.d. dosing. Substantial experience suggests that bleeding risk is low with this regimen, even in surgical populations. The major advantages of UFH are that the dose is unaffected by renal function and it can easily be reversed in cases of unanticipated bleeding.

Low-molecular-weight heparins (LMWHs), a heterogeneous group of drugs derived by partial depolymerization of heparin, present another option for prophylaxis. The two LMWHs in most widespread use in the United States are enoxaparin and dalteparin. Like UFH, both of these LMWHs are administered subcutaneously for DVT prophylaxis. They possess certain theoretical advantages over UFH, such as a reduced incidence of laboratory demonstrated heparin-induced thrombocytopenia (HIT) during routine use. Two large meta-analyses compared UFH to LMWH for VTE prevention and demonstrated no significant difference in VTE prevention between the two; however, one analysis did show a small reduction in bleeding complications with LMWH. A recent, large randomized controlled trial in critically ill patients in Australia failed to show any differences between dalteparin and UFH in terms of both VTE prevention and bleeding complications, although there was a trend toward less HIT with dalteparin. The typical dose of dalteparin is 5,000 IU subcutaneously daily, while enoxaparin can be administered subcutaneously, dosed either 30 mg twice daily or 40 mg daily. One distinct difference between UFH and LMWH is that caution must be taken when using LMWH in patients with renal failure; a lower dose of enoxaparin, 30 mg/day, should be used if the GFR is less than 30 mL/minute.

Fondaparinux is the first entirely synthetic anticoagulant whose structure is based on the active site of heparin and LMWH. The mechanism of action is similar to heparin-based anticoagulants. The data for fondaparinux for VTE prophylaxis in medical patients are based on comparisons with placebo only. Clinical trials have not been reported comparing fondaparinux's safety and efficacy to UFH or LMWHs in a wide range of clinical situations. After orthopedic and general surgery procedures, it appears that fondaparinux, 2.5 mg administered subcutaneously every 24 hours, is comparable to the LMWHs for prophylaxis.

Warfarin is an alternative, effective drug for prophylaxis in high-risk patients such as after orthopedic surgery or traumas. Vitamin K antagonists such as warfarin are not recommended for VTE prophylaxis in hospitalized medical patients. For orthopedic surgery, one approach is to begin prior to surgery with low doses (1–2 mg/day), then escalate to a therapeutic range after surgery. Another is to begin warfarin only after surgery, finally achieving the desired prothrombin range (International Normalized Ratio [INR]: 2.0–3.0) after several days.

Several synthetic oral anticoagulants have recently become available. These include rivaroxaban (a specific inhibitor of activated factor X), dabigatran (a direct thrombin inhibitor active against both free and clot-bound thrombin) and apixaban (also a specific inhibitor of activated factor X). These agents have all shown promise in randomized controlled trials compared against enoxaparin in patients undergoing hip or knee surgery. They appear to be at least non-inferior to enoxaparin in this specific population of orthopedic patients in terms of prevention of VTE, with a small but significant trend toward lower associated bleeding risk. However, there are two major disadvantages to the use of these newer medications. First, there are no specific antidotes if clinically relevant bleeding develops. This is a major limitation to the utility of these drugs for VTE prophylaxis, especially in hospitalized medical patients whose risk of bleeding may be more unpredictable than in orthopedic patients. Second, the increased cost of these newer agents compared to UFH and the LMWHs for minimal incremental benefit must be considered. Cost-effectiveness studies may clarify the latter concern.

Among other options, aspirin, dipyridamole, sulfinpyrazone, and other antiplatelet drugs have not been shown to be useful for prophylaxis of venous thrombosis. Reports regarding the value of intravenous infusion of low-molecular-weight dextran are mixed, placing this polymer in the category of "probably effective." Dextran does carry the potential risk of volume overload and allergic reactions.

MECHANICAL PROPHYLAXIS

In patients who are at high risk for VTE, but in whom anticoagulation is contraindicated, there are several forms of mechanical prophylaxis that can be considered. These include compression stockings, sequential compression devices, and inferior vena cava filter placement. While none of these have been proven to be as effective as the pharmacologic agents, they do reduce the risk of VTE, specifically PE, without increased risk of bleeding.

Graded compression stockings can be used in all settings to reduce the risk of proximal DVT. There are two lengths of stockings available: knee-high and thigh-high. In the CLOTS trial, knee-high stockings were compared with thigh-high stockings in patients with stroke. There was an increased incidence of proximal DVT in the knee-high stockings compared to that in the thigh-high stockings; however, an increase in mild skin breakdown was seen in the thigh-high group. For this reason, we favor use of the thigh-high stockings only in patients who cannot be anticoagulated and in whom we are able to ensure the stockings are applied properly. The nursing staff should be trained in proper application of the stockings and should also assess for skin breakdown on a daily basis. The added value of compression stockings in patients receiving pharmacologic prophylaxis is unknown and exposes the patient to increased risk of skin breakdown.

Intermittent pneumatic compressive devices prevent venous stasis by inflating a cuff for several seconds each minute. Some compress the calf alone; others compress the calf and thigh sequentially. There seems to be little difference in efficacy between the two. Although it is unclear if different pressures and speed of intermittent cuff inflation lead to improved prophylactic efficacy, it is clear that the pattern of rhythmic inflation is helpful. While intermittent compressive devices are safe, effective, and well tolerated, the only trials to support the use of these devices are in postoperative surgical patients. No comparative clinical trials have established the efficacy of intermittent compression devices in hospitalized, medical patients; however, this deficiency in the literature alone should not prevent their use in this population, especially in patients unable to receive pharmacologic prophylaxis. The only contraindications to their use are the presence of active venous thrombosis (which should be ruled out prior to their application if suspected), limb ischemia from arterial insufficiency, or the presence of circumstances that prevent their application (e.g., a cast in place). The devices should be applied promptly (e.g., preoperatively) and maintained during the risk period. This approach has particular value in those patients for whom antithrombotic drugs are contraindicated (e.g., neurosurgical, head trauma, and known hemorrhagic diathesis). As with elastic stockings, the added value of compression devices to pharmacologic prophylaxis is unknown.

Finally, a small group of patients who are at high risk for VTE but with absolute contraindications to anticoagulation, such as trauma or hemorrhagic stroke, may benefit from placement of an inferior vena caval (IVC) filter. The value of prophylactic IVC filter placement, even in these groups, remains extremely controversial and is best considered for each case individually. Removable IVC filters for this indication have the advantage that a filter can be withdrawn once it is safe to anticoagulate the patient.

CONCLUSION

Several pharmacologic and mechanical methods are available to prevent VTE. The exact prophylactic "recipe" appropriate for each patient depends on the risks associated in the particular clinical situation. Many studies have been performed to compare different methods and drug regimens in VTE prophylaxis. Although these comparative trials may provide useful clinical guidance, they should be interpreted with some care, considering each trial's sponsorship and scientific rigor. For example, the comparator medication should have been dosed optimally (or, in the case of mechanical modalities, optimal devices/methods should have been employed). The limitations of these studies have been translated to weaker endorsements of specific prophylactic regimens in the most recent guidelines for VTE prevention prepared by both the American College of Physicians and American College of Chest Physicians.

Regardless of the specific regimen selected, it is clear that prophylaxis should be considered carefully for all patients at risk of VTE. The reasons, if any, for withholding prophylaxis should be documented and reconsidered periodically. Because prevention of DVT is the best means of preventing PE and death due to embolism, and because the vast majority of venous thrombi occur in hospitalized patients to whom a prophylactic option easily can be applied, widespread use of prophylactic options can considerably reduce the incidence of DVT and PE. Further developments in this field hold the promise of safely preventing it even further, perhaps to the point of eliminating it entirely.

FURTHER READING

1. Kahn SR, Lim W, Dunn AS, et al. Prevention of VTE in nonsurgical patients. *Chest.* 2012;141(2 suppl):e195S–e226S.

   The most recent ACCP guidelines on VTE prevention in nonsurgical patients has acknowledged the weakness of the literature and no longer differentiates between unfractionated heparin and the low molecular weight heparin.

2. The PROTECT Investigators for the Canadian Critical Care Trials Group and the Australian and New Zealand Intensive Care Society Clinical Trials Group. Dalteparin versus unfractionated heparin in critically ill patients. *N Engl J Med.* 2011;364(14):1305–1314.

   In this study conducted by the PROTECT investigators in Australia, Canada, and New Zealand demonstrated UFH was equal to dalteparin in preventing proximal DVTs in critically ill patients.

3. Lederle FA, Zylla D, MacDonald R, et al. Venous thromboembolism prophylaxis in hospitalized medical patients and those with stroke: a background review for an American College of Physicians Clinical Practice Guideline. *Ann Intern Med.* 2011;155(9):602–615.

   The ACP conducted an exhaustive review of the literature with excellent external validity.

4. CLOTS (Clots in Legs Or sTockings after Stroke) Trial Collaboration. Thigh-length versus below-knee stockings for deep venous thrombosis prophylaxis after stroke: a randomized trial. *Ann Intern Med.* 2010;153(9):553–562.

   The CLOTS2 trial demonstrated less proximal DVT with thigh length compression stockings compared to knee length in patients with stroke.

5. Decousus H, Tapson VF, Bergmann J-F, et al. Factors at admission associated with bleeding risk in medical patients. *Chest.* 2011;139(1):69–79.

   The IMPROVE study group conducted a multivariate analysis to determine the factors associated with bleeding risk in patients receiving pharmacologic prophylaxis for VTE.

6. Barbar S, Noventa F, Rossetto V, et al. A risk assessment model for the identification of hospitalized medical patients at risk for venous thromboembolism: the Padua Prediction Score. *J Thromb Haemost.* 2010;8(11):2450–2457.

   This Italian group created a risk assessment model to determine the risk for VTE in hospitalized medical patients then internally validated their model.

7. Gruber VF, Saldeen T, Brokup B. Incidence of fatal post-operative pulmonary embolism after prophylaxis with dextran-70 and low-dose heparin: an international multicentre study. *Br Med J.* 1980;1:69.

   Dextran-70 was effective in this well-done study; other reports, both positive and negative, leave the efficacy question unresolved.

8. Kakkar VV, Corrigan TP, Fossard DP. Prevention of post-operative embolism by low-dose heparin: an international multi-center trial. *Lancet.* 1975;2:45.

   A large trial documenting a reduction in incidence of DVT, PE, and lethal PE in patients treated with low-dose heparin versus controls.

9. Moser KM, LeMoine JR. Is embolic risk conditioned by location of deep venous thrombosis? *Ann Intern Med.* 1981;94:439.

   The answer to the questions posed in articles 4 and 5 seems to be "yes"; those with thrombi extending into above-knee veins are at high embolic risk.

10. Effect of aspirin on postoperative venous thrombosis: report of the Steering Committee of a trial sponsored by the Medical Research Council. *Lancet.* 1972;2:441.

    This article is one of many reports in which aspirin was not effective.

11. Salzman EW, Ploetz J, Bettmann M, et al. Intraoperative external pneumatic calf compression to afford long-term prophylaxis against deep vein thrombosis in urologic patients. *Surgery.* 1980;87:239.

    One of a large number of reports indicating the efficacy of this prophylactic option.

12. Sevitt S, Gallagher NG. Prevention of venous thrombosis and pulmonary embolism in injured subjects: a trial of anti-coagulant prophylaxis with phenindione in middle-aged and elderly patients with fractured femoral necks. *Lancet.* 1959;2:981.

    References 8 and 9 are carefully done landmark studies establishing the efficacy of prothrombinopenic drugs as prophylactic agents in these patient groups. The positive results, based on vein and lung dissection, are not open to debate, a rare event in the thromboembolic literature.

13. Turpie AG, Gallus A, Beattie WS, et al. Prevention of venous thrombosis in patients with intracranial disease of intermittent pneumatic compression of the calf. *Neurologia.* 1977;27:435.

    This prophylactic option was effective in patients with neurologic disease.

14. Collins R, Scrimgeour A, Yusuf S, et al. Reduction in fatal pulmonary embolism and venous thrombosis by perioperative administration of subcutaneous heparin. *N Engl J Med.* 1988;318:1162.

    An exhaustive review of the many studies regarding prophylaxis with heparin in patients at risk. The authors conclude that the value of this approach has been clearly established in multiple surgical subgroups.

15. Clark-Pearson DL, Synan IS, Hinshaw WM, et al. Prevention of postoperative venous thromboembolism by external pneumatic calf compression in patients with gynecologic malignancy. *Obstet Gynecol.* 1984;63:92.

    The study concludes that application of this device significantly reduces the incidence of postoperative DVT in these patients.

16. Francis CW, Marder VJ, Evarts CM, et al. Two-step warfarin therapy. *JAMA.* 1983;249:374.

    This approach proved effective, and with low bleeding risk, in patients undergoing hip and knee replacement.

17. Francis CW, Pellegrini VD, Marder VJ, et al. Comparison of warfarin and external pneumatic compression in prevention of venous thrombosis after total hip replacement. *JAMA.* 1992;267:2911.

    Both approaches were effective in reducing the frequency of DVT.

18. Levine MN, Hirsh J, Gent M, et al. Prevention of deep vein thrombosis after elective hip replacement: a randomized trial comparing low molecular weight heparin with standard unfractionated heparin. *Ann Intern Med.* 1991;114:543.

    Low-molecular-weight heparin is as effective as standard heparin in prophylaxis of these patients.

19. Huisman MV, Büller HR, ten Cate JW, et al. Serial impedance plethysmography for suspected deep venous thrombosis in outpatients. *N Engl J Med*. 1986;314:823.

    Excellent study demonstrating that, unless DVT suspects have or develop positive impedance plethysmography (indicating thrombosis in popliteal vein and above), outcomes are excellent without treatment. Thus, without treatment, thrombi that remain calf limited pose no significant embolic risk.

20. Oster G, Tuden RL, Colditz GA. Prevention of venous thromboembolism after general surgery: cost-effectiveness analysis of alternative approaches to prophylaxis. *Am J Med*. 1987;82:889.

    Prophylaxis not only reduces morbidity and mortality but also is cost effective.

21. Moser KM. Venous thromboembolism: state of the art. *Am Rev Respir Dis*. 1990;141:235.

    A review of multiple aspects of venous thromboembolism, heavily referenced.

22. Kakkar VV, Cohen AT, Edmonson RA, et al. Low molecular weight versus standard heparin for prevention of venous thromboembolism after major abdominal surgery. *Lancet*. 1993;341:259.

    The two drugs were of equal efficacy.

23. Eriksson BI, Ekman S, Lindbratt S, et al. Prevention of thromboembolism with use of recombinant hirudin: results of a double-blind, multicenter trial comparing the efficacy of desirudin (Revasc) with that of unfractionated heparin in patients having a total hip replacement. *J Bone Joint Surg Am*. 1997;79:326–333.

    Hirudin performed well as a prophylactic agent in this trial, compared to low-dose heparin.

24. Samama MM, Cohen AT, Darmon JY, et al; for Prophylaxis in Medical Patients with Enoxaparin Study Group. A comparison of enoxaparin with placebo for the prevention of venous thromboembolism in acutely ill medical patients. *N Engl J Med*. 1999;341:793–800.

    Moderately high doses of enoxaparin compared favorably to placebo in this patient population, although its performance compared to higher dose prophylactic heparin is unknown.

25. Philbrick JT, Becker DM. Calf deep venous thrombosis: a wolf in sheep's clothing? *Arch Intern Med*. 1988;148:2131.

    A review suggesting that calf-limited DVT, followed to ensure that it does not extend, is of no significant morbid or embolic risk.

26. Anderson FA Jr, Wheeler HB, Goldberg RJ, et al. Physician practices in the prevention of venous thromboembolism. *Ann Intern Med*. 1991;115:591.

    Although the value of prophylaxis is established, this report indicates that it is still not adequately applied by physicians.

70

Thromboembolic Disease: Therapy

Mary Elmasri and Timothy A. Morris

Management of venous thromboembolism (VTE) should be guided by the primary goals of treatment, namely, to prevent and minimize serious sequelae. These include: (1) death or dyspnea, chest pain, and hemodynamic instability from pulmonary emboli (PE); (2) leg discomfort from deep vein thrombosis (DVT); and (3) long-term recurrence of VTE or other problems such as postphlebitic leg swelling and pulmonary hypertension.

It is important to note that no form of anticoagulation reduces embolic risk or enhances thrombus resolution *directly*. Treated DVT patients remain at embolic risk until the DVT either dissolves or organizes; consequently, embolization occurring in the first few days of therapy does not reflect "drug failure." The only evidence of anticoagulation failure is thrombus growth or development of a new thrombus during therapy. Furthermore, approximately 50% of patients with above-knee acute DVT have already had an asymptomatic PE; thus, it is important not to misinterpret the presence of preexisting emboli discovered during the course of treatment as evidence of recurrent thromboembolic disease.

A DVT confined to calf veins typically does not require anticoagulant therapy because it is associated with a low rate of clinically important sequelae. In contrast, a DVT occurring in the proximal veins (i.e., the popliteal, femoral, common femoral, or higher veins) is more dangerous and does require treatment. Both compression ultrasound and impedance plethysmography (IPG) are convenient, reliable ways to make this distinction, although IPG is used far less frequently. However, 15% to 20% of calf-limited thrombi may propagate into the proximal veins within 2 weeks of presentation; thus, serial testing within this timeframe may ensure that a proximal DVT is detected and treated promptly.

The goals of anticoagulation in the acute treatment of VTE are to diminish the amount of vascular obstruction and prevent embolization. In the case of hemodynamically significant PE, inhibiting the release of vasoactive substances into the pulmonary circulation and optimizing right ventricular (RV) function is also an important goal of immediate anticoagulation. Anticoagulation decreases ongoing thrombosis by inactivating a variety of clotting factors, most importantly thrombin and factor Xa. This inactivation of the coagulation system inhibits thrombus growth and allows the fibrinolytic system to proceed unopposed. Anticoagulation, therefore, indirectly speeds the resolution of VTEs and reduces the size of potential emboli.

In the acute stage, the milieu within and around the thrombi contains a high concentration of activated clotting enzymes. In the initial phase of treatment, the enzymes (particularly thrombin or activated factor X, also called "Xa") must be inactivated to halt the self-perpetuating thrombotic process on the clot's surface. Antithrombin (historically called "antithrombin III") irreversibly inactivates these enzymes. Enhancement of antithrombin is the basis for parenteral therapy with heparin and heparin-like anticoagulants. The options include intravenous unfractionated heparin (UFH) as well as subcutaneous UFH, low molecular weight heparin (LMWH), and fondaparinux. Although clinical data are relatively sparse, most experts agree that at least 5 days of parenteral anticoagulation are necessary for the initial phase of treatment.

Clinical trials have failed to demonstrate clear or consistent superiority of any one type of anticoagulation. A literature review suggests that UFH, LMWH, and fondaparinux are all comparable in their efficacy and safety and any may be used for the acute parenteral phase of anticoagulation for acute DVT or PE. The choice between agents depends in large part on the relative cost and ease of administration, with the subcutaneous route permitting more mobility and the possibility of outpatient management. The 9th edition ACCP guidelines for antithrombotic treatment of VTEs recommend LMWH or fondaparinux over intravenous UFH and subcutaneous UFH for the parenteral phase of anticoagulation (Grade 2B and Grade 2C recommendations, respectively, apparently influenced by ease of administration). The risk of heparin-induced thrombocytopenia is about the same with UFH and the LMWHs. However, when subcutaneous absorption is in question or the patient is being considered for thrombolytic therapy, the ACCP recommends the use of intravenous UFH.

The key to the parenteral phase of anticoagulation is achieving therapeutic dosing quickly. The recommended intravenous UFH regimen is weight-based dosing of intravenous UFH at 80 units/kg bolus followed by a continuous infusion of 18 units/kg/hour. When compared to less aggressive treatment regimens, the weight-based regimen is more effective in terms of mortality and recurrence. The individual anticoagulant response to intravenous UFH varies widely, so it is useful to monitor intravenous UFH with the activated partial thromboplastin time (aPTT). A precise therapeutic range for aPTT has never been established unequivocally, but most experts recommend an aPTT during continuous intravenous infusion of heparin of 1.5 to 2.5 times the patient's baseline aPTT. Although the 1.5- to 2.5-times relative range for aPTT can help identify gross over- or under-dosage, it is unlikely to precisely define a therapeutic range. The beneficial effects observed clinically with the 1.5- to 2.5-times range may reflect the appropriate *dose* of heparin rather than the aPTT test result itself. One clinical implication of this finding is that high-dose UFH subcutaneous regimens, with or without aPTT monitoring, are at least as safe and effective as intravenous regimens.

LMWH is prepared by the depolymerization of UFH and shares many properties with it. Like UFH, all LMWHs also bind antithrombin; however, because of shorter length, they favor inactivation of Xa more than thrombin. LMWHs have longer half-lives than UFH. They are cleared via the kidneys so should be used cautiously in patients with renal failure. The three formulations of LMWH currently approved in the United States are enoxaparin, dalteparin, and tinzaparin. Dalteparin is currently only FDA-approved for the treatment of VTE in cancer patients. All are given in a fixed, weight-adjusted dose either once or twice daily. Although not identical in their pharmacokinetics or anticoagulant properties, no particular LMWH has been found to be clinically superior.

Fondaparinux is a synthetic polysaccharide with similar active antithrombin binding sites as UFH and LMWH. Because of its small size, it enhances antithrombin-mediated inactivation of Xa exclusively. Fondaparinux has almost complete bioavailability with a longer half-life than LMWH. It may accumulate to dangerous levels in patients with renal insufficiency because of its near-total renal clearance. It is given subcutaneously once daily at a dose of 7.5 mg for patients with a body weight of 50 to 100 kg, 5 mg for patients weighing less than 50 kg, and 10 mg for patients weighing greater than 100 kg.

Rivaroxaban is a synthetic inhibitor of Xa that can be used in the acute phase of VTE treatment. It differs from the parenteral agents (UFH, LMWH, and fondaparinux) in two substantial ways. First, it is a direct inhibitor that does not depend on the body's antithrombin to inactivate thrombi. Second, it is well absorbed when given orally. For these reasons, it can be used to treat VTE in the acute as well as long-term phases. The acute phase of VTE treatment with rivaroxaban lasts for 3 weeks, as opposed to the shorter acute phase used with parenteral agents.

Long-term anticoagulation after the acute phase of treatment is necessary to prevent recurrence of VTE. The options for long-term anticoagulation include UFH, LMWH, vitamin K antagonists (warfarin), direct Xa inhibitors (e.g., rivaroxaban), and direct thrombin inhibitors (e.g., dabigatran, discussed below). Vitamin K antagonists are the most commonly used agents for long-term anticoagulation. Clinical trials comparing LMWH to vitamin K antagonists have not shown substantial differences in outcome, with the exception of cancer patients who do better with LMWH. Because of the substantial cost of LMWH and the discomfort and inconvenience of subcutaneous administration, vitamin K antagonists (warfarin in particular) remain the treatment of choice for most patients.

Vitamin K antagonists can be started early in the course of VTE treatment, often on the same day as parenteral therapy. Parenteral anticoagulation is typically continued for a minimum of 5 days and until the International Normalized Ratio (INR) is greater than 2.0 for at least 24 hours. The recommended therapeutic INR range for the duration of long-term treatment is 2.0 to 3.0.

Rivaroxaban is a safe and effective therapeutic option for long-term as well as acute treatment of VTE (discussed above). Another option for long-term use is dabigatran, a direct thrombin inhibitor. Like rivaroxaban, dabigatran is well absorbed orally. An advantage of both rivaroxaban and dabigatran is their pharmacokinetic consistency, which alleviates the need for drug monitoring such as the INR monitoring necessary with warfarin. However, there are some important differences between the two. Dabigatran is not used for the acute phase of VTE treatment, but exclusively for long-term treatment. In healthy volunteers, rivaroxaban could be reversed with prothrombin complex concentrate (a human-plasma-derived intravenous product with high concentrations of thrombin, factor X, factor VII, and factor IX). Dabigatran appears not to be reversed by prothrombin complex concentrate, but it may be removed by hemodialysis. However, clinical experience with reversing either agent during therapy is lacking.

The appropriate type and duration of long-term anticoagulation therapy should be tailored to the clinical situation. Patients at high risk for recurrence, characterized by having unresolved or ongoing risk factors for VTE, are likely to require prolonged (possibly lifelong) anticoagulation. Biological phenomena such as deficiencies in antithrombin, protein C, and protein S, as well as the antiphospholipid syndrome, strongly predispose VTE patients to recurrence. Clinical risk factors include immobility, heart failure, persistent venous obstruction, and malignancy. On the other end of the spectrum are patients with VTE because of transient risk factors. Those patients require no more than 3 months of therapy, provided that the original risk factor(s) have subsided (e.g., the broken leg has healed and the patient is fully ambulatory). Patients with VTE that was not provoked by transient risk factors have moderately high rates of recurrence, perhaps because of uncharacterized risk factors. After 3 to 6 months of long-term anticoagulation appropriate for nearly all patients with VTE, those with unprovoked VTE may benefit from longer or even life-long therapy. Although various algorithms and testing strategies appear promising, the duration of therapy for unprovoked VTE is best individualized to the patient's particular risks of recurrence and bleeding.

The major complication of anticoagulation is hemorrhage. It was initially hoped that LMWH would be safer than UFH, but this has not borne out in clinical studies; all available forms of anticoagulation carry a similar risk of bleeding. In fact, host factors appear to be far more important than the type and dose of anticoagulation in determining bleeding risk. These include age (especially beyond the sixth decade), presence of unsuspected or known bleeding sites (e.g., stomach, bowel, and kidney), uremia, and demonstrable hemostatic defects (e.g., thrombocytopenia). Available data indicate that bleeding risk is very low among patients who do not have a significant coexistent disease or coagulopathy.

Approaches specific to DVT therapy have been proposed, but are not commonly used. Surgery (e.g., thrombectomy, ligation) has no role. Systemic administration of thrombolytic agents (e.g., streptokinase, urokinase, tissue plasminogen activator) may decrease the risk of post-thrombotic syndrome, but is associated with significant increase in major bleeding such as intracranial hemorrhage. Catheter-directed thrombolysis has been studied in patients with iliofemoral DVT. In selected cases and specialized clinical settings, catheter-directed thrombolysis may decrease the risk of post-thrombotic syndrome and improve outcomes. However, this procedure is still under investigation and is not applicable for most cases of DVT. Future studies with new or existing thrombolytic agents and strategies may modify these views.

The treatment of PE in very stable patients is generally identical to DVT, but several issues require extra consideration. The most important is recognizing that outpatient subcutaneous treatment regimens for PE are only applicable to very stable patients. Less healthy patients merit hospital admission. Additional therapeutic issues specific to PE include: (1) the importance of the initial dose of heparin and the dosage regimen during the first 24 hours, (2) the need for cardiopulmonary supportive measures, (3) the role of caval filters and surgery, and (4) the role of thrombolytic agents.

The initial anticoagulant dose during acute treatment may be important to the outcome of patients with PE. Pharmacologically active peptides released from platelets within PE may contribute to the initial severity of the cardiopulmonary symptoms by inducing pulmonary vasoconstriction. Adequate levels of heparin inactivate thrombosis on the clot surface, inhibit platelet aggregation, and subsequently retard the release of vasoconstrictive agents. On the basis of these data, we recommend prompt initiation of a therapeutic heparin dose, followed by a continuous infusion. Dose adjustment is generally the same as for DVT, but with special attention to avoiding low doses or during the first 1 to 2 days of therapy. In most cases, of PE, careful attention to anticoagulation results in excellent clinical outcomes.

In some cases, cardiopulmonary supportive measures may be indicated for PE treatment, including administration of oxygen if arterial hypoxemia is present. Systemic hypotension, if present, is usually due to acute RV ischemia and failure. Animal experiments suggest that an important mechanism of RV ischemia is low myocardial perfusion pressure (coronary pressure – RV pressure) occurring as the right heart "strains" to overcome massive pulmonary artery obstruction. For that reason, we prefer systemic vasoconstrictive agents, such as phenylephrine, to raise arterial pressure (and coronary pressure) during PE-associated shock.

Massive PE may require a more aggressive approach, particularly during the first few days of heparin therapy when heparin cannot prevent a recurrence. In this situation, death may be caused by additional embolization of lower limb DVT that occurs while the patient is already hemodynamically compromised. Multiple procedures are available to prevent recurrent embolism of lower limb DVTs. Our current choice is limited to the insertion of an inferior vena caval filter. These devices are relatively easy to insert, do not interfere with caval blood flow, and have an excellent (95%) record of long-term patency. It is, for us, the "standard" against which other devices and approaches should be measured. When a recurrence may be fatal in the setting of massive PE, we consider filter placement to be a life-saving procedure.

The role of thrombolytic agents in management of PE is unclear. The choice of patients who might benefit from thrombolytics must be made on the basis of indirect information rather than by comparative clinical trials. Multiple studies have established that these agents promote more rapid embolic resolution than heparin alone. Positive effects on morbidity and mortality have not been demonstrated; in addition, the degree of embolic resolution after the first week of anticoagulation is about the same without thrombolytic therapy. Thrombolytic agents are costly and carry significant risks for adverse consequences. We believe that such agents should be used only in the management of patients with massive embolism and persistent hypotension and only by physicians quite familiar with the drugs.

Acute pulmonary embolectomy (by thoracotomy, suction catheter, or balloon catheter) is an aggressive procedure that is performed at some institutions. In our view, it is rarely warranted because medical therapy is so successful, patient selection is so difficult, and the results of acute embolectomy are so unimpressive. Conceivably, there are special situations in which this surgery is possible (massive embolism failing to respond promptly to medical therapy and the diagnosis is certain). However, the procedure carries a very high mortality and we do not recommend it in most cases.

For follow-up after the immediate treatment period, the use of lung scans in patients with above-knee DVT (to rule out asymptomatic embolism) and in patients with PE (to evaluate resolution) merits comment. Often, in patients with DVT, pleuritic chest pain or other embolic symptoms appear several days after admission, and a scan demonstrates defects. In our experience, these defects were usually present on the admission scan and, therefore, do not merit a change in therapy. Without the admission scan, such decisions are much more difficult. A follow-up scan during PE treatment not only provides evidence of satisfactory embolic resolution but also alerts the physician to the possibility that the patient may require close follow-up to rule out chronic thromboembolic pulmonary hypertension.

FURTHER READING

1. Alpert JS, Smith R, Carlson J, et al. Mortality in patients treated for pulmonary embolism. *JAMA.* 1976;236:1477.

   An interesting study that implies, among other things, that embolectomy is not likely to impact on the mortality associated with PE.

2. Basu D, Gallus A, Hirsh J, et al. A prospective study of the value of monitoring heparin treatment with the activated partial thromboplastin time. *N Engl J Med.* 1972;287:324.

   Well-designed study discussing the optimum heparin regimen and the value of monitoring the dose with the partial thromboplastin time. Compare with references 7 and 20.

3. Bentley PG, Kakkar VV, Scully MF, et al. An objective study of alternative methods of heparin administration. *Thromb Res.* 1980;18:177.

   Another approach to heparin administration.

4. Bonnameau XH, Banga JD, Bluhmki E, et al. Double-blind, randomized comparison of systemic continuous infusion of 0.25 versus 0.50 mg/kg/24 h of alteplase over 3 to 7 days for treatment of deep venous thrombosis in heparinized patients: results of the European thrombolysis with rt-PA in venous thrombosis trial. *Thromb Haemost.* 1992;67:306.

   Trial was discontinued because of low efficacy and excessive bleeding.

5. Brandjes DPM, Heijboer H, Büller HR, et al. Acenocoumarol and heparin compared with acenocoumarol alone in the initial treatment of proximal vein thrombosis. *N Engl J Med.* 1992;327:1485.

   Initiation of therapy with heparin is advisable.

6. Brill-Edwards P, Ginsberg JS, Johnston M, et al. Establishing a therapeutic range for heparin therapy. *Ann Intern Med.* 1993;119:104.

   The variability of reagents used for the aPTT test can influence the heparin dose significantly. The authors suggest an alternative (but not generally available) monitoring approach.

7. Crotty GM, Bynum LJ, Wilson JE III. Heparin therapy in venous thromboembolism. *Clin Res.* 1978;26:135A.

   Well-designed study that proposes guidelines for heparin use that differ from those in references 2 and 20.

8. Fedullo PF, Moser KM, Moser KS, et al. 111-Indium labelled platelets: effect of heparin on uptake by venous thrombi and relationship to the activated partial thromboplastin time. *Circulation.* 1982;66:632.

   In dogs, maintaining an aPTT above 1.5 times the control does prevent venous thrombus growth, as measured by prevention of platelet accretion to the thrombus.

9. Fihn SD, McDonell M, Martin D, et al. Risk factors for complications of chronic anticoagulation. *Ann Intern Med.* 1993;118:511.

   By closely monitoring the prothrombin time ratio, safety and efficacy of chronic anticoagulation can be enhanced. Bleeding risk is highest during the first several months of therapy.

10. Hirsh J. Oral anticoagulant drugs. *N Engl J Med.* 1991;324:1865.

11. Hirsh J. Heparin. *N Engl J Med.* 1991;321:1565.

    References 10 and 11 provide detailed reviews of the actions, therapeutic uses, and new developments with regard to heparin and oral anticoagulant drugs.

12. Hommes DW, Bura A, Mazzolai L, et al. Subcutaneous heparin compared with continuous intravenous heparin administration in the initial treatment of deep vein thrombosis: a meta-analysis. *Ann Intern Med.* 1992;116:279.

    This meta-analysis concluded that subcutaneous heparin, with or without monitoring, was a bit more effective and safer than monitored, continuous intravenous therapy.

13. Huisman MV, Buller HR, ten Cate JW, et al. Unexpected high prevalence of pulmonary embolism in patients with deep venous thrombosis. *Chest.* 1989;95:498.

    When treating DVT, one is often treating PE as well; in this series, 51% of patients with DVT—with no symptoms of embolism—had a "high probability" lung scan.

14. Hull R, Delmore T, Carter C, et al. Adjusted subcutaneous heparin versus warfarin sodium in the long-term treatment of venous thrombosis. *N Engl J Med.* 1982;306:189.

    Efficacy and safety are quite similar with an upward adjustment in heparin dose and a downward adjustment in warfarin "range."

15. Marder VJ. The use of thrombolytic agents: choice of patient, drug administration, laboratory monitoring. *Ann Intern Med.* 1979;90:802.

    An informative review written by a proponent of this form of therapy.

16. Moser KM. Venous thromboembolism: state of the art. *Am Rev Respir Dis.* 1990;141:235.

    A detailed review of many aspects of the subject.

17. Nelson PH, Moser KM, Stoner C, et al. Risk of complications during intravenous heparin therapy. *West J Med.* 1982;136:189.

A study and review indicating that coexistent disease, not heparin dose, is the major determinant of hemorrhagic risk.

18. Research Committee of the British Thoracic Society. Optimal duration of anticoagulation for deep vein thrombosis and pulmonary embolism. *Lancet.* 1992;340:873.

   Although arbitrary durations can be suggested, as in this study, establishing specific criteria for individual patients is a preferable approach.

19. Rosenberg RD. Heparin action. *Circulation.* 1974;49:603.

   An excellent comment on how heparin works.

20. Salzman EW, Deykin D, Shapiro RM, et al. Management of heparin therapy: a controlled prospective study. *N Engl J Med.* 1975;292:1046.

   Well-designed study that reaches conclusions differing from those in references 2 and 7.

21. Hull R, Hirsh J, Jay R, et al. Different intensities of anticoagulation in the long-term treatment of proximal venous thrombosis. *N Engl J Med.* 1982;307:1676.

22. Huisman MV, Büller HR, ten Cate JW. Utility of impedance plethysmography in the diagnosis of recurrent deep-vein thrombosis. *Arch Intern Med.* 1988;148:681.

   The IPG test can be used effectively to determine whether DVT has recurred and, therefore, additional treatment is necessary. In 67% of patients with proximal DVT, IPG reverts to negative at 3 months, 85% at 6 months and 95% at 12 months.

23. Kirchmaier CM, Wolf H, Scheafer H, et al; for the Certoparin-Study Group. Efficacy of a low molecular weight heparin administered intravenously or subcutaneously in comparison with intravenous unfractionated heparin in the treatment of deep venous thrombosis. *Int Angiol.* 1998;17:135–145.

24. Meyer G, Brenot F, Pacouret G, et al. Subcutaneous low-molecular-weight heparin fragmin versus intravenous unfractionated heparin in the treatment of acute non massive pulmonary embolism: an open randomized pilot study. *Thromb Haemost.* 1995;74:1432–1435.

25. Fiessinger JN, Lopez-Fernandez M, Gatterer E, et al. Once-daily subcutaneous dalteparin, a low molecular weight heparin, for the initial treatment of acute deep vein thrombosis. *Thromb Haemost.* 1996;76:195–199.

26. Lindmarker P, Holmstrom M; for the Swedish Venous Thrombosis Dalteparin Trial Group. Use of low molecular weight heparin (dalteparin), once daily, for the treatment of deep vein thrombosis: a feasibility and health economic study in an outpatient setting. *J Intern Med.* 1996;240:395–401.

27. Luomanmeaki K, Grankvist S, Hallert C, et al. A multicentre comparison of once-daily subcutaneous dalteparin (low molecular weight heparin) and continuous intravenous heparin in the treatment of deep vein thrombosis. *J Intern Med.* 1996;240:85–92.

28. de Valk HW, Banga JD, Wester JW, et al. Comparing subcutaneous danaparoid with intravenous unfractionated heparin for the treatment of venous thromboembolism: a randomized controlled trial. *Ann Intern Med.* 1995;123:1–9. See comments.

29. Levine M, Gent M, Hirsh J, et al. A comparison of low-molecular-weight heparin administered primarily at home with unfractionated heparin administered in the hospital for proximal deep vein thrombosis. *N Engl J Med.* 1996;334:677–681.

30. Hull RD, Raskob GE, Pineo GF, et al. Subcutaneous low-molecular-weight heparin compared with continuous intravenous heparin in the treatment of proximal-vein thrombosis. *N Engl J Med.* 1992;326:975–982. See comments.

31. Prandoni P, Lensing AW, Beuller HR, et al. Comparison of subcutaneous low-molecular-weight heparin with intravenous standard heparin in proximal deep-vein thrombosis. *Lancet.* 1992;339:441–445.

32. Koopman M, Prandoni P, Piovella F. Treatment of venous thrombosis with intravenous unfractionated heparin administered in the hospital as compared with subcutaneous low-molecular-weight heparin administered at home. *N Engl J Med.* 1996;334:682–687.

33. Lopaciuk S, Meissner AJ, Filipecki S, et al. Subcutaneous low molecular weight heparin versus subcutaneous unfractionated heparin in the treatment of deep vein thrombosis: a Polish multicenter trial. *Thromb Haemost.* 1992;68:14–18.

34. Simonneau G, Sors H, Charbonnier B, et al; for the THESEE Study Group. A comparison of low-molecular-weight heparin with unfractionated heparin for acute pulmonary embolism. Tinzaparine ou Heparine Standard: Evaluations dans l'Embolie Pulmonaire. *N Engl J Med.* 1997;337:663–669.

References 23 to 34 describe randomized controlled trials of subcutaneous LMWHs to intravenous unfractionated heparin for the treatment of DVT or PE. Taken as a whole, the trials demonstrate no differences in efficacy, safety, or complications (i.e., thrombocytopenia) between the two types of regimens.

35. Buller HR, Davidson BL, Decousus H, et al. Subcutaneous fondaparinux versus intravenous unfractionated heparin in the initial treatment of pulmonary embolism. *N Engl J Med.* 2003;349:1695–1702.

36. Buller HR, Davidson BL, Decousus H, et al. Fondaparinux or enoxaparin for the initial treatment of symptomatic deep venous thrombosis: a randomized trial. *Ann Intern Med.* 2004;140:867–873.

References 35 and 36 show that the synthetic anticoagulant fondaparinux is comparable (but not superior) in safety and efficacy to heparin and LMWH for the treatment of stable PE and DVT, respectively.

37. Bauersachs R, Berkowitz SD, Brenner B, et al. Oral rivaroxaban for symptomatic venous thromboembolism. *N Engl J Med.* 2010;363(26):2499–2510.

38. Buller HR, Prins MH, Lensin AW, et al. Oral rivaroxaban for the treatment of symptomatic pulmonary embolism. *N Engl J Med.* 2012;366(14):1287–1297.

Rivaroxaban is safe and effective for the acute and long-term treatment of DVT (ref. 37) and PE (ref. 38). The acute treatment lasts for three weeks and uses higher doses than long-term treatment.

39. Schulman S, Kearon C, Kakkar AK, et al. Dabigatran versus warfarin in the treatment of acute venous thromboembolism. *N Engl J Med.* 2009;361(24):2342–2352.

Dabigatran was safe and effective for follow-up treatment of VTE, but was not used for the acute phase of treatment.

40. Eerenberg ES, Kamphuisen PW, Sijpkens MK, et al. Reversal of rivaroxaban and dabigatran by prothrombin complex concentrate: a randomized, placebo-controlled, crossover study in healthy subjects. *Circulation.* 2011;124(14):1573–1579.

In healthy human volunteers, prothrombin complex concentrate reversed the laboratory indicators of anticoagulation after rivaroxaban administration but not after dabigatran.

41. Decousus H, Leizorovicz A, Parent F, et al; for the Prevention du Risque d'Embolie Pulmonaire par Interruption Cave Study Group. A clinical trial of vena caval filters in the prevention of pulmonary embolism in patients with proximal deep-vein thrombosis. *N Engl J Med.* 1998;338(7):409–415.

42. Decousus H. Eight-year follow-up of a randomized trial investigating vena cava filters in the prevention of PE in patients presenting a proximal DVT: the PREPIC trial. *J Thromb Haemost.* 2003;(suppl 1):OC440.

References 41 and 42 provide the rationale for IVC filter placement to prevent short-term occurrence of PE during acute VTE, which, in the presence of unstable PE, could be disastrous. In reference 41, IVC filters in addition to anticoagulation prevented acute PE (1.1% incidence) better than anticoagulation alone (4.8% incidence; odds ratio, 0.22; 95% CI, 0.05–0.90). Although the filters were associated with more recurrent DVTs in the short-term, the long-term follow-up (ref. 42) showed an equal amount of VTE between the groups, with the filter group maintaining a lower incidence of PE.

43. Stein PD, Matta F, Keyes DC, et al. Impact of vena cava filters on in-hospital case fatality rate from pulmonary embolism. *Am J Med.* 2012;125(5):478–484.

In this retrospective study, patients with acute PE who received IVC filters did better than those who were treated without them.

44. Konstantinides S, Geibel A, Heusel G, et al. Heparin plus alteplase compared with heparin alone in patients with submassive pulmonary embolism. *N Engl J Med.* 2002;347(15):1143–1150.

45. Dalen JE, Alpert JS, Hirsh J. Thrombolytic therapy for pulmonary embolism: is it effective? Is it safe? When is it indicated? *Arch Intern Med.* 1997;157:2550–2556.

46. Wan S, Quinlan DJ, Agnelli G, et al. Thrombolysis compared with heparin for the initial treatment of pulmonary embolism: a meta-analysis of the randomized controlled trials. *Circulation.* 2004;110(6):744–749.

References 44 to 46 emphasize the lack of data supporting improved outcome for most patients with PE treated with thrombolytics. In addition, the increased incidence of intracranial bleeding and other serious bleeding with thrombolytics argues against their routine use in PE patients.

71 Chronic Thromboembolic Pulmonary Hypertension

Peter F. Fedullo and William R. Auger

Chronic thromboembolic pulmonary hypertension (CTEPH) represents an aberrant outcome that occurs in a minority of patients following an acute or recurrent episode of pulmonary embolism (PE). Estimates of disease prevalence vary and range from 0.6% to 3.8%. In the largest published study, a cohort screening study involving 866 survivors of acute PE, 4 patients (0.6%) were ultimately diagnosed with CTEPH.

The pathophysiologic events leading to CTEPH are not entirely understood. Although anatomic resolution of acute embolism is often incomplete, sufficient resolution occurs in the majority of patients to restore normal hemodynamics and functional status. Incomplete thrombus resolution and hemodynamic recovery following an acute thromboembolic event, even with appropriate antithrombotic therapy, can occur in some patients. It is also apparent that many patients with CTEPH have had an asymptomatic or misdiagnosed thromboembolic event. Because appropriate antithrombotic therapy was not initiated at the time of the initial embolic event, it is possible that endogenous fibrinolytic mechanisms were overcome by the age, extent, or location of the obstructing embolus.

Despite extensive investigation, identifying a thrombophilic tendency or a defect in fibrinolytic activity has been elusive in most patients with established chronic thromboembolic disease. The presence of a lupus anticoagulant or anticardiolipin antibodies can be established in 10% to 24% of CTEPH patients. The frequency of protein S or C deficiency, factor V Leiden mutation, and the prothrombin 20210G mutation have not consistently been found to be more common in CTEPH than in the general population. In terms of medical conditions, CTEPH has been associated with myeloproliferative syndromes as well as chronic inflammatory states, chronic ventriculoatrial shunts, splenectomy, recurrent episodes of venous thromboembolism, and chronic indwelling central venous catheters.

The diagnosis of CTEPH usually is not made until the degree of pulmonary hypertension is advanced. As a result, the exact hemodynamic evolution of the disease has not been established. The symptomatic history has been well described. A patient may carry on relatively normal activities following a pulmonary embolic event, whether clinically apparent or occult, and even when extensive pulmonary vascular occlusion has occurred. Following an asymptomatic period, which may range from months to years, exertional dyspnea worsens and hypoxemia and right ventricular failure ensue. The basis for this asymptomatic ("honeymoon") period followed by gradual hemodynamic and symptomatic decline has only recently been elucidated.

The progressive nature of the pulmonary hypertension in the majority of patients with chronic thromboembolic disease does not appear to be the result of recurrent embolic events or *in situ* thrombosis, as initially postulated. The increase in pulmonary artery pressures arises from two different sources: a decrease in the cross-sectional area of the pulmonary vascular bed associated with the unresolved thromboembolic component of the disease, and the development over time of a distal, small-vessel arteriopathy pathologically indistinct from that seen in a wide range of pulmonary hypertensive disorders. It appears that these secondary pulmonary hypertensive changes, perhaps induced by high pulmonary artery pressures or flows, result in an incremental increase in right ventricular afterload, progressive pulmonary hypertension, and, ultimately, right ventricular failure.

Progressive dyspnea is a complaint common to all patients with CTEPH. The subjective complaint of dyspnea must be considered in the context of the patient's usual lifestyle. The sensation of dyspnea and development of exercise intolerance are more troubling and lead to earlier evaluation in patients who are normally active than in those who live a sedentary lifestyle. Later in the course of the disease, exertional chest pain, near-syncope or syncope, and lower extremity edema may develop.

Although a history of documented thromboembolism may be absent, many patients provide a history consistent with an acute embolic event such as an episode of "pleurisy," lower extremity "muscle strain," or prolonged, atypical "pneumonia." Alternatively, they may describe a hospitalization or surgical procedure from which they never fully recovered.

Diagnostic delay occurs commonly, particularly in the absence of an acute history of venous thromboembolism. Progressive dyspnea and exercise intolerance from CTEPH are often erroneously attributed to coronary artery disease, cardiomyopathy, interstitial lung disease, asthma, deconditioning, or psychogenic dyspnea.

The nonspecific and often subtle clinical presentation of CTEPH especially early in the course of the disease demands that a high level of suspicion be maintained in patients presenting with unexplained dyspnea. Careful consideration should be given to prior medical conditions and the circumstances surrounding the onset of dyspnea and/or exercise intolerance. In retrospect, patients without a documented history of venous thromboembolism often provide a history consistent with that diagnosis, such as an episode of pneumonia or an operative procedure with persistent symptoms and functional impairment. Findings on physical examination may be subtle early in the course, thereby contributing to the diagnostic delay. Prior to the development of significant right ventricular hypertrophy or overt right ventricular failure, abnormalities can be limited to a widening of the second heart sound or a subtle accentuation of its pulmonic component. In time, more obvious findings of pulmonary hypertension and right ventricular dysfunction develop, which may include a right ventricular heave, jugular venous distension, prominent A and V wave venous pulsation, fixed splitting of S2, a right ventricular S4 or S3, a murmur of tricuspid regurgitation, hepatomegaly, ascites, and peripheral edema. A distinctive physical finding in certain patients with chronic thromboembolic disease is the presence of flow murmurs over the lung fields. These subtle bruits, which appear to originate from turbulent flow through partially obstructed or recanalized pulmonary arteries, are high pitched and blowing in quality, heard over the lung fields rather than the precordium, accentuated during inspiration, and frequently heard only during periods of breath-holding. Their importance lies in their not having been described in primary pulmonary hypertension, which is the most common alternative diagnostic possibility. The flow murmurs, however, are not unique to chronic thromboembolic disease and may be encountered in congenital stenotic lesions of the pulmonary vasculature, and in major-vessel pulmonary vasculitides.

The diagnostic approach is relatively straightforward once an abnormality of the pulmonary vascular bed has been considered as a basis for the patient's complaints. The goals of diagnostic evaluation are: (1) to establish the presence and degree of pulmonary hypertension; (2) to define its etiology; and (3) to determine if major vessel thromboembolic disease is present and accessible to surgical intervention. Findings on standard laboratory tests are nonspecific, depending on when in the natural history of the disease they are obtained, and reflect the hemodynamic and gas exchange consequences of the thromboembolic obstruction and the accompanying cardiac dysfunction. The chest radiograph is often normal, although it may demonstrate one or more of the following findings that suggest the diagnosis: (1) enlargement of both main pulmonary arteries or asymmetry in the size of the central pulmonary arteries, (2) areas of hypoperfusion or hyperperfusion, (3) evidence of old pleural disease, unilaterally or bilaterally, or (4) evidence of right ventricular hypertrophy. Pulmonary function testing is often within normal limits, although approximately 20% of patients demonstrate a mild-to-moderate restrictive abnormality. The majority of patients have a reduction in the single breath diffusing capacity for carbon monoxide (D_{LCO}); however, a normal value does not exclude the diagnosis. When a spirometric abnormality is present (reflecting either restrictive or obstructive disease), the degree of the abnormality is almost always less impressive than the patient's gas exchange abnormalities, symptomatic complaints, and degree of pulmonary hypertension. Although the arterial Po_2 may be within normal limits, the alveolar–arterial oxygen gradient is typically widened, and the majority of patients have a decline in arterial Po_2 with exercise. Dead space ventilation (Vd/Vt) is often elevated at rest and increases with exercise.

Echocardiography commonly provides the initial objective evidence for pulmonary hypertension. Findings include evidence of right atrial and right ventricular enlargement, abnormal septal position and motion related to the right ventricular pressure and volume overload, and evidence of pulmonary hypertension as determined from the tricuspid regurgitant jet.

Ventilation–perfusion lung scanning provides an excellent noninvasive means of distinguishing between potentially operable major-vessel thromboembolic pulmonary hypertension and small-vessel pulmonary hypertension. In chronic thromboembolic disease, at least one (and, more commonly, several) segmental or larger mismatched ventilation–perfusion defects are present. In primary pulmonary hypertension, perfusion scans are either normal or exhibit a "mottled" appearance characterized by subsegmental defects. However, it is important to recognize that the ventilation–perfusion scan often understates the actual *extent* of central pulmonary vascular obstruction. Channels through or partial flow around partially recanalized or organized central obstructing lesions allow the radioisotopic agent to reach the periphery of the lung. Depending on the distribution of flow, these areas may appear normal or as relatively hypoperfused "grey zones." Ventilation–perfusion scanning, therefore, is capable of suggesting the potential presence of chronic thromboembolic obstruction, but it is unable to determine the magnitude, location, or proximal extent of the disease, information critical to the question of surgical accessibility.

Right-heart catheterization and pulmonary angiography are essential to determine the degree of pulmonary hypertension, to exclude competing diagnoses, and to define the surgical accessibility of the obstructing thrombotic lesions. If hemodynamic measurements at rest demonstrate only modest degrees of pulmonary hypertension, measurements should be obtained following a short period of exercise. In patients with chronic thromboembolic obstruction sufficient to abolish normal compensatory mechanisms, exercise-related increases in cardiac output will be accompanied by an excessive elevation in pulmonary artery pressure.

Five distinct angiographic patterns different from those encountered in acute embolism have been described that correlate with the finding of organized thromboembolic material at the time of thromboendarterectomy: (1) defects with a pouch configuration, (2) pulmonary artery webs or bands, (3) intimal irregularities, (4) abrupt narrowing of the major pulmonary arteries, and (5) obstruction of lobar or segmental vessels at their point of origin, with complete absence of blood flow to pulmonary segments normally perfused by those vessels. In experienced hands, pulmonary angiography can be performed safely, even in patients with severe pulmonary hypertension. The use of nonionic contrast media, provision of supplemental oxygen to avoid hypoxemia, and minimizing contrast volume with separate proximal pulmonary artery injections (i.e., avoiding right ventricular injections) are some of the technical safeguards necessary to prevent adverse outcomes in the evaluation of this patient population.

Computed tomography (CT) can be useful in the evaluation of competing diagnostic possibilities, such as pulmonary artery sarcoma, fibrosing mediastinitis, and extrinsic vascular compression related to malignancies or inflammatory disease. Large vessel pulmonary arteritis can also mimic certain of the angiographic findings of chronic thromboembolic disease. Arch aortography may be useful if this diagnosis is being considered.

A variety of abnormalities may be appreciated on helical CT scans obtained in patients with CTEPH, including right ventricular enlargement, chronic thromboembolic material within dilated central pulmonary arteries, bronchial artery collateral flow, and mosaic attenuation of the pulmonary parenchyma. The detection of central disease by CT scanning does not necessarily imply that the patient represents an operative candidate. A syndrome of primary pulmonary hypertension with secondary, central pulmonary artery thrombosis has been described, a situation in which surgical intervention is contraindicated.

A positive CT or magnetic resonance (MR) angiogram can be used as a basis for surgical intervention in selected patients. Technologic advances in both MR and CT scanning, their three dimensional capabilities, and the lack of radiation exposure and ability to provide hemodynamic information in the case of MR imaging suggest that they may play an expanded role in the future. However, until further comparative and outcome studies have been performed, their wholesale substitution for conventional angiography does not yet appear warranted.

Several other essential issues must be considered prior to surgery. Placement of an inferior vena cava filter should be considered prior to surgery given the risk of embolic recurrence, both over the long term and especially during the high-risk perioperative period when bleeding complications may contraindicate the administration of even prophylactic doses of anticoagulation. Coronary angiography should also be considered preoperatively for those at risk of coronary artery disease. Coronary artery bypass surgery, if necessary, can be performed without significant additional operative risk at the time of the pulmonary thromboendarterectomy (PTE).

The decision to proceed to PTE in patients suffering from CTEPH is based upon both objective and subjective factors, which are carefully defined during the preoperative evaluation. The first and most important criterion for potential surgical intervention is the accessibility of the thrombi, as defined by angiography and angioscopy. Present surgical techniques allow removal of chronic thrombi whose proximal location extends to the main, lobar, and segmental arteries. Those that begin more distally are not typically subject to endarterectomy. Failure to remove sufficient embolic material to lower pulmonary vascular resistance, especially in patients with severe pulmonary hypertension and right ventricular dysfunction, may result in inability to wean the patient from cardiopulmonary bypass at the time of thromboendarterectomy and, if the patient does survive, is associated with a negative long-term outcome. The second criterion involves the presence of hemodynamic or ventilatory impairment as a consequence of the chronic thromboembolic pulmonary vascular obstruction. The majority of operated patients have a pulmonary vascular resistance in excess of 300 dynes/sec/cm^5, at rest or with exercise. Occasional patients, especially those with involvement of one main pulmonary artery, have significant exercise impairment due to high minute ventilatory demands, without substantially altered pulmonary hemodynamics. The third criterion involves the presence and severity of comorbid conditions, such as severe parenchymal lung disease, which may adversely affect outcome. Although the presence of other disease processes does not represent an absolute contraindication to the procedure, the risks imposed by any coexistent condition and its potential effects on long-term outcome are carefully reviewed with the patient before a surgical decision is made. Age by itself is not a contraindication to the procedure. Patients up to 84 years of age, if they are otherwise fit, have successfully undergone PTE.

The surgical option is also considered in patients with exercise-associated pulmonary hypertension related to their chronic thromboembolic disease. Because this hemodynamic response reproduces events during the patient's activities of daily living, it may reflect the true work load of the right ventricle. Furthermore, given what is now suspected about the pathophysiologic mechanisms of the disease, it is possible that the exercise-related augmentation of pressure and flow over a sufficient period of time will result in progressive levels of pulmonary hypertension.

Although a thoracotomy approach to CTEPH has been utilized in the past, sternotomy with cardiopulmonary bypass and periods of circulatory arrest currently represent the procedure of choice. The most critical need for sternotomy arises from the bilateral nature of the disease process. Sternotomy allows access to both pulmonary arteries and assures more complete removal of the chronically obstructing material. The use of cardiopulmonary bypass allows periods of complete circulatory arrest, which provides the bloodless operative field essential for meticulous lobar and segmental dissections. Finally, the presence of bronchial artery collateral flow and pleural adhesions makes a transthoracic approach difficult.

Thromboendarterectomy bears no resemblance to acute pulmonary embolectomy. The procedure is a true endarterectomy, requiring careful dissection of chronic endothelialized material from the native intima to restore pulmonary arterial patency. Establishing the correct plane is essential and requires a considerable degree of surgical experience and expertise. Too deep a plane will result in perforation of the vessel; too superficial a plane will not result in an adequate endarterectomy.

Periods of circulatory arrest are limited to 20-minute intervals. With experience, the entire unilateral endarterectomy can usually be accomplished within this time. At the completion of the bilateral endarterectomy, circulation is reestablished and the patient rewarmed. The atrial septum is routinely inspected, since an atrial septal defect or persistent foramen ovale is seen (and subsequently repaired) in approximately 25% of cases. If additional procedures are required, such as coronary bypass grafting or valve replacement, they are performed during the rewarming period.

Careful postoperative management is essential for a successful outcome following PTE. Although pulmonary hemodynamics improve immediately in the majority of patients, the postoperative course can be complex. In addition to complications common to other forms of cardiac surgery (e.g., arrhythmias, atelectasis, wound infection, pericardial effusions, delirium), patients undergoing PTE often experience three unique postoperative conditions capable of significantly impairing gas exchange and hemodynamic stability: pulmonary artery "steal," reperfusion pulmonary edema, and persistent pulmonary hypertension.

Pulmonary artery "steal" represents a postoperative redistribution of pulmonary arterial blood flow away from previously well-perfused segments and into the newly endarterectomized segments. Although the basis for this phenomenon remains speculative, it is likely related to the temporary development of differential resistances and the loss of normal vasoregulation in the pulmonary vascular bed following thromboendarterectomy. Long-term follow-up has demonstrated that pulmonary vascular steal resolves in the majority of patients.

Reperfusion pulmonary edema appears to represent a form of high-permeability lung injury acute respiratory distress syndrome (ARDS), which is limited to those areas of lung from which proximal thromboembolic obstructions have been removed. It may appear up to 72 hours after surgery and is highly variable in severity, ranging from a mild form of edema resulting in postoperative hypoxemia to an acute, hemorrhagic and fatal complication. When associated with pulmonary artery steal, reperfusion pulmonary edema can represent a significant challenge in terms of postoperative gas exchange since pulmonary blood flow is directed toward edematous, noncompliant areas of lung, which contribute poorly to gas exchange.

Management of reperfusion edema, as with other forms of acute lung injury, is supportive until resolution occurs. As is the case in patients with ARDS, low volume ventilatory strategies are used routinely. The judicious use of inverse ratio ventilation has proven useful in improving ventilation/perfusion relationships and gas exchange when conventional ventilatory support has failed. Nitric oxide, delivered at a concentration of 20 ppm, has also proven beneficial in improving gas exchange, although its effect on mortality remains unclear. Finally, extracorporeal support has been utilized successfully when conventional measures fail.

Patients posing the most difficult management problem in the postoperative period are those with persistent pulmonary hypertension following thromboendarterectomy. This outcome results from either distal, surgically inaccessible thromboembolic disease or to a secondary, small vessel arteriopathy, and is associated with poor short-term and long-term outcomes. Unless right ventricular afterload is substantially reduced at the time of surgery, even patients with well-compensated right ventricular function prior to the procedure may experience postoperative hemodynamic instability and a low output state as a result of the depressant effects of cardiopulmonary bypass, deep hypothermia, acidosis, and hypoxemia.

The early intensive care management goals for the patient with persistent pulmonary hypertension and right ventricular failure following attempted thromboendarterectomy should be directed toward minimizing systemic oxygen consumption, optimizing right ventricular preload, and providing aggressive inotropic support. The use of afterload reduction in this patient population is fraught with difficulty. Pulmonary vascular resistance is commonly fixed, and attempts at pharmacologic manipulation of right ventricular afterload (sodium nitroprusside, calcium channel blockers, epoprostenol) may simply decrease systemic blood pressure and right coronary artery perfusion pressure. Inhaled nitric oxide at a concentration of 20 to 40 ppm is theoretically ideal for this circumstance since it has negligible systemic effects. Experience with this intervention in the setting of persistent postoperative pulmonary hypertension, however, has been disappointing.

At the University of California, San Diego, the operative and perioperative mortality rate in the 196 patients who underwent PTE prior to 1990 was 15.8%. Between 1994 and 1998, in-hospital mortality in the 500 patients operated on during this time period was 8.8%, declining further to 4.4% for the 500 patients operated on between 1998 and 2002. Mortality rate over the last 500 cases has fallen to 2.2%. During this latter time frame, the major causes of death were related to reperfusion pulmonary edema and to residual postoperative pulmonary hypertension and right ventricular failure when PTE failed to achieve substantial improvement in pulmonary hemodynamics. Other centers involved with this procedure have experienced the same learning curve. The need for a coordinated, multidisciplinary team to manage the care of these patients cannot be emphasized too strongly. Experience and expertise in the evaluative, surgical, and postoperative aspects of care are essential to minimize the substantial morbidity and mortality associated with the surgical correction of this disease state.

Among survivors of thromboendarterectomy, the immediate hemodynamic improvement observed has been dramatic, with marked reductions in pulmonary artery pressures and pulmonary vascular resistance. Echocardiography demonstrates a decrease in right atrial and right ventricular chamber size, normalization of the interventricular septum, and improvement or resolution of tricuspid regurgitation. This improvement is reflected in the patient's postoperative physical examination and symptomatic status.

The long-term hemodynamic and symptomatic outcomes have been equally dramatic. Symptomatic improvement continues for periods as long as 9 to 12 months following surgery. This long-term improvement probably involves resolution of the patients' postoperative anemia and deconditioned state, as well as improvement in the ventilation/perfusion balance as the postoperative pulmonary artery steal resolves. In addition, resolution of the pulmonary hypertensive changes within the pulmonary vascular bed, suggested by preliminary scan and angiographic data, further reduces right ventricular afterload. The majority of patients who were initially in NYHA Class III or IV status preoperatively return to NYHA Class I or II status and are able to resume normal activities. One follow-up of 308 patients surveyed a mean of 3.3 years after surgery found that 62% of patients who were unemployed prior to thromboendarterectomy had returned to work.

Lung transplantation remains a therapeutic alternative for patients not deemed candidates for PTE based on the location and/or extent of their thromboembolic disease, and for patients who have undergone PTE with an inadequate hemodynamic outcome not responsive to medical therapy. Candidates have usually failed medical therapy as well and satisfy the other standard guidelines for transplantation. There are currently no data on how CTEPH patients fare following lung transplantation compared to other categories of patients.

Disease-modifying therapies developed for use in idiopathic pulmonary arterial hypertension (IPAH), including prostacyclin analogs, endothelin receptor antagonists, and phosphodiesterase-5 inhibitors have been studied in patients with CTEPH. Potential indications for medical therapy in CTEPH include: (1) surgically accessible CTEPH in patients who elect not to undergo surgery for personal choice or when comorbidities are so substantial as to exclude the patient from consideration of PTE, (2) distal chronic thromboembolic disease or limited central disease that is so disproportionate to the severity of the pulmonary hypertension that the surgical mortality risk of PTE is prohibitive, (3) use as a preoperative therapeutic "bridge" to surgery in patients with severe right ventricular dysfunction, and (4) management of persistent pulmonary hypertension following PTE.

In terms of the role of pulmonary hypertension-specific medical therapies, it is worth reiterating that PTE remains the definitive intervention for CTEPH. The hemodynamic and symptomatic benefits from medical therapy, although often positive, are modest in comparison to those resulting from PTE. A decision to forego PTE and to utilize medical therapy should be made only after a comprehensive evaluation has been performed, only for defined indications, and only after consultation with a center experienced in the management of this disease process.

Lifelong anticoagulation is strongly recommended after PTE. Thromboembolic recurrence can occur when anticoagulation is discontinued or maintained at a subtherapeutic level. Reoperative PTE is feasible with a perioperative risk comparable to primary PTE.

In summary, experience over the past 30+ years has demonstrated that CTEPH represents a potentially treatable form of pulmonary hypertension, and that PTE, when performed at a center experienced in the management of these patients, is capable of restoring severely compromised patients to near-normal or normal hemodynamic and symptomatic status.

FURTHER READING

1. Auger WR, Fedullo PF. Chronic thromboembolic pulmonary hypertension. *Semin Respir Crit Care Med.* 2009;30:471–483.

   Comprehensive review of chronic thromboembolic disease and its evaluation and management.

2. Klok FA, van Kralingen KW, van Dijk AP, et al. Prospective cardiopulmonary screening program to detect chronic thromboembolic pulmonary hypertension in patients after acute pulmonary embolism. *Haematologica.* 2010;95:970–975.

   In a cohort screening study involving 866 survivors of acute pulmonary embolism, four patients were ultimately diagnosed with CTEPH (confirmed by right-heart catheterization) for a cumulative incidence of CTEPH of 0.57%.

3. Wartski M, Collignon M-A. Incomplete recovery of lung perfusion after 3 months in patients with acute pulmonary embolism treated with antithrombotic agents. *J Nucl Med.* 2000;41:1043–1048.

   Residual perfusion scan abnormalities after 3 months were observed in 66% of patients experiencing an acute embolic event, with 8% of patients having defects greater than 50% of the total pulmonary vascular bed.

4. Miniati M, Monti S, Bottai M, et al. Survival and restoration of pulmonary perfusion in a long-term follow-up of patients after pulmonary embolism. *Medicine.* 2006;85:253–262.

Lung perfusion scan continued to demonstrate abnormalities in 35% of patients one year after the acute event, although the degree of pulmonary vascular obstruction was less than 15% in 90% of the patients.

5. Stein PD, Matta F, Musani MH, et al. Silent pulmonary embolism in patients with deep venous thrombosis: a systematic review. *Am J Med.* 2010;123:426–431.

Silent pulmonary embolism is diagnosed in 32% of patients with venous thrombosis.

6. Riedel M, Stanek V, Widimsky J, et al. Longterm follow-up of patients with pulmonary thromboembolism: late prognosis and evolution of hemodynamic and respiratory data. *Chest.* 1982;81:151–158.

Pulmonary hypertension occurred most frequently in patients with occult embolism. Pulmonary hypertension progressed further in patients with mean pulmonary artery pressure greater than 30 mmHg.

7. Wolf M, Soyer-Neumann C, Parent F, et al. Thrombotic risk factors in pulmonary hypertension. *Eur Respir J.* 2000;15:395–399.

Incidence of prothrombotic tendencies in CTEPH patients.

8. Bonderman D, Turecek PL, Jakowitsch J, et al. High prevalence of elevated clotting factor VIII in chronic thromboembolic pulmonary hypertension. *Thromb Haemost.* 2003;90:372–376.

CTEPH patients had significantly higher FVIII levels than controls.

9. Moser KM, Bloor CM. Pulmonary vascular lesions occurring in patients with chronic major vessel thromboembolic pulmonary hypertension. *Chest.* 1993;103:685–692.

A description of the small-vessel changes that occur in patients with CTEPH.

10. Morris TA, Auger WR, Ysrael MZ, et al. Parenchymal scarring is associated with restrictive spirometric defects in patients with chronic thromboembolic pulmonary hypertension. *Chest.* 1996;110:399–403.

Of patients referred for thromboendarterectomy, 22% had a restrictive ventilatory pattern. The presence of parenchymal scarring was highly associated with lung restriction.

11. Ryan KL, Fedullo PF, Davis GB, et al. Perfusion scan findings understate the severity of angiographic and hemodynamic compromise in chronic thromboembolic pulmonary hypertension. *Chest.* 1988;93:1180–1185.

Perfusion scans consistently understated the degree of pulmonary artery obstruction as defined by pulmonary angiography.

12. van der Plas MN, Reesink HJ, Roos CM, et al. Pulmonary endarterectomy improves dyspnea by the relief of dead space ventilation. *Ann Thorac Surg.* 2010;89:347–352.

Dead-space ventilation is increased in CTEPH and correlates with hemodynamic severity of disease and symptomatic dyspnea.

13. Pitton MB, Duber C, Mayer E, et al. Hemodynamic effects of nonionic contrast bolus injection and oxygen inhalation during pulmonary angiography in patients with chronic major-vessel thromboembolic pulmonary hypertension. *Circulation.* 1996;94:2485–2491.

Pulmonary angiography can be performed safely in patients with severe pulmonary hypertension secondary to chronic thromboembolic disease.

14. Auger WR, Fedullo PF, Moser KM, et al. Chronic major-vessel thromboembolic pulmonary artery obstruction: appearance at angiography. *Radiology.* 1992;182:393–398.

Angiographic patterns encountered in CTEPH.

15. Thistlethwaite PA, Kaneko K, Madani MM, et al. Techniques and outcomes of pulmonary endarterectomy surgery. *Ann Thorac Cardiovasc Surg.* 2008;14:274–282.

Discussion of the updated surgical approach and outcome in 1,100 patients undergoing thromboendarterectomy.

16. Olman MA, Auger WR, Fedullo PF, et al. Pulmonary vascular steal in chronic thromboembolic pulmonary hypertension. *Chest.* 1990;98:1430–1434.

A description of the pulmonary artery steal phenomenon occurring after thromboendarterectomy.

17. Levinson R, Shure D, Moser KM. Reperfusion pulmonary edema after pulmonary artery thromboendarterectomy. *Am Rev Respir Dis.* 1986;134:1241–1245.

Original description of reperfusion pulmonary edema occurring after thromboendarterectomy.

18. Corsico AG, D'Armini AM, Cerveri I, et al. Long-term outcome after pulmonary endarterectomy. *Am J Resp Crit Care Med.* 2008;178:419–424.

    Long-term survival and cardiopulmonary function recovery is excellent in most patients undergoing thromboendarterectomy.

19. Archibald CJ, Auger WR, Fedullo PF, et al. Long-term outcome after pulmonary thromboendarterectomy. *Am J Respir Crit Care Med.* 1999;160:523–528.

    Long-term symptomatic, quality-of-life, and functional follow-up in 308 patients undergoing thromboendarterectomy.

20. Condliffe R, Kiely DG, Gibbs JS, et al. Improved outcomes in medically and surgically treated chronic thromboembolic pulmonary hypertension. *Am J Respir Crit Care Med.* 2008;177:1122–1127.

    Long-term prognosis for patients with persistent pulmonary hypertension 3 months after thromboendarterectomy is good.

21. Becattini C, Manina G, Busti C, et al. Bosentan for chronic thromboembolic pulmonary hypertension: findings from a systematic review and meta-analysis. *Thromb Res.* 2010; 126:e51–e56.

    Bosentan therapy is associated with an improvement of hemodynamics and probably exercise capacity in patients with CTEPH.

22. Bresser P, Pepke-Zaba J, Jais X, et al. Medical therapies for chronic thromboembolic pulmonary hypertension. *Proc Am Thorac Soc.* 2006;3:594–600.

    Comprehensive review of medical therapies for chronic thromboembolic disease.

23. Suntharalingam J, Treacy CM, Doughty NJ, et al. Long-term use of sildenafil in inoperable chronic thromboembolic pulmonary hypertension. *Chest.* 2008;134:229–236.

    Pilot study that suggests benefit of sildenafil in CTEPH.

24. Reichelt A, Hoeper MM, Galanski M, et al. Chronic thromboembolic pulmonary hypertension: evaluation with 64-detector row versus digital subtraction angiography. *Eur J Radiol.* 2009;71:49–54.

    Comparison of 64-detector row with digital subtraction angiography in the preoperative evaluation of patients with CTEPH.

Unusual Forms of Embolism

Peter F. Fedullo

Because the lung receives all of the blood flow returned from the venous system, the pulmonary vascular bed serves as a "sieve" for all particulate substances entering the venous blood and is the first vascular bed to be exposed to any toxic substance injected intravenously. As a result of its strategic position, the pulmonary vascular bed is, therefore, exposed to a wide variety of potentially obstructing and injurious agents.

SCHISTOSOMIASIS

Among such agents, the most common worldwide, though not in the United States, is schistosomiasis. Schistosomiasis is caused by one of a variety of blood flukes, *Schistosoma haematobium* (Africa and Middle East), *S. japonicum* (Japan, China, Philippines), *S. mansoni* (Africa, Arabia, South America), *S. mekongi* (Laos, Thailand), and *S. intercalatum* (Africa) being among the most common. Limited data suggest that cardiopulmonary schistosomiasis is seen most often in *S. mansoni* and *S. Japonicum* infection.

Infection occurs after contact with water containing the infective stage of the parasite, the cercaria. The cerceria penetrate unbroken skin and subcutaneous tissue and migrate through the lungs and then to the portal vein, probably by an intravascular route. The maturing schistosomes pair in the portal vein and then migrate to the venules of the mesentery, bladder, or ureters and begin to deposit eggs, many of which are subsequently swept back to the liver.

During acute infection (Katayama fever), nonspecific influenza-like symptoms, abdominal pain, lymphadenopathy, hepatosplenomegaly, and blood eosinophilia associated with fleeting chest radiographic abnormalities can occur.

Pulmonary hypertension occurs in less than 5% of infected patients. Cor pulmonale related to schistosomal infection usually does not occur in the absence of concomitant liver schistosomal liver disease because the liver is involved, usually quite extensively, before pulmonary involvement. Pulmonary vascular obstruction appears to be induced by two mechanisms: anatomic obstruction by the organism itself and by an intense, granulomatous, inflammatory vasculitic response to shunted and embolized schistosomal eggs. In endemic areas, schistosomal disease is the most common cause of cor pulmonale.

The premortem diagnosis of cardiopulmonary schistosomiasis depends on the detection of viable schistosomal ova in stool, urine, or tissue (rectal mucosa or lung) along with evidence of hepatic fibrosis and pulmonary hypertension. Currently utilized serologic tests only indicate past or present infection, although promising serologic markers capable of differentiating acute from chronic disease are being investigated. Treatment with praziquantel can effectively eradicate schistosomal infections in the acute phase of the disease with minimal toxicity. However, chronic cardiopulmonary manifestations are not likely to be reversible given the fibrotic changes that are present.

AIR EMBOLISM

An increasingly common form of nonthrombotic embolism in the United States is venous air embolism. The increasing frequency reflects the wide variety of invasive surgical and medical procedures now available, broad use of indwelling central venous catheters, use of positive pressure ventilation with high levels of positive end expiratory pressure, and the frequency of thoracic and other forms of trauma. The simple inadvertent transection or loss of closure of a large-bore intravenous catheter, particularly in the jugular or subclavian vein, can result in ingress of substantial quantities of air. Air bubbles enter the pulmonary vascular bed and, from there, can enter the arterial system and be diffusely distributed throughout the body by way of either an intracardiac shunt (atrial septal defect, patent foramen ovale) or, more likely, through microvascular pulmonary shunts. Direct arterial gas embolism has been reported with transthoracic diagnostic procedures with inadvertent entry into a pulmonary vein.

The lethal volume of injected air in humans is estimated to be in the range of 100 to 500 mL. Physiologic consequences include an abrupt rise in pulmonary artery pressure. Non-cardiogenic pulmonary edema may develop, lung compliance falls, and hypoxemia ensues. The elevated pulmonary artery pressure may result in elevated right atrial pressure and subsequent paradoxical embolization. Gas entry into the systemic circulation results in ischemia of the affected organ.

The symptoms of venous air embolism are variable and nonspecific, and may include alterations in sensorium, chest pain, dyspnea, or a sense of impending doom. These and other consequences appear to be due to two phenomena: actual lodgment of the bubbles in capillary beds that interfere with nutrient supply to the affected organs, and the formation of platelet-fibrin aggregates, creating diffuse microthrombi. Thrombocytopenia may be seen as a consequence of this latter event. The most serious consequences result from cerebral or coronary artery air embolism, the severity of the consequences depending upon the rate and volume of air gaining access to the circulation.

The best approaches to air embolism are prevention and early detection. Aggressive treatment is essential and should consist of measures designed to restore flow and promote reabsorption of the intravascular air. Measures designed to restore flow include patient positioning (Trendelenburg position with the left side down), removal of air through central venous catheters or direct needle aspiration, and closed chest cardiac massage. Measures designed to increase absorption include the use of 100% oxygen and the institution of hyperbaric oxygen therapy as early as possible. Recovery following delayed institution of hyperbaric oxygen has been reported. Utilizing such aggressive measures, mortality from venous air embolism has been reduced dramatically.

FAT EMBOLISM

Another reasonably frequent and dramatic form of nonthrombotic embolism is fat embolism. By far, the most common inciting event is traumatic fracture of long bones, with incidence rising with the number of fractures. However, orthopedic procedures and trauma to other fat-laden tissues (e.g., fatty liver) occasionally can be followed by the same syndrome. Although considerably less common, fat embolism syndrome has been reported following both liposuction and lipoinjection procedures.

A rather characteristic syndrome follows entry of neutral fat into the vascular system, consisting of the onset of dyspnea, hypoxemia, petechiae, and mental status changes. Seizures and focal neurologic deficits have been described. There is a variable lag time of 24 to 72 hours in the onset of the syndrome following the inciting event; rarely, cases occur within 12 hours or as late as 2 weeks after the event.

The variability in incidence of the syndrome after apparently comparable injuries has not been well-defined; neither has the reason for the delay in clinical presentation been explained. The pathophysiologic consequences appear to derive from two events: (1) actual vascular obstruction by neutral particles of fat and (2) the injurious effects of free fatty acids released by the action of lipases on the neutral fat. The latter effect is probably more important, causing diffuse vasculitis with leakage from cerebral, pulmonary, and other vascular beds. The time necessary to produce toxic intermediaries may explain the delay from the inciting event to clinical presentation.

The diagnosis of fat embolism syndrome is a clinical one suggested by the onset of dyspnea, neurologic abnormalities, petechiae, and fever in the proper clinical context. Chest imaging studies may demonstrate bilateral infiltrates, ground glass opacities, and centrilobular and subpleural nodules. Petechiae, typically distributed over the head, neck, anterior chest, and axillae are present in only 20% to 50% of cases. Their absence, therefore, should not preclude consideration of the disease. No laboratory test is diagnostic of the syndrome. Fat can be demonstrated in the serum of a majority of fracture patients with evidence of fat embolism syndrome. The finding of lipid-laden cells in bronchoalveolar lavage fluid appears to occur commonly in patients with traumatic injuries, irrespective of the presence of fat embolism syndrome.

Although a variety of treatments have been suggested (e.g., intravenous ethanol, albumin, dextran, heparin), none has proven effective. The role of corticosteroid therapy to prevent the onset of fat embolism syndrome after an inciting event remains controversial. Supportive treatment, including mechanical ventilatory support when necessary, is the primary approach, and survival is now the rule with meticulous support.

AMNIOTIC FLUID EMBOLISM

Another special form of embolism is amniotic fluid embolism, a rare but unpredictable and catastrophic complication of pregnancy that represents the third leading cause of maternal mortality. This disorder occurs during or after delivery when amniotic fluid gains access to uterine venous channels and, therefore, to the pulmonary and systemic circulations. The delivery may be either spontaneous or by cesarean section and is usually uneventful. Most cases occur during labor, but delayed onset of symptoms up to 48 hours after delivery can occur. Although specific risk factors have not yet been identified, advanced maternal age, multiparity, premature placental separation, fetal death, and meconium staining of amniotic fluid have been associated with increased risk of amniotic fluid embolism.

Amniotic fluid embolism syndrome is primarily a clinical diagnosis. There is, unexpectedly, sudden onset of severe respiratory distress, cyanosis, hypotension, cardiovascular collapse, and, often, disseminated intravascular coagulation. Occasionally, seizure activity occurs. It has been postulated that there is a biphasic pattern of hemodynamic disturbance: an initial period of pulmonary hypertension, commonly seen in animal models, followed by left ventricular dysfunction and cardiogenic shock. Patients who survive the first several hours develop noncardiogenic pulmonary edema coincident with improvement in left ventricular dysfunction.

Amniotic fluid does contain particulate materials that can cause pulmonary vascular obstruction, but the major pathogenetic mechanism of the syndrome remains uncertain. Amniotic fluid does have thromboplastic activity that leads to extensive fibrin deposition in the lung vasculature and, occasionally, in other organs. As a consequence of fibrin deposition, a severe consumptive coagulopathy develops, including marked hypofibrinogenemia and thrombocytopenia. Following the acute event, an enhanced fibrinolytic state often occurs.

The diagnosis of amniotic fluid embolism is based on a compatible clinical picture, often enhanced by finding amniotic fluid components in the pulmonary circulation. The presence of squamous cells in pulmonary arterial blood, once considered pathognomonic, has proven to be a nonspecific finding. Serological assays and immunohistochemical staining techniques have been described as having high sensitivity for amniotic fluid embolism. Validation will be required prior to being introduced into clinical practice.

Although various forms of therapy have been suggested (e.g., antifibrinolytic agents such as aminocaproic acid, cryoprecipitate), the best approach is supportive. Pulmonary artery catheterization is essential to monitor left ventricular function and volume status and to guide the appropriate utilization of inotropic and vasoactive agents. Even in the setting of aggressive supportive measures, however, maternal mortality has approached 80%.

SEPTIC EMBOLISM

Septic embolism is another special disorder that, unfortunately, is also increasing in frequency owing to widespread intravenous drug abuse and the expanding use of indwelling intravenous catheters. Previously, septic embolism was almost exclusively a complication of septic pelvic thrombophlebitis due to both septic abortion and postpuerperal uterine infection. However, almost any venous structure can be involved, either as a focus of primary infection or from intravascular or contiguous spread, for example, septic cavernous sinus thrombosis resulting from meningitis, sinusitis, or facial cellulitis; septic portal vein thrombosis resulting from diverticulitis or liver abscess; and septic tonsillar or internal jugular vein thrombosis (Lemierre syndrome) resulting from oropharyngeal infection. Increasingly common causes are those related to intravenous drug use and those that are iatrogenic; namely, infections secondary to indwelling catheters inserted for a variety of diagnostic or therapeutic purposes.

Microscopically, septic phlebitis consists of purulent material admixed with fibrin thrombus. Embolization from such material does occur and can result in obstruction of small pulmonary vessels, but the major consequence is pulmonary infection. Characteristically, the chest roentgenogram displays scattered pulmonary infiltrates that undergo cavitation. An increasing number of such infiltrates develops over periods of hours to a few days. Symptoms and signs include a septic temperature course, dyspnea, cough, pleuritic chest pain, and hemoptysis. Initial treatment consists of appropriate antimicrobial drugs. If an indwelling catheter is the source of the infection, it should be removed. If there is not a prompt response to this regimen, surgical isolation of the septic vein, if present, should be considered. The role of systemic anticoagulation remains uncertain. Endocarditis may complicate septic phlebitis, or mimic it, particularly in drug addicts.

TUMOR EMBOLISM

Involvement of the pulmonary vascular bed by tumor cells is not unusual, given the frequency with which circulating tumor cells can be identified in patients with a wide range of malignancies and the frequency with which tumor emboli are discovered as an incidental finding at autopsy. Tumor embolism becomes clinically apparent, however, in only a minority of patients with malignancy.

Microvascular tumor embolism is associated with a wide range of malignancies, the most common sites of origin being the breast, lung, prostate, stomach, and liver. Tumor embolism of large fragments occurs rarely and may mimic acute thromboembolic disease. In this setting, survival following tumor embolectomy has been reported.

The clinical presentation of microvascular tumor embolism is typically subacute and involves progressive dyspnea, tachycardia, and tachypnea. Jugular venous distention, a prominent P2, tricuspid regurgitation or a right-sided S3 may be present on physical examination if the extent of pulmonary vascular obstruction is sufficient to cause pulmonary hypertension.

The development of pulmonary hypertension is a common accompaniment of symptomatic, microvascular tumor embolism and remains a major cause of mortality. Pulmonary hypertension appears to result from both obliteration of the pulmonary vascular bed by an admixture of tumor cells and thrombus as well as the development of medial hypertrophy, intimal fibrosis, and fibrinoid necrosis encountered in other variants of pulmonary hypertension.

Hypoxemia and a compensated respiratory alkalosis are commonly present. The chest radiograph is most often normal but focal or diffuse infiltrates, which may be fleeting, have been described. Ventilation–perfusion scanning most commonly demonstrates a mottled appearance or peripheral, subsegmental defects; segmental or larger defects, indistinguishable from those associated with thromboembolic embolism, may occur in those rare instances of large-vessel involvement. Computed tomography may demonstrate peripheral, wedge-shaped defects consistent with infarcts; a pattern of multifocal dilatation and beading of the peripheral pulmonary arteries has been described. Tree-in-bud opacities may also be present. In the setting of pulmonary hypertension, echocardiographic findings will reflect that diagnosis and include evidence of right atrial and right ventricular hypertrophy, abnormal septal position and motion, and a tricuspid regurgitant envelope consistent with elevated pulmonary artery pressures.

Pulmonary angiographic findings are most commonly normal. Delayed vascular filling, pruning, and tortuosity, similar to that seen in other forms of small-vessel pulmonary hypertension, may be encountered. The angiographic findings in large fragment tumor embolism may be indistinguishable from those seen in acute thromboembolic disease.

Pulmonary microvascular cytology on specimens aspirated through a wedged pulmonary artery catheter may demonstrate malignant cells. Positive cytologies, however, can also be obtained in the setting of lymphangitic carcinomatosis. It should also be emphasized that the misidentification of megakaryocytes obtained in this manner has been reported to lead to false-positive results.

Although diagnosis by transbronchial biopsy has been reported, diagnostic confirmation may require open-lung biopsy. Before proceeding to that step, however, it must be stressed that the impact of early diagnosis on outcome is uncertain. This intervention should only be considered in the setting of a primary malignancy for which effective chemotherapeutic options are available.

The differential diagnosis of tumor embolism includes thrombotic embolism, parenchymal metastasis, lymphangitic carcinomatosis, malignant pericardial effusion, and chemotherapy-related lung toxicity. The premortem diagnosis is often one of exclusion. Parenchymal metastasis, lymphangitic carcinomatosis, and chemotherapy-related lung toxicity can be differentiated from tumor embolism by findings on high resolution computed tomography.

Differentiation of tumor embolism from thrombotic embolism may be somewhat more problematic, especially if there is large-vessel involvement. Under most circumstances, however, pulmonary angiography is capable of differentiating thrombotic embolism from microvascular tumor embolism.

OTHER EMBOLI

Because of its sieve function, the lung may also be embolized on occasion by a wide variety of other materials. Trophoblastic tissue can escape the uterus and lodge in the pulmonary circulation during pregnancy or in the setting of malignant trophoblastic disease. After head trauma, brain tissue has been found in the lungs; the same is true of liver cells following abdominal trauma and of bone marrow after cardiopulmonary resuscitation.

Finally, in this era of intravenous drug abuse, noninfectious vasculitic–thrombotic complications are being seen with increasing frequency, in association with the intravenous use of drugs intended for oral use. Medications implicated with pulmonary complications include methylphenidate hydrochloride, oral opiates (pentazocine, meperidine), and antihistamines. Particulate and irritant drug carriers (e.g., talc and cellulose) and occasionally the drugs themselves may cause vascular inflammation and secondary thrombosis. The clinical presentation may be diverse and includes lower lobe emphysema, diffuse interstitial fibrosis, and progressive massive fibrosis. Repetitive insults may lead to severe and irreversible pulmonary hypertension. In many intravenous drug users, perfusion scans demonstrate segmental or smaller defects. Distinguishing these defects from those due to venous thromboembolism may be difficult.

The diagnosis is often suggested by the clinical history. Radiographic findings include small, diffuse, well-defined nodular densities. These nodules can progress and massive fibrosis may ensue. Lower lobe emphysematous changes may also be present. Diagnostic confirmation often requires lung biopsy, either open or transbronchial. The prognosis is poor, with progressive pulmonary disease being the rule.

FURTHER READING

1. Jorens PG, Van Marck E, Parizel PM. Nonthrombotic pulmonary embolism. *Eur Respir J.* 2009;34:452–474.

   Comprehensive, well-referenced review.

2. Montagnana M, Cervellin G, Franchini M, et al. Pathophysiology, clinics and diagnostics of non-thrombotic pulmonary embolism. *J Thromb Thrombolysis.* 2011;31:436–444.

   Comprehensive, well-referenced review.

3. Han D, Lee KS, Franquet T, et al. Thrombotic and non-thrombotic pulmonary arterial embolism: spectrum of imaging studies. *Radiographics.* 2003;23:1521–1539.

   Reviews radiologic findings in both thrombotic and nonthrombotic pulmonary embolism.

4. Kolosionek E, Crosby A, Harhay MO, et al. Pulmonary vascular disease associated with schistosomiasis. *Expert Rev Anti Infect Ther.* 2010;8:1467–1473.

   Concise review of the cardiopulmonary manifestations of schistosomal disease.

5. Palmer PE. Schistosomiasis. *Semin Roentgenol.* 1998;33:6–25.

   Review with emphasis on radiographic manifestations of schistosomal disease.

6. Mirski MA, Lele AV, Fitzsimmons L, et al. Diagnosis and treatment of vascular air embolism. *Anesthesiology.* 2007;106:164–177.

   Comprehensive, well-referenced review.

7. Tibbles PM, Edelsberg JS. Hyperbaric-oxygen treatment. *N Engl J Med.* 1996;334:1642–1648.

   Review of the indications for hyperbaric-oxygen treatment, including air embolism.

8. Morris WP, Butler BD, Tonnesen AS, et al. Continuous venous air embolism in patients receiving positive end-expiratory pressure. *Am Rev Respir Dis.* 1993;147:1034–1037.

   Description of three patients in whom continuous air embolism in the inferior vena cava that persisted for days was detected. The bubbles appeared to arise from splanchnic veins, and they were associated with barotrauma and positive airway pressure.

9. Alvaran SB, Tuong JK, Graff TE, et al. Venous air embolism: comparative merits of external cardiac massage, intracardiac aspiration, and left lateral decubitus position. *Anesth Analg.* 1978;57:166–170.

   In an animal model of venous air embolism, intracardiac aspiration was not superior to either external cardiac massage of left lateral decubitus position despite the shorter resuscitation time.

10. Bou-Assaly W, Pernicano P, Hoeffner E. Systemic air embolism after transthoracic lung biopsy: a case report and review of the literature. *World J Radiol.* 2010;2:193–196.

    World literature review of gas embolism associated with transthoracic needle procedures.

11. Ely EW, Hite RD, Baker AM, et al. Venous air embolism from central venous catheterization: a need for increased physician awareness. *Crit Care Med.* 1999;27:2113–2117.

    Awareness of venous air embolism or its prevention did not correlate with the level of physician training, experience, or specialty.

12. Wysoki MG, Covey A, Pollak J, et al. Evaluation of various maneuvers for prevention of air embolism during central venous catheter placement. *J Vasc Interv Radiol.* 2001;12:764–766.

Valsalva maneuver is superior to breath-hold and humming for increasing central venous pressure during central line placement.

13. Johnson MJ, Lucas GL. Fat embolism syndrome. *Orthopedics*. 1996;19:41–48.

    Review of the classic and current literature on fat embolism syndrome with regard to its causes, pathophysiology, clinical presentation, diagnosis, and treatment.

14. Roger N, Xzaubet A, Agusti C, et al. Role of bronchoalveolar lavage in the diagnosis of fat embolism syndrome. *Eur Respir J*. 1995;8:1275–1280.

    BAL oil red O positive macrophages were frequently observed in trauma patients irrespective of the presence of fat embolism syndrome.

15. Habashi NM, Andrews PL, Scalea TM. Therapeutic aspects of fat embolism syndrome. *Injury*. 2006;37(suppl 4):S68–S73.

    Concise review of the management of fat embolism syndrome.

16. Bederman SS, Bhandari M, McKee MD, et al. Do corticosteroids reduce the risk of fat embolism syndrome in patients with long bone fractures? A meta-analysis. *Can J Surg*. 2009;52:386–393.

    Corticosteroids may be beneficial in preventing the fat embolism syndrome and hypoxia but not mortality in patients with long bone fractures.

17. Conde-Agudelo A, Romero R. Amniotic fluid embolism: an evidence-based review. *Am J Obstet Gynecol*. 2009;201:445.e1– 445.e13.

    Comprehensive review of the pathophysiology, clinical presentation, diagnosis, and therapy of amniotic fluid embolism.

18. Clark SL, Montz FJ, Phelan JP. Hemodynamic alterations associated with amniotic fluid embolism: a reappraisal. *Am J Obstet Gynecol*. 1985;151:617–621.

    Presentation of a model of hemodynamic changes accompanying amniotic fluid embolism that incorporates both experimental and clinical observations.

19. Clark SL, Hankins GD, Dudley DA, et al. Amniotic fluid embolism: analysis of the national registry. *Am J Obstet Gynecol*. 1995;172:1158–1167.

    In a review of 61 cases of amniotic fluid embolism, maternal mortality was 61%, with neurologically intact survival seen in only 15% of women. Of fetuses in utero at the time of the event, only 39% survived.

20. Julander I. Staphylococcal septicaemia and endocarditis in 80 drug users. *Scand J Infect Dis*. 1983;41:49–54.

    Descriptive report of 80 patients with staphylococcal sepsis. Endocarditis was documented or suspected in 65% of patients.

21. Raad I, Hanna H, Maki D. Intravascular catheter-related infections: advances in diagnosis, prevention and management. *Lancet Infect Dis*. 2007;7:645–657.

    Comprehensive, well-referenced review.

22. Oim GM, Jeffrey RB Jr, Ralls PW, et al. Septic thrombophlebitis of the portal vein: CT and clinical observations. *J Comput Assist Tomogr*. 1989;13:656–658.

    Review of the CT and clinical findings in seven patients with septic thrombosis of the portal vein.

23. Ebright JR, Pace MT, Niazi AF. Septic thrombosis of the cavernous sinuses. *Arch Intern Med*. 2001;161:2671–2676.

    Mortality has decreased from 80% to 100% in the preantibiotic era to 20% to 30%.

24. Kniemeyer HW, Grabitz K, Buhl R, et al. Surgical treatment of septic deep venous thrombosis. *Surgery*. 1995;118:49–53.

    In complicated cases of septic deep vein thrombosis without improvement after conservative management, venous thrombectomy can be a lifesaving procedure.

25. Plemmons RM, Dooley DP, Longfield RN. Septic thrombophlebitis of the portal vein (pylephlebitis): diagnosis and management in the modern era. *Clin Infect Dis*. 1995;21:1114–1120.

    Case report and review of the literature.

26. Browne CE, Stettler RW, Twickler D, et al. Puerperal septic pelvic thrombophlebitis: incidence and response to heparin therapy. *Am J Obstet Gynecol*. 1999;181:143–148.

Women given heparin in addition to antimicrobial therapy for septic thrombophlebitis did not have a better outcome than did those for whom antimicrobial therapy alone was continued.

27. Kubik-Huch RA, Hebisch G, Huch R, et al. Role of duplex color Doppler ultrasound, computed tomography, and MR angiography in the diagnosis of septic puerperal ovarian vein thrombosis. *Abdom Imaging.* 1999;24:85–91.

Magnetic resonance angiography is recommended in patients with inconclusive duplex color Doppler ultrasound findings and persistent suspicion for septic puerperal ovarian vein thrombosis

28. Karkos PD, Asrani S, Karkos CD, et al. Lemierre's syndrome: a systematic review. *Laryngoscopy.* 2009;119:1552–1559.

Comprehensive, well-referenced review.

29. Roberts KE, Hamele-Bena D, Saqu A, et al. Pulmonary tumor embolism: a review of the literature. *Am J Med.* 2003;115:228–232.

Comprehensive, well-referenced review of pulmonary tumor embolism.

30. Goldhaber SZ, Dricker E, Buring JE, et al. Clinical suspicion of autopsy-proven thrombotic and tumor pulmonary embolism in cancer patients. *Am Heart J.* 1987;114:1432–1435.

Of 73 patients with solid malignant tumors and PE, 56 had major thrombotic PE and 17 had major tumor embolism to the lungs. Of the 56 with cancer and thrombotic PE, 45% had the correct diagnosis suspected antemortem. By contrast, in only 6% of patients with tumor embolism was the diagnosis made correctly antemortem.

31. Shepard JA, Moore EH, Templeton PA, et al. Pulmonary intravascular tumor emboli: dilated and beaded peripheral pulmonary arteries at CT. *Radiology.* 1993;187:797–801.

Description of the chest CT scan findings in four patients with intravascular tumor emboli.

32. Marchiori E, Lourenco S, Gasparetto TD, et al. Pulmonary talcosis: imaging findings. *Lung.* 2010;188:165–171.

Description of the clinical and radiologic findings in patients with pulmonary talcosis.

73

Pulmonary Hypertension: Pathogenesis and Etiology

Amy L. Firth and Jason X.-J. Yuan

Establishing an accurate diagnosis of pulmonary hypertension (PH) is essential for proficient management of the disease. Indeed, several distinct cardiopulmonary diseases are encompassed by PH. Each requires an in-depth knowledge of the normal pulmonary vasculature and the pathophysiological progression of the disease.

The pulmonary vascular bed is normally a high-flow, low-resistance and low-pressure system that transports blood to the pulmonary capillaries; here, oxygen is taken up by the venous blood and excess carbon dioxide is unloaded through the blood–gas barrier. The complex branching structure of pulmonary vessels from the main pulmonary artery to small resistance vessels is described by three models: the Weibel model, the Strahler model, and the diameter-defined Strahler model. Regardless of the model used, the total resistance in the pulmonary vascular bed is dependent upon the intraluminal diameter, or cross-sectional area, of the pulmonary arteries. A reduction in this diameter can result from three fundamental pathologic processes: vasoconstriction, obstruction, and obliteration.

Pulmonary artery pressure (PAP) is calculated as a product of cardiac output (CO) and pulmonary vascular resistance (PVR), represented by the formula PAP = CO × PVR. While PAP is known to vary with age, the mean PAP is approximately 20 mmHg. It might be expected that during intense exercise there would be a large increase in PAP due to the increase in CO, but only a small increase is observed as the compliance of the pulmonary vascular wall compensates by increasing the cross-sectional area of the vessels through vasodilation and recruitment of previously unperfused vessels. The major cause of elevated PVR in PH patients is a decrease in pulmonary arterial wall compliance (e.g., an increase in vascular wall stiffness due to vascular remodeling is the major cause of elevated PVR in PH patients). In the early stages of PH, it is common for PAP and PVR to be normal under resting conditions; however, when blood flow increases, there is a notable increase in PAP. Resting PH ensues as the disease progresses. To sustain the increase in PAP, an increase in the musculature of the right ventricle is necessary. Right ventricular hypertrophy is thus an indicative feature of sustained PAP in PH. If the right ventricular afterload is high enough, right-sided heart failure develops, manifesting as resting dyspnea, jugular venous distension, hepatic congestion, ascites, and dependent edema.

It cannot be understated that PH, in whichever form it may present clinically, is a phenomenon comprising many unique but interrelated mechanisms at a cellular level. The arterial remodeling itself can encompass activation and proliferation of an array of cell types including endothelial cells, fibroblasts, myofibroblasts, and vascular smooth muscle cells (SMC). Pulmonary vasoconstriction, generally associated with chronic exposure to hypoxia, eventually leads to hypertrophy of the medial SMC layer of the artery, compromising the integrity of the vessel lumen. Consequences unfold and vascular wall tension will increase, leading to further proliferation and intimal scarring. Intimal lesions/fibrosis are common to most forms of PH. The pulmonary vascular bed integrity is maintained by a fine balance between apoptosis and proliferation; when either of these processes is compromised, arteriopathic changes occur in the pulmonary vasculature.

During the 4th World Symposium on PH held in 2008 in Dana Point, CA, experts in the field decided to modify the clinical classification of PH previously established in 2003 at the 3rd World Symposium held in Venice. The current classification is summarized in Table 73-1. Correctly distinguishing the pathogenesis of PH is of upmost importance when it comes to discerning the most effective treatment régime for the patient. The new classification system has been associated with notable improvements in the quality and efficacy of clinical care for PH patients. Class I, known as pulmonary arterial hypertension (PAH), encompasses idiopathic and hereditary PAH, among others. Patients with a mean PAP greater than 25 mmHg without evidence of increased wedge pressure, parenchymal lung disorders, or thromboembolic disease are considered to have PAH. Historically, idiopathic pulmonary arterial hypertension (IPAH, previously known as primary pulmonary hypertension) occurs without demonstrable etiology. Secondary PH, on the other hand, develops as a complication of other diseases. The hereditable nature of PAH is usually due to mutations in the bone morphogenetic protein receptor type 2 gene (*BMPR2*) or, less commonly, members of the transforming growth factor-β superfamily, namely activin-like kinase 1 (ALK1) and endoglin (ENG). The latter two are associated with hereditary hemorrhagic telangiectasia. While approximately 20% of patients with IPAH and 70% of those with hereditary PAH have heterozygous germline mutations in *BMPR2*, they a have variable lifetime penetrance of about 10% to 20% and, even if identified, there are no known preventative measures.

As mentioned previously, PAH is a common, often rare but life-threatening secondary complication of other conditions, most notably connective tissue diseases, HIV infection, portal hypertension (portopulmonary hypertension or PoPH), and congenital heart disease. PoPH has a prevalence of about 5% to 6% of patients with decompensated liver disease in which significant vascular remodeling increases PAP and PVR. A definitive diagnosis typically requires right heart catheterization. Furthermore, liver cirrhosis can also be complicated by hepatopulmonary syndrome (HPS) caused by intrapulmonary arteriovenous shunting with resultant hypoxemia. While HPS remains refractory to treatment, PoPH is responsive to vasodilators and improvement in pulmonary hemodynamics. Using PAH-specific therapies such as endothelin receptor antagonists may overcome the contraindication for liver transplantation. HIV-related PAH is of

TABLE 73-1	Revised Nomenclature of Pulmonary Hypertension

Class 1: Pulmonary Arterial Hypertension (PAH)

1.1. Idiopathic PAH
1.2. Hereditable
    1.2.1. *BMPR2*
    1.2.2. ALK1, endoglin (with/without hereditary hemorrhagic telangiectasia)
    1.2.3. Unknown
1.3. Drug- and toxin-induced
1.4. Associated with...
    1.4.1. Connective tissue diseases
    1.4.2. HIV infection
    1.4.3. Portal hypertension
    1.4.4. Congenital heart diseases
    1.4.5. Schistosomiasis
    1.4.6. Chronic hemolytic anemia
1.5. Persistent pulmonary hypertension of the newborn (PPHN)
1.6. Pulmonary veno-occlusive disease (PVOD) and/or pulmonary capillary hemangiomatosis (PCH)

Class 2: Pulmonary Hypertension owing to Left Heart Disease

2.1. Systolic dysfunction
2.2. Diastolic dysfunction
2.3. Valvular disease

Class 3: Pulmonary Hypertension owing to Lung Diseases and/or Hypoxia

3.1. Chronic obstructive pulmonary disease (COPD)
3.2. Interstitial lung disease
3.3. Other pulmonary diseases with mixed restrictive and obstructive patterns
3.4. Sleep-disordered breathing
3.5. Alveolar hypoventilation disorders
3.6. Developmental abnormalities

Class 4: Chronic Thromboembolic Pulmonary Hypertension (CTEPH)

Class 5: Pulmonary Hypertension with Unclear Multifactorial Mechanisms

5.1. Hematologic disorders: myeloproliferative disorders, splenectomy
5.2. Systemic disorders: sarcodosis, pulmonary Langerhans cell
    Histiocytosis: lymphangioleiomyomatosis, neurofibromatosis, vasculitis
5.3. Metabolic disorders: glycogen storage disease, Gaucher disease, thyroid disorders
5.4. Others: tumoral obstruction, fibrosing mediastinitis, chronic renal failure on dialysis

unknown etiology and can be associated with both early and late stages of immunodeficiency. Theories for pathogenesis currently focus on smooth muscle and endothelial cell injury postulated to be due to elevated levels of cytokines (e.g., ET-1, IL-6, and PDGF). The appetite suppressant fenfluramine was withdrawn from the market in 1997 due to its association with PAH. More recently (1998–2009), the fenfluramine derivative Benfluorex (on the market since 1976) has also been associated with PAH and valve disorders; these contraindications are currently being formally assessed.

While PAH may be associated with a variety of conditions, response to therapy and pathophysiological abnormalities remain somewhat consistent, with a spectrum of microvascular lesions observed in the small resistance arteries. Despite the cellular and molecular pathways being currently undefined, these lesions include medial hypertrophy, intimal fibrosis, plexiform lesions (endothelial outgrowths from the pulmonary arteriole intima into the lumen at branches in the pulmonary arteries), and microthrombotic lesions.

Another form of IPAH is pulmonary veno-occlusive disease (PVOD) and/or pulmonary capillary hemangiomatosis (PCH). Prognosis for these diseases is still bleak (<2 years) despite significant recent advancements in understanding and treatment. The main histopathological hallmark of the disease is widespread fibrous intimal proliferation, predominantly involving the pulmonary venules and small veins. PVOD mimics other forms of PAH and is clinically impossible to distinguish. Treatment with pulmonary vasodilators is possible; however, these often precipitate pulmonary edema due to increasing pulmonary blood flow with "fixed" outflow (pulmonary vein) obstruction. It is also worth noting that elevation in pulmonary venous pressure can occur with any disorder impairing pulmonary venous outflow, including systolic and diastolic left ventricular dysfunction, mitral stenosis, and, less commonly, disorders of the pericardium or pulmonary veins themselves. Similar pathogenesis is observed with mild PH, augmented by vasoconstriction and, when sustained, hypertrophy and intimal proliferation. At this point, treating the elevated pulmonary venous pressure (e.g., repair of mitral stenosis) should still be considered.

Persistent pulmonary hypertension of the newborn (PPHN) develops when PVR remains elevated after birth. Right-to-left shunting of blood through fetal circulatory pathways occurs and PVR remains elevated due to pulmonary hypoplasia, maldevelopment, and poor adaptation of the pulmonary arteries and vascular bed. Potential therapeutic targets currently being pursued include inhibition of phosphodiesterase-5 activity (Sildenafil), activation of guanylate cyclase (BAY 41-2272), and recombinant human vascular endothelial growth factor (rhVEGF), administered by intrapulmonary infusion.

Chronic obstructive pulmonary disease (COPD), interstitial lung disease, and widespread parenchymal destructive processes (tuberculosis) are parenchymal pulmonary diseases directly associated with the development of PH. The prevalence of PH in patients with advanced COPD is high; it usually presents with moderate severity (mean PAP are typically <40 mmHg) and progresses slowly. Hypoxemia is believed to be the major cause of PH in COPD; this leads to vascular remodeling characterized by intimal proliferation of poorly differentiated SMCs and the deposition of elastic and collagen fibers. The disease manifests with impairment of endothelial function in the earliest stages leading to decreased vasodilator release (e.g., NO). PH is an under-recognized complication of interstitial lung diseases (ILD), which most commonly include connective tissue disease-related ILD, sarcoidosis, idiopathic pulmonary fibrosis, and pulmonary Langerhans cell histiocytosis. Diagnosis can be difficult and often overlooked as the clinical presentation is fairly nonspecific; associated pathologies include pulmonary vasoconstriction, pulmonary vascular remodeling, vascular inflammation, perivascular fibrosis, and thrombotic angiopathy.

In obstructive sleep apnea (OSA), PH can cause functional limitation and increased mortality; however, it usually presents in a milder form induced by hypoxemia, hypercapnia, or acidosis. This applies similarly to other hypoventilation syndromes, including central alveolar hypoventilation and obesity–hypoventilation syndrome. Structural changes in the pulmonary vasculature are rare and current treatment options are restricted to treatment of the underlying diseases. Clinical trials have been proposed for newer vasodilator drugs, which may improve the prognosis.

Chronic thromboembolic pulmonary hypertension (CTEPH) is a serious complication of acute venous pulmonary embolism (PE). It is a distinct entity characterized by obstruction of large, elastic (main, lobar, and segmental) pulmonary arteries by chronic, unresolved, organized PE. PH thus arises due to the blockade of the pulmonary artery. CTEPH is discussed in more detail in Chapter 71.

FURTHER READING

1. Cicalini S, Chinello P, Petrosillo N. HIV infection and pulmonary arterial hypertension. *Expert Rev Respir Med.* 2011;5:257–266.

   Detailed current review encompassing epidemiology, pathogenesis, clinical presentation, diagnostic approach, and available treatments for HIV-associated PAH.

2. Melgosa MT, Ricci GL, Garcia-Pagan JC, et al. Acute and long-term effects of inhaled iloprost in portopulmonary hypertension. *Liver Transpl.* 2010;16:348–356.

   Comparative study of the effect of iloprost in patients with PoPH. Pulmonary vasodilation was observed without significant effects on hepatic hemodynamics. The study outcome suggests the need for a randomized, controlled clinical trial.

3. Maclean MR, Dempsie Y. The serotonin hypothesis of pulmonary hypertension revisited. *Adv Exp Med Biol.* 2010;661:309–322.

   A nice review describing the role of serotonin in the pathobiology of PAH.

4. Sajkov D, McEvoy RD. Obstructive sleep apnea and pulmonary hypertension. *Prog Cardiovasc Dis.* 2009;51:363–370.

   A comprehensive review of the development of sleep apnea-associated PH.

5. Abe K, Toba M, Alzoubi A, et al. Formation of plexiform lesions in experimental severe pulmonary arterial hypertension. *Circulation.* 2010;121:2747–2754.

   A detailed study on the development of an animal model to study the genesis, hemodynamic effects, and reversibility of plexiform and other occlusive lesions in PAH.

6. Upton PD, Davies RJ, Trembath RC, et al. Bone morphogenetic protein (BMP) and activin type II receptors balance BMP9 signals mediated by activin receptor-like kinase-1 in human pulmonary artery endothelial cells. *J Biol Chem.* 2009;284:15794–15804.

   Indepth study that provides evidence suggesting that a differential signaling may contribute to the contrasting pathologies of hereditary hemorrhagic telangiectasia and PAH. A critical role of type II receptors in balancing BMP9 signaling via ALK1 was emphasized.

7. Steinhorn RH, Kinsella JP, Pierce C, et al. Intravenous sildenafil in the treatment of neonates with persistent pulmonary hypertension. *J Pediatr.* 2009;155:841–847, e841.

   Intravenous (IV) sildenafil, an inhibitor of cyclic guanosine monophosphate-specific phosphodiesterase, was well tolerated, and sustained improvement in oxygenation was observed in near-term and term newborns with PPHN.

8. Boutet K, Frachon I, Jobic Y, et al. Fenfluramine-like cardiovascular side-effects of benfluorex. *Eur Respir J.* 2009;33:684–688.

   This study presents reports of five cases of severe PAH and one case of valvular heart disease occurring in patients exposed to benfluorex.

9. Proceedings of the 4th World Symposium on Pulmonary Hypertension, February 2008, Dana Point, California, USA. *J Am Coll Cardiol.* 2008;54:S1–S117.

   Updated classification of PH.

10. Humbert M, Montani D, Perros F, et al. Endothelial cell dysfunction and cross talk between endothelium and smooth muscle cells in pulmonary arterial hypertension. *Vascul Pharmacol.* 2008;49:113–118.

    Summarizes the role of several mediators in smooth muscle cell proliferation and endothelial cell function and this in the development of pulmonary vascular hypertrophy and structural remodeling in PAH.

11. Farrow KN, Lakshminrusimha S, Reda WJ, et al. Superoxide dismutase restores eNOS expression and function in resistance pulmonary arteries from neonatal lambs with persistent pulmonary hypertension. *Am J Physiol Lung Cell Mol Physiol.* 2008;295:L979–L987.

    This study highlights a significant improvement in eNOS function and levels of available BH(4) in response to recombinant human SOD, which may prove to be useful in the treatment of PPHN in newborn infants.

12. Murray F, Patel HH, Suda RY, et al. Expression and activity of cAMP phosphodiesterase isoforms in pulmonary artery smooth muscle cells from patients with pulmonary hypertension: role for PDE1. *Am J Physiol Lung Cell Mol Physiol.* 2007;292:L294–L303.

    This study studies the role of specfic PDE isoforms in decreased cAMP and increased proliferation of PASMC in patients with PH. Indeed, PDE1 isoforms may be novel targets for the treatment of both primary and secondary PAH.

13. Mandegar M, Remillard CV, Yuan JX. Ion channels in pulmonary arterial hypertension. *Prog Cardiovasc Dis.* 2002;45:81–114.

    An indepth summary of the role of ion channels in the pathogenesis of PAH.

14. Arbustini E, Morbini P, D'Armini AM, et al. Plaque composition in plexogenic and thromboembolic pulmonary hypertension: the critical role of thrombotic material in pultaceous core formation. *Heart.* 2000;88:177–182.

    A comparative study concluding that CTEPH is associated with atherosclerotic plaques with glycophorin-rich pultaceous cores, and plexogenic pulmonary hypertension with fibrous plaques.

15. Hirose S, Hosoda Y, Furuya S, et al. Expression of vascular endothelial growth factor and its receptors correlates closely with formation of the plexiform lesion in human pulmonary hypertension. *Pathol Int.* 2000;50:472–479.

    VEGF and its receptors are shown to be upregulated and closely correlate with the development of plexiform lesions suggesting that VEGF expressed by SMC may activate the endothelial cells and lead to the formation of plexiform lesions.

16. Fishman AP. Changing concepts of the pulmonary plexiform lesion. *Physiol Res.* 2000;49:485–492.

    Although a little older, this review provides a good pathological analysis of the plexiform lesions associated with PH.

74 Pulmonary Hypertension: Diagnosis and Treatment

David Poch and Jess Mandel

The main challenges in the diagnosis of pulmonary hypertension are: (1) including pulmonary hypertension in the initial differential diagnosis and (2) completing a thorough diagnostic evaluation that establishes its presence. Historical information is usually nonspecific and patients frequently are misdiagnosed with more common conditions, such as asthma or heart failure. As an example, dyspnea on exertion is present in virtually all patients with pulmonary hypertension and may be the only presenting symptom. Other common symptoms include cough (30%), easy fatigability (25%), chest pain (21%), and hemoptysis (10%). These nonspecific symptoms often appropriately suggest other, more common, diagnostic considerations (asthma, coronary artery disease, psychogenic dyspnea) rather than pulmonary hypertension. More specific historical information, such as a history of anorectic drug use or childhood heart murmurs, should arouse suspicion for a specific pulmonary hypertensive disorder.

Findings on physical examination can be relatively subtle. Signs of pulmonary hypertension can include murmurs of tricuspid regurgitation or pulmonic insufficiency, accentuation of the pulmonic component of the second heart sound (P_2), fixed splitting of S_2, and a left parasternal lift, indicative of right ventricular hypertrophy. With more advanced disease, pedal edema, hepatomegaly, and jugular venous distension may be appreciated. One notable physical examination finding observed in some patients with chronic thromboembolic pulmonary hypertension (CTEPH) is the presence of pulmonary artery flow murmurs. These are bruits auscultated over the lung fields, heard best during breath holding at mid-inspiration. These sounds indicate flow through partially occluded central pulmonary arteries and are highly suggestive of chronic large-vessel pulmonary embolic disease.

Chest radiography frequently is unrevealing. If pulmonary hypertension is severe, enlargement of the right ventricle and pulmonary arteries is apparent. Chest radiography, however, can be useful in documenting secondary causes of pulmonary hypertension such as interstitial lung disease or chronic obstructive pulmonary disease (COPD). One notable radiographic finding is the presence of interstitial edema (Kerley B lines) in the setting of right ventricular failure and pulmonary artery enlargement. This constellation of x-ray findings should raise suspicion for pulmonary veno-occlusive disease.

In patients in whom pulmonary hypertension is suspected, echocardiography is a very useful initial test that is likely to be abnormal in the presence of moderate or severe pulmonary hypertension. Two-dimensional echocardiography demonstrates varying degrees of right atrial and right ventricular enlargement. Paradoxical movement of the interventricular septum indicates right ventricular pressure overload. Doppler echocardiography can also estimate the pulmonary artery systolic pressure (PASP) using the velocity of a tricuspid regurgitant jet (almost always present) and the formula $PASP = 4 \times v^2 + right atrial pressure$.

The 2008 Dana Point classification of pulmonary hypertension includes five major categories:

1. Pulmonary arterial hypertension (PAH)
   a. Idiopathic
   b. Heritable
   c. Drug and toxin associated (e.g., fenfluramine, cocaine)
   d. Associated with collagen vascular disease, congenital systemic to pulmonic shunts, portal hypertension, HIV, drugs and toxins, schistosomiasis, and others
   e. Associated with significant venous or capillary involvement: pulmonary veno-occlusive disease, pulmonary capillary hemangiomatosis
2. Pulmonary hypertension due to left-sided heart disease
3. Pulmonary hypertension associated with lung diseases or hypoxemia (e.g., COPD, interstitial lung disease, sleep-disordered breathing, alveolar hypoventilation disorders, chronic exposure to high altitude, developmental abnormalities)
4. Pulmonary hypertension caused by chronic thromboembolic disease (CTEPH)
5. Pulmonary hypertension with unclear multifactorial mechanisms (e.g., sarcoidosis, histiocytosis X, lymphangiomatosis, Gaucher disease).

Once a patient is identified as having a reasonable likelihood of pulmonary hypertension, additional tests are required to establish the diagnosis and determine which type of disease is present. These tests include: (1) echocardiography to exclude the presence of congenital heart disease (atrial septal defect, ventricular septal defect, patent ductus arteriosus) and left-sided heart disease (valvular or ventricular dysfunction), (2) pulmonary function testing to determine if significant obstructive or restrictive lung disease is present, (3) ventilation–perfusion scanning and possibly pulmonary angiography to identify CTEPH, (4) arterial blood gas analysis to evaluate for a hypoventilation syndrome, (5) polysomnography, if clinically indicated, and (6) chest radiography and high-resolution computed tomography scanning if the diagnosis of interstitial lung disease–associated pulmonary hypertension is contemplated.

With these noninvasive studies, multiple disorders can be excluded and patients with PAH can be identified. Further studies to identify conditions associated with PAH include liver function tests, HIV serology, and antinuclear antibody titer (collagen vascular disease). Patients should also be questioned regarding a family history of pulmonary hypertension, a history of anorexigen use, or a history of use of stimulant drugs (e.g., methamphetamines, cocaine). Right heart catheterization should be done to confirm the diagnosis and exclude an elevated pulmonary capillary wedge pressure indicative of left atrial hypertension, assess disease severity, and determine whether vasoreactivity is present.

The outcome of patients with untreated idiopathic PAH is quite unfavorable. In the National Institutes of Health Registry of such patients before modern treatments were available, median survival from the time of recognition was 2.9 years. Factors associated with a worse prognosis include severity of right ventricular failure (high right atrial pressure, low cardiac index), poor functional class, and poor exercise capacity as assessed by a 6-minute walk test.

Because the subset of patients with PAH that is responsive to vasodilators has a much better prognosis, it is critical to determine the ability of the pulmonary vascular bed to vasodilate in response to pharmacologic agents such as epoprostenol, inhaled nitric oxide, or adenosine; longer acting agents should not be used. An acute fall in mean pulmonary arterial pressure of at least 10 mmHg and to a final value less than 40 mmHg without reduction in cardiac output identifies a subgroup that may do well on long-term calcium channel blockers. Unfortunately, less than 10% of patients fall into this acute "vasoreactive" subgroup.

Since the late 1990s, effective medical therapy has been available for most patients with PAH. Therapies currently available in the United States include:

- Epoprostenol, an intravenous prostacyclin analog ("prostenoid") requiring continuous administration
- Treprostinil, a prostacyclin analog that can be administered intravenously, subcutaneously, or via the inhaled route
- Iloprost, an inhaled prostacyclin analog
- Bosentan and ambrisentan, oral endothelin antagonists
- Sildenafil and tadalafil, oral phosphodiesterase-5 inhibitors

The choice of treatment depends upon the severity of the pulmonary hypertension and the side effects and complication profile of the medications. Continuous intravenous prostenoid (e.g. epoprostenol) therapy is invasive, has numerous side effects, and requires an indwelling catheter for administration. However, it is considered the most effective treatment and is generally felt to be the drug of choice in PAH patients who are World Health Organization (WHO) functional class IV. Of interest is that the beneficial effects of prostenoids are noted even in the absence of favorable acute hemodynamic responses to the agent, suggesting non-vasodilator effects such as advantageous pulmonary vascular remodeling.

Bosentan and ambrisentan, orally administered endothelin receptor antagonists, have also been shown to improve hemodynamics and exercise capacity in patients with PAH. The agents are generally well tolerated, with their most important complications being hepatotoxicity (usually reversible) and teratogenicity.

Sildenafil and tadalafil are orally administered phosphodiesterase-5 inhibitors that have been shown to improve exercise capacity in patients with PAH. They are generally well tolerated, but can produce life-threatening hypotension if combined with nitrates.

Therapies currently under investigation include orally available prostacyclin receptor agonists, inhaled nitrates, and tyrosine kinase inhibitors. Additional studies are also underway examining the impact of upfront combination therapy with two or more of the approved drug classes listed above. It is not yet certain whether this combined approach offers benefit over sequential addition of therapies.

In addition to the primary treatments described, warfarin is recommended based upon retrospective data indicating a significant survival benefit in idiopathic PAH. Diuretics are frequently required to control symptoms such as hepatic congestion and lower extremity edema. Diuretics, however, must be used with caution because excessive reduction in blood volume can adversely affect the preload-dependent right ventricle and lead to systemic hypotension. Digoxin is considered to be of limited benefit at best.

Other supportive measures occasionally considered for patients with progressive right ventricular failure include low-dose inotropic therapy and balloon septostomy. Inotropic support with low-dose dopamine, dobutamine, or milrinone can improve cardiac output and symptoms, and has been used long-term in a small number of patients. Balloon septostomy creates a small atrial septal defect that allows blood, albeit deoxygenated, to reach the left ventricle, thereby improving cardiac output and, in many cases, oxygen delivery. However, hypoxemia and decompensation may result. The size of the defect created appears to be critical in balancing improvement in cardiac output against severe hypoxemia.

Lung and heart–lung transplantation are reserved for patients who do not show significant improvement and stabilization with medical therapy. This is best assessed through evaluation of posttreatment hemodynamic data in combination with a 6-minute walk distance and functional class. Double-lung transplantation is preferred over single-lung transplantation in pulmonary hypertension; heart–lung transplantation is generally reserved for complex congenital heart abnormalities that cannot be corrected at the time of lung transplantation. Successful transplantation results in marked hemodynamic and functional improvement. However, beneficial long-term outcomes with lung transplantation are tempered by the high morbidity of the procedure and a mean posttransplantation survival of less than 8 years.

FURTHER READING

1. Aguilar RV, Farber HW. Epoprostenol (prostacyclin) therapy in HIV-associated pulmonary hypertension. *Am J Respir Crit Care Med.* 2000;162:1846.

   Six consecutive patients with HIV-associated PAH underwent treatment with epoprostenol and were followed for 12 to 47 months. Hemodynamics improved significantly between baseline and 1 year, and functional class improved in all patients.

2. Badesch DB, Tapson VF, McGoon MD, et al. Continuous intravenous epoprostenol for pulmonary hypertension due to the scleroderma spectrum of disease. *Ann Intern Med.* 2000;132:425.

   In 111 patients with scleroderma-associated PAH, those treated with intravenous epoprostenol had significantly improved hemodynamics, functional class, and exercise capacity versus conventionally treated patients, and showed a trend toward less Raynaud phenomenon and fewer digital ulcers.

3. Barst RJ, Rubin LJ, Long WA, et al; for the PPH Study Group. A comparison of continuous intravenous epoprostenol (prostacyclin) with conventional therapy for primary pulmonary hypertension. *N Engl J Med.* 1996;334:296.

   A landmark study demonstrating the efficacy of continuous prostacyclin in improving both exercise capacity and survival in PPH.

4. Barst RJ, Gibbs JS, Ghofrani HA, et al. Updated evidence-based treatment algorithm in pulmonary arterial hypertension. *J Am Coll Cardiol.* 2009;54:S78–S84.

   An authoritative patient-centered, evidence-based guideline on the management of pulmonary hypertension.

5. Benza RL, Gomberg-Maitland M, Miller DP, et al. The REVEAL Registry risk score calculator in patients newly diagnosed with pulmonary arterial hypertension. *Chest.* 2012;141:354–362.

   Based upon a large registry cohort, the authors present an algorithm to calculate risk for adverse outcomes among patients with PAH.

6. Channick RN, Simonneau G, Sitbon O, et al. Effects of the dual endothelin-receptor antagonist bosentan in patients with pulmonary hypertension: a randomized placebo-controlled study. *Lancet.* 2001;358:1119.

   Demonstrates the benefits of bosentan in the treatment of PAH, with improved 6-minute walk distance and hemodynamics in bosentan-treated patients versus those receiving placebo.

7. D'Alonzo GE, Barst RJ, Ayres SM, et al. Survival in patients with primary pulmonary hypertension: results from a national prospective registry. *Ann Intern Med.* 1991;115:343.

   Documents poor survival in untreated PPH (median survival 2.9 years), which is strongly influenced by hemodynamics such as right atrial pressure, mean pulmonary artery pressure, and cardiac index.

8. Frank H, Mlczoch J, Huber K, et al. The effect of anticoagulant therapy in primary and anorectic drug-induced pulmonary hypertension. *Chest.* 1997;112:714.

   This and other retrospective studies suggest a survival benefit for PAH patients receiving anticoagulation.

9. Galiè N, Olschewski H, Oudiz RJ, et al. Ambrisentan for the treatment of pulmonary arterial hypertension: results of the ambrisentan in pulmonary arterial hypertension, randomized, double-blind, placebo-controlled, multicenter, efficacy (ARIES) study 1 and 2. *Circulation.* 2008;117:3010–3019.

   Ambrisentan, a selective endothelin-1 A-type receptor antagonist, was shown in a randomized, double-blind fashion to improve exercise tolerance in patients with PAH.

10. Galiè N, Ghofrani HA, Torbicki A, et al. Sildenafil citrate therapy for pulmonary arterial hypertension. *N Engl J Med.* 2005;353:2148–2157.

    This double-blind placebo-controlled trial showed the effectiveness of oral sildenafil in improving exercise tolerance among patients with PAH.

11. McLaughlin VV, Shillington A, Rich S, et al. Survival in primary pulmonary hypertension. The impact of epoprostenol therapy. *Circulation.* 2002;106:1477–1482.

    Intravenous epoprostenol improves long-term survival versus predicted survival, with outcome dependent on posttreatment variables, including functional class, hemodynamics, and exercise capacity.

12. Mukerjee D, St George D, Coleiro B, et al. Prevalence and outcome in systemic sclerosis associated pulmonary arterial hypertension: application of a registry approach. *Ann Rheum Dis.* 2003;62:1088.

Seven hundred twenty-two patients with scleroderma were screened for PAH by echocardiogram and PFTs; those with suspicious findings underwent catheterization. Twelve percent (89/722) showed evidence of pulmonary hypertension by right-heart catheterization, confirming the high risk of disease in this patient population.

13. Olschewski H, Simonneau G, Galiè N, et al. Inhaled iloprost for severe pulmonary hypertension. *N Engl J Med.* 2002;347:322.

    This placebo-controlled trial evaluated inhaled iloprost, a prostacyclin analog, in the treatment of pulmonary hypertension, including PPH, anorexigens-associated, scleroderma-associated, and nonoperable CTEPH. At 12 weeks, patients receiving iloprost (2.5–5.0 μg, 6–9 times daily) showed greater improvement in 6-minute walk distance, hemodynamics, and functional class versus placebo.

14. Raymond RJ, Hinderliter AL, Willis PW, et al. Echocardiographic predictors of adverse outcomes in primary pulmonary hypertension. *J Am Coll Cardiol.* 2002;39:1214.

    Pericardial effusion, right atrial enlargement, and septal displacement predict adverse outcomes in patients with advanced PAH.

15. Rich S, Kaufmann E, Levy PS, et al. The effect of high doses of calcium channel-blockers on survival in primary pulmonary hypertension. *N Engl J Med.* 1992;327:76.

    The first study to demonstrate improved survival in PPH patients who responded acutely to high-dose calcium channel blockers and were then continued on these agents.

16. Rothman A, Sklansky MS, Lucas VW, et al. Atrial septostomy as a bridge to lung transplantation in patients with severe pulmonary hypertension. *Am J Cardiol.* 1999;84:682.

    Twelve patients with severe pulmonary hypertension were treated with graded balloon dilation to make a small atrial septal defect. Mean oxygen delivery improved, and six patients had clinical improvement, five of whom subsequently underwent lung transplantation.

17. Rubin LJ, Badesch DB, Barst RJ, et al. Bosentan therapy for pulmonary arterial hypertension. *N Engl J Med.* 2002;346:896.

    Second and larger placebo-controlled trial of bosentan. Confirmed the findings of the earlier study showing improvement in 6-minute walk distance, WHO class, and Borg dyspnea index in the bosentan-treated patients.

18. Sastry BK, Narasimhan C, Reddy NK, et al. Clinical efficacy of sildenafil in primary pulmonary hypertension: a randomized, placebo controlled, double-blind, crossover study. *J Am Coll Cardiol.* 2004;43:1149.

    In this study, 22 patients received either placebo or sildenafil (25–100 mg tid, based on body weight) for 6 weeks, and were then crossed over to the other treatment (placebo or sildenafil) for an additional 6 weeks. Sildenafil led to improved exercise time, cardiac index, and quality-of-life scores.

19. Setaro JF, Cleman MW, Remetz MS, et al. The right ventricle in disorders causing pulmonary venous hypertension. *Cardiol Clin.* 1992;10:165.

    An excellent review article describing the physiologic and clinical consequences of pulmonary venous hypertension.

20. Simonneau G, Barst RJ, Galie N, et al. Continuous subcutaneous infusion of treprostinil, a prostacyclin analogue, in patients with pulmonary arterial hypertension. *Am J Respir Crit Care Med.* 2002;165:800.

    Showed improved hemodynamics and 6-minute walk distance in treprostinil-treated patients versus placebo. Improvement was greater with higher treprostinil dose achieved.

21. Simonneau G, Robbins IM, Beghetti M, et al. Updated clinical classification of pulmonary hypertension. *J Am Coll Cardiol.* 2009;54:S43–S54.

    Provides the most recent classification scheme for pulmonary hypertension, derived from the 2008 Dana Point international conference.

22. Sitbon O, Humbert M, Nunes H, et al. Long-term intravenous epoprostenol infusion in primary pulmonary hypertension: prognostic factors and survival. *J Am Coll Cardiol.* 2002;40:780.

    Prospective study of 178 class III/IV PPH patients undergoing treatment with epoprostenol. Persistence of WHO functional class III/IV symptoms, failure to show a decrease in TPR of at least 30%, and any history of right-ventricular failure were all independent predictors of mortality when analyzed by multivariate analysis.

23. Task Force for Diagnosis and Treatment of Pulmonary Hypertension of European Society of Cardiology (ESC) and the European Respiratory Society (ERS), endorsed by the International Society of Heart and Lung Transplantation (ISHLT). Guidelines for the diagnosis and treatment of pulmonary hypertension. *Eur Respir J.* 2009;34:1219–1263.

Comprehensive European guidelines for the diagnosis and treatment of pulmonary hypertension.

Lung Transplantation

Marisa Magaña and Gordon L. Yung

Lung transplantation has a relatively short history: the first successful human single and double lung transplants were performed in 1983 and 1986, respectively. Organ availability remains the major obstacle to the number of lung transplants, with only 15% to 20% of all potential donors' lung(s) being suitable for transplant. With better donor management and better public awareness, there has been a small but steady increase in the number of patients receiving lung transplantation, despite an increasing number of double lungs over single lung transplants (which would, theoretically, result in a decrease in the total number of patients receiving lung transplant). In 2011, 1,822 adult lung transplants were performed in 60 adult and 3 pediatric transplant centers in the United States, including one living donor transplant. Compared to a total of 3,519 lung transplants reported from 178 centers worldwide to the International Society of Heart and Lung Transplantation in 2010, the United States continues to lead the world in this treatment. Encouragingly, the median posttransplant survival has increased from 4.7 years in the 1990s to 5.7 years for the past decade.

The most common indications for lung transplantation worldwide are chronic obstructive pulmonary disease (COPD) (including α-1 antitrypsin deficiency, ~40%), interstitial lung disease (including idiopathic pulmonary fibrosis [IPF], ~27%), and cystic fibrosis (~17%). Other less common indications, each constituting approximately 1% to 3% of all cases, include pulmonary arterial hypertension (PAH), sarcoidosis, bronchiectasis, and lymphangioleiomyomatosis. In addition, 1% to 2% of all lung transplants were performed in patients who had a previous lung transplant, usually due to chronic rejection (bronchiolitis obliterans). In the United States, due to a new prioritizing allocation system established in 2005 that favors interstitial lung disease, the proportion of patients with this group of conditions approaches that of patients with COPD.

PATIENT SELECTION

Because of limited organ availability, there are often conflicts during recipient selection between individual patient needs and societal benefits. For example, "high risk" patients who might benefit from transplant but who have a low chance of posttransplant survival may be denied transplant in favor of other patients with a better chance of survival. In addition, in developed countries, where rationing of resources is not a normal societal expectation, physicians may face significant ethical dilemmas. For example:

1. Should patients be allowed to have repeat transplants for a second or third time, even though they are sicker than others who have not had their first one?
2. Should a 25-year-old patient with cystic fibrosis (a disease he or she has no control over) who is the sole source of income for a family with young children be chosen over a 78-year-old retired individual with COPD who was a life-long smoker?

3. Should there be limits on the number of transplants for foreign nationals, including illegal immigrants, when there are not enough organs for legal residents/citizens?

Exclusion Criteria

Ethical issues and society considerations aside, selection of patients should be based primarily on potential benefits for the patient, either in terms of improved survival, quality of life or both. The significant perioperative and postoperative risks for morbidity and mortality, as well as the scarcity of donor organs, necessitates a vigorous selection process for suitable recipients that is critical to successful outcomes that benefit the largest number of patients for the longest period of time. The ideal patient should be healthy enough to undergo the surgery safely with the least risk of postoperative complications (both immediate and long-term), yet sick enough (i.e., high expected mortality and sufficiently impaired quality of life) to justify the considerable risks. Every patient is, therefore, required to undergo an extensive evaluation to determine transplant candidacy. This includes a detailed history and physical examination, testing for latent infections or organ dysfunction, cardiac and pulmonary function testing, imaging with chest radiograph and CT scan, as well as a careful psychosocial assessment.

Although every transplant center has its own guidelines regarding recipient selection, there is a general consensus that patients with the following conditions should not be considered for transplant until these issues are resolved: active tobacco, drug, or alcohol abuse; severe psychiatric illness that impairs the patient's ability to comply with medical care; documented current history of medical nonadherence; lack of a significant social support system; active infection with hepatitis B or C, especially with histologic evidence of liver disease; untreatable advanced dysfunction of another major organ; significant chest wall/spinal deformities; and recent malignancy with the exception of nonmelanoma skin cancers. It is important to recognize that experience in lung transplants is still relatively limited and some of the "conventional" practices and guidelines are constantly being challenged and undergoing change. For example, most transplant centers still consider infection with HIV to be an absolute contraindication; however, with advances in antiviral therapies, it is possible that patients with HIV or chronic viral hepatitis may be candidates in the future if these infections can be treated successfully. Age is considered a relative contraindication due to evidence of worse outcomes in patients over the age of 65 years. However, increasingly, there is an emphasis on physiologic age, so that if a patient over 65 years is physically strong and healthy aside from the lung disease, consideration can be given to transplantation. In fact, in 2011, more than 25% of all lung transplants in United States were performed on patients older than 64 years. Long-term outcome data on lung transplants in "elderly" patients are inconclusive, but it is likely that, even in well-selected patients, long-term (5 year) survival of patients over 70 years of age would be significantly worse that those younger than 65 years. Finally, selected patients with multi-organ failure may have successful multi-organ transplants, most commonly heart–lung and lung–kidney transplants.

Other conditions may increase posttransplant mortality and should also be taken into account when considering a patient's transplant candidacy, including: symptomatic osteoporosis, poor functional status with poor potential for rehabilitation, hemodynamic instability, and active and untreated extrapulmonary infections.

Although patients with cystic fibrosis and pan-resistant *Pseudomonas aeruginosa* have worse transplant outcomes than those with sensitive strains, they are similar to non–cystic fibrosis patients, presumably due to the younger age of this population. Thus, one may argue that colonization with pan-resistant *P. aeruginosa* should not preclude transplantation. On the other hand, patients colonized with *Burkholderia cepacia type III* have significantly decreased 1 year survival posttransplant, prompting some centers to consider colonization with this organism a contraindication to transplantation.

Selected patients on chronic home ambulatory ventilator support have comparable survival outcomes, but those with acute respiratory failure requiring mechanical ventilation and urgent lung transplant generally have significantly worse outcomes. Extreme high or low body weight ($\pm20\%$–30% of ideal body weight) is associated with worse outcome; aggressive approaches, including dietary restriction or placement of a feeding tube, are often necessary. Some centers use a body mass index of 30 as a "cut-off" for transplant consideration, although one should also take into account the distribution of fat and relative muscle/fat proportion in making the final decision. Increasingly, gastroesophageal reflux disease (GERD) has been associated with worse transplant outcomes due to its association with chronic lung rejection, and some transplant centers now recommend definitive surgical treatment in severe cases either prior to, or soon after, lung transplantation.

Inclusion Criteria

To select the right patients, physicians should consider several factors:

1. *Survival after transplant:* While no one can accurately predict how long an individual patient will live after a transplant, the most comprehensive data are available from the annual report from the Registry of the International Society of Heart and Lung Transplantation. In the 2012 report of self-reported data of almost 33,000 lung transplants performed between 1994 to 2010, the average survival after lung transplant was about 5½ years (single lung: 4.6 years, double lung: 6.7 years). The survival difference in single versus double lung transplant may, in part, be a result of selection bias: most older patients, who would be expected to have shorter posttransplant survival, typically receive single rather than double lung transplants. Similar survival data have also been reported in the United States by the Scientific Registry for Transplant Recipients (which operates under the Department of Health and Human Services to collect all transplant data in the United States). Different diagnoses may also have different transplant outcomes, in part because of age at the time of transplant. The shortest survival is associated with IPF (4.5 years). Previously, idiopathic PAH had the lowest 1-year survival, but this has improved to an average of 4.9 years. Patients with COPD have an average posttransplant survival of 5.3 years, while those with the similar disease of emphysema due to $\alpha 1$ antitrypsin deficiency survive an average of 6.3 years. Patients with cystic fibrosis have the longest average survival of 7.4 years. It is likely that age and, possibly, single versus double lung transplant plays a significant role in the reported differences in survival.

2. *Survival without transplant:* To evaluate the benefits of transplant, one should compare posttransplant survival to the expected survival of patients without transplant. To achieve this goal, one has to estimate individual patient survival without transplant. Because most lung diseases are associated with a wide range of survival, it is important for transplant physicians to take into account an individual patient's condition and disease progression, and not simply look at the average survival for each disease. For example, a patient with COPD who quit smoking 20 years previously and has had stable lung function for the past 5 years may have significantly better survival than another patient with $\alpha 1$ antitrypsin deficiency and similar pulmonary function tests, but who just quit smoking only 6 months earlier. Similarly, a patient with pulmonary hypertension who has not yet received optimal medical therapy might have a very different prognosis than another patient with similar pulmonary hemodynamics, but who was already receiving maximal medical therapy. Guidelines were developed in 2006 by the International Society for Heart and Lung Transplantation (Table 75-1), which provide a framework for patient selection for lung transplant, but these

---

TABLE 75-1	Guidelines for Selected Diseases

Chronic Obstructive Pulmonary Disease

Referral guidelines

BODE[a] index >5

Transplantation guidelines

BODE index of 7–10 or at least one of the following:

• History of hospitalization for exacerbation associated with acute hypercapnia ($Pco_2 > 50$ mmHg)

- Pulmonary hypertension or cor pulmonale or both despite oxygen therapy
- FEV_1 < 20% predicted and either D_{LCO} < 20% predicted or homogenous distribution of emphysema

Cystic Fibrosis
Referral guidelines

- FEV_1 < 30% predicted or a rapid decline in FEV_1, particularly in female patients
- Exacerbation requiring ICU stay
- Increasing frequency of exacerbations requiring antibiotics
- Refractory and/or recurrent pneumothorax
- Recurrent hemoptysis not controlled by embolization

Transplantation guidelines

- Oxygen-dependent respiratory failure
- Pulmonary hypertension
- Hypercapnia

Idiopathic Pulmonary Fibrosis
Referral guidelines

- Histologic or radiographic evidence of usual interstitial pneumonitis (UIP) regardless of vital capacity
- Histologic evidence of fibrotic nonspecific interstitial pneumonitis (NSIP)

Transplantation guidelines

Histologic or radiographic evidence of UIP and any of the following:

- D_{LCO} < 39% predicted
- 10% or greater decline in FVC during 6 mo of follow-up
- Pulse oximetry <88% during a 6-min walk test. Honeycombing on HRCT (fibrosis score >2)

Histologic evidence of NSIP and any of the following:

- D_{LCO} < 35% predicted
- 10% or greater decline in FVC or 15% decrease in D_{LCO} during 6 mo of follow-up

Primary Pulmonary Hypertension
Referral guidelines

- NYHA functional class III or IV, regardless of current treatment
- Rapidly progressive disease

Transplantation guidelines

- Persistent NYHA class III or IV symptoms despite maximal medical therapy
- Failing therapy with intravenous epoprostenol or equivalent
- Low (<350 m) or declining 6-min walk test; cardiac index <2 L/min/m²
- Right atrial pressure >15 mmHg

Adapted from the ISHLT 2006 Guidelines for the Selection of Lung Transplant Candidates.

[a]The BODE index is a multidimensional grading system that predicts mortality from COPD on the basis of body-mass Index, airflow obstruction, dyspnea, and exercise capacity.

do not substitute for an individual physician's judgment, especially with regard to disease progression and consideration of quality of life. Because different countries may have very different systems of prioritizing organ allocation, and waiting time can vary considerably among different transplant centers in the same country, it is important for physicians to work with their local transplant centers to optimize the timing for transplant referrals.

LUNG ALLOCATION SCORE

In May 2005, a new system of lung allocation was implemented in the United States under the administration of the United Network of Organ Sharing (UNOS). On the basis of several variables, a patient receives a lung allocation score (LAS) that determines his or her ranking on the organ distribution lists. Available organs are then prioritized according to location, blood type, and LAS ranking of patients on the waiting list. The LAS, normalized between 0 and 100, incorporates a common set of variables that combines the predicted risk of death within 1 year while on the waiting list and the predicted likelihood of (1-year) survival after transplantation. A higher score indicates greater urgency and need for transplantation.

The introduction of the LAS has led to many changes in the allocation of lungs as well as the outcomes in the transplant patient population. The number of patients on the waiting list has decreased significantly and, more importantly, the waiting time from listing to transplantation has decreased dramatically. From 1998 to 2002, prior to the implementation of the LAS, the average wait time for lung transplant was 1,000 days; in 2007, this had dropped to 141 days. Patients with the highest LAS (>45 points) can now expect to wait approximately 1 to 2 months, compared to about 9 months for those with a lower score (<25). Wait-list mortality has also decreased from 15% prior to LAS to 11% after its inception. In addition, the type of patients receiving transplantation has changed as well. Prior to the LAS, the most common indication for lung transplantation was COPD; in the post-LAS era, IPF has become most common, accounting for approximately 33% of all lung transplants in 2007. Finally, the proportion of lung transplant patients with cystic fibrosis has increased from 16% to 20% following implementation of the LAS.

With the exception of idiopathic pulmonary hypertension, wait-list mortality has decreased for most lung conditions following implementation of the LAS. This and other evidence suggest that the LAS may underestimate disease severity in patients with PAH. Ongoing efforts are in place to review and refine the current system. Finally, recent data suggest a trend toward higher posttransplant mortality after implementation of LAS. The explanation for this trend is not clear. Possibly, it indicates that sicker patients are being transplanted, or that there is a need for a better method for calculating the LAS.

DONOR SELECTION

It is clear that proper donor selection and optimal organ preservation improve transplant outcomes. After being accepted on the waiting list, patients are matched with donors according to their ABO blood group and lung size. Donor organs are routinely evaluated for function and to exclude active or latent infections. Traditional donor criteria include the following: age less than or equal to 55 years, ABO compatibility, chest radiograph with clear lung fields or with only minimal abnormalities, PaO_2 greater than or equal to 300 on 100% FIO_2 and PEEP of 5.0 cm H_2O, tobacco history less than or equal to 20 pack years, absence of significant chest trauma, no evidence of significant aspiration or sepsis, and no prior cardiopulmonary surgery. The decision to use marginal donor lungs should be made only after careful consideration, supported by informed consent from the individual patient. It has become apparent that these criteria may be too stringent and contributing to the current shortage of donor organs; many centers have reported comparable outcomes with donor lungs that do not fit all of the traditional donor criteria. The traditional donor criteria, therefore, serve more as guidelines and not strict selection criteria. Each potential donor has to be considered on a case-by-case basis.

More recently, several devices have been developed for *ex vivo* transportation of explanted lung blocs at near-body temperature, while the organs continue to receive blood or fluid perfused through a closed circuit as well as ventilation through a transport ventilator. This has the potential of extending the distance and time that an explanted organ can remain viable without the prolonged ischemic injury that current organ preservation methods can cause (ice cold perfusion solution to suspend organ cellular function). Preliminary data have been encouraging and even suggest the possibility of improved lung function with this method of *ex vivo* perfusion.

Approximately 8.6% of donors are classified as high-risk donors by the Public Health Service and Center for Disease Control, meaning that the donor participated in behaviors that placed him/her at high risk of acquiring certain infectious diseases, specifically HIV and hepatitis B and C. When a donor is classified high risk, the transplant team is required to obtain special informed consent prior to proceeding with surgery with respect to the risk of transmission of these infectious diseases. This classification was first defined decades ago to avoid inadvertent transfer of infections such as HIV or viral hepatitis through the donor organ. With the availability of newer DNA polymerase chain reaction (PCR) testing, this category of high-risk donor may soon become obsolete.

TYPE OF TRANSPLANT

There are three types of lung transplantation: single lung (SLT), bilateral (sequential) lung (BLT), and living donor transplantation. Heart–lung transplantation is seldom performed now and is most often used in cases of pulmonary hypertension related to severe congenital cardiac anomalies. The type of transplantation performed depends primarily on the underlying disease, associated conditions (e.g., age, degree of secondary pulmonary hypertension, bronchiectasis or active lung infections, previous thoracic or pleural surgeries, and comorbid conditions), and institutional practice. Because of the limited number of suitable donors and decreased operative morbidity, SLT is preferred whenever feasible. It is also technically the simplest and can usually be performed via a thoracotomy without cardiopulmonary bypass. The disadvantages of SLT are that the recipients are left with one diseased lung, generally have poorer results on pulmonary function testing even after recovery, and may have shorter posttransplant survival. However, patients with successful SLT have little functional disability in almost all normal daily activities.

BLT is performed either through an anterior thoracosternotomy (clam-shell incision) or bilateral thoracotomies and is usually reserved for patients at risk of recurrent pulmonary infections if the native lung is left behind. BLT is therefore recommended for all patients with cystic fibrosis or suppurative lung diseases. When SLT is performed in patients with PAH or severe secondary PH, most of the cardiac output flows through the transplanted lung leading to a high incidence of pulmonary edema in the allograft. Therefore, patients with PAH or severe secondary PH generally undergo bilateral lung transplantation.

There are some data suggesting slightly better long-term outcomes in patients with COPD from BLT compared with SLT. However, in patients with IPF, studies have not demonstrated any consistent mortality benefit for BLT over SLT. Therefore, the decision to perform BLT or SLT in patients with COPD or IPF is usually center and case-dependent. Finally, as long as there is a significant organ shortage, the ethics of giving one donor's lungs to one versus two recipients in order to provide a small additional survival benefit should also be considered.

Because of the shortage of donors, living donor transplantation was used in the late 1990s until 2005. Most cases were performed on pediatric patients with cystic fibrosis, with the donors being close family members. Two donors are required, each donating the lower lobe of one lung (right lower lobe and left lower lobe) to the respective chest cavity of the recipient. This procedure has the advantage of allowing extensive donor evaluation and can potentially improve HLA matching. Criteria for living donor transplant recipients should be the same as for other types of lung transplantation; the procedure should not be performed as a rescue operation for patients *in extremis*. Aside from the technical difficulties, there are ethical considerations of subjecting two healthy adults to surgery that does not directly benefit their own health. Since the implementation of LAS, the need of living donor transplantation has decreased significantly. Between 2006 and 2011, only one to four patients annually received this form of transplant in the United States.

POSTTRANSPLANT COMPLICATIONS

Primary Graft Dysfunction

In approximately 10% to 30% of patients, primary graft dysfunction (PGD) develops in the postoperative period. PGD is a form of acute lung injury that occurs within the first 72 hours immediately after surgery. It is thought to be related to ischemia–reperfusion injury; various risk factors related to the donor and organ preservation, recipient characteristics, and injuries from operation are thought to play a role. A grading system based on the Pao_2/Fio_2 ratio has been used to assess severity at the following time points; immediately postoperative within 6, 24, 48, and 72 hours. Severe PGD, grade 3 ($Pao_2/Fio_2 < 200$) carries significant short- and long-term morbidity and mortality. Christie et al. demonstrated that patients with grade 3 PGD at 72 hours had significantly higher all-cause 30-day mortality of 63% compared to 9% in patients without any PGD. In addition, multiple studies have demonstrated an association between PGD and the development of bronchiolitis obliterans syndrome (BOS), even years later. The mechanism of how PGD causes BOS is unclear. BOS is the major obstacle to better long-term survival after lung transplantation. There is no definitive treatment of this condition and the main therapy is supportive care while awaiting recovery.

Acute Rejection

Acute rejection occurs in 30% to 40% of transplant recipients. Unlike PGD, it usually occurs after the first 5 to 7 days following transplant, and is rare after the first year. Symptoms may be nonspecific and include fever, dyspnea, and cough and are often associated with chest radiograph opacities. The gold standard for diagnosis is pathologic examination of tissue, usually obtained by transbronchial biopsy. Bronchoscopy also allows for the evaluation of infectious etiologies, especially cytomegalovirus (CMV), which can sometimes mimic acute rejection. Histologically, acute rejection is characterized by lymphocytic perivascular inflammation which may also contain lymphocytic bronchiolitis.

A grading system for acute rejection, based on the severity of perivascular inflammation, has been developed, although the relation of grade to treatment response and long-term prognosis has not been clearly demonstrated. Treatment generally consists of high-dose pulse IV corticosteroids followed by an oral prednisone taper. Most patients respond well to this therapy; those unresponsive to first-line therapy may require other treatments that may include antilymphocyte antibodies, plasmapheresis, or other immunosuppressants. Most cases of acute rejection are thought to be cellular in origin, involving T-lymphocytes, although increasingly the entity of B-cell or antibody-mediated response (often related to donor-specific antibodies) is being recognized as a cause of rejection. The occurrence of acute rejection, especially episodes with histologically proven lymphocytic bronchiolitis, is well recognized to be a risk factor for the development of chronic rejection, prompting some centers to treat the condition aggressively and follow with repeated lung biopsies, even in asymptomatic patients. Whether early treatment can prevent the subsequent development of chronic rejection is not clear.

Anastomotic Complications

In the early era of lung transplantation, anastomotic dehiscence was one of the most feared complications. The incidence has since decreased significantly through improved surgical techniques and with the avoidance of sirolimus within the first 6 weeks posttransplant. Sirolimus use in the postoperative period has been associated with a 40% to 60% risk of anastomotic dehiscence due to poor wound healing. For this reason, it must be avoided in the early postoperative period.

Anastomotic stenosis is a common complication usually occurring between 9 and 12 months posttransplant. When recognized early, it can often be managed with serial balloon dilation and, in more severe cases, placement of an airway stent. In some cases, laser removal of granulation tissue may also be needed. In our experience, silicone or hybrid (silicone and metal) stents result in the least complications, and can be removed with permanent "cure" after 9 to 12 months in most cases. Use of pure metal stents is generally discouraged due to the propensity for granulation tissue formation and the difficulty in removing them at a later date. However, because of the need for rigid bronchoscopy for silicone stent placement, many centers do not have the expertise and prefer metal stents due to the ease of placement. Currently, hybrid (metal-silicone) stents are being developed that may be placed with a flexible bronchoscopy.

Infection

Infections are a major cause of both early and late deaths in lung transplant recipients and are considered to be the most common cause of death within the first year post–lung transplant. Bacterial infections are frequent in the early postoperative period. Infections with *Pseudomonas* spp., followed by *Staphylococcus aureus,* are the most common causes of death during the first 3 months after transplant. Fungal infections, predominately from *Aspergillus* spp., can occur both early and late after lung transplantation. As a result, many centers use antifungal prophylaxis. However, the choice of antifungal drug, dose, and length of prophylaxis has not been standardized. In some centers located in endemic fungal areas, long-term antifungal prophylaxis has been proposed. CMV was previously a common cause of viral infection, especially in the first year after transplant, and has been associated with an increased risk of developing chronic rejection. Since the development of effective oral anti-CMV prophylaxis that allows for long-term suppressive therapy, this complication is now uncommon. However, the optimal duration of CMV prophylaxis has not been clearly established. CMV seronegative patients who receive an organ from a seropositive donor are at the greatest risk of developing CMV illness; these patients should receive prophylaxis for at least 6 months. However, a recent study comparing a 12- versus 3-month course of valganciclovir in patients who are either donor or recipient CMV-positive demonstrated significantly decreased incidence of CMV disease (4% vs. 32%) without significant increase in drug side effects, suggesting that perhaps longer courses of prophylaxis should be employed.

Chronic Rejection

Chronic allograft rejection presents as progressive small airway obstruction. Histologically, biopsies demonstrate changes of obliterative bronchiolitis. Because repeated open lung biopsies are not practical, and transbronchial biopsies often yield inconclusive results, the term "bronchiolitis obliterans syndrome" has been accepted as a surrogate term for chronic rejection. Once other conditions that may cause airway obstructions are excluded (such as anastomotic stenosis), diagnosis of chronic rejection (or BOS) can safely be made when a progressive obstructive pattern is seen on pulmonary function tests. BOS does not usually occur within the first 6 months of transplant; however, once it develops, most cases progress without intervention. Approximately 40% of patients develop BOS by 5 years after transplant and it remains the most common cause of death for patients beyond the first year. Multiple treatments have been tried with varying success. These include a change in the existing immunosuppressive regimen, addition of Azithromycin and/or Sirolimus, and use of anti-CD 52 antibodies (Alemtuzumab). Several small case series have also reported success with the use of extracorporeal photopheresis in BOS. Other centers have reported success in preventing progressive BOS after transplant with successful surgical treatment of gastroesophageal reflux. Unlike acute rejection, chronic rejection does not respond to corticosteroids. Re-transplantation remains the only effective, though controversial, treatment option for patients with severe BOS that would allow significant functional recovery.

Most other long-term complications after transplantation are related to the use of immunosuppressive therapy and include: osteoporosis, hypertension, hyperlipidemia, diabetes, renal insufficiency (with 2%–3% of patients requiring long-term dialysis and <1% undergoing kidney transplant 5 years post–lung transplant), myelosuppression, and malignancy (especially skin cancer and lymphoproliferative disease).

In summary, lung transplantation is still a developing area of pulmonary medicine. Selection of appropriate patients continues to change over time as organ availability improves. The task of equitably prioritizing patients according to needs and outcomes remains challenging. Even after almost three decades we still do not have a unified approach to selection and management of patients. Interestingly, no drug has been approved by the Food and Drug Administration for lung transplantation. As long as there is a significant organ shortage, ethical issues will remain an area of conflict between a transplant physician's obligation to individual patients versus society.

FURTHER READING

1. Kotloff RM, Thabut G. Lung transplantation. *Am J Respir Crit Care Med.* 2011;184(2): 159–171.

   Excellent and up-to-date overview of lung transplantation, with sufficient details for most clinicians.

2. Orens JB, Estenne M, Arcasoy S, et al. International guidelines for the selection of lung transplant candidates: 2006 update—a consensus report from the Pulmonary Scientific Council of the International Society for Heart and Lung Transplantation. *J Heart Lung Transplant.* 2006;25: 745–755.

   Guidelines for timing of referral and transplantation by common disease types.

3. Takahashi SM, Garrity ER. The impact of the lung allocation score. *Semin Respir Crit Care Med.* 2010;31:108–114.

   An excellent, comprehensive review of the impact of the new lung allocation score.
   One of the most comprehensive reviews of all aspects of lung transplantation.

4. Christie JD, Edwards LB, Kucheryavaya AY, et al. The Registry of the International Society for Heart and Lung transplantation: 29th adult lung and heart-lung transplant report—2012. *J Heart Lung Transplant.* 2012;31(10):1087–1095.

   A yearly update with current statistics on survival and analysis of risk factors of heart and lung transplantations performed worldwide. Results are reported according to the type of transplantation.

5. Sundaresan S, Semenkovich J, Ochoa L, et al. Successful outcome of lung transplantation is not compromised by the use of marginal donor lungs. *J Thorac Cardiovasc Surg.* 1995;109: 1075–1079.

   Forty-four lung transplantations with "marginal donor lungs" showed comparable short-term results to controls.

6. Christie JD, Sager JS, Kimmel SE, et al. Impact of primary graft failure on outcomes following lung transplantation. *Chest.* 2005;127:161–165.

   A retrospective review of 255 lung transplant patients and outcomes following primary graft dysfunction.

7. Lee JC, Christie JD, Keshavjee S. Primary graft dysfunction: definition, risk factors, short- and long-term outcomes. *Semin Respir Crit Care Med.* 2010;31:161–171.

   Thorough review of PGD and its etiology and effect on lung transplant outcomes.

8. Shennib H, Massard G. Airway complications in lung transplantation. *Ann Thorac Surg.* 1994;57:506–511.

   Review of airway complications after lung transplantation showed 2% to 3% fatal cases and 7% to 14% late stricture. The authors also propose a classification of airway complications.

9. Novick RJ, Stitt LW, Al-Kattan K, et al; for the Pulmonary Retransplantation Registry. Pulmonary retransplantation: predictors of graft function and survival in 230 patients. *Ann Thorac Surg.* 1998;65:227–234.

   Survival of 230 patients after retransplantation of lungs was 47%, 40%, and 33% at 1, 2, and 3 years after surgery, respectively. Although survival was better in ambulatory, nonventilated patients, results were still inferior to statistics from first-time transplants.

10. Kaiser LR, Pasque MK, Trulock EP, et al. Bilateral sequential lung transplantation: the procedure of choice for double-lung replacement. *Ann Thorac Surg.* 1991;52:438–445.

    This study demonstrated the efficacy and safety of sequential lung transplantation over the old en bloc double-lung technique, and is now the procedure of choice for double lung transplantation.

11. Guilinger RA, Paradis IL, Dauber JH, et al; The importance of bronchoscopy with transbronchial biopsy and bronchoalveolar lavage in the management of lung transplant recipients. *Am J Respir Crit Care Med.* 1995;152:2037–2043.

    Retrospective analysis of 1,124 bronchoscopies in 161 lung transplant patients showed unsuspected rejection and infection in 25% cases, of which 68% occurred in the first 6 months.

12. Sundaresan RS, Trulock EP, Mohanakumar T, et al. Prevalence and outcome of bronchiolitis obliterans syndrome after lung transplantation. *Ann Thorac Surg.* 1995;60:1341–1347.

    High incidence of bronchiolitis obliterans with significant mortality. Most common presentation was decline in spirometric flow rates.

13. Ettinger NA, Bailey TC, Trulock EP, et al. Cytomegalovirus infection and pneumonitis: impact after isolated lung transplantation. *Am Rev Respir Dis.* 1993;147:1017–1023.

    High incidence of CMV pneumonitis after transplantation, especially in CMV-positive donors. Only one-third cases of CMV pneumonitis had chest radiograph changes.

14. Palmer SM, Limaye AP, Banks M, et al. Extended valganciclovir prophylaxis to prevent cytomegalovirus after lung transplantation: a randomized, controlled trial. *Ann Intern Med.* 2010;152:761–769.

    A randomized controlled clinical trial comparing 3 versus 12 months of CMV prophylaxis with valganciclovir in 136 lung transplant recipients. Longer prophylaxis resulted in a significantly decreased incidence of CMV disease, 4% versus 32%.

15. Sanchez PG, D'Ovidio F. Ex-vivo lung perfusion. *Curr Opin Organ Transplant.* 2012;17(5):490–495. doi:10.1097/MOT.0b013e328357f865.

    A nice summary of the current status of ex-vivo perfusion for explanted lungs, even though there are still ongoing studies.

16. Annual report from Organ Procurement and Transplantation Network. http://optn.transplant.hrsa.gov/data/annualReport.asp.

    This is a website of the US Organ Procurement and Transplantation Network, including up-to-date national, local, and individual transplant center statistics.

Pulmonary Manifestations of Sickle Cell Disease

Marisa Magaña and Jess Mandel

INTRODUCTION

Sickle cell disease (SCD) is a hemoglobinopathy that has multisystem deleterious effects. It is one of the most common autosomal recessive genetic disorders worldwide. It occurs as a result of a single base pair substitution in the β-subunit of hemoglobin, which results in the production of hemoglobin-S. In response to various stressors such as hypoxemia, oxidative stress, and cellular dehydration, sickle hemoglobin (HbS) polymerizes, resulting in structural abnormalities of the red blood cell, including characteristic sickle forms. This structural abnormality of the red blood cell results in the two main pathophysiologic processes of SCD: (1) occlusion of vascular beds with resulting ischemia–reperfusion injury and (2) hemolytic anemia.

Pulmonary complications of SCD commonly result in significant morbidity and mortality. An estimated 25% to 85% of deaths in SCD are related to pulmonary complications. Acute chest syndrome (ACS) is the most common cause of mortality in these patients and is a frequent cause of hospital admissions. Pulmonary hypertension is an increasingly recognized complication of SCD and is also associated with mortality. In addition, patients often have significant reactive airway disease and may develop chronic lung disease as a sequela of SCD.

ACUTE CHEST SYNDROME

ACS is characterized by a new pulmonary infiltrate, fever, chest pain, dyspnea, and wheezing or cough in a patient with SCD. This complication is the second most common cause (behind painful vaso-occlusive crises) for SCD patients to be admitted to the hospital and is the number one cause of admission to the ICU and death in patients with SCD. A key 2000 study evaluated 671 episodes of ACS in 538 patients and demonstrated that more than one-half of the patients were admitted for other reasons such as pain crises and before developing clinical signs of ACS an average of 2 to 3 days after admission. On the basis of this observation, there is speculation that vaso-occlusive crises are likely to be a prodrome of ACS. Patients who developed ACS had an average hospital length of stay of 10.5 days; 22% developed neurologic complications, 13% developed respiratory failure requiring mechanical ventilation, and there was a mortality rate of 9% in patients above 20 years of age. Interestingly, 81% of the patients who developed respiratory failure requiring mechanical ventilation recovered. Older patients (age >20 years) were more likely to develop complications and die in this study.

Several causes of ACS have been proposed. It is likely they all play a role in certain clinical situations; however, in almost half of cases no clear cause for ACS can be found. Known causes of ACS include infection with respiratory pathogens, fat embolism related to bone marrow infarction, sequestration of sickled cells in the pulmonary vasculature, and bronchospasm. Once one of these processes develops, it initiates a cycle of steps: further endothelial damage, worsened ventilation/perfusion matching, additional local hypoxemia, and further sickling of red blood cells and propagation of the cycle. Despite an aggressive diagnostic algorithm, a definite etiology is found in a minority of ACS episodes. In addition, investigators have noted that a high complication rate (up to 13% in the study referenced above) occurred during diagnostic bronchoscopy, with eight patients requiring intubation. They concluded that aggressive diagnostic modalities should be reserved for patients who are not responding to standard therapy.

The diagnosis of fat embolism can be made from bronchoscopy with bronchioloaleolar lavage or from induced sputum with oil red O-staining of macrophages, although these findings are more specific than sensitive. Some studies suggest that patients with evidence of fat embolism as the etiology of ACS have a slightly worse clinical course, with more pain and neurologic complications. However, because treatment of ACS does not differ when fat embolism is a primary cause, the importance of its diagnosis is uncertain at this time.

Treatment for ACS is predominantly supportive. *Chlamydia pneumoniae* (11%), *Mycoplasma pneumoniae* (8%), respiratory syncytial virus (4%), and *Streptococcus pneumoniae* (2%) are common respiratory pathogens isolated. Early empiric treatment of potential respiratory pathogens with antibiotics is recommended, usually with a third generation cephalosporin and either a macrolide or respiratory fluoroquinolone. In addition to antibiotic therapy, hydration, oxygen, red cell or exchange transfusion, aggressive pain control, and incentive spirometry are all important parts of the treatment of ACS. A component of reactive airway disease is frequently present and should be treated aggressively with bronchodilators.

PULMONARY ARTERIAL HYPERTENSION

In recent years pulmonary hypertension (PH) has been increasingly recognized as a complication of the hemolytic anemias and as a risk factor for death in patients with SCD. Pulmonary hypertension is defined as a mean pulmonary artery pressure (PAP) greater than or equal to 25 mmHg at rest. Various studies have suggested that from 20% to 30% of patients with SCD have PH. The presence of PH is associated with increased mortality; in one study, the 22-month mortality rate was as high as 40%. However, most of these studies used an echocardiographic diagnosis of PH, which is not as accurate as cardiac catheterization. In a group of 192 patients with SCD evaluated by echocardiogram, 32% had evidence of PH as defined by a tricuspid regurgitant (TR) jet velocity of greater than 2.5 m/second. Right heart catheterization was performed in 18 of the 195 patients and there was a correlation with the echocardiographic diagnosis of PH and hemodynamics by right heart catheterization, with a mean PAP in the cohort of 34 ± 2.7 mmHg. These data are similar to published retrospective reviews, which estimate the echocardiographic prevalence of PH in SCD between 20% and 40%. There is evidence to suggest that when a TR jet velocity of greater than 2.5 m/second was present, it was associated with an increased risk of death (rate ratio 10.1) when compared to patients with a TR velocity of less than 2.5 m/second.

The etiology of PH in SCD is likely multifactorial. It appears to be associated with the severity of the hemolytic anemia and some studies have suggested that left heart disease may play a role in its development. In the study by Gladwin et al., when echocardiographic variables associated with diastolic dysfunction were analyzed in a logistic regression model, they were not associated with a risk of death; therefore the authors concluded that because PH was associated with an increased risk of death, PH was likely independent of diastolic dysfunction. Interestingly, in the Gladwin et al. study, the mean pulmonary artery wedge pressure was 17.2 ± 1.2 mmHg, suggesting that perhaps left heart disease may have been contributing in some of the cases that underwent right heart catheterization.

There is substantial data that demonstrate the presence of increased mortality when PH exists. Therefore, patients with SCD should be screened for PH with echocardiogram. However, to confirm the presence of PH and determine the etiology, right heart catheterization should be performed prior to the initiation of any treatment for PH. Hypoxemia, thrombosis, and volume status may all influence TR velocity. Therefore, it is important that screening for PH be done in the steady state.

In addition to the degree of hemolytic anemia and left heart disease, the following mechanisms have been proposed as potential causes or contributing factors to the development of PH in patients with SCD: hypoxemia, iron overload, HIV infection, and thromboembolic disease. Interestingly, the frequency of ACS and vaso-occlusive crises does not seem to be related to the development of PH in SCD. The exact pathophysiology of hemolysis-induced pulmonary hypertension has not been clearly elucidated but is thought to be related to relative NO depletion due to non–red cell-contained hemoglobin from hemolysis. In addition, hemolysis causes release of arginase, which degrades arginine, the main substrate for NO generation. These two processes combined lead to decreased effects of NO, including pulmonary vasodilation. Unfortunately, studies that have evaluated therapeutics aimed at increasing NO levels have failed to show a consistent clinical benefit. As an example, a pilot study by Morris et al. investigated the effects of oral arginine supplementation in SCD patients with PH and found a statistically significant reduction in PAP measured by echocardiogram. However, this was not reproducible in a different study by Little et al. On the basis of the depleted NO hypothesis, the use of sildenafil in SCD-related PH has been tried as well. The Walk-Pulmonary Hypertension and Sickle Cell Disease with Sildenafil Therapy (Walk-PHaSST) study attempted to evaluate the safety and efficacy of sildenafil in SCD patients with Doppler-proven PH. This study was terminated early after enrollment of 74 out of 132 patients due to increased adverse events in the treatment arm, consisting mainly of painful vaso-occlusive crises. On the basis of this trial and pending further data, sildenafil is not recommended as first-line therapy for PH in patients with SCD.

Preliminary data suggest that bosentan may be effective and well-tolerated in SCD patients with Doppler-defined PH. However, further studies in more patients are needed before the therapy can be advocated on a broad scale.

ASTHMA

In children the prevalence of asthma in SCD is similar to that in age- and race-matched controls. However, children with SCD with a diagnosis of asthma are more likely to have episodes of ACS and vaso-occlusive pain crises than SCD patients without asthma. The relationship between asthma and SCD in adults is not well-established. In adults, the presentation of ACS and asthma may have significant clinical overlap and the prevalence of asthma in adults is lower, making it more difficult to study. However, the possibility of asthma should be investigated, diagnosed, and aggressively treated if potentially present.

CHRONIC LUNG DISEASE IN SCD

Chronic lung disease in SCD encompasses a variety of pulmonary disorders that have not been well-characterized in adults. The largest cross-sectional study evaluating lung function in adults with SCD included 310 adult African American SCD patients who were in a steady clinical state at least 4 weeks after a vaso-occlusive crisis. It found that 90% of patients had abnormal pulmonary function tests and the most common abnormalities were a restrictive defect occurring (74%) and low diffusing capacity (13%). An obstructive defect either alone or in combination with restriction was uncommon, occurring in 3% of patients. Interestingly, half of the patients with restrictive defects had a decreased total lung capacity but normal spirometry, suggesting that spirometry alone may not be a good screening test in these patients. Patients in this study did not undergo routine imaging to look for the presence of interstitial lung disease (ILD). Therefore, the etiology of these findings is unclear and may be related to undiagnosed ILD or extrapulmonary causes. There was no echocardiographic screening done to determine whether the patients with an isolated low diffusing capacity had PH. Other studies have shown that some patients with SCD and a restrictive pulmonary defect have a fibrotic interstitial disease that contributes to morbidity and mortality. More comprehensive and longitudinal studies are needed to determine the incidence, natural history, and clinical significance of these findings.

In addition, sleep-disordered breathing has been reported in a large fraction of adults and children with SCD. Therefore, these patients should undergo polysomnography or, at least, evaluation for nocturnal desaturation as this has clearly been linked with increased vaso-occlusive crises and neurologic events in SCD patients.

INFECTION

The role of infection in ACS has already been discussed. This section will focus upon infection in the functionally asplenic SCD patient not related to ACS. By the time patients with SCD reach adulthood, they are functionally asplenic due to repeated episodes of vaso-occlusion and infarction in the spleen. The spleen plays a critical role in the clearance of infection, especially encapsulated bacteria. Therefore, SCD patients are at significantly increased risk of infection with these organisms, most notably *S. pneumoniae* and *Haemophilus influenzae* type B. Prior to the introduction of preventive measures (see below), children with SCD were 30 to 600 times more likely to develop invasive pneumococcal disease. This has dropped significantly, but both children and adults who develop infection with these bacteria have a significantly increased risk of mortality. For this reason, any sign of infection should be treated aggressively with empiric antibiotics.

Two measures have significantly decreased invasive pneumococcal infection: antibiotic prophylaxis and pneumococcal vaccination. Children who are functionally asplenic should receive daily bacterial prophylaxis until the age of 5 with penicillin or erythromycin to prevent invasive pneumococcal disease. There are conflicting data regarding the use of prophylactic antibiotics in older children. The United States guidelines do not recommend its use after the age of 5, while the British guidelines recommend its use until the age of 16 and state that lifelong use is optional.

Vaccinations are particularly important in this group. Adults should receive the pneumococcal polyvalent vaccine and be revaccinated 5 years later according to the CDC. Some European agencies recommend these individuals receive revaccination every 5 years. In addition, they should receive *H. influenza* B conjugate vaccine, if not given in childhood, as well as the meningococcal C conjugate vaccine. Yearly influenza vaccination is also indicated.

Osteomyelitis occurs more commonly in SCD patients, likely because of repeated vaso-occlusion and infarction. *Salmonella typhimurium* is the most common etiology in SCD patients with osteomyelitis, in contrast to *Staphylococcus aureus* in patients without SCD.

FURTHER READING

1. Rees DV, Williams TN, Gladwin MT. Sickle-cell disease. *Lancet.* 2010;376:2018–2031.

   A general review on all aspects of SCD.

2. Minter KR, Gladwin MT. Pulmonary complications of sickle cell anemia: a need for increased recognition, treatment, and research. *Am J Respir Crit Care Med.* 2001;164:2016.

   A concise review of the pulmonary manifestations of SCD and pathogenesis. Review of the literature on deaths related to pulmonary causes in SCD.

3. Vij R, Machado RF. Pulmonary complications of hemoglobinopathies. *Chest.* 2010;138:973–983.

   An excellent and comprehensive review on pulmonary complications of hemoglobinopathies mostly focused on SCD.

4. Vichinsky EP, Neumayr LD, Earles AN, et al, Causes and outcomes of the acute chest syndrome in sickle cell disease. *N Engl J Med.* 2000;342:1855.

   Landmark, multicenter study evaluating etiology and outcomes of ACS. The management of these patients is also addressed.

5. Platt OS. The acute chest syndrome of sickle cell disease. *N Engl J Med*. 2000;342:1904–1907.

6. Castro O, Brambilla DJ, Thorington B, et al. The acute chest syndrome in sickle cell disease: incidence and risk factors. *Blood*. 1994;89:643.

   Details from the Cooperative Study of Sickle Cell Disease, involving 3,751 patients, with 19,867 years of follow-up.

7. Vichinsky E, Williams R, Das M, et al. Pulmonary fat embolism: a distinct cause of severe acute chest syndrome in sickle cell disease. *Blood*. 1994;83:3107.

   Twelve of 27 patients with ACS had lipid-laden macrophages on bronchoalveolar lavage. Those with evidence of fat embolism had a distinct clinical course, with a higher frequency of concomitant bone pain and neurologic symptoms and longer hospitalization

8. Lechapt E, Habibi A, Bachir D, et al. Induced sputum versus bronchoalveolar lavage during acute chest syndrome in sickle cell disease. *Am J Respir Crit Car Med*. 2003;168:1373–1377.

   Detection of Oil Red O-stained macrophages in induced sputum samples correlated with samples obtained from BAL, and the authors conclude that sputum induction is a safe and useful test for the detection of fat embolism in patients with ACS.

9. Gladwin MT, Sachdev V, Jison ML, et al. Pulmonary hypertension as a risk factor for death in patients with sickle cell disease. *N Engl J Med*. 2004;350:886.

   Large, prospective, controlled study demonstrating that pulmonary hypertension as defined echocardiographically is common in adults with SCD and carries an increased risk for death.

10. Bunn HF, Nathan DG, Dover GJ, et al. Pulmonary hypertension and nitric oxide depletion in sickle cell disease. *Blood*. 2010;116(5):687–692.

11. Bachir D, Parent F, Hajji L, et al. Prospective multicentric survey on pulmonary hypertension (PH) in adults with sickle cell disease [abstract]. *Blood*. 2009;114(11) 572. ASH Annual Meeting Abstracts.

    Prospective evaluation of 379 patients with SCD, 96 had echocardiographic evidence of PH and were evaluated by RHC. There was no PH in 72/96 of these patients. They conclude that the PH is relatively rare in patients with SCD and that echocardiogram is not a reliable diagnostic tool.

12. Machado RF, Barst RJ, Martyr SE, et al. Safety and efficacy of sildenafil therapy for Doppler-defined pulmonary hypertension in patients with sickle cell disease: preliminary results of the Walk-PHaSST clinical trial [abstract]. *Blood*. 2009;114:571.

    Trial was stopped early due to increased episodes of painful vaso-occlusive episodes in the treatment arm. Based on this trial, sildenafil is not recommended as first-line therapy for SCD patients with PH.

13. Morris CR, Morris SM, Hagar W, et al. Arginine therapy: a new treatment for pulmonary hypertension in sickle cell disease? *Am J Respir Crit Care Med*. 2003;168:63.

    Pulmonary artery pressure based on echocardiography decreased by a mean 15.2% after 5 days of treatment with oral L-arginine in 10 patients.

14. Little JA, Hauser KP, Martyr SE, et al. Hematologic, biochemical, and cardiopulmonary effects of L-arginine supplementation or phosphodiesterase 5 inhibition in patients with sickle cell disease who are on hydroxyurea therapy. *Eur J Haematol*. 2009;82:315–321.

15. Minniti CP, Machado RF, Coles WA, et al. Endothelin receptor antagonists for pulmonary hypertension in adult patients with sickle cell disease. *Br J Haematol*. 2009;147:737–743.

16. Barst RJ, Mubarak KK, Machado RF, et al. Exercise capacity and hemodynamics in patients with sickle cell disease with pulmonary hypertension treated with bosentan: results of the ASSET studies. *Br J Haematol*. 2010;149(3):426–435.

    The goal of this study was to evaluate the efficacy of bosentan in Doppler-defined PH in SCD. The study was stopped early due to slow enrollment and only enrolled 26 patients; therefore, outcome analysis could not be performed. Bosentan appeared to be well tolerated in these patients.

17. Klings ES, Wyszynski DF, Nolan VG, et al. Abnormal pulmonary function in adults with sickle cell anemia. *Am J Respir Crit Care Med*. 2006;173:1264–1269.

    Large study (2,061 patients) evaluating various parameters related to SCD and their effect on lung function in adults.

18. Haupt HM, Moore GW, Bauer TW, et al. The lung in sickle cell disease. *Chest*. 1982;81:332.

    An autopsy study of 72 patients with advanced SCD. The main pulmonary findings were alveolar wall necrosis secondary to vascular obstruction, focal parenchymal scars, and necrotic bone marrow emboli.

19. Bhalla M, Abboud MR, McLoud TC, et al. Acute chest syndrome in sickle cell disease: CT evidence of microvascular occlusion. *Radiology.* 1993;187:45.

In this thin section CT study, 9 of 10 patients with ACS were found to have small vessel attenuation in the lung, consistent with microvascular obstruction, surrounded by areas of ground-glass infiltrate.

20. Bellet PS, Kalinyak KA, Shukla R, et al. Incentive spirometry to prevent acute pulmonary complications in sickle cell diseases. *N Engl J Med.* 1995;333:699.

Of patients with ACS, 39.5% had evidence of thoracic bone infarcts; in these patients, hospital duration and the development of pulmonary complications were significantly reduced by the use of incentive spirometry when compared with controls.

21. Booth C, Inusa B, Obara SK. Infection in sickle cell disease: a review. *Int J Infect Dis.* 2010;14:e2–e12.

A comprehensive review of infections in SCD patients.

22. Davies JM, Barnes R, Milligan D. Update of guidelines for the prevention and treatment of infection in patients with an absent or dysfunctional spleen. *Clin Med.* 2002;2:440–444.

Guidelines regarding prophylactic antibiotics and vaccinations for functionally asplenic or asplenic patients. Pneumococcal revaccination is recommended every 5 years. Antibiotic prophylaxis with erythromycin or penicillin is recommended for the prevention or invasive pneumococcal disease.

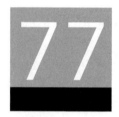

Cystic Fibrosis

Douglas J. Conrad

Cystic fibrosis (CF) is a systemic disease characterized by acute and chronic sinusitis, progressive bronchiectasis, and pancreatic malabsorption. In the past, patients with CF rarely survived through childhood and were cared for almost exclusively by pediatricians. However, aggressive treatment and newer therapies have dramatically improved prognosis: The predicted median age of survival of CF patients currently is approximately 38 years in North America. Mild or atypical forms of CF are diagnosed in adults because of recent advances in diagnostic technology. For these reasons, primary care providers and adult pulmonologists diagnose and manage CF patients more frequently now than in previous years.

ETIOLOGY AND PATHOPHYSIOLOGY

The CF gene and the most common mutations associated with the disease were identified in 1989. These data characterized the CF gene product, a protein termed the *cystic fibrosis transmembrane conductance regulator* (CFTR). CF is inherited as an autosomal recessive. Mutations in the *CFTR* gene are common in the general population (1:29 in North American Caucasians), but the incidence varies significantly in different ethnic populations. Carriers of a single mutated *CFTR* allele are minimally symptomatic but may have an increased incidence of pancreatitis and allergic rhinitis. The life expectancy of carriers with *CFTR* mutations is normal.

The CFTR protein is located primarily on the apical membranes of epithelial cells of the respiratory, hepatobiliary, and pancreatic tracts, as well as in the crypts of the large intestine and sweat gland ducts. It forms a large, regulated pore in the apical cell membrane, which functions as a chloride channel but also transports other anions including bicarbonate. Dysfunction of CFTR-dependent ion transport is believed to be responsible for the pulmonary manifestations of CF. The "hydration hypothesis" states that ion transport by CFTR in airway epithelial cells is critical for maintaining hydration and normal function of the airway lining fluid, including the secreted mucus. When these processes are disturbed, the mucociliary clearance mechanism is diminished and bacteria form a chronic polymicrobial biofilm, which elicits a strong innate immune response. Neutrophil proteases stimulate submucosal gland hypertrophy and secretion and eventually cause a breakdown of the airway wall support leading to bronchiectasis. In addition, the neutrophils leave large quantities of cellular DNA, dramatically increasing airway secretion viscosity and further impairing airway clearance. Respiratory failure occurs as a result of a self-perpetuating cycle of inflammation and decreased airway clearance. The bronchiectasis is progressive and leads to respiratory failure in 80% of patients with CF.

Additional studies indicate that the pathophysiology of CF in the gastrointestinal tract and pulmonary systems also involves bicarbonate transport. In these studies, bicarbonate transport is critical for the deployment of mucus over these epithelia. Mutations in *CFTR* lead to abnormal mucus deployment, mucus plugging, and eventually, end organ dysfunction in the pancreatic and hepatobiliary ducts and intestinal obstruction in the lower gastrointestinal tract.

CLINICAL PRESENTATION

Patients with CF present with a wide variety of respiratory and gastrointestinal complaints that are typically evident in childhood. The more common manifestations include nasal polyps; sinusitis; bronchospasm; recurrent bronchitis or pneumonia; airway colonization with *Staphylococcus aureus, Haemophilus influenza,* or *Pseudomonas aeruginosa*; steatorrhea; pancreatic malabsorption; meconium ileus; failure to thrive; rectal prolapse; distal intestinal obstructive syndrome; and hepatic cirrhosis with portal hypertension. Undiagnosed adults frequently present with recurrent bronchitis (in a nonsmoker), asthma associated with the radiographic evidence of diffuse bronchiectasis, chronic sinusitis, allergic bronchopulmonary aspergillosis (ABPA), airway bacterial colonization with atypical mycobacteria or mucoid *P. aeruginosa,* cirrhosis, idiopathic pancreatitis, or male infertility.

The physical examination is nonspecific but includes findings consisted with chronic sinusitis and obstructive lung disease. Chest examination reveals an increased chest anteroposterior diameter, with decreased diaphragmatic excursion. Diffuse rales and rhonchi are common in most patients and prominent in the apices. Breath sounds are occasionally normal in patients with mild disease. Digital clubbing is frequent. Most patients have pancreatic insufficiency and, thus, have some degree of protein–calorie malnutrition.

Taken individually, the findings on history and physical examination are nonspecific; however, the particular combination of sinusitis, diffuse bronchiectasis, pancreatic malabsorption with malnutrition, obstructive colonopathy, and male infertility is very specific for CF. Although primary ciliary dysfunction and other immunoglobulin deficiencies syndromes mimic some of the pathophysiologic consequences, they are not usually associated with gastrointestinal symptoms. More extensive use of genetic testing has identified patients with milder disease.

DIAGNOSTIC LABORATORY CONFIRMATION

A diagnosis of CF is made after a confirming laboratory study performed in patients with a consistent clinical picture. The sweat chloride test remains the standard in the laboratory confirmation of CF. This test should be performed by experienced laboratory personnel in accredited labs. Pilocarpine iontophoresis is used to stimulate secretion of sweat, which is collected, weighed, and analyzed for its chloride and sodium concentrations. A chloride concentration greater than 60 mEq/L is diagnostic of CF, with most positive tests falling in the 90 to 110 mEq/L range. All positive or indeterminate results (values between 40 and 60 mEq/L) should be repeated at least once. Since the identification of the gene for CF in 1989, more than 1,500 disease-causing mutations have been identified. Several commercial laboratories now offer complete sequencing of the *CFTR* gene. Combined *CFTR* sequencing and sweat chloride testing may be particularly helpful in evaluating patients with atypical presentations.

MANAGEMENT

Management of CF is focused on: (1) maintaining optimal nutritional status, (2) promoting airway clearance of inflammatory cells, (3) decreasing bacterial colonization, and (4) minimizing the impact of respiratory and gastrointestinal complications, particularly pulmonary exacerbations.

Management of progressive, chronic bronchiectasis focuses on decreasing the frequency of pulmonary exacerbations by diminishing airway inflammation and promoting airway clearance. Antibiotics are used to decrease the level of bacterial colonization. Although chronic antibiotic suppressive therapy with anti-staphylococcal antibiotics was demonstrated to be not tremendously useful, this practice is being reconsidered in the context of dramatic increase in methicillin-resistant *S. aureus* infections. Inhaled anti-pseudomonal antibiotics have a long history of utility in CF. Inhaled tobramycin at doses up to 300 mg twice daily every other month improves lung function and health-related quality of life and decreases absenteeism. Similar data exist for inhaled aztreonam lysate. In upcoming years, inhaled fluoroquinolones and other aminoglycosides are likely to be other approved alternatives. In general, inhaled antibiotics are best used as chronic, suppressive therapy and are less useful during acute exacerbations, particularly in patients with advanced lung disease.

Several pharmacologic therapies may improve airway clearance and reduce airflow obstruction. The concentration of DNA in respiratory secretions of patients with CF is high and dramatically increases the viscosity of the sputum and impairs its clearance. Aerosolized recombinant human deoxyribonuclease (DNase), a pancreatic-derived enzyme that degrades DNA, may be inhaled to diminish the effect DNA has on respiratory secretion viscosity. Clinical studies have demonstrated improvement in pulmonary function, decreased use of antibiotics, and subjective improvement in symptoms with inhaled DNase. Similarly, inhaled 7% hypertonic saline has also improved lung function and decreased the time to pulmonary exacerbation.

A great deal of clinical investigation has focused on anti-inflammatory therapy in CF. The use of steroids in CF is controversial largely because of the long-term risk of adverse effects. Corticosteroids are generally not used in the chronic outpatient management of CF patients, but are helpful in selected patients with severe lung disease and bronchospasm. Chronic use of nonsteroidal anti-inflammatory drugs, specifically ibuprofen, does preserve lung function; however, these effects were most prominent in children and in patients with mild lung function abnormalities. Several randomized clinical trials in pediatric and adult CF patients have demonstrated that the anti-inflammatory effects of macrolides, particularly azithromycin, improve pulmonary function, decrease antibiotic use, and improve quality of life.

Chest physiotherapy is the major mechanical means of augmenting airway clearance. This is typically delivered manually or with a mechanical percussor two to four times per day. Other airway clearance techniques, such as autogenic drainage, positive expiratory pressure masks, and flutter valves, can be helpful. Finally, chest physiotherapy vests generate shearing forces and dislodge inspissated airway secretions and are very useful for most CF patients.

Many providers encourage patients to perform strenuous aerobic exercise daily. Exercise improves cardiovascular conditioning, promotes airway clearance, and, importantly, benefits patients psychologically. Patients who perform routine aerobic exercise may also be more sensitive to a decline in their performance, which can be an early indicator of pulmonary illness requiring therapy.

Lung transplantation is an option for some patients with severely depressed lung function whose lifestyles have been significantly limited by the disease (see Chapter 71). Lung transplant candidates should be selected carefully, with consideration given to other medical comorbidities, psychosocial support, and patient motivation. Most centers that perform lung transplantation for patients with CF report a 1-year survival rate of approximately 80% and a 4-year survival rate of 50%.

Chronic sinusitis is evident in most patients with the disease; symptoms are managed initially with antibiotics and topical steroids. Although conservative management can be helpful, many patients are eventually referred for surgical polypectomies, sinus antrectomies, and tissue debridement. This aggressive therapy frequently relieves symptoms and, in some cases, is associated with improvement in pulmonary function.

Pancreatic malabsorption and protein–calorie malnutrition should be managed aggressively. Thorough reviews of daily caloric intake and monitoring of body weight are important to maintaining nutritional goals. Fat-soluble vitamins (vitamins A, D, E, and K) are not readily absorbed through the gastrointestinal tract of patients with CF. These vitamin levels should be monitored annually and dietary supplements should be provided. Adequate pancreatic enzyme replacement is the key to maintaining nutritional status and avoiding symptoms of pancreatic malabsorption. As a general rule, most patients who have insufficient pancreatic function require between 1,000 and 2,000 U/kg body weight per meal of lipase activity. In patients who are compliant with the nutritional regimen but whose body weight remains less than 80% of ideal body weight, the oral diet should be augmented with nocturnal gastrostomy tube feedings of nutritional supplements.

RESPIRATORY COMPLICATIONS

The most common cause of a hospital admission is a pulmonary exacerbation of infectious bronchiectasis. Patients often present with worsening exertional capacity, diminished pulmonary function, and increased cough and sputum production. Inpatients are typically treated with two antibiotics targeting organisms observed in sputum cultures. *In vitro* sensitivity data may help guide the antibiotic selection; however, clinical improvement is frequently observed even when the cultured bacteria have demonstrated significant *in vitro* resistance. In most cases, patients are treated empirically with two anti-pseudomonal antibiotics and an antibiotic targeting *S. aureus* if it is present in airway secretions. In addition to antibiotics, patients typically receive aggressive chest physiotherapy four times daily and frequent bronchodilators. Pancreatic malabsorption is treated the same as in the outpatient setting. Although home IV antibiotic administration is an option for treating pulmonary exacerbations in some patients, these patients must be carefully selected. Those who are most likely to have successful outcomes with outpatient IV antibiotics typically have had good responses to antibiotics in the past, are very motivated, and have adequate support in the home. IV antibiotics should be continued as long as the patient's clinical status is improving, which typically takes 10 to 14 days. If stabilization occurs before reaching the patient's functional baseline, then changing antibiotic therapy based on antibiotic sensitivities may be considered.

The use of mechanical ventilation to treat respiratory failure is particularly controversial. All decisions regarding mechanical ventilatory support should be individualized. Some patients who are cooperative and motivated may respond temporarily to noninvasive ventilatory support. In general, patients who develop respiratory failure despite optimal treatment should not be mechanically ventilated because of the progressive nature of this disease. However, patients who have not received optimal therapy or who have respiratory failure secondary to reversible complications (e.g., hemoptysis, pneumothorax, etc.) should be considered for mechanical ventilation.

Massive hemoptysis (>250 mL/24 hours) is not uncommon in patients with CF. Most patients can be treated conservatively, using supportive measures such as IV antibiotics, oxygen supplementation, temporary suppression of cough, avoidance of chest physiotherapy during active bleeding, transfusions of platelets or packed red blood cells, when appropriate, and the correction of any clotting abnormalities with either vitamin K or fresh frozen plasma. Occasionally, these measures are inadequate because of progressive respiratory failure or ongoing bleeding. In these cases, medical stabilization should be followed with bronchial arterial embolization, which typically controls bleeding quickly. Surgery is very rarely needed for control, but may be considered if embolization does not control life-threatening bleeding and the patient is an adequate surgical candidate.

Pneumothorax occurs frequently in patients with severe lung disease caused by CF. Conservative therapy with oxygen supplementation, antibiotics, and bronchodilators is usually successful in patients with small, asymptomatic pneumothoraces. In patients with larger, symptomatic or nonresolving pneumothoraces, a more aggressive approach is warranted. Chest tube drainage is frequently successful in reexpanding the lung and allows the option of chemical pleurodesis. Pleurodesis, either chemical or surgical, should be avoided if the patient is to be considered for lung transplantation in the future.

ABPA is a hypersensitivity reaction to aspergillus in the airway and occurs in 5% to 20% of patients with CF. In most instances, patients with ABPA exacerbations are treated with corticosteroid courses and antifungal therapy. Atypical mycobacterial infections are an emerging problem in CF patients. In many cases, the mycobacteria cause progressive airway destruction and volume loss. Standard therapy for macrolide sensitive isolates typically includes prolonged courses of clarithromycin, ethambutol, and rifampin. For recurrences or resistant isolates, infectious disease consultation can be useful.

NONRESPIRATORY COMPLICATIONS

Occasionally, patients with CF develop an obstructive colonopathy such as meconium ileus or distal intestinal obstructive syndrome. Frequently, they complain of constipation and right-sided abdominal pain. This abdominal pain needs to be distinguished from peptic ulcer disease, cholelithiasis, pancreatitis, colitis, or appendicitis. Initial management should include administration of pancreatic enzymes, along with mild laxatives and an increase in dietary fiber. Gastrografin enemas may help to relieve the obstruction in some cases; surgery is needed occasionally.

CF-related diabetes (CFRD) is common in adults with CF and is diagnosed either by an abnormal 2-hour oral glucose tolerance test or persistent elevation of fasting serum glucose values. Patients with untreated diabetes may have significant problems with gaining weight and preserving lung functions. Clinicians are increasingly treating CFRD more aggressively with insulin to assist in the treatment of nutritional therapy and to preserve lung function.

Other important nonrespiratory complications that occur frequently include bone disease (osteopenia/osteoporosis), chronic depression and anxiety, and infertility. The reader is referred to other resources that address these critical issues.

ONGOING RESEARCH

CF is an area of active clinical research. Some of the more promising areas of research are aimed at developing inhaled antibiotics, identifying novel anti-inflammatory agents. Modulators of epithelial anion transport are a primary focus of recent translational investigation. The results of recent clinical trials and approval of Kalydeco™ for patients with at least one copy of the *CFTR* G551D confirmed the approach of using small bioavailable molecules to correct the consequences of a single *CFTR* mutation. Investigations targeting therapies for nonsense mutations, mutations affecting *CFTR* mRNA splicing and "corrector" therapies are currently in early phase investigation. Successful therapy for CF is likely to involve multiple therapies targeting the pathophysiologic process at several steps.

FURTHER READING

1. Lazarowski ER, Boucher RC. Purinergic receptors in airway epithelia. *Curr Opin Pharmacol.* 2009;9(3):262–267.
2. Quinton PM. Role of epithelial HCO_3^- transport in mucin secretion: lessons from cystic fibrosis. *Am J Physiol Cell Physiol.* 2010;299(6):C1222–C1233.

   Two important reviews covering basic pathophysiologic issues associated with cystic fibrosis.

3. Kerem B, Rommens JM, Buchanan JA, et al. Identification of the cystic fibrosis gene: genetic analysis. *Science.* 1989;245:1073.
4. Riordan JR, Rommens JM, Kerem B, et al. Identification of the cystic fibrosis gene: cloning and characterization of complementary DNA. *Science.* 1989;245:1066.
5. Rommens JM, Iannuzzi MC, Kerem B, et al. Identification of the cystic fibrosis gene: chromosome walking and jumping. *Science.* 1989;245:1059.

   References 3, 4, and 5 are the classic articles identifying the cystic fibrosis gene, the most common disease-causing mutations and the initial characterization of the gene product CFTR.

6. Elkins MR, Robinson M, Rose BR, et al; for the National Hypertonic Saline in Cystic Fibrosis (NHSCF) Study Group. A controlled trial of long-term inhaled hypertonic saline in patients with cystic fibrosis. *N Engl J Med.* 2006;354(3):229–240.
7. Saiman L, Marshall BC, Mayer-Hamblett N, et al. Azithromycin in patients with cystic fibrosis chronically infected with *Pseudomonas aeruginosa. JAMA.* 2003;290:1749–1756.

8. Fuchs HJ, Borowitz DS, Christiansen DH, et al; for the Pulmozyme Study Group. Effect of aerosolized recombinant human DNase on exacerbations of respiratory symptoms and on pulmonary function in patients with cystic fibrosis. *N Engl J Med.* 1994;331:637. See also comments.
9. Konstan MW, Byard PJ, Hoppel CL, et al. Effect of high-dose ibuprofen in patients with cystic fibrosis. *N Engl J Med.* 1995;332:848. See also comments.
10. Ramsey BW, Pepe MS, Quan JM, et al; for the Cystic Fibrosis Inhaled Tobramycin Study Group. Intermittent administration of inhaled tobramycin in patients with cystic fibrosis. *N Engl J Med.* 1999;340:23.
11. Retsch-Bogart GZ, Quittner AL, Gibson RL, et al. Efficacy and safety of inhaled aztreonam lysine for airway pseudomonas in cystic fibrosis. *Chest.* 2009;135(5):1223–1232.

References 6 through 11 are important clinical research trials establishing the roles for rhDNase I, hypertonic saline, ibuprofen, inhaled antibiotics, and azithromycin in the chronic care of patients with cystic fibrosis.

12. Flume PA, Mogayzel PJ Jr, Robinson KA, et al. Cystic fibrosis pulmonary guidelines: treatment of pulmonary exacerbations. *Am J Respir Crit Care Med.* 2009;180:802–808.
13. Flume PA, Mogayzel PJ, Robinson KA, et al; for the Clinical Practice Guidelines for Pulmonary Therapies Committee. Cystic fibrosis pulmonary guidelines: pulmonary complications: hemoptysis and pneumothorax. *Am J Respir Crit Care Med.* 2010;182:298–306.
14. Stenbit AE, Flume PA. Pulmonary exacerbations in cystic fibrosis. *Curr Opin Pulm Med.* 2011;17:442–447.
15. Hoffman LR, Ramsey BW. Cystic fibrosis therapeutics: the road ahead. *Chest.* 2013;143(1):207–213.

References 12 to 15 are excellent detailed summaries of current clinical practice guidelines and a review of therapies currently under investigation.

Disorders of the Thoracic Spine

Thuy K. Lin and Justin C. Reis

The thoracic volume is determined by the height of the thoracic spine and the width and depth of the rib cage. Disorders that distort the chest wall or cause chest wall restriction can compromise respiratory function. The most common disorders are scoliosis, kyphosis, kyphoscoliosis, and ankylosing spondylitis.

SCOLIOSIS/KYPHOSIS/KYPHOSCOLIOSIS

Scoliosis is characterized by a lateral curvature of the spinal column with rotation of the vertebrae. Its severity is defined by the angle between the tangents of the most inclined vertebral plateau, also known as the Cobb angle. The greater the Cobb angle, the shorter the hemithorax on the concave side of the curve. Kyphosis is defined by anteroposterior angulation of the spine. Scoliosis is usually associated with a component of kyphosis, but kyphosis can occur in isolation. Kyphoscoliosis is characterized by distortion of the thoracic cage, which can cause impairment of lung growth. Respiratory symptoms are usually mild unless: (1) the Cobb angle is greater than 100°, (2) scoliosis occurs prior to age 9, or (3) the patient has kyphoscoliosis. Congenital kyphosis, kyphoscoliosis, and scoliosis are all part of a spectrum of spinal deformities due to developmental vertebral anomalies.

Eighty percent of kyphoscoliosis begins in childhood and is idiopathic; the rest are due to neuromuscular diseases (e.g., poliomyelitis, syringomyelia, neurofibromatosis), congenital defects of the spine, vertebral disease (e.g., tuberculosis, tumor, osteomalacia), and thoracic disease (e.g., emphysema, thoracoplasty). Idiopathic kyphoscoliosis is more common in women (4:1) and is usually not as severe compared to the deformities of poliomyelitis, tuberculosis, and congenital spine defects. Infantile scoliosis (onset 0 to 3 years) and juvenile scoliosis (onset 4 to 9 years) are more likely to be associated with Cobb angles greater than 100°, fused or absent ribs, rotation of the spine with secondary rib deformity, or restriction of rib motion. Pulmonary development involves growth of new alveoli until 5 to 8 years of age. Any bony abnormality that reduces thoracic volume during this time may affect lung size. Individuals who reach skeletal maturity with a vital capacity of less than 45% of predicted (using arm span to determine predicted height) have an increased risk of respiratory failure when their lung function starts to decline from the age of 35 onward. However, studies of patients followed for 50 to 60 years demonstrate that the more common adolescent scoliosis is rarely a cause of mortality.

Patients with kyphoscoliosis are subject to a variety of mechanical factors, which eventually contribute to alveolar hypoventilation. With progressive disease, total lung capacity (TLC), vital capacity (VC), and functional residual capacity (FRC) can become reduced, mainly due to reductions in chest wall compliance and alterations in the mid-position of the thoracic cage. The degree of pulmonary restriction and gas exchange impairment is highly correlated with the angle of scoliosis. In 1975, Kafer established a correlation between the degree of scoliosis and TLC, VC, FRC, and residual volume. The degree of scoliosis (higher Cobb angle) was negatively correlated with alveolar ventilation (VA) and VC and positively correlated with the physiological dead space/tidal volume ratio (VD/VT). Deformity above T10 is associated with a greater degree of respiratory impairment. At rest, minute ventilation is reduced due to diminished tidal volume. With exercise, the mechanical effects of the chest wall deformity are of greater significance and hypoventilation is more marked.

Mild kyphoscoliosis has a good prognosis. Pulmonary rehabilitation may improve pulmonary function and exercise capacity. Jones et al. performed 6-minute walk tests on six patients with moderate-to-severe kyphoscoliosis (mean Cobb angle 79°) and reported that oxygen therapy relieved symptoms of dyspnea and improved desaturation, but did not increase the 6-minute walk distance, in contrast to patients with chronic obstructive pulmonary disease (COPD). Supplemental oxygen may alleviate vasoconstriction associated with pulmonary hypertension secondary to regional or global alveolar hypoventilation. Patients with respiratory failure can benefit from noninvasive positive pressure ventilation, which increases lung compliance, decreases the work of breathing, and allows fatigued respiratory muscles to rest.

Surgery in adults with established kyphoscoliosis has questionable benefits and can result in significant complications. Gitelman et al. performed a retrospective review of 49 patients with adolescent idiopathic scoliosis who underwent corrective surgical procedures. Over 10 years, pulmonary function tests showed that the group who underwent corrective chest wall surgery had no change in forced vital capacity (FVC) and forced expiratory volume in 1 second (FEV$_1$), but demonstrated a significant decrease in percent-predicted FVC. The group that underwent posterior spinal fusion/instrumentation with iliac crest bone graft and no thoracic cage disruption had a significant increase in both FVC and FEV$_1$, but no change in percent-predicted values.

Indications for surgery in young patients include (1) progression of disease despite good external brace care, (2) deformity that is too advanced to respond to external bracing, (3) scoliosis greater than 50°, (4) intractable pain, (5) nonalignment of occiput over sacrum, and (6) psychiatric disturbances. Surgical treatment for progressive congenital kyphosis or kyphoscoliosis is indicated at an early age, not only to prevent severe spinal deformity and possible neurologic complications but also to prevent the adverse effects on lung development and function caused by constriction of the thoracic cage and impairment of diaphragmatic movement.

ANKYLOSING SPONDYLITIS

Ankylosing spondylitis (AS) is a chronic inflammatory disease affecting joints of the axial skeleton with secondary fibrosis and ossification of the ligamentous structures of the spine, sacroiliac joints, and rib cage. It predominately affects males aged 20 to 40 years. Approximately 90% of patients with AS are positive for the HLA-B27 antigen. Ankylosing spondylitis can affect the tracheobronchial tree and pulmonary parenchyma, and is associated with several unique pulmonary manifestations, including fibrobullous, fibrocystic, and pleural chest wall disease.

Ankylosing spondylitis causes fixation of the chest wall through fusion of the costovertebral joints and ankylosis of the thoracic spine. Clinical manifestations include intermittent low back pain or stiffness, weight loss, anorexia, and fever. Chest wall pain, typically with inspiration, has been noted in more than 60% of patients. Dyspnea, though relatively uncommon, can be associated with pulmonary or cardiovascular involvement. Severe respiratory symptoms are rare as long as diaphragmatic function is normal. Patients will often manifest only mild restriction on pulmonary function tests with decrease in TLC and VC. Reduction in VC, if present, is primarily due to diminished thoracic cage compliance.

Approximately 1% of patients with ankylosing spondylitis develop pulmonary parenchymal disease, usually in the form of apical fibrobullous or fibrocavitary disease. Apical fibrobullous disease generally presents in adulthood, with an average interval of 15 years or more between the onset of arthritic manifestations and the development of pulmonary abnormalities. Apical fibrosis, unless extensive or secondarily infected by bacteria or fungi, is typically asymptomatic. In more advanced disease, cough, sputum production, or dyspnea may develop. Hemoptysis is more likely to occur in those with bronchiectasis or intracavitary mycetoma. An increased incidence of spontaneous pneumothoraces and obstructive sleep apnea has also been reported.

The mechanism responsible for the apical fibrobullous pulmonary changes is unknown. Proposed causes include reduced ventilation to the upper lobes due to chest wall rigidity, altered mechanical stresses on the lung apices, repeated pulmonary infections, and/or primary airway inflammation. Fungal and/or mycobacterial superinfections have been reported in up to one-third of patients with upper lobe cystic and cavitary disease. Prior thoracic irradiation has been implicated, although apical changes are also present in those who have not undergone radiation therapy. Recurrent aspiration pneumonitis secondary to esophageal muscle dysfunction has been suggested as well.

Chest radiographic findings may mirror the severity of the clinical involvement. Chest radiography initially shows a nodular or reticular pattern in the apical or subapical lung zones. These abnormalities may initially be asymmetric, but many patients eventually develop bilateral disease. Pulmonary parenchymal disease is typically progressive. Nodules often coalesce into larger opacities; cyst formation, cavitation, and fibrosis are seen with more advanced cases. Upward retraction of hilar structures is due to upper lobe volume loss. Computed tomography (CT) of the chest, particularly high-resolution techniques, is highly sensitive in defining the extent of airway and pulmonary parenchymal changes and in detecting intracavitary pulmonary mycetomas. CT is also useful in identifying pleural thickening, volume loss, cavitation, and bronchiectasis.

Treatment is primarily preventative and supportive. Anti-inflammatory therapy has not been shown to influence the pulmonary manifestations of the underlying disease. No treatment has been shown to alter the clinical course of apical fibrobullous disease. Management of respiratory complications of ankylosing spondylitis is mainly related to treating pulmonary superinfections using antifungal or antimicrobial agents. Surgical excision of fibrocystic disease is rarely indicated except for major hemoptysis from an aspergilloma. Several preliminary reports on the use of tumor necrosis factor (TNF) blockers in ankylosing spondylitis suggest short-term improvement in disease activity ratings and quality-of-life measures; however, improvements in pulmonary function tests and respiratory symptoms have not been assessed consistently.

In summary, disorders of the thoracic spine like scoliosis, kyphosis, kyphoscoliosis, and ankylosing spondylitis can affect respiratory function and cause dyspnea. Respiratory failure is rare unless the disease is severe.

FURTHER READING

1. Ayhan-Ardic FF, Oken O, Yorgancioglu ZR, et al. Pulmonary involvement in lifelong non-smoking patients with rheumatoid arthritis and ankylosing spondylitis without respiratory symptoms. *Clin Rheumatol.* 2006;25:213–218.

   Study demonstrating HRCT as a sensitive tool in detecting interstitial lung disease (ILD) in patients with rheumatoid arthritis and AS with no signs and symptoms of pulmonary involvement.

2. Bergofsky EH, Turino GM, Fishman AP. Cardiorespiratory failure in kyphoscoliosis. *Medicine.* 1959;38:263–317.

   An excellent review of kyphoscoliosis.

3. Boulware DW, Weissman DN, Doll NJ. Pulmonary manifestations of the rheumatic diseases. *Clin Rev Allergy.* 1985;3:249–267.

   Review article of the clinicopathologic pulmonary presentations of rheumatic diseases.

4. Braun J, Brandt J, Listing J, et al. Two year maintenance of efficacy and safety of infliximab in the treatment of ankylosing spondylitis. *Ann Rheum Dis.* 2005;64:229–234.

   Infliximab as a reasonable therapeutic option in the regression and stabilization of symptoms due to AS.

5. Dos Santos Alves VL, Stirbulov R, Avanzi O. Impact of a physical rehabilitation program on the respiratory function of adolescents with idiopathic scoliosis. *Chest.* 2006;130:500–505.

   Rehabilitation program improves FVC, FEV$_1$, inspiratory capacity, expiratory reserve volume, and 6-minute walk test in patients with idiopathic scoliosis.

6. Fenlon HM, Casserly I, Sant SM, et al. Plain radiographs and thoracic high-resolution CT in patients with ankylosing spondylitis. *AJR Am J Roentgenol.* 1997;168:1067–1072.

   Study with comparison of abnormalities seen on HRCT in patients with AS to those found on plain radiograph. Prospective study, but only 26 patients.

7. Franssen MJAM, van Herwaarden CLA, van de Putte LBA, et al. Lung function in patients with ankylosing spondylitis: a study of the influence of disease activity and treatment with nonsteroidal anti-inflammatory drugs. *J Rheumatol.* 1986;13:936–940.

   Small study looking at lung function in patients with AS treated with two different nonsteroidal anti-inflammatory drugs; determining that vital capacity is not an appropriate variable for the evaluation of short-term therapy in AS.

8. Gitelman Y, Lenke LG, Bridwell KH, et al. Pulmonary function in adolescent idiopathic scoliosis relative to the surgical procedure. *Spine.* 2011;36:1665–1672.

   This is a retrospective review looking at the long-term effect of pulmonary function in 49 patients who had surgical correction of adolescent idiopathic scoliosis.

9. Hunninghake GW, Fauci AS. Pulmonary involvement in the collagen vascular diseases. *Am Rev Respir Dis.* 1979;119:471–503.

   Comprehensive review of the various effects of collagen vascular diseases on the respiratory system.

10. Jessamine AG. Upper lobe fibrosis in ankylosing spondylitis. *Can Med Assoc J.* 1968;98:25–29.

   One of the first articles to describe the unique finding of apical fibrosis in patients with poorly controlled AS.

11. Jones DJM, Paul EA, Bell JH, et al. Ambulatory oxygen therapy in stable kyphoscoliosis. *Eur Respir J.* 1995;8:819–823.

   A small study showing that patient with moderate to severe kyphoscoliosis had desaturation on exercise and had symptoms improvement on oxygen; however, oxygen did not affect walking distance.

12. Kafer ER. Idiopathic scoliosis: mechanical properties of the respiratory system and ventilator response to carbon dioxide. *J Clin Invest.* 1975;55:1153–1163.

   This article reviews the effects of scoliosis (angle) and age on lung volumes, elastic properties of the respiratory system, and the ventilatory response to carbon dioxide.

13. Kafer ER. Idiopathic scoliosis: gas exchange and the age dependence of arterial blood gases. *J Clin Invest.* 1976;58:825–833.

   This article examines the gas exchange and arterial blood gas abnormalities among patients with scoliosis, and the correlation of these abnormalities with age and severity of deformity.

14. Kanathur N, Lee-Chiong T. Pulmonary manifestations of ankylosing spondylitis. *Clin Chest Med.* 2010;31:547–554.

   Recent review highlighting the diagnosis, management of complications, and prognosis of pulmonary disease in patients with AS.

15. Lee CC, Lee SH, Chang IJ, et al. Spontaneous pneumothorax associated with ankylosing spondylitis. *Rheumatology.* 2005;44:1538–1541.

   Review of the incidence and clinical characteristics of spontaneous pneumothorax in patients with AS.

16. Lee-Chiong TL Jr. Pulmonary manifestations of ankylosing spondylitis and relapsing polychondritis. *Clin Chest Med.* 1998;19:747–757.

Review of the literature comparing the pulmonary manifestations of AS to relapsing polychondritis.

17. McMaster MJ, Glasby MA, Singh H, et al. Lung function in congenital kyphosis and kyphoscoliosis. *J Spinal Disord Tech.* 2007;20:203–208.

A study looking at 41 patients with congenital kyphosis and kyphoscoliosis shows increasing severity of kyphosis, above T10, was associated with a significant increase in respiratory impairment.

18. Romaker AM. Chest wall and neuromuscular disorders: disorders of the thoracic spine. In: Bordow RA, Ries AL, ed. *Manual of Clinical Problems in Pulmonary Medicine.* 6th ed. Philadelphia, PA: Lippincott Williams & Wilkins; 2005:427–430.

This current review is based on this prior edition with new updates.

19. Rosenow E, Strimlan CV, Muhm JR, et al. Pleuropulmonary manifestations of ankylosing spondylitis. *Mayo Clin Proc.* 1977;52:641–649.

Of 2,080 patients with AS, 28 (1.3%) had typical chest roentgenograms; 5 of 28 (18%) had aspergillomas; 3 had transient exudative pleural effusions with normal glucose levels.

20. Rumancik WM, Firooznia H, Davis MS, et al. Fibrobullous disease of the upper lobes: an extraskeletal manifestation of ankylosing spondylitis. *J Comput Tomogr.* 1984;8:225–229.

Article reviewing some characteristic radiographic findings of AS and ways to help differentiate these from pulmonary tuberculosis and intracavitary pulmonary mycetoma.

21. Solak O, Fidan F, Dundar U, et al. The prevalence of obstructive sleep apnea syndrome in ankylosing spondylitis patients. *Rheumatology.* 2009;48:433–435.

The prevalence of obstructive sleep apnea syndrome in AS patients with a disease duration less than 5 years was 11.8% and its prevalence in AS patients with a disease duration of greater than or equal to 5 years was 35.7%.

22. Souza AS Jr, Muller NL, Marchiori E, et al. Pulmonary abnormalities in ankylosing spondylitis. *J Thorac Imaging.* 2004;19:259–263.

Small study in radiographic journal examining the various findings on plain radiograph and inspiratory and expiratory HRCT.

23. Tanoue LT. Pulmonary involvement in collagen vascular disease: a review of the pulmonary manifestations of the Marfan syndrome, ankylosing spondylitis, Sjögren's syndrome, and relapsing polychondritis. *J Thorac Imaging.* 1992;7:62.

Comprehensive discussion of pulmonary involvement in four diseases: the Marfan syndrome, AS, Sjögren syndrome, and relapsing polychondritis.

24. Tardif C, Sohier B, Derenne JP. Control of breathing in chest wall diseases. *Monaldi Arch Chest Dis.* 1993;48(1):83–86.

Review on how the respiratory system compensates for kyphoscoliosis.

25. van der Heijde D, Kivitz A, Schiff MH, et al. Efficacy and safety of adalimumab in patients with ankylosing spondylitis: results of a multicenter, randomized, double-blind, placebo-controlled trial. *Arthritis Rheum.* 2006;54:2136.

Adalimumab was well-tolerated during the 24-week study period and was associated with a significant and sustained reduction in the signs and symptoms of active AS.

Disorders of the Diaphragm

Tony S. Han

The diaphragm is the principal muscle of respiration during quiet breathing. It also serves as the barrier between the thoracic and abdominal compartments. Proper integrity of the diaphragm is important in maintaining negative pressure within the thoracic cavity. Disorders of the diaphragm include paralysis, weakness, eventration, herniation, and rupture.

PARALYSIS OF THE DIAPHRAGM

Paralysis is the most important clinical condition affecting the diaphragm. It can be discovered incidentally but often presents with dyspnea on exertion or dyspnea when in the supine position. The right and left phrenic nerves originate from the third, fourth, and fifth cervical roots. They run in the lateral compartment of the neck, enter the thorax posteriorly, and then run anteriorly over the pericardium to finally innervate the hemidiaphragms. Cooling of the heart during cardiac surgery can damage the phrenic nerves or diaphragm leading to paralysis. Paralysis usually occurs on the left side and is often temporary. The overall incidence is about 2%. Other causes of paralysis include tumor invasion, surgical section, trauma, and post-viral neuropathy. Often, the exact etiology is unknown. Rare causes include neck irradiation, hypothyroidism, post-polio syndrome, acid maltase deficiency, Guillain–Barré syndrome, systemic lupus erythematosus, and malnutrition. Bilateral diaphragmatic paralysis is usually the result of cervical spinal cord trauma. Bilateral involvement is also seen with generalized neuromuscular disorders such as amyotrophic lateral sclerosis.

Patients with diaphragmatic paralysis present with dyspnea on exertion and orthopnea. Other conditions such as obstructive lung disease, congestive heart failure, thromboembolic disease, and pulmonary arterial hypertension must be excluded. Symptoms can be progressive and lead to significant disability. Sometimes the dyspnea is worse with immersion in water due to increased pressure on the abdomen. With diaphragmatic paralysis, the intercostal and the accessory muscles become the chief muscles of inspiration. Orthopnea occurs due to the effect of hydrostatic pressure of abdominal contents on the diaphragm and decreasing vital capacity. Also, there may be paradoxical elevation of the paralyzed hemidiaphragm during inspiration, which compromises ventilation. On physical examination, patients with bilateral diaphragmatic paralysis often show prominent activity of the accessory muscles of inspiration (i.e., intercostals, scalene, and sternocleidomastoids), because their inspiration results primarily from elevation of the rib cage by these muscles. Patients often favor the upright position, from which they can fixate their pectoral girdle and use their pectoral muscles to elevate the chest wall and breathe more efficiently. When supine, they may display a classic paradoxical inward motion of the anterior abdominal wall during quiet inspiration. Percussion of the chest wall before and after inspiration may reveal decreased excursion of the hemidiaphragms.

Chest radiographs may show elevation of the paralyzed hemidiaphragm. This finding is sensitive (0.90) but not specific (0.44). Thus, many patients found to have incidental elevation of the hemidiaphragm on chest radiograph have normal lung function. Pulmonary function testing in diaphragmatic paralysis reveals a reduced forced vital capacity (FVC) and reduced forced expiratory volume in 1 second (FEV_1) with preserved FEV_1/FVC ratio. In addition, total lung capacity (TLC), vital capacity, inspiratory capacity, and maximal inspiratory pressure are all reduced. Unilateral paralysis reduces TLC and maximal inspiratory pressure by 20% to 25%. A low inspiratory capacity that decreases still further in the supine position suggests diaphragmatic paralysis.

The definitive diagnosis of diaphragmatic paralysis has traditionally rested on fluoroscopic demonstration of diminished, absent, or paradoxical upward motion during normal inspiration. The "sniff maneuver" with a closed mouth is used to enhance this paradoxical upward movement during a quick inspiration. With unilateral disease, the normal diaphragm moves downward while the paralyzed diaphragm moves paradoxically upward. In cases of bilateral paralysis, the diaphragms may move together and appear to be functioning normally (though not in the appropriate direction during inspiration and expiration), thus producing a false-negative fluoroscopic result. A more comprehensive evaluation can be made by inserting balloon catheters to record gastric and esophageal pressures to measure transdiaphragmatic pressure (Pdi). Pdi should increase with inspiration and the abdomen should move outward. The failure to increase Pdi, or the generation of greater Pdi by inward motion of the abdomen, suggests diaphragmatic paralysis. Magnetic phrenic nerve stimulators applied to the neck coupled with these pressure measurements have been used to definitively diagnose paralysis. Absence of pressure change in response to nerve stimulation is diagnostic. Recent studies have also suggested using two-dimensional B-mode ultrasound to assess diaphragm function. An ultrasound transducer is placed in the eighth or ninth intercostals space in the midaxillary line. Diaphragmatic thickness is measured at functional residual capacity and TLC to indicate the degree of thickening. Less than a 20% change in thickness may indicate diaphragmatic paralysis.

Patients with diaphragmatic paralysis may be at higher risk for sleep disordered breathing, particularly during REM sleep. Compared to typical obstructive sleep apnea patients, their respiratory events seem to be primarily central hypopneas associated with more severe oxyhemoglobin desaturation. This is apparently due to respiratory muscle fatigue and mechanical disadvantage. It may be worthwhile to pursue sleep testing, particularly if the patient has significant daytime symptoms.

Diaphragmatic paralysis not related to spinal injury may improve spontaneously over a period of months to years. Treatment of diaphragmatic paralysis with pacing may be indicated in central paralysis when the phrenic nerve and diaphragmatic muscle are preserved. Electrodes are surgically implanted around the phrenic nerve, and electronic signals are generated using an external radio-wave source worn by the patient. Following installation of such a pacing device, weeks or months may be required to achieve full effect if diaphragmatic atrophy has antedated pacing.

Recovery of diaphragmatic paralysis over 6 to 12 months has been described in cases of thermal injury during cardiac surgery. If there is no improvement after 12 to 24 months, surgical plication of the hemidiaphragm is a viable option for patients with significant dyspnea. The thin flaccid diaphragm is made taut with nonresorbable sutures to improve lung mechanics. The procedure can be performed either through video-assisted thoracoscopy (VATS) or thoracotomy. Long-term follow-up at 4 to 6 years indicate sustained improvement in symptoms and lung function. Alternatively, in unilateral diaphragmatic paralysis associated with brachial plexus neuritis, a few patients have responded well to valacyclovir therapy with improvement within 4 to 6 weeks.

EVENTRATION OF THE DIAPHRAGM

Eventration in the purest sense is a congenital malformation consisting of failure of muscular development of all or part of the diaphragm. It is associated with other malformations such as hypoplastic lungs, transposition of the viscera, and chest wall and spinal abnormalities and is a surgical emergency. In common use, the term "eventration" has been used to describe chronic elevation of the hemidiaphragm from any cause including diaphragmatic paralysis. On chest roentgenogram, eventration is apt to be confused with a diaphragmatic hernia or pleuropericardial cyst. It has poor specificity for hemidiaphragm paralysis, especially if the patient is asymptomatic.

HERNIATION OF THE DIAPHRAGM

Herniation of abdominal contents through the diaphragm can occur through regions of congenital defect or weakness, including the esophageal hiatus, the posterolateral or pleuroperitoneal foramen of Bochdalek (in infants), and the retrosternal (parasternal) foramen of Morgagni (any age). Hiatal hernia (via the esophageal hiatus) is relatively common in adults. It is usually asymptomatic, but can cause retrosternal burning and pain, which are aggravated by lying flat and relieved by antacids. Occasionally, hiatal hernia can be associated with nocturnal aspiration and recurrent pneumonia.

Herniation through the posterolateral aspect of the diaphragm (foramen of Bochdalek) is the most common and serious hernia in infants. It usually presents as an acute respiratory emergency at or shortly after birth and requires immediate surgical repair.

Herniation through the foramen of Morgagni is more common in adults and is often asymptomatic. Obesity is an important predisposing factor. On chest roentgenogram, the abnormal shadow appears retrosternally, usually along the right sternal border, and can mimic a pericardial cyst.

TEARS AND RUPTURE OF THE DIAPHRAGM

Tears or rupture of the diaphragm can occur with blunt or penetrating trauma. Use of single-point, lap-belt restraint systems in high-speed motor vehicle accidents is associated with diaphragmatic rupture. Herniation of the abdominal contents can cause respiratory distress and substernal pain. This injury can be missed in the unconscious trauma victim until an upright chest roentgenogram shows absence of the affected diaphragmatic outline or until computed tomography is obtained.

DIAPHRAGM FATIGUE

Diaphragmatic fatigue is a common clinical problem in patients requiring mechanical ventilation. It occurs when the energy expenditure of the diaphragm exceeds the capacity of the blood supply to provide oxygen and nutrients. An increase in the fraction of the maximal contractile pressure developed by the diaphragm during a breath and the fraction of ventilatory time spent in inspiration (i.e., with the diaphragm contracting) both independently increase the likelihood of diaphragmatic fatigue. The multiple of these two fractions, which is called the *tension time index*, predicts the development of fatigue when the value exceeds 0.15. Mechanical ventilation may induce atrophy and diaphragmatic dysfunction predisposing it to fatigue. The blood flow to the diaphragm is also an important determinant of fatigue. The threshold for fatigue is reduced under hypotensive or hypoxemic conditions.

Muscle rest is the primary therapy for respiratory muscle fatigue; however, a number of agents, most notably aminophylline, increase diaphragmatic contractility and endurance in the experimental setting. The significance of these findings for therapy of clinical respiratory muscle fatigue remains uncertain, but the complications of these agents probably outweigh their clinical utility in patients with respiratory muscle fatigue.

FUNCTIONAL DISORDERS OF THE DIAPHRAGM

The most common functional disorder of the diaphragm is the mechanical disadvantage that results from an extreme degree of hyperinflation with severe airways obstruction or advanced emphysema. During the course of chronic obstructive pulmonary disease (COPD), the diaphragm is displaced inferiorly and flattened out, thereby reducing the pressure that can be generated as the diaphragm contracts. Some adaptation of the diaphragm occurs with emphysematous change to make the diaphragm more fatigue-resistant, but mechanical disadvantage is more important than fatigue in causing ventilatory limitation. Lung volume reduction procedures can reduce lung volume in selected patients, restoring mechanical advantage to the diaphragm and improving exercise tolerance.

Other functional diaphragmatic disorders include hiccup (singultus) and diaphragmatic flutter. Hiccup is usually a benign disorder that results from repetitive, abrupt inspiratory spasm of the diaphragm, with associated closure of the glottis. It commonly follows transient diaphragmatic irritation, such as with gastric distention caused by aerophagia or overeating. Treatment of acute gastritis can be an effective means of reducing the frequency of hiccups. Protracted episodes may follow upper abdominal surgery, cardiac surgery, or inferior myocardial infarction. Hiccup can also be associated with mediastinitis, tumor invasion, pericarditis, pleuritis, gastritis, and peritonitis. In patients with cardiac pacemakers, hiccup can signal perforation of the right ventricle by the pacing electrode.

Diaphragmatic flutter (respiratory myoclonus or Leeuwenhoek disease) is a rare disorder characterized by dyspnea associated with frequent diaphragmatic contractions (~100/minute) superimposed on the normal respiratory excursion and by prominent epigastric pulsations. The attacks are paroxysmal. Diphenylhydantoin may be helpful.

SUMMARY

Disorders of the diaphragm can be an important unrecognized cause of exertional dyspnea. Although immediate treatment is not recommended in most cases, recognition of diaphragmatic paralysis is important to determine prognosis. Initial evaluation should include a careful physical exam of the chest wall, lung function testing, chest radiographs, and, possibly, fluoroscopy. Severe or persistent cases may be amenable to surgical treatment.

FURTHER READING

1. Bellemare F, Grassino A. Evaluation of human diaphragm fatigue. *J Appl Physiol*. 1982;53:1196–1206.

   The fraction of maximal contraction and the time spent in inspiration influences the endurance time; a tension time index of 0.15 or greater predicts fatigue.

2. Baltzan MA, Scott AS, Wolkove N. Unilateral hemidiaphragm weakness is associated with positional hypoxemia in REM sleep. *J Clin Sleep Med*. 2012;8(1):51–58.

   Sleep disordered breathing is observed in five patients with unilateral diaphragm paralysis and no previous obstructive sleep apnea.

3. Canbaz S, Turgut N, Halici U, et al. Electrophysiological evaluation of phrenic nerve injury during cardiac surgery—a prospective, controlled, clinical study. *BMC Surg*. 2004;4:2.

   Prospective study of phrenic nerve injury in 78 patients undergoing cardiac surgery. Three weeks after surgery, left phrenic nerve function was absent in 5 of 49 patients who underwent hypothermic cardiopulmonary bypass. None of the 29 patients undergoing normothermic surgery for coronary artery bypass grafting or peripheral vascular surgery developed phrenic nerve injury.

4. Celli B. The diaphragm and respiratory muscles. *Chest Surg Clin N Am*. 1998;8:207–224.

   A good review of the functional anatomy and function of the diaphragm in the context of the other respiratory muscles.

5. Chervin RD, Guilleminault C. Diaphragm pacing for respiratory insufficiency. *J Clin Neurophysiol*. 1997;14:369–377.

   A review of diaphragm pacing by electrical stimulation of the phrenic nerve, outlining the preoperative evaluation and procedures for surgical implantation.

6. Chetta A, Rehman AK, Moxham J, et al. Chest radiography cannot predict diaphragm function. *Respir Med*. 2005;99:39–44.

   Prevalence of diaphragmatic dysfunction based on phrenic nerve stimulation tests was 24% among chest radiographs with elevation of the diaphragm.

7. Crausman RS, Summerhill EM, McCool FD. Idiopathic diaphragmatic paralysis: Bell's palsy of the diaphragm? *Lung*. 2009;187(3):153–157.

   Three patients with unilateral paralysis of the diaphragm improved in 4 to 6 weeks after valacyclovir treatment, suggesting a possible viral etiology.

8. Criner G, Cardova FC, Leyenson V, et al. Effect of lung volume reduction surgery on diaphragm strength. *Am J Respir Crit Care Med*. 1998;157:1578–1585.

   Lung volume reduction surgery significantly improves diaphragm strength that is associated with a reduction in lung volumes and an improvement in exercise performance.

9. De Troyer A, Leeper JB, McKenzie DK, et al. Neural drive to the diaphragm in patients with severe COPD. *Am J Respir Crit Care Med*. 1997;155:1335–1340.

   Patients with severe COPD have an increased neural drive not only to the rib cage inspiratory muscles but also to the diaphragm. The reduced inspiratory expansion of the abdomen in severe COPD results predominantly from mechanical factors in stable, severe COPD.

10. Dureuil B, Matuszczak Y. Alteration in nutritional status and diaphragm muscle function. *Reprod Nutr Dev*. 1998;38:175–180.

    In cachectic subjects, the diaphragm muscle mass and thickness are reduced in proportion to the reduction in body weight. Respiratory muscle strength and endurance are reduced more severely than the weight loss. This finding suggests that malnutrition induces a reduction in muscular mass that is associated with a decrease in contractility.

11. Freeman RK, Van Woerkom J, Vyverberg A, et al. Long-term follow-up of the functional and physiologic results of diaphragm plication in adults with unilateral diaphragm paralysis. *Ann Thorac Surg*. 2009;88(4):1112–1117.

    Forty-one patients showed improvement in lung function parameters of about 20% at a mean follow-up interval of 57 months following surgical plication. Thirty-seven of 41 showed symptomatic improvement as well.

12. Fromageot C, Lofaso F, Annane D, et al. Supine fall in lung volumes in the assessment of diaphragmatic weakness in neuromuscular disorders. *Arch Phys Med Rehabil*. 2001;82:123–128.

    Measurement of changes in vital capacity and maximal inspiratory pressure from sitting to supine positions was helpful in detecting diaphragmatic weakness.

13. Hughes PD, Polkey MI, Harrus ML, et al. Diaphragm strength in chronic heart failure. *Am J Respir Crit Care Med.* 1999;160:529–534.

Mild reduction in diaphragm strength occurs in chronic heart failure, possibly because of an increased proportion of slow fibers, but overall strength of the respiratory muscles remains well preserved.

14. Johnson BD, Babcock MA, Suman OE, et al. Exercise induced diaphragmatic fatigue in healthy humans. *J Physiol.* 1993;460:385–405.

Significant diaphragmatic fatigue can be caused by the ventilatory requirements imposed by heavy endurance exercise. The magnitude of the fatigue and the likelihood of its occurrence increase as the relative intensity of the exercise exceeds 85% $\dot{V}PO_{2max}$.

15. LaRoche C, Carroll N, Moxham J, et al. Clinical significance of severe isolated diaphragm weakness. *Am Rev Respir Dis.* 1988;138:862–866.

All patients studied had normal resting gas exchange, and nocturnal hypercapnia did not develop. Dyspnea with exertion and orthopnea were common to all patients.

16. Lando Y, Boiselle PM, Shade D, et al. Effect of lung volume reduction surgery on diaphragm length in severe chronic obstructive pulmonary disease. *Am J Respir Crit Care Med.* 1999;159:796–805.

Lung volume reduction surgery leads to a significant increase in diaphragm length, especially in the area of apposition of the diaphragm with the rib cage. Diaphragm lengthening after this surgery is most likely the result of a reduction in lung volume. Increases in diaphragm length after surgery correlate with post-operative improvements in diaphragm strength, exercise capacity, and maximal voluntary ventilation.

17. Laghi F, Jubran A, Topeli A, et al. Effect of lung volume reduction surgery on neuromechanical coupling of the diaphragm. *Am J Respir Crit Care Med.* 1998;157:475–483.

Lung volume reduction surgery improves diaphragmatic function greater than can be accounted for by a decrease in operating lung volume, and enhances diaphragmatic neuromechanical coupling.

18. Laghi F, D'Alfonso N, Tobin MJ. Pattern of recovery from diaphragmatic fatigue over 24 hours. *J Appl Physiol.* 1995;79:539–546.

Induction of diaphragmatic fatigue with an experimental protocol produced marked decrease in diaphragmatic contractility that persisted for at least 24 hours, suggesting that prolonged rest may be necessary for full recovery of diaphragmatic muscle strength after development of fatigue.

19. Levine S, Kaiser L, Leferovich J, et al. Cellular adaptations in the diaphragm in chronic obstructive pulmonary disease. *N Engl J Med.* 1997;337:1799–1806.

Severe COPD increases the slow-twitch characteristics of the muscle fibers in the diaphragm, an adaptation that increases resistance to fatigue.

20. Maish MS. The diaphragm. *Surg Clin North Am.* 2010;90:955–968.

A concise review of anatomy and congenital disorders from a surgical perspective.

21. Mihos P, Potaris K, Gakidis J, et al. Traumatic rupture of the diaphragm: experience with 65 patients. *Injury.* 2003;34:169–172.

Descriptive case series of 65 patients with traumatic diaphragmatic rupture over 11 years in a trauma center in Greece. Rupture was left-sided in 66%, right-sided in 32%, and bilateral in 2%. Blunt trauma accounted for 80% of cases. Emphasizes importance of high index of suspicion and early diagnosis, which can be missed in the acute trauma setting despite use of CT scanning.

22. Mouroux J, Venissac N, Leo F, et al. Surgical treatment of diaphragmatic eventration using video-assisted thoracic surgery: a prospective study. *Ann Thorac Surg.* 2005;79:308–312.

A series of 12 patients with mostly traumatic or iatrogenic paralysis undergo successful minimally invasive plication.

23. Oh KS, Newman B, Bender TM, et al. Radiologic evaluation of the diaphragm. *Radiol Clin North Am.* 1988;26:355–364.

One of those "everything you wanted to know but were afraid to ask" reviews. Especially good on congenital and traumatic disorders of the diaphragm.

24. Phillips JR, Elderidge FL. Respiratory myoclonus (Leeuwenhoek's disease). *N Engl J Med.* 1973;289:1390–1395.

Clinical features as well as pulmonary function test, electrocardiographic, and electromyography findings are presented. Still the best review of this rare disorder.

25. Reber A, Nylund U, Hedenstierna G. Position and shape of the diaphragm: implications for atelectasis formation. *Anaesthesia.* 1998;53:1054–1061.

Compared with conscious, spontaneous breathing, mechanical ventilation decreases the inspiratory displacement of the dependent part of the diaphragm. This change in movement of the diaphragm can play an additional role in atelectasis formation.

26. Roussos C. Function and fatigue of respiratory muscles. *Chest.* 1985;88:124S–132S.

Blood flow to respiratory muscles is relatively high and fixed even in the presence of cardiac failure, a point to be remembered when timing interventions such as intubation and mechanical ventilation in cardiac patients.

27. Ruel M, Deslauriers J, Maltais F. The diaphragm in emphysema. *Chest Surg Clin N Am.* 1998;8:381–399.

Concise review of pathophysiology and surgical treatment options of diaphragmatic dysfunction related to hyperinflation in emphysema.

28. Steier J, Jolley CJ, Seymour J, et al. Sleep-disordered breathing in unilateral diaphragm paralysis or severe weakness. *Eur Respir J.* 2008;32:1479–1487.

Eleven patients with diaphragmatic paralysis underwent polysomnogram with transesophageal EMG. Mean respiratory disturbance index was 26 in REM sleep.

29. Steier J, Kaul S, Seymour J, et al. The value of multiple tests of respiratory muscle strength. *Thorax.* 2007;62:975–980.

A combination of maximal inspiratory pressure and nasal sniff pressure led to greater diagnostic precision in diaphragmatic weakness. Adding Pdi-improved precision further, but was more invasive.

30. Tsao BE, Ostrovskiy DA, Wilbourn AJ, et al. Phrenic neuropathy due to neuralgic amyotrophy. *Neurology.* 2006;66:1582–1584.

Seventeen of 33 patients diagnosed with idiopathic phrenic neuropathy had clinical features of neuralgic amyotrophy.

31. Versteegh MI, Braun J, Voigt PG, et al. Diaphragm plication in adult patients with diaphragm paralysis leads to long-term improvement of pulmonary function and level of dyspnea. *Eur J Cardiothorac Surg.* 2007;32(3):449–456.

Twenty-two patients followed for a mean of 4.9 years demonstrate improvement in supine vital capacity from 53% to 73% as well as improvement in dyspnea scores.

32. Weksler B, Ginsberg RJ. Tumors of the diaphragm. *Chest Surg Clin N Am.* 1998;8:441–447.

A review of primary tumors of the diaphragm, most of which are benign.

Neuromuscular Diseases and Spinal Cord Injury

Russell J. Miller and John Scott Parrish

NEUROMUSCULAR DISEASES

Neuromuscular disorders can affect multiple aspects of respiratory function. This heterogeneous group includes disorders affecting motor neurons (e.g., poliomyelitis, amyotrophic lateral sclerosis, Guillain–Barré syndrome [GBS]), neuromuscular junctions (e.g., myasthenia gravis, Eaton–Lambert syndrome, botulism), and skeletal muscles (e.g., muscle dystrophy, drug-induced myopathy, polymyositis). Although the pathophysiology of these diseases can vary greatly, the expected morbidity is relatively predictable and directly related to respiratory insufficiency. There are three major muscle groups required for ventilation: inspiratory, expiratory, and bulbar muscles. The inspiratory muscles, with primary responsibility for normal tidal breathing, include the diaphragm, external intercostals, and accessory muscles, such as the sternocleidomastoid and scalene, which are used in stressed inhalation. Expiration is normally a passive process, but forced expiration used with coughing, exercise, or spirometry testing is performed primarily by the abdominal and internal intercostal muscles. The bulbar muscles are responsible for cough, swallowing, and airway protection.

Hypoventilation

Hypoventilation in neuromuscular disorders is primarily related to respiratory muscle weakness as reflected by pulmonary function tests (PFT) demonstrating reduction in vital capacity (VC), tidal volume, and minute ventilation. Hypoventilation may be further complicated by stiffening of the chest wall leading to decreased thoracic compliance. With exertion, patients will often develop a rapid shallow breathing pattern as a mechanism to maintain minute ventilation as a result of reduced ability to generate adequate tidal volumes. Respiratory muscle fatigue from this pattern of breathing can result in air hunger and hypercapnia from increased dead space ventilation. Dyspnea at rest and air hunger are actually late findings in many of the neuromuscular diseases due to the patient's adjustment to sedentary lifestyle associated with the underlying disorder. Pulmonary function testing is typically characterized by restriction, although the pattern varies depending on which muscles are affected (inspiratory and/or expiratory). VC can be reduced either due to a loss of inspiratory capacity (reduced total lung capacity), expiratory reserve volume (elevated residual volume), or both. Functional residual capacity (FRC), the end-tidal lung volume representing the balance of static lung and chest wall elastic recoil, may be unaffected. The gold standard for evaluation of diaphragmatic strength is measurement of trans-diaphragmatic pressure, but this requires the use of an esophageal balloon, is somewhat invasive, and is not commonly used. Other less-invasive tests for assessing respiratory muscle weakness include the maximum inspiratory pressure (MIP) and maximum expiratory pressure (MEP). To perform these tests, the patient is encouraged to inspire or expire with maximal effort against an occluded external airway from residual volume (MIP) or from total lung capacity (MEP). The maximum pressure generated is recorded with a manometer. The MIP and MEP can be abnormal early in the course of disease, even when the static lung volumes are normal. These maneuvers, however, can be technically difficult. A normal MIP and MEP is useful in excluding clinically significant respiratory muscle weakness, but values are often falsely low and hence lack specificity. The VC obtained during routine, upright spirometry may miss or underestimate significant diaphragmatic weakness since restrictive changes are most pronounced in the supine position. Daytime hypercapnia ($Pco_2 > 45$) is an ominous sign and usually predicts development of overt respiratory failure.

Chronic hypoventilation in patients with neuromuscular disease is typically treated with noninvasive ventilatory support. Although tracheostomy is a tempting means to aid daytime hypoventilation, the complications of chronic invasive ventilation often outweigh the benefits. These complications include increased risk of developing ventilator-associated infections and reduced quality of life. In patients with intact bulbar muscle function, inspiratory and expiratory muscle support can be provided with intermittent noninvasive ventilation. The most commonly used method of noninvasive positive pressure ventilation for daytime use is through a mouth piece attached to either a bi-level pressure or portable volume ventilator. Patients can receive ventilator-assisted breaths as needed by creating a lip seal around the mouth piece and making a "sipping" effort to trigger the ventilator. Alternatively, positive pressure ventilation can be administered with a nasal interface that provides the advantage of delivering continuous ventilation; however, mouth air leaks and skin breakdown are significant problems that can limit its effectiveness.

Airway Clearance and Secretions

Respiratory infections in patients with neuromuscular disorders are common and result from a combination of inability to generate adequate cough and recurrent aspiration. Coughing, an essential protective mechanism that helps to clear mucus-trapped particles and maintain patent airways, produced by a short, deep inspiration followed by forceful exhalation against a transiently closed glottis. Neuromuscular weakness can impair cough through several mechanisms. Reduced lung expansion and/or force of exhalation results in inability to generate the intrathoracic pressures necessary to achieve adequate airway clearance. Patients with isolated bulbar dysfunction will have impaired cough due to inability to adequately clear upper airway secretions and protect the airway from aspiration. Patients with abnormal cough may not be symptomatic until they develop respiratory infection. Peak cough flow can be measured easily with a peak flow meter connected to a mouthpiece. A peak cough flow of less than 160 L/minute has been shown to correlate with extubation failure in patients with neuromuscular disease. In non-ventilated patients, baseline peak cough flow less than 270 L/minute is associated with a reduction in peak cough flow to less than 160 L/minute during respiratory infections. Abdominal thrust-assist maneuvers performed by caregivers can aid in airway clearance in patients with expiratory muscle weakness. With inspiratory muscle weakness breath stacking maneuvers can help patients obtain inflation volumes necessary to generate an adequate cough. A variety of commercial devices are also available to aid in airway clearance by augmenting mechanical insufflation and exsufflation. These devices include the "pneumobelt," which provides intermittent abdominal pressure, and mechanical in-exsufflators (MI-E), which simulate a normal cough by delivering positive-pressure insufflation followed by expulsive exsufflation through a nasal mask. In patients with bulbar dysfunction, these simple therapies are of limited value, and tracheostomy may be indicated when persistent hypoxemia develops due to inability to clear airway secretions.

Sleep-Related Problems

Sleep-related breathing problems are common in patients with neuromuscular diseases and generally precede awake manifestations of overt respiratory failure. Normal rapid eye movement (REM) sleep results in reduced activity of the intercostal and accessory muscles of respiration causing a drop in minute ventilation with an associated decrease in oxyhemoglobin saturation and rise in carbon dioxide. Causes of this physiologic sleep-induced hypoventilation include loss of a "wakefulness drive" (from reduced chemoreceptor and mechanoreceptor responsiveness) and concurrent pharyngeal muscle relaxation, which increases upper airway resistance. Patients with neuromuscular impairment are at risk for upper airway obstruction (obstructive sleep apnea), exaggerated sleep-related hypoventilation, or both, depending on the relative strength of the pharyngeal dilator muscles and diaphragm. Patients with diaphragmatic paralysis tend to hypoventilate during sleep, while patients with predominantly bulbar weakness are more likely to develop upper airway obstruction. In these patients, nocturnal hypercapnia often precedes and predicts the development of daytime hypercapnia and subsequent ventilatory failure.

Predictors of nocturnal hypoventilation in patients with neuromuscular diseases include daytime sleepiness (assessed with standard questionnaires such as the Epworth Sleepiness Scale) and daytime supine inspiratory VC of less than 60% predicted. It should be noted, however, that in 15% of patients with neuromuscular disease unsuspected nocturnal hypoventilation can be found during polysomnography. Use of nocturnal positive pressure ventilation in patients with neuromuscular disease has been shown to produce sustained daytime effects including normalization of Pco_2 and improved medical quality of life and survival. It is not completely clear why noninvasive nocturnal ventilation has such profound effects. Proposed mechanisms include improved ventilatory mechanics, resting fatigued muscles, and improvement of the blunted chemoreceptor response to hypercapnia, which occurs secondary to sleep deprivation.

Guillain–Barré Syndrome

The most common acute neuropathy to affect the respiratory system is GBS, with an annual incidence of 1 to 3 per 100,000 persons. Patients typically present with ascending motor weakness (although sensory symptoms may also be present to a lesser degree), often following a viral respiratory or gastrointestinal illness. Areflexia, increased cerebrospinal fluid protein without leukocytosis, and electromyogram evidence of demyelination establish the diagnosis. Respiratory compromise is common, and mechanical ventilation is required in approximately

30% of patients. The rate of progression may be dramatic, with acute respiratory failure occurring within 24 to 48 hours of symptom onset. Serial bedside measurements of the VC provide objective data on which to base intubation and ventilatory assistance decisions. A VC of less than 30 mL/kg compromises cough, and atelectasis with hypoxemia may develop when the VC falls below 25 mL/kg. Intubation should be strongly considered when the VC reaches 15 mL/kg, especially when there is clinical evidence of fatigue or difficulty handling secretions. Other supportive treatments include IV fluids, electrolyte and nutrition management, physical therapy including passive joint movement, meticulous skin care with frequent turning or use of specialized beds, and deep venous thrombosis prophylaxis. Intravenous immunoglobulin and plasmapheresis have been shown to be equally efficacious; combining treatments appear to confer no additional benefit. Approximately 20% of patients experience autonomic complications such as dysrhythmias and volatile blood pressures. Over two-thirds of all patients with GBS recover with only minor neurologic deficits.

Amyotrophic Lateral Sclerosis

Amyotrophic Lateral Sclerosis (ALS) is a progressive and fatal degenerative disease of both upper and lower motor neurons with an annual incidence in the United States of 0.7 to 2.5 cases per 100,000 persons. It typically affects adults over 40 years of age with the most frequent onset in the seventh decade of life. A large majority of cases occur sporadically with no known risk factors, though approximately 10% of patients with ALS have a familial form. Patients typically present with limb weakness. Respiratory impairment occurs in the more advanced stages of disease and is the most common cause of morbidity and mortality. Treatment of ALS is aimed at improving quality of life; there are very few interventions that impact survival. The only pharmacologic therapy available is the sodium channel antagonist riluzole, which has been shown to slow the natural progression of disease and delay the onset of ventilator dependence by months. Patients who tolerate and can use noninvasive positive pressure ventilation (NPPV) may experience improvement in quality of life. NPPV should be strongly considered when patients develop early signs of respiratory insufficiency based on either the presence of symptoms, a reduction of VC to less than 50% predicted, or hypercapnia ($Pco_2 > 45$ mmHg). For patients with bulbar involvement, NPPV plays a limited role and has not been shown to provide any consistent benefit. Nevertheless, a trial should probably be offered, given the lack of other therapeutic options. Tracheostomy has been shown to improve survival in ALS; however, quality of life is typically worse than in patients who receive noninvasive ventilation. Patient desire for invasive ventilator support, including intubation and tracheostomy, should be addressed early in the course of the disease. As the disease progresses, palliative support such as narcotics and benzodiazepines can be utilized to reduce air hunger and anxiety.

SPINAL CORD INJURY

More than 200,000 patients in the United States have significant spinal cord injury and approximately 10,000 new injuries occur each year. The anatomic level of spinal cord injury is critical in determining respiratory system impairment. When intubation is required in such patients, it is the standard of care to perform manual in-line stabilization and, if possible, awake fiberoptic intubation to avoid further spinal cord damage. High cervical cord lesions (C1–C2) cause complete paralysis of all muscles of respiration and result in respiratory arrest and need for immediate ventilatory support. Middle cervical cord lesions (C3–C5) cause variable loss of phrenic nerve function and the prognosis improves with lower lesions: 40%, 14%, and 11% of C3, C4, and C5 lesions, respectively, are chronically ventilator-dependent. Lower cervical (C6–C8) and upper thoracic lesions (T1–T6) spare the diaphragm and neck accessory muscles, but chest wall (intercostal muscles) and abdominal muscle functions are lost. The nadir of lung function occurs immediately after a spinal cord injury due to flaccid paralysis of the affected respiratory muscles. In the acute setting, the chest wall contracts instead of expands during inspiration, resulting in a substantial (up to 70%) reduction in maximal inspiratory forces. After several months, the intercostal and abdominal muscles become spastic, no longer collapse with inspiration, and VC improves to approximately 60% of predicted pre-injury levels. VC will typically improve over the first year after injury with most of the improvement occurring during the first 5 weeks. In patients with injuries at C3 and above, need for long-term ventilatory support is nearly universal and early tracheostomy is recommended to facilitate ICU discharge. Patients with injury at C6 or below requiring intubation can often be extubated without requiring tracheostomy. The major limitation to extubation in these patients is related to impaired cough and inability to clear airway secretions. Transition to bi-level noninvasive ventilation following extubation has been shown to reduce need for reintubation. In patients who require reintubation, subsequent extubation attempts are unlikely to be unsuccessful and early tracheostomy is recommended. Another potentially catastrophic pulmonary complication of spinal cord injury is venous thromboembolism. The ACCP Antithrombotic and Thrombolytic Therapy, 9th edition recommends a combination of pharmacologic and mechanical thromboprophylaxis with pneumatic compression or graded compression stockings when not contraindicated by lower extremity injury. The guidelines also recommend that vena cava filters not be utilized for primary venous thromboprophylaxis.

Although the majority of respiratory care in spinal cord injury is supportive, there are therapeutic interventions that have shown promise. Electric pacing of the diaphragm with implanted electrodes is an option for patients with intact phrenic nerves; however, this is a costly procedure and not widely available. Therapeutic hypothermia immediately after injury and stem cell transplantation to delay and reverse deficits in spinal cord injury are current areas of investigation.

Chronic management issues in spinal cord injury include prevention of pneumonia, atelectasis, and respiratory failure. Despite preservation of the cough reflex, loss of innervation to the expiratory muscles leads to ineffective cough. To overcome this deficiency, intensive resistive training of the inspiratory muscles can mildly increase maximal voluntary ventilation (MVV) and MIP, and, in some patients, reduce elements of sleep-disordered breathing, such as hypercapnia and nocturnal desaturation. Manually assisted cough techniques have been shown to increase peak cough expiratory flow and mucous clearance. Placement in the supine position (as opposed to upright) is an important mechanical factor for quadriplegics. In the supine position, passive pressure from the abdominal contents helps to position the diaphragm optimally; this effect is lost in the upright position because of the flaccid abdominal wall.

FURTHER READING

1. Ambrosino N, Carpene N, Gherardi M. Chronic respiratory care for neuromuscular diseases in adults. *Eur Respir J.* 2009;34:444–451.

   Excellent review of respiratory care management issues related to patients with neuromuscular diseases. Provides an in-depth review of the use of noninvasive mechanical ventilation in this group of patients. Has 84 references.

2. Bach J. Invited review: noninvasive respiratory management of high level spinal cord injury. *J Spinal Cord Med.* 2012;35(2):72–80.

   Detailed review of the use of noninvasive ventilation for the management of patients with respiratory failure associated with spinal cord injury. Has 33 references.

3. Boitano L. Management of airway clearance in neuromuscular disease. *Respir Care.* 2006;51(8): 913–922.

   Thorough review of the pathophysiology and management of neuromuscular disease associated cough insufficiency. Has 57 references.

4. Bourke SC, Gibson GJ. Sleep and breathing in neuromuscular disease. *Eur Respir J.* 2002;19: 1194–1201.

   Good review of normal breathing and muscle function during sleep in normal individuals and patients with neuromuscular weakness. Individual disorders including isolated diaphragmatic paralysis, ALS, Duchenne muscular dystrophy, myotonic dystrophy, and myasthenia gravis are reviewed.

5. Branco B, Plurad D, Green DJ, et al. Incidence and clinical predictors for tracheostomy after cervical spinal cord injury: a national trauma databank review. *J Trauma.* 2011;70:111–115.

   A retrospective review of 5,265 patients in the National Trauma Databank who sustained a cervical spinal cord injury. Intubation on scene or emergency department, complete CSCI at C1–C4 or C5–C7 levels, ISS > 16, facial fracture, and thoracic trauma were independently associated with the need for tracheostomy.

6. Brown R, DiMarco A. Respiratory dysfunction and management in spinal cord injury. *Respir Care.* 2006;51(8):853–868.

   A good review of the pathophysiology and management options available for patients with spinal cord injury associated respiratory dysfunction.

7. Carratu P, Spicuzza L, Cassano A, et al. Early treatment with noninvasive positive pressure ventilation prolongs survival in amyotrophic lateral sclerosis patients with nocturnal respiratory insufficiency. *Orphanet J Rare Dis.* 2009;4:10.

   A retrospective review of 28 patients with ALS and a forced vital capacity (FVC) less than 75% who were offered NPPV. The 16 patients who were treated with NPPV had slower rate of decline in FVC and an increased one year survival rate as compared to the 12 patients who refused NPPV.

8. Chatwin M, Ross E, Hart N, et al. Cough augmentation with mechanical insufflation/exsufflation in patients with neuromuscular disorders. *Eur Respir J.* 2003;21:502–508.

   Peak cough flows were compared at baseline and using three augmentation techniques: standard physiotherapy-assisted cough; cough after noninvasive positive pressure inhalation; exsufflation-assisted cough; and combination insufflation/exsufflation-assisted cough. Neuromuscular patient peak cough flows were highest with insufflation/exsufflation. Insufflation/exsufflation consists of positive pressure to achieve maximal lung inflation followed by an abrupt shift to negative pressure, thereby simulating the flow changes characteristic of a spontaneous cough.

9. Dicpinigaitis PV, Grimm DR, Lesser M. Cough reflex sensitivity in subjects with cervical spinal cord injury. *Am J Respir Crit Care Med.* 1999;159:1660–1662.

   Small trial demonstrating that sensitivity of cough reflex is preserved in spinal cord injury. Given intact reflex, ineffective cough is likely caused by loss of innervation of the respiratory muscles.

10. Dietrich W, Levi A, Wang M, et al. Review: hypothermic treatment for acute spinal cord injury. *Neurotherapeutics.* 2011;8:229–239.

    State-of-the-art review of the data supporting the use of this therapy. Has 102 references.

11. Gelinas DF. Pulmonary function screening. *Semin Neurol.* 2003;23:89–96.

    Review of the utility, advantages, and disadvantages of pulmonary function tests in neuromuscular disease.

12. Just N, Bautin N, Danel-Brunaud V, et al. The Borg Dyspnea Score: a relevant clinical marker of inspiratory muscle weakness in amyotrophic lateral sclerosis. *Eur Respir J.* 2010;35:353–360.

    The results of this study involving 72 patients with ALS suggest that the Borg Dyspnea Scale may be a useful clinical tool for the early detection of ventilatory failure in this group of patients.

13. Katz S, Gaboury I, Keilty K, et al. Nocturnal hypoventilation: predictors and outcomes in childhood progressive neuromuscular disease. *Arch Dis Child.* 2010;95:998–1003.

    In this study of 46 children with neuromuscular disease, 15% were found to have clinically unsuspected nocturnal hypoventilation. Clinical predictors of nocturnal hypoventilation included reduced FVC, forced expiratory volume in 1 second, and the presence of scoliosis.

14. Langevin B, Petitjean T, Philit F, et al. Nocturnal hypoventilation in chronic respiratory failure (CRF) due to neuromuscular disease. *Sleep.* 2000;23:S204–S209.

    Ventilatory drive during sleep is decreased because of loss of a behavioral stimulus. Concurrently, upper airway muscle tone decreases, resistance increases, and respiratory load compensation is compromised. REM sleep is a particularly vulnerable time because ventilation completely depends on an intact diaphragm; patients with diaphragmatic weakness may profoundly desaturate.

15. Lanini B, Misuri G, Gigliotti F, et al. Perception of dyspnea in patients with neuromuscular disease. *Chest.* 2001;120:402–408.

16. Lyall RA, Donaldson N, Fleming T, et al. A prospective study of quality of life in ALS patients treated with noninvasive ventilation. *Neurology.* 2001;57:153–156.

    Prospective cohort study of 16 ALS patients found improvement in the "vitality" domain of the SF-36 questionnaire despite overall disease progression. Other functional domain measures fell with disease progression in both treated patients and a control group; therefore, the authors rejected the hypothesis that improved quality of life obtained from ventilatory assistance would be negated by increasing disability afforded by prolonged survival.

17. Mangera Z, Panesar G, Makker H. Practical approach to management of respiratory complications in neurological disorders. *Int J Gen Med.* 2012;5:255–263.

General overview of management issues for patients with respiratory impairment associated with neuro-muscular disorders. Has 30 references.

18. Markstrom A, Sundell K, Lysdahl M, et al. Quality-of-life evaluation of patient with neuromuscular and skeletal diseases treated with noninvasive and invasive home mechanical ventilation. *Chest.* 2002;122:1695–1700.

    Home ventilator patients reported good overall health as measured by three different questionnaires. Patients with tracheostomy seemed to do better than noninvasively ventilated patients; however, the authors pointed out that the marked disparity in management routines and social support (monthly versus annual follow-up) may explain the difference.

19. Mehta S, Hill NS. State of the art: noninvasive ventilation. *Am J Respir Crit Care Med.* 2001;163:540–577.

    Exhaustive overview of the role of noninvasive ventilation in acute and chronic respiratory failure.

20. Piper A. Sleep abnormalities associated with neuromuscular disease: pathophysiology and evaluation. *Semin Respir Crit Care Med.* 2002;23:211–219.

    A simple relationship between awake pulmonary function tests and sleep-related breathing events does not exist. The importance of studying neuromuscular patients during REM sleep is emphasized.

21. Radunovic A, Mitsumoto H, Leigh P. Clinical care of patients with amyotrophic lateral sclerosis. *Lancet Neurol.* 2007;6:913–925.

    Extensive review of all aspects of the care of patients with ALS. Provides an in-depth review of the respiratory management for this group of patients. Has 142 references.

22. Schönhofer B, Sortor-Leger S. Equipment needs for noninvasive mechanical ventilation. *Eur Respir J.* 2002;20:1029–1036.

    Reviews the important equipment-related issues for noninvasive mechanical ventilation, including ventilator selection, ventilator settings, interfaces, leak management, humidification, oxygen supplementation, and medication nebulization.

23. Simonds A. Recent advances in respiratory care for neuromuscular disease. *Chest.* 2006;130:1879–1886.

    Overview of respiratory care for patients with neuromuscular disorders. Has 38 references.

24. Suarez A, Pessolano F, Monteiro S, et al. Peak flow and peak cough flow in the evaluation of expiratory muscle weakness and bulbar impairment in patients with neuromuscular disease. *Am J Phys Med Rehabil.* 2002;81:506–511.

    Seventy-nine patients with ALS and Duchenne muscular dystrophy were studied. Results suggest that cough flow–peak expiratory flow may be useful to monitor expiratory muscle weakness and bulbar involvement in these patients.

25. The Plasma Exchange/Sandoglobin Guillain–Barré Trial Group. Randomized trial of plasma exchange, intravenous immunoglobulin, and combined treatments in Guillain–Barré syndrome. *Lancet.* 1997;349:225–230.

    Multicenter, randomized trial of 383 patients demonstrated that IV immunoglobulin and plasmapheresis are equally efficacious when given within the first 2 weeks after onset of neuropathic symptoms; the combination of both treatments did not confer additional benefit.

26. Toussaint M, Steens M, Soudon P. Lung function accurately predicts hypercapnia in patients with Duchene muscular dystrophy. *Chest.* 2007;131:368–375.

    One hundred fourteen patients with Duchenne muscular dystrophy were studied. Results demonstrate the value of VC in predicting the development of hypercapnia in this group of patients. VC less than 1,820 mL was associated with the development of nocturnal hypercapnia, while a VC less than 680 mL was associated with increased risk of diurnal hypercapnia.

27. Tow AM, Graves DE, Carter RE. Vital capacity in tetraplegics twenty years and beyond. *Spinal Cord.* 2001;39:139–144.

    VC in tetraplegics decreases with age and duration of spinal cord injury, regardless of age of injury, gender, or severity of injury.

28. Vazquez-Sandoval A, Huang E, Jones S. Hypoventilation in neuromuscular disease. *Semin Respir Crit Care Med.* 2009;30:348–358.

    Thorough review of respiratory failure in neuromuscular diseases. Has 107 references.

29. Wang AY, Jaeger RJ, Yarkony GM, et al. Cough in spinal cord injured patients: the relationship between motor level and peak expiratory flow. *Spinal Cord.* 1997;35:299–302.

    Demonstration of a direct relationship between motor level and peak expiratory flow produced during coughing.

30. Wang TG, Wang YH, Tang FT, et al. Resistive inspiratory muscle training in sleep-disordered breathing of traumatic tetraplegia. *Arch Phys Med Rehabil.* 2002;83:491–496.

    Home-based resistive inspiratory muscle training for 6 weeks can mildly enhance MVV and MIP and, in some, reduce some elements of sleep disordered breathing (end tidal co_2 and nocturnal desaturation).

31. Winslow C, Rozovsky J. Effect of spinal cord injury on the respiratory system. *Am J Phys Med Rehabil.* 2003;82:803–814.

    Review of epidemiology and pathophysiology of acute and chronic spinal cord injury.

32. Yuki N, Hartung H. Medical progress Guillain–Barré syndrome. *N Engl J Med.* 2012;366: 2294–2304.

    Current review of the pathophysiology and management of GBS. Has 85 references.

81 Sleep Apnea, Alveolar Hypoventilation, and Obesity-Hypoventilation

Kathleen Sarmiento and José S. Loredo

SLEEP-DISORDERED BREATHING

The spectrum of sleep-disordered breathing ranges from intermittent snoring, which is primarily a nuisance, to obesity-hypoventilation syndrome (OHS), which is associated with severe morbidity and high mortality. In between these two extremes are disorders of gradually increasing impact on morbidity and mortality, including chronic snoring, upper airway resistance syndrome (UARS), and sleep apnea. More recently, continuous positive airway pressure (CPAP)-emergent central apnea (complex sleep apnea syndrome) has been described in patients with unequivocal obstructive sleep apnea (OSA) who develop central apnea when exposed to CPAP.

OSA is the most common form of sleep-disordered breathing seen in the sleep laboratory. Both children and adults may be affected; however, the prevalence of obstructive apnea is highest in middle-aged men. In 1993, the prevalence of symptomatic OSA in the middle-age working population was 4% in men and 2% in women and the prevalence of asymptomatic sleep apnea was 24% in men and 9% in women. However, with the rise in obesity in the last 20 years, the prevalence of OSA is higher, especially in patients with cardiovascular or metabolic disorders ($\geq 50\%$). OSA is characterized by repetitive upper airway obstructions during sleep. The immediate consequences of OSA include microarousals from sleep, full awakenings, hypoxemia, hypercapnia, increased systemic and pulmonary pressures, nocturia due to increased atrial natriuretic peptide levels, and sleep fragmentation. The most common presenting symptoms are excessive daytime somnolence and chronic loud snoring. However, it is not uncommon for the OSA patient to present with complaints of daytime fatigue, decreased cognitive function, sexual dysfunction, depression, and even sleep maintenance insomnia due to frequent nocturnal awakenings. Loud snoring, choking spells, abnormal motor activity during sleep, and, more specifically, observed apneas often are noted by the bed partner. These patients also have higher rates of automobile accidents than the general population. In children OSA often presents with snoring and hyperactivity and can be misdiagnosed as attention-deficit hyperactivity disorder.

The etiology of OSA is not well understood. However, obesity, upper airway narrowing, loss of upper airway motor tone during sleep, abnormalities of central control of ventilation, high CO_2 sensitivity, and cardiac dysfunction have been implicated. Major risk factors for OSA include obesity (strongest), upper airway abnormalities, male gender, increasing age, a family history of OSA, and menopause in women. There are strong epidemiologic and experimental evidence-linking OSA with the development of systemic hypertension and other cardiovascular complications. The mechanism for this association is unclear, but chronic intermittent hypoxia and frequent arousals leading to hyperactivity of chemoreceptors and the sympathetic nervous system may be involved. Current evidence suggests that untreated OSA causes systemic hypertension, and its treatment reduces blood pressure.

There are three basic types of sleep-disordered breathing: (1) apnea, 90% or more decrease in airflow greater than or equal to 10 seconds; (2) hypopnea, 30% reduction in airflow greater than or equal to 10 seconds accompanied by 4% oxygen desaturation or, alternately, 50% reduction in airflow greater than or equal to 10 seconds accompanied by 3% oxygen desaturation or an arousal; and (3) respiratory effort related arousals (RERAs), the UARS.

Three types of apnea have been described: (1) obstructive apnea, in which oronasal airflow is blocked and diaphragmatic efforts continue; (2) central apnea, in which diaphragmatic and intercostal muscle activity cease; and (3) mixed apnea, obstructive apnea with an initial central component. In most symptomatic patients with sleep apnea, all three types of apnea are found, but, by far, obstructive events predominate. The syndromes of obstructive and mixed sleep apnea are clinically similar and, therefore, are grouped together. UARS differs in that oxyhemoglobin desaturation and obvious apneas or hypopneas are not evident in the standard polysomnogram. However, airflow limitation associated with crescendo snoring often terminates in an arousal; RERAs can be observed if a pressure transducer is used to measure airflow. The gold standard for diagnosing RERAs is by measuring esophageal pressure during sleep; this is seldom performed clinically.

On physical examination, 70% of patients are overweight or obese; it is not unusual to find them dozing in the waiting room. Hypertrophy of the tonsils and adenoids appears to be the major mechanism of the upper airway obstruction in children but not in adults. Malformations of the jaw and maxilla, such as retrognathia, micrognathia, narrow high-arching palate (long face syndrome), and large tori of the palate and the jaw, are noted occasionally. More commonly, the adult sleep apnea patient presents with erythematous, enlarged and edematous soft palate and uvula, prominent tonsillar pillars, drapelike soft palate, macroglossia with scalloping, and Mallampati class 3 to 4 oropharyngeal opening, resulting in oropharyngeal crowding and reduced caliber. However, in some patients the physical examination may be entirely normal. Despite having a narrow oropharyngeal opening, airway obstruction during the waking state is absent secondary to neuromuscular compensation. During sleep, this neuromuscular compensation is lost, predisposing the patient to upper airway obstruction. In the waking state, pulmonary function tests, arterial blood gases, and ventilatory response to carbon dioxide are usually normal, unless the separate effects of morbid obesity or another disease are present. Systemic hypertension is present in up to 50% of patients. Pulmonary arterial hypertension may occur in up to 40% of cases of uncomplicated OSA; however, this is generally not clinically significant.

The diagnosis of the sleep apnea syndromes can be most accurately made by documenting apneic episodes with polysomnography (type 1 study), which measures EEG, oculogram, oronasal airflow, chin and tibialis anterior electromyogram, ventilatory effort, heart rate, and arterial oxygen saturation. More recently, unattended cardiorespiratory sleep recordings (type 3 studies) have been recommended for patients with a high likelihood of OSA after clinical assessment by a sleep specialist. To be considered significant, apneic episodes must last at least 10 seconds and occur repetitively. The Apnea/Hypopnea Index (AHI) is used to determine the severity of sleep apnea. The AHI represents the number of apneas plus hypopneas per hour of sleep. An AHI less than 5 is considered normal, while an AHI greater than or equal to 30 is considered severe.

The pathophysiology and hemodynamic consequences of the sleep apnea syndromes have been studied extensively. During an obstructive episode, the posterior wall of the hypopharynx collapses and the strap muscles of the neck become hypotonic as documented by electromyographic recordings. As the apneic episode continues, hypercapnia and hypoxemia develop. Progressive increases in negative intrathoracic pressure develop with increasing efforts to breathe against the obstruction. Systemic and pulmonary hypertension, sinus bradycardia, and a variety of arrhythmias and conduction disturbances may occur. A loud snort may signal the end of the obstruction and correlates with an EEG pattern of arousal from sleep. Subsequently, abnormalities of gas exchange and hemodynamics resolve rapidly, unless repetitive apneic episodes occur, a frequent situation in severely affected individuals.

Treatment of OSA patients should always include behavioral interventions: weight reduction, smoking cessation, and avoidance of alcohol, sedatives, sleep deprivation, and sleeping in the supine position. Weight reduction to optimum levels can be curative in some cases. However, even modest weight reduction may result in significant reductions in sleep apnea severity. More recently, in small randomized clinical trials, physical exercise, even without weight reduction, and playing the didgeridoo have been shown to decrease AHI by about 25% to 50%. Patients with positional sleep apnea (supine AHI >10/hour and nonsupine AHI <10/hour) may benefit from sleeping in the lateral position, which can be achieved with antisnore shirts, bumper belts, or specialized pillows. Pharmacological therapy for sleep apnea has been disappointingly ineffective in reducing AHI. Nocturnal nasal oxygen therapy can improve arterial oxygen saturation during sleep in OSA, but it does not significantly change the AHI. CPAP is the most effective treatment for sleep apnea. CPAP maintains upper airway patency during sleep by creating a pneumatic splint. In most cases, it can effectively control sleep apnea, reduce arousals, and reverse oxyhemoglobin desaturation. CPAP is usually well tolerated. Complications are mild, usually associated with mask-fit problems. In rare cases, aerophagia can be problematic. CPAP remains a cumbersome therapy despite significant technological advances, including integrated heated humidifiers, auto-CPAP, bi-level positive airway pressure (PAP) modalities, expiratory pressure relief, and ultraquiet blowers. However, with proper introduction and follow-up, CPAP compliance can be significantly higher than the usually quoted 50% nightly use after 4 months of therapy. Overnight CPAP titration in the laboratory is still the preferred method of identifying the optimal pressure level to treat OSA. However, in selected patients, a trial of auto-CPAP at home with minimal pressure estimated from a CPAP prediction formula may be effective and practical in treating OSA and controlling the night-to-night variability of AHI. Oral appliances provide an alternative to CPAP in patients with mild to moderate sleep apnea, although these are not as effective as CPAP in controlling apneic events. Many types of appliances are available; the most effective are those that are adjustable and advance the jaw, increasing upper airway patency. Temporomandibular joint pain is a common complaint from the use of an oral appliance. Surgical procedures that increase upper airway size (e.g., uvulopalatopharyngoplasty) have been found to effectively eliminate snoring, but frequently fail to control sleep apnea, especially when sleep apnea is severe. Except in highly selected cases, uvulopalatopharyngoplasty is no longer recommended to treat OSA. Unfortunately, there is no way to predict which patients will benefit from surgical treatment. Extensive surgery to advance the entire mouth forward (maxillary mandibular advancement) has been as successful as CPAP in controlling sleep apnea in highly selected populations; however, convalescence can be prolonged, frequently resulting in prolonged facial numbness and cosmetic changes. More recently, several minimally invasive operations have been proposed to treat OSA in patients intolerant of CPAP. These include radiofrequency volume reduction of the base of the tongue and genioglossus advancement surgery, in combination with the pillar procedure. However, this type of surgical intervention has not been evaluated systematically. Hypoglossal nerve stimulation to treat OSA remains experimental. Improving upper airway muscle tone during sleep corrects part of the pathophysiology of OSA. In some studies, the AHI has decreased by 50% with hypoglossal nerve stimulation during sleep. Tracheotomy is a last resort for patients with life-threatening conditions exacerbated by untreated OSA and who are not able to use CPAP. Tracheotomy is consistently effective in relieving signs and symptoms of OSA; however, its morbidity makes it a rarely used procedure. Finally, an effort should be made to identify associated conditions that may worsen sleep apnea (e.g., hypothyroidism, use of testosterone, alcohol or sedatives before sleep). Correcting these can sometimes cure or improve sleep apnea. In children, removal of obstructing tonsils and adenoids is usually curative, although the rise in obesity in children has somewhat reduced the effectiveness of this procedure.

Pure central sleep apnea is often associated with advanced age, CNS disorders, congestive heart failure, and sleeping at high altitude. It may be associated with high sensitivity to carbon dioxide, conditions that promote hypocapnia, and chronic opioid therapy. Oral acetazolamide and nasal CPAP have both been partially successful in treating patients with central sleep apnea. Supplemental oxygen may also be beneficial, especially in central sleep apnea associated with high altitude. More recently, adaptive servo-ventilation therapy has been effective in controlling central sleep apnea, especially when associated with Cheyne–Stokes ventilation in patients with heart failure. Successful treatment can result in improved cardiac function.

ALVEOLAR HYPOVENTILATION

Alveolar hypoventilation is defined as an elevation in $Paco_2$ greater than 45 mmHg due to a reduction in minute ventilation. A rise in alveolar Pco_2 will lead to a decrease in alveolar Po_2 and result in hypoxemia. Alveolar hypoventilation can occur with several disorders, referred to as the hypoventilation syndromes. Although hypercapnia and hypoxemia can be evident during wakefulness, these are usually more severe during deep sleep in most cases of alveolar hypoventilation.

The syndrome of primary alveolar hypoventilation (Ondine curse) is a rare disorder characterized by hypercapnia and hypoxemia that develops mostly in young adult males without abnormalities of the lung parenchyma, chest wall, respiratory muscle function, or voluntary control of ventilation. Central alveolar hypoventilation is a term used when alveolar hypoventilation is caused by an identified CNS process such as destructive lesions in the medullary chemoreceptor. Congenital central hypoventilation is a rare disorder of ventilation control diagnosed in early childhood and may have a familial component. In all cases of primary alveolar hypoventilation, there is a failure of the central autonomic regulation of ventilation and inability to integrate the neural input from peripheral chemoreceptors. Invariably, these children have multisystem involvement, with significant developmental problems and common occurrence of congenital megacolon.

Clinical manifestations of alveolar hypoventilation include lethargy, somnolence, and morning headaches. Dyspnea is remarkably absent unless congestive heart failure supervenes. Apnea during sleep is often prominent. Cyanosis with a normal alveolar–arterial O_2 gradient is the most common physical finding and can usually be reversed by voluntary hyperventilation. Polycythemia and cor pulmonale are present in 50% of cases. Although hypercapnia and hypoxemia at rest are noted in the vast majority, arterial blood gases may occasionally be normal; unexplained metabolic alkalosis may be a clue to previous chronic hypercapnia. Pulmonary function tests reveal normal lung volumes and flow rates; however, diminished or absent ventilatory response to carbon dioxide inhalation may be greatly diminished. Ventilatory response to hypoxia is frequently impaired as well. Breath-holding time is often prolonged, and exercise may result in worsening of hypoxemia and hypercapnia due to impaired chemoreceptor response.

Several forms of therapy have been proposed. Respiratory stimulants are generally ineffective. Rocking beds or mechanical ventilatory assistance (bi-level PAP via a nasal mask) has been useful in severe cases, particularly at night when the hypoventilation is most severe. Nocturnal phrenic nerve pacing has been described as safe and effective therapy and may be the treatment of choice in severely affected individuals. However, noninvasive ventilation (NIV) is the most common therapy for congenital central hypoventilation syndrome, usually through a tracheotomy.

OBESITY-HYPOVENTILATION SYNDROME

The OHS was originally described as the "Pickwickian syndrome" by Burwell and Robin, named after a character in Dickens's *The Pickwick Papers* ("the fat boy Joe") who was obese and continually falling asleep. It is characterized by daytime hypercapnia ($Paco_2 > 45$ mmHg), obesity (BMI > 30), and alveolar hypoventilation not explained by neuromuscular, mechanical, or metabolic reasons. Nearly 90% of patients with this syndrome also have OSA. Not all obese individuals develop alveolar hypoventilation. Prevalence of OHS is unknown, but is thought to affect only a minority of obese individuals. The only clear risk factor for the development of OHS is morbid obesity (BMI > 40).

The etiology of the OHS is complex, probably resulting from an imbalance between ventilatory drive and ventilatory load. Currently, there are no data supporting an inherited mechanism for decreased ventilatory drive in OHS. Factors depressing ventilation and gas exchange in these patients include (1) obesity with its increased work of breathing and interference with the mechanical efficiency of ventilation, (2) heart failure, (3) diffuse airway obstruction, and (4) OSA, especially when severe. Patients with OHS have a high risk of mortality and morbidity; sudden unexpected death is common.

The findings on history and physical examination define this syndrome. Patients are severely hypersomnolent and fall asleep at the most inappropriate times. Though snoring is not a universal finding, these patients often have a long history of loud and disruptive snoring. On physical examination, patients are obese, often greater than 50% above predicted weights. They may have a ruddy complexion or cyanosis due to hypoxemia and secondary erythrocytosis; short, thick neck; enlarged uvula; and a small oropharyngeal opening. They may have crackles or wheezes on chest examination and demonstrate hepatomegaly, peripheral edema, and other findings of right-heart failure.

Chest radiographs show an enlarged heart and small lung fields with pulmonary congestion. Electrocardiograms often demonstrate right-atrial and ventricular enlargement. Arterial blood gases show hypoxemia and hypercapnia, with a widened alveolar–arterial oxygen gradient. However, these patients can voluntarily hyperventilate and normalize their Pco_2. Approximately one-half of these patients have erythrocytosis. Spirometry demonstrates decreased forced vital capacity (FVC) and forced expiratory volume in 1 second (FEV_1); some patients also have evidence of superimposed airway obstruction, that is, FEV_1/FVC less than 75%. The total lung capacity (TLC) is 20% smaller and the maximal voluntary ventilation (MVV) is 40% lower than that of patients with simple obesity. Tests of ventilatory control show a diminished response to both hypercapnia and hypoxemia. Polysomnography demonstrates moderate to severe OSA, often with prolonged and severe hypoxemia in the large majority. Only a minority of patients demonstrate pure OHS.

OHS patients should be evaluated thoroughly and treated to avoid serious complications such as pulmonary arterial hypertension, cor pulmonale, acute ventilatory decompensation, and sudden death. Clinical evaluation should include a careful history and complete physical examination, arterial blood gases, spirometry, maximal inspiratory and expiratory pressures, thyroid function tests, and overnight polysomnography. This evaluation should focus on any conditions that could contribute to persistent daytime hypoventilation, such as hypothyroidism, severe OSA, or respiratory muscle weakness. In addition, one should consider other sources of ventilatory impairment, such as left-ventricular heart failure, sedative and narcotic medications, and diffuse airway disease.

There are no established guidelines on the treatment of OHS. The primary goal of therapy is to correct the obvious pathologic derangements. Therapy should focus on reducing ventilatory loads and increasing ventilatory drive. Weight loss invariably results in improvement in hypoventilation and clinical symptoms. Unfortunately, permanent weight loss in these patients is difficult and may require bariatric surgery. Respiratory stimulants such as acetazolamide and high-dose progesterone are not well-studied in OHS; their long-term clinical utility is unknown. The risk of deep-venous thrombosis and pulmonary embolism is high in these obese patients; when nonambulatory, prophylactic measures should be taken with the use of subcutaneous heparin or lower extremity intermittent compression stockings. Sedatives, alcohol, and other ventilatory depressants should be avoided. Nocturnal and daytime oxygen supplementation must be used with caution in order to avoid further ventilatory depression and worsening hypercapnia. Approximately 50% of OHS patients will require supplemental oxygen in addition to PAP therapy. The goal is to maintain an Sao_2 of at least 88% to avoid pulmonary vasospasm and pulmonary hypertension. Correcting upper airway obstruction and hypoventilation during sleep is important in the treatment of OHS. CPAP alone is effective in correcting OSA in mild OHS and has been shown to improve daytime symptoms and hypercapnia in some OHS patients. However, in severely decompensated OHS, NIV, most commonly bi-level PAP, should be used. NIV can effectively correct both upper airway obstruction and nocturnal hypoventilation in OHS. Expiratory positive airway pressure (EPAP) should be started at 5 cm H_2O and titrated to abolish obstructive apneas, hypopneas, and snoring. Inspiratory positive airway pressure (IPAP) should be started at 5 cm H_2O above the EPAP and titrated to correct Pco_2 and increase Sao_2 to greater than or equal to 92%. Typically, IPAP needs to be 8 to 10 cm H_2O above EPAP to effectively control hypoventilation during sleep and avoid hyperventilation. Supplemental oxygen may be needed to maintain Sao_2 greater than or equal to 92%. Average volume assured pressure support (AVAPS) is a newer form of auto adjusting NIV that that targets preset minute ventilation and tidal volumes by adjusting pressure support. In a recent study, AVAPS was shown to be as effective as fixed bi-level PAP in treating patients with OHS. Tracheotomy alone can correct the upper airway obstruction in OHS and, in preliminary studies, was reported to also improve daytime hypoventilation. However, tracheotomy generally requires the addition of mechanical ventilation during sleep to control worsened hypoventilation experienced by OHS patients. Since the advent of NIV to treat OHS, tracheotomy is only used in life-threatening situations or when NIV is not available or contraindicated.

FURTHER READING
Sleep Apnea

1. Young T, Palta M, Dempsey J, et al. The occurrence of sleep disordered breathing among middle-aged adults. *N Engl J Med.* 1993;328:1230–1235.

   In a random sample of working adults, 2% of women and 4% of men had a clinically important degree of sleep apnea. Twenty-four percent of men and 9% of women had sleep apnea by laboratory criteria.

2. Lurie A. Obstructive sleep apnea in adults: epidemiology, clinical presentation, and treatment options. *Adv Cardiol.* 2011;46:1–42.

   The prevalence of OSA is much higher (≥50%) in patients with cardiac or metabolic disorders than in the general population.

3. Morgenthaler TI, Kagramanov V, Hanak V, et al. Complex sleep apnea syndrome: is it a unique clinical syndrome? *Sleep.* 2006;29(9):1203–1209.

   Some patients with obstructive sleep apnea hypopnea syndrome have elimination of obstructive events but emergence of problematic central apneas or Cheyne–Stokes breathing pattern when exposed to CPAP. Significance of syndrome has not been well characterized.

4. Umlauf MG, Chasens ER, Greevy RA, et al. Obstructive sleep apnea, nocturia and polyuria in older adults. *Sleep.* 2004;27:139–144.

   Subjects with higher Apnea–Hypopnea Index had higher atrial natriuretic peptide levels and greater nocturia.

5. Findley L, Levinson M, Bonnie R. Driving performance and automobile accidents in patients with sleep apnea. *Clin Chest Med.* 1992;13:427–435.

   A review of the studies demonstrating poor driving performance and high automobile accident rates in drivers with untreated sleep apnea. Legal and liability questions are also addressed.

6. Gottlieb DJ, Vezina RM, Chase C, et al. Symptoms of sleep-disordered breathing in 5-year-old children are associated with sleepiness and problem behaviors. *Pediatrics.* 2003;112:870–877.

   Children with symptoms of sleep-disordered breathing had more parent-reported daytime sleepiness and problem behaviors (hyperactivity, inattention, aggressiveness), suggestive of attention-deficit hyperactivity disorder.

7. Mezzanote WS, Tangel DJ, White DP. Waking genioglossal electromyogram in sleep apnea patients versus normal controls (a neuromuscular compensatory mechanism). *J Clin Invest.* 1992;89:1571–1579.

   Obstructive sleep apnea patients demonstrate neuromuscular overcompensation during wakefulness to maintain a patent upper airway. This overcompensation is lost during sleep, predisposing them to upper airway obstruction.

8. Wilkinson V, Malhotra A, Nicholas CL, et al. Discharge patterns of human genioglossus motor units during sleep onset. *Sleep*. 2008;31(4):525–533.

   Fifty percent of genioglossus inspiratory motor units drop out at sleep onset.

9. Norman D, Loredo JS, Nelesen RA, et al. Effects of continuous positive airway pressure versus supplemental oxygen on 24-hour ambulatory blood pressure. *Hypertension*. 2006;47(5): 840–845.

   This was a randomized, double-blind, placebo-controlled study comparing the effects of 2 weeks of CPAP versus sham-CPAP versus supplemental nocturnal oxygen on 24-hour ambulatory blood pressure in 46 patients with moderate-to-severe OSA. Only CPAP therapy resulted in a significant reduction in daytime mean arterial and diastolic blood pressure, and nighttime mean systolic and diastolic blood pressure.

10. Iber C, Ancoli-Israel S, Chesson A, et al; for the American Academy of Sleep Medicine. *The AASM Manual for the Scoring of Sleep and Associated Events: Rules, Terminology and Technical Specifications.* 1st ed. Westchester, IL: American Academy of Sleep Medicine; 2007.

    The criteria for scoring hypopneas are not universally accepted. The American Academy of Sleep Medicine has proposed a recommended and an alternate criteria, both of them require physiological changes (oxygen desaturation or an arousal) to qualify as a respiratory event.

11. Resnick HE, Redline S, Shahar E, et al. Diabetes and sleep disturbances: findings from the Sleep Heart Health Study. *Diabetes Care*. 2003;26:702–709.

    Diabetics had higher prevalence of periodic breathing, which is associated with abnormalities in the central control of ventilation. Diabetes may be a risk factor for obstructive sleep apnea.

12. Javaheri S. A mechanism of central sleep apnea in patients with heart failure. *N Engl J Med*. 1999;341:949–954.

    This study concludes that enhanced sensitivity to carbon dioxide may predispose patients with heart failure to the development of central sleep apnea.

13. Sharabi Y, Dagan Y, Grossman E. Sleep apnea as a risk factor for hypertension. *Curr Opin Nephrol Hypertens*. 2004;13:359–364.

    A review of the epidemiological data and other factors that link obstructive sleep apnea to the development of hypertension and the benefits of treatment.

14. Guilleminault C, Chowdhuri S. Upper airway resistance syndrome is a distinct syndrome. *Am J Respir Crit Care Med*. 2000;161:1412–1413.

    An excellent review of the physiological and clinical evidences for the upper airway resistance syndrome.

15. Sajkov D, Wang T, Saunders NA, et al. Daytime pulmonary hemodynamics in patients with obstructive sleep apnea without lung disease. *Am J Respir Crit Care Med*. 1999;159:1518–1526.

    Pulmonary arterial hypertension is common in obstructive sleep apnea; however, in most cases, the systolic pulmonary pressures are only mildly elevated.

16. Kansanen M, Vanninen E, Tuunainen A, et al. The effect of a very low-calorie diet-induced weight loss on the severity of obstructive sleep apnoea and autonomic nervous function in obese patients with obstructive sleep apnoea syndrome. *Clin Physiol*. 1998;18:377–385.

    Weight loss with a very low calorie diet in 15 obese patients resulted in significant improvement of sleep apnea and favorable effects on blood pressure and baroreflex sensitivity.

17. Kline CE, Crowley EP, Ewing GB, et al. The effect of exercise training on obstructive sleep apnea and sleep quality: a randomized controlled trial. *Sleep*. 2011;34(12):1631–1640.

    A 12-week 150 minutes/week intervention of moderate-intensity aerobic activity, followed by resistance training twice/week, versus stretching resulted in significant reduction of AHI despite no change in weight.

18. Loredo JS, Ancoli-Israel S, Dimsdale JE. Effects of CPAP vs placebo-CPAP in sleep quality. *Chest*. 1999;116:1545–1549.

    CPAP was an effective therapy to correct the respiratory disturbance index (RDI), oxyhemoglobin desaturation, and arousals in obstructive sleep apnea. However, CPAP was not as effective in correcting sleep architecture abnormalities after one week of treatment.

19. Morgenthaler TI, Aurora RN, Brown T, et al; for the Standards of Practice Committee of the AASM. Practice parameters for the use of autotitrating continuous positive airway pressure devices

for titrating pressures and treating adult patients with obstructive sleep apnea syndrome: an update for 2007. An American Academy of Sleep Medicine report. *Sleep*. 2008;31(1):141–147.

Auto-PAP devices may be used for unattended treatment and to determine a fixed CPAP treatment pressure for patients with moderate to severe OSA without significant comorbidities (congestive heart failure, chronic obstructive pulmonary disease, central sleep apnea syndromes, or hypoventilation syndromes).

20. Eastwood PR, Barnes M, Walsh JH, et al. Treating obstructive sleep apnea with hypoglossal nerve stimulation. *Sleep*. 2011;34(11):1479–1486.

Hypoglossal nerve stimulation partially reversed the low upper airway muscle activity during sleep that is part of the pathophysiology of OSA. Hypoglossal nerve stimulation has significantly reduced AHI, but it remains an experimental procedure.

21. Marklund M, Stenlund H, Franklin KA. Mandibular advancement devices in 630 men and women with obstructive sleep apnea and snoring: tolerability and predictors of treatment success. *Chest*. 2004;125:1270–1278.

A prospective study of the use of a jaw advancement device in mild sleep disordered breathing. The authors concluded that jaw advancement devices are recommended for women with sleep apnea, men with supine-dependent sleep apnea, and for snorers without sleep apnea.

22. Sher AE, Schechtman KB, Piccirillo JF. The efficacy of surgical modifications of the upper airway in adults with obstructive sleep apnea syndrome. *Sleep*. 1996;19:156–177.

A meta-analysis: only 41% of patients undergoing uvulopalatopharyngoplasty responded with a reduction of the RDI to less than <20.

23. Li KK, Riley RW, Powell NB, et al. Maxillomandibular advancement for persistent obstructive sleep apnea after phase I surgery in patients without maxillomandibular deficiency. *Laryngoscope*. 2000;110:1684–1688.

Maxillomandibular advancement surgery was effective in correcting obstructive sleep apnea after failure of uvulopalatopharyngoplasty.

24. Riley RW, Powell NB, Li KK, et al. An adjunctive method of radiofrequency volumetric tissue reduction of the tongue for OSAS. *Otolaryngol Head Neck Surg*. 2003;129:37–42.

Radiofrequency volumetric reduction of the base of the tongue was effective in decreasing sleep apnea severity by more than 50% in sleep apnea patients with isolated tongue base obstruction.

25. Walker JM, Farney RJ, Rhondeau SM, et al. Chronic opioid use is a risk factor for the development of central sleep apnea and ataxic breathing. *J Clin Sleep Med*. 2007;3(5):455–461.

A retrospective study showing that chronic opioid therapy was associated with dose-related central sleep apnea and ataxic breathing, especially at high doses.

26. Aurora RN, Chowdhuri S, Ramar K, et al. The treatment of central sleep apnea syndromes in adults: practice parameters with an evidence-based literature review and meta-analyses. *Sleep*. 2012;35(1):17–40.

Adaptive servo-ventilation therapy is effective in controlling central sleep apnea in heart failure and results in improvement of cardiac function.

Primary Hypoventilation and Obesity Hypoventilation Syndromes

27. Vanderlaan M, Holbrook CR, Wang M, et al. Epidemiologic survey of 196 patients with congenital central hypoventilation syndrome. *Pediatr Pulmonol*. 2004;37:217–229.

In this survey, congenital central hypoventilation was associated with multisystem involvement among all participants; 16.3% had congenital megacolon; 61.7% of the children had a tracheotomy. Use of noninvasive ventilation was common.

28. Krachman S, Criner GJ. Hypoventilation syndromes. *Clin Chest Med*. 1998;19:139–155.

An excellent and succinct review of the hypoventilation syndromes.

29. Bickelmann AG, Burwell CS, Robin ED, et al. Extreme obesity associated with alveolar hypoventilation: a Pickwickian syndrome. *Am J Med*. 1956;21:811–818.

A classic case report.

30. Kessler R, Chaouat A, Schinkewitch P, et al. The obesity-hypoventilation syndrome revisited: a prospective study of 34 consecutive cases. *Chest*. 2001;120:369–376.

In this series, pure obesity hypoventilation syndrome was rare. It was usually associated with obstructive sleep apnea. Patients with obesity hypoventilation syndrome had severe diurnal hypoxemia, and 58% had pulmonary hypertension as compared with 9% for patients with sleep apnea alone.

31. Rapoport DM, Garay SM, Epstein H, et al. Hypercapnia in the obstructive sleep apnea syndrome: a re-evaluation of the Pickwickian syndrome. *Chest.* 1986;89:627–635.

    Successful treatment of sleep apnea corrected daytime hypercapnia in approximately one-half of patients with obstructive sleep apnea and daytime hypercapnia.

32. Koenig SM. Pulmonary complications of obesity. *Am J Med Sci.* 2001;321:249–279.

    A review of the effects of obesity on pulmonary function, morbidity and mortality.

33. Masa JF, Celli BR, Riesco JA, et al. The obesity hypoventilation syndrome can be treated with noninvasive mechanical ventilation. *Chest.* 2001;119:1102–1107.

    Use of bilevel positive pressure ventilation for 4 months during sleep was effective in reversing the respiratory failure of obesity hypoventilation syndrome and improving symptoms.

34. Mokhlesi B, Kryger MH, Grustein RR. Assessment and management of patients with obesity hypoventilation syndrome. *Proc Am Thorac Soc.* 2008;15:218–225.

    A review of the epidemiology, clinical presentation, and practical recommendations for the treatment of patients with OHS.

35. Murphy PB, Davidson C, Hind MD, et al. Volume targeted versus pressure support non-invasive ventilation in patients with super obesity and chronic respiratory failure: a randomized controlled trial. *Thorax.* 2012;67:717–734.

    Autotitrating AVAPS and fixed pressure support were compared with the primary outcome of daytime arterial P_{CO_2} at 3 months. There was improvement in both groups, not significantly different.

Silicosis

Richard D. Drucker

Silicosis is a fibrotic disease of the lungs caused by inhalation of free crystalline silica (silicon dioxide). Silica is a ubiquitous material that is a major component of the earth's crust. The three major crystalline forms associated with lung injury are quartz, cristobalite, and tridymite. Quartz is the most common silica and is found in most rocks, including granite and sandstone. Cristobalite and tridymite are associated with high temperatures, are naturally found in lava, and can be produced from other forms of silica by exposure to high temperatures. These are termed *free silica,* in contrast to silicates, which are crystals of silicon dioxide complexed with inorganic cations such as calcium, iron, magnesium, or aluminum. Silicates such as asbestos, talc, and mica are also capable of inducing lung injury.

The classic occupations at risk for silicosis are mining (quarrying, tunneling), manufacturing (glass, pottery, porcelain, abrasives), and sandblasting. The development of disease is related to the duration, concentration, and structure of the free silica dust in the environment as well as each individual's susceptibility to silica inhalation, which is incompletely characterized. Only a minority of workers at risk actually develop silicosis. The prevalence of silicosis appeared to be decreasing following introduction of improved dust control in the 1970s, but the prevalence recently has increased for unknown reasons.

The exact pathogenic mechanism of pulmonary silicosis is unclear, but there is abundant evidence that the pulmonary alveolar macrophage plays an important role in mediating lung damage. It is hypothesized that crystalline free silica interacts with water to form oxygen radicals that injure the alveolar macrophage. The macrophages release cytokines such as tumor necrosis factor, interleukin-1, and arachidonic acid metabolites. The resulting proliferation of type II pneumocytes, fibroblasts, and collagen eventually cause pulmonary fibrosis.

The classic pathologic lesion of silicosis is the hyaline nodule, consisting of concentric whorls of connective tissue and an acellular central zone containing free silica. The middle zone has fibroblasts and collagen, and the peripheral zone contains macrophages, fibroblasts, and free silica. The nodules are scattered throughout the lungs with predominance in the upper lobes. Simple nodules rarely compress airways or blood vessels, but larger coalescent masses in the advanced stage of silicosis can involve these structures. Regional lymphadenopathy and pleural adhesions are common, particularly in more severe cases of silicosis.

The three major clinical presentations of silicosis are chronic silicosis, accelerated silicosis, and acute silicosis. Chronic and accelerated silicoses present with similar symptoms and radiographs except that chronic silicosis becomes clinically apparent only decades after exposure to free silica, while accelerated silicosis becomes clinically apparent sooner and typically after exposure to heavy concentrations of silica. Radiographic abnormalities characteristically occur prior to the development of symptoms such as cough, sputum production, and dyspnea on exertion. Acute silicosis (silicoproteinosis) develops within 6 to 24 months of massive exposure to free silica. It tends to have a fulminant course consisting of cough, weight loss, rapidly progressive dyspnea, and early death. Histologically, the alveoli are filled with a PAS–positive acellular material like that seen in pulmonary alveolar proteinosis. The lungs of people exposed to free silica, whether or not silicosis is present, also may demonstrate pathologic evidence of emphysema or chronic bronchitis. Extrapulmonary involvement (kidney and liver) also has been described in acute silicosis.

There are several patterns of radiographic abnormalities in silicosis. Simple silicosis frequently is associated with reticular and nodular patterns. The nodules range from 1 mm to less than 10 mm in meter, predominate in the upper lobes, and usually have sharp margins. Hilar adenopathy is common and may predate the parenchymal findings. Five percent of the lymph nodes contain characteristic "eggshell calcification," a finding that once was considered pathognomonic of silicosis; however, it also has been reported in sarcoidosis and tuberculosis. Progressive massive fibrosis (also termed conglomerate or complicated silicosis) is characterized by densities that are 10 mm or larger in diameter and often seem to coalesce into larger masses. In chronic silicosis, the involvement is primarily in the upper lobes, in contrast to the lower and middle lobe predominance in the accelerated variant. Retraction is common in the involved lobes, with compensatory overexpansion of the remaining lobes. Superimposed mycobacterial disease should be suspected in the presence of cavitation, pleural thickening, or rapid increase in nodule size. In acute silicosis, the chest roentgenogram has either a diffuse alveolar filling pattern similar to pulmonary alveolar proteinosis or, less commonly, a reticulonodular pattern.

Pulmonary function abnormalities in silicosis are variable. Asymptomatic patients with simple silicosis may demonstrate no abnormality but may also show an accelerated loss of lung function. Patients with progressive massive fibrosis show restriction, obstruction, or a mixed pattern. Reductions in diffusing capacity, compliance, and arterial oxygenation with exercise have been shown in patients with advanced stages of silicosis. Some studies have suggested an association between obstructive pulmonary physiology and silica exposure in the absence of radiographic evidence of silicosis.

Silicosis has been associated with the development of lung cancer, mycobacterial disease, and collagen vascular disease. In 1996, the International Agency for Research on Cancer classified crystalline silica as a group I carcinogen. There also is an increased incidence of connective tissue diseases in patients with silicosis. Particularly prevalent are systemic sclerosis, rheumatoid arthritis, and systemic lupus erythematosus. Clinically, the course of the connective tissue disease is similar whether or not silicosis is present; however, the clinical course of silicosis is less favorable in those patients who also have a connective tissue disease. In silicosis, there is an increased incidence of hypergammaglobulinemia, antinuclear antibodies, rheumatoid factor, and circulating immune complexes. There is no demonstrated correlation, however, between these serologic abnormalities and the clinical, radiographic, or physiologic presentation of the silicotic patient. Patients with silicosis have an increased incidence of tuberculous and nontuberculous mycobacterial infections. Tuberculosis has been found in up to one-third of South African gold miners with silicosis. It is important for the clinician to have a high index of suspicion for possible tuberculosis in patients with silicosis.

The diagnosis of silicosis is based on a history of significant exposure to free silica, characteristic radiographic abnormalities, and the absence of another disease that is more likely to account for the findings. Biopsy is indicated only in patients with atypical radiographs or in a medicolegal situation such as a compensation case involving multiple dust exposures. Hyaline nodules in various stages of development are characteristic. Doubly refractile particles can be seen with polarizing light microscopy, but these particles are not diagnostic of silicosis. In certain cases, X-ray energy spectrometry or scanning electron microscopy is needed for diagnosis.

Management is aimed at disease prevention by limiting free silica exposure and by removing patients with silicosis from further exposure. Preventative efforts have resulted in reduced mortality rates over the past few decades. Unfortunately, there is no proven effective treatment for silicosis. The efficacy of corticosteroids is unproved, although an uncontrolled clinical trial has shown short-term improvement in chronic silicosis and a case report has shown improvement in acute silicosis. The use of whole-lung lavage in silicosis has been employed successfully to remove dust, but the clinical utility is not yet proven. Patients with a significantly reactive tuberculin skin test should receive isoniazid chemoprophylaxis.

FURTHER READING

1. Ziskind M, Jones RW, Weill H, et al. Silicosis. *Am Rev Respir Dis.* 1976;113:643.

   A classic comprehensive review article.

2. Rimal B, Greenberg A, Rom W. Basic pathogenic mechanisms in silicosis: current understanding. *Curr Opin Pulm Med.* 2005;11:169.

   A review of the molecular and cellular mechanisms in silicosis.

3. Centers for Disease Control and Prevention. Silicosis, mortality, prevention, and control—United States, 1968–2002. *Morb Mortal Wkly Rep.* 2005;54:401.

   A silicosis statistics over three decades.

4. International Agency for Research on Cancer. Silica, some silicates, coal dust and para-aramid fibrils. *IARC Monogr Eval Carcinog Risks Hum.* 1996;68:1.

   A report that classifies silica as a class I carcinogen.

5. Buechner H, Ansari A. Acute silico-proteinosis. *Dis Chest.* 1969;55:274.

   This article describes sandblasters who have acute silicosis and a symptomatology similar to pulmonary alveolar proteinosis.

6. Bailey W, Brown M, Buechner HA, et al. Silico-mycobacterial disease in sandblasters. *Am Rev Respir Dis.* 1974;110:115.

   Association of mycobacterial and other granulomatous diseases in patients with accelerated silicosis.

7. Davies J. Silicosis and tuberculosis among South African goldminers—an overview of recent studies and current issues. *S Afr Med J.* 2001;91:562.

   A discussion of the relationship between silicosis and tuberculosis.

8. Doll N, Stankus RP, Hughes J, et al. Immune complexes and autoantibodies in silicosis. *J Allergy Clin Immunol.* 1981;68:281.

   An investigation of the humoral immune system in 53 patients with silicosis.

9. Dee P, Suratt P, Winn W. The radiographic findings in acute silicosis. *Radiology.* 1978;126:359.

   A spectrum of radiographic findings is described.

10. Hertzberg V, Rosenman KD, Reilly MJ, et al. Effect of occupational silica exposure on pulmonary function. *Chest.* 2002;122:721.

    An epidemiologic study showing an association between pulmonary function test abnormalities and estimated silica exposure.

11. Mason G, Abraham JL, Hoffman L, et al. Treatment of mixed-dust pneumoconiosis with whole lung lavage. *Am Rev Respir Dis.* 1982;126:1102.

    A case report of a patient treated with whole-lung lavage.

12. Sharma S, Pande J, Verma K, et al. Effect of prednisolone treatment in chronic silicosis. *Am Rev Respir Dis.* 1991;143:814.

    An uncontrolled study in patients with chronic silicosis of corticosteroid effects on lung function and bronchoalveolar lavage.

Coal Workers' Pneumoconiosis

William G. Hughson

Coal workers' pneumoconiosis, formerly called *anthracosis* or *anthracosilicosis,* exists in two forms: simple and complicated. Simple coal workers' pneumoconiosis is diagnosed by a history of exposure to coal dust and chest radiographs showing an increased profusion of small, round parenchymal densities (categories 0, 1, 2, and 3 as rated by the International Labor Office system for grading radiographs for pneumoconiosis). Complicated coal workers' pneumoconiosis is known as *progressive massive fibrosis.* The diagnosis of progressive massive fibrosis requires densities larger than 1 cm in diameter; some authorities require lesions larger than 2 cm.

Bronchial stenosis associated with black pigmentation of the overlying mucosa was thought to be complication of tuberculosis. However, this condition has now been reported where tuberculosis was excluded, and the term *anthracofibrosis* is used to describe it. The stenosis and associated postobstructive atelectasis can mimic lung cancer.

PATHOPHYSIOLOGY

The basic pathologic lesion in simple coal workers' pneumoconiosis is the *coal macule.* This is a collection of coal dust-laden macrophages, reticulin, and collagen located within the walls of respiratory bronchioles and adjacent alveoli. Macules range in size from 1 to 5 mm in diameter and are located predominantly in the upper lobes. As the number of macrophages grows, fibrosis increases, creating micronodules (<7 mm) and macronodules (7–20 mm). A zone of focal emphysema is usually seen around macules and nodules, possibly caused by mechanical traction on adjacent parenchyma or digestion of alveolar walls by proteolytic enzymes released from macrophages. A tendency is seen for nodules to cluster and eventually to coalesce to produce progressive massive fibrosis lesions. There is some evidence that coal workers may be at risk for chronic interstitial pneumonia, even when coal workers' pneumoconiosis is not present.

PATHOGENESIS

The pathogenesis of coal workers' pneumoconiosis is unclear. Silica in coal dust was thought to be the cause; it is now recognized that coal workers' pneumoconiosis is a pathologic entity distinct from silicosis, although the two conditions can coexist. Coal is composed predominantly of elemental carbon and varying amounts of minerals, metals, and organic compounds. Electrically charged surface radicals on coal dust damage biologic membranes. Regional differences in the frequency and severity of coal workers' pneumoconiosis may be caused by the content of Fe^{2+} and the buffering capacity of the dust. Higher (hardness)-rank coals are associated with increased risk of simple coal workers' pneumoconiosis and progressive massive fibrosis. Anthracite is the highest rank, followed by bituminous and lignite. Experimentally, high-rank coals are cleared more slowly from the lungs and are more cytotoxic. The attack rate for progressive massive fibrosis rises with increasing total lung dust; progressive massive fibrosis usually occurs in the setting of advanced simple coal workers' pneumoconiosis (categories 2 and 3). Increased silica content of inhaled dust also increases the incidence of progressive massive fibrosis. Historically, tuberculosis has been considered as a risk factor for progressive massive fibrosis; its role has diminished in recent decades, although this organism should always be sought in a patient with expanding upper-lobe lesions. Cavitation of progressive massive fibrosis lesions usually results from tissue necrosis, not tuberculosis. Coal miners do not have a greater incidence of tuberculosis compared with the general population.

The pulmonary macrophage plays a central role in the pathogenesis of coal workers' pneumoconiosis by releasing inflammatory factors, recruiting polymorphonuclear leukocytes into the lung, and stimulating fibroblast production of collagen. A number of immunologic abnormalities have been found in miners with coal workers' pneumoconiosis. Their causative role, if any, is unknown and their prevalence has varied in different studies. Miners with coal workers' pneumoconiosis have elevated serum levels of IgA, IgG, C3, antinuclear antibodies, rheumatoid factor, and α_1-proteinase inhibitor; similar findings are seen in other forms of pneumoconiosis.

No clear correlation is found between serologic factors and the risk or severity of coal workers' pneumoconiosis except for rheumatoid pneumoconiosis (Caplan syndrome), which describes coal miners with rheumatoid arthritis. The characteristic radiographic features of rheumatoid pneumoconiosis are rapidly enlarging, evenly distributed nodules ranging in size from 0.3 to 5.0 cm in diameter, occurring in lungs that otherwise show little evidence of pneumoconiosis. Microscopically, the active lesions are similar to subcutaneous rheumatoid nodules; vasculitis is a common feature. Coal mining does not predispose to rheumatoid arthritis.

REGULATIONS AND RISK OF COAL WORKERS' PNEUMOCONIOSIS

The risk of development and progression of coal workers' pneumoconiosis increases with cumulative dust exposure. Most affected miners worked before 1969, when the Federal Coal Mine Health and Safety Act (known as the *Coal Act*) was passed. It required that a coal worker's exposure to respirable dust be maintained at or below 2 mg/m³. The Federal Mine Safety and Health Act of 1977 (known as the *Mine Act*) consolidated all federal health and safety regulations of the mining industry under a single statutory scheme, and created the Mine Safety and Health Administration for enforcement. The prevalence of coal workers' pneumoconiosis in coal miners decreased dramatically from the 1970s until 2000, but has increased since then. New mining techniques and machinery have increased coal production, and miners now spend about 25% more time underground than they did in the 1980s. The risk of coal workers' pneumoconiosis and progressive massive fibrosis is much greater in small mines with fewer than 50 miners, raising concern about poor dust control and increased silica exposure due to the mining of thinner coal seams. New cases of coal workers' pneumoconiosis and progressive massive fibrosis are still occurring, raising the issue of whether the current exposure limit is too high or if enforcement is inadequate. The National Institute for Occupational Safety and Health has recommended a reduction in the exposure limit to 1 mg/m³.

IMPAIRMENT AND DISABILITY

The issue of impairment and disability caused by coal workers' pneumoconiosis is controversial. Most authorities agree that clinically significant pulmonary impairment does not occur in nonsmoking patients with simple coal workers' pneumoconiosis, although small reductions in spirometric values are common. Conversely, progressive massive fibrosis is associated with significant morbidity and premature death. Cough and sputum production, often described as industrial bronchitis, usually have little effect on lung function in the absence of smoking. Cigarette smoking, although responsible for most pulmonary impairment among coal miners, does not increase the incidence of simple coal workers' pneumoconiosis or the risk of progression to progressive massive fibrosis. Coal dust causes emphysema even in nonsmokers, and may be the major cause of respiratory morbidity in miners who do not have progressive massive fibrosis. The Mine Act and Black Lung Benefits Program established guidelines for rating disability based on reduction of the forced expiratory volume in 1 second (FEV_1) and maximal voluntary ventilation. Decrements in spirometric values are based on a miner's height, but not age, and do not consider the effects of smoking. Should a miner have either a normal ventilatory capacity or a slight decrement, that person can still qualify for benefits if the PaO_2 is reduced below a certain level with an alveolar–arterial oxygen gradient greater than 45 mmHg breathing-room air at rest. Exercise testing is not included in the rating system.

Today, the life expectancy of a coal worker approximates that of the general population. Excess deaths are seen for nonmalignant respiratory disease, accidents, and possibly stomach cancer. Approximately 4% of coal worker deaths are directly attributable to pneumoconiosis, usually progressive massive fibrosis; most studies have not shown an excess mortality for simple coal workers' pneumoconiosis. These excess deaths are counterbalanced by decreased mortality from lung cancer and ischemic heart disease. Employed populations typically have morbidity and mortality rates 10% to 20% lower than the general population, which contains individuals disabled by chronic diseases. This deficit of disease is referred to as the *healthy worker effect*. Cor pulmonale and right-ventricular hypertrophy do not occur in the absence of cigarette smoking or progressive massive fibrosis. No specific treatment exists for coal workers' pneumoconiosis except limiting dust exposure.

FURTHER READING

1. Attfield MD, Kuempel ED. Mortality among U.S. underground coal miners: a 23-year follow-up. *Am J Ind Med.* 2008;51:231–245.

   Mortality from all causes was similar to the general public, but there was a doubling of risk from non-malignant respiratory diseases, particularly pneumoconiosis. There was no increased risk of lung cancer or stomach cancer.

2. Brichet A, Tonnel AB, Brambilla E, et al. Chronic interstitial pneumonia with honeycombing in coal workers. *Sarcoidosis Vasc Diffuse Lung Dis.* 2002;19:211–219.

   Describes a possible association between chronic interstitial pneumonia and coal dust exposure, with or without associated coal workers' pneumoconiosis.

3. Cohen R, Velho V. Update on respiratory disease from coal mine and silica dust. *Clin Chest Med.* 2002;23:811–826.

   A good review article.

4. Fisher BE. Between a rock and a healthy place. *Environ Health Perspect.* 1998;106:A544–A546.

   A review of legislation and agencies intended to prevent coal workers' pneumoconiosis.

5. Goodwin S, Attfield M. Temporal trends in coal workers' pneumoconiosis prevalence. Validating the National Coal Study results. *J Occup Environ Med.* 1998;40:1065–1071.

   Prevalence of coal workers' pneumoconiosis and progressive massive fibrosis has diminished with time, but new cases still occur despite current exposure standard for coal dust of 2 mg/m³. National Institute for Occupational Safety and Health has recommended reducing the exposure limit for coal dust to 1 mg/m³.

6. Henneberger PK, Attfield MD. Respiratory symptoms and spirometry in experienced coal miners: effects of both distant and recent coal mine dust exposures. *Am J Ind Med.* 1997;32:268–274.

   Frequency of respiratory symptoms decreased after the US Coal Mine Health and Safety Act of 1969, but 2 mg/m³ standard did not eliminate coal workers' pneumoconiosis.

7. Huang X, Fournier J, Koenig K, et al. Buffering capacity of coal and its acid-soluble Fe^{2+} content: possible role in coal workers' pneumoconiosis. *Chem Res Toxicol.* 1998;11:722–729.

   Frequency of coal workers' pneumoconiosis is greater when coal has high acid-soluble Fe^{2+}, and low buffering capacity, which may explain regional differences in frequency and severity of coal workers' pneumoconiosis.

8. Laney AS, Attfield MD. Coal workers' pneumoconiosis and progressive massive fibrosis are increasingly more prevalent among workers in small underground coal mines in the United States. *J Occup Environ Med.* 2009;67:428–431.

   Risk of coal workers' pneumoconiosis and progressive massive fibrosis is greater in mines with fewer than 50 workers. This may be due to poor dust control, lax enforcement of regulations, and the mining of thinner coal seams leading to greater exposure to silica and other dusts.

9. Joyce S. Major issues in miner health. *Environ Health Perspect.* 1998;106:A538–A543.

   An excellent review of miner health problems and legislation to prevent coal workers' pneumoconiosis.

10. Kuempel ED, Wheeler MW, Smith RJ, et al. Contributions of dust exposure and cigarette smoking to emphysema severity in coal miners in the United States. *Am J Respir Crit Care Med.* 2009;180:257–264.

    Emphysema severity was significantly increased in coal miners compared with nonminers even in nonsmokers.

11. McCunney RJ, Morfield P, Payne S. What component of coal causes pneumoconiosis? *J Occup Environ Med.* 2009;51:462–471.

    This review article concludes the active agent within coal dust is iron, and that silica is not important in the pathogenesis of coal workers' pneumoconiosis.

12. Naccache J-M, Monnet I, Nunes H, et al. Anthracofibrosis attributed to mixed mineral dust exposure: report of three cases. *Thorax.* 2008;63:655–657.

Three cases of bronchial stenosis with black pigmentation in the overlying mucosa where tuberculosis was excluded.

13. Prince TS, Frank AL. Causation, impairment, disability: an analysis of coal workers' pneumoconiosis evaluations. *J Occup Environ Med.* 1996;38:77–82.

The relationship of exposure, impairment, and awarded disability in coal workers' pneumoconiosis is unclear in many cases. Miners with normal radiographs and spirometry often receive compensation.

14. Tomas LHS. Emphysema and chronic obstructive pulmonary disease in coal miners. *Curr Opin Pulm Med.* 2011;17:123–125.

Emphysema and COPD can develop independent of smoking status in coal miners, and risk is related to cumulative exposure to respirable coal dust.

15. Vallyathan V, Brower PS, Green FH, et al. Radiographic and pathologic correlation of coal workers' pneumoconiosis. *Am J Respir Crit Care Med.* 1996;154:741–748.

Compares whole lung sections with radiographic findings. Radiographs were insensitive to minimal coal workers' pneumoconiosis lesions, but correlated fairly well to pathology with International Labor Office (generally referred to as ILO) ratings of 0/1 or greater. For progressive massive fibrosis lesions, radiographic and pathologic findings often did not correlate.

16. Wade WA, Petsonk EL, Young B, et al. Severe occupational pneumoconiosis among West Virginia coal miners: 138 cases of progressive massive fibrosis compensated between 2000 and 2009. *Chest.* 2011;139(6):1458–1462. doi:10.1378/chest.10-1326.

Most of the miners with progressive massive fibrosis had worked after the current federal dust regulations were implemented, suggesting the current standard is inadequate, enforcement is inadequate, or both.

17. Wynn GJ, Turkington PM, O'Driscoll BR. Anthracofibrosis, bronchial stenosis with overlying anthracotic mucosa: possibly a new occupational lung disorder. *Chest.* 2008;134:1069–1073.

Endobronchial pigmentation with airway narrowing was initially described as a complication of tuberculosis. The term anthracofibrosis was coined to describe this condition in patients without tuberculosis.

84 Asbestos-Related Disease

William G. Hughson

The term *asbestos* refers to a group of naturally occurring, fibrous hydrated silicates that share characteristics of heat and chemical resistance. *Chrysotile,* or serpentine asbestos, is characterized by curvilinear fibrils. The other types have straight fibers, and are referred to as *amphibole asbestos.* The most important amphiboles are amosite and crocidolite. Asbestos has been used for multiple purposes, including textiles, thermal insulation, building materials, and friction products such as brake linings.

The risk of asbestos-related disease is related to the amount of exposure, described using the term *fiber/cc-year,* which is the amount of asbestos that would be inhaled by working for a year in an atmosphere where the time-weighted average level of asbestos was 1 fiber/cc of air. The *year* in this term is a working year (8 hours/day for 250 days), and only fibers longer than 5 μm are counted. Historically, exposure levels were very high. For example, insulators working in shipyards and commercial construction were exposed to approximately 10 fibers/cc. Exposures for chrysotile miners and textile workers were in the range of 10 to 100 fibers/cc. In contrast, automobile mechanics doing brake repair had an average exposure of 0.1 fibers/cc. The threshold limit value for asbestos was 5 million particles per cubic foot (~15 fibers/cc) until 1968. Since then, it has been progressively lowered to the current permissible exposure limit of 0.1 fiber/cc.

The risk of asbestos-related disease is also related to fiber type. Chrysotile asbestos is cleared rapidly from the lungs. In contrast, amphibole asbestos is retained to a much greater extent. As a result, the risk of disease in chrysotile-exposed populations is lower on a fiber/cc-year basis. For example, the chrysotile miners and millers of Quebec had little evidence of increased mortality up to a cumulative exposure of approximately 1,000 fiber/cc-years. In contrast, the risk of mesothelioma from crocidolite or amosite is increased by exposures in the range of 2 to 5 fiber/cc-years. Approximately 90% of the asbestos used in North America was chrysotile. Amosite was used primarily in insulation products, and crocidolite was used mainly for asbestos cement. In Europe and Australia, amphibole use was more common. Those areas have experienced a much higher rate of asbestos-related malignancies.

Although the high exposure levels of the 1900s are a thing of the past, the widespread use of asbestos-containing construction materials has led to concern that occupants of public buildings and schools may be harmed. Asbestos fibers are present in the air of many buildings, typically in the range of 0.001 to 0.0001 fibers/cc. Most are chrysotile, and there is no evidence that the general public is at increased risk from these environmental or background levels of exposure. There have been reports of family members developing asbestos-related diseases caused by exposure to fibers brought home on the clothes of asbestos workers. Most of those cases involved amphibole asbestos, and lung tissue analysis has demonstrated that the family members had lung tissue concentrations similar to people with occupational exposures.

Regulatory agencies such as the Occupational Safety and Health Agency and Environmental Protection Agency (EPA) use a linear no-threshold model for risk assessment. An inevitable consequence of this model is that any level of asbestos exposure, no matter how small, can be calculated to cause some degree of risk. However, there is ample evidence that low levels of exposure, particularly to chrysotile asbestos, do not cause an increased risk of asbestos-related disease. For example, residents in the Quebec chrysotile mining townships were exposed to ambient levels between 0.1 and 3 fibers/cc prior to 1970. The estimated lifetime exposure at these levels would be approximately 25 fiber/cc-years. There is no evidence of increased lung cancer risk in the townships, and almost all the reported cases of mesothelioma had either occupational exposure in the mining industry, or lived with family members who were employed in the industry. The EPA's model significantly overestimated the risk of lung cancer and mesothelioma in the Quebec mining townships.

The term *asbestosis* refers to parenchymal fibrosis caused by asbestos, and is characterized by the presence of interstitial fibrosis and an increased number of asbestos ferruginous bodies and uncoated asbestos fibers in lung tissue. The ferruginous body is an asbestos fiber coated with proteinaceous iron-staining material; it is visible on light microscopy. Using lung digestion techniques, uncoated fibers can be identified and counted. Patients with asbestosis typically have concentrations of ferruginous bodies and uncoated fibers that are 100 to 1,000 times higher than the general population. Asbestosis usually begins subpleurally in the lung bases. As the disease progresses, it can involve both lungs diffusely as a fine fibrosis. In the final stages, the lungs can acquire a cystic honeycomb appearance and can be indistinguishable radiographically from other forms of severe interstitial fibrosis.

Patients with asbestosis usually present with dyspnea on exertion, and may have a nonproductive cough. A clinical diagnosis of asbestosis requires an appropriate exposure history. Asbestosis requires a high level of exposure, and is now a rare disease. The latency period (the number of years from the initial exposure) is 20 years or longer for most patients. Chest radiographs show an increased profusion of bibasilar irregular densities. The American Thoracic Society (ATS) criteria for a diagnosis of asbestosis require a rating of 1/0 or higher using the International Labor Office (ILO) system. It is possible, though uncommon, to have histologic evidence of asbestosis in a patient with a normal chest radiograph. Other criteria include a restrictive pattern on the pulmonary function tests, reduction in the diffusing capacity for carbon monoxide, and the presence of rales. High-resolution, thin-section computed tomography (CT) scans with supine and prone views may demonstrate interstitial disease in the presence of normal, equivocal, or mild parenchymal abnormalities on chest radiographs.

Exercise testing is useful in identifying the cause of dyspnea in patients with relatively normal pulmonary function. The level of dyspnea often does not correlate with a single pulmonary function test value or with a specific radiographic profusion score. The degree of impairment and disability should be noted according to subjective and objective criteria established by the ATS and the American Medical Association.

Pleural disease or *pleural fibrosis* is the most common form of asbestos-related pulmonary injury. It occurs at relatively low levels of exposure, far less than is required for asbestosis. Pathologically, localized areas of pleural scarring (the pleural plaque) are seen. Calcification can occur, and is an index of chronicity rather than severity. Pleural plaques viewed on a plain chest radiograph are usually bilateral and involve the middle and lower thirds of the thoracic cage. They are often seen on the diaphragm. Pleural plaques are generally found on the parietal pleural surface, but can occur on the visceral pleura and mediastinum. Usually, pleural plaques do not lead to abnormal lung function; however, studies of groups of workers with plaques have shown a mild but statistically significant decrement in vital capacity and forced expiratory volume in 1 second (FEV_1). Extensive pleural plaques can cause restrictive lung disease. Diffuse pleural thickening is distinct from localized pleural plaques, with fibrosis of the visceral and parietal pleura. If extensive and severe enough, it results in lung entrapment and can lead to severe impairment and ventilatory failure. The most likely cause of benign diffuse pleural thickening is an initial asbestos-related pleural effusion. Pleural effusions caused by asbestos are exudative, and may be chronic and recurrent. Infection and malignancy must be excluded before attributing the effusion to asbestos.

Rounded atelectasis is a benign finding characterized by localized pleural thickening and entrapment of adjacent lung tissue. Before advances in CT scanning made the characteristic appearance readily identifiable, biopsy was often necessary to distinguish this process from mesothelioma and lung cancer.

Populations with high levels of exposure to asbestos have an increased risk of lung cancer. For example, the insulators described by Selikoff had a relative risk of approximately 5-fold if they did not smoke regularly. Insulators who smoked had a risk of 50- to 90-fold compared with nonsmoking members of the general public because of a synergistic interaction between the risk of asbestos and smoking. Subsequent studies by Kipen and others demonstrated that the insulators who developed lung cancer also had asbestosis. Although there is some controversy on this subject, the preponderance of data suggest that the risk of lung cancer is increased when clinical or pathologic asbestosis is present, and that asbestos exposure alone does not increase the risk in the absence of pulmonary fibrosis. Approximately two-thirds of asbestos-related lung cancers occur in the lower lobes, in contrast to the predominantly upper-lobe distribution of most lung cancers. The distribution of cell types is similar to smoking-related lung cancers, and is not helpful in identifying tumors caused by asbestos. Many studies do not control adequately for smoking. Because blue-collar workers smoke more than the general population, failure to control for smoking can lead to the erroneous conclusion that occupational exposures are causing an increased risk of lung cancer.

Mesothelioma is a rare tumor, arising in the pleura and peritoneum. Approximately 75% of men and 10% of women with mesothelioma have a history of occupational exposure to asbestos. Some cases have been reported in family members of asbestos workers. Fiber type is very important in the etiology of mesothelioma. Although chrysotile can cause mesothelioma, it does so rarely, and only after levels of exposure similar to those necessary to cause asbestosis. In contrast, amphibole asbestos causes mesothelioma at low doses. There is no evidence that the general public is at increased risk of mesothelioma because of ambient levels of asbestos.

No specific therapy exists for asbestos-related pleural or pulmonary disease. Every effort should be made to eliminate smoking. Other measures include early treatment of lung infections, influenza and pneumonia vaccinations, careful surveillance, and treatment of complications of respiratory failure.

FURTHER READING

1. Banks DE, Shi R, McLarty J, et al. American College of Chest Physicians consensus statement on the respiratory health effects of asbestos. *Chest*. 2009;135:1619–1627.

   An interesting paper showing the spectrum of opinions concerning the health effects of asbestos.

2. Camus M, Siemiatycki J, Meek B. Nonoccupational exposure to chrysotile asbestos and the risk of lung cancer. *N Engl J Med*. 1998;338:1565–1571.

   The EPA's model overestimated the risk of lung cancer by at least a factor of 10 in the chrysotile mining areas of Quebec.

3. Camus M, Siemiatycki J, Case BW, et al. Risk of mesothelioma among women living near chrysotile mines versus US EPA asbestos model: preliminary findings. *Ann Occup Hyg*. 2002;46 (suppl):95–98.

   The EPA's model overestimated the risk of mesothelioma by a factor of about 100 in the chrysotile mining areas of Quebec.

4. Case BW, Camus M, Richardson L, et al. Preliminary findings for pleural mesothelioma among women in the Quebec chrysotile mining regions. *Ann Occup Hyg*. 2002;46(suppl):128–131.

   Most of the women diagnosed with mesothelioma had occupational exposures, or lived with employees who worked in the industry.

5. Cugell DW, Kamp DW. Asbestos and the pleura: a review. *Chest*. 2004;125:1103–1117.

   A comprehensive review article.

6. Graham GW, Berry G. Mesothelioma and asbestos. *Regul Toxicol Pharmacol*. 2008;52:S223–S231.

   Pure chrysotile probably does not cause mesothelioma. Amphibole asbestos is a potent cause of mesothelioma.

7. Greillier L, Astoul P. Mesothelioma and asbestos-related pleural diseases. *Respiration*. 2008;76:1–15.

   A comprehensive review article describing benign and malignant pleural diseases caused by asbestos.

8. Guidotti TL, Miller A, Christiani D, et al. Diagnosis and initial management of nonmalignant diseases related to asbestos. *Am J Respir Crit Care Med*. 2004;170:691–715.

   A position paper of the ATS.

9. Hodgson JT, Darnton A. The quantitative risks of mesothelioma and lung cancer in relation to asbestos exposure. *Ann Occup Hyg*. 2000;44:565–601.

   A review of epidemiologic studies. The risk of lung cancer and mesothelioma is greater for amphibole asbestos than for chrysotile.

10. Kipen HM, Lilis R, Suzuki Y, et al. Pulmonary fibrosis in asbestos insulation workers with lung cancer: a radiological and histopathological evaluation. *Br J Ind Med*. 1987;44:96–100.

    An important study of 138 insulators with lung cancer demonstrating that all had pathological evidence of asbestosis, and chest radiographs with an ILO rating of 1/1 or greater identified the excess number of lung cancers. Subsequent reports of 415 cases demonstrated that 99% had pathological asbestos, and virtually all were smokers or ex-smokers.

11. Lanphear BP, Buncher CR. Latent period for malignant mesothelioma of occupational origin. *J Occup Med*. 1992;34:718–721.

    Latent period for mesothelioma is 20 years or longer in 96% of cases.

12. Lee DJ, Fleming LE, Arheart KL, et al. Smoking rate trends in U.S. occupational groups: the 1987 to 2004 National Health Interview Survey. *J Occup Environ Med*. 2007; 49:75–81.

    Smoking is more common in blue-collar workers than in the general public.

13. Liddell FDK, McDonald AD, McDonald JC. The 1891–1920 birth cohort of Quebec chrysotile miners and millers: development from 1901 and mortality to 1992. *Ann Occup Hyg*. 1997;41:13–36.

    Heavily exposed miners and millers had little evidence of increased mortality with cumulative exposures to 1,000 fiber/cc-years.

14. Price B, Ware A. Time trend of mesothelioma incidence in the United States and projection of future cases: an update based on the SEER data for 1973 through 2005. *Crit Rev Toxicol*. 2009;39:576–588.

Estimated 2,400 cases of mesothelioma in the United States in 2008. Projected 68,000 cases between 2008 and 2042.

15. Roggli VL, Sanders LL. Asbestos content of lung tissue and carcinoma of the lung: a clinicopathologic correlation and mineral fiber analysis of 234 cases. *Ann Occup Hyg.* 2000;44:109–117.

Cases with asbestosis had markedly elevated asbestos levels in the lungs, most of which were amphiboles. An amphibole burden sufficient to cause lung cancer is usually accompanied by histologic evidence of asbestosis.

16. Roggli VL, Sharma A, Butnor KJ, et al. Malignant mesothelioma and occupational exposure to asbestos: a clinicopathological correlation of 1445 cases. *Ultrastruct Pathol.* 2002;26:55.

Commercial amphiboles are responsible for most mesotheliomas in the United States.

17. Selikoff IJ, Hammond EC. Asbestos and smoking. *JAMA.* 1979;242:458.

Insulators who smoked had a 50- to 90-fold increased risk of lung cancer.

Work-Related Asthma

William G. Hughson

Asthma is a disorder of lung function characterized by widespread obstruction of the airways that (1) varies in severity; (2) is reversible, either spontaneously or as a result of treatment; and (3) is not caused by cardiovascular disease. Work-related asthma is the broad term that refers to asthma that is induced *or* exacerbated by inhalation exposures in the workplace and includes both occupational asthma and work-exacerbated asthma. Occupational asthma is *caused by* exposure to airborne dusts, gases, vapors, or fumes in the working environment. Work-exacerbated asthma refers to asthma *triggered by* various work-related factors in workers known to have pre-existing or concurrent asthma.

ETIOLOGY

Asthma is a common disease. Approximately 10% of people are diagnosed with asthma during their lifetime (i.e., the incidence of asthma). Some cases resolve, but approximately 5% of the population has active asthma (i.e., the prevalence of asthma). Approximately 10% to 15% of cases of adult asthma is either caused or exacerbated by workplace exposures. The frequency of work-related asthma varies widely among occupations and within industries at different levels of exposure. The true occurrence of work-related asthma is probably greater than reported because affected workers often terminate their employment, leaving unaffected survivors. This type of self-selection is common in studies of working individuals that compare morbidity and mortality rates to those of the general population. Employed populations typically have morbidity and mortality rates 10% to 20% lower than the general population, which contains individuals disabled by chronic diseases. This deficit of disease is referred to as the *healthy worker effect.* Because asthma is common in the general population and the clinical findings in work-related asthma are identical to those of non–work-related asthma, the clinical challenge is to understand the nature and degree of workplace exposures and to make a temporal association between the asthma and occupation. Diagnosis can be difficult, given the inherent variability of asthma and the fact the patient can have early, late, dual, or recurrent late onset of symptoms.

PATHOGENESIS

The pathogenetic mechanisms of work-related asthma can be classified as reflex, inflammatory, pharmacologic, and allergic. *Reflex bronchoconstriction* involves irritant receptors in the airway that are stimulated by agents such as cold air, inert dust particles, gases, and fumes. The reaction does not involve immune mechanisms and is nonspecific. Many patients have a history of pre-existing asthma. *Inflammatory bronchoconstriction* begins as a nonspecific reaction following inhalation of high concentrations of nonspecific irritants. Most individuals recover, but a few develop chronic asthma. This condition is often referred to as *reactive airways dysfunction syndrome* (RADS). Vocal-cord dysfunction characterized by hoarseness, cough, and dyspnea is also caused by irritant exposures, and can be mistaken for asthma. *Pharmacologic bronchoconstriction* occurs when agents in the work environment exert a specific pharmacologic effect on the lung. An example is cholinesterase inhibition by organophosphate pesticides causing bronchoconstriction because of excessive parasympathetic stimulation.

Allergic bronchoconstriction is the most common cause of occupational asthma. Susceptible workers develop IgE or IgG antibodies following exposure to workplace antigens such as animal or plant proteins. If high-molecular-weight compounds are responsible (e.g., baker's asthma), individuals who are atopic become sensitized more readily than workers who are nonatopic. However, atopy is not a predisposing factor when low-molecular-weight compounds are involved (e.g., isocyanate manufacturing). Sensitization takes time, and the latency period between exposure and the onset of symptoms can be weeks to years. Several hundred workplace agents have been shown to cause occupational asthma, and the list grows every year. Cigarette smoking doubles the risk of occupational asthma, possibly by recruiting inflammatory cells into the lung where they are available to react with irritants and sensitizers.

DIAGNOSIS

When considering work-related asthma as a diagnosis, two questions must be answered: (1) does this patient actually have asthma and (2) is the asthma related to work. The general approach to diagnosing asthma is discussed elsewhere in this manual (see Chapter 63). Methods for answering the second question include a detailed clinical and occupational history, physical examination, chest radiographs, pulmonary function tests, inhalation challenge tests, and immunologic tests.

The clinical history of the patient with work-related asthma typically reveals shortness of breath, chest tightness, cough, and wheezing at work or within several hours after leaving work. Respiratory symptoms are often accompanied by rhinitis or conjunctivitis. Recurrent attacks of *bronchitis* are often reported. Improvement on weekends, vacations, or when away from work is an important clue. Patients who develop symptoms immediately after exposure or whenever they work with the same material usually recognize a causal relationship. However, a large number of substances, particularly low-molecular-weight organic and inorganic compounds, may give rise to late asthmatic reactions. Nocturnal attacks of dyspnea and cough may be the only manifestation of work-related asthma; thus, be aware that the onset of symptoms may not be simultaneous with workplace exposure. Key elements influencing the pattern of symptoms and airflow obstruction seen in workers with work-related asthma are the recovery time and the effects of cumulative exposures. Some individuals improve rapidly after leaving work, and recovery is virtually complete before the next workday. Such workers show a similar deterioration during each shift. At the other extreme are those who need more than 2 days to recovery. Repeated exposures over several weeks, even with weekends off, result in a steady deterioration of pulmonary function. Clinical features can be indistinguishable from chronic obstructive lung disease because of nonoccupational causes. The reactive nature of the disease can be masked by a fixed reduction in expiratory flow rates seemingly unrelated to work activities. In such cases, the true relationship between the patient's occupation and asthma becomes apparent only after prolonged cessation of exposure allows sufficient time for recovery of normal pulmonary function. When the patient finally returns to work, the simultaneous reappearance of symptoms and airflow obstruction makes the link obvious.

The occupational history is crucial for the diagnosis of work-related asthma. Obtain a detailed description of the patient's work practices, including the agents used, protective equipment such as respirators and gloves, and the adequacy of ventilation. In addition to the patient's own work, information concerning other processes and chemicals used by coworkers should be obtained; bystander exposures can cause reactions in sensitized individuals. It is often helpful to ask whether coworkers have similar problems. Patients usually have only limited knowledge of the agents they use. Material safety data sheets should be obtained from the employer, who is legally required to provide them to the worker. If the clinician is careful to avoid a confrontational situation, the employer or the workers' compensation insurance company may provide industrial hygiene data concerning the nature and degree of exposures. Site visits are often helpful, and the clinician must be prepared to search the medical literature to complete the assessment.

The physical examination may reveal conjunctivitis, rhinitis, and wheezing; however, these signs are often absent, particularly when the patient has been away from work for some time. The chest radiographs are usually normal in patients with work-related asthma, although parenchymal infiltrates and hyperinflation may be seen.

Pulmonary function tests should demonstrate expiratory obstruction and hyperinflation, with improvement following inhalation of bronchodilator medication. However, variability of airway obstruction is a key feature of asthma, and pulmonary function tests may be normal. In this situation, the demonstration of bronchial hyperreactivity depends on provocation tests using methacholine, histamine, cold air, or exercise as a stimulus. These nonspecific promoters of bronchial hyperreactivity cannot identify a workplace cause. The gold standard for diagnosing occupational asthma in the pulmonary laboratory is a specific inhalation challenge using the suspected agent. However, it is often difficult to select the correct chemical from among many used in the typical, complicated workplace environment. In addition, practical difficulties exist to administering the correct concentration of the agent and few facilities have sophisticated environmental chambers. Pre- and postshift pulmonary function tests may demonstrate expiratory obstruction after workplace exposures. Another approach is serial measurement of peak flow rates. The patient is provided with an inexpensive flow meter and maintains a diary during the workweek, evenings, and weekends. At least 2 weeks of observation is needed. This requires considerable patient cooperation, and the results of self-administered tests are often suspect in the setting of potential litigation and secondary gain. Some authors have recommended serial measurements of bronchial hyperreactivity using methacholine before and after work shifts; decreased provocative dose following exposure is supportive of work-related asthma.

Skin tests and serology may be useful in identifying specific sensitization. However, selection and preparation of agents for skin testing is difficult, and nonspecific irritation can lead to false-positive findings. Antibody assays are available for only a limited number of workplace chemicals; positive serology indicates previous exposure, but is not diagnostic of asthma caused by that agent. Skin tests and serology may suggest the cause of work-related asthma but are not definitive.

TREATMENT

The treatment of work-related asthma is identical to that for non–work-related asthma. Emphasis should be placed on avoidance of the agent responsible in sensitized individuals and reduction in exposure to nonspecific irritants. The prognosis of patients with work-related asthma is guarded. More than 50% remain symptomatic one year after removal from exposure. The clinician is often asked to define disability caused by work-related asthma. This requires a careful assessment of the degree of airflow obstruction and bronchial hyperreactivity and whether the patient could return to work with certain restrictions or job modifications. If return to work is not feasible, vocational rehabilitation is required. These decisions require input from the clinician, patient, employer, and the agency responsible for administering workers' compensation claims.

FURTHER READING

1. Banks DE. Use of the specific challenge in the diagnosis of occupational asthma: a "gold standard" test or a test not used in current practice of occupational asthma? *Curr Opin Allergy Clin Immunol.* 2003;3:101–107.

   Discusses the difficulty of specific inhalation challenge tests, including the lack of fellowship training and the limited number of centers with inhalation chambers.

2. Burge S. Recent developments in occupational asthma. *Swiss Med Wkly.* 2010;140:128–132.

   A concise review article.

3. Castano R, Malo J-L. Occupational rhinitis and asthma: where do we stand, where do we go? *Curr Allergy Asthma Rep.* 2010;10:135–142.

   Occupational rhinitis and asthma often coexist. Good discussion of mechanisms and approaches to diagnosis.

4. Chan-Yeung M. Christie Memorial lecture. Occupational asthma—the past 50 years.. *Can Respir J.* 2004;11:21–26.

   Provides an interesting historical perspective on our understanding of occupational asthma.

5. Cowl CT. Occupational asthma: review of assessment, treatment and compensation. *Chest.* 2011;139:674–681.

   A good review which includes discussion of impairment, disability, workers compensation, and insurance systems.

6. Hendrick DJ. Recognition and surveillance of occupational asthma: a preventable illness with missed opportunities. *Br Med Bull.* 2010;95:175–192.

   An excellent review article.

7. Jeal H, Jones M. Allergy to rodents: an update. *Clin Exp Allergy.* 2010;40:1593–1601.

   Approximately 10% of animal handlers develop rhinitis, conjunctivitis, or asthma.

8. Malo J-L, L'Archeveque J, Castellanos L, et al. Long-term outcomes of acute irritant-induced asthma. *Am J Respir Crit Care Med.* 2009;179:923–928.

   Approximately 80% of patients with RADS will be symptomatic and have abnormal lung function a decade after the acute irritant exposure.

9. McHugh MK, Symanski E, Pompeii LA, et al. Prevalence of asthma by industry and occupation in the U.S. working population. *Am J Ind Med.* 2010;53:463–475.

   Describes prevalence of asthma in various working groups. Miners, healthcare workers and teachers are high-risk populations.

10. Rachiotis G, Savani R, Brant A, et al. Outcome of occupational asthma after cessation of exposure: a systematic review. *Thorax.* 2007;62:147–152.

    Complete symptomatic recovery from occupational asthma occurred in only 32% of patients followed for an average of 33 months.

11. Stoughton T, Prematta M, Craig T. Assessing and treating work-related asthma. *Allergy Asthma Clin Immunol.* 2008;4:164–171.

    An excellent review article.

12. Tarlo SM, Balmes J, Balkisson R, et al. Diagnosis and management of work-related asthma. American College of Chest Physicians consensus statement. *Chest.* 2008;134:1S–41S.

    A detailed review article which outlines the current state-of-the-art for work-related asthma.

13. Tarlo SM, Cartier A, Lemiere C. Work-related asthma: a case-based guide. *Can Respir J.* 2009;16:e57–e61.

    A concise article describing key points in diagnosing work-related asthma.

14. Tarlo SM, Liss GM. Prevention of occupational asthma. *Curr Allergy Asthma Rep.* 2010;10:278–286.

    A good review of strategies to reduce the risk of work-related asthma.

15. Tarlo SM, Liss GM, Blanc PD. How to diagnose and treat work-related asthma: key messages for clinical practice from the American College of Chest Physicians consensus statement. *Pol Arch Med Wewn.* 2009;119:660–666.

    Clearly written and practical review for the clinician.

16. Vandenplas O. Asthma and rhinitis in the workplace. *Curr Allergy Asthma Rep.* 2010;10:373–380.

    A good discussion of research in last 5 years.

17. Zock J-P, Vizcaya D, Le Moual N. Update on asthma and cleaners. *Curr Opin Allergy Clin Immunol.* 2010;10:114–120.

    Cleaning workers have an increased risk of work-related asthma due to sensitization and irritant effects of cleaning agents.

Pulmonary Injury in Burn Patients

86

Bruce M. Potenza

The diagnosis and treatment of pulmonary problems encountered in patients with severe burn injuries may be challenging. Pulmonary injury may occur as a sole entity or in combination with cutaneous burn injury. Approximately 30% of patients with cutaneous burns will have an associated pulmonary injury. The presence of smoke inhalation with a cutaneous burn may increase mortality by 20% to 50% depending upon the size of the burn. Eighty percent of all burn fatalities result from smoke inhalation, with most occurring in house fires and at night. Care for patients with smoke inhalation ranges from supplemental oxygen and β-agonist nebulizers to advanced ventilator management and bronchoscopy. The course of pulmonary support in burn patients is different from that for general medical and surgical patients requiring respiratory assistance. This is, in part, due to the pathophysiology of inhalation injury compounded by the long hospital course associated with a large burn.

INHALATION INJURY

Exposure to smoke and flame in an enclosed area such as a home, automobile, industrial building, tank, or silo is the major risk factor for smoke inhalation injury. In a closed-space fire, the oxygen concentration of the atmosphere may be 10% or less depending upon the fire characteristics. The toxic byproducts of combustion are confined, resulting in high concentrations of carbon monoxide (CO), aldehydes, ammonia, hydrogen (chloride, cyanide, and sulfide), phosgene, and sulfur dioxide. Some of these gases, which are heavier than air, settle at the lower levels of the enclosed space increasing the exposure of a victim who is crawling to escape the fire or is lying unconscious. In addition, more particulates tend to be released during a fire in a closed space and act as a vehicle to deposit the toxic byproducts of combustion deep into the respiratory tract. Industrial inhalation injuries may occur without a fire when workers are exposed to noxious aerosolized chemicals in a confined space. Often, these patients become unconscious due to the prolonged exposure.

Clinical signs and symptoms of inhalation injury may include facial, neck, and upper torso cutaneous burns; singed eyebrows, nasal and scalp hair; and soot in the nares, mouth, or hypopharynx. The patient may exhibit a change in voice (hoarseness or high-pitched) or stridor. Additional findings may include tachypnea, hypoxemia, and the presence of carboxyhemoglobin. Bronchoscopic confirmation of airway injury includes soot deposition, respiratory epithelial edema, hyperemia, ulceration, sloughing, or hemorrhage.

Inhalation injury is composed of three separate pathophysiologic mechanisms: injury due to particulate matter, toxic byproducts of combustion, and direct thermal injury. Any one or all three mechanisms may be involved in any patient. Inhalation injury due to particulate matter (smoke and soot) depends upon the size of the particles that are deposited in different anatomic areas. Larger particles are deposited proximally in the nares, concha, and hypopharynx. Smaller particulates are transmitted into the trachea and bronchioles. These smaller particles adhere to the respiratory epithelium and tend to incite or exacerbate reactive airway problems best treated with β-agonists and supplemental oxygen. It is usually a self-limiting process, but, in patients with a long exposure time, intubation and bronchoscopy to evaluate the airways and facilitate airway clearance may be indicated. Particulate matter that is adherent to the lower respiratory epithelium may take 24 to 48 hours to fully clear in moderate cases and up to 3 days in severe smoke inhalation.

The classic model for inhalation injury due to toxic byproducts of combustion is CO poisoning. Other frequent byproducts include cyanide, hydrogen chloride or sulfide, ammonia, and formaldehyde. Cyanide poisoning is difficult to diagnose, since there is no readily available laboratory test to confirm the diagnosis in real time. The presence of a persistent anion gap acidosis and elevated serum lactate is supportive evidence of cyanide poisoning.

Treatment for CO poisoning is high-flow oxygen. CO has a 200- to 250-fold higher affinity to bind hemoglobin than oxygen. The half-life of CO is 320 minutes on room air (21% F_{IO_2}), but can be reduced to 90 minutes at 100% F_{IO_2}. Most hospital and paramedic pulse oximeters cannot differentiate oxyhemoglobin and carboxyhemoglobin. Therefore, a patient with a high CO level may still have a high oxygen saturation level measured by the pulse oximeter. The correct oxygen saturation can be determined from the arterial blood gas and is often significantly lower. The actual CO level can be measured from an arterial or venous blood sample. It is our policy (extrapolated to the prehospital area) to place all patients with a history of fire exposure in a closed-space environment on high-flow 100% oxygen until the oxygen saturation and CO levels are validated by a blood gas.

Patients with high CO levels may be candidates for hyperbaric oxygen therapy to reduce serum CO levels but, more importantly, reduce central nervous system levels of CO. Long-term cognitive deficits are seen in 10% of patients with CO poisoning; hyperbaric therapy may reduce this. Three "dives" in a hyperbaric chamber are typically completed within the first 24 hours of exposure in patients with CO levels greater than or equal to 25%. Care must be taken in the burn patients to ensure that they are sufficiently hemodynamically stable to undergo hyperbaric treatment. If unstable, the dive should not be attempted. Cyanide poisoning is treated with hydroxycobalamin (CYANOKIT®) and, if this is not available, amyl nitrate.

Direct thermal injury is the least common form of smoke inhalation and represents an injury that occurs with a very intense heat source or with lesser heat and long exposure. These injuries result in airway edema; respiratory epithelial sloughing or ulceration; and copious production of thick, tenacious sputum. Intubation and bronchoscopic evaluation and aggressive pulmonary toilet are indicated in these patients. Secondary postobstructive pneumonia and acute respiratory disease syndrome (ARDS) is not uncommon in these individuals.

CHRONIC OBSTRUCTIVE PULMONARY DISEASE AND FACIAL BURNS

A special situation in the burn unit is the patient with chronic obstructive pulmonary disease (COPD) on supplemental oxygen who has been smoking and suffers a flash burn to the face and nares. This usually results in a small, 1% to 2% total body surface area (TBSA) partial thickness burn that does not require grafting. The mucosa of the nose, however, often is burned and results in edema and sloughing. This makes the act of breathing more difficult and uncomfortable requiring these patients to breathe predominantly through their mouth. They may develop severe rhinorrhea and epithelial sloughing and require aggressive external pulmonary toilet. Admission for 24 to 48 hours is usual and permits serial burn wound care to the face as well as good pulmonary toilet—intubation or mechanical ventilation usually is not required as the actual burn injury is small, superficial, and does not extend distal to the nasal or hypopharyngeal tissue. Nevertheless, they are prone to develop pneumonia as a late complication within a week of the burn injury, so it is very important to follow these patients carefully after discharge.

INTUBATION

The control and maintenance of the airway in a burn-injured patient is a high priority and may be quite challenging. Direct burn injury to the face and upper airway may create a critical situation where intubation and mechanical ventilation are lifesaving. Edematous oral, pharyngeal, and supraglottic tissue may complicate airway control. Traditional landmarks may be distorted and the ability to preoxygenate such patients tends to be limited. One must be prepared to secure an airway with direct laryngoscopy and an endotracheal tube or establish an airway surgically with an emergent cricothyroidotomy.

Burns distant to the face may result in edema leading to the loss of the airway during the resuscitation phase of patient care. This is due to edema in the oral, hypopharyngeal, and supraglottic areas. Constant reevaluation of the nonintubated patient is prudent during the first 24 hours of a large TBSA burn. If airway problems are anticipated, early intubation may be indicated. Some patients may have no smoke inhalation, yet will require intubation to protect their airway during the resuscitation phase of the burn injury. The best action is to anticipate the need for an airway before the need becomes critical.

The decision to intubate the burn patient and obtain airway control is supported by the presence of severe respiratory distress, severe dyspnea, stridor, chest wall retractions, extensive facial or neck burns, or central nervous system depression (Glasgow Coma Scale <8). Relative indications for intubation include tachypnea, moderate dyspnea, minor facial burns, and the presence of a large greater than 40% TBSA burn where resuscitation fluid may result in late airway edema.

Adjuncts to direct laryngoscopy include intubation under direct visualization with the bronchoscope and use of the GlideScope. A laryngeal mask airway (LMA) may serve as a "rescue airway," but is not a definitive airway and will not protect the airway in the long term. As supraglottic and hypopharyngeal edema increase during a larger resuscitation, the patency of the airway will diminish. Yet, in an emergency situation, an LMA might provide an airway until a permanent or surgical airway is established. A surgical airway may be difficult to obtain if the patient already has massive cervical edema from the burn resuscitation. The strategy to overcome this problem is to make a large transverse incision and then retract the edematous soft tissue out of the surgical field. This will facilitate direct palpation of the crucial anatomic landmarks to complete the procedure successfully.

Increasing facial edema during the resuscitation phase will require the bedside nurse and respiratory therapist to constantly monitor and adjust the tension in the endotracheal ties. As facial edema increases the ties need to be loosened and often a soft guard for the corners of the mouth will be needed underneath the tracheostomy ties. Soft materials such as hydrocolloids can be used to provide padding underneath the endotracheal ties to prevent pressure necrosis of the underlying facial tissue. As the facial edema decreases the ties will need to be tightened. The use of two endotracheal ties during the facial edema phase can be utilized, with one tracheostomy tie over the ears and another under the ears as the massive facial edema is often asymmetrical. The time a burn patient spends on a ventilator is different from that for other medical or surgical patients. It is often governed by ongoing treatment of the burn wounds (large painful bandage changes, excision, grafting, and reconstruction) rather than the inhalation injury itself. In larger burns an elective tracheostomy may be considered due to the needs for multiple surgical procedures and for sedation and analgesia during wound care.

PULMONARY TOILET AND AIRWAY PATENCY

In the nonintubated burn patient, increasing burn size limits patient movement and ambulation. Sedation and analgesia for wound care often compromise normal pulmonary toilet and physiotherapy in these patients. In order to combat this problem, aggressive pulmonary toilet including frequent coughing, turning, elevation of head of bed, incentive spirometry, and chest physiotherapy should be utilized as indicated. Aggressive pulmonary physiotherapy to manage secretions in the intubated burn patient is essential to maintain airway patency and prevent pulmonary complications. Patients with inhalation injury have compromised pulmonary mechanics and diminished ciliary motion and secretion clearance. Atelectasis, consolidation, and distal airway obstruction are continuous problems in these patients. Complications such as acute oxygen desaturation, endotracheal tube plugging, postobstructive pneumonia, and ventilator-associated pneumonia may occur.

In the intubated patient with a large burn or inhalation injury, secretion control and pulmonary toilet can be greatly enhanced with fiberoptic bronchoscopy. The normal indications for fiberoptic bronchoscopy for other ICU patients should be broader in burn patients. The efficacy of blind, in-line endotracheal suctioning is often not sufficient for secretion clearance. Often, the suction catheter will be inserted into the right main-stem bronchus leaving the left main-stem bronchus, as well as distal airways, without adequate pulmonary toilet. The secretions tend to be very viscous, contributing to airway obstruction, atelectasis, inspissation, and pneumonia. Bronchoscopic pulmonary toilet offers a directed procedure for irrigation of soot and secretions, suctioning, and therapy to difficult distal airways. Ventilator prevention bundles, including elevation of the head of the bed to 30°, and oral care should be implemented.

Use of aerosolized nebulizer therapy may include β_2-agonists, mucolytic agents, and anticoagulants. β_2-Agonists have both bronchodilator and anti-inflammatory properties. They also decrease the release of inflammatory mediators from pulmonary mast cells decreasing microvascular permeability. Mucolytics include *N*-acetylcysteine or dornase alpha. Nebulized heparin, solely or in combination with *N*-acetylcysteine, has been used at some burn centers as a mediator of the procoagulant activity seen in combined burn and smoke inhalation.

It is important to realize that management of a mechanically ventilated burn patient entails some very important differences compared with typical patients in medical or surgical intensive care. Within the first 3 days, management of a patient with a large burn greater than 40% to 50% TBSA is very different from that of other patients due to the large volume of fluid required for resuscitation. For example, a 70-kg male with a 50% TBSA burn receiving a Parkland resuscitation of 4 mL/kg/percent TBSA will be given almost 20 L of fluid in the first 24 hours. The capillary leak phenomena seen with burn shock will result in an increase in both vascular and alveolar permeability, resulting in fluid leak into the interstitial pulmonary space as well as the alveoli. Oxygenation and ventilation may be compromised with decreased lung compliance, higher airway pressures, and worsening ventilation–perfusion ($\dot{V}/\dot{Q}$) mismatch and gas exchange. Managing these patients on the ventilator is a dynamic process.

PNEUMONIA IN A BURN PATIENT

Pneumonia in the intubated burn patient may be difficult to diagnose. The combination of burn and trauma results in additional pathophysiologic manifestations that make the diagnosis of pneumonia challenging. The usual signs and symptoms of pneumonia are frequently present without solid evidence of pulmonary infection. Patients with large burns often have elevated temperature, in part due to pyrogen and cytokines released from the burn tissue itself and not related to any infectious process. An elevated white blood cell count of 12,000 to 18,000 is common in patients with significant burn injuries. This leukocytosis may decrease slightly after complete excision of the burned tissue, but often remains elevated in the immediate perioperative period, in part due to stress and the various cytokines and pyogens released during the excision. Left shift in the differential may be due to physiologic stress from surgery or resuscitation. Pulmonary infiltrates on chest radiograph may represent actual infection, simple atelectasis or consolidation, fluid from resuscitation, and airway obstruction secondary to secretion plugging.

Quantitative cultures can assist in identifying and determining the concentrations of microorganisms to help determine whether or not this represents colonization or active pulmonary infection. One can also follow absolute colony counts over time to help with the diagnosis of pneumonia. Increasing quantitative culture counts in the presence of a rising white count, increased sputum, and fever may favor the initiation of antibiotic therapy. The total length of antibiotic coverage is a very difficult decision in burn patients, but, in general, pulmonary infection strategies prevail. Inhalation injury in the burn patient requires a unique perspective and approach as the underlying burn management, and not just the respiratory status, often dictates the pulmonary management strategy.

FURTHER READING

1. Bourdeaux C, Manara A. Burns and smoke inhalation. *Anaesth Intensive Care Med.* 2008;9:404–408.

   An excellent pathophysiology review of inhalation injury and management strategies.

2. Baruchin O, Yoffe B, Baruchin AM. Burns in inpatients by simultaneous use of cigarettes and oxygen therapy. *Burns.* 2004;30:836–838.

   Describes the problem of patients on chronic oxygen therapy causing facial burns while attempting to smoke a cigarette.

3. Cancio L. Airway management and smoke inhalation injury in the burn patient. *Clin Plast Surg.* 2009;36(4):555–567.

   One of the best reviews of care of the burn patient with inhalation injury.

4. Cyanokit. Columbia, MD: Meridian Medical Technologies. http://www.cyanokit.com/. Accessed January 11, 2013.

   This is a company website delineating the mechanism of action of hydroxocobalamin in cyanide poisoning.

5. Desai MH, Mlcak R, Richardson J, et al. Reduction in mortality in pediatric patients with inhalation injury with aerosolized heparin/acetylcystine therapy. *J Burn Care Rehabil.* 1998;19:210–212.

Describes the use of inhaled heparin and n-acetylcysteine in patients with inhalation injury to ameliorate the difficulty with secretions and cellular debris in the smaller airways.

6. Eckert MJ, Wade TE, Davis KA, et al. Ventilator-associated pneumonia after combined burn and trauma is caused by associated injuries and not the burn wound. *J Burn Care Res.* 2006;27(4):457–462.

This paper examined the relationship between pneumonia in burn patients with combined trauma and burns and found that the burn injury was not an independent factor developing pneumonia. While the major factor seemed to be the associated traumatic injuries, it is well known that the presence of a cutaneous burn of greater than 20% is a risk factor for pneumonia by itself.

7. Edelman DA, White MT, Tyburski JG, et al. Factors affecting prognosis of inhalation injury. *J Burn Care Res.* 2006;27:848–853.

One of the prime factors increasing patient ventilator days, ICU days, and mortality was an increasing cutaneous burn size in patient with inhalation injury. In patients with a greater than 50% TBSA burn, the incidence of inhalation injury was 63%. In patients without inhalation injury, the mortality rate was 3%, and in those with inhalation injury, it was 20%.

8. Edelman DA, Khan N, Kempf K, et al. Pneumonia after inhalation injury. *J Burn Care Res.* 2007;28:241–246.

This paper is a good paper examining the association of pneumonia in burn patients. The rate of pneumonia in patients with inhalation injury was 27%. Pneumonia developed twice as often in a burn patient with inhalation injury versus no inhalation injury. If a patient had a TBSA greater than 20%, he or she was more likely to develop pneumonia and had a higher mortality rate than those patients with less than 20% TBSA or no cutaneous burn.

9. Fidkowski CW, Fuzaylov G, Sheridan RL, et al. Inhalation burn injury in children. *Paediatr Anaesth.* 2009;19(suppl 1):147–154.

This is a good paper on inhalation injury and management strategies for the care of pediatric patients.

10. Latenser BA. Critical care of the burn patient: the first 48 hours. *Crit Care Med.* 2009; 37(10):2819–2826.

This is an overview of the initial management of the burn patient for the nonburn surgeon. It is a good primer for medical personnel taking care of a burn patient.

11. Mlcak RP, Suman OE, Herndon DN. Respiratory management of inhalation injury. *Burns.* 2007;33:2–13.

An excellent pathophysiology review of inhalation injury and management strategies.

12. Mosier MJ, Gamelli RL, Halerz MM, et al. Microbial contamination in burn patients undergoing urgent intubation as part of their early airway management. *J Burn Care Res.* 2008;29(2):304–310.

This paper describes the findings of early bronchoscopy and the microbiologic activity of the airway in patient with inhalation injury—17.6% of patients had no growth on bronchoalveolar lavage, 29.7% had normal flora, 3.5% had less than 100,000 cfu, and 16% had greater than 100,000 cfu.

13. Moisier MJ, Pham TN. American burn association practice guidelines for prevention, diagnosis, and treatment of ventilator-associated pneumonia in burn patients. *J Burn Care Res.* 2009;30:910–928.

This paper describes the common modalities to prevent ventilator-associated pneumonia in mechanically ventilated patients and how these may apply to burn patients (with and without inhalation injury). It is a good review of consensus pathways, including ventilator bundles, silver endotracheal tube, selective decontamination, glucose control, and other modalities.

14. Nugent N, Herndon DN. Diagnosis and treatment of inhalation injury. In: Herndon DN, ed. *Total Burn Care.* 3rd ed. Philadelphia, PA: Saunders Elsevier; 2007:262–271.

A general chapter concerning inhalation injury.

15. Palmieri T. Use of beta agonists in inhalation injury. *J Burn Care Res.* 2009;30:156–159.

Describes the utility of β-agonists as a treatment for acute lung injury and ARDS in burn patients.

16. Toon MH, Maybauer MO, Greenwood JE, et al. Management of acute smoke inhalation injury. *Crit Care Resusc.* 2010;12(1):53–65.

A very good overview of inhalation injury and pathophysiology.

17. Traber DL, Herndon DN, Enkhabaatar P, et al. The pathophysiology of inhalation injury. In: Herndon DN, ed. *Total Burn Care*. 3rd ed. Philadelphia, PA: Saunders Elsevier; 2007:248–261.

 A very good chapter on inhalation injury in a premier burn textbook.

18. Weaver LK, Hopkins RO, Chan KJ, et al. Hyperbaric oxygen for acute carbon monoxide poisoning. *N Engl J Med*. 2002;347(14):1057–1067.

 Reviews the pathophysiology of CO poisoning and addresses the studies on the incidence of developing neuropsychological symptoms post CO poisoning. The adjusted odds ratio of 0.45 was demonstrated in patients who underwent three hyperbaric oxygen dives in 24 hours compared to normobaric untreated patients.

19. Weaver LK, Valentine KJ, Hopkins RO. Carbon monoxide poisoning: risk factors for cognitive sequelae and the role of hyperbaric oxygen. *Am J Respir Crit Care Med*. 2007;176:491–497.

 Describes the utility of hyperbaric oxygen in patients with CO poisoning if symptomatic, CO levels greater than 25% and age greater than 35 years.

Hypersensitivity Pneumonitis
Dominic A. Munafo, Jr.

ETIOLOGY

Hypersensitivity pneumonitis (HP), also known as *extrinsic allergic alveolitis*, results from an exaggerated immunologic response to various inhaled biologic and chemical antigens. Most cases of HP occur through occupational, environmental, or avocational exposures. Examples of HP include the classic farmer's lung (thermophilic actinomycetes in moldy hay), pigeon breeder's lung (serum proteins in pigeon droppings), bagassosis (bagasse in sugarcane), maple bark disease (fungi in moldy bark), hot-tub lung (mycobacteria), and humidifier lung (amoebae in humidifier water). Additional antigens include a wide range of animal and insect proteins, molds from wind instruments, and chemicals such as isocyanates and anhydrides. New inciting antigens are reported regularly in the literature. Inhaled antigens are typically 1 to 5 μm in diameter; therefore, the site of lung injury is the distal airway and alveolus. An antigen's ability to trigger an immune response depends on its solubility, resistance to digestion by macrophages, and properties as an immunologic adjuvant. Prevalence rates vary widely (0.5%–30%) in an exposed population and appear to depend on intensity and duration of exposure as well as antigen type and host susceptibility. In studies conducted on exposed farmers, the estimated prevalence was 0.5% to 3%. HP is more prevalent among pigeon breeders than among farmers, perhaps in part because of the more chronic nature of the exposure in pigeon breeding.

PRESENTATION

Although HP classically has been categorized as acute, subacute, or chronic in presentation, these distinctions were not substantiated by a cluster analysis of patients performed by the HP Study Group. They found that most patients fit into one of two clusters and suggested that patients be considered as having either active or residual disease based on clinical evaluation, pulmonary function tests and high-resolution computed tomography (HRCT). The study group further concluded that the assumption that patients move temporally from acute to subacute and finally chronic disease in sequence had not been clearly established. Therefore, the group recommended that classifications of acute, subacute, and chronic not be used. This newly suggested classification will require prospective validation.

Active disease occurs after a previous sensitizing exposure to a particular antigen. Approximately 4 to 8 hours following reexposure, the individual experiences the abrupt onset of a flu-like syndrome. Symptoms typically include nonproductive cough, fever, chills, dyspnea, myalgias, and malaise. The most prominent physical findings are tachypnea, tachycardia, and bibasilar inspiratory crackles. Wheezing is uncommon. Symptoms typically peak within 24 hours and remit spontaneously within 72 hours. Symptoms recur with subsequent exposures, and the severity depends on the intensity and duration of exposure as well as a particular individual's sensitivity. Chronic exposure to lower levels of antigen may be accompanied by mild or absent symptoms and disease progression can be insidious. Continued exposure is associated with increasing dyspnea, cough, anorexia, and weight loss.

Residual disease refers to the end-stage findings of emphysematous change or fibrosis present long after the acute inflammatory reaction has dissipated. Inspiratory crackles and resting hypoxemia would be characteristic.

DIAGNOSIS

The diagnosis of HP is suggested by a history that relates symptoms to exposure, but may be particularly difficult in those patients with chronic low-level exposure. Most of the signs and symptoms of disease are nonspecific. Numerous recommendations have been made as to the appropriate diagnostic criteria; however, most have not been validated. The HP Study Group published a logistic regression model that identified six significant predictors of HP: (1) exposure to a known offending antigen, (2) precipitating antibodies to the offending antigen, (3) recurrent symptoms, (4) inspiratory crackles on examination, (5) symptoms within 4 to 8 hours of exposure, and (6) weight loss. Depending on a patient's particular constellation of findings, the probability of HP can be predicted by the model.

Laboratory findings are largely nonspecific. IgG serum precipitating antibodies to the offending antigen are present in most patients, but only a fraction actually develop disease. IgA and IgM antibodies may also be seen. Immunoglobulin levels are usually elevated in both serum and bronchoalveolar lavage fluid (BALF); however, IgE levels remain normal. The presence of antibodies is not diagnostic of disease but only indicates previous significant exposure.

Leukocytosis with a left shift typically accompanies acute episodes. Eosinophilia is uncommon and should suggest the possibility of another diagnosis. BALF shows a dramatic increase in the number of T lymphocytes recovered. Although the percentage of alveolar macrophages recovered is markedly reduced, the absolute number of macrophages is elevated. BALF findings are not diagnostic of HP but rather serve to support the diagnosis and help to rule out other processes. A normal BALF lymphocyte count would only be found in residual disease.

Histologically, a neutrophilic alveolitis in the first 24 hours gives way to an intense peribronchial inflammatory infiltrate of lymphocytes, plasma cells, macrophages, and giant cells. Noncaseating granulomas are often seen in the interstitium. In residual disease, both granulomas and interstitial fibrosis are seen. The fibrotic patterns seen include elements suggestive of usual interstitial pneumonia and nonspecific interstitial pneumonia. Bronchiolitis obliterans is found frequently (25%–50%) with or without organizing pneumonia (15%–25%). Vasculitis is not present.

Chest radiographic findings of HP are highly variable. Initially, radiographs may be normal (20%–30%) or show bilateral, ill-defined alveolar and interstitial nodular infiltrates. The distribution can be patchy or diffuse, with some predilection for the lower lobes. Hilar adenopathy and pleural effusions are rare. In residual disease, the chest radiograph shows a reticulonodular pattern with interstitial fibrosis, honeycombing, and loss of lung volume. The fibrotic changes are often more prominent in the upper lobes and periphery of the lung. HRCT is more sensitive than chest radiography in demonstrating the characteristic centrilobular nodules and emphysematous changes; however, its sensitivity and specificity appear to vary, depending on disease severity and chronicity.

Pulmonary function tests during an acute episode usually show a restrictive defect. Mild to moderate hypoxemia, hypocapnia, and a decrease in the diffusing capacity of the lung for carbon monoxide (D$_{LCO}$) are often present. As many as 60% of patients may demonstrate a positive methacholine challenge. Patients who experience recurring attacks most commonly develop airway obstruction and a persistent decrement in D$_{LCO}$. Progressive restriction secondary to interstitial fibrosis may also be seen. Early cessation of exposure leads to gradual resolution of the pulmonary function abnormalities over days to weeks. In advanced disease, progressive pulmonary insufficiency, chronic hypoxemia, and cor pulmonale may develop. Inhalation challenge, either in a laboratory setting or by returning the patient to the site of exposure, may yield supportive information; however, standardized protocols for inhalation challenge have not been developed. In the absence of an identifiable cause and in more chronic presentations, lung biopsy may be necessary to define the pathology and rule out other possibilities. Skin tests are not helpful. Differential diagnosis in the acute setting includes atypical and viral pneumonia, collagen vascular disease, lymphocytic interstitial pneumonia, organic dust toxic syndrome, and other acute inhalational injuries. In patients who wheeze, consider occupational asthma, allergic bronchopulmonary aspergillosis, and byssinosis. Miliary tuberculosis, sarcoidosis, fungal infection, eosinophilic granuloma, and idiopathic pulmonary fibrosis can mimic residual HP. As many as 10% of referrals to some tertiary centers for idiopathic pulmonary fibrosis demonstrate pathology suggestive of HP. Therefore, a detailed exposure history in a patient with interstitial lung disease is essential.

PATHOPHYSIOLOGY

The immunologic mechanisms responsible for HP are complex and remain incompletely understood. Although both humoral and cellular immunity are involved, recent investigations indicate that cell-mediated immunity is likely the more consequential. The acute alveolitis seen hours after antigen exposure is thought secondary to precipitation of immune complexes in the alveoli and interstitium. This type III immune response activates complement, resulting in an increase in vascular permeability and recruitment of additional inflammatory cells. Activated macrophages secrete a variety of proinflammatory cytokines, including tumor necrosis factor-α (TNF-α;), macrophage inflammatory protein-1α (MIP-1α), interleukin-1β (IL-1β), IL-8, and IL-12. MIP-1α is chemotactic for $CD8^+$ T cells. A murine model of HP has shown that interferon-γ (IFN-γ) is essential in the formation of granulomatous inflammation. IL-10 inhibits expression of IFN-γ and appears to mitigate the inflammatory response to antigen. Conversely, IL-12 enhances IFN-γ production, thus promoting granulomatous inflammation. Additional factors that may enhance the lymphocytic inflammation include increased expression of the adhesion molecule L-selectin by lymphocytes in BALF and the observation that HP lymphocytes demonstrate decreased apoptosis. Bronchus-associated lymphoid tissue can also serve as a site of induction and amplification of the local immune response. These data, coupled with studies showing adoptive transfer of HP using TH1-type cells, have been taken to suggest that differences in regulation of this type IV immune response may help explain the varying clinical presentations of disease. However, recent data suggest that the frequently seen elevation of $CD8^+$ T cells may reflect more active disease, and an expansion of the $CD4^+$ subset and movement toward a TH2 phenotype in the more chronic phases of disease. Lastly, there is evidence that the apoptotic pathways of epithelial cells may be activated and that epithelial apoptosis may be an important profibrotic event in the development of residual HP. Overall, no single immune mechanism can fully explain the constellation of findings in HP. Multiple mechanisms appear to be necessary.

Interestingly, common respiratory viruses have been found in the lower airways of patients with HP with increased frequency. A murine model suggests that a preceding viral infection can augment the inflammatory response in HP. Approximately 80% to 95% of HP patients are nonsmokers. Smoking may be immunosuppressive and therefore confer some degree of protection. Nicotine has been found to reduce IL-1 and TNF-α release from alveolar macrophages in a murine model. In addition, smokers have a lower incidence of antibody production. A significant active smoking history speaks against a diagnosis of HP.

TREATMENT

The mainstay of therapy is avoiding exposure to the offending antigen. A less-desirable alternative is the use of a mask or other filtration technique to substantially reduce or prevent exposure. The symptoms of active and progressive disease can be indolent. Thus, if continued exposure is unavoidable, close follow-up with pulmonary function tests and radiographic studies is essential to assess disease activity. Oral corticosteroids remain the cornerstone of therapy. The use of corticosteroids in the acute setting often speeds recovery and decreases symptoms. In addition, some patients treated with corticosteroids develop less radiographic evidence of fibrosis. To date, however, no clear evidence indicates that corticosteroids have a beneficial effect on lung function. Patients should be advised to avoid antigen exposure to the greatest extent possible.

PROGNOSIS

The prognosis of HP is quite variable. Some patients with farmer's lung may tolerate continued exposure without persistent symptoms or disease progression. However, other patients with pigeon breeder's lung have developed progressive disease despite complete antigen avoidance. Chronic low-level exposures appear to confer a worse prognosis than short-term intermittent exposures. The presence of fibrosis on lung biopsy has been associated with reduced survival.

FURTHER READING

1. Hodnett PA, Naidich DP. Fibrosing interstitial lung disease: a practical HRCT based approach to diagnosis and management and review of the literature. *Am J Respir Crit Care Med.* 2013;188(2):141–149.

   Describes how to best use HRCT in the diagnosis and management of chronic interstitial lung diseases such as chronic HP.

2. Lota HK, Keir GJ, Hansell DM, et al. Novel use of rituximab in hypersensitivity pneumonitis refractory to conventional treatment. *Thorax.* 2013;68(8):780–781.

   Rituximab is a chimeric anti-CD20 monoclonal antibody. The CD20 protein is expressed on mature B cells. A dramatic reduction in the number of CD20 B cells might alter B-cell-mediated antigen presentation and subsequently reduce T cell activation and antibody production.

3. Lacasse Y, Girard M, Cormier Y. Recent advances in hypersensitivity pneumonitis. *Chest.* 2012;142(1):208–217.

   An excellent review of HP presentations, pathophysiology, treatment, and prognosis. Addresses the differing definitions and classifications of HP.

4. Jinta T, Miyazaki Y, Kishi M, et al. The pathogenesis of chronic hypersensitivity pneumonitis in common with idiopathic pulmonary fibrosis: expression of apoptotic markers. *Am J Clin Pathol.* 2010;134:613.

   Demonstrates that apoptotic epithelial cells are seen in chronic HP and postulates that they play a role in the chronic fibrotic process.

5. Lacasse Y, Selman M, Costabel U, et al. Classification of hypersensitivity pneumonitis: a hypothesis. *Int Arch Allergy Immunol.* 2009;149:161.

   Cluster analysis data from the HP Study Group suggesting that HP is best classified into active and residual disease rather than the classical acute, subacute, and chronic.

6. Barrera L, Mendoza F, Zuniga J, et al. Functional diversity of T-cell subpopulations in subacute and chronic hypersensitivity pneumonitis. *Am J Respir Crit Care Med.* 2008;177:44.

   Suggests that CD8$^+$ T cells are more prominent during acute disease and CD4$^+$ T cells accompany chronic disease with a shift toward a TH2 phenotype.

7. Blanchet MR, Israel-Assayag E, Cormier Y. Inhibitory effect of nicotine on experimental hypersensitivity pneumonitis in vivo and in vitro. *Am J Respir Crit Care Med.* 2004;169:903.

   A murine model demonstrating the inhibitory effect of nicotine on the immune response.

8. Vourlekis JS, Schwarz MI, Cherniack RM, et al. The effect of pulmonary fibrosis on survival in patients with hypersensitivity pneumonitis. *Am J Med.* 2004;116:662.

   A study of 72 HP patients with fibrosis on lung biopsy who exhibited increased mortality.

9. Lacasse Y, Selman M, Costabel U, et al. Clinical diagnosis of hypersensitivity pneumonitis. *Am J Respir Crit Care Med.* 2003;168:952.

   Details the HP Study Group's prediction rule and the six significant predictors of HP.

10. Laflamme C, Israel-Assayag E, Cormier Y. Apoptosis of bronchoalveolar lavage lymphocytes in hypersensitivity pneumonitis. *Eur Respir J.* 2003;21:225.

    Pulmonary lymphocytes from patients with HP showed decreased apoptosis compared to normal controls. This promotes accumulation of lymphocytes in the lung.

11. Navarro C, Mendoza F, Barrera L, et al. Up-regulation of L-selectin and E-selectin in hypersensitivity pneumonitis. *Chest.* 2002;121:354.

    L-selectin is upregulated in HP and may enhance lymphocytic inflammation.

12. Suda T, Chida K, Hayakawa H, et al. Development of bronchus-associated lymphoid tissue in chronic hypersensitivity pneumonitis. *Chest.* 1999;115:357.

    Reports the presence of bronchus-associated lymphoid tissue in three of five patients with chronic HP. The authors postulate that this tissue plays an important role in the mucosal immune response.

13. Dakhama A, Hegele RG, Laflamme G, et al. Common respiratory viruses in lower airways of patients with acute hypersensitivity pneumonitis. *Am J Respir Crit Care Med.* 1999;159:1316.

    An interesting report using polymerase chain reaction to document the presence of influenza A in the BALF of 6 of 13 patients with HP; two of six controls also had evidence of virus. The ultimate significance of this finding has yet to be determined.

14. Erkinjuntti-Pekkanen R, Rytkonen H, Kokkarinen JI, et al. Long-term risk of emphysema in patients with farmer's lung and matched control farmers. *Am J Respir Crit Care Med.* 1998;158:662.

    A 14-year follow-up study of patients with HP. The study documents an increased risk of developing emphysema using pulmonary function tests and HRCT. Interestingly, no increase in fibrosis was seen in patients with HP compared with matched controls.

15. Erkinjuntti-Pekkanen R, Kokkarinen JI, Tukiainen HO, et al. Long-term outcome of pulmonary function in farmer's lung: a 14-year follow-up with matched controls. *Eur Respir J.* 1997;10:2046.

    A persistent decrement in D$_{LCO}$ was the most important sequela of farmer's lung disease. Chronic farmer's lung disease can lead to an obstructive pulmonary defect.

16. Schuyler M, Gott K, Cherne A, et al. Th1 CD4$^+$ cells adoptively transfer experimental hypersensitivity pneumonitis. *Cell Immunol.* 1997;177:169.

    Reviews the cytokine profile of T$_H$1 and T$_H$2 subsets. Documents that CD4$^+$ cells with a T$_H$1 profile can adoptively transfer experimental HP in a murine model.

17. Gudmundsson G, Hunninghake GW. Interferon-γ is necessary for the expression of hypersensitivity pneumonitis. *J Clin Invest.* 1997;99:2386.

    Interferon-deficient (knockout) mice did not develop granulomatous inflammation in response to inhaled antigen.

18. Hansell DM, Wells AU, Padley SP, et al. Hypersensitivity pneumonitis: correlation of individual CT patterns with functional abnormalities. *Radiology.* 1996;199:123.

    The analysis of thin-section CT in 22 patients demonstrated that the most commonly found pattern was decreased attenuation and mosaic perfusion. Ground-glass opacification and nodules were also commonly seen. The radiographic appearance was thought suggestive of bronchiolitis.

19. Yoshizawa Y, Miyake S, Sumi Y, et al. A follow-up study of pulmonary function tests, bronchoalveolar lavage cells, and humoral and cellular immunity in bird fancier's lung. *J Allergy Clin Immunol.* 1995;96:122.

    This 5-year follow-up study in five patients documents the variability of the course of bird fancier's lung. The patients demonstrated persistence of sensitized lymphocytes and continued antibody production. Despite antigen avoidance, these patients should be followed closely for evidence of disease progression.

20. Lynch DA, Rose CS, Way D, et al. Hypersensitivity pneumonitis: sensitivity of high-resolution CT in a population-based study. *AJR Am J Roentgenol.* 1992;159:469.

    A population-based study of 31 symptomatic patients, 11 of whom met diagnostic criteria for HP. HRCT scanning was more sensitive than chest radiography. Of the 11 patients, 5 had abnormal CT scans, but only 1 had an abnormal chest radiograph.

21. Kokkarinen JI, Tukiainen HO, Terho EO. Effect of corticosteroid treatment on the recovery of pulmonary function in farmer's lung. *Am Rev Respir Dis.* 1992;145:3.

    A double-blind, randomized, placebo-controlled trial in 36 patients with acute farmer's lung, using 8 weeks of systemic corticosteroids. At 1 month, the corticosteroid group showed a significantly higher D$_{LCO}$. At 3 months, 6 months, 1 year, and 5 years, no significant differences were seen in any of the measures of pulmonary function.

22. Monkare S. Influence of corticosteroid treatment on the course of farmer's lung. *Eur J Respir Dis.* 1983;64:283.

    A prospective study of no steroids (in less severe cases) versus 4 and 12 weeks of therapy in 93 Finnish farmers. Treatment had no significant effect on the course of lung function; however, steroids improved acute symptoms and decreased fibrotic changes on chest radiographs.

88 Drowning and Diving Accidents

Ian R. Grover

Accidental drowning occurs in all age groups, but is most common in children aged 1 to 4 years. Despite a recent decline in the number of deaths, drowning remains the second leading cause of injury-related death for children aged 1 to 14 years, and the sixth leading cause of accidental death for all age groups. In adults, alcohol is the most important single factor contributing to drowning incidents. US statistics from 2007 show there were 3,443 unintentional drowning-related deaths, and approximately 70,000 episodes of drowning where the victim survived. A recent decline in the number of fatalities may reflect better prevention because of enhanced private pool safety.

Previous reports and studies used conflicting nomenclature to refer to drowning victims. Cases were divided into freshwater and saltwater drowning, and they were also divided into drowning (victims died within 24 hours of the incident) and near-drowning (survived for at least 24 hours after the incident). In 2003, the American Heart Association published the "Recommended Guidelines for Uniform Reporting of Data From Drowning" that removes the different classifications and simplifies the reporting of drowning cases. Drowning is now defined as "a process resulting in primary respiratory impairment from submersion/immersion in a liquid medium." Implicit in this definition is that a liquid/air interface is present at the entrance of the victim's airway, preventing the victim from breathing air. The victim may live or die after this process, but whatever the outcome, he or she has been involved in a "drowning incident."

PATHOPHYSIOLOGY

Historically, the pathophysiology of drowning was attributed to an electrolyte disturbance induced by aspiration of fluid. However, current data suggest aspiration-related hypoxemia as the major pathophysiologic abnormality. The earlier notion that death could result from drowning without aspiration was based on misinterpretation of seminal documents. In 10% to 15% of drowning cases, hypoxemia appeared to be secondary to simple asphyxia. In these cases, termed *dry drowning,* with little or no aspiration, the hypothesis was that reflex laryngospasm prevented aspiration. However, no experimental evidence supports this hypothesis. Most experts believe that dry drowning does not occur and that other causes for in-water fatalities should be sought, such as sudden cardiac death. The sine qua non of drowning is the aspiration of fluid.

The hypoxemia observed in drowning cases is related to aspiration. The exact volume of fluid aspirated by victims remains unclear but animal experiments that seem to duplicate human injury require fluid in the range of 1 to 10 mL/kg. The mechanism of hypoxemia depends on the nature of the fluid aspirated. In seawater aspiration, osmotic and irritative effects from sand, diatoms, algae, and other particles provoke an exudative response. This exudate fills alveoli and results in ventilation/perfusion ($\dot{V}/\dot{Q}$) mismatch and hypoxemia. In freshwater aspiration, pulmonary surfactants are also lost from the lung, leading to focal collapse, ($\dot{V}/\dot{Q}$) mismatch, and hypoxemia. When water is instilled into the trachea of experimental animals, pathologic studies reveal damage to alveolar and endothelial cells, as well as disruption of the capillary basement membrane.

CLINICAL MANIFESTATIONS

The clinical manifestations of drowning vary with the duration and severity of the hypoxemia. The neurologic presentation reflects the degree of cerebral anoxia. Pulmonary injury ranges from mild, manifesting as cough and mild shortness of breath, to severe, presenting with extreme dyspnea, pulmonary edema, and acute respiratory distress syndrome.

Laboratory studies generally reveal hypoxemia, metabolic acidosis, and, perhaps, superimposed respiratory acidosis. Minor changes in electrolytes are seen frequently; however, clinically significant alterations in serum sodium or potassium are distinctly unusual in drowning in either freshwater or seawater. Chest radiographs may display a spectrum of abnormalities, ranging from patchy infiltrates to dense pulmonary edema. Rarely, massive particulate aspiration can also occur. It has been hypothesized that the pulmonary edema occasionally seen in drowning victims is caused by negative pressure inspiration (attempting to breathe against a closed glottis) or to neurogenic factors.

MANAGEMENT

The management of drowning patients is mainly supportive. Arterial blood gases should be monitored frequently and mechanical ventilatory support should be instituted if acute respiratory failure and refractory hypoxemia develop. Patients with acute respiratory failure may require high ventilator pressures to provide adequate oxygenation and ventilation, reflecting the marked reduction in pulmonary compliance. The application of positive end–expiratory pressure (PEEP) during mechanical ventilation reduces morbidity and mortality. In most cases, ventilatory support is necessary for only a short time. Less invasive methods of ventilatory support such as nasal continuous positive airway pressure and bi-level positive airway pressure may reduce the need for intubation and the risks associated with mechanical ventilation. The routine administration of hypertonic or hypotonic intravenous fluids is not warranted. The use of antibiotics in the drowning victim is usually restricted to those who develop fever, new pulmonary infiltrates, or purulent secretions. Prophylactic antibiotics do not improve mortality or decrease morbidity. Most pulmonary infections in drowning victims are secondary to hospital-acquired organisms; prophylactic antibiotics may only select more resistant organisms. Rarely, the victim may aspirate water that is heavily contaminated with a known organism. Prophylactic antibiotics may be appropriate in this situation.

Routine bronchoscopy to search for particulate matter causing airway obstruction is generally unnecessary. Adrenocortical steroids are not indicated to treat the lung injury associated with near drowning. Experimental evidence strongly suggests that steroids do not improve the long-term outcome or short-term morbidity. One uncontrolled report (four cases), however, suggests high-dose steroids may be beneficial in drowning victims who present with pulmonary edema. The use of surfactants to treat drowning victims has been reported recently. It is unclear whether such therapy alters the outcome. In an experimental model, surfactant therapy did not offer any benefit over traditional supportive approach.

COMPLICATIONS

Pneumothorax, lung abscess, and empyema occasionally complicate the course in drowning patients if severe respiratory failure occurs. Hypothermia at the time of the immersion incident can also complicate the picture. Although renal failure and disseminated intravascular coagulation have been reported, they are probably sequelae of prolonged acidosis, hypoxemia, and hypotension, rather than specific complications of near drowning.

PROGNOSIS

The victim's prognosis primarily depends on the extent and duration of the hypoxemic episode. Age and prior illnesses can be modifying factors. Epidemiologic data do not support the hypothesis that cold-water immersion improves the prognosis of the drowning victim. However, in rare, well-documented cases, victims who fully recover after prolonged submersion in cold water have been reported. Many empiric studies have attempted to better define prognostic factors for the drowning victim. Unfortunately, no factors seem to be completely reliable. In general, patients who present with a normal chest radiograph or normal mental status are likely to survive without sequelae.

Most large studies indicate that 5% to 10% of all victims suffer varying degrees of permanent neurologic dysfunction, although some suggest a higher percentage with long-term neurologic sequelae. Not surprisingly, those who sustain a cardiorespiratory arrest persisting to the time of presentation in an emergency room have a poor chance of survival and a high incidence of neurologic sequelae. However, children who sustain a "cardiorespiratory arrest" that responds to first aid measures at the scene of the accident do not necessarily have a poor prognosis. In the late 1970s after a small experience of drowning victims with a high percentage of long-term neurologic sequelae, it was suggested that the incidence of neurologic dysfunction following near-drowning episodes could be lowered by aggressive attempts at cerebral salvage. This *HYPER therapy* included barbiturate coma, controlled hyperventilation, diuretics, paralysis, intentional hypothermia, and adrenocortical steroids. The rationale for this therapy was to lower intracranial pressure (ICP), reduce cerebral edema, and lower cerebral oxygen demand in order to prevent further (secondary) neurologic damage. This mode of therapy presumes that further damage occurs after the initial anoxic insult and that further damage can be prevented by these measures.

Unfortunately, after more than two decades of experience, it is not clear that morbidity and mortality have changed appreciably with this mode of therapy. The largest study, performed by the group that originally advocated this therapy, reported a 7% incidence of neurologic morbidity. This was not appreciably different from multiple studies performed before the advent of this therapy. Additionally, although very high ICP is associated with poor outcome, other studies suggest that normal ICP does not ensure neurologic recovery and that HYPER therapy does not necessarily prevent elevation of ICP. Indeed, it appears that elevation of ICP is the result, not the cause, of brain injury. Certainly, most authorities agree that if this therapy is indicated at all, it should be reserved for the most severely affected patients in whom ICP is being monitored, and then only in an intensive care unit setting that is staffed, equipped, and experienced with this therapy. Even in such a setting, the aspects of this therapy that are associated with significant morbidity should be reserved for victims whose ICP cannot be controlled by other more conventional means (e.g., head elevation, osmotic diuretics).

The decision to admit the drowning victim to the hospital is somewhat controversial. Any victim with significant respiratory symptoms, an abnormal chest radiograph, or abnormal arterial oxygenation (signs or symptoms suggesting aspiration) should be admitted to the hospital, because pulmonary damage may not reach its peak for several hours after the accident. It is less clear whether patients who have suffered solely a loss of consciousness and present with normal neurologic function and no cardiopulmonary signs or symptoms require hospital admission.

SPECIAL CIRCUMSTANCES
Scuba Diving

In scuba diving accidents, the most common cause of death reportedly is drowning. However, problems exist with data collection. Barotraumatic systemic gas embolism may, in fact, be a more common cause of death. The physiologic mechanism is related to Boyle's law, which states that in a closed system the product of pressure and volume remains constant at a given temperature ($P_1V_1 = P_2V_2$). If a submerged diver fills his or her lungs from a compressed gas source and then rises in the water column, that gas must expand because of the reduction in barometric pressure. If the egress of gas is blocked (i.e., a closed glottis), intrapulmonary blood vessels can rupture, allowing gas to enter the pulmonary venous circulation resulting in systemic embolism. The most common symptoms are attributable to embolization of air in the cerebral vessels. Sudden unconsciousness with subsequent aspiration can then occur. The expanding gas can also dissect through the interstitium of the lung to the hila, producing pneumomediastinum and subcutaneous emphysema at the base of the neck. Rarely, pneumothorax may occur. Treatment of pulmonary barotrauma is supportive unless air embolism develops. In that case, recompression is indicated. A variety of hematologic and biochemical abnormalities have also been reported from arterial gas embolism. Pulmonary barotrauma with cerebral air embolism is seen only in divers breathing from a compressed gas source. Swimmers who descend below the surface following inspiration to total lung capacity initially compress the gas in their chest. On surfacing, that gas expands, but it does not expand to a volume greater than the initial total lung capacity, and therefore, barotrauma does not occur.

Decompression sickness also affects divers but rarely causes pulmonary problems. Shortness of breath occurs in fewer than 1% of cases. Most patients present with limb pain or spinal cord lesions. These patients also require recompression therapy. The pathophysiology of decompression sickness is related to absorption of an inert gas (nitrogen) with subsequent reduction in barometric pressure sufficient to generate a gas phase within the tissues. The precise pathophysiologic mechanisms of the different forms and presentations of decompression sickness are still unclear. Prophylaxis for deep venous thrombosis in paralyzed divers may be problematic because hemorrhage into the spinal cord secondary to bubble damage is thought to be a mechanism involved in the generation of paralytic symptoms. As a result, these patients must be monitored extremely carefully if heparin prophylaxis is not administered.

Although not generally reported in diving fatality statistics, there is strong evidence that intentional hyperventilation prior to breath-hold diving is associated with drowning episodes. Hyperventilation reduces the partial pressure of arterial carbon dioxide ($PaCO_2$) so that the breath-hold break point is prolonged sufficiently for hypoxemia to occur before the individual is forced to breathe. Hypoxemia, in turn, may cause the individual to lose consciousness, resulting in a drowning incident.

Submersion-Induced Pulmonary Edema

Another interesting phenomenon is swimming- or submersion-induced pulmonary edema (SIPE) that usually occurs with strenuous swimming activities, especially in cold water. It appears to have many features similar to exertional pulmonary edema. The pathophysiologic mechanism resulting in SIPE is not currently known. It is known, however, that it is not caused by aspiration or negative pressure inspiration against a closed glottis. It has been postulated that the effects of immersion in water, especially cold water, lead to an increase in central vascular volume, redistribution of pulmonary blood flow, and change in lung volumes. When these changes occur with an increased cardiac output from heavy exertion, it may expose the pulmonary capillary bed to high pressures. This high pressure may cause extravasation of fluid by hydrostatic forces and stress failure of pulmonary capillaries, resulting in pulmonary edema and frank hemorrhage.

These patients then present with dyspnea, cough, hypoxemia, tachypnea, and hemoptysis. Chest radiographs show an infiltrate or frank pulmonary edema. These patients occasionally require admission for observation and supportive treatment. Recovery is usually quite rapid, and diuretics are generally not required.

FURTHER READING

1. Anker AL, Santora T, Spivey W. Artificial surfactant administration in an animal model of near drowning. *Acad Emerg Med.* 1995;2:204.

   No benefit is seen of surfactant administration over standard ventilation in this animal model of near drowning.

2. Bates ML, Farrell ET, Eldridge MW. The curious question of exercise-induced pulmonary edema. *Pulm Med.* 2011;2011:1–7.

   An excellent review article looking at exercise-induced pulmonary edema and SIPE.

3. Bell TS, Ellenberg L, McComb JG. Neuropsychological outcome after severe pediatric near drowning. *Neurosurgery.* 1985;17:604.

   Children who recover from even severe near-drowning episodes generally show average cognitive functioning and only mild gross motor and coordination deficits.

4. Brubank AO, Neuman TS. *Bennett and Elliott's Physiology and Medicine of Diving.* 5th ed. Philadelphia, PA: Elsevier; 2003.

   A comprehensive, well-written text regarding the physiology of diving and diving medicine.

5. Bohn DJ, Biggar WD, Smith CR, et al. Influence of hypothermia, barbiturate therapy, and intracranial monitoring on morbidity and mortality after near drowning. *Crit Care Med.* 1986;14:529.

   Essentially, a retraction of their earlier work advocating HYPER therapy.

6. Bove AA, Davis JC. *Diving Medicine.* 4th ed. Philadelphia, PA: WB Saunders; 2004.

   An excellent, well-written introductory text to all aspects of diving medicine.

7. Calderwood H, Modell J, Ruiz B. Ineffectiveness of steroid therapy for treatment of fresh water and near drowning. *Anesthesiology.* 1975;43:642.

   Strong evidence that steroids are not routinely useful in cases of near drowning.

8. Conn AW, Edmonds J, Barker G. Cerebral resuscitation in near drowning. *Pediatr Clin North Am.* 1979;26:691.

   An uncontrolled study suggesting decreased long-term morbidity in patients aggressively treated for anoxic encephalopathy.

9. DeNicola LK, Falk JL, Swanson ME, et al. Submersion injuries in children and adults. *Crit Care Clin.* 1997;13:477.

   A comprehensive review of near drowning (125 references).

10. Dubowitz DJ, Blumi S, Arcinue E, et al. MR of hypoxic encephalopathy in children after near drowning: correlation with quantitative proton MR spectroscopy and clinical outcome. *Am J Neuroradiol.* 1998;19:1617.

    An attempt to use magnetic resonance imaging as an aid to prognosis in nearly drowned children.

11. Ender PT, Dolan MJ. Pneumonia associated with near drowning. *Clin Infect Dis.* 1997;25:896.

    A review of the bacteriology of pneumonias associated with near-drowning episodes (102 references).

12. Golden F, Tipton MJ, Scott RC. Immersion, near drowning and drowning. *Br J Anaesth.* 1997;79:214.

    A comprehensive review of the pathophysiology and treatment of near drowning and drowning, especially in cold water.

13. Gonzalez-Rothi RJ. Near drowning: consensus and controversies in pulmonary and cerebral resuscitation. *Heart Lung.* 1987;16:474.

    A comprehensive review of the problem of cerebral resuscitation in the near-drowning victim (62 references).

14. Grausz H, Amend WJ, Early LE. Acute renal failure in seawater near drowning. *JAMA.* 1971;217:207.

    Concludes that acute renal failure represents acute tubular necrosis secondary to the combination of hypoxemia and hypotension.

15. Huckabee HCG, Craig PL, Williams JM. Near drowning in frigid water: a case study of a 31-year-old woman. *J Int Neuropsychol Soc.* 1996;2:256.

    A case study describing neurologically intact survival after 30 minutes of submersion in cold water.

16. Idris AH, Berg RA, Bierens J, et al. Recommended guidelines for uniform reporting of data from drowning: the "Utstein style." *Circulation.* 2003;108:2565–2574.

    Guidelines developed to reduce confusion and discrepancies involved in the reporting and researching of drowning cases.

17. Lavelle JM, Show KN. Near drowning: is emergency department cardiopulmonary resuscitation or intensive care unit cerebral resuscitation indicated? *Crit Care Med.* 1993;21:368.

    A discussion of 54 pediatric cases showing no apparent benefit of cerebral resuscitation, but approximately 5% of victims arriving at emergency department requiring cardiopulmonary resuscitation (CPR) and cardiotonic drugs went on to full recovery.

18. Lund KL, Mahon RT, Tanen DA, et al. Swimming-induced pulmonary edema. *Ann Emerg Med.* 2003;41:251.

    A discussion of three cases of SIPE.

19. Martin CM, Barrett O. Drowning and near drowning: a review of 10 years' experience in a large army hospital. *Mil Med.* 1971;136:439.

    No clinically significant hemoconcentration or hemodilution was noted; no difference in clinical or radiographic recovery occurred in those given antibiotics or steroids.

20. Modell JH, Bellefleur M, Davis JH. Drowning without aspiration: is this an appropriate diagnosis? *J Forensic Sci.* 1999;44:1119.

    An excellent review article looking at animal drowning studies to determine if the entity of "dry drowning" is a possibility.

21. Modell JH. Drowning. *N Engl J Med.* 1993;328:253.

    A classic review article authored by the researcher who defined much of our understanding of the pathophysiology of drowning (53 references).

22. Modell J, Davis J. Electrolyte changes in human drowning victims. *Anesthesiology.* 1969; 30:414.

    One of several classic articles refuting the importance of electrolyte changes in drowning victims.

23. Modell J, Graves S, Ketover A. Clinical course of 91 consecutive near drowning victims. *Chest.* 1976;70:231.

    A large series, now mostly of historical interest.

24. Modell J, Calderwood HW, Ruiz BC, et al. Effect of ventilatory patterns on arterial oxygenation after near drowning in seawater. *Anesthesiology.* 1974;40:376.

    Suggests PEEP should be used in victims of near drowning in seawater.

25. Neuman TS. Arterial gas embolism and decompression sickness. *News Physiol Sci.* 2002;17:77.

    A summary of the pathophysiology and treatment of arterial gas embolism and decompression sickness (14 references).

26. Nichter MA, Everett PB. Childhood near drowning: is cardiopulmonary resuscitation always indicated? *Crit Care Med.* 1989;17:993.

    Of 93 pediatric near-drowning cases, two-thirds requiring CPR went on to intact survival; however, all patients requiring cardiotonic drugs in association with CPR either died or had severe neurologic damage.

27. Nussbaum E, Maggi JC. Pentobarbital therapy does not improve neurologic outcome in nearly drowned, flaccid-comatose children. *Pediatrics.* 1988;81:630.

    Discusses 31 patients in sequential treatment groups.

28. Orlowski JP. Drowning, near drowning, and ice water submersions. *Pediatr Clin North Am.* 1987;34:75.

    A good review with a fine section on ice water submersion (53 references).

29. Pearn J. The management of near drowning. *Br Med J.* 1985;291:1447.

    Although somewhat dated, still an interesting review (107 references).

30. Pearn J. Neurological and psychometric studies in children surviving fresh water immersion accidents. *Lancet.* 1977;1:7.

    Indicates good long-term neurologic outcome of children receiving CPR at the time of rescue.

31. Pearn J, Nixon J, Wilkey I. Freshwater drowning and near drowning accidents involving children: a five-year total population study. *Med J Aust.* 1976;2:942.

    An excellent, epidemiologic review.

32. Peterson B. Morbidity of children near drowning. *Pediatrics.* 1977;59:364.

    Neurologic outcome of children still requiring CPR on arrival in the emergency room is dismal.

33. Schench H, McAniff JJ. *United States Underwater Fatality Statistics, 1970–1981.* Kingston, RI: University of Rhode Island. NOAA Report No. URI-SSR-83-16.

    Describes all scuba fatalities in the United States during the years 1970 to 1981 and is the only complete epidemiologic report of its kind. An annual report is published yearly as well.

34. Schilling UM, Bortolin M. Drowning. *Minerva Anestesiol.* 2011;77(4):1–9.

    This is an excellent overview of drowning cases, pathophysiology, and treatment in the emergency department.

35. Shupak A, Weiler-Ravell D, Adir Y, et al. Pulmonary oedema induced by strenuous swimming: a field study. *Respir Physiol.* 2000;121:25.

    A prospective study that looked at the incidence and recurrence rate of strenuous SIPE in healthy young men in a fitness-training program.

36. Slade JB Jr, Hattori T, Ray CS, et al. Pulmonary edema associated with scuba diving. *Chest.* 2001;120:1686.

    A case report of eight scuba divers who developed pulmonary edema after diving.

37. Sladen A, Zander H. Methylprednisolone therapy for pulmonary edema following near drowning. *JAMA.* 1971;215:1793.

    Weak evidence that steroids may be of benefit in patients presenting with pulmonary edema.

38. Smith RM, Neuman TS. Elevation in serum CK in divers with arterial gas embolism. *N Engl J Med.* 1994;330:19.
39. Smith RM, Neuman TS. Abnormal serum biochemistries in association with arterial gas embolism. *J Emerg Med.* 1997;15:285.

    These two articles are representative of several delineating the laboratory abnormalities seen in victims of arterial gas embolism.

40. Spack L, Gedeit R, Splaingard M, et al. Failure of aggressive therapy to alter outcome in pediatric near drowning. *Pediatr Emerg Care.* 1997;13:98.

    The most recent article demonstrating that the currently available aggressive therapies do not alter outcome.

41. Staudinger T, Bankier A, Strohmaier W, et al. Exogenous surfactant therapy in a patient with adult respiratory distress syndrome after near drowning. *Resuscitation.* 1997;35:179.

    The most recent of several case reports using surfactant to treat near-drowning victims.

42. Suominen PK, Korpela RE, Silfvast TG, et al. Does water temperature affect outcome of nearly drowned children. *Resuscitation.* 1997;35:111.

    The only recent article to examine the effect of water temperature on outcome. The data seem to indicate cold water near drownings do no better than others and that duration of immersion is the critical factor.

43. Swann HG, Bruce M. The cardiorespiratory and biochemical events during rapid anoxic death, VI: fresh water and sea water drowning. *Tex Rep Biol Med.* 1949;7:604.
44. Swann HG, Brucer M, Moore C, et al. Fresh water and sea water drowning: a study of the terminal cardiac and biochemical events. *Tex Rep Biol Med.* 1947;5:423.

    References 39 and 40 are the basis for 15 years of misunderstanding concerning the pathophysiology of near drowning.

45. van Berkel M, Bierens JJ, Lie RL, et al. Pulmonary oedema, pneumonia and mortality in submersion victims: a retrospective study in 125 patients. *Intensive Care Med.* 1996;22:101.

    A retrospective series of 125 victims that evaluates the development of pulmonary edema and the need for hospitalization in near-drowning victims.

46. Zuckerman GB, Gregory PM, Santos-Domaini SM. Predictors of death and neurologic impairment in pediatric submersion injuries. *Arch Pediatr Adolesc Med.* 1998;152:134.

    The most recent of many articles trying to determine factors that can be used to make prognoses on nearly drowned children. Contains 34 references, most of which are to other articles relating to the prognosis of near-drowning victims.

89 Radiation-Induced Lung Disease

Lindsay G. Jensen, Mark M. Fuster, and Ajay P. Sandhu

BACKGROUND

Radiotherapy for thoracic neoplasms often includes normal lung tissue within the field, creating a risk of radiation-induced lung injury. Reports on the frequency of radiation-induced lung injury after radiotherapy for lung cancer, breast cancer, esophageal cancer, and Hodgkin disease vary widely depending upon whether the study assesses radiographic or clinical features. Post radiation changes are common and occur in the majority of patients in some studies; however, clinical symptoms occur in a much smaller proportion of patients. Although the increasing use of conformal radiation therapy (RT) techniques can limit normal-tissue exposure, radiation-induced lung injury is an important consideration during radiotherapy planning and treatment.

PATHOPHYSIOLOGY

Radiation creates reactive oxygen and nitrogen species which damage cell proteins, membranes, and DNA. The exact pathophysiology of radiation injury is incompletely understood, but involves damage to endothelial cells as well as type I and II pneumocytes.

The acute phase of radiation pneumonitis is characterized by endothelial cell changes, swelling of the basement membrane, interstitial edema, variable capillary occlusion, and presence of inflammatory cells. There is an initial increase in surfactant due to release of surfactant-containing lamellar bodies from type II pneumocytes, followed by decreased surfactant and hyaline membrane change. Sloughing endothelial cells and increased capillary permeability result in capillary obstruction and accumulation of proteinaceous exudate in alveoli, impairing gas exchange.

Inflammatory cells in the acute phase of radiation pneumonitis induce a cytokine cascade, which ultimately mediates a host response characterized by fibrosis. Cytokines including transforming growth factor-β (TGF-β), tumor necrosis factor-α (TNF-α), interleukin-6 (IL-6), and IL-1 play an important role, and their serum levels have been studied as potential predictors of radiation pneumonitis. Late injury, occurring 6 months or more after RT, is characterized by fibrosis and thickening of vessel walls and alveolar septa. TGF-β in particular is thought to be involved in the development of chronic fibrosis by increasing synthesis of collagen and fibronectin.

The likelihood of developing radiation-induced lung injury depends on total dose, dose per fraction, concurrent chemotherapy, total lung volume irradiated, location of tumor, history of chest irradiation, and pre-existing lung disease. Older age and large gross tumor volume (GTV) may increase risk. Smokers may have a decreased risk of developing radiation pneumonitis. Studies have shown conflicting results on whether abnormal pulmonary function tests (PFTs) at baseline can predict for radiation pneumonitis. Dose per fraction and total lung dose have been shown to be particularly important, and higher total doses can be delivered without inducing lung injury when smaller fraction sizes are used. In large single doses, the frequency of radiation pneumonitis increases rapidly with fraction size above 7.5 Gy. Using smaller fraction sizes of 1.8 to 2 Gy, the estimated whole lung doses resulting in a 5% and 50% probability of a complication within 5 years are approximately 17.5 and 24.5 Gy, respectively. Several studies evaluating dose–volume parameters have sought to establish the relationship between radiation pneumonitis and V_{DOSE}, which is defined as the percent of lung volume (V) receiving greater than or equal to a specified dose in Gray (DOSE). No single dose parameter can reliably predict for lung damage, but mean lung dose (MLD) above 20 Gy and V_{13}, V_{20}, and V_{30} above 40%, 25% to 30%, and 10% to 15%, respectively, appear to increase probability of symptomatic radiation pneumonitis.

Predicting radiation pneumonitis as a function of dose is an area of active research. A review of studies reporting dose–volume parameters, normal-tissue complication probability (NTCP) models, and MLD found that most models had only fair to poor accuracy in predicting likelihood of radiation pneumonitis. Predictive models to determine risk for radiation-induced lung injury based on large patient datasets have also not proven to be effective when applied to other datasets.

Chemotherapy with drugs that are toxic to the lung can exacerbate the effects of radiation pneumonitis. Bleomycin is the most well-known of these compounds, but Adriamycin (doxorubicin), busulfan, paclitaxel, cisplatin, dactinomycin, vincristine, cyclophosphamide, mitomycin, gemcitabine, and other chemotherapeutic agents may also contribute to radiation-induced lung injury. Sequential, rather than concurrent, administration of chemotherapy drugs may decrease lung injury. Certain chemotherapeutic agents have also been reported to cause a "recall pneumonitis," where signs and symptoms of radiation pneumonitis occur in the previously irradiated field within hours of receiving the chemotherapeutic drug. This response can occur months after the completion of radiotherapy.

CLINICAL PRESENTATION

Radiation-induced lung disease can be divided into two stages: acute radiation pneumonitis and chronic radiation fibrosis.

Acute Radiation Pneumonitis

Damage to lung tissue begins within days of radiation exposure, but radiation pneumonitis usually becomes symptomatic after 1 to 3 months. Early onset is associated with a worse clinical course. The most common symptom of radiation pneumonitis is dyspnea, but cough, fever, and chest pain can also occur. Cough is typically minimally productive, occasionally with streaky hemoptysis. Chest pain may be vague or pleuritic in nature. Physical exam is usually normal, but crackles, pleural, or pericardial rub may be heard. Signs of consolidation may also be noted in the affected lung area. Acute radiation pneumonitis can rarely progress to fulminant respiratory failure and death.

Chronic Radiation Fibrosis

Chronic fibrosis usually develops 6 months or more after radiotherapy and stabilizes by 2 years. Fibrosis likely occurs to some degree in all patients receiving radiation to the lung, but it is often asymptomatic. Dyspnea is the most common symptom. In severe cases of fibrosis, pulmonary hypertension and cor pulmonale may develop. Physical findings may include inspiratory crackles, elevated hemidiaphragms, cyanosis, clubbing, and elevated venous pressure.

Radiographic Changes

Radiographic changes for both early and late pulmonary injury are more common than clinical symptoms. Acute radiation pneumonitis typically presents as hazy opacity on chest radiography. Radiation changes can have a sharp edge corresponding to the shape of the radiation port, but this may be less pronounced as more patients are treated with conformal radiotherapy fields. Later findings include septal thickening and air bronchograms. Radiation fibrosis appears within the irradiated area as a linear interstitial pattern, dense fibrotic strands with occasional dense consolidation, volume loss, and traction bronchiectasis. Pleural thickening may also be seen. CT is more sensitive than plain radiography in assessing structural lung changes, which include (in order of severity) increased density, patchy consolidation, and solid consolidation. MRI may be particularly useful in differentiating radiation pneumonitis from recurrent disease.

While radiographic findings are confined to the irradiated area, a bilateral lymphocytic alveolitis has been described outside of the radiation field. Bronchoalveolar lavage in patients undergoing unilateral breast irradiation shows increased lymphocytes and neutrophils compared to controls, with no difference in number between the irradiated and nonirradiated sides. It is unclear if the degree of lymphocytosis correlates with symptoms of radiation pneumonitis.

Functional imaging studies can also aid in the diagnosis and quantification of lung injury. Increasing fludeoxyglucose positron emission tomography (FDG-PET) uptake following radiotherapy appears to correlate with maximum degree of clinical radiation pneumonitis. FDG-PET uptake following radiotherapy also increases with radiation dose, but there is a significant variation in the magnitude of increase, indicating possible differences in the underlying biologic response between patients. Single photon emission computed tomography (SPECT) shows decreased ventilation and perfusion 3 to 4 months after RT with some studies reporting partial recovery of function occurring at 18 months.

PFTs are variable in radiation-induced lung injury and are particularly difficult to evaluate in lung cancer patients who may have abnormal PFTs at baseline. The diffusion capacity of carbon monoxide is more consistently decreased than other parameters. Decreased forced expiratory volume in 1 second (FEV_1) is also fairly common. Total lung capacity and vital capacity may decrease as a result of fibrosis. In some cases, PFTs may improve when tumor shrinkage decreases obstruction. The most common laboratory findings associated with radiation pneumonitis are polymorphonuclear leukocytosis and elevated erythrocyte sedimentation rate.

Differential diagnosis for radiation-induced lung injury includes infection, pericarditis, drug toxicity, pulmonary emboli, exacerbation of baseline lung disease, recurrent tumor, or lymphangitic tumor spread. Radiation-induced lung injury is usually scored using the National Cancer Institute Common Terminology Criteria for Adverse Events, Radiation Therapy Oncology Group (RTOG) scale, or Southwest Oncology Group (SWOG) scale. All are 5-point scales where 1 is minimal or asymptomatic and 5 is death, but reported grade of toxicity has been shown to vary depending on which scale is used.

COMPLICATIONS

Pleural effusion, pneumothorax, bronchial stenosis, and tracheoesophageal fistula are uncommon complications of thoracic radiation. Pleural effusions are typically small and occur in the same time frame as other radiographic findings of acute pneumonitis. Bronchial stenosis has been reported mainly in patients receiving endobronchial brachytherapy, but can occur after high-dose external beam radiotherapy.

Bronchiolitis obliterans organizing pneumonia (BOOP) is an inflammatory reaction that can occur after thoracic radiotherapy. Symptoms are similar to those of radiation pneumonitis, including cough and dyspnea, but BOOP can be differentiated from radiation pneumonitis by the presence of affected lung tissue outside of the radiotherapy field and migratory infiltrates on chest radiograph or CT. BOOP is uncommon, occurring in 2.5% of patients in breast cancer series, and can present months to years after the completion of radiotherapy. Symptoms of BOOP are typically responsive to corticosteroids, but recur more frequently than classic radiation pneumonitis symptoms when corticosteroids are withdrawn.

PREVENTION AND TREATMENT

A number of compounds have been evaluated for their potentially protective effects on the lung during and after RT. Amifostine is a free-radical scavenger that has shown protective effects against pneumonitis in several randomized trials. The largest randomized study did not show a significant effect, but has been criticized for the schedule of drug administration. Pentoxyfylline, which inhibits TNF-α and platelet aggregation and increases microvascular blood flow, was also associated with a moderate decrease in radiation pneumonitis in one small randomized trial. Angiotensin II converting enzyme inhibitors (ACE-I) and angiotensin receptor blockers (ARB) may decrease risk of radiation-induced lung injury, according to animal studies and retrospective clinical findings. A recent randomized trial of berberine found decreased incidence of early and late radiation-induced lung injury. None of these medications are currently approved for the prevention of radiation-induced lung injury. Other compounds including taurine, genistein, statins, and gefitinib have shown potential for reducing pulmonary inflammation or fibrosis in animal models.

Treatment for radiation-induced lung injury is mainly supportive. Radiographic disease without clinical symptoms does not require treatment. Dyspnea and cough can be treated with bronchodilators and cough suppressants. Fever, if it occurs, can be treated with antipyretics, while infection may be investigated and is occasionally empirically treated. Patients with more severe radiation-induced lung injury may require supplemental oxygen.

Corticosteroids are the most effective treatment for radiation pneumonitis, with as many as 80% of patients showing improvement in symptoms. Steroids can be given at doses of 60 mg for at least 2 weeks and should be tapered. Rapid withdrawal of steroids may result in worsening symptoms. Prophylactic steroids have not been shown to be effective in preventing radiation pneumonitis. Non-steroidal anti-inflammatory drugs may also improve symptoms. Antibiotics do not play a role in the treatment of radiation pneumonitis and should not be given unless the patient has a known infection. Nevertheless, infection may occasionally be difficult to exclude, and a high index of suspicion is warranted.

CONFORMAL TECHNIQUES IN RADIOTHERAPY

The use of conformal radiotherapy techniques to treat thoracic neoplasms has increased significantly during the last decade. Intensity modulated radiation therapy (IMRT) and stereotactic body radiation therapy (SBRT) are two conformal radiotherapy techniques that can deliver a high dose to tumor while decreasing the dose to surrounding normal structures.

Several dosimetric planning studies in lung cancer treatment have shown improved target conformity and decreased dose to lung parenchyma with conformal techniques as compared to conventional radiotherapy. A large study comparing CT/3DCRT with 4DCT/IMRT treatment for treatment of lung cancer found decreased grade greater than or equal to 3 radiation pneumonitis and similar disease control with 4DCT/IMRT.

SBRT is a focal, high-dose therapy typically delivered in five fractions or less, which can be used to treat medically inoperable lung cancer. Clinical outcomes studies of SBRT in the lung have shown improved survival and excellent tumor control compared to conventional radiotherapy. Concern exists that high doses per fraction may increase the risk of toxicity in exposed normal tissue, particularly for patients with tumor in the proximal bronchial tree, but clinical reports of toxicity have varied. Two large retrospective review of SBRT for non–small-cell lung carcinoma (NSCLC) reported only 1% to 2.4% of patients experiencing grade greater than or equal to 3 toxicity. Two prospective trials to evaluate toxicity and outcomes of SBRT found high rates of local control with moderate grade greater than or equal to 3 toxicity (15%–16%). SBRT is still relatively new to clinical practice, and larger, prospective studies will be needed to establish toxicity profiles.

FUTURE DIRECTIONS

Ongoing studies of conformal radiotherapy techniques will further our knowledge of optimal treatment planning and also help to clarify risk factors for radiation pneumonitis. Preliminary functional imaging studies using SPECT and FDG-PET have indicated that these imaging modalities may be helpful in identifying active lung regions before treatment in order to spare them in treatment planning. Levels of TGF-β, IL-1, IL-6, intercellular adhesion molecule-1 (ICAM-1), and Krebs von den Lungen-6 (KL-6) may be useful biomarkers to identify patients who are more likely to develop radiation-induced lung injury. Recent studies have found genotype variations in single nucleotide polymorphisms of certain genes may also be useful in predicting individual susceptibility to lung injury. Several protective agents during radiotherapy have shown initial promising results, but further evidence is needed before they can be used in routine clinical practice.

FURTHER READING

1. Movsas B, Raffin JA, Ebstein AH, et al. Pulmonary radiation injury. *Chest.* 1997;111:1061.

   A review of clinical syndromes and pathophysiology of classic radiation pneumonitis, as well as modern radiation planning strategies and key factors predisposing to radiation pneumonitis.

2. Liao Z, Travis L, Komaki R. Radiation treatment-related lung damage. In: Pass H, Carbone D, Johnson D, et al, eds. *Principles and Practice of Lung Cancer.* Philadelphia, PA: Lippincott Williams & Wilkins; 2011:601–642.

   A detailed review of the mechanisms, risk factors, dose–volume relationships, and prediction models for radiation-induced lung injury.

3. Mehta V. Radiation pneumonitis and pulmonary fibrosis in non–small-cell lung cancer: pulmonary function, prediction, and prevention. *Int J Radiat Oncol Biol Phys.* 2005;63:5–24.

   A review of risk factors, dosimetric parameters, and biochemical markers for radiation pneumonitis. Discusses potential benefits of evolving radiotherapy strategies and cytoprotective medications.

4. McDonald S, Rubin P, Phillips TL, et al. Injury to the lung from cancer therapy: clinical syndromes, measurable endpoints, and potential scoring systems. *Int J Radiat Oncol Biol Phys.* 1995;31:1187.

   A detailed summary of the effects of thoracic radiation on lung cell types at various time points after radiation. The article also illustrates the role of TGF-β in multicellular interactions initiating and sustaining the fibrogenic process.

5. Ghafoori P, Marks L, Vujaskovic C. Radiation-induced lung injury assessment, management, and prevention. *Oncology.* 2008;22:37–47.

   A review of mechanisms, effects, imaging findings, prediction, and prevention methods for radiation-induced lung injury.

6. Morgan GW, Breit SN. Radiation and the lung: a reevaluation of the mechanisms mediating pulmonary injury. *Int J Radiat Oncol Biol Phys.* 1995;31:361.

   Includes discussion of the steep dose–response relationship between thoracic irradiation and radiation pneumonitis. The review also discusses the nonclassic bilateral lymphocytic alveolitis response as a generalized hypersensitivity response to radiation-damaged lung.

7. Vogelius IR, Bentzen SM. A literature-based meta-analysis of clinical risk factors for development of radiation induced pneumonitis. *Acta Oncol.* 2012;1:975–983.

    A meta-analysis including 419 to 2,167 patients for each variable found older age, mid-lower lung tumors, comorbidity, and sequential chemotherapy to be significant risk factors for radiation pneumonitis. Smoking was found to be protective.

8. Palma DA, Senan S, Tsujino K, et al. Predicting radiation pneumonitis after chemoradiation therapy for lung cancer: an international individual patient data meta-analysis. *Int J Radiat Oncol Biol Phys.* 2013;85:444–450.

    A meta-analysis using a training dataset of 557 patients, found V20 and carboplatin/paclitaxel chemotherapy to predict for symptomatic (grade ≥2) pneumonitis, which was also true in validation dataset (n = 279).

9. Zhang XJ, Sun JG, Sun J, et al. Prediction of radiation pneumonitis in lung cancer patients: a systematic review. *J Cancer Res Clin Oncol.* 2012;138:2103–2116.

    A meta-analysis of approximately 20 potential risk factors for radiation pneumonitis, including 200 to 2,100 patients for each variable. They found chronic lung disease, tumor located in the middle or lower lobe, without pre-RT surgery, RT combined with chemotherapy, plasma end/pre-RT TGF-β1 ratio greater than or equal to 1, and GTV to be predictive of grade greater than or equal to 2 radiation pneumonitis.

10. Wang J, Cao J, Yuan S, et al. Poor baseline pulmonary function may not increase the risk of radiation-induced lung toxicity. *Int J Radiat Oncol Biol Phys.* 2013;85:798–804.

    Evaluated 260 patients from two institutions and found that poor baseline DLCO, FEV$_1$, and FVC did not significantly increase the risk of developing symptomatic radiation-induced lung toxicity.

11. VanDyk J, Keane TJ, Kan S, et al. Radiation pneumonitis following large single-dose irradiation: a reevaluation based on absolute dose to lung. *Int J Radiat Oncol Biol Phys.* 1981;7:461.

    Describes the incidence of radiation pneumonitis in a group of 303 patients, based on absolute dose to lung. The onset of pneumonitis occurred at approximately 7.5 Gy.

12. Emami B, Lyman J, Brown A, et al. Tolerance of normal tissue to therapeutic irradiation. *Int J Radiat Oncol Biol Phys.* 1991;21:109–122.

    Provides cumulative doses resulting in 5% and 50% probability of complication at 5 years.

13. Constine LS, Milano MT, Friedman D. Late effects of cancer treatment on normal tissues. In: Halperin EC, Perez CA, Brady LW, eds. *Principles and Practice of Radiation Oncology.* 5th ed. Philadelphia, PA: Lippincott Williams & Wilkins; 2008:319–355.

    Discusses time course, risk factors, diagnosis, pathophysiology, and clinical syndromes of radiation-induced lung injury.

14. Rodrigues G, Lock M, D'Souza D, et al. Prediction of radiation pneumonitis by dose–volume histogram parameters in lung cancer—a systematic review. *Radiother Oncol.* 2004;71: 127–138.

    A review of 12 studies of V$_{DOSE}$, MLD, and NTCP as predictors of pneumonitis. Concluded that the association between dose parameters and radiation pneumonitis has been demonstrated in the literature, but no ideal metric has been found.

15. Bradley JD, Hope A, El Naqa I, et al. A nomogram to predict radiation pneumonitis, derived from a combined analysis of RTOG 9311 and institutional data. *Int J Radiat Oncol Biol Phys.* 2007;69:985–992.

    Used clinical, dosimetric, and tumor location data from Washington University (n = 219) and RTOG 9311 (n = 129) datasets to create predictive models for radiation pneumonitis. Found both models were poor in predicting radiation pneumonitis in the other dataset, but that combined model performed well.

    A general review of radiation-induced lung injury.

16. Davis SD, Yankelevitz DF, Henschke CL, et al. Radiation effects on the lung: clinical features, pathology, and imaging findings. *AJR Am J Roentgenol.* 1992;159:1157.

    A review focusing on imaging findings.

17. Kocak Z, Evans ES, Zhou SM, et al. Challenges in defining radiation pneumonitis in patients with lung cancer. *Int J Radiat Oncol Biol Phys.* 2005;62:635–638.

Prospectively evaluated 318 lung cancer patients for RT-induced lung injury. Forty-seven patients had grade greater than or equal to 2 pneumonitis symptoms. Of these, 28% had confounding factors, medical factors making definitive diagnosis of radiation pneumonitis difficult.

18. Mac Manus MP, Ding Z, Hogg A, et al. Association between pulmonary uptake of fluoro-deoxyglucose detected by positron emission tomography scanning after radiation therapy for non–small-cell lung cancer and radiation pneumonitis. *Int J Radiat Oncol Biol Phys.* 2011;80:1365–1371.

Performed FDG-PET in 88 patients and compared grade of PET pneumonitis with clinical pneumonitis and found significant correlation.

19. Guerrero T, Johnson V, Hart J, et al. Radiation pneumonitis: local dose versus [18F]-fluorodeoxy-glucose uptake response in irradiated lung. *Int J Radiat Oncol Biol Phys.* 2007;68:1030–1035.

Measured FDG-PET uptake in 36 esophageal cancer patients. Found that a linear relationship existed but that it varied substantially between patients, indicating a possible variation in biologic response to radiation.

20. Speiser BL, Spratling L. Radiation bronchitis and stenosis secondary to high dose rate endobronchial irradiation. *Int J Radiat Oncol Biol Phys.* 1993;85:589.

Radiation bronchitis and stenosis are clinical entities that are identified in patients undergoing bronchial brachytherapy.

21. Miller KL, Shafman TD, Anscher MS, et al. Bronchial stenosis: an underreported complication of high-dose external beam radiotherapy for lung cancer? *Int J Radiat Oncol Biol Phys.* 2005;61:64–69.

Assessed 103 patients treated with twice daily radiotherapy at doses of 70.8 to 86.4 Gy, found clinically significant bronchial stenosis in 8 patients.

22. Katayama N, Sato S, Katsui K, et al. Analysis of factors associated with radiation-induced bronchiolitis obliterans organizing pneumonia syndrome after breast-conserving therapy. *Int J Radiat Oncol Biol Phys.* 2009;73:1049.

Evaluated 702 women treated with breast conservation therapy at seven institutions and evaluated potential predictive factors, finding age greater than 50 and use of concurrent endocrine therapy to be associated with BOOP.

23. King TE. BOOP: an important cause of migratory pulmonary infiltrates? [editorial]. *Eur Respir J.* 1995;8:193.

Pearl editorial on case reports of migratory BOOP resulting from thoracic irradiation.

24. Graves PR, Siddiqui F, Anscher MS, et al. Radiation pulmonary toxicity: from mechanisms to management. *Semin Radiat Oncol.* 2010;20:201–207.

A review of molecular and cellular events, symptoms, strategies for prevention, and experimental methods for prevention.

25. Komaki R, Lee JS, Milas L, et al. Effects of amifostine on acute toxicity from concurrent chemotherapy and radiotherapy for inoperable non–small-cell lung cancer: report of a randomized comparative trial. *Int J Radiat Oncol Biol Phys.* 2004;58:1369.

Promising use of a radioprotective agent (and free-radical scavenger) in a human trial.

26. Movsas B, Scott C, Langer C, et al. Randomized trial of amifostine in locally advanced non–small-cell lung cancer patients receiving chemotherapy and hyperfractionated radiation: Radiation Therapy Oncology Group Trial 98-01. *J Clin Oncol.* 2005;23:2145–2154.

Two hundred forty-three patients with NSCLC randomized to amifostine vs. placebo during radiotherapy. Primary endpoint of the study was esophagitis. Grade greater than or equal to 3 pneumonitis occurred in 16.7% of placebo arm and 8% of amifostine arm, with P = NS.

27. Ozturk B, Egehan I, Atavci S, et al. Pentoxifylline in prevention of radiation-induced lung toxicity in patients with breast and lung cancer: a double-blind randomized trial. *Int J Radiat Oncol Biol Phys.* 2004;58:213–219.

Forty breast and lung cancer patients randomized to pentoxifylline or placebo. PFT changes, radiologic findings of lung damage, and LENT-SOMA scores indicated a possible protective effect of pentoxifylline.

28. Kharofa J, Gore E. Symptomatic radiation pneumonitis in elderly patients receiving thoracic irradiation. *Clin Lung Cancer.* 2013;14(3):283–287.

Reviewed 256 patients and found higher incidence of grade greater than or equal to 2 radiation pneumonitis in patients greater than or equal to 70 (or 4.52, P = 0.001) and lower incidence in the patients taking ACE inhibitors during treatment (or 0.22, P = 0.02).

29. Liao ZX, Komaki RR, Thames HD Jr, et al. Influence of technologic advances on outcomes in patients with unresectable, locally advanced non–small-cell lung cancer receiving concomitant chemoradiotherapy. *Int J Radiat Oncol Biol Phys.* 2010;76:775–781.

    Compares outcomes for 496 NSCLC patients treated with 4DCT/IMRT and CT/3DCRT. Found significantly lower toxicity and V20 in 4DCT/IMRT group with similar disease control.

30. Fakiris AJ, McGarry RC, Yiannoutsos CT, et al. Stereotactic body radiation therapy for early-stage non–small-cell lung carcinoma: four-year results of a prospective phase II study. *Int J Radiat Oncol Biol Phys.* 2009;75:677–682.

    Four-year results for 70 patients treated with SBRT for NSCLC, three-year local control overall survival, and cancer specific survival were 88.1%, 42.7%, and 81.7%, respectively. Grade greater than or equal to 3 toxicity occurred 15.7% (11/70) of patients.

31. Nath SK, Sandhu AP, Kim D, et al. Locoregional and distant failure following image-guided stereotactic body radiation for early-stage primary lung cancer. *Radiother Oncol.* 2011;99:12–17.

    Forty-eight patients treated with SBRT for NSCLC. Two-year local control was 95%. Grade 3 toxicity occurred in only one patient and was nonpulmonary.

32. Timmerman R, Paulus R, Galvin J, et al. Stereotactic body radiation therapy for inoperable early stage lung cancer. *JAMA.* 2010;303:1070–1076.

    Results of RTOG 0236, a multicenter prospective trial to evaluate the efficacy and toxicity of SBRT to treat inoperable small-cell lung cancer. Excluded patients with involvement of proximal bronchial tree. Found grade 3 or greater pulmonary or upper respiratory tract toxicity in approximately 16% (9/55) of patients.

33. Barriger RB, Forquer JA, Brabham JG, et al. A dose–volume analysis of radiation pneumonitis in non–small-cell lung cancer patients treated with stereotactic body radiation therapy. *Int J Radiat Oncol Biol Phys.* 2012;83:457–462.

    A single institution review of 251 patients treated with SBRT for NSCLC. Low rates of grade 3 (2%) and grade 4 (0.4%) toxicity. Found MLD and V20 to be predictive of radiation pneumonitis.

34. Baker R, Han G, Sarangkasiri S, et al. Clinical and dosimetric predictors of radiation pneumonitis in a large series of patients treated with stereotactic body radiation therapy to the lung. *Int J Radiat Oncol Biol Phys.* 2013;85:190–195.

    Evaluated 240 patients treated with SBRT for lung tumors, incidence of grade greater than or equal to 2 and greater than or equal to 3 pneumonitis were 11% and 1%, respectively. In multivariate analysis, female gender, pack-years smoking, and larger gross internal tumor volume were predictive of radiation pneumonitis.

35. Pang Q, Wei Q, Xu T, et al. Functional promoter variant rs2868371 of HSPB1 is associated with risk of radiation pneumonitis after chemoradiation for non–small-cell lung cancer. *Int J Radiat Oncol Biol Phys.* 2013;85(5):1332–1339.

    Evaluated risk of radiation pneumonitis in 146 patients based on genotypes of single nucleotide polymorphisms HSPB1 protein and found risk to be significantly higher in one of the genotypes. This was also true in a validation data set of 125 patients.

Sarcoidosis

Xavier Soler

Sarcoidosis is a multisystem granulomatous disease of undetermined etiology with a variable clinical presentation and course that ranges from an incidental radiographic finding in an asymptomatic individual to life-threatening illness. The epidemiology of sarcoidosis remains problematic because of its variable presentation and insensitive and nonspecific diagnostic tests. In the United States, sarcoidosis has a higher prevalence among African-Americans, especially women. Several epidemiologic studies have demonstrated temporal, seasonal, and geographic clustering of sarcoidosis cases, suggesting a common etiologic origin. Possible agents have been identified as a cause for sarcoidosis, although none has been definitely confirmed. There is increasing evidence to suggest that infectious agents are involved. Genome-wide scans (GWAS) have identified candidate genes, and cytokine dysregulation has been demonstrated. However, the criteria for diagnosis have not changed. Sarcoidosis remains a diagnosis of exclusion best supported by a tissue biopsy specimen demonstrating noncaseating granulomas in a patient with compatible clinical and radiologic features.

The immunopathogenesis of sarcoidosis remains unclear. It is likely due to a complex interplay to exposure to one or more exogenous antigens, environmental conditions, and host immunologic responses. Reports of case-clustering, increased susceptibility in certain occupations and environmental exposures (e.g., work in agriculture, exposure to mold, mildew, musty odors, or pesticides), and transmission via organ transplant all support this theory. After the World Trade Center disaster, firefighters exposed to dust exhibited a higher-than-expected incidence of sarcoidosis that was clinically and phenotypically distinct from that in the general population. Reduced risk has been associated with allergic responses and tobacco use. GWAS has identified non-HLA candidate susceptibility genes commonly involved in host-immune response, such as butyrophilin-like 2 (BTNL2). It has become increasingly well recognized that polymorphisms within various chemical mediators of inflammation contribute to the immunopathogenesis of sarcoidosis. In the United States, African-Americans are affected more frequently and generally have chronic and more severe disease. Familial clustering of sarcoidosis is common.

The ACCESS (A Case Control Etiologic Study of Sarcoidosis) study collected data on 704 patients with newly diagnosed, biopsy-proven sarcoidosis and control subjects matched by age, sex, race, and geographic area and found that cases were five times more likely than control subjects to report an affected sibling or parent. Also, polymorphisms in the promoter region of tumor necrosis factor-α (TNF-α) have been associated with Löfgren syndrome, a form of sarcoidosis characterized by erythema nodosum, hilar adenopathy, uveitis, and a good prognosis. Insertion/deletions in the promoter region of angiotensin-1 converting enzyme have also been identified. The importance of TNF has been validated in studies documenting the effectiveness of biologic TNF antagonists in treating some patients with sarcoidosis. Reduced numbers of natural killer T (NKT) cells have been found in sarcoid blood and bronchoalveolar lavage (BAL) fluid.

There are data suggesting that bacteria, such as *Mycobacteriun Tuberculosis* or *Propionibacterium acnes*, may be involved in causing the disease. It is quite possible that the triggering antigen varies depending on ethnicity, geographic location, and individual genetic background. Also, strongly polarized T helper cell (TH) 1 immune responses are present more frequently. The immune response may precipitate a cascade of events leading to granuloma formation involving (1) exposure to the antigen; (2) presentation of the antigen (by macrophages via HLA class II molecules to T lymphocytes); and (3) immune effector cells promoting the development of noncaseating granulomas, the pathologic hallmark of sarcoidosis. The release of cytokines, such as interleukin-2 (IL-2) and interferon-γ, by activated CD4 T lymphocytes (indicating a TH-1 immunologic response) eventually leads to enhanced fibroblast replication and granuloma formation. Despite the increased local immunologic activity, cutaneous anergy is commonly present.

The diagnosis of sarcoidosis is never certain, although it may be established by clinical correlation of nonspecific symptoms with biochemical, radiologic, and pathologic confirmation. Sarcoidosis is usually underdiagnosed. The clinical presentation ranges from asymptomatic to life-threatening organ involvement. A common feature of this disease is its multiorgan involvement, including respiratory (cough, chest pain, and dyspnea), musculoskeletal (arthralgia and myalgia), ocular (visual changes and pain), and skin manifestations (erythema nodosum, nodules, plaques, and papules). There is no gold standard for diagnosis. Certain nonspecific clinical features are typical of sarcoidosis including bilateral hilar adenopathy, Löfgren syndrome (erythema nodosum coupled with bilateral hilar adenopathy and often fever and/or arthritis), Heerfordt syndrome (uveitis, parotitis, and fever), and gallium-67 scan uptake in the parotid and lacrimal glands (panda sign) along with right paratracheal and bilateral hilar areas (lambda sign). Unless one of the special clinical situations previously described is present, the diagnosis usually requires histologic confirmation and exclusion of alternative causes. Cough and dyspnea are the most common respiratory complaints. The heart can be affected in 1% to 4% of cases and cardiac sarcoidosis is potentially sudden and life-threatening. Erythema nodosum is seen occasionally with the typical presentation of bilateral hilar adenopathy and generally indicates a good prognosis. Pleural disease occurs uncommonly and can be associated with pleural effusions. Between 30% and 60% of patients are asymptomatic and present with incidental findings on chest radiographs.

The chest radiograph is staged as follows:

- *Stage 0*, normal;
- *Stage 1*, bilateral hilar adenopathy;
- *Stage 2*, bilateral hilar adenopathy with pulmonary infiltrate;
- *Stage 3*, pulmonary infiltrates without hilar adenopathy; and
- *Stage 4*, pulmonary fibrosis.

Currently, no reliable prognostic biomarkers have been identified. Pathologically, the most commonly involved organ systems are the lungs, peripheral lymphatics, liver, heart, skin, eye, spleen, salivary glands, joints, and bone. A reduction in diffusion capacity is the most common abnormality on pulmonary function testing (PFT). This is often accompanied by a restrictive pattern, although airflow obstruction can be found in approximately 30% of patients. Hypoxemia may be present at rest and during exercise. Changes on serial PFTs may be useful in identifying candidates for therapy and further follow-up. Laboratory tests are generally not helpful. Levels of angiotensin-1 converting enzyme are often increased, but this finding is not specific and should not be used for screening. Chest CT remains controversial for routine assessment. Magnetic resonance imaging with gadolinium and nuclear imaging have been evaluated to aid in the diagnosis, monitor disease activity, and determine the optimal site for biopsy. Studies with positron emission tomography (PET) technology have proven valuable in locating occult sites of active disease. BAL can be used as an adjunctive measure to support the diagnosis (increased number of CD4 cells and elevated CD4/CD8 ratio). When tissue diagnosis is required, biopsy of an involved site is almost always diagnostic. The histologic picture is not pathognomonic; therefore, diseases such as tuberculosis, fungal infection, beryllium exposure, drug reactions, and local sarcoid-like reactions must be excluded. Endobronchial ultrasound and transbronchial needle aspiration (EBUS-TBNA) allow localization and aspiration of hilar and mediastinal lymph nodes, often eliminating the need for more invasive procedures, such as mediastinoscopy.

Most patients with sarcoidosis do not require therapy; many experience spontaneous remission. Recently, a more symptom-oriented approach in deciding to initiate or maintain therapy has been suggested to reduce secondary-drug side effects. Systemic long-term therapy may be necessary when significant organ involvement or systemic symptoms are present. Urgent indications include ocular, myocardial, and central nervous system involvement. Other relative indications include persistent hypercalcemia, disfiguring cutaneous lesions, symptomatic respiratory disease, thrombocytopenia, and severe constitutional symptoms. Asymptomatic individuals with stable lung infiltrates are not usually treated. Corticosteroids remain the drugs of choice with significant functional impairment, but sustained treatment may result in disabling side effects that may be reduced by using steroid-sparing agents such as methotrexate or azathioprine. Most therapeutic regimens use prednisone (0.5 mg/kg/day), with tapered doses over a period of 6 months or longer until a response is observed. In the presence of a positive tuberculin reaction or complete anergy, it may be reasonable to start isoniazid concomitantly with corticosteroids. Exacerbations can occur when prednisone is decreased below 15 mg/day. Therapy is best monitored by symptom resolution and not by blood tests or imaging techniques. Inhaled corticosteroids may be used in mild cases, but their role is still unclear. Azathioprine may be used in corticosteroid-resistant sarcoidosis. Chloroquine, intradermal steroids, methotrexate, and retinoids appear to be effective in managing skin disease. Topical steroids may be effective in treating uveitis. TNF inhibitors (i.e., infliximab and etanercept) are being investigated for the treatment of refractory sarcoidosis. Phosphodiesterase-5 inhibitors, prostaglandin analogs, and endothelin antagonists have been used in treating sarcoidosis-associated pulmonary hypertension. However, their efficacy is unknown. The indication for surgical intervention in certain forms of sarcoidosis, particularly sinonasal, remains controversial, and it is not usually recommended. Organ transplantation has been used successfully, but noncaseating granulomas may recur. The prognosis of sarcoidosis is generally favorable. The majority of patients with pulmonary involvement resolve within 1 to 2 years. However, some patients gradually decline and may die from pulmonary involvement.

FURTHER READING

1. Morgenthau AS, Iannuzzi MC. Recent advances in sarcoidosis. *Chest.* 2011;139(1):174–182.

   A review of all aspects of sarcoidosis, including imaging, genetic evaluation, and current treatment options.

2. Baughman RP, Nagai S, Balter M, et al. Defining the clinical outcome status (COS) in sarcoidosis: results of WASOG Task Force. *Sarcoidosis Vasc Diffuse Lung Dis.* 2011;28(1):56–64.

   A task force effort to define clinical phenotypes of the disease on the basis of a clinical outcomes status assessment.

3. Baughman RP, Culver DA, Judson MA. A concise review of pulmonary sarcoidosis. *Am J Respir Crit Care Med.* 2011;183(5):573–581.

   A comprehensive state-of-the-art review of clinical aspects of sarcoidosis, including etiology, laboratory findings, diagnosis, and treatment.

4. Tremblay A, Stather DR, Maceachern P, et al. A randomized controlled trial of standard vs endobronchial ultrasonography-guided transbronchial needle aspiration in patients with suspected sarcoidosis. *Chest.* 2009;136(2):340–346.

   A randomized control trial comparing the diagnostic yield of EBUS-TBNA with TBNA in 50 patients with mediastinal adenophathy and suspected sarcodosis. Results demonstrated that EBUS-TBNA was superior compared to TBNA alone in diagnosing sarcoidosis.

5. Kim JS, Judson MA, Donnino R, et al. Cardiac sarcoidosis. *Am Heart J.* 2009;157(1):9–21.

   A comprehensive review of this rare but potentially fatal condition seen in some patients.

6. Victorson DE, Cella D, Judson MA. Quality of life evaluation in sarcoidosis: current status and future directions. *Curr Opin Pulm Med.* 2008;14(5):470–477.

   A review of health-related quality of life as a measure of relevant clinical information to assess patient status.

7. Rossman MD, Thompson B, Frederick M, et al. HLA and environmental interactions in sarcoidosis. *Sarcoidosis Vasc Diffuse Lung Dis.* 2008;25(2):125–132.

   A study of detailed environmental histories and high-resolution HLA class II typing in 476 cases, along with interactions of genetic predisposition and environmental exposure.

8. Judson MA, Baughman RP, Costabel U, et al. Efficacy of infliximab in extrapulmonary sarcoidosis: results from a randomised trial. *Eur Respir J.* 2008;31(6):1189–1196.

   The authors found that infliximab may be beneficial compared with placebo in extrapulmonary sarcoidosis in patients already receiving corticosteroids.

9. Moller DR. Potential etiologic agents in sarcoidosis. *Proc Am Thorac Soc.* 2007;4(5):465–468.

   A study and review about possible etiologies of sarcoidosis. The authors concluded that Mycobacterium tuberculosis catalase-peroxidase protein was a tissue antigen and target of the adaptative immune response in sarcoidosis, and, therefore, a possible etiology in a subset of patients.

10. Garwood S, Judson MA, Silvestri G, et al. Endobronchial ultrasound for the diagnosis of pulmonary sarcoidosis. *Chest.* 2007;132(4):1298–1304.

    A study of 50 patients to assess EBUS-TBNA as an emerging tool to diagnose mediastinal sarcoidosis. The authors concluded that EBUS-TBNA was a safe and minimally invasive diagnostic procedure.

11. Handa T, Nagai S, Miki S, et al. Incidence of pulmonary hypertension and its clinical relevance in patients with sarcoidosis. *Chest.* 2006;129(5):1246–1252.

    A study investigating the frequency of pulmonary hypertension using doppler echocardiography in 246 Japanese sarcoid patients.

12. Baughman RP, Drent M, Kavuru M, et al. Infliximab therapy in patients with chronic sarcoidosis and pulmonary involvement. *Am J Respir Crit Care Med.* 2006;174(7):795–802.

    The authors found significant improvement with infliximab suggesting its potential use in some severe and symptomatic cases.

13. Rybicki BA, Hirst K, Iyengar SK, et al. A sarcoidosis genetic linkage consortium: the Sarcoidosis Genetic Analysis (SAGA) study. *Sarcoidosis Vasc Diffuse Lung Dis.* 2005;22(2):115–122.

    A study intended to identify chromosomal regions that may harbor sarcoidosis susceptibility genes and identify environmental factors among African-Americans.

14. Newman LS, Rose CS, Bresnitz EA, et al. A case control etiologic study of sarcoidosis: environmental and occupational risk factors. *Am J Respir Crit Care Med.* 2004;170(12):1324–1330.

    A study intended to identify environmental and occupational exposures associated with sarcoidosis in 706 patients. The authors did not identify a single, predominant cause but several exposures associated with sarcoidosis risk.

15. Judson MA, Baughman RP, Thompson BW, et al. Two year prognosis of sarcoidosis: the ACCESS experience. *Sarcoidosis Vasc Diffuse Lung Dis.* 2003;20(3):204–211.

    A cohort of 215 patients across the United States underwent clinical evaluation at baseline and two years later. Factors associated with improved or worse outcome over 2 years were identified.

16. Paramothayan S, Jones PW. Corticosteroid therapy in pulmonary sarcoidosis: a systematic review. *JAMA.* 2002;287(10):1301–1307.

    An extensive literature review of the use of oral and inhaled corticosteroids in pulmonary sarcoidosis.

17. Mana J. Magnetic resonance imaging and nuclear imaging in sarcoidosis. *Curr Opin Pulm Med.* 2002;8(5):457–463.

    An excellent review of the different imaging modalities and their limitations in both intra- and extrathoracic sarcoidois, with emphasis on MRI.

18. Eishi Y, Suga M, Ishige I, et al. Quantitative analysis of mycobacterial and propionibacterial DNA in lymph nodes of Japanese and European patients with sarcoidosis. *J Clin Microbiol.* 2002;40(1):198–204.

    The authors analyzed 108 lymph nodes with sarcoidosis, 65 with tuberculosis, and 86 in controls for possible etiological links between sarcoidosis and suspected bacterial species in Europe and Japan.

19. Schurmann M, Reichel P, Muller-Myhsok B, et al. Results from a genome-wide search for predisposing genes in sarcoidosis. *Am J Respir Crit Care Med.* 2001;164(5):840–846.

    A GWAS analysis to identify chromosomal regions that contribute to the risk of sarcoidois.

20. Baughman RP, Teirstein AS, Judson MA, et al. Clinical characteristics of patients in a case control study of sarcoidosis. *Am J Respir Crit Care Med.* 2001;164(10, pt 1):1885–1889.

    Using the ACCESS sarcoidosis assessment system, the authors evaluated organ involvment in 736 patients and found that the initial presentation of sarcoidosis was related to gender, ethnicity, and age.

21. Baughman RP, Ohmichi M, Lower EE. Combination therapy for sarcoidosis. *Sarcoidosis Vasc Diffuse Lung Dis.* 2001;18(2):133–137.

    The authors discussed methods for implementing corticosteroid and alternative therapies to relieve and control disabling symptoms.

22. Johns CJ, Michele TM. The clinical management of sarcoidosis. A 50-year experience at the Johns Hopkins Hospital. *Medicine (Baltimore)*. 1999;78(2):65–111.

    A review of Johns Hopkins Sarcoid Clinic experience over the past 50 years, with discussion of diagnostic tools, treatment indications, follow-up, and unusual manifestations, including extrathoracic manifestations of sarcoidosis.

23. Hunninghake GW, Costabel U, Ando M, et al. ATS/ERS/WASOG statement on sarcoidosis. American Thoracic Society/European Respiratory Society/World Association of Sarcoidosis and other Granulomatous Disorders. *Sarcoidosis Vasc Diffuse Lung Dis*. 1999;16(2):149–173.

    Sarcoidosis is descriptively defined by the International Conference on Sarcoidosis. This article also reviews the clinical and radiologic diagnosis of sarcoid in addition to reviewing the etiology and genetics.

24. Kantrow SP, Meyer KC, Kidd P, et al. The CD4/CD8 ratio in BAL fluid is highly variable in sarcoidosis. *Eur Respir J*. 1997;10(12):2716–2721.

    Findings indicated that BAL-derived CD4:CD8 ratios failed to distinguish the presence of sarcoidosis among 86 patients with biopsy-proven disease, with a low sensitivity for this disease.

25. Moller DR, Forman JD, Liu MC, et al. Enhanced expression of IL-12 associated with Th1 cytokine profiles in active pulmonary sarcoidosis. *J Immunol*. 1996;156(12):4952–4960.

    The authors investigated the immunophathogenesis of sarcoidosis and idiopathic pulmonary fibrosis in BAL.

26. Levinson RS, Metzger LF, Stanley NN, et al. Airway function in sarcoidosis. *Am J Med*. 1977;62(1):51–59.

    In 18 patients with sarcoidosis, the authors found that airway dysfunction is common.

27. Beekman JF, Zimmet SM, Chun BK, et al. Spectrum of pleural involvement in sarcoidosis. *Arch Intern Med*. 1976;136(3):323–330.

    Results of this study demonstrate that clinical involvement of the pleura in sarcoidosis remains an unusual entity, but histologic involvment is more common than generally appreciated.

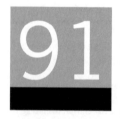

Granulomatosis with Polyangiitis (Wegener Granulomatosis)

Justin P. Stocks and Michael Tripp

Granulomatosis with polyangiitis (GPA), formerly known as Wegener granulomatosis (WG), is an idiopathic systemic vasculitis that may involve any organ system, but most frequently involves the upper respiratory tract, lungs, and kidneys. In a 2010 consensus statement, the American College of Rheumatology, the American Society of Nephrology, and the European League Against Rheumatism recommended changing the name of Wegener granulomatosis to shift the emphasis from an eponym-based label to a more disease-descriptive nomenclature.

GPA is a rare entity with an estimated annual incidence of 11.3 per million population. The estimated prevalence of GPA in the United States is 3.0 per 100,000 persons, with an equal male/female ratio. Caucasians are affected predominantly, comprising up to 95% in epidemiological studies. A class of autoantibodies known as antineutrophil cytoplasmic antibodies (ANCA) is closely associated with GPA and likely contributes to the pathogenesis of these disorders. Up to 90% of patients with GPA have involvement of the upper or lower respiratory tracts. Upper respiratory symptoms in GPA include chronic sinusitis, rhinorrhea, epistaxis, sinus pain, otitis media, and nasal or oral ulcerations. Tracheal involvement can lead to stenosis, obstruction, and stridor. Pulmonary symptoms may include cough, pleuritic chest pain, dyspnea, or hemoptysis. GPA can present as fulminating pulmonary hemorrhage leading to hypoxic respiratory failure or as acute lung injury with a systemic inflammatory response syndrome in 50% to 75% of acutely ill patients. Conversely, up to one-third of patients with pulmonary involvement may be asymptomatic. Other manifestations of GPA include arthralgias or myalgias, mono- or polyarthritis, constitutional symptoms, neurologic symptoms including mononeuritis multiplex, skin lesions, and pericarditis.

The diagnosis of GPA is made by a combination of clinical, radiographic, serological, and histopathological findings on biopsy. The presence of two or more American College of Rheumatology classification criteria (abnormal urinary sediment, characteristic chest radiograph abnormalities, oral ulcers or nasal discharge, and granulomatous inflammation on biopsy) has a sensitivity of 88% and a specificity of 92%. ANCA serologies are indicated in all patients. Pulmonary function abnormalities are nonspecific but may reveal an obstructive pattern, reflecting airway stenosis, or a reduction in carbon monoxide diffusion capacity (D_{LCO}) and lung volumes related to significant parenchymal disease. The definitive diagnosis of GPA is confirmed by tissue biopsy. Samples from the upper respiratory tract may demonstrate necrotizing granulomatous inflammation but have a sensitivity as low as 44% to 53%. In the presence of impaired renal function or active urinary sediment, renal biopsy can demonstrate a characteristic pattern of segmental necrotizing glomerulonephritis and is less invasive than surgical lung biopsy. Bronchoscopic abnormalities are nonspecific and may be found in up to 80% of patients with GPA; alveolar hemorrhage, sublgottic stenosis, and tracheobronchial and laryngeal inflammation are the most frequent findings. In one large bronchoscopic study of 197 patients with GPA, segmental stenosis and airway inflammation were most common and predominated in the right lung. Transbronchial lung biopsy is of limited usefulness in the diagnosis of pulmonary GPA, but it is valuable for excluding infection and evaluating hemoptysis. Nonspecific elevations in either neutrophils or lymphocytes have been described in alveolar lavage samples with no pathognomonic CD4/CD8 ratio. Progressively, hemorrhagic lavage aliquots may be seen in alveolar hemorrhage with associated hemosiderin-laden macrophages. Surgical lung biopsy is the gold standard for diagnosis of pulmonary GPA and may demonstrate a plethora findings, including, most commonly, neutrophilic microabscesses with necrosis, polymorphic granulomas with giant cells, angiitis with eccentric focal parietal crescent-shaped microabscesses, geographic necrosis surrounded by palisading histiocytes, and alveolar hemorrhage.

Radiographic findings in pulmonary GPA span a spectrum, including consolidation, solitary or multiple nodules that may cavitate, pleural effusions, parenchymal bands, and focal or diffuse ground-glass opacities. Computed tomography (CT) is superior to conventional chest radiography for detecting and characterizing pulmonary opacities. Lung nodules occur in 40% to 70% of patients, usually bilateral without segmental predilection, multiple in number, and with cavitation in up to 25% to 50% of cases. High-Resolution CT (HRCT) findings of nodules and areas of parenchymal opacification have been correlated directly with disease activity in multiple studies. Unilateral or bilateral pleural effusions may occur in up to 12% of patients. Enlarged mediastinal lymph nodes have been seen in 0% to 15% of patients, but bronchiectasis, honeycombing, pleural thickening, and pneumothorax are rare. Tracheobronchial stenosis may be appreciated on HRCT. Sinus radiographs may demonstrate air–fluid levels.

Renal involvement occurs in up to 80% of patients with GPA. Microscopic hematuria and red cell casts may be seen on urinalysis. Renal biopsies can demonstrate varying degrees of inflammation, from focal or segmental glomerulitis to rapidly progressing necrotizing glomerulonephritis. Immunofluorescence shows this to be a "pauci-immune" glomerulonephritis, with absent or minimal immunoglobulin deposits. Glomerulonephritis may precede pulmonary GPA by a period of months to years.

GPA is associated with a class of autoantibodies to specific antigens in neutrophils (ANCA) that are present in several forms of systemic vasculitis, including Churg–Strauss syndrome, polyarteritis nodosa, and microscopic polyangiitis. Two patterns of indirect immunofluorescence have been described: a diffuse cytoplasmic (cANCA) and a perinuclear pattern (pANCA). The specific antigens involved have been identified. Proteinase 3 (PR3) is the usual target of cANCA, and myeloperoxidase (MPO) is the most common target of pANCA. Approximately 90% of patients with active GPA are ANCA positive. The cANCA associated with GPA is almost always an anti-PR3 antibody. Therefore, it is prudent to confirm a finding of cANCA by a specific ELISA assay for anti-PR3 or anti-MPO. Up to 10% of patients with GPA do not have evidence of ANCA. Titers of ANCA correlate weakly with disease activity in two-thirds of patients.

Standard therapy is combination treatment with cyclophosphamide and prednisone. An initial oral dose of cyclophosphamide (2 mg/kg/day) is usually given in combination with prednisone (1 mg/kg/day). Prednisone is then tapered over 3 months to 0.25 mg/kg/day and continued for at least 1 year. Fulminant or life-threatening disease has been treated with higher doses of steroids, including pulse doses of intravenous methylprednisolone (up to 1,000 mg/day for 3 days), as well as higher doses of cyclophosphamide (up to 15 mg/kg intravenously). Plasmapheresis (40–60 mL/kg for 4–7 treatments) has been used to manage renal disease requiring dialysis and has been recommended in patients with severe pulmonary hemorrhage. Patients receiving cyclophosphamide and prednisone are at risk for *Pneumocystis jiroveci* pneumonia, and prophylactic therapy with cotrimoxazole is recommended.

Remission is reflected by the absence of clinical symptoms, inactive urinary sediment, and resolution of radiographic abnormalities; ANCA may be reduced or eliminated. Following remission, most authorities advocate continuing therapy for at least 12 months at lower doses. Cyclophosphamide therapy is associated with significant adverse effects, including hemorrhagic cystitis, increased risk of bladder cancer, myelodysplasia, and lymphoproliferative disorders. Alternative agents such as azathioprine, low-dose methotrexate, cotrimoxazole, mycophenolate mofetil, and leflunomide have shown efficacy for maintaining remission when administered with continued low-dose prednisone. Relapses of GPA are treated by resuming or increasing doses of cyclophosphamide and prednisone until clinical remission is attained. Monthly pulse cyclophosphamide therapy results in higher relapse rates with no effect on morbidity or mortality compared to a daily oral regimen. Fulminant relapses may require the reinstitution of induction therapy. While the anti-tumor necrosis factor agent etanercept has not been shown to be effective for remission, infliximab has shown benefit for the treatment of GPA. The anti-CD20 monoclonal rituximab is being investigated for benefit in GPA.

In summary, GPA is a multisystem disease with several life-threatening pulmonary manifestations. The diagnosis can be made with a combination of serology, clinical examination, and findings obtained through standard pulmonary procedures. Treatment should be started with immune suppression immediately and aggressively for pulmonary conditions such as alveolar hemorrhage and necrotizing granulomas. Less-fulminant presentations such as sinus inflammation and tracheal stenosis may be the first signs of disease. The prognosis of GPA is guarded and depends upon prompt recognition, treatment, and surveillance of relapses, which may require repeat induction therapy. The overall median survival of patients with GPA exceeds 20 years. GPA patients are best managed with a team of physicians to include rheumatologists, nephrologists, and pulmonologists who are familiar with the complex pathophysiology of GPA and management with chronic immunosuppressant medications.

FURTHER READING

1. Falk RJ, Gross WL, Guillevin L, et al. Granulomatosis with polyangiitis (Wegener's): an alternative name for Wegener's granulomatosis. *Arthritis Rheum*. 2011;63:863–864.

   Rationale and recommendations for changing name of Wegner granulomatosis to granulomatosis with polyangiitis.

2. Watts RA, Mooney J, Skinner J, et al. The contrasting epidemiology of granulomatosis with polyangiitis (Wegener's) and microscopic polyangiitis. *Rheumatology*. 2012;51(5):926–931.

   A large prospective epidemiological study in Europe evaluating incidence of GPA and microscopic polyangiitis.

3. Cotch MF, Hoffman GS, Yerg DE, et al. The epidemiology of Wegener's granulomatosis. *Arthritis Rheum*. 1996;39:87–92.

   Epidemiology of GPA in the United States of America including prevalence and mortality.

4. Stevic R, Jovanović D, Obradović LN, et al. Wegener's granulomatosis: clinic-radiological finding at initial presentation. *Coll Antropol*. 2012;36:505–511.

   A retrospective Serbian review of 37 GPA patient records and initial clinical and radiographic findings.

5. Khan AM, Jariwala S, Appel D, et al. Wegener's granulomatosis: predicting mortality/morbidity in those with pulmonary manifestations. *Chest.* 2008;134:(4 Meeting Abstracts):p128003.

   A retrospective review evaluating presenting symptoms, initial presentations, morbidity and mortality of 20 patients with GPA admitted to the intensive care unit.

6. Klein LW, Polychronopolus VS, Golbin JM, et al. Frequency and location of tracheobronchial lesions in Wegener granulomatosis. *Chest.* 2008;134:(4 Meeting Abstracts):s13002.

   A chart review of 197 patients at Mayo Clinic diagnosed with GPA and associated bronchoscopic findings. Seventy-one percent of patients had abnormal bronchoscopies. Tracheal inflammation, subglottic stenosis, and alveolar hemorrhage were the most common abnormal findings on bronchoscopy.

7. Ananthakrishnan L, Sharma N, Kanne JP. Wegener's granulomatosis in the chest: high-resolution CT findings. *AJR Am J Roentgenol.* 2009;192:676–682.

   An excellent review of spectrum of HRCT findings in GPA with associated frequencies and numerous pictures.

8. Zycinska K, Wardyn KA, Zycinski Z, et al. Association between clinical activity and high-resolution tomography findings in pulmonary Wegener's granulomatosis. *J Physiol Pharmacol.* 2008;59:833–838.

   A cohort study of GPA disease activity correlating with HRCT findings in 66 patients.

9. Reuter M, Schnabel A, Wesner F, et al. Pulmonary Wegener's granulomatosis: correlation between high-resolution CT findings and clinical scoring of disease activity. *Chest.* 1998;114:500–506.

   A pilot study of 73 GPA patients correlating disease activity with specific HRCT abnormalities.

10. Martinez F, Chung JH, Digumarthy SR, et al. Common and uncommon manifestations of Wegener's granulomatosis at chest CT: radiologic-pathologic correlation. *Radiographics.* 2012;32:51–69.

    Published online (doi:10.1148/rg.321115060). Excellent review of common and rare radiographic manifestations of GPA.

11. Manna R, Cadoni G, Ferri E, et al. Wegener's granulomatosis: an update on diagnosis and therapy. *Expert Rev Clin Immunol.* 2008;4:481–485.

    A review article of GPA diagnosis and therapy.

12. Leavitt RY, Fauci AS, Bloch DA, et al. The American College of Rheumatology 1990 criteria for the classification of Wegener's granulomatosis. *Arthritis Rheum.* 1990;33:1101–1107.

13. Jennette JC, Falk RJ, Andrassy K, et al. Nomenclature of systemic vasculitides. *Arthritis Rheum.* 1994;37:187–192.

    Chapel Hill consensus criteria.

14. Watts R, Lane S, Hanslik T, et al. Development and validation of a consensus methodology for the classification of the ANCA-associated vasculitides and polyarteritis nodosa for the epidemiological studies. *Ann Rheum Dis.* 2007;66:222–227.

    A validation of an updated algorithm for the diagnosis of GPA.

15. Polychronopoulos VS, Prakash UB, Golbin JM, et al. Airway involvement in Wegener's granulomatosis. *Rheum Dis Clin North Am.* 2007;33:755–775.

    A comprehensive review of PFTs and associated airway abnormalities in patients with pulmonary GPA.

16. Borner U, Landis BN, Banz Y, et al. Diagnostic value of biopsies in identifying cytoplasmic antineutrophil cytoplasmic antibody-negative localized Wegener's granulomatosis presenting primarily with sinonasal disease. *Am J Rhinol Allergy.* 2012;26:475–480.

    A retrospective review of 82 GPA patients with nasal biopsies. The sensitivity of nasal biopsy was 44% for patients with generalized GPA.

17. Traveis WD, Hoffman GS, Leavitt RY, et al. Surgical pathology of the lung in Wegener's granulomatosis. *Am J Surg Pathol.* 1991;15:315–333.

    A retrospective review of surgical lung pathology in 87 lung biopsies from 67 GPA patients with frequencies of pathognomic and uncommon findings.

18. Harper L, Morgan MD, Walsh M, et al. Pulse versus daily oral cyclophosphamide for induction of remission in ANCA-associated vasculitis: long-term follow-up. *Ann Rheum Dis.* 2012;71:955–960.

    Pulse cyclophosphamide was associated with almost 40% relapse rate compared to 20% relapse in patients treated with oral daily cyclophosphamide.

19. Csernok E. Anti-neutrophil cytoplasmic antibodies and pathogenesis of small vessel vasculitidies. *Autoimmun Rev.* 2003;2:158.

   A review of work to date establishing that ANCA are directly involved in the pathogenesis of WG and related disorders.

20. DeGroot K, Reinhold-Keller E, Tatsis E, et al. Therapy for the maintenance of remission in sixty-five patients with generalized Wegener's granulomatosis: methotrexate versus trimethoprim/sulfamethoxazole. *Arthritis Rheum.* 1996;39:2052–2061.

   Methotrexate maintained remissions in 86% of patients compared to 58% given trimethoprim–sulfamethoxazole.

21. Fauci AS, Haynes BF, Katz P, et al. Wegener's granulomatosis: prospective clinical and therapeutic experience with 85 patients for 21 years. *Ann Intern Med.* 1983;98:76.

   Reports the National Institutes of Health (NIH) experience and confirms the efficacy of cyclophosphamide as a potentially curative agent.

22. Hoffman G, Kerr GS, Leavitt RY, et al. Wegener granulomatosis: an analysis of 158 patients. *Ann Intern Med.* 1992;116:488.

   A long-term follow-up of the NIH trials, confirming the benefit of cyclophosphamide, but raising concerns about the frequency of relapse and toxicity of treatment.

23. Jayne D, Rasmussen N, Andrassy K, et al. A randomized trial of maintenance therapy for vasculitis associated with antineutrophil cytoplasmic antibodies. *N Engl J Med.* 2003;349:36.

   Documents the efficacy of azathioprine as maintenance therapy after induction of remission. Of patients receiving azathioprine, 15.5% suffered relapses.

24. Kyndt X, Reumaux D, Bridoux F, et al. Serial measurements of antineutrophil cytoplasmic antibodies in patients with systemic vasculitis. *Am J Med.* 1999;106:527.

   The predictive value of a rise in cANCA for a subsequent relapse of WG was only 28%.

25. Langford C, Talar-Williams C, Barron KS, et al. Use of a cyclophosphamide-induction methotrexate maintenance regimen for the treatment of Wegener's granulomatosis: extended follow-up and rate of relapse. *Am J Med.* 2003;114:463.

   Methotrexate given for maintenance therapy was well tolerated but had a 52% rate of relapse.

26. Ognibene F, Shelhamer JH, Hoffman GS, et al. *Pneumocystis carinii* pneumonia: a major complication of immunosuppressive therapy in patients with Wegener's granulomatosis. *Am J Respir Crit Care Med.* 1995;151:795.

   Six percent of patients treated for WG developed P. carinii pneumonia.

27. Reinhold-Keller E, Beuge N, Latza U, et al. An interdisciplinary approach to the care of patients with Wegener's granulomatosis: long-term outcome in 155 patients. *Arthritis Rheum.* 2000;43:1021.

   A review of patients treated with cyclophosphamide and prednisone; complete remission occurred in 83 of 155. Drug toxicity was a significant problem, especially when total cyclophosphamide dose equaled 100 g.

28. Stegemen CA, Tervaert JWC, deJong PE, et al. Trimethoprim-sulfamethoxazole for the prevention of relapses of Wegener's granulomatosis. *N Engl J Med.* 1996;335:16.

   Eighty-one patients were randomized to receive either trimethoprim-sulfamethoxazole (TMP/SMX) or placebo. The relative risk of relapse for patients given SPM/SMX was 0.40 over 24 months.

29. Schnabel A, Holl-Ulrich K, Dalhoff K, et al. Efficacy of transbronchial biopsy in pulmonary vasculitides. *Eur Respir J.* 1997;10:2738.

   Transbronchial biopsy had a low yield in WG, but bronchoscopic biopsy of upper airway lesions was useful. Biopsy of upper respiratory tract lesions had the highest yield in WG.

30. Seo P, Stone J. The antineutrophil cytoplasmic antibody-associated vasculitides. *Am J Med.* 2004;117:39.

   A comprehensive review of clinical manifestations, diagnosis, and treatment of WG and other ANCA-associated diseases.

92 Goodpasture Syndrome

Omar H. Mohamedaly

Goodpasture syndrome refers to the pulmonary–renal syndrome of diffuse alveolar hemorrhage (DAH) and glomerulonephritis. The term often is used interchangeably with Goodpasture disease, although, strictly speaking, the term *disease* should be restricted to the presence of circulating or tissue-bound antiglomerular basement membrane antibody (AGBMA), while the term *syndrome* may be applied to any pathogenesis. The term AGBMA disease may be more appropriate and, to avoid confusion, will be used in this chapter.

Interestingly, the original description of the eponymous syndrome by American pathologist Ernest Goodpasture at Vanderbilt University in 1919 was likely referring to a vasculitis rather than what we now refer to as AGBMA disease. It was the case of an 18-year-old man who died 6 weeks after influenza infection and was found to have DAH, glomerulonephritis, splenic infarcts, and vasculitis of the small bowel. This case report does highlight salient features that have been shown to be important in AGBMA disease.

As the term AGBMA disease implies, it is an autoimmune disorder resembling a type II hypersensitivity reaction. The AGBMA itself, first identified in 1965, is now known to target the noncollagenous-1 (NC1) domain of the α3 chain of type IV collagen. Expression of the α3 chain is highest in glomerular and alveolar basement membranes, which explains the clinical syndrome of DAH and glomerulonephritis in AGBMA disease. α3 Chain expression is also found, though at much lower levels, in renal tubular basement membranes, choroid plexus, cochlea, and retina.

AGBMA disease is a rare disease with a reported incidence of about one patient per million population. It may, however, be responsible for up to 20% of all cases of rapidly progressive glomerulonephritis. Prevalence data are difficult to assess. A bimodal distribution has been described with slight male predominance in younger patients in the third decade and equal sex distribution to a slight female predominance in older patients in the sixth and seventh decades. The younger group is more likely to present with the full pulmonary–renal syndrome, while older patients tend to have disease limited to the kidneys.

In about 60% to 80% of cases, pulmonary and renal diseases present simultaneously; however, pulmonary disease may appear up to 12 months prior to renal disease. In about 5% to 10% of cases, lung involvement occurs alone. It is worth noting, though, that even in the absence of overt renal disease, AGBMA deposits are often found in the glomeruli if kidney biopsy is performed.

Pulmonary symptoms are most common on presentation, including hemoptysis, cough, and/or dyspnea. The degree of hemoptysis varies considerably; it can be minimal or life-threatening. Glomerulonephritis rarely manifests with hypertension and gross hematuria. Fatigue related to renal failure is more common. Fever may be present, especially in the context of antecedent flu-like symptoms or upper respiratory tract infection. However, other systemic symptoms such as malaise, weight loss, arthralgia, and myalgia should raise suspicion for vasculitis.

Laboratory evaluation may reveal iron-deficiency anemia related to alveolar hemorrhage. Urinary sediment is active with microscopic hematuria, nonnephrotic range proteinuria, and, occasionally, erythrocyte casts or dysmorphic erythrocytes. Serum creatinine is often elevated. Complement levels are normal; reduced C3 and/or C4 should point to vasculitis or alternative diagnoses as the cause of the pulmonary–renal syndrome. Circulating AGBMA can be detected in greater than 90% of patients presenting with AGBMA disease. Positive antineutrophil cytoplasmic antibody (ANCA) titers may be found in up to 30% of cases.

Imaging tends to be nonspecific. Chest radiographs often show diffuse symmetric airspace opacities and, less commonly, asymmetric, focal, or interstitial opacities. Pleural effusions are rare in the absence of concomitant volume overload or infection. Pulmonary infiltrates usually resolve over days. Occasionally, the chest radiograph can be normal despite a history of hemoptysis. Chest computed tomography is reportedly more sensitive for DAH than plain radiography and can demonstrate ground-glass opacities and consolidation, though such findings are hardly specific for DAH.

During active alveolar hemorrhage, pulmonary function tests reveal an increase in the diffusing capacity of the lung for carbon monoxide (DLCO), reflecting the presence of abundant erythrocytes in the alveolar space creating a large diffusion sink for CO to which hemoglobin has a high affinity. An increase in DLCO above 30% of predicted normal has been suggested as an indicator of widespread intra-alveolar hemorrhage. Such an increase may precede clinical and radiographic changes and can, therefore, be used in monitoring for recurrence of DAH.

AGBMA titers do not always correlate with disease activity, though they are generally useful for monitoring. Higher levels are thought to indicate more severe renal disease. The most commonly used assay is an enzyme-linked immunosorbent antibody (ELISA) assay which has a sensitivity of 70% to 100% depending on the specific antigen used. Assays using native or recombinant human α3 (IV) antigen substrates have a reported sensitivity of 95% to 100% and specificity of 91% to 100%. Confirmatory Western blot is performed at many centers.

The pathogenicity of AGBMA was demonstrated in a classic experiment in which antibodies isolated from serum or renal eluate samples of patients with Goodpasture syndrome induced glomerulonephritis in recipient monkeys. Interestingly, in some animal models AGBMA leads to renal but not pulmonary disease. After identification of the epitope as the α3 (IV) chain with its cDNA mapped to chromosome 2q35-37, it was cloned and shown to induce expression of the protein bound by AGBMA when transfected into cells. These antibodies are typically of the IgG 1 or 3 subclass and less commonly of the IgA or IgM class. They do not bind native cross-linked α-3,4,5 hexamers until they are dissociated. Autoreactive T cells have also been implicated in the pathogenesis of AGBMA disease. T cells specific for the NC1 domain of the α3 (IV) chain have been found at higher frequency in patients with AGBMA disease than in controls. There is also growing evidence that effector T cells may contribute directly to injury and that $CD4^+$ $CD25^+$ regulatory T cells may facilitate the autoimmune response seen in AGBMA disease.

The inciting factor triggering the autoimmune response remains unknown. A combination of environmental and genetic factors is most likely. Temporal association between development of AGBMA disease and various infections and exposures suggests the role for some injurious stimulus that exposes previously concealed basement membrane epitopes that either stimulate an autoimmune response or, more likely, are attacked by already circulating autoreactive antibodies and T cells. The association with influenza infection, first described by Goodpasture himself, has subsequently been reported in larger series. Other upper respiratory tract infections, hydrocarbon exposure, and tobacco use have all been implicated as well. In one study, 100% of smokers with AGBMA disease developed both DAH and glomerulonephritis, whereas only 20% of nonsmokers developed DAH, suggesting that direct pulmonary insult is needed to precipitate DAH in AGBMA disease. Similarly, there are reports of AGBMA disease occurring rarely after lithotripsy or in the presence of urinary tract infection or other glomerulonephritis conditions. Genetic predisposition is suggested by the presence of HLA-DR2 and HLA-B7 in 90% and 60% of AGBMA disease patients, respectively. HLA-DRw15, a subtype of DR2, and DR4 in particular increase the risk of AGBMA disease. Disease susceptibility is most likely conferred by a common 6-amino acid motif found in these antigens, which are uncommon in blacks who have a lower incidence of the disease. DR1 and DR7 portend a lower risk of AGBMA disease.

On histopathological examination, lung biopsy specimens typically demonstrate bland pulmonary hemorrhage with intra-alveolar erythrocytes and hemosiderin-laden macrophages. Much less commonly, pulmonary capillaritis may be seen. Alveolar wall necrosis as seen in pulmonary vasculitis is uncommon. Kidney biopsy reveals focal segmental necrotizing glomerulonephritis with crescent formation. Immunofluorescence reveals the pathognomonic finding of uninterrupted linear deposition of IgG along the glomerular basement membrane. In 60% to 70% of biopsies, linear C3 deposition is also seen. Similar appearance on immunofluorescence can be found in lung biopsies as well, though these are more technically challenging to demonstrate. Typical staining can be found in kidney biopsies even in the absence of overt renal disease.

Treatment strategies are aimed at removing circulating antibodies as well as preventing new antibody formation. Isolated DAH responds to corticosteroids, though glomerulonephritis is typically resistant to corticosteroid monotherapy. The mainstay of therapy is the combination of plasmapheresis, corticosteroids, and immunosuppressives. Plasmapheresis is typically performed daily or every other day for 2 to 3 weeks with volumes of 3 to 6 L per session. The only randomized controlled trial was a small study in which two of eight patients receiving plasmapheresis progressed to dialysis dependence, compared with six of nine patients who were not plasmapheresed. The benefit, however, seemed to correlate with the serum creatinine level and percent of crescents found on renal biopsy. Nevertheless, the biological plausibility of AGBMA removal with plasmapheresis, as well as observations that AGBMA titers, declines more rapidly in patients receiving a plasmapheresis in addition to corticosteroids, and immunosuppressives (compared with those receiving corticosteroids and immunosuppressives alone) led to the recommendation of plasmapheresis for all patients with AGBMA disease.

Corticosteroids are typically administered with an initial pulse dose (methylprednisolone 15–30 mg/kg/day to a max of 1,000 mg/day for 3 days) followed by prednisone 1 mg/kg/day to a maximum of 60 to 80 mg/d. The immunosuppressive agent most often used is cyclophosphamide at 2 mg/kg/day; the dose is usually capped at 100 mg/day in elderly patients to avoid drug toxicity. Daily cyclophosphamide therapy is favored over intermittent intravenous dosing, since durable remissions are more likely with daily therapy. Once remission is achieved, steroids can be tapered gradually and a less toxic immunosuppressive agent, such as azathioprine, may be substituted for cyclophosphamide. Maintenance therapy is generally continued for 6 to 9 months, though larger series suggest that 2 to 3 months may be sufficient, given the low risk of recurrence. AGBMA titers are usually measured every 1 to 2 weeks during therapy until they are negative on two occasions. Expert opinion suggests monitoring for 6 months thereafter to ensure continued remission. Case reports of treatment with rituximab and mycophenolate mofetil also have been published. Newer therapies include immunoadsorption and T-cell targeting techniques. Immunoadsorption involves the use of a sepharose-coupled sheep-antihuman IgG column that has been shown to be of benefit when added to immunosuppression in one case report. T-cell targeted therapy is still in the animal model stage; a fusion protein that blocks the CD28-B7 costimulatory pathway for T-cell activation was shown to prevent crescentic glomerulonephritis in a murine model. Renal transplantation is necessary when there is no recovery of renal function; it is typically delayed until AGBMA has been undetectable for 9 to 12 months. Recurrence of AGBMA disease is responsible for 14% of graft failures.

The prognosis of AGBMA disease has improved from the originally described 80% mortality at 6 months. However, the overall 5-year survival is still low at 50%. Certain prognostic factors portend different mortality risks. The two most important such factors are serum creatinine and the extent of crescent formation on renal biopsy. Values under 3 mg/dL and 30%, respectively, are associated with better outcomes. The presence of greater than 90% crescents on biopsy is almost always associated with poor renal and overall patient outcome. Similarly, immediate hemodialysis, defined as the need for dialysis within the first 72 hours of disease presentation, is a poor prognostic factor. In one large retrospective review of 71 patients, those with a Cr of less than 5.7 mg/dL had a patient and renal survival of 100% and 95%, respectively, at one year and 84% and 74%, respectively, at final follow-up (median 90 months). If Cr was more than 5.7 mg/dL, but there was no immediate need for dialysis, patient and renal survival were 83% and 82%, respectively, at one year and 72% and 69%, respectively, at final follow-up. Immediate dialysis conferred the worst prognosis, with patient and renal survival at 65% and 8%, respectively, at one year and 36% and 5%, respectively, at final follow-up. DAH, on the other hand, resolved in 90% of patients. Relapses are uncommon, reported at 2% in one center's experience, and may be associated with smoking and hydrocarbon exposure. ANCA positivity is of unclear significance; a role in pathogenesis seems unlikely, given the fact that it occurs in no more than 30% of AGBMA disease cases, though a recent case-control study demonstrated the presence of ANCA positivity years prior to the development of clinical AGBMA disease. From a prognostic standpoint, patients with AGBMA disease who are ANCA positive seem to have better prognosis, though current episode of ANCA-related vasculitis is seen commonly in such patients.

FURTHER READING

1. Goodpasture EW. The significance of certain pulmonary lesions in relation to the etiology of influenza. *Am J Med Sci.* 1919;158:863–870.

   The original report of a patient with DAH, glomerulonephritis, splenic infarcts, and small bowel vasculitis after influenza infection. This was likely a vasculitis rather than true AGBMA disease, but remains the reason Dr. Goodpasture is credited with the pulmonary–renal syndrome.

2. Stanton MC, Tange JD. Goodpasture's syndrome. *Aust N Z J Med.* 1958;7:132–144.

   The first use of the term Goodpasture syndrome.

3. Cashman SJ, Pusey CD, Evans DJ. Extraglomerular distribution of immunoreactive Goodpasture antigen. *J Pathol.* 1988;155:61–70.

   The distribution of the α3 (IV) chain in extraglomerular tissues.

4. Pusey CD. Anti-glomerular basement membrane disease. *Kidney Int.* 2003;64:1535–1550.

   A great review that is particularly strong on the research into the pathogenesis of AGBMA disease.

5. Wilson CB, Dixon FJ. Anti-glomerular basement membrane antibody-induced glomerulonephritis. *Kidney Int.* 1973;3:74–89.

   A classic review article of AGBMA glomerulonephritis summarizing state of knowledge at the time.

6. Segelmark M, Hellmark T. Autoimmune kidney diseases. *Autoimmun Rev.* 2010;9:366–371.

   A review article of four immune-mediated types of glomerulonephritis: AGBMA disease, IgA nephritis, membranous nephropathy, and membranoproliferative glomerulonephritis.

7. Lazor R, Bigay-Gamé L, Cottin V, et al. Alveolar hemorrhage in anti-basement membrane antibody disease: a series of 28 cases. *Medicine (Baltimore).* 2007;86:181–193.

   A retrospective review of 28 cases of AGMBA disease. Tobacco and other inhalational exposures were common. Renal outcome was excellent in patients with predominant pulmonary involvement. Of interest, D_{LCO} was increased in only 25% of patients with alveolar hemorrhage. Bronchoalveolar lavage was most sensitive for detection of alveolar hemorrhage.

8. Lahmer T, Heemann U. Anti-glomerular basement membrane antibody disease: a rare autoimmune disorder affecting the kidney and lung. *Autoimmun Rev.* 2012;12:169–173.

   Another good review article of AGBMA disease.

9. Kluth DC, Rees AJ. Anti-glomerular basement membrane disease. *J Am Soc Nephrol.* 1999;10:2446–2453.

   A good review article of AGBMA disease with a section on recurrence and description of AGBMA disease after renal transplantation in patients with Alport disease.

10. Ewan PW, Jones HA, Rhodes CG, et al. Detection of intrapulmonary hemorrhage with carbon monoxide uptake: appreciation in Goodpasture's syndrome. *N Engl J Med.* 1976;295:1391–1396.

    An early description of the role of D_{LCO} measurement in detection of pulmonary hemorrhage and its use for monitoring purposes. This study also describes the ratio of CO uptake to clearance using the radioisotope $C^{15}O$ during breath holding to differentiate between Goodpasture syndrome patients with and without pulmonary hemorrhage.

11. Primack SL, Miller RR, Müller NL. Diffuse pulmonary hemorrhage: clinical, pathologic, and imaging features. *AJR Am J Roentgenol.* 1995;164:295–300.

    A good review of the clinical, pathologic, and radiographic features of diffuse pulmonary hemorrhage as well as treatment of common causes.

12. Lerner RA, Glassock RJ, Dixon FJ. The role of anti-glomerular basement membrane antibody in the pathogenesis of human glomerulonephritis. *J Exp Med.* 1967;126:989–1004.

    A description of a classic experiment in which AGBMA eluted from patients' kidneys was shown to induce glomerulonephritis in recipient monkeys.

13. Pedchenko V, Bondar O, Fogo AB, et al. Molecular architecture of the Goodpasture autoantigen in anti-GBM nephritis. *N Engl J Med.* 2010;363:343–354.

    An ELISA-based study of the epitopes bound by circulating and kidney-bound AGBMA suggesting conformational changes in the quaternary structure of the α-3,4,5-NC1 hexamer that exposes epitopes selectively recognized and bound by AGBMA, specifically α3-NC1 and α4-NC1 monomers.

14. Salama AD, Pusey CD. Immunology of anti-glomerular basement membrane disease. *Curr Opin Nephrol Hypertens.* 2002;11:279–286.

A good review of the molecular pathogenesis of AGBMA disease focusing on the humoral and cellular immune mechanisms involved in disease initiation and perpetuation.

15. Queluz TH, Pawlowski I, Brunda MJ, et al. Pathogenesis of an experimental model of Goodpasture's hemorrhagic pneumonitis. *J Clin Invest.* 1990;85:1507–1515.

An interesting animal model study of the role of cytokines in the pathogenesis of pulmonary hemorrhage in Goodpasture syndrome, presumably by increasing alveolar endothelial permeability and thus granting circulating AGBMA access to the alveolar basement membrane. Naïve mice with normal lungs had no pulmonary hemorrhage when injected with rabbit AGBMA alone, but did have the pathologic findings of Goodpasture hemorrhagic pneumonitis when pretreated with human recombinant IL-2 and IFN-α. Interestingly, the synergy of both IL-2 and IFN-α was required in this murine model.

16. Donaghy M, Rees AJ. Cigarette smoking and lung haemorrhage in glomerulonephritis caused by autoantibodies to glomerular basement membrane. *Lancet.* 1983;2:1390–1393.

A case-control study of patients with glomerulonephritis caused by AGBMA. Thirty-seven of 37 smokers compared to 2/10 nonsmokers had pulmonary hemorrhage with no significant difference in the titers of circulating AGBMA. In one patient, resumption of smoking was followed by recurrence of pulmonary hemorrhage.

17. Fisher M, Pusey CD, Vaughan RW, et al. Susceptibility to anti-glomerular basement membrane disease is strongly associated with HLA-DRB1 genes. *Kidney Int.* 1997;51:222–229.

An analysis of the HLA-DRB and DQB alleles inherited by 82 patients demonstrating a hierarchy of association of DRB1 genes with AGBMA disease: susceptibility alleles (DRB1*15, DRB1*04), neutral alleles (DRB1*03), and protective alleles (DRB1*07). Further sequencing localized the segment conferring susceptibility or protection to the second peptide binding region of the HLA class II antigen binding groove.

18. Phelps RG, Rees AJ. The HLA complex in Goodpasture's disease: a model for analyzing susceptibility to autoimmunity. *Kidney Int.* 1999;56:1638–1653.

A thorough analysis of the HLA associations with Goodpasture disease and examination of the molecular mechanisms (including antigen-HLA interaction and antigen presentation to T cells) that could account for the observed HLA associations.

19. Litwin CM, Mouritsen CL, Wilfahrt PA, et al. Anti-glomerular basement membrane disease: role of enzyme-linked immunosorbent assays in diagnosis. *Biochem Mol Med.* 1996;59:52–56.

A comparison of two ELISA assays to indirect immunofluorescence for the measurement of AGBMA. Sensitivity was high at 93.3% for one ELISA assay, but much lower at 63.3% for the other.

20. Sinico RA, Radice A, Corace C, et al. Anti-glomerular basement membrane antibodies in the diagnosis of Goodpasture syndrome: a comparison of different assays. *Nephrol Dial Transplant.* 2006;21(2):397–401.

A comparison of performance characteristics of four immunoassay-based AGBMA kits. All assays showed sensitivities between 94.7% and 100%, but specificity varied significantly between 90.9% and 100%. Higher specificity was observed in a fluorescence immunoassay that uses a recombinant antigen.

21. Merkel F, Kalluri R, Marx M, et al. Autoreactive T-cells in Goodpasture's syndrome recognize the N-terminal NC1 domain on alpha 3 type IV collagen. *Kidney Int.* 1996;49:1127–1133.

First report of the involvement of autoreactive T cells in the pathogenesis of Goodpasture syndrome. T cells from patients and controls were isolated and stimulated by purified native or recombinant type IV collagen proteins and synthetic oligopeptides. Clones specific to the NC1 domain of α3 chain of type IV collagen were found in patients, but not in controls.

22. Salama AD, Chaudhry AN, Ryan JJ, et al. In Goodpasture's disease, CD4+ T cells escape thymic deletion and are reactive with the autoantigen a3(IV)NC1. *J Am Soc Nephrol.* 2001;12:1908–1915.

An interesting study on the role of autoreactive T cells in the pathogenesis of Goodpasture syndrome. Immunohistochemistry and RT-PCR were used to demonstrate expression of the Goodpasture antigen in normal human thymus. The frequency of circulating autoreactive T cells in patients and controls was then assessed using limiting dilution analyses and found to be higher in patients during active disease and decreasing over time, consistent with the observed low frequency of recurrence.

23. Lombard CM, Colby TV, Elliott CG. Surgical pathology of the lung in anti-basement membrane antibody-associated Goodpasture's syndrome. *Hum Pathol.* 1989;20:445–451.

A report of surgical lung biopsies from five patients with AGBMA disease. Pulmonary capillaritis and alveolar hemorrhage were seen in four biopsies; diffuse alveolar damage was the dominant finding in the fifth biopsy specimen.

24. Abboud RT, Chase WH, Ballon HS, et al. Goodpasture's syndrome: diagnosis by transbronchial lung biopsy. *Ann Intern Med.* 1978;89:635–638.

A case report of a 28-year-old man with hemoptysis and pulmonary infiltrates whose transbronchial lung biopsy showed RBCs, iron-containing alveolar macrophages, and normal basement membranes with positive linear staining for IgG. Renal biopsy showed similar immunofluorescent staining despite the absence of clinical renal involvement.

25. Zimmerman SW, Varanasi UR, Hoff B. Goodpasture's syndrome with normal renal function. *Am J Med.* 1979;66:163–171.

Two case reports of patients with Goodpasture syndrome presenting predominantly with pulmonary hemorrhage but minimal renal manifestations (microscopic hematuria in both, transient protein-uria in one) with normal creatinine. Renal biopsies in both patients showed linear IgG deposition on immunofluorescence.

26. Keogh AM, Ibels LS, Allen DH, et al. Exacerbation of Goodpasture's syndrome after inadvertent exposure to hydrocarbon fumes. *Br Med J.* 1984;288:188.

A case report of a 16-year-old girl who developed Goodpasture syndrome after exposure to hydrocarbon fumes at her job as a bank teller with disease recurrence after exposure to hydrocarbon-containing insect repellant spray.

27. Jindal KK. Management of idiopathic crescentic and diffuse proliferative glomerulonephritis: evidence-based recommendations. *Kidney Int Suppl.* 1999;70:33–40.

An evidence-based review of the treatment options for several diseases associated with crescentic glomerulonephritis, including the data behind the 2-week course of plasmapheresis and 2 months of treatment with corticosteroids and cyclophosphamide for AGBMA disease.

28. Levy JB, Turner AN, Rees AJ, et al. Long-term outcome of anti-glomerular basement membrane antibody disease treated with plasma exchange and immunosuppression. *Ann Intern Med.* 2001;134:1033–1042.

A retrospective review of all patients with AGBMA disease treated with plasmapheresis, prednisolone, and cyclophosphamide—stratified patient and renal survival based on entry serum creatinine levels above versus below 5.7 mg/dL.

29. Johnson JP, Moore J Jr, Wilson CB, et al. Therapy of anti-glomerular basement membrane an-tibody disease: analysis of prognostic significance of clinical, pathologic and treatment factors. *Medicine (Baltimore).* 1985;64:219–227.

A small case-control study of patients with AGBMA disease receiving immunosuppression alone or with plasmapheresis showing more rapid clearing of AGBMA titers and improvement in serum creatinine with combination therapy. However, subgroup analysis showed better outcome prediction based on de-gree of crescent involvement on initial renal biopsy and entry serum creatinine level.

30. Arzoo K, Sadeghi S, Liebman HA. Treatment of refractory antibody mediated autoimmune disor-ders with an anti-CD20 monoclonal antibody (rituximab). *Ann Rheum Dis.* 2002;61:922–924.

Three case reports of successful treatment of refractory autoimmune conditions with rituximab; one of the case reports is of a patient with Goodpasture syndrome presenting with hemoptysis and hematuria refractory to cyclophosphamide, prednisone, and plasmapheresis.

31. Garcia-Canton C, Toledo A, Palomar R, et al. Goodpasture's syndrome treated with mycopheno-late mofetil. *Nephrol Dial Transplant.* 2000;15:920–922.

A case report of a patient with Goodpasture syndrome whose DAH relapsed several times despite conven-tional therapy and responded to mycophenolate mofetil.

32. Laczika K, Derfler K, Soleiman A, et al. Immunoadsorption in Goodpasture's syndrome. *Am J Kidney Dis.* 2000;36:392–395.

A case report of a patient with Goodpasture syndrome and advanced hemodialysis-dependent renal failure whose renal function recovered with initiation of immunoadsorption in conjunction with immunosuppression.

33. Reynolds J, Tam FW, Chandraker A, et al. CD28-B7 blockade prevents the development of experimental autoimmune glomerulonephritis. *J Clin Invest.* 2000;105:643–651.

    Animal model data suggesting utility of CD28-B7 blockade in preventing crescentic glomerulonephritis.

34. Kalluri R, Meyers K, Mogyorosi A, et al. Goodpasture syndrome involving overlap with Wegener's granulomatosis and anti-glomerular basement membrane disease. *J Am Soc Nephrol.* 1997;8:1795–1800.

    A case report of a patient presenting with what was thought to be Wegener granulomatosis based on cANCA positivity, pulmonary nodules, and acute renal failure, but who was later found to have AGBMA and a renal biopsy consistent with Goodpasture disease. Discussion of the role of those autoantibodies in the pathogenesis of rapidly progressive glomerulonephritis.

35. Levy JB, Hammad T, Coulthart A, et al. Clinical features and outcome of patients with both ANCA and anti-GBM antibodies. *Kidney Int.* 2004;66:1535–1540.

    A retrospective chart review of patients with positive ANCA and AGMBA serologies, demonstrated poor prognosis and rare recovery from renal failure in such patients.

36. Olson SW, Arbogast CB, Baker TP, et al. Asymptomatic autoantibodies associate with future anti-glomerular basement membrane disease. *J Am Soc Nephrol.* 2011;22:1946–1952.

    A case-control study using serum samples from the Department of Defense Serum Repository demonstrated anti-MPO and PR3 positivity years before onset of clinical AGBMA disease.

93 Idiopathic Pulmonary Hemosiderosis
William L. Ring

ETIOLOGY

Idiopathic pulmonary hemosiderosis (IPH) is a rare disease of unclear etiology and pathogenesis characterized by the abnormal collection of hemosiderin in the lungs. It is primarily a disease of the first decade of life, but may be diagnosed in adults. Equal gender distribution is seen, and at least some cases seem to have a genetic predisposition. A number of reports have noted an association between celiac disease and IPH, and in some cases, treatment of the celiac disease seemed to improve the course of the IPH. However, a pathogenetic link between celiac disease and IPH remains controversial. Some reports have suggested that IPH may be associated with low socioeconomic status, toxic exposure (insecticides, hydrocarbons), seasonal clustering (spring and fall), viral agents, or diet (cow's milk allergy). Exacerbations of IPH have been reported with and after pregnancy. Despite these associations, the etiology of IPH remains obscure.

PRESENTATION

The presentation of IPH is highly variable. Iron-deficiency anemia and recurrent or chronic pulmonary symptoms (e.g., cough, hemoptysis, and dyspnea) characterize IPH. Patients may present with hemoptysis, which tends to be episodic. Although hemoptysis can be massive, it is often mild and can be absent despite significant intrapulmonary bleeding. Intrapulmonary bleeding may initially be clinically silent. Iron-deficiency anemia can overshadow clinical or roentgenographic pulmonary abnormalities. Chronic cough, fatigue, dyspnea, and pallor are frequent. Occasionally, pulmonary hypertension develops.

DIAGNOSIS

The diagnosis of IPH is one of exclusion and generally requires ruling out coagulopathy, hemodynamic abnormalities (congestive heart failure, mitral stenosis), and infection, as well as systemic disorders such as vasculitis, immune-complex disease, or antibasement membrane antibody disease.

CLINICAL FINDINGS

Chest radiographs in IPH are generally abnormal and demonstrate diffuse parenchymal infiltrates. At the time of acute hemorrhage, chest radiographs may show diffuse mottled densities, which are particularly prominent in the perihilar regions and lower lung fields. After 2 to 3 days, consolidation is replaced by a reticular pattern that resolves over 10 to 14 days. With repeated bleeding episodes, progressive interstitial changes can develop into a pattern of interstitial fibrosis, which can become massive. Hilar lymph nodes may be enlarged, particularly during acute episodes. Computed tomography (CT) findings confirm the chest roentgenogram findings. Magnetic resonance imaging may specifically diagnose a new hemorrhage because of the paramagnetic effect of ferric iron. Pulmonary function studies show a restrictive pattern, with elevation of the carbon monoxide diffusing capacity during an episode of bleeding. A transient obstructive component also may be present.

The histologic findings are nonspecific, but an open-lung biopsy is often required to exclude other diagnoses. The dominant histopathologic features are intra-alveolar hemorrhage and hemosiderin-laden macrophages. Hyperplasia of the alveolar epithelium and variable degrees of fibrosis can be seen, but vasculitis, necrosis, and granuloma formation are absent. Immunofluorescent stains are negative for immune deposits at the basement membranes, and inflammatory changes are minimal.

TREATMENT AND PROGNOSIS

The prognosis of IPH is highly variable, ranging from decade-long periods of remission to sudden death from massive hemoptysis. The median survival is reported to be approximately 3 years after diagnosis, although more recent studies support a much better prognosis. Treatment of IPH is immune suppression with otherwise supportive care. The results of therapy are difficult to interpret because of the natural variation in the clinical course of disease and the small number of patients reported. No controlled therapeutic trials have been conducted. Corticosteroids remain the primary line of treatment, supported by other immunosuppressant agents, particularly azathioprine, chloroquine, and 6-mercaptopurine, based largely on clinical improvement in a number of case reports and retrospective studies. Case reports suggest that long-term treatment with moderate doses of inhaled steroids after stabilization with systemic steroids may help to control IPH. While lung transplantation has been performed for IPH, there is at least one report of rapid recurrence of IPH in the transplanted lung.

FURTHER READING

1. Soergel KH, Sommers SC. Idiopathic pulmonary hemosiderosis and related syndromes. *Am J Med.* 1962;32:499.

   A classic description of IPH.

2. Leatherman JW, Davies SF, Hoidal JR. Alveolar hemorrhage syndromes: diffuse microvascular lung hemorrhage in immune and idiopathic disorders. *Medicine (Baltimore).* 1984;63:343.

   An excellent review of all alveolar hemorrhage syndromes, including IPH.

3. Le Clainche L, Le Bourgeois M, Fauroux B, et al. Long-term outcome of idiopathic pulmonary hemosiderosis in children. *Medicine (Baltimore).* 2000;79:318.

   A detailed description of 15 patients, including symptoms, chest radiographs, pulmonary function studies, CT scans, response to treatment, and follow up between 10 and 25 years.

4. Cassimos CD, Chryssanthopoulos C, Panagiotidou C. Epidemiologic observations in idiopathic pulmonary hemosiderosis. *J Pediatr.* 1983;102:698.

An epidemiologic survey of 30 children from northern Greece. The incidence of newly diagnosed cases decreased with improved living conditions and prohibition of certain insecticides, suggesting that environmental factors may contribute to the pathogenesis.

5. Gencer M, Ceylan E, Bitiren M, et al. Two sisters with idiopathic pulmonary hemosiderosis. *Can Respir J.* 2007;14:490.

Typical report of family members with IPH; in this report both diagnosis were made in adults. Suggests familial factors may contribute to the etiology of IPH.

6. Khemiri M, Ouederni M, Khaldi F, et al. Screening for celiac disease in idiopathic pulmonary hemosiderosis. *Gastroenterol Clin Biol.* 2008;32:745.

A report of screening 10 patients with IPH for celiac disease, with 30% positive, all of whom improved markedly with treatment of the celiac disease, suggesting an etiologic link between celiac disease and IPH.

7. Helman D, Sullivan A, Kariya ST, et al. Management of idiopathic pulmonary haemosiderosis in pregnancy: report of two cases. *Respirology.* 2003;8:398.

Review of the treatment of IPH during pregnancy.

8. Buschman DL, Ballard R. Progressive massive fibrosis associated with idiopathic pulmonary hemosiderosis. *Chest.* 1993;104:293.

A case report of a patient diagnosed with IPH during pregnancy at age 30 years, who over the next 23 years developed massive pulmonary fibrosis, felt to be secondary to the IPH.

9. Akyar S, Ozbek SS. Computed tomography findings in idiopathic pulmonary hemosiderosis. *Respiration.* 1993;60:63.

A case report on the CT findings in a patient with IPH.

10. Rubin GD, Edwards DK III, Reicher MA, et al. Diagnosis of pulmonary hemosiderosis by MR imaging. *AJR Am J Roentgenol.* 1989;152:573.

Suggests magnetic resonance imaging may have a role in the diagnosis of occult pulmonary hemorrhage.

11. Kabra SK, Bhargava S, Lodha R, et al. Idiopathic pulmonary hemosiderosis: clinical profile and follow up of 26 children. *Indian Pediatr.* 2007;44:333.

Reports the experience at a university hospital in India, treated initially with steroids and hydroxychloroquine and followed by inhaled corticosteroids, with possible improved survival.

12. Saeed MM, Woo MS, MacLaughlin EF, et al. Prognosis in pediatric idiopathic pulmonary hemosiderosis. *Chest.* 1999;1116:721.

A US retrospective review of 17 patients with IPH. Reports a 5-year survival of 86%, which they felt was due to long-term immunosuppression therapies, including steroids, hydroxychloroquine, and azathioprine.

13. Lui XQ, Ke ZY, Huang LB, et al. Maintenance therapy with dose-adjusted 6-mercaptopurine in idiopathic pulmonary hemosiderosis. *Pediatr Pulmonol.* 2008;43:1067.

A study of 15 patients, suggests that 6-mercaptopurine can be an effective treatment of IPH.

14. Tutor JD, Eid NS. Treatment of idiopathic pulmonary hemosiderosis with inhaled flunisolide. *South Med J.* 1995;88:984.

A case report of treating an adult with inhaled flunisolide 750 µg twice per day, after weaning off systemic corticosteroids, associated with at least 4 years of remission.

15. Calabrese F, Giacometti C, Rea F, et al. Recurrence of idiopathic pulmonary hemosiderosis in a young adult patient after bilateral single-lung transplantation. *Transplantation.* 2002;74:1643.

A report of recurrence of IPH in the transplanted lung 3 years after lung transplantation.

94 Idiopathic Interstitial Pneumonias

Gordon L. Yung and Cecilia M. Smith

In the 1940s, the term "idiopathic (diffuse) interstitial pneumonias" (IIP) was used to describe a general, ill-defined category of interstitial lung diseases of unknown origin. Subsequently, several different classifications were proposed. In the late 1990s, the term IIP was adopted to categorize and define various types of interstitial lung diseases of unclear etiology. The new classification was developed largely due to new understanding of distinct histological subtypes that were previously grouped together under the general umbrella of idiopathic pulmonary fibrosis (IPF).

CLASSIFICATION

Under the current classification, IIP is divided into seven subgroups (Table 94-1). The term "unclassifiable interstitial pneumonia" is applied when histological changes on surgical biopsy are nonspecific and do not fit with any of these subgroups. It is likely that further changes will occur in the future as we better understand these subgroups.

Adoption of this new classification by the general medical community has been slow, partly because of some misconceptions:

1. The histological features, even in surgical (open) lung biopsy specimens, are not unique to each subtype. Other "nonidiopathic" lung conditions may share similar histological changes.

TABLE 94-1	Classification of Idiopathic Interstitial Pneumonias	
Clinical Diagnosis	**Pathologic Diagnosis**	**Examples of Associated Conditions**
IPF	UIP	Smoking, gastro–esophageal reflux disease, wood working, CTD, sarcoidosis, HP
NSI P	NSIP	CTDs, drug toxicity, HIV, HP, slowly healing diffuse alveolar damage (DAD), relapsing organizing pneumonia, occupational exposure, immunodeficiency (mainly HIV infection), graft-versus-host disease (GVHD)
DIP	Respiratory bronchiolitis with airspace macrophage infiltration	Smoking, Langerhan cell histiocytosis
RB-ILD	Respiratory bronchiolitis	Smoking
Acute interstitial pneumonia	DAD	IPF, CTDs, drugs and toxins, ARDS, pneumonia (atypical or viral), acute HP
COP	Organizing pneumonia	Lung infection, drugs and substance abuse, radiation, CTDs, sarcoidosis, radiofrequency ablation, lymphomatoid granulomatosis, Wegener granulomatosis, tumor, pulmonary infarcts, systemic inflammatory diseases, malignancies
LIP	Cellular infiltrates with nodular lymphoid aggregates	Sjögren's, SLE, RA, AIDS, common variable immunoglobulin deficiency

In other words, it is important to exclude other systemic conditions by clinical and laboratory criteria before making a definitive diagnosis of IIP.

2. Some IIP subtypes may coexist in the same pathologic specimen, implying that some of these conditions may share common pathologic mechanisms, whereas others may represent distinct entities. For example, up to one-third of specimens with features of usual interstitial pneumonia (UIP, the histological description of IPF) may have coexisting changes consistent with nonspecific interstitial pneumonia (NSIP). Patients with IPF also may experience an acute exacerbation of their lung condition with development of changes consistent with acute interstitial pneumonia in biopsy or autopsy specimens.

CLINICAL, RADIOGRAPHIC, AND HISTOLOGIC FEATURES
Idiopathic Pulmonary Fibrosis

IPF, also known as cryptogenic fibrosing alveolitis, is the most common form of IIP, accounting for roughly half of all cases. The true incidence of IPF is not known, as many cases remain undiagnosed or misdiagnosed. One reasonable estimate suggests an annual incidence of about 30,000 to 40,000 new cases in the United States and a prevalence of about 80,000 to 100,000 cases. Most cases occur sporadically, although approximately 10% of patients have a positive family history. Despite intensive research, understanding of this condition remains incomplete. Use of animal models does not translate to humans, as the unique histological and radiographic equivalent of IPF has never been duplicated in laboratory specimens. Unfortunately, IPF often is mistaken by many to be synonymous with any interstitial pulmonary fibrosis that does not have a clear etiology (hence "idiopathic"). The diagnosis of IPF sometimes causes significant stress in patients because the older medical literature widely available on the Internet frequently quoted an average survival of 2 to 2½ years after diagnosis. We now know that survival is quite variable; it is not uncommon for patients, especially those with atypical features and earlier diagnosis, to survive much longer. A lone report noted better survival in IPF patients who have atypical computed tomography (CT) scan findings as compared to those patients with "classical" changes. Other studies suggest that mortality may be linked to the extent of honeycombing. Therefore, it is important to adhere to strict diagnostic criteria to avoid confusion and unnecessary anxiety for patients. It also is clear that, although the clinical disease course of IPF is usually one of progressive worsening, the pace of change is not necessarily linear. Some patients can have relatively stable lung function for up to 7 to 10 years, although the usual clinical course is that of a relatively slow decline interspersed with acute exacerbations at irregular intervals. Typically, patients experience significant and permanent loss of lung function following each exacerbation; it is not uncommon to not survive an exacerbation. A definitive diagnosis of IPF only can be made by the presence of (a) appropriate clinical features and laboratory findings *and* (b) either classical radiographic changes on chest CT or distinct histological changes on surgical lung biopsy specimens.

1. *Clinical and laboratory findings:* Unlike most other IIPs, patients with IPF tend to be older, often presenting in their 60s or 70s and rarely before the age of 50 years. There is a male predominance (approximately two-thirds) and which is more apparent in older patients. There also is an association with cigarette smoking (ex- or current), gastro–esophageal reflux disease, and a history of exposure to wood or metal dust. Up to 20% of patients have a family history of pulmonary fibrosis, suggesting an element of genetic predisposition, at least in some patients. Typically, patients present with one of the following: (i) insidious onset and progressive shortness of breath and dry cough; (ii) persistent cough and shortness of breath after an episode of respiratory tract infection; or (iii) incidental findings of interstitial changes on chest radiograph. Clinical examination can offer important clinical clues; the presence of "Velcro"-like crackles at lung bases and finger clubbing strongly suggests a diagnosis of IPF.

2. *Radiographic changes:* Chest X-ray changes are never diagnostic of IPF or, indeed, of any of the IIPs. Because of convenience and relative low radiation dose, chest X-ray may be used as a screening tool in instances of acute change in respiratory symptoms. Chest CT scan offers the potential ability to differentiate various forms of IIP. When all the classical radiographic changes are present, a diagnosis of IPF can be made with more than over 90% confidence

without the need for lung biopsy. The classical changes considered diagnostic of IPF include the following:

a. Peripheral honeycombing

b. Irregular reticular opacities

c. Traction bronchiectasis

d. Minimal ground-glass changes

e. Subpleural, posterior, lower lobe predominance

3. Only a relatively small proportion of patients with IPF have all of the classic features. In clinical practice a probable diagnosis can be made with the presence of peripheral honeycombing in a subpleural distribution and the absence of any significant ground-glass changes.

4. *Histological changes:* IPF demonstrates a pattern of histological changes called UIP. It is important to recognize that similar changes can occur in lung specimens of several lung conditions, such as sarcoidosis, scleroderma, and rheumatoid arthritis (RA). Diagnostic criteria include the presence of noninflammatory fibrosis with "temporal heterogeneity" (varying degree and stages of fibrosis, interspersed with relatively uninvolved lung parenchyma), fibroblastic foci, and no evidence of significant inflammatory cells or granuloma. Of note, fibroblastic foci are areas where fibrotic tissue is generated; the number of foci correlates with survival. These changes can be obscured by end-stage fibrosis so to improve diagnostic yields at least two biopsy specimens should be obtained, including one sample from a relatively uninvolved area of the lungs. There are some inherent risks associated with lung biopsy, especially when there is no Food and Drug Administration (FDA)-approved treatment for the condition. It is, therefore, reasonable to consider forgoing the biopsy procedure if the results would not affect clinical management or if a clinical diagnosis can reasonably be made without histology.

5. *Pulmonary function tests:* IPF exemplifies the classical changes of a restrictive pattern on pulmonary function tests. Lung volumes, especially vital capacity (VC) and total lung capacity (TLC), are reduced. In addition, the forced vital capacity (FVC) and forced expiratory volume in 1 second (FEV_1) are both reduced with relative preservation of the ratio of FEV_1/FVC. The diffusing capacity for carbon monoxide (DLco) is perhaps the most sensitive indicator of disease progression, although it has a relatively poor specificity. Both FVC and FEV_1 have been linked to survival. In one study, the change in FVC and DLco over a 6-month period provided accurate prediction of 2-year survival.

Although there is no uniform explanation of the unique clinical, radiographic, and histological changes in IPF, one can propose a possible model of pathogenesis. Recent studies have suggested that the presence of either telomerase mutation or telomere abnormalities may contribute to the pathogenesis of IPF. Telomeres are repetitive sequences of DNA elements found at the end of chromosomes; their length (and function) may shorten with aging and smoking. They appear to play a crucial role in cell division and, possibly, tissue repair processes. This, and other genetic changes, may explain why IPF tends to occur later in life and is associated with smoking (which more commonly causes airway injury and disease, rather than interstitial injury), and why the condition often accelerates after exacerbations associated with chest infections, when fibrosis develops in areas not involved in the infection. It has been hypothesized that the initial injury may be due to negative pressure exerted on the surface of the lungs during forced inspiration and cough, and not due to the infection itself. This pathogenesis model supports the findings that early IPF affects peripheral (subpleural) parts of the lungs, where stress/force is usually maximal during cough and inspiration. It also supports the clinical impression that IPF patients with significant cough tend to progress more rapidly, and would explain why those with a history of smoking, wood and dust exposure, and gastro–esophageal reflux disease are at higher risks of IPF (conditions associated with increased cough). Finally, this theory may explain why treatments targeted to various pathways of fibrosis have been relatively unsuccessful, even though these same pathways are shared by other forms of fibrosis that respond to antifibrotic therapies.

Nonspecific Interstitial Pneumonia

The term NSIP is both a clinical and histological diagnosis. It is the second most common form of IIP, comprising about one quarter of all cases. Patients with NSIP can present at any age.

In many cases, extrapulmonary manifestations suggesting underlying rheumatologic conditions develop years after the onset of lung disease.

When referring to NSIP, it is important to specify whether the term refers to a clinical diagnosis (a subtype of IIP) or a pathologic diagnosis by biopsy, in which case several underlying conditions should be considered. The idiopathic form of NSIP generally occurs in middle-age females in their 40s and 50s with no significant history of smoking. Up to one-third of cases have a subacute presentation of respiratory symptoms. Some of these patients have nonspecific serological markers of connective tissue diseases (CTDs) and may eventually develop clinical features of conditions such as scleroderma, RA, or others of these conditions. Three types of NSIP are generally identified: cellular, fibrotic, and mixed (coexisting cellular and fibrotic changes), depending on the presence or absence of significant interstitial inflammatory changes. In general, cellular NSIP with significant inflammatory changes has a better chance of responding to immunosuppressive therapy and better overall survival. Fibrotic NSIP behaves clinically more like UIP/IPF, in both prognosis and a poor response to treatment. In fact, up to 75% of NSIP patients may show stabilization or improvement with treatment.

Most cases of NSIP demonstrate nonspecific radiographic interstitial changes with or without ground-glass attenuation. Early cases of cellular NSIP may show ground-glass attenuation with a bibasilar distribution, whereas fibrotic NSIP may demonstrate ground-glass attenuation along with reticular lines. Traction bronchiectasis can occur in both NSIP and UIP and reflects chronicity that is more common in fibrotic NSIP and UIP. The extent of ground-glass opacities found on CT scan in NSIP presumably reflects the degree of inflammation and has been associated with the likelihood of a positive treatment response and longer survival. Unlike UIP, honeycombing is rare. Also, unlike IPF, there are no specific radiographic changes that are diagnostic of NSIP. Recently, demonstration of subpleural sparing of radiographic interstitial changes on CT scan has been suggested as having a high specificity for the diagnosis of NSIP. Further validation of this pathologic–radiographic association is needed before one can confidently make a diagnosis of NSIP without lung biopsy. In general, flexible bronchoscopy with transbronchial biopsy or bronchoalveolar lavage (BAL) is not useful in the diagnosis of UIP or NSIP. The major indication for performing flexible bronchoscopy includes the need to rule out alternative diagnoses such as sarcoidosis and coexisting infections. An elevation of lymphocytes over 30% in BAL fluid supports a diagnosis of NSIP over UIP.

Histologic diagnosis by surgical lung biopsy remains the gold standard and should be obtained whenever possible. NSIP is characterized by relatively uniform mononuclear inflammatory infiltrates and interstitial fibrosis, with relatively few areas of normal parenchyma (i.e., temporal and spatial homogeneity). As is the case with UIP, it is important to exclude other histologic findings such as granulomatous disease that also can result in NSIP-like changes. Coexisting findings of organizing pneumonia is common, but not a predominant feature in NSIP (<10% of cross sectional lung area).

Acute Interstitial Pneumonia

Much less is known about acute interstitial pneumonia, which was first described in 1935 as Hamman–Rich syndrome. Like other IIPs, it can occur in isolation or with other conditions, but it is the only form of acute or subacute IIP that presents with acute respiratory failure without an apparent inciting event such as sepsis. Other than the lack of an identifiable precipitating cause, its clinical and radiographic features are similar to acute respiratory distress syndrome (ARDS) with rapid onset and progressive shortness of breath and respiratory failure. Prodromal symptoms occur in some patients 1 to 2 weeks prior to the onset of shortness of breath, raising the possibility that an infectious agent may be a precipitating factor. In some cases, it occurs associated with an acute exacerbation of IPF, although how the two conditions are related is unclear.

Radiographic changes in acute interstitial pneumonia include diffuse, rapidly progressive ground-glass opacities and consolidation. In some cases, the initial degree of hypoxemia may be out of proportion to the radiographic changes. Over time, bronchial dilatation may also be observed. Histologic changes involve diffuse alveolar damage, often associated with fibroblastic proliferation and interstitial fibrosis. Two stages are described: an exudative phase characterized by the presence of interstitial edema, hyaline membranes, acute interstitial inflammation, and varying degree of hemorrhage; and, a later organizing phase with type II pneumocyte hyperplasia and organizing fibrosis, mostly within the alveolar septa. Unlike most of the other IIPs, transbronchial biopsies can provide sufficient tissue for diagnosis, although, in clinical practice, the rapidity of disease progression often makes even this procedure risky. Perhaps because of the rapidly progressive clinical course from the exudative to organizing phase, treatment is often unsuccessful with mortality greater than 60%; most deaths occur within 6 months of presentation.

Cryptogenic Organizing Pneumonia

Under the new classification, cryptogenic organizing pneumonia (COP) has replaced the term bronchiolitis obliterans organizing pneumonia (BOOP). As the old name suggests, there are two components of the disease—small airway obstruction and alveolar space inflammation. Histologic diagnosis depends on the demonstration of "buds" of granulation tissue (mixture of fibroblasts and myofibroblasts within a loose network of connective matrix) within the lumen of distal airways and alveolar spaces.

Patients present at any ages, but more commonly in the sixth to seventh decade of life, with an equal male to female ratio. Common features include cough, shortness of breath, and bilateral crackles on physical examination. Although listed under the category of IIP, more than half of these cases are preceded by a viral-like illness. Other conditions also have been associated with this disease process, including chemotherapy, CTD, and radiation therapy. Unlike other IIPs, the clinical presentation, prognosis, treatment response, and relapse rates between idiopathic and secondary forms of COP are similar, raising the question of whether idiopathic COP truly exists independently. Pulmonary function tests generally show a mixed restrictive and obstructive pattern, with disproportionally reduced D$_{LCO}$.

Early radiographic changes in COP can be subtle and it is not uncommon for the initial chest X-ray to be normal despite significant respiratory symptoms. Most CT scans in this condition demonstrate one of three patterns, in decreasing frequency: (1) bilateral patchy infiltrates (alveolar opacities cases), (2) diffuse infiltrative opacities involving subpleural (may be triangular in shape) and/or peribronchovascular parenchyma, and (3) solitary focal nodule or mass. In addition, approximately 12% to 20% of COP cases demonstrate a reversed halo sign (also called "atoll sign" or "fairy ring sign") on CT scan. The reversed halo sign is defined by a central, round area of ground-glass opacity with a surrounding ring ("halo") or crescent of consolidation. The ground-glass changes correspond to alveolar inflammation and the peripheral consolidation represents organizing pneumonia in the alveolar ducts. It has been suggested that a nodular appearance of the ring represents granuloma and suggests a secondary cause of COP. Although the latter radiographic change was initially described as specific to COP, other conditions have now been reported to show the same changes.

In the appropriate clinical and radiographic setting, surgical lung biopsy may not be necessary for diagnosis of COP. Since the disease appears to originate from the distal airways and alveoli, transbronchial biopsy may yield a diagnosis in two-thirds of cases. Some suggest that, in cases of a nondiagnostic CT scan, the addition of BAL may be helpful when lymphocytosis and foamy macrophages are found.

Corticosteroid therapy is the best treatment option. The outcome of patients suffering from COP is good; up to 80% of patients will be cured. Relapse and mortality rates after 1 year of follow-up have been reported as 37.8% and 9.4%, respectively.

Desquamative Interstitial Pneumonia

Desquamative interstitial pneumonia (DIP) is a relatively uncommon form of IIP, comprising less than 10% of all cases. More than 90% of patients are male, and they often present in the fourth and fifth decades of life. Most patients (>90%) are smokers; those without a smoking history, especially females, often have an associated CTD such as systemic lupus erythematosus (SLE) or RA.

In early disease, the chest radiograph can be normal, although ground-glass opacities are often seen on CT scan. As the disease progresses, small cystlike lesions may develop and, later on, honeycombing changes can occur. The disease appears to have a significant inflammatory component, with BAL showing elevated eosinophil counts in many patients. Definitive diagnosis usually requires surgical lung biopsy and is characterized by the diffuse accumulation of widespread large numbers of pigmented macrophages in alveolar spaces associated with interstitial inflammation and/or fibrosis. Patients often respond well to corticosteroids with preservation or improvement in lung function. Because of the association with smoking, these patients should be strongly urged to quit smoking. Mortality from DIP has been reported between 6% and 30%, with the majority of deaths in patients who presented late in the course of illness.

Respiratory Bronchiolitis-Associated Interstitial Lung Disease

Respiratory bronchiolitis, first described in 1974, is a common autopsy finding in smokers. However, a small number of patients develop associated interstitial lung disease (RB-ILD). These patients, typically in their 30s to 50s, are generally asymptomatic or present with mild nonspecific respiratory symptoms of mild chronic cough or shortness of breath on exertion. All of these patients have a significant history of first (rarely second)-hand cigarette smoke exposure (>30 pack-year history); two-thirds are male.

Because of the significant overlap in clinical, radiographic, and histological features between RB-ILD and DIP, these two conditions are considered to represent a spectrum of the same disease process with RB-ILD representing the early stage of disease. However, it is likely that distinct underlying genetic or other factors are required for the development of DIP from RB-ILD. Clinically, it is also important to differentiate the two conditions: death directly from RB-ILD is rarely reported, even though the mortality from DIP has been reported to be between 6% and 30%.

Radiographic changes of RB-ILD can be subtle and nonspecific and include nonbranching ground-glass opacities associated with evenly distributed, ill-defined, centrilobular (micro) nodules, often with some degree of upper-lobe predominance. In some patients, nonspecific interstitial changes on CT scan are seen and thought to represent significant bronchiolar inflammation with secondary nonspecific fibrosis in the adjacent alveolar septa. Although the finding of micronodules may allow one to separate RB-ILD from DIP, similar radiographic changes can also be seen in NSIP, DIP, and acute or subacute hypersensitivity pneumonitis (HP). Histologically, RB-ILD is characterized by the prominent presence of yellow–brown pigmented macrophages within respiratory bronchioles and adjacent alveoli. Most patients with RB-ILD have mild symptoms that often, but not always, improve after smoking cessation. Rarely, steroids may be prescribed, but mortality from the disease is rare.

Lymphoid Interstitial Pneumonia

Idiopathic lymphoid interstitial pneumonia (LIP) is probably very rare, though the true incidence is not known. Although classified under IIP, it also is considered part of the spectrum of pulmonary lymphoproliferative disorders, a group of diseases that is characterized by uncontrolled proliferation of lymphoid cells. It is likely that these lymphoid cells originate from native pulmonary lymphoid tissue (bronchial mucosa-associated lymphoid tissue, MALT), and can cause pathological conditions ranging from simple benign small airway lymphoid aggregates to malignant lymphoma. LIP generally refers to a nonmalignant form of diffuse polyclonal lymphoid proliferation that progresses from airways into pulmonary parenchyma. Despite earlier concerns, LIP is probably not a precursor of lymphoma, but represents a locally invasive form of benign lymphoproliferative disorder limited to the lung parenchyma. Similar to other types of IIP, no clear etiology has been found in the idiopathic form of LIP. Secondary forms of LIP are typically associated with immune disorders such as CTDs. In some cases, HIV or Ebstein–Barr virus DNA has been found in the lymphoid cells. Unlike other IIPs, LIP often occurs more commonly in children. In adults, it is often associated with autoimmune disease (particularly Sjögren's) or HIV. Adult patients are typically between 40 to 60 years of age, with a female predominance and usually present with progressive cough and shortness of breath. The clinical course is quite variable and occasionally is fatal. Pulmonary function tests typically show a restrictive pattern with disproportionately low DLco.

Radiographic changes are often nonspecific. The most common features include uniform or patchy areas of bilateral ground-glass opacity and poorly defined centrilobular nodules, with or without subpleural nodules. In most cases, interlobular and peribronchovascular thickening as well as mediastinal lymphadenopathy also are present. In about two-third of cases, thin-wall cystic air spaces of variable size are noted. This last feature is thought to be due to bronchiolar stenosis and obstruction caused by peribronchiolar lymphocytic infiltration. Because clinical and radiographic changes are nonspecific, biopsy is often required for diagnosis. Histologically, LIP is characterized by a diffuse inflammatory alveolar infiltrate comprised of mainly T lymphocytes, plasma cells, and histiocytes, often with loosely formed nonnecrotizing epithelioid granulomas.

APPROACH TO DIAGNOSIS OF IIP

All patients suspected of IIP should have a detailed clinical history, including past history of occupational, drug, tobacco, and other toxic exposures. Signs and symptoms suggestive of a more systemic illness should also be noted. Wheezing and hemoptysis are uncommon in IIP and when present suggests an alternative diagnosis, the development of secondary bronchiectasis, or a superimposed infection. Digital clubbing should raise the possibility of IPF, although it also can occur in later stages of sarcoidosis and HP. It is important to remember that many radiographic and histologic changes of IIPs can occur in other conditions, including various CTDs. Pulmonary involvement in these conditions may precede other clinical features by many years. Another common condition that mimics IIP is HP. A detailed history of exposure to avian, fungal, and atypical mycobacteria should be obtained.

Imaging Studies

Standard chest radiographs are neither sensitive nor specific enough for the diagnosis and follow-up of patients with IIPs. Therefore, all patients suspected of IIPs should have a high resolution CT scan of the chest. In early cases, both prone and supine images may help to distinguish early interstitial changes from dependent atelectasis. Although many cases of IIP do not have diagnostic CT changes, there are a few exceptions: some cases of IPF may show classic changes as noted previously; subpleural sparing of peripheral basal interstitial changes may point to a diagnosis of NSIP; and in the appropriate clinical setting, a CT scan may be highly suggestive of COP. Other forms of IIP, however, usually require tissue confirmation for definitive diagnosis.

Gallium scan and fludeoxyglucose-positron emission tomography (FDG-PET) scans are generally not useful, unless specific alternative diagnoses, such as malignancy, are suspected.

Serologic Testing

Because of the strong association with various rheumatologic conditions, serologic testing is often performed. The extent of testing depends on clinical suspicion. Detailed testing should be considered especially in a younger, female patient. Typical serologic tests include antinuclear antibody (ANA) (and double stranded DNA (ds-DNA)), rheumatoid factor, cyclic citrullinated peptide (CCP), creatine phosphokinase (CPK) and aldolase, antimyositis panel (including anti-Jo-1 antibodies), extractable nuclear antigen (ENA) panel (anti-Scl-70, anti-Ro, and anti-La), and antineutrophil cytoplasmic antibodies (ANCA). Unfortunately, many patients with IIP present with positive serologic markers without corresponding clinical features to support a specific diagnosis. Some of these patients may develop new extrapulmonary clinical findings of CTDs years after the initial pulmonary presentation, while others with initial negative serologic tests may subsequently develop positive tests later. A HP panel should also be considered in patients with appropriate history or radiographic changes. In the case of COP, the use of serum procalcitonin may be useful in differentiating infective from noninfective causes.

Flexible Bronchoscopy, BAL, and Transbronchial Biopsy

The role of bronchoscopy, BAL, and transbronchial biopsy for diagnosis remains controversial. Both IPF/UIP and NSIP cannot be diagnosed through this route alone, since both diagnoses require demonstration of architectural changes in a larger specimen. However, unique features in other IIPs may be seen in transbronchial biopsies, as discussed previously. Some physicians have proposed using differential cell counts to determine diagnosis and the likelihood of response to corticosteroid and other immunosuppressive therapy, but most have not found this approach to be useful. The most consistent use of bronchoscopy appears to be in excluding infection and malignancies, as well as for confirming specific lung conditions such as DIP and sarcoidosis.

Surgical Lung Biopsy

For most patients, a surgical lung biopsy obtained via video-assisted thoracoscopic surgery (VATS) is the "gold standard" for diagnosis. When IPF and NSIP are suspected, it is important to take samples from locations away from those of advanced fibrosis, where normal architecture may be completely destroyed. The benefits of surgical biopsy should also be weighed against potential risks, which may include accelerated decline in pulmonary function postbiopsy. In IPF, where effective therapy is lacking, a definitive diagnosis may not offer a therapeutic advantage, other than providing potential prognostic indicators.

Other Tests

Baseline full pulmonary function tests, including DLCO, should be obtained. A significant obstructive component should alert physicians to an alternative diagnosis other than IIP. Other tests commonly performed include echocardiography to exclude cardiac causes of dyspnea and cough as well as pulmonary hypertension, an exercise tests to evaluate oxygen desaturation and need for supplemental oxygen, and, if appropriate, a sleep study to rule out sleep apnea that may increase oxygen needs and cause early and severe pulmonary hypertension.

TREATMENT
Specific Therapy

There is no specific treatment for IPF that is approved in the United States by the FDA. However, a new drug, pirfenidone, has shown promise in several large prospective randomized clinical trials. Its use has been approved in other countries, including Japan, the European Union, Canada, and China. A multinational prospective randomized study is currently underway in the United States and other countries to further evaluate this drug's efficacy; results are expected to be available in 2014. Use of N-acetyl cysteine remains controversial. Despite an earlier report of success in a small number of IPF patients, recent data showed contrary results, especially when combined with low-dose prednisone.

For other IIPs, the first-line treatment is typically corticosteroid therapy, usually oral prednisone at an initial dose of 0.5 to 1 mg/kg daily. The optimal duration of treatment is not known. Only about 20% to 30% of NSIP patients respond to steroid therapy, most commonly those with the cellular type of NSIP. Acute interstitial pneumonia, however, rarely responds to any treatment. In part because many patients with non-IPF types of IIP have an underlying CTD, it is reasonable to use a steroid sparing agent such as azathioprine or mycophenolate (sodium or mofetil) in patients who do not respond to steroid therapy, or those who respond but require high-dose therapy (typically more than 10–20 mg prednisone daily). Other immunosuppressive drugs, such as cyclophosphamide, have been used with limited and variable success.

Supportive Care and Pulmonary Rehabilitation

An important strategy of managing IIP is to adopt an aggressive strategy to avoid and treat chest infections. This may be particularly important in IPF patients, since mechanical injury from coughing may contribute to lung injury and subsequent fibrosis. Strategies generally include use of mucolytics, cough suppressants, early antibiotics, and treatment of gastro–esophageal reflux disease. Other important measures include patient education with hand hygiene, and up-to-date immunization for patients and their household members.

Many IIP patients reported significant benefits from participating in a pulmonary rehabilitation program, including improvement in symptoms (e.g., dyspnea) and exercise tolerance. In addition, many programs help to evaluate and educate patients for selecting optimal oxygen delivery systems. It is likely that the high prevalence of pulmonary hypertension in IIP patients may, in part, be related to repeated and prolonged periods of hypoxemia. Aggressive use of supplemental oxygen may improve or slow down the development of pulmonary hypertension and cor pulmonale.

Lung Transplantation

For many IIP patients, lung transplantation remains the only option for improving lung function and extending survival. For instance, typical IPF patients have an average survival of about 4 years, and 30% to 50% of patients with LIP die within 5 years of diagnosis. Because of the risks of transplantation, as well as limited organ availability, it is important to carefully balance the risks and potential benefits of transplantation for each patient. Within each subgroup of IIP, patient response to therapy and disease progression can be highly variable, and an individualized approach to assess the benefit of transplant benefit is important. Additional information is available in the chapter on lung transplantation.

FURTHER READING

1. American Thoracic Society, European Respiratory Society. American Thoracic Society/European Respiratory Society international multidisciplinary consensus classification of the idiopathic interstitial pneumonias. *Am J Respir Crit Care Med.* 2002;165(2):277–304.

   A good starting point for understanding the basics of IIP classification. Updates are expected.

2. Travis WD, Hunninghake G, King TE Jr, et al. Idiopathic nonspecific interstitial pneumonia: report of an American Thoracic Society project. *Am J Respir Crit Care Med.* 2008;177(12):1338–1347.

   A comprehensive report looking at NSIP.

3. Nathan SD, Shlobin OA, Weir N, et al. Long-term course and prognosis of idiopathic pulmonary fibrosis in the new millennium. *Chest.* 2011;1:221–229.

   A more detailed look at how IPF is not a uniform disease, but one with varying outcomes. Data based on different clinical trials using new therapies. Although the trials often failed to demonstrate efficacy of therapy, they nevertheless provide good information on the natural course of IPF.

4. Raghu G, Collard HR, Egan JJ, et al. An official ATS/ERS/JRS/ALAT statement: idiopathic pulmonary fibrosis: evidence-based guidelines for diagnosis and management. *Am J Respir Crit Care Med.* 2011;183(6):788–824.

   A comprehensive review of IPF, based on more recent data.

5. Ohshimo S, Bonella F, Cui A, et al. Significance of bronchoalveolar lavage for the diagnosis of idiopathic pulmonary fibrosis. *Am J Respir Crit Care Med.* 2009;179(11):1043–1047.

   One of the few studies looking at the role of BAL in IPF, based on the modern IIP classification. Small study but data are summarized well.

6. Kinder BW, Wells AU. The art and science of diagnosing interstitial lung diseases. *Am J Respir Crit Care Med.* 2009;179(11):974–975.

   A good review of the difficulties in ILD diagnosis.

7. Flaherty KR, Toews GB, Travis WD, et al. Clinical significance of histological classification of idiopathic interstitial pneumonia. *Eur Respir J.* 2002;19:275–283.

   A comprehensive review of clinical and histologic correlations in IIP.

8. Lee HY, Lee KS, Jeong YJ, et al. High-resolution CT findings in fibrotic idiopathic interstitial pneumonia with little honeycombing: serial changes and prognostic implications. *AJR Am J Roentgenol.* 2012;199(5):982–989.

   A retrospective analysis of 154 patients with early UIP or NSIP, showing that, over time, the overall extent of parenchymal changes on CT scan correlate with survival.

9. Larsen BY, Colby TV. Update for pathologists on idiopathic interstitial pneumonias. *Arch Pathol Lab Med.* 2012;136(10):1234–1241.

   A very good review of histologic changes of different types of IIP.

10. Poletti V, Romagnoli M. Current status of idiopathic nonspecific interstitial pneumonia. *Semin Respir Crit Care Med.* 2012;33(5):440–449.

    A comprehensive review of NSIP.

11. King TE Jr, Tooze JA, Schwarz MI, et al. Predicting survival in idiopathic pulmonary fibrosis: scoring system and survival model. *Am J Respir Crit Care Med.* 2001;164:1171–1181.

    A retrospective analysis of 238 biopsy-confirmed IPF patients. Survival was related to age, length of smoking, clubbing, CT scan changes, pulmonary arterial hypertension, and lung physiology at rest and during exercise.

12. Jegal Y, Kim DS, Shim TS, et al. Physiology is a stronger predictor of survival than pathology in fibrotic interstitial pneumonia. *Am J Respir Crit Care Med.* 2005;171:639–644.

    A retrospective analysis of 179 patients with either IPF or NSIP. Results demonstrated that short-term physiologic changes by PFTs (FVC) may be more important in predicting survival than radiographic changes on CTs.

13. Kawabata Y, Takemura T, Hebisawa A, et al; for the Desquamative Interstitial Pneumonia Study Group. Desquamative interstitial pneumonia may progress to lung fibrosis as characterized radiologically. *Respirology.* 2012;17:1214–1221.

    One of the largest studies on long-term follow-up of DIP. The results were not limited to radiologic progression, but also provide data on BAL findings of high lactate dehydrogenase, IgG, and eosinophils.

14. Cottin V, Cordier JF. Cryptogenic organizing pneumonia. *Semin Respir Crit Care Med.* 2012;33(5):462–475.

    A recent comprehensive report on COP.

15. Jara-Palomares L, Gomez-Izquierdo L, Gonzalez-Vergara D, et al. Utility of high-resolution computed tomography and BAL in cryptogenic organizing pneumonia. *Respir Med.* 2010;104(11):1706–1711.

    The study provides data about the ability to make a diagnosis of COP based on CT scan findings and BAL, without surgical lung biopsy. BAL findings were relatively specific (89%) but had low sensitivity.

16. Walsh SL, Roberton BJ. Images in thorax: the atoll sign. *Thorax.* 2010;65:1029–1030.

    A succinct review on interpretation of the atoll sign.

17. Drakopanagiotakis F, Paschalaki K, Abu-Hijleh M, et al. Cryptogenic and secondary organizing pneumonia: clinical presentation, radiographic findings, treatment response, and prognosis. *Chest.* 2011;139(4):893–900.

    A review of 61 patients with biopsy-proven COP, looking at clinical and radiographic presentation, BAL changes, relapse rate, and mortality.

18. Nakanishi M, Demura Y, Mizuno S, et al. Changes in HRCT findings in patients with respiratory bronchiolitis-associated interstitial lung disease after smoking cessation. *Eur Respir J.* 2007;29(3):453–461.

    Improvement in clinical symptoms, CT changes, and DLCO after smoking cessation in five patients with RB-ILD.

19. Niewoehner DE, Kleinerman J, Rice DB. Pathologic changes in the peripheral airways of young cigarette smokers. *N Engl J Med.* 1974;291:755–758

    An early study suggesting the presence of respiratory bronchiolitis in asymptomatic young cigarette smokers.

20. Yousem SA, Colby TV, Gaensler EA. Respiratory bronchiolitis–associated interstitial lung disease and its relationship to desquamative interstitial pneumonia. *Mayo Clin Proc.* 1989;64:1373–1380.

    A small report emphasizing histologic similarities between RB-ILD and DIP.

21. Heyneman LE, Ward S, Lynch DA, et al. Respiratory bronchiolitis, respiratory bronchiolitis–associated interstitial lung disease, and desquamative interstitial pneumonia: different entities or part of the spectrum of the same disease process? *AJR Am J Roentgenol.* 1999;173:1617–1622.

    This report emphasizes the similarities in CT scan findings in DIP and RB-ILD.

22. Wells AU, Nicholson AG, Hansell DM, et al. Respiratory bronchiolitis-associated interstitial lung disease. *Semin Respir Crit Care Med.* 2003;24(5):585–594.

    A good and comprehensive review of RB-ILD.

23. Swigris JJ, Berry GJ, Raffin TA, et al. Lymphoid interstitial pneumonia: a narrative review. *Chest.* 2002;122(6):2150–2164.

    A great review of LIP.

24. Hare SS, Souza CA, Bain G, et al. The radiological spectrum of pulmonary lymphoproliferative disease. *Br J Radiol.* 2012;85(1015):848–864.

    A comprehensive review of radiographic changes in various pulmonary lymphoproliferative disorders.

25. Cha SI, Fessler MB, Cool CD, et al. Lymphoid interstitial pneumonia: clinical features, associations and prognosis. *Eur Respir J.* 2006;28(2):364–369.

    A review of 15 LIP patients, most of those secondary, over a 14-year period.

26. Ferreira A, Garvey C, Connors GL, et al. Pulmonary rehabilitation in interstitial lung disease: benefits and predictors of response. *Chest.* 2009;135(2):442–447.

    A retrospective review of 113 patients with IIP who underwent pulmonary rehabilitation. Improvements were noted in dyspnea, mood (depression), and 6-minute walk distance. Improvement in walk distance was greater in those with initially low walk distance.

Pulmonary Manifestations of Rheumatoid Arthritis

Frank D. Bender

Rheumatoid arthritis (RA) is a systemic inflammatory disorder whose pulmonary effects can be grouped into eight categories: (1) pleural disease, (2) interstitial pneumonitis, (3) drug-related pulmonary disease, (4) pulmonary nodules, (5) airways disease, (6) pulmonary vascular disease, (7) apical fibrocavitary disease, and (8) miscellaneous effects. Although frequently present as distinct entities, more than one manifestation can occur simultaneously or in sequence in an individual with rheumatoid disease.

PLEURAL DISEASE

Pleural disease is the most frequent pulmonary manifestation; it occurs as pleurisy in 20% of cases or as pleural effusion in 3% to 5%. In addition, asymptomatic pleural involvement is probably common, because autopsy series show pleural fibrosis or pleural effusion in approximately 50% of patients with RA. Despite the fact that RA itself is more common among women, pleural disease has a striking predominance for middle-aged men. It can occur at any time during the course of the RA; in 20% of cases, however, it immediately precedes or occurs at the onset of arthritis. The presence of pleural disease appears to bear no definite relationship to the activity of the arthritis or to the titer of rheumatoid factor but correlates to some extent with the presence of subcutaneous nodules. Pathologically, the pleura shows chronic (mononuclear cell) inflammation; pleural or subpleural rheumatoid nodules may occasionally be seen.

Symptoms, which are usually minimal, are absent at least one-third of the time. When present, symptoms can include pleuritic pain or cough. Rarely, a large effusion causes dyspnea, especially in individuals with underlying parenchymal lung disease. Fever is uncommon. The chest roentgenogram reveals pleural thickening or effusion, which is unilateral in 80% of cases with a right-sided predominance.

A diagnostic thoracentesis is indicated to rule out other etiologies such as malignancy or infection. The pleural fluid is characteristically a yellow-green color, although long-standing effusions may have an opalescent or milky quality from cholesterol crystals. Rheumatoid effusions are exudative and have elevated protein levels and lactate dehydrogenase levels frequently above 1,000 U/L. The pH and glucose levels are low. The glucose is less than 50 mg/dL in 80% of cases and is less than 25 mg/dL in 66% of patients. The pleural fluid glucose fails to rise during intravenous infusions of glucose—a characteristic that distinguishes rheumatoid effusions from low glucose effusions caused by other diseases. The hyaluronidase level may be elevated. The differential cell count is usually lymphocytic, but granulocytes can predominate if the thoracentesis is done early on in the inflammatory process. Rheumatoid factor is present in higher concentrations than in the serum, but this is a nonspecific finding that occurs in effusions from other causes as well. Complement levels in pleural fluid can be sharply reduced in comparison with blood levels, a finding that distinguishes rheumatoid effusions and effusions secondary to systemic lupus erythematosus from those of other causes. A characteristic pleural fluid cytologic triad of elongated macrophages, giant multinucleated macrophages, and granular cell debris is felt to be diagnostic and should be sought. Mesothelial cells are nearly always absent. Pleural biopsy may be required to rule out malignancy or infection.

The pleural effusions in RA tend to resolve spontaneously over the course of several months and frequently leave residual pleural thickening. Rarely, such thickening is sufficient to cause significant lung restriction and lead to consideration of pleural decortication. If the pleural disease causes significant dyspnea or other symptoms, therapeutic options include (1) nonsteroidal anti-inflammatory drugs, (2) drainage by thoracentesis or chest tube, (3) a trial of oral or intrapleural corticosteroids if the effusion recurs, and (4) pleurodesis. Approximately 20% of RA-associated pleural effusions are persistent. Most of these, however, resolve within 1 to 5 years. Empyema has been reported to complicate rheumatoid pleural effusion, possibly because of impaired local defense mechanisms in conjunction with necrosis of a subpleural necrobiotic nodule. Systemic steroids, if used, could contribute to or mask the presence of an empyema, and those undergoing this treatment should be monitored carefully.

INTERSTITIAL PNEUMONITIS

Interstitial pneumonitis, historically and clinically indistinguishable from the idiopathic variety, occurs with greater-than-expected frequency in patients with RA. Conversely, 15% to 20% of patients with idiopathic interstitial pneumonitis either have a positive rheumatoid factor or develop symmetric polyarthritis consistent with RA during their clinical course. As with pleural disease, men are overrepresented. Interstitial pneumonitis precedes the onset of arthritis in 20% of patients. Patients are generally seropositive, but the activity of the arthritis bears no relationship to the occurrence or severity of the interstitial pneumonitis.

The exact incidence of interstitial pneumonitis in RA is unclear. Characteristic roentgenographic findings of interstitial pneumonitis, a diffuse reticulonodular infiltrate with basilar predominance, occurred in 1.6% in a series of 516 patients with RA. Other series show characteristic plain chest film abnormalities in up to 6% of patients. High-resolution computed tomography (HRCT) is more sensitive than a plain chest roentgenogram in detecting interstitial disease. Various series report interstitial abnormalities in 10% to 60% of patients. Pulmonary function test abnormalities indicating characteristically restriction and reduced diffusing capacity abnormalities occur frequently. One report describes abnormal pulmonary function in 41% of an unselected series of patients with RA, the majority of whom had no pulmonary symptoms. The carbon monoxide diffusing capacity (DLco) is believed to be more sensitive than spirometry and lung volume determination in detecting interstitial disease. A recent study concluded that a diffusing capacity less than 54% of predicted at presentation is a sensitive predictor of progressive interstitial lung disease.

With a combination of imaging techniques, physiologic testing, and bronchoalveolar lavage, abnormalities suggesting interstitial lung disease can be seen in up to 58% of patients with recent onset RA. In 14%, the changes are clinically significant. Cigarette smoking is an important risk factor in the development and progression of interstitial disease. Patients should be counseled regarding smoking cessation. Serologic testing for circulating levels of KL-6 (a MUC1 mucin) has been proposed as a sensitive marker for active rheumatoid interstitial pneumonitis as well as other forms of interstitial lung disease.

Nonproductive cough, exertional dyspnea, and easy fatigability are the most frequent symptoms. Clinical stability may be present for years, or, rarely, a rapid progression toward respiratory failure is seen. Examination reveals characteristic fine "Velcro" bibasilar crepitation. Subcutaneous nodules occur in most cases, and finger clubbing is quite common. Symptomatic individuals demonstrate hypoxemia (worsened by exercise), diminished DLco, and reduced static lung volumes. The course of rheumatoid interstitial pneumonitis is variable.

The decision to treat rheumatoid-associated interstitial disease is based on the initial severity of symptoms and of physiologic impairment, as well as on the rate of deterioration over time. No controlled studies exist to guide treatment options. Initial treatment is usually with corticosteroids plus an immunosuppressive agent: cyclophosphamide or aziothioprine. Mycophenolate may have a role in treatment, although the series reporting a benefit had a small number of patients. Oxygen is given for hypoxemia. When appropriate, referral for lung transplantation may be considered. A poor prognosis for patients with RA hospitalized for evaluation or treatment of interstitial pneumonitis has been reported, with a median survival of 3.5 years and a 5-year survival of 39%.

DRUG-RELATED PULMONARY DISEASE

The possibility of drug-induced interstitial pneumonitis and of other pulmonary reactions to treatment must be kept in mind when evaluating patients with RA. Methotrexate causes pulmonary reactions in 1% to 5% of patients. An acute hypersensitivity interstitial pneumonitis is most common. Other reactions include pleuritis, hilar adenopathy, and nodules. Eosinophilia may be seen in up to 50%. Cough not associated with interstitial disease can occur, and which is thought felt to be an irritant effect of methotrexate. Risk factors for the development of methotrexate-associated pulmonary toxicity include advanced age, diabetes, low serum albumin, preexisting interstitial abnormalities, and previous adverse reactions to disease-modifying antirheumatic drugs. Low-dose methotrexate is not associated with the development of chronic interstitial lung disease. Opportunistic infections may occur.

Gold can produce interstitial pneumonitis. Factors that can help in distinguishing gold-induced interstitial pneumonitis from rheumatoid-associated interstitial disease are a female predominance, the presence of a skin rash or fever, low titers of rheumatoid factor, a lymphocytosis in bronchoalveolar lavage fluid, and gold-specific chest CT findings. With both methotrexate and gold, treatment of pulmonary toxicity involves withdrawal of the drug and administration of corticosteroids.

Ibuprofen has been associated with hypersensitivity pneumonitis, pleural effusions, and exacerbation of asthma. Corticosteroids are associated with opportunistic pulmonary infections that can resemble an interstitial pneumonitis.

Antitumor necrosis factor-α (anti-TNF-α) drugs, etanercept, infliximab, and adalimumab, have been associated with rapidly progressive, often fatal pulmonary fibrosis. They also raise the risk of opportunistic infections, particularly mycobacterial and fungal infections. *Mycobacterium tuberculosis* is more frequent. Infection may occur early in the treatment and present with extrapulmonary disease.

Leflunomide has been associated with fatal exacerbation of interstitial lung disease, pulmonary nodules, diffuse alveolar hemorrhage, and alveolar proteinosis.

In general, the evaluation and management of possible drug-related pulmonary toxicity requires (1) excluding progression of rheumatoid interstitial disease and infection; (2) withdrawing the potentially offending drug (and not rechallenging); and (3) treating with corticosteroids, as appropriate.

Bronchoscopy with lavage and/or open-lung biopsy should be considered in cases (1) of rapidly progressive interstitial disease; (2) where concern exists regarding drug-induced disease or opportunistic lung infection; or (3) of unexplained fever.

PULMONARY NODULES

Necrobiotic nodules in the lung parenchyma, either single (34% of cases) or multiple (66%), can occur at any time during the course of RA. They sometimes occur coincident with an exacerbation of joint symptoms. Necrobiotic nodules are more common in men and correlate with the presence of subcutaneous nodules. Histologically identical to subcutaneous rheumatoid nodules, they are characterized by palisading epithelial cells surrounding a central core of fibrinoid necrosis. These lesions tend to be asymptomatic unless they become very large, when they can cause compressive symptoms. They infrequently undergo cavitation, at which time minimal hemoptysis may be present. Few become infected. Nodules can rupture into the pleural space, resulting in bronchopleural fistulas, pleural effusions, pneumothoraces, or pyopneumothoraces. On chest radiographs, the nodules appear as rounded, homogenous densities 0.3 to 7.0 cm in diameter, typically located in the peripheral lung fields. They can persist unchanged, cavitate, or resolve spontaneously; frequently, they wax and wane with disease activity. Although reports attest to steroids hastening their resolution, most nodules require no specific therapy; however, a single nodule requires the same evaluation as any solitary pulmonary nodule.

Caplan syndrome was initially described as the appearance of nodular pulmonary opacities in coal miners with simple pneumoconiosis who had symmetric polyarthritis consistent with rheumatoid disease, a positive rheumatoid factor, or both. The syndrome has subsequently been described in individuals with occupational exposure to silicates, asbestos, iron, and aluminum powder. Histologically, the nodules resemble necrobiotic nodules except that a zone of inflammatory cells containing the offending dust is interposed between the palisading epithelial cells and the central necrosis. The nodules tend to occur in crops, which may herald the onset or worsening of arthritis symptoms. Roentgenographically, the nodules are multiple, 0.5 to 5.0 cm in diameter, and peripherally located. They frequently undergo cavitation and occasionally calcify. No specific therapy currently exists.

AIRWAYS DISEASE

Upper airways involvement in RA most commonly affects the cricoarytenoid joint. Up to 75% of patients may have abnormalities recognized with laryngoscopy and CT scan. Symptoms may be mild and chronic; however, an acute presentation with stridor may require emergent airway management. In addition, C1–C2 subluxation which can occur with neck hyperextension during oral endotracheal intubation can produce quadriplegia. The use of smaller endotracheal tubes and possibly fiber optic intubation may reduce the risks of laryngeal complications with surgery. Vocal cord nodules and obstructive sleep apnea may also be seen.

Distal airways involvement in RA can manifest as small airways disease with expiratory airflow obstruction, bronchiolitis obliterans with organizing pneumonia (BOOP), obliterative bronchiolitis, follicular bronchiolitis, or bronchiectasis.

Small airways disease resulting in expiratory airflow obstruction occurs in 16% to 30% of nonsmokers and 60% of smokers with RA. Airflow obstruction is caused by a peribronchiolar mononuclear cell infiltration, which can progress to an obliterative bronchiolitis. Small airways disease is associated with the presence of rheumatoid factor in high titer, rheumatoid nodules, keratoconjunctivitis sicca (Sjögren syndrome), and specific human leukocyte antigen alloantigens.

Pathologically, BOOP is defined as granulation tissue in terminal bronchioles with distal organizing pneumonia. BOOP is associated with restrictive pulmonary function tests, cough, fever, weight loss, dyspnea, and bilateral pulmonary infiltrates. Corticosteroids are useful for treatment.

Obliterative bronchiolitis is pathologically a constrictive peribronchiolar fibrosis involving small airways. Despite the similar sounding name, this disorder is pathologically and prognostically distinct from BOOP. Obliterative bronchiolitis is associated with obstructive pulmonary function tests, female gender, more advanced rheumatoid disease, use of gold and penicillamine, and Sjögren syndrome. Rapidly progressive dyspnea with cough is seen. Corticosteroids are used in treatment.

Follicular bronchiolitis is characterized by lymphocytic infiltrates with hyperplastic lymphoid follicles along bronchioles. Clinically, patients have dyspnea with cough and, sometimes, fever. Pulmonary function tests may show a mixed obstructive and restrictive pattern with a reduced diffusing capacity.

Bronchiectasis is seen in 35% of patients on HRCT scan and may reflect the result of small airways disease and recurrent infections.

PULMONARY VASCULAR DISEASE

Severe pulmonary vascular involvement in RA is rare. Several cases of progressive pulmonary hypertension with resultant cor pulmonale have been reported in young women with long-standing RA. Although lung tissue from individuals with rheumatoid interstitial pneumonitis occasionally contains a minor component of vasculitis, lung histology from these women predominantly reveals pulmonary arteritis with fibrotic intimal proliferation and medial hypertrophy within small muscular pulmonary arteries and negligible interstitial pneumonitis. Whether such cases represent a distinct variant of rheumatoid lung disease rather than a coincidental association of pulmonary arteritis with RA remains unclear. Patients with this syndrome have a poor prognosis. They present and behave similarly to those with primary pulmonary hypertension.

Pulmonary hypertension (pulmonary artery systolic pressure of 30 mmHg or more by Doppler echocardiography) was detected in 31% of a group of patients with RA. Two-thirds of this group had no clinical evidence of heart disease or pulmonary function test abnormalities.

Pulmonary capillaritis and diffuse alveolar hemorrhage have been described, but they are rare. Secondary pulmonary hypertension from interstitial pneumonitis can occur.

APICAL FIBROCAVITARY DISEASE

Apical fibrocavitary lesions have been described in a very small number of patients with RA. A recent report suggested that this is a clinically distinct pattern of lung involvement in RA. Clinically, the lesions may suggest tuberculosis and look similar to the apical pulmonary lesions seen in ankylosing spondylitis. Pathologically, cavitary necrobiotic nodules (clinically unsuspected) and interstitial fibrosis are seen.

MISCELLANEOUS

Other pulmonary conditions seen in patients with RA include malignancies with an increased incidence of bronchogenic carcinoma and lymphoma. Amyloid can produce interstitial infiltrates or pulmonary nodules. Reduced respiratory muscle strength and endurance and a reduced aerobic capacity are described. Dyspnea, a result of muscle weakness, may be due to RA myositis, vasculitis, or treatment drugs: corticosteroids, D-penicillamine, or hydroxychloroquine. RA is also associated with an increased risk of deep vein thrombosis.

FURTHER READING

1. Vourlekis JS, Brown KK. Thoracic complications of RA. PCCU lesson 17, vol 14. http://www .chestnet.org/education/online/pccu/vol14.

   A well-referenced recent review article. An excellent resource.

2. Dedhia HV, DiBartolomeo A. Rheumatoid arthritis. *Crit Care Clin.* 2002;18:841–854.

   A review article with an emphasis on ICU care and airway management.

3. Tanoue LT. Pulmonary manifestations of rheumatoid arthritis. *Clin Chest Med.* 1998;4:667.

   An excellent, concise, well-referenced review article. A definitive source.

4. Anaya JM, Diethelm L, Ortiz LA, et al. Pulmonary involvement in rheumatoid arthritis. *Semin Arthritis Rheum.* 1995;24:242.

   A comprehensive review article.

5. Helmers R, Galvin J, Hunninghake G. Pulmonary manifestations associated with rheumatoid arthritis. *Chest.* 1991;100:235.

   A concise, well-referenced review article.

6. Winterbauer RH, DePaso W, Lambert J. Pulmonary disease in rheumatoid arthritis patients. *J Respir Dis.* 1989;10:35.

   A clinically oriented review article.

7. Sahn SA. The pleura. *Am Rev Respir Dis.* 1988;138:184.

   A state-of-the-art review of pleural effusion with a well-referenced section on rheumatoid pleural involvement. A definitive source.

8. Saag KG, Kolluri S, Koehnke RK, et al. Rheumatoid arthritis lung disease: determinants of radiographic and physiologic abnormalities. *Arthritis Rheum.* 1996;39:1711.

   Concludes that smoking is an independent predictor of radiographic and physiologic abnormalities suggestive of interstitial lung disease in RA.

9. Gabbay E, Tarala R, Will R, et al. Interstitial lung disease in recent onset rheumatoid arthritis. *Am J Respir Crit Care Med.* 1997;156:528.

10. Dawson JK, Fewins HE, Desmond J, et al. Predictors of progression of HRCT diagnosed fibrosing alveolitis in patients with RA. *Ann Rheum Dis.* 2002;61:517–521.

    They found a low diffusing capacity (<54% predicted) progression.

11. Vassallo R, Matteson E, Thomas CF Jr. Clinical response of RA-associated pulmonary fibrosis to tumor necrosis factor-a inhibition. *Chest.* 2002;122:1093–1096.

    In this case report, infliximab treatments stabilized deteriorating pulmonary function and improved cough, dyspnea, and fatigue.

12. Oyama T, Kohno N, Yokoyama A, et al. Detection of interstitial pneumonitis in patients with rheumatoid arthritis by measuring circulating levels of KL-6, a human MUC1 mucin. *Lung.* 1997;175:379.

    This report associates active interstitial pneumonitis with an elevated serum KL-6 level. Potentially, a very useful test.

13. Ohnishi H, Yokoyama A, Kondo K, et al. Comparative study of KL-6, surfactant protein-A, surfactant protein-D, and monocyte chemoattractant protein-1 as serum markers for interstitial lung diseases. *Am J Respir Crit Care Med.* 2002;165:378–381.

    Of the markers studied, KL-6 is the best marker for interstitial lung disease. Twelve of the 33 patients with interstitial lung disease had collagen vascular diseases.

14. Hakala M. Poor prognosis in patients with rheumatoid arthritis hospitalized for interstitial lung fibrosis. *Chest.* 1988;93:114.

    A unique clinical analysis of one end of the spectrum of rheumatoid interstitial lung disease.

15. Kremer JM, Alarcón GS, Weinblatt ME, et al. Clinical laboratory, radiographic, and histopathologic features of methotrexate-associated lung injury in patients with rheumatoid arthritis: a multicenter study with literature review. *Arthritis Rheum.* 1997;40:1829.

    An important review article.

16. Ohosonc Y, Okano Y, Kameda H, et al. Clinical characteristics of patients with rheumatoid arthritis and methotrexate induced pneumonitis. *J Rheumatol.* 1997;12:2299.

    This retrospective review defines risk factors for methotrexate pulmonary toxicity.

17. Dawson JK, Graham DR, Desmond J, et al. Investigation of the chronic pulmonary effects of low-dose methotrexate in patients with RA: a prospective study incorporating HRCT scanning and pulmonary function tests. *Rheumatology (Oxford).* 2002;41:262–267.

18. Keane J, Gershon S, Wise RP, et al. Tuberculosis associated with infliximab, a tumor necrosis factor alpha-neutralizing agent. *N Engl J Med.* 2001;345:1098–1104.

    One must be aware of the potential for opportunistic infection with this drug. M. tuberculosis *is the most common.*

19. Tomioka R, King TE Jr. Gold-induced pulmonary disease: clinical features, outcomes and differentiation from rheumatoid lung disease. *Am J Respir Crit Care Med.* 1997;155:1011.

    A clinically oriented article.

20. Perez T, Remy-Jardin M, Cortet B. Airways involvement in rheumatoid arthritis: clinical, functional and HRCT findings. *Am J Respir Crit Care Med.* 1998;157:1658.

    This study indicates that HRCT appears to be more sensitive than pulmonary function tests for detecting small airways disease.

21. Begin R, Massé S, Cantin A, et al. Airways disease in a subset of non-smoking rheumatoid patients. *Am J Med.* 1983;72:743.

    Further evidence of the bronchiolitis of RA and its possible autoimmune basis.

22. Frank ST, Weg JG, Walsh RE, et al. Pulmonary dysfunction in rheumatoid disease. *Chest.* 1973;63:27.

    In this series, 41% had reduced diffusing capacity, including 50% of those with normal chest X-ray films.

23. Geddes DM, Webley M, Brewerton DA, et al. a-1-Antitrypsin phenotypes in fibrosing alveolitis and rheumatoid arthritis. *Lancet.* 1977;2:1049.

    A highly significant increase in the frequency of MZ phenotype was found in patients with fibrosing alveolitis, both with and without RA—but not in patients with RA without lung involvement.

24. Geddes DM, Corrin B, Brewerton DA, et al. Progressive airway obliteration in adults and its association with rheumatoid disease. *Q J Med.* 1977;46:427.

    Six patients with RA and rapidly progressive obstructive airways disease are described; four were nonsmokers. Chest roentgenograms showed hyperinflation without infiltrates, and histologic examination revealed bronchiolitis obliterans.

25. Caplan A. Certain unusual radiological appearances in the chest of coal miners suffering from rheumatoid arthritis. *Thorax.* 1953;8:29.

    An initial description of rheumatoid pneumoconiosis.

26. Rubin EH, Gordon M, Thelmo WL. Nodular pleuropulmonary rheumatoid disease. *Am J Med.* 1967;42:567.

    A review of nonpneumoconiotic rheumatoid lung disease. Subpleural necrobiotic-type nodules and persistent bronchopleural fistula were seen.

27. Dawson JK, Goodson NG, Graham DR, et al. Raised pulmonary artery pressures measured with Doppler echocardiography in RA patients. *Rheumatology (Oxford)*. 2000;39:1320–1325.

Mild pulmonary hypertension was seen in 31% of RA patients.

28. Schwarz MI, Zamora MR, Hodges TN, et al. Isolated pulmonary capillaritis and diffuse alveolar hemorrhage in rheumatoid arthritis and mixed connective tissue disease. *Chest.* 1998;113:1609.

First reported cases of diffuse alveolar hemorrhage in RA.

29. Morikawa J, Kitamura K, Habuchi Y, et al. Pulmonary hypertension in a patient with rheumatoid arthritis. *Chest.* 1988;93:876.

A case report and literature review of the rare association of pulmonary arteritis and RA.

30. Kay JM, Banik S. Unexplained pulmonary hypertension with pulmonary arteritis in rheumatoid disease. *Br J Dis Chest.* 1977;71:53.

Describes a young woman with RA and pulmonary vasculitis, and reviews the related literature.

31. Yue CC. Apical fibro-cavitary lesions of the lung in rheumatoid arthritis: review of 2 cases and review of the literature. *Am J Med.* 1986;81:741.

A good, clinically oriented report of this unusual condition.

32. Mellemkjaer L, Linet MS, Gridley G, et al. Rheumatoid arthritis and cancer risk. *Eur J Cancer.* 1996;324:1753.

A positive association was seen between RA and non-Hodgkin lymphoma, Hodgkin disease, and lung cancer. There was a negative association between RA and colorectal cancer.

33. Cimen B, Deviren SD, Yorgacloglu ZR. Pulmonary function tests, aerobic capacity, respiratory muscle strength, and endurance of patients with RA. *Clin Rheumatol.* 2001;20:168–173.

Reduced respiratory muscle strength, endurance, and aerobic capacity were seen in this study of 25 RA patients with normal pulmonary function tests.

34. Lofgren RH, Montgomery WW. Incidence of laryngeal involvement in rheumatoid arthritis. *N Engl J Med.* 1962;267:193.

Describes features of cricoarytenoid involvement in RA.

35. Artin-Ozerkis D, Gaffo AL, Alarcón GS. Pulmonary manifestations of rheumatoid arthritis. *Clin Chest Med.* 2010;31:451.

A current, comprehensive, well-referenced review article.

36. Kelly C, Saravanan V. Treatment strategies for a rheumatoid arthritis patient with interstitial lung disease. *Expert Opin Pharmacother.* 2008;9(18):3221.

An excellent authoritative review of current and possible future treatment options.

37. Matta F, Singala R, Yaekoub AY, et al. Risk of venous thromboembolism with rheumatoid arthritis. *J Thromb Haemost.* 2009;101(1):134.

RA patients are felt to be at increased risk of venous thrombosis.

38. Kim E, Dillon K, McGlothan K, et al. Rheumatoid arthritis-associated interstitial lung disease: the relevance of histopathology and radiographic pattern. *Chest.* 2009;136(5):1397.

A discussion of the diagnostic and management approach to RA-associated interstitial lung disease based on the high-resolution chest CT pattern.

39. Nesheiwat J, Dillon K, McGlothan K, et al. An elderly man with rheumatoid arthritis and dyspnea. *Chest.* 2008;135(4):1090.

A case report of leflunomide pulmonary toxicity with a good discussion of the workup.

96 The Lungs in Systemic Lupus Erythematosus, Systemic Sclerosis, Polymyositis, Dermatomyositis, and Mixed Connective Tissue Disease

Cecilia M. Smith and Gordon L. Yung

SYSTEMIC LUPUS ERYTHEMATOSUS

Systemic lupus erythematosus (SLE) commonly affects the lungs and pleura. Manifestations of SLE that directly affect the respiratory system include (1) pleuritis with or without pleural effusions; (2) acute lupus pneumonitis; (3) chronic interstitial pneumonitis and interstitial fibrosis; (4) hemorrhagic alveolitis with or without hemoptysis; (5) bronchiolitis obliterans with organizing pneumonia (BOOP); (6) diaphragm–respiratory muscle dysfunction; (7) upper airway dysfunction; (8) pulmonary hypertension with or without thromboembolic disease; (9) less commonly, diffuse lung disease findings of organizing pneumonia (OP), diffuse alveolar damage (DAD), or acute fibrinous and organizing pneumonia (AFOP); and (10) risk for lung cancer. The indirect effects of SLE on the lungs arise from predisposition to infection; in fact, pneumonia is the most frequent cause of infiltrates in patients with lupus.

Pleuritis and accompanying pleuritic chest pain, with or without effusions, are the most common pulmonary manifestations of SLE, occurring in 50% to 75% of patients, with a slightly higher male predominance. It can occur at any time during the clinical course and is the initial manifestation in approximately one-third of cases. The effusions are generally small and bilateral, but can be massive, unilateral, or associated with a pericardial effusion. The exudative fluid can be clear or serosanguineous, and the pH can be high or low; however, the glucose is usually greater than 56 mg/dL, which is useful in distinguishing it from a rheumatoid effusion. Cell counts reveal predominantly polymorphonuclear cells. Total hemolytic complement and serum antinuclear antibody (ANA) titers can be variable, but pleural fluid ANA titers greater than 1:320 strongly support the diagnosis of SLE pleuritis. Lupus erythematosus cells in the pleural fluid are diagnostic. Although most pleural effusions resolve completely with steroid therapy, some residual pleural thickening can persist.

The incidence of interstitial pneumonitis in SLE is controversial, depending on whether clinical, pulmonary function testing, or histologic findings are used as the criteria for diagnosis. Histologic changes display a spectrum similar to idiopathic interstitial pneumonitis, ranging from interstitial mononuclear infiltration to extensive fibrosis. The presence of anti-Sm antibodies in the serum significantly correlates with lung fibrosis. Clinically, acute lupus pneumonitis often presents with the sudden appearance of fever (as high as 104°F) and a nonproductive cough, which can progress rapidly to frank respiratory failure. Histology reveals a florid mononuclear cell infiltrate, interstitial thickening, alveolitis, and vasculitis. Several series report findings of immune complexes and complement within the alveolar walls, the pulmonary arterioles, and small vessels.

In contrast to other collagen vascular diseases such as rheumatoid arthritis and scleroderma, chronic interstitial pneumonitis and interstitial fibrosis are uncommon in SLE. In one report, fibrosis was observed in fewer than 3% of patients with lupus. Patients with fibrosis tend to be older (45–50 years) and have had a prolonged duration of disease before the development of chronic lung disease. The histologic findings include evidence of (1) chronic or recurrent pneumonitis, (2) interstitial and alveolar fibrosis, and (3) immunoglobulin and complement deposition in the alveolar septae. The nail-fold capillary density is a useful physical finding, because it correlates with the extent of gas exchange deficiency. Both acute and chronic lupus pneumonitis may clear radiographically. However, they can also progress to advanced interstitial fibrosis and honeycomb lung. Even after improvement in symptoms and radiographic appearance, decreased diffusing capacity of lung for carbon monoxide (DLCO) and restrictive defects in pulmonary function often persist.

Pulmonary alveolar hemorrhage is a relatively rare presenting feature of SLE. It occurs predominantly in women and is associated with the presence of lupus nephritis. In the correct setting, the combination of anemia, dyspnea associated with hypoxemia, and new radiographic chest infiltrate may suggest its presence. Mortality approaches 50% and is even higher in patients who have required mechanical ventilation, have received cyclophosphamide (perhaps indicating more advanced disease), or have a nosocomial infection. Pathology usually shows a small vessel capillaritis, arteriolitis, and venulitis. Immune complex deposition in a granular pattern distinguishes the pathology of diffuse alveolar hemorrhage (DAH) in SLE from Goodpasture's (linear distribution).

A relatively common histologic finding in open-lung biopsy specimens is cryptogenic organizing pneumonia (COP), which includes characteristic plugs of granulation tissue within small airways and alveolar ducts in conjunction with inflammatory changes of the bronchioles and pulmonary parenchyma. The usual associated clinical presentation is nonspecific, and patients may show a restrictive ventilatory defect. Diagnosis requires thoracoscopic or open-lung biopsy, and the pathologic changes tend to respond to steroid treatment.

Physiologic studies include the importance of diaphragmatic and respiratory muscle weakness as a cause of dyspnea and a restrictive ventilatory defect in some patients with SLE. A condition known as *shrinking lung syndrome* consists of dyspnea with chest radiograph findings of small lung volumes, elevated hemidiaphragms, and basilar atelectasis. Maximal inspiratory pressure and maximal expiratory pressure measurements demonstrate inspiratory and expiratory respiratory muscle weakness as the basis for the restrictive ventilatory defects. Comparing the movement of the two hemidiaphragms by fluoroscopy is not useful because both tend to be affected. Transdiaphragmatic pressure during active breathing, measured by esophageal and gastric balloons, confirms the presence of diaphragmatic weakness. Most patients do not have diffuse muscle weakness; therefore, random muscle biopsy is of little utility. The pathogenesis remains unclear and the optimal therapy for this syndrome has not been established. This is also associated with pleurisy. Pleurisy with pleuritic chest pain was present at the time of evaluation in 65% of 77 patients reported.

Although upper airway involvement is uncommon in SLE, hypopharyngeal ulceration, laryngeal inflammation, epiglottitis, and subglottic stenosis have been reported. These manifestations of SLE may result in complications during endotracheal intubation.

Pulmonary hypertension with cor pulmonale, which can be seen with or without associated pulmonary emboli, is significantly correlated with the antiphospholipid syndrome. In one series of 24 patients who had pulmonary hypertension, 68% had a lupus anticoagulant or anticardiolipin antibody. The cause of pulmonary hypertension in SLE can vary among patients. Possible causes include (1) small vessel arteriopathy, (2) chronic large vessel thromboembolic disease, and (3) secondary hypertension caused by end-stage parenchymal fibrosis. In many patients, the pathologic findings in the pulmonary vascular bed are indistinguishable from primary pulmonary hypertension. Raynaud phenomenon is almost uniformly seen in cases not associated with parenchymal lung disease. Vasculitis and immune deposits are seen in SLE with or without the development of pulmonary hypertension. On the other hand, thromboembolism occurs in up to 25% of patients with SLE and is a major cause of death. Most patients with thromboembolism are treated with life-long anticoagulation. Thromboendarterectomy for chronic pulmonary thromboembolic disease has been successful in lupus patients.

Less common to rare manifestations include OP and DAD. AFOP has histopathology features of intra-alveolar fibrin deposition associated with OP. There are overlap features with

DAD, OP, and AFOP. Thoracoscopic or open-lung biopsy is required to differentiate these histopathologic findings.

Acute reversible hypoxemia has been described in patients with lupus associated with normal chest radiographs and widened A–a oxygen gradients. Patients generally present with pleuritic chest pain, dyspnea, and chest discomfort. Vital capacity and D$_{LCO}$ are significantly reduced. The syndrome appears to respond to corticosteroids, which improve oxygenation. The cause may be related to transient, complement-mediated aggregation, and neutrophil activation within the pulmonary vasculature.

There is a link between SLE and an increased risk of lung cancer. In one review of 30 cases, 75% were female with a median age of 61 (range 21–91) years. The histologic distribution of the cell types of lung cancers from SLE patients was similar to that of lung cancer patients in the general population. In this group, 71% were smokers and only 20% were exposed to immunosuppressive therapies.

Pulmonary function abnormalities are common, occurring in 70% to 80% of patients with SLE-associated lung disease even in the absence of symptoms and radiographic abnormalities. The most common abnormalities are decreased D$_{LCO}$ and reduced lung volumes. Airway obstruction is unusual. Hypoxemia at rest or with exercise is present frequently. Concomitant renal dysfunction is seen frequently with lupus-associated pulmonary disease.

The management of pulmonary involvement in SLE is generally supportive. Corticosteroids appear to be the most useful drugs, with other agents such as cyclophosphamide, azathioprine, or mycophenolate mofetil added according to the severity of organ involvement. Therapies focusing on B- and T-cell functions by rituximab (anti-CD20 monoclonal antibody) or infliximab (tumor necrosis factor-α blockade) are also being evaluated in ongoing studies. Even if the patient responds to therapy, pulmonary involvement is a poor prognostic sign; respiratory syndromes in SLE have been associated with a 2-fold increased risk of death at 1 year. Pulmonary hypertension associated with SLE is responsive to each type of pulmonary vasodilator therapy as reported in the literature. For patients with pulmonary hypertension associated with pulmonary thromboemboli, treatment is directed for pulmonary embolic disease, acute or chronic.

SYSTEMIC SCLEROSIS

Systemic scleroderma (SSc) is one form of scleroderma that involves internal organs as well as the characteristic skin disorder, which typically undergoes serial changes from the edematous phase to induration and skin thickening and tightness. Eventually, pitting scars and acrosclerosis can also occur in the fingers. The other form of this disease is localized to skin and adjacent tissues (morphea, linear scleroderma). Systemic sclerosis is further categorized into five subsets based on the extent and distribution of the skin involvement, plus the pattern of internal organs involved: diffuse cutaneous, limited cutaneous, sine scleroderma, environmentally induced scleroderma, and overlap syndrome with other collagen vascular diseases.

The two most common subsets of SSc are diffuse cutaneous and limited cutaneous. The disease is considered to be either diffuse or limited based on the extent and distribution of skin involvement plus internal organs affected.

Diffuse cutaneous systemic sclerosis (dcSSc) is associated with diffuse, often rapidly progressive, skin involvement of the chest, abdomen, shoulders and upper arms, and internal organ injuries due to fibrosis and/or ischemic vascular disease. Raynaud phenomenon generally is followed rapidly by the onset of skin and other systemic changes. Internal organ involvement with renal disease, interstitial pulmonary fibrosis, GI (esophageal dysmotility), and myocardial disease can occur early and be significant, and overall prognosis is generally poor.

Limited cutaneous systemic sclerosis (lcSSc) differs from dcSSc in that the skin involvement is generally *limited* to the hands and distal forearms as well as the face and neck, and there is often prolonged delay in the appearance of internal organ manifestations. Limited cutaneous SSc is associated with vascular manifestations such as telangiectasia and calcinosis; in its full form, it is often associated with the CREST syndrome. The CREST syndrome consists of (1) *c*alcinosis cutis, (2) *R*aynaud phenomenon, (3) presence or absence of *e*sophageal dysfunction, (4) *s*clerodactyly, and (5) *t*elangiectasias. Raynaud phenomenon may be present for an extensive period of time before diagnosis.

The other subsets of SSc include sine scleroderma, which is a rare form with the presence of internal organ disease without skin involvement; environmentally induced scleroderma, with the manifestations of scleroderma precipitated by exposure to a chemical agent (e.g., vinyl chloride or pesticides); and overlap syndrome including features of scleroderma as well as manifestations of other collagen vascular diseases.

Systemic sclerosis commonly affects the lung. Lung pathology is second in frequency to esophageal disease, and pulmonary complications are the most frequent cause of death, making early detection of lung involvement an important predictor of survival. Pulmonary pathology is found in approximately 90% of patients at autopsy.

The most common lung abnormalities include interstitial lung disease and pulmonary arterial hypertension (PAH). The most common pattern of diffuse lung disease is nonspecific interstitial pneumonitis (NSIP). This pattern is seen in up to 75% of patients with SSc-associated interstitial lung disease. It is more frequent in dcSSc (approximately 40%) than in lcSSc (approximately 35%). A small subset of these patients evolves to end-stage pulmonary fibrosis, with histopathology consistent with findings of usual interstitial pneumonia (UIP).

PAH occurs in up to 40% of patients with systemic sclerosis. PAH occurs in both diffuse and limited forms of disease but is seen 10 times more commonly in the limited cutaneous form of systemic sclerosis. PAH can occur with or without interstitial pulmonary fibrosis. When PAH develops, it can lead to cor pulmonale and right-sided heart failure.

Other pulmonary conditions associated with systemic sclerosis include aspiration pneumonitis associated with esophageal dysmotility, airway disease, hypoventilation due to neuromuscular weakness, extrinsic pulmonary restrictive physiology due to chest wall involvement of cutaneous skin disease, pleural effusions, pneumothorax, and lung cancer.

Patients with scleroderma have significantly higher risk for lung cancer than the general population. Scleroderma patients who smoke have a 7-fold higher risk as compared to nonsmoking scleroderma patients, and nonsmoking scleroderma patients have a 5-fold higher risk for developing lung cancer as compared to age- and gender-matched subsets of the general population. This appears to be similar for both diffuse cutaneous as well as limited cutaneous forms of systemic sclerosis.

Although the lung is commonly affected, respiratory symptoms are rarely the presenting complaint. Dyspnea on exertion is the most common pulmonary symptom, followed by a nonproductive or minimally productive cough. Pleuritic chest pain and pleural effusions are rare. Lung examination reveals basilar inspiratory crackles. Signs of pulmonary hypertension may be present, depending on the severity of the disease. The finding of digital ulcers is associated with interstitial lung disease but not PAH.

Pulmonary function studies are abnormal in most patients; decreased D_{LCO} is the most common finding, followed by reduced lung volumes and airway obstruction. Chest roentgenograms reveal interstitial infiltrates in approximately one-third of patients. The echocardiogram with estimated pulmonary arterial pressures can screen for the development of PAH. However, if abnormal, a right-heart catheterization is required to diagnose PAH. An exercise echocardiogram may need to be performed to elicit abnormal elevation in pulmonary artery pressure.

There is no specific laboratory test for systemic sclerosis; the diagnosis is based on a constellation of clinical and laboratory findings. Raynaud phenomenon and sclerotic skin changes occur in over 90% of these patients at various times of the disease, and about 80% will eventually develop some degree of esophageal dysmotility. Various autoantibodies have been associated with systemic sclerosis, but the incidence varies widely, with many autoantibodies developing late in the course of the disease. ANA, typically of a speckled fluorescence but also nucleolar, is found in more than 90% of patients with scleroderma. Several "scleroderma-specific" antibodies demonstrate specificity of 70% to 80%, but poor sensitivities of less than 20%. In general, anti-DNA topoisomerase I (Scl-70), anti-U3 ribonucleoprotein (anti–U3-RNP), and anti-RNA polymerase I, II, and III antibodies are associated with diffuse scleroderma and renal crisis, whereas anticentromere antibody (ACA) is positive in 25% to 30% of all systemic sclerosis patients and up to 70% to 80% of patients with lcSSc. Patients who are ACA positive have been noted to have a decreased frequency of interstitial fibrosis and restrictive lung disease, but are prone to develop PAH and esophageal disease. On the other hand, anti–Scl-70 antibodies are associated with diffuse skin involvement, visceral organ involvement, interstitial lung disease, and a greater risk of cancer. Finally, anti-PM/Scl tends to be found in those with scleroderma/polymyositis overlap syndrome.

Because of the lack of specific markers for diagnosis, and the lag time for the development of full disease manifestations, a recently proposed scheme was developed for early diagnosis of systemic sclerosis. A diagnosis of systemic sclerosis should be considered in patients with a combination of Raynaud phenomenon, "puffy fingers," and positive antinuclear antibodies. This should then be followed by nail-fold capillaroscopy (for abnormal capillary dilation and/or dropout) and blood tests for scleroderma-specific antibiotics. A diagnosis of systemic sclerosis is made if either test is positive.

The age distribution and gender predominance of pulmonary involvement reflect those of systemic sclerosis in general: most patients are in the fourth to sixth decades with a 3:1 female predominance.

It is believed that a multifactorial complex pathologic process involving hyperproliferative lung fibroblasts from increased expression of transcription factor Sp1, endothelial injury, and impaired vasodilation plays a role in promoting and advancing pulmonary fibrosis. As fibrosis progresses, severe pulmonary architectural distortion occurs, which is associated with bronchiectasis and the formation of cystic air spaces of up to 1 to 2 cm in diameter in a subpleural distribution. Rupture of these cysts can result in spontaneous pneumothorax. Pulmonary hypertension can also develop in association with the interstitial lung process. Radiographic (HRCT scan) evidence of fine basilar reticular or reticulonodular changes is usually accompanied by restrictive pulmonary function defects. Reduced DLco may be the first indication of pulmonary involvement and has been found to be quite sensitive. In the absence of radiographic or ventilatory defects, significant dyspnea with a low DLco suggests the presence of pulmonary vascular disease.

The incidence of PAH in scleroderma ranges from 6% to 60%, depending on the test used to diagnose PAH. Additionally, the presence of autoantibodies to antitopoisomerase 1 is associated with severe pulmonary vascular disease. The pathogenesis of PAH is believed to be secondary to inflammatory and fibrogenic pathways in blood vessels and the heart. Fibrosis and perivascular cellular infiltration with activated T cells in the pulmonary arteries lead to pulmonary hypertension and cor pulmonale. Left-ventricular failure, secondary to systemic hypertension or cardiomyopathy, is frequently coexistent. Isolated PAH has a worse prognosis than PAH secondary to fibrosis, with a poor prognosis and 2-year survival of 40%. Early diagnosis and treatment are critical.

Pleuritis is present histologically in up to 85% of patients at autopsy, but is only symptomatic in 16% of patients with scleroderma. Clinically significant effusions are uncommon. Pleural effusions or pleural thickening occur as a result of scleroderma involving the pleura or secondary to congestive heart failure from cardiac involvement. Reexpansion of the lung after thoracentesis is usually slow because of decreased lung compliance and recurrence is common, often requiring pleurodesis.

Aspiration pneumonitis can occur because of esophageal dysfunction, which can contribute to the development of chronic pneumonitis. Respiratory muscle dysfunction without generalized weakness has been reported to occur, similar to the phenomenon described in SLE.

A 2-fold increased incidence of bronchogenic carcinoma has been observed with systemic sclerosis, relative to the normal population. Older patients, diffuse disease, presence of pulmonary fibrosis, and antitopoisomerase 1 antibody have been associated with an increased risk of cancer in scleroderma.

Low vitamin D levels have been found in patients with systemic sclerosis. In one study, systemic sclerosis patients with low vitamin D levels demonstrated more severe disease. In another study, patients with systemic sclerosis, compared to matched healthy controls, had lower vitamin D levels. It may be beneficial to measure vitamin D levels and replace as necessary. However, the impact on the course of this disease is unknown.

No therapeutic regimens exist to reverse the interstitial pulmonary fibrotic disease at an early stage. There have been several studies evaluating the role of cyclophosphamide therapy for pulmonary fibrosis associated with systemic sclerosis with both the oral and intravenous routes of administration. A common finding from these different studies is stabilization in improvement of lung function at the completion of the treatment phase of up to 1 year, but effectiveness in maintaining the gains achieved may vary. Some studies reported sustained improvement in lung function after 2 and 3 years off therapy, while another reported decline in function after 1 year off therapy. Cyclophosphamide was also found to improve health-related quality of life parameters after 1 year of therapy. Another study evaluated the use of cyclophosphamide initially followed by subsequent treatment with azathioprine to sustain the improvements of the initial therapy. Mycophenolate mofetil is also being studied for its effectiveness in treatment of pulmonary fibrosis associated with systemic sclerosis. The results of two independent small studies for mycophenolate mofetil appeared promising with improvement or trend to improvement in lung function after 1 year of therapy. Mycophenolate mofetil improves the cutaneous changes of this disease.

Treatment of PAH needs to be given early due to the severity of this progressive disease in patients with systemic sclerosis. Oxygen, oral pulmonary vasodilator therapy, and/or prostacyclin analogs have demonstrated effectiveness in reducing pulmonary artery pressures and improving cardiac output and exercise capacity. Many authors advocate the addition of warfarin anticoagulation, based on its apparent efficacy in the treatment of primary pulmonary hypertension.

Lung transplantation may be an option for some patients with systemic sclerosis. One center's experience compared outcomes of two groups of transplanted patients with systemic sclerosis or idiopathic pulmonary fibrosis (IPF). The 1-year all-cause mortality did not differ between the two patient groups. The incidence of acute rejection was higher in the systemic sclerosis group, but chronic rejection, infection, and pulmonary function showed no difference. Transplantation may be an option but will need to be an individualized decision based on extent and severity of other organ involvement.

POLYMYOSITIS

Polymyositis (PM) is an inflammatory, autoimmune myopathy characterized by proximal muscle weakness. *Dermatomyositis* (DM) is similar to PM and additionally involves the skin with a characteristic heliotrope rash. Pulmonary involvement has been reported in up to 10% of patients and is a significant cause of mortality. Both conditions have a 2:1 female predominance with a peak incidence in the fifth and sixth decades. The syndromes associated with PM and DM can be loosely separated into the following categories: (1) adult PM, (2) adult DM, (3) childhood PM or DM, (4) PM or DM associated with malignancy, and (5) PM or DM associated with a preestablished collagen vascular disease.

The syndrome may affect the lung in any of the following ways: (1) primary interstitial pneumonitis with progression to fibrosis; (2) pulmonary hypertension secondary to interstitial lung disease or pulmonary vascular disease; (3) recurrent aspiration pneumonitis secondary to esophageal muscle dysmotility; (4) respiratory muscle weakness with resultant hypoventilation, atelectasis, and pneumonia; (5) spontaneous pneumomediastinum; and (6) COP.

The pulmonary component of PM or DM can precede the muscle symptoms by years. When interstitial pneumonitis precedes muscle manifestations, the diagnosis can be missed because of the focus on the pulmonary disease. The presence of serum antibody to histidyl-tRNA-synthetase (anti–Jo-1) significantly correlates with interstitial lung disease in up to 75% of patients. The discovery of this antibody in a patient with isolated pulmonary interstitial lung disease may be helpful in predicting the future development of PM or DM.

The antisynthetase syndrome consists of interstitial lung disease, arthritis, myositis, fever, mechanic's hands, and Raynaud phenomenon in the presence of antisynthetase autoantibody, most commonly anti–Jo-1. Other antisynthetase autoantibodies are also believed to be associated with this clinical presentation.

Two other forms of respiratory involvement can occur as complications of therapy: (1) opportunistic infection secondary to immunosuppressive drugs and (2) drug-induced lung changes secondary to cytotoxic therapy for the muscle component of the disease.

Spontaneous pneumomediastinum is a rare complication of PM/DM. Up to 25% of patients in one series died within 1 month of occurrence. Pneumomediastinum can occur prior to DM diagnosis or with no or minimum muscle involvement. Severe pulmonary disease was present prior to the onset of the pneumomediastinum.

PM/DM is recognized to be associated with malignancies. Common cancers associated with PM/DM include ovarian, lung, pancreatic, breast, and stomach. A rarer occurrence is the association with hematologic malignancies, including acute myelocytic leukemia. Interstitial lung disease is less commonly seen in PM/DM associated with malignancy.

The pathologic findings differ between patients with acute, symptomatic interstitial lung disease and those with a more subacute or chronic presentation. In the acute presentation, patients may present with cough, fever, and dyspnea with or without skin or muscle findings. The chest radiographic study reveals diffuse mixed alveolar interstitial infiltrates. The clinical course is similar to Hamman–Rich syndrome. Pathologic findings include NSIP, usual interstitial pneumonitis, COP, or DAD with focal alveolar hemorrhage. Small vessel vasculitis (pulmonary capillaritis) was recently reported in several patients with PM, where pulmonary and muscle symptoms presented simultaneously. With the chronic presentation, pathology usually is consistent with usual interstitial pneumonitis. The pathogenesis of the muscle and pulmonary manifestations of the disease is thought to involve T-cell activation by muscle autoantigens, resulting in a release of interleukin-2 and γ-interferon. Subsequent promotion of macrophages and a cytokine called *macrophage inflammatory protein* lead to eventual tissue injury.

Clinically, respiratory symptoms are absent in up to 40% of patients with roentgenographic or histologic pulmonary changes. When symptoms occur, patients may present with dyspnea, dysphagia, or nonproductive cough. Examination of the lungs of patients with interstitial lung disease characteristically reveals fine, late inspiratory crackles (described as "Velcro-like") in a bibasilar distribution. Roentgenographically, the disease manifests as lower-lobe reticulonodular infiltrates with an associated alveolar-filling component in 20% of patients. Pleural involvement is rare. Pulmonary function studies typically show a restrictive pattern caused by either interstitial changes or respiratory muscle weakness. Commonly, a reduced DLco is also found.

Routine laboratory findings are nonspecific. The sedimentation rate is usually elevated, whereas antinuclear antibodies and rheumatoid factor are negative. Serum levels of muscle enzymes (creatine kinase and aldolase) are elevated in most cases.

Response to therapy varies, depending on the histologic features. COP is most responsive to steroids, whereas DAD has, to date, been associated with uniformly poor prognosis. However, studies of different therapies are ongoing. Corticosteroids can be used alone, or in combination with cyclophosphamide or azathioprine for parenchymal lung disease. A small series of patients with DM and acute/subacute interstitial pneumonia was treated with cyclosporine and prednisolone at different dosing of the cyclosporine. The group with combined prednisolone and cyclosporine started in the early days of lung disease manifestation had lower mortality from respiratory failure. A series of monthly intravenous cyclophosphamide plus oral prednisolone for chronic progressive interstitial pneumonia had improved symptoms, pulmonary function tests, and HRCT scan findings. Rituximab, an anti-CD20 monoclonal antibody targeting B cells, has been used in inflammatory myositis, DM more commonly but also PM. The most common manifestations of disease include skin and muscle weakness. The drug has been well tolerated with good response. The most common complication was respiratory infections.

MIXED CONNECTIVE TISSUE DISEASE

Mixed connective tissue disease (MCTD) has clinical and laboratory characteristics of SLE, PM/DM, and scleroderma. The distinguishing feature of MCTD is an antibody to extractable nuclear antigen (anti–nRNP-Ab) or ribonuclease-sensitive ribonucleoprotein (sn-RNP). Dilutions of sn-RNP greater than 1:10,000 are considered confirmatory of MCTD. Controversy continues regarding whether MCTD is a distinct entity from the other collagen vasculitides.

The incidence of pulmonary involvement in MCTD is approximately 85% ($n = 34$), of which 73% are asymptomatic. Pleural effusion (25%–50%), interstitial pneumonitis, pulmonary vasculitis, pulmonary artery hypertension, pulmonary thromboembolic disease, aspiration pneumonia, and hypoventilatory failure can occur. Presenting symptoms include exertional dyspnea, nonproductive cough, pleuritic chest pain, and fever. Clubbing is not seen. Of the asymptomatic patients with MCTD, 75% have evidence of pulmonary involvement on chest radiograph or pulmonary function studies. There is no significant HRCT scan finding that distinguishes MCTD from any of the other collagen vascular diseases, but interlobular septal thickening in the lower lobes predominates. Correlation with HLA-DR3 and interstitial pulmonary fibrosis has been observed in one small study.

Histopathology of the lung in interstitial lung disease associated with MCTD is similar to IPF. Additionally, a proliferative vasculopathy is associated with MCTD, characterized by intimal thickening with medial muscular hypertrophy of the pulmonary arteries and arterioles, which correlates with the presence of pulmonary hypertension.

Radiographically, bilateral basilar interstitial opacities, right ventricular hypertrophy, and pulmonary artery enlargement can be seen. Pulmonary function abnormalities include decreased D_{LCO} (up to 67% of patients) and reduced lung volumes (50% of patients). Small airway obstruction is seen early and is an indication of functional impairment.

It had been reported that the pulmonary disease of MCTD is benign and responds to steroid therapy with improvement shown on the chest roentgenogram and pulmonary function studies. A few reports, however, describe progressive pulmonary disease and rapid deterioration despite steroid therapy. Renal disease and Raynaud phenomenon is associated with a higher mortality rate. Some long-term follow-up studies show evolution of MCTD toward other connective tissue diseases (SLE, progressive systemic sclerosis, and rheumatoid arthritis). The overall prognosis is estimated to be similar to that seen in patients with SLE.

FURTHER READING
Lupus Erythematosus

1. Ford HJ, Roubey RAS. Pulmonary manifestations of the antiphospholipid antibody syndrome. *Clin Chest Med.* 2010;31:537–545.

   Vascular and pulmonary parenchymal involvement associated with antiphospholipid antibody syndrome with pulmonary thromboembolism and pulmonary hypertension being the most common manifestations.

2. Prabu A, Patel K, Yee CS, et al. Prevalence and risk factors for pulmonary arterial hypertension in patients with lupus. *Rheumatology (Oxford).* 2009;48(12):1506–1511.

   A large cohort of lupus patients followed in nontertiary centers was studied for the prevalence of PAH, which was 4.2%. Lupus anticoagulant was found to be a significant association.

3. Kamen DL, Strange C. Pulmonary manifestations of systemic lupus erythematosus. *Clin Chest Med.* 2010;31:479–488.

   A review of the various forms of SLE-associated lung disease.

4. Toya SP, Tzelepis GE. Association of the shrinking lung syndrome in systemic lupus erythematosus with pleurisy: a systematic review. *Semin Arthritis Rheum.* 2009;39(1):30–37.

   Pleural disease as well as diaphragmatic muscle weakness plays a role in this phenomenon.

5. Bin J, Bernatsky S, Gordon C, et al. Lung cancer in systemic lupus erythematosus. *Lung Cancer.* 2007;56(3):303–306.

6. Bernatsky S, Boimin JF, Joseph L, et al. Mortality in systemic lupus erythematosus. *Arthritis Rheum.* 2006;54(8):2550–2557.

7. Oudiz RJ, Schilz RJ, Barst RJ, et al. Treprostinil, a prostacyclin analogue, in pulmonary arterial hypertension associated with connective tissue disease. *Chest.* 2004;126(2):420–427.

8. Garcia-Carrasco M, Jimenez-Hernandez M, Escarcega RO, et al. Use of rituximab in patients with systemic lupus erythematosus: an update. *Autoimmun Rev.* 2009;8(4):343–348.

9. Hassoun PM. Pulmonary arterial hypertension complicating connective tissue diseases. *Semin Respir Crit Care Med.* 2009;30:429–439.

10. Wahl D, Guillemin F, de Maistre E, et al. Risk for venous thrombosis related to antiphospholipid antibodies in systemic lupus erythematosus—a meta-analysis. *Lupus.* 1997;6:467–473.

11. Flaherty K, Colby TV, Travis WD, et al. Fibroblastic foci in usual interstitial pneumonia, idiopathic versus collagen vascular disease. *Am J Respir Crit Care Med.* 2003;167:1410–1415.

12. Rojas-Serrano J, Pedroza J, Regalado J, et al. High prevalence of infections in patients with systemic lupus erythematosus and pulmonary hemorrhage. *Lupus.* 2008;17(4):295–299.

13. Pope J. An update in pulmonary hypertension in systemic lupus erythematosus–do we need to know about it? *Lupus.* 2008;17(4):274–277.

14. Swigris JJ, Olson AL, Fischer A, et al. Mycophenolate mofetil is safe, well tolerated, and preserves lung function in patients with connective tissue disease-related interstitial lung disease. *Chest.* 2006;130(1):30–36.

15. Badsha H, Teh CL, Kong KO, et al. Pulmonary hemorrhage in systemic lupus erythematosus. *Semin Arthritis Rheum.* 2004;33(6):414–421.

Systemic Sclerosis

16. Hudson M, Fritzler MJ, Baron M, et al. Systemic sclerosis: establishing diagnostic criteria. *Medicine (Baltimore).* 2010;89(3):159–165.

    The Canadian Scleroderma Research Group Registry evaluated over 1,000 scleroderma patients to learn clues with sensitivity for the diagnosis of SSc. The sensitivity of the establishing diagnosis is 97% with the presence of Raynaud phenomenon, skin involvement, visible telangiectasias, and at least one SSc-related autoantibodies.

17. Tyndall AJ, Bannert B, Vonk M, et al. Causes and risk factors for death in systemic sclerosis: a study from the EULAR Scleroderma Trials and Research (EUSTAR) database. *Ann Rheum Dis.* 2010;69(10):1809–1815.

    The cause of death was investigated on a cohort of 234 patients. Fifty-five percent of deaths were attributed directly to SSc. The SSc-related deaths included 35% due to pulmonary fibrosis, 26% to pulmonary hypertension, and 26% due to cardiac causes.

18. Tashkin DP, Elashoff R, Clements PJ, et al. Cyclophosphamide versus placebo in scleroderma lung disease. *N Engl J Med.* 2006;354(25):2655–2666.

    A multicenter, double-blind, randomized, placebo-controlled trial to assess the effect of oral cyclophosphamide on lung function in patients with pulmonary fibrosis associated with SSc. One year on therapy provided a significant benefit on lung function that was maintained through 24 months.

19. Shitrit D, Amital A, Peled N, et al. Lung transplantation in patients with scleroderma: case series, review of the literature, and criteria for transplantation. *Clin Transplant.* 2009;23(2):178–183.

20. Goldin JG, Lynch DA, Strollo DC, et al. High-resolution CT scan findings in patients with symptomatic scleroderma-related interstitial lung disease. *Chest.* 2008;134(2):358–367.

21. Steen V, Chou M, Shanmugam V, et al. Exercise-induced pulmonary arterial hypertension in patients with systemic sclerosis. *Chest.* 2008;134(1):146–151.

22. Koutroumpas A, Ziogas A, Alexiou I, et al. Mycophenolate mofetil in systemic sclerosis-associated interstitial lung disease. *Clin Rheumatol.* 2010;29(10):1167–1168.

23. Avouac J, Wipff J, Kahan A, et al. Effects of oral treatments on exercise capacity in systemic sclerosis-related pulmonary arterial hypertension: a meta-analysis of randomized controlled trials. *Ann Rheum Dis.* 2008;67(6):808–814.

24. Tashkin DP, Elashoff R, Clements PJ, et al. Effects of 1-year treatment with cyclophosphamide on outcomes at 2 years in scleroderma lung disease. *Am J Respir Crit Care Med.* 2007;176(10):1026–1034.

25. Khanna D, Yan X, Tashkin DP, et al. Impact of oral cyclophosphamide on health-related quality of life in patients with active scleroderma lung disease: results from the scleroderma lung study. *Arthritis Rheum.* 2007;56(5):1676–1684.

26. Domiciano DS, Bonfa E, Borges CT, et al. A long-term prospective randomized controlled study of non-specific interstitial pneumonia (NSIP) treatment in scleroderma. *Clin Rheumatol.* 2011;30(2):223–229.

27. Hant FN, Silver RM. Biomarkers of scleroderma lung disease: recent progress. *Curr Rheumatol Rep.* 2011;13(1):44–50.

28. Manno R, Boin F. Immunotherapy of systemic sclerosis. *Immunotherapy.* 2010;2(6):863–878.

29. LePavec J, Launay D, Mathai SC, et al. Scleroderma lung disease. *Clin Rev Allergy Immunol.* 2011;40(2):104–116.

30. Hsu E, Shi H, Jordan RM, et al. Lung tissues in patients with systemic sclerosis have gene expression patterns unique to pulmonary fibrosis and pulmonary hypertension. *Arthritis Rheum.* 2011;63(3):783–794.

31. Bussone G, Mouthon L. Interstitial lung disease in systemic sclerosis. *Autoimmun Rev.* 2011;10(5):248–255.

32. Arnson Y, Amital H, Agmon-Levin N, et al. Serum 25-OH vitamin D concentrations are linked with various clinical aspects in patients with systemic sclerosis: a retrospective cohort study and review of the literature. *Autoimmun Rev.* 2011;10(8):490–494. doi:10.1016/j.autrev.2011.02.002.

33. Hudson M, Lo E, Lu Y, et al. Cigarette smoking in patients with systemic sclerosis. *Arthritis Rheum.* 2011;63(1):2230–2238.

34. Christmann RB, Wells AU, Capelozzi VL, et al. Gastroesophageal reflux incites interstitial lung disease in systemic sclerosis: clinical, radiologic, histopathologic, and treatment evidence. *Semin Arthritis Rheum.* 2010;40(3):241–249.

35. Swartz JS, Chatterjee S, Parambil JG. Desquamative interstitial pneumonia as the initial manifestation of systemic sclerosis. *J Clin Rheumatol.* 2010;166:284–286.

36. Mouthon L, Berezne A, Guillevin L, et al. Therapeutic options for systemic sclerosis related interstitial lung diseases. *Respir Med.* 2010;104(suppl 1):S59–S69.

37. Sweiss NJ, Jushaw L, Thenappan T, et al. Diagnosis and management of pulmonary hypertension in systemic sclerosis. *Curr Rheumatol Rep.* 2010;12(1):8–18.

38. Mathai SC, Hassoun PM. Therapy for pulmonary arterial hypertension associated with systemic sclerosis. *Curr Opin Rheumatol.* 2009;21(6):642–648.

39. Lynch DA. Lung disease related to collagen vascular disease. *J Thorac Imaging.* 2009;24(4):299–309.

40. Hachulla E, Launay D, Yaici A, et al. Pulmonary arterial hypertension associated with systemic sclerosis in patients with functional class II dyspnoea: mild symptoms but severe outcome. *Rheumatology (Oxford).* 2010;49(5):940–944.

41. Launay D, Sitbon O, Le Pavec J, et al. Long-term outcome of systemic sclerosis-associated pulmonary arterial hypertension treated with bosentan as first-line monotherapy followed or not by the addition of prostanoids or sildenafil. *Rheumatology (Oxford).* 2010;49(3):490–500.

42. Badesch DB, McGoon MD, Barst RJ, et al. Longterm survival among patients with scleroderma-associated pulmonary arterial hypertension treated with intravenous epoprostenol. *J Rheumatol.* 2009;36(10):2244–2249.

43. Badesch DB, Hill NS, Burgess G, et al. Sildenafil for pulmonary arterial hypertension associated with connective tissue disease. *J Rheumatol.* 2007;34(12):2417–2422.

44. Pontifex EK, Hill CL, Roberts-Thomson P. Risk factors for lung cancer in patients with scleroderma: a nested case-control study. *Ann Rheum Dis.* 2007;66(4):551–553.

45. Al-Dhaher FF, Pope JE, Ouimet JM. Determinants of morbidity and mortality of systemic sclerosis in Canada. *Semin Arthritis Rheum.* 2010;39:269–277.

Polymyositis/Dermatomyositis

46. Kalluri M, Sahn SA, Oddis CV, et al. Clinical profile of anti-PL-12 autoantibody: cohort study and review of the literature. *Chest.* 2009;135:1550–1556.

A focused discussion on the antisynthetase antibodies, which are associated with the antisynthetase syndrome. Clinical findings and the strong association with interstitial lung disease are reviewed.

47. Kalluir M, Oddis CV. Pulmonary manifestations of the idiopathic inflammatory myopathies. *Clin Chest Med.* 2010;31:501–512.

A clinicopathologic review of the pulmonary presentations of PM.

48. Connors GR, Christopher-Stine L, Oddis CV, et al. Interstitial lung disease associated with the idiopathic inflammatory myopathies: what progress has been made in the past 35 years? *Chest.* 2010;138:1464–1474.

A review of pathogenesis, clinical presentation, diagnostic testing, biomarkers, and therapies. A diagnostic and management algorithm provides guidance in the care of these patients.

49. Rios FR, Callejas RJL, Sanchez CD, et al. Rituximab in the treatment of dermatomyositis and other inflammatory myopathies: a report of 4 cases and review of the literature. *Clin Exp Rheumatol.* 2009;27(6):1009–1016.

50. Fathi M, Vikgren J, Boijsen M, et al. Interstitial lung disease in polymyositis and dermatomyositis: longitudinal evaluation by pulmonary function and radiology. *Arthritis Rheum.* 2008;59:677–685.

51. Richards TJ, Eggebeen A, Gibson K, et al. Characterization and peripheral blood biomarker assessment of anti-Jo-1 antibody-positive interstitial lung disease. *Arthritis Rheum.* 2009;60:2183–2192.

52. Douglas WW, Tazelaar HD, Hartman TE, et al. Polymyositis-dermatomyositis associated interstitial lung disease. *Am J Respir Crit Care Med.* 2001;164:1182–1185.

53. Tillie-Leblond I, Wislez M, Valeyre D, et al. Interstitial lung disease and anti-Jo-1 antibodies: difference between acute and gradual onset. *Thorax.* 2008;63:53–59.

54. Arakawa H, Yamada J, Kurihara Y, et al. Nonspecific interstitial pneumonia associated with polymyositis and dermatomyositis: serial high-resolution CT findings and functional correlation. *Chest.* 2003;123:1096–1103.

55. LeGoff B, Cherin P, Cantagrel A, et al. Pneumomediastinum in interstitial lung disease associated with dermatomyositis and polymyositis. *Arthritis Rheum.* 2009;61:108–118.

56. Teixeira A, Cherin P, Demoule A, et al. Diaphragmatic dysfunction in patients with idiopathic inflammatory myopathies. *Neuromuscul Disord.* 2005;15:32–39.

57. Kotani T, Makino S, Takeuchi T, et al. Early intervention with corticosteroids and cyclosporine A and 2-hour postdose blood concentration monitoring improves the prognosis of acute/subacute interstitial pneumonia in dermatomyositis. *J Rheumatol.* 2008;35(2):254–259.

58. Yamasaki R, Yamada H, Yamasaki M, et al. Intravenous cyclophosphamide therapy for progressive interstitial pneumonia in patients with polymyositis/dermatomyositis. *Rheumatology (Oxford).* 2007;46(1):124–130.

Mixed Connective Tissue Disease

59. Hant FN, Herpel LBM, Silvery RM. Pulmonary manifestations of scleroderma and mixed connective tissue disease. *Clin Chest Med.* 2010;31:433–449.

A review of the pulmonary manifestations of MCTD, therapeutic options, and prognosis.

60. Vegh J, Szodoray P, Kappelmayer J, et al. Clinical and immunoserological characteristics of mixed connective tissue disease associated with pulmonary arterial hypertension. *Scand J Immunol.* 2006;64:69–76.

Autoantibodies associated with the presence of PAH were studied in 197 patients. Differences in patient demographics and mortality were assessed in patients with and without the presence of PAH.

61. Devaraj A, Wells AU, Hansell DM. Computed tomographic imaging in connective tissue diseases. *Semin Respir Crit Care Med.* 2007;28:389–397.

A review of the spectrum of findings of the chest in connective tissue diseases, including MCTD.

62. Lundberg IE. Cardiac involvement in autoimmune myositis and mixed connective tissue disease. *Lupus.* 2005;14:708–712.

63. Burdt MA, Hoffman RW, Deutscher SL, et al. Long-term outcome in mixed connective tissue disease: longitudinal clinical and serologic findings. *Arthritis Rheum.* 1999;42:899–909.

64. Bull TM, Fagan KA, Badesch DB. Pulmonary vascular manifestations of mixed connective tissue disease. *Rheum Dis Clin North Am.* 2005;31:451–464.

65. Bodolay E, Szekanecz Z, Devenyi K, et al. Evaluation of interstitial lung disease in mixed connective tissue disease (MCTD). *Rheumatology (Oxford).* 2005;44:656–661.

66. Fagundes MN, Caleiro MT, Navarro-Rodriguez T, et al. Esophageal involvement and interstitial lung disease in mixed connective tissue disease. *Respir Med.* 2009;103:854–860.

67. Horiki T, Fuyuno G, Ishii M, et al. Fatal alveolar hemorrhage in a patient with mixed connective tissue disease presenting polymyositis features. *Intern Med.* 1998;37:554–560.

97 Pulmonary Langerhans Cell Histiocytosis

Cecilia M. Smith and Gordon L. Yung

Pulmonary Langerhans cell histiocytosis (PLCH), also known as histiocytosis X, is a diffuse interstitial lung disease characterized histologically by a predominance of differentiated cells of the monocytes/macrophage lineage. The term PLCH is preferred over other names such as eosinophilic granuloma or Langerhans cell granulomatosis. These are both misnomers because the pathologic lesions contain few, if any, eosinophils and do not form true granulomas. PLCH shares a spectrum of disease with Letterer–Siwe disease and Hand–Schüller–Christian disease. The latter two diseases have characteristic ages of onset (typically childhood), are more severe, and affect multiple organs including bone and, occasionally, soft tissues with infiltration of atypical histiocytes. Although PLCH was initially described as a disease of bone, isolated lung disease and multisystem involvement are well described.

The incidence and prevalence of PLCH are unknown. However, it is diagnosed rarely, even at centers that specialize in diffuse interstitial pulmonary disease. PLCH may occur at any age. It has been reported as early as infancy (3 months of age) and up to the seventh decade; however, most cases are diagnosed in young adulthood, between 20 and 40 years of age. PLCH was previously believed to affect men more than women, but recent data do not support a gender predilection. Women tend to develop the disease at a later age than men. Caucasians appear to be affected more commonly than those of African and Asian descent. There is no associated occupational predisposition. The most striking demographic feature of the disease is its strong association with current or past tobacco use. Fewer than 5% of patients are lifelong nonsmokers.

CLINICAL PRESENTATION

Although patients with PLCH often present with pulmonary (cough, dyspnea, chest pain) or constitutional (fever, weight loss) symptoms, some present with asymptomatic radiographic findings. The most common abnormal radiographic presentation is spontaneous pneumothorax. Hemoptysis may occasionally occur, but this should prompt a search for opportunistic infections (especially *Aspergillus* spp.) or associated tumor. Painful bony lesions may precede lung involvement and result in pathologic fracture as a presenting symptom. There are no diagnostic findings on bone radiographs. Diabetes insipidus may occur as a result of hypothalamic involvement and probably portends a poor prognosis. Airway involvement, pleural effusion, and lymphadenopathy are distinctly uncommon manifestations.

The physical examination is often normal. Crackles and finger clubbing are uncommon; however, in advanced disease, evidence of pulmonary hypertension with associated right-heart failure may be present. Laboratory evaluation is typically normal. Peripheral eosinophilia is not associated with PLCH. Although spirometry and static lung volumes are often normal, obstructive or restrictive patterns may be seen and the diffusing capacity of the lung for carbon monoxide (D_{LCO}) is characteristically reduced. Obstructive airway disease with hyperinflation occurs in a minority of patients with advanced cystic disease. There is usually exercise intolerance with activity limitation out of proportion to pulmonary function impairment. Resting room air arterial blood gas measurements are typically normal until disease is advanced, but exercise testing may reveal gas exchange abnormalities as well as a reduction in maximum oxygen consumption and workload.

DIAGNOSIS

The diagnosis of PLCH is strongly suggested by typical findings on the chest radiograph and high-resolution computed tomography (HRCT) scan. Specifically, small (2–12 mm) stellate nodules, upper-lobe reticulonodular opacities, and cysts or honeycombing favoring the upper lung zones are strongly suggestive. Differential diagnosis of similar radiologic findings might include lymphangioleiomyomatosis, tuberous sclerosis, hypersensitivity pneumonitis, chronic eosinophilic pneumonia, sarcoidosis, and end-stage idiopathic pulmonary fibrosis. In the appropriate clinical setting (i.e., young smokers), these findings may be pathognomonic. HRCT scanning can detect disease not readily apparent on the chest radiograph and is extremely useful in monitoring disease progression and response to therapy. Radiographic findings include upper lung zone predominance characteristically sparing the costophrenic angles, reticulonodular opacities, ill-defined or stellate nodules (2–12 mm size), upper-zone cysts, and honeycomb lung with preservation of lung volume. Patients with costophrenic angle involvement are more likely to experience disease progression and have an unfavorable prognosis.

The Langerhans cell, the pathologic cell type involved in PLCH, is derived from the monocyte/macrophage lineage and is characterized by pale cytoplasm and a large nucleus with prominent nucleoli. Pentalaminar cytoplasmic inclusions seen on electron microscopy are known as Birbeck granules or X bodies, and are considered pathognomonic. Immunohistochemical stains are positive for S100 and CD1a. These cells are normally found scattered in the dermis, lung, pleura, and reticuloendothelial system. Small numbers may also be seen in the pulmonary parenchyma of patients with idiopathic pulmonary fibrosis. Immunostaining and identification of the S100 protein or CD1a receptor on pathologic specimens usually obviate the need for electron microscopy.

In a minority of patients with PLCH (15%), the diagnosis can be established on the basis of appropriate radiographic studies and clinical history. In the absence of the classic findings, it is necessary to obtain tissue. Bronchoalveolar lavage (BAL) is usually insufficient, although recovery in the lavage fluid of more than 5% Langerhans cells is strongly suggestive. Transbronchial biopsy specimens may provide adequate tissue for analysis and is reported to be diagnostic in 10% to 40% of patients. However, the small sample size and potential for sampling error may yield false-negative results. Video-assisted thoracoscopic surgery or open-lung biopsy provides larger specimens under direct visualization and is the most definitive diagnostic procedures.

Histopathologic specimens show an accumulation of Langerhans cells, tissue inflammation, fibrosis, and cystic spaces. Inflammatory lesions (cellular infiltrates) are centered around bronchioles, arterioles, and venules early in the disease course giving the characteristic stellate appearance. The cellular infiltrate consists of Langerhans cells mixed with neutrophils, lymphocytes, and scattered eosinophils. Eosinophils are not a prominent component of the inflammatory process, and well-formed granulomas are rare. Areas of desquamative interstitial pneumonia (pseudodesquamative interstitial pneumonia) and respiratory bronchiolitis (smoker's bronchiolitis) may also be seen. End-stage fibrosis may occur. In these cases, the typical histopathology may no longer be present, replaced by acellular tissue findings that may be difficult to distinguish from other forms of end-stage pulmonary fibrosis with findings of fibrosis, honeycombing, and cystic lesions.

TREATMENT

Initial therapy should consist of smoking cessation. Clinical and radiographic resolution has been well described with this intervention alone. Patients who continue to smoke can expect gradual progression of disease. Corticosteroids and cytotoxic agents (vinblastine, methotrexate, cyclophosphamide, and chlorodeoxyadenosine) have failed to produce any benefit. Only patients with prominent nodular opacities respond to glucocorticoid therapy. Despite the lack of documented efficacy, systemic corticosteroids continue to be used in patients with progressive pulmonary disease, perhaps only because of the lack of any other effective treatment. Radiation therapy is highly effective for isolated bone lesions, but has been disappointing with respect to pulmonary lesions. Recurrent pneumothorax has been treated effectively with medical and surgical pleurodesis. Lung transplantation has been successful in patients with isolated end-stage lung disease, but PLCH has also been shown to recur in the transplanted lung.

The natural history of PLCH is extremely variable: some patients experience complete remission, and others progress to end-stage lung disease. Median survival is reported to be 12 years from the time of diagnosis. Almost 50% of deaths are from respiratory failure. Factors suggesting a worse prognosis include extremes of age at diagnosis, low forced expiratory volume in 1 second (FEV_1), and low D_{LCO}, presence of pulmonary arterial hypertension, and presence of isolated lung disease. Patients with PLCH are at an increased risk of developing both malignant and nonmalignant tumors. These include bronchogenic carcinoma and pulmonary carcinoid tumors, as well as hematologic malignancies (both Hodgkin and non-Hodgkin lymphoma). Recurrent spontaneous pneumothorax occurs in up to 25%. Associated malignancy follows only respiratory failure as cause of death in patients with PLCH. Patients may also develop pulmonary hypertension out of proportion to the degree of pulmonary fibrosis. Pulmonary hypertension is associated with increased mortality that may be responsive to systemic corticosteroids. Diabetes insipidus is usually responsive to chemotherapy, but patients may require long-term desmopressin replacement. Patients with radiographic sparing of the costophrenic angles are more likely to remain stable or improve.

Additional information for both patients and providers is available through the Histiocytosis Association of America (www.histio.org; 1-800-548-2758).

FURTHER READING

1. Lazor R, Etienne-Mastroianni B, Khouatra C, et al. Progressive diffuse pulmonary Langerhans cell histiocytosis improved by cladribine chemotherapy. *Thorax.* 2009;64:274–275.

   A description of the cellular proliferation triggered by an inhaled agent, its location as bronchiolocentric granulomas that advance to cysts, and the predominantly upper lung zone findings of histiocytic granulomas and cyst lesions are characteristic of Langerhans cell histiocytosis.

2. Aerni MR, Aubry MC, Myers JL, et al. Complete remission of nodular pulmonary Langerhans cell histiocytosis lesions induced by 2-chlorodeoxyadenosine in a non-smoker. *Respir Med.* 2008;102: 316–319.

   A report of a patient responding to 2-chlorodeoxyadenosine. While steroids and immunosuppressive agents have been used with advancing disease, efficacy is unclear.

3. Beasley MB. Smoking-related small airway disease—a review and update. *Adv Anat Pathol.* 2010;17:270–276.

   Reviews the spectrum of histologic findings and pathogenesis of smoking-related small airway disease.

4. Nagarjun Rao R, Moran CA, Suster S. Histiocytic disorders of the lung. *Adv Anat Pathol.* 2010;17(1):12–22.

   A review of pulmonary histiocytic proliferations of uncertain histogenesis, which includes pulmonary Langerhans cells histiocytosis.

5. Arico M, Girschikofsky M, Genereau T, et al. Langerhans cell histiocytosis in adults: report from the International Registry of the Histiocyte Society. *Eur J Cancer.* 2003;39:2341–2348.

   One of the largest patient data collections. Data on 274 patients from 13 countries. This paper presents demographic data, prognostic factors, and treatment. Highest mortality was reported in patients who had only localized pulmonary disease, yet remained good with a 87.5% probability of survival at 5 years post diagnosis.

6. Sundar KM, Gosselin MV, Chung HL, et al. Pulmonary Langerhans cell histiocytosis: emerging concepts in pathobiology, radiology and clinical evolution of disease. *Chest.* 2003;123:1673–1683.

   An excellent review with specific attention to etiology and pathologic basis of eosinophilic granuloma and radiologic modalities for monitoring disease.

7. Vassallo R, Ryu JH, Schroeder DR, et al. Clinical outcomes of pulmonary Langerhans'-cell histiocytosis in adults. *N Engl J Med.* 2002;346:484–490.

   A 4-year follow-up of a cohort of 102 patients. There were 33 deaths, 15 due to respiratory failure. Six hematologic cancers diagnosed. Median survival is 12.5 years. Survival significantly worse than predicted based on actuarial tables of the general population. Poor prognostic indicators included low FEV_1, high residual volume, and low D_{LCO}. Respiratory failure accounts for significant number of deaths.

8. Mendez JL, Nadrous HF, Vassallo R, et al. Pneumothorax in pulmonary Langerhans' cell histiocytosis (PPLCH). *Chest.* 2004;125:1028–1032.

   A retrospective review of 102 adults with pneumothorax in pulmonary Langerhans cell histiocytosis assessing frequency, recurrence, and management of pneumothorax. Pneumothorax occurred in 16% and was recurrent in 63% of those patients. No pneumothoraces recurred after chest tube evacuation and pleurodesis.

9. Dacic S, Trusky C, Bakker A, et al. Genotypic analysis of pulmonary Langerhans' cell histiocytosis. *Hum Pathol.* 2003;34:1345–1349.

   A comparative genotypic analysis using loss of heterozygosity of tumor-suppressor genes. Results indicated that the putative tumor suppressor genes may lie on chromosomes 9, 22, or both.

10. Suzuki M, Betsuyaku T, Suga M, et al. Pulmonary Langerhans' cell histiocytosis presenting with an endobronchial lesion. *Intern Med.* 2004;43:227–230.

    An atypical presentation of eosinophilic granuloma. A case report of concomitant parenchymal and endobronchial evidence of eosinophilic granuloma, both of which spontaneously resolved.

11. Vassallo R, Ryu JH. Pulmonary Langerhans' cell histiocytosis. *Clin Chest Med.* 2004;25:561–571.

    A review of this uncommon cause of interstitial lung disease, occurring predominantly in adult cigarette smokers. The disease can be mild to severe with single organ to extensive organ involvement and high mortality. Pulmonary involvement is more common in adults.

12. Tazi A. Adult pulmonary Langerhans' cell histiocytosis. *Eur Respir J.* 2006;27:1272–1285.

    An overview of clinical presentation and diagnostic tests. A description of HRCT scan findings, which is a combination of nodules, cavitated nodules, and thick and thinned walled cysts that predominate in the upper lobes. BAL can provide Langerhans cells but have low sensitivity. Biopsy with Langerhans cell granulomas is required for diagnosis.

13. Gotz G, Fighter J. Langerhans'-cell histiocytosis in 58 adults. *Eur J Med Res.* 2004;9:510–514.

    Data collected on adult patients demonstrating a predominance in single organ involvement (72%) and 28% with multisystem involvement. Osseous and cutaneous focus seen predominantly outside lung involvement. Eighty-eight percent of patients are current or ex-smokers.

14. Chaowalit N, Pellikka PA, Decker PA, et al. Echocardiographic and clinical characteristics of pulmonary hypertension complicating pulmonary Langerhans cell histiocytosis. *Mayo Clin Proc.* 2004;79:1269–1275.

    Pulmonary hypertension is associated with higher mortality. There is an inverse relationship between forced vital capacity and estimated pulmonary artery systolic pressure.

15. Canuet M, Kessler R, Jeung MY, et al. Correlation between high-resolution computed tomography findings and lung function in pulmonary Langerhans cell histiocytosis. *Respiration.* 2007;74:640–646.

    No correlation found between lung nodular profusion score and lung function or gas exchange parameters. The score of cystic extent correlated with FEV_1 and PaO_2. Predominant cystic pattern had highest grade of dyspnea, lowest FEV_1, and lowest PaO_2 than nodular or mixed pattern disease.

16. Vassallo R, Ryu JH. Tobacco smoke-related diffuse lung diseases. *Semin Respir Crit Care Med.* 2008;29(6):643–650.

    Cigarette smoking–associated interstitial lung diseases are reviewed. Both a bronchiolar and interstitial inflammation results from tobacco smoke inhalation.

17. Attili AK, Kazerooni EA, Gross BH, et al. Smoking-related interstitial lung disease: radiologic-clinical-pathologic correlation. *Radiographics.* 2008;28(5):1383–1396.

    Overlap of spectrum of histopathology in smoking-related conditions. The correlation of clinical, radiologic, and pathologic data is needed for identification of specific entity.

Neurofibromatosis, Lymphangioleiomyomatosis, and Tuberous Sclerosis

Cecilia M. Smith and Gordon L. Yung

NEUROFIBROMATOSIS

Neurofibromatosis type 1 (NF1, von Recklinghausen disease) is characterized by cutaneous neurofibromas, café-au-lait spots, Lisch nodules of the iris, and various other systemic manifestations. Von Recklinghausen disease, an autosomal dominant dysplasia of ectoderm and mesoderm with a variable clinical expression, appears in all races, with a prevalence of 1 in 3,000 live births. The *NF1* gene is located on chromosome 17. In 30% to 50% of patients, there is no family history of the disease. The lungs and thorax are involved by cutaneous and subcutaneous neurofibromas on the chest wall, kyphoscoliosis, ribbon deformity of the ribs, thoracic neoplasms, and interstitial lung disease (ILD).

Interstitial pneumonitis occurs in a subset of patients with NF1. In a review of the literature, there were 64 patients with NF1 who had diffuse lung disease (DLD). Some authors state that 7% to 20% of adults with *NF1* have ILD. The mean age of patients with NF1 and DLD was 50 years, with more males than females. Most patients report dyspnea as a complaint. The cause of the pneumonitis remains obscure. Pathologically, it is grossly and microscopically indistinguishable from idiopathic interstitial pneumonia. The lung surface is often studded with bullae of varying sizes with striking upper-lobe predominance; a honeycombed appearance is common on sectioning. Histologic specimens show diffuse interstitial fibrosis and architectural disruption, with extensive alveolar destruction and cystic changes. Hyperplasia of neurolemma cells of intrapulmonary nerves has been described.

Dyspnea of insidious onset is often the presenting manifestation, although discovery in an asymptomatic individual through an incidental chest roentgenogram may occur. Cough occurs in approximately one-third of patients and chest pain in 5%. Chest radiographs in 63 patients revealed bullous lung disease in 73%, predominantly in the upper lobes. Basilar linear densities were present in 63% and honeycombing in 13%. HRCT scans revealed bullae (50%), reticular abnormalities (50%), ground-glass abnormality (37%), cysts (25%), and emphysema (25%). In one study, HRCT scans in 6 nonsmokers with NF1 demonstrated 2- to 18-mm thin wall cysts, upper-lobe predominant patchy ground-glass densities, and centrilobular micronodules. Lung cysts were located in the central or subpleural regions, or both. There was no radiologic evidence of lung fibrosis, honeycombing, or severe bullous disease. The chest radiograph may initially reveal only accentuated interstitial markings or diffusely mottled, ill-defined infiltrates. The infiltrates usually progress over years to a coarse linear or reticulated pattern and bulla formation. Interstitial fibrosis is usually symmetric with a basal predominance. Bullae form diffuse fibrobullous interstitial disease. Other thoracic manifestations of this disease include paravertebral neurofibroma, lateral meningocele, kyphoscoliotic vertebral deformity, and cutaneous neurofibroma. Physiologic measurements reveal a combination of restrictive and obstructive defects, diminished carbon monoxide diffusing capacity (DLCO), and hypoxemia (initially limited to exercise).

The diagnosis is generally obvious because the neurocutaneous manifestations almost invariably precede the interstitial pneumonitis. Rarely, biopsy is necessary to exclude another infiltrative pulmonary process. The course is variable and often slowly progressive. No specific therapy currently exists for pulmonary fibrosis associated with NF1.

Rarely, patients develop progressive respiratory failure with pulmonary hypertension (PH) leading to death. PH, when it occurs, has a late onset and female predominance and can occur late in the course of pulmonary disease. However, NF1-associated PH also can occur in patients with mild or absent parenchymal lung disease. Precapillary plexiform pulmonary arteriopathy is seen in NF1-associated PH, similar to idiopathic pulmonary arterial hypertension. Dyspnea and symptoms of right-heart failure are major symptoms leading to the diagnosis of PH. Conventional treatment with oxygen, diuretics, and anticoagulation should be considered. Treatment with pulmonary vasodilator medications, phosphodiesterase type 5 inhibitors, endothelin receptor antagonists, and prostanoids have each been used in patients with NF1-associated PH, but the role of these medications is not clear. The response to these medications has varied. It has been reported that there has been a limited response with poor outcome. In one small series of seven patients, five patients died within 3 years of presentation.

Emphasis on early referral for lung transplantation assessment in eligible patients should be stressed. Often, referral is appropriate early in the course of the patient's disease presentation.

Other thoracic manifestations include severe scoliosis and neurofibromas of the posterior or superior mediastinum. Neurofibromas arise from nerve sheaths in the sympathetic chain, vagus, and intercostal and intrapulmonary nerves. These tumors are commonly found adjacent to the spinal column. Neurofibromas can present in the tongue, larynx, trachea, and bronchi and cause airway obstruction. Patients may also have a hoarse voice, difficulty swallowing, or a deviated trachea. Neurogenic tumors involving the lung are rare, although multiple neurofibromas of varying size can occur. Hypoxemia can be caused by right-to-left shunts within these tumors. These tumors are usually benign, but malignant change can occur. The development of carcinoma can be a complication of the diffuse interstitial disease.

LYMPHANGIOLEIOMYOMATOSIS

Lymphangioleiomyomatosis or lymphangiomatosis (LAM) is a rare, progressive cystic pulmonary disorder with female predominance. LAM occurs in approximately 30% of women with the tuberous sclerosis complex (TSC) as well as in women without tuberous sclerosis (sporadic LAM, S-LAM). There is proliferation and infiltration of pulmonary interstitial smooth muscle cells with cystic destruction within the lungs. LAM frequently involves other organs (e.g., the kidneys, retroperitoneal or abdominal lymph nodes, liver, uterus, and pancreas) in addition to the lungs and can also be associated with abdominal and thoracic lymphatic spread with lymphadenopathy and abdominal tumors. Renal angiomyolipomas have been reported in 30% to 50% of patients with LAM. The incidence of meningioma is increased in women with LAM.

LAM occurs almost exclusively in women of childbearing age, in whom the disease can progress either rapidly or slowly to respiratory failure and death. There are rare cases of LAM diagnosed in males with TSC. In one series of 29 men with TSC, a retrospective review of CT scans of the chest was performed to assess the frequency of cystic lung disease. Thirty-eight percent (11/29) of the men had findings of four or more cysts present. The mean age was 46.3 years. None experienced a pneumothorax or chylothorax.

Over the last decade, there have been advances in the basic science of LAM. LAM and TSC are caused by mutations in one or the other of the tuberous sclerosis genes, TSC1 or TSC2. These genes control cell growth, cell survival, and cell motility through the Akt/mammalian target of rapamycin (mTOR) signaling pathway. Encoded proteins, hamartin or tuberin, are either deficient or dysfunctional, which results in loss of regulation of signals. The activation of mTOR kinase and S6 kinase leads to inappropriate cellular proliferation, migration, and invasion. Its incidence in young women, exacerbations during pregnancy, and associated steroid receptors in the lung, coupled with the known effect of estrogen and progesterone on smooth muscle, suggests that hormonal interactions are important in its pathogenesis, though these mechanisms are not well understood.

The hallmarks of pathology in LAM are nodular and tortuous masses of smooth muscle and epithelioid cells around bronchovascular structures that extend into the interstitium, without significant fibrosis. Diffuse cystic dilatation of terminal airspaces is a unique feature, ranging in size from subcentimeter to several centimeters in diameter. Grossly, the pleura is thickened, and large thick-walled cystic airspaces give rise to a honeycombed appearance of the lungs. Hilar, mediastinal, and retroperitoneal lymph nodes are often enlarged and spongy, and the thoracic duct is distended with lymph. Chylothorax can be present because of lymphatic rupture. Microscopically, a striking nodular proliferation of smooth muscle is seen within the pleura and alveolar walls, as well as in and around the walls of bronchioles, venules, and lymphatics. Immunohistochemistry stains assist in confirming the diagnosis with positive melanocytic and muscle markers. These smooth muscle cells exhibit melanoma-related marker, HMB45 immunoreactivity, distinct from other causes of smooth muscle proliferation. HMB45, a monoclonal antibody, also reacts with angiomyolipomas, clear cell tumors of the lung, and melanoma cells.

Bronchiolar obstruction from smooth muscle proliferation leads to air trapping, resulting in destruction of alveolar septa and honeycombed cystic spaces, especially at the lung bases. Ultra-structural studies of lung biopsy specimens demonstrate degradation of elastic fibers in areas of smooth muscle accumulation, which may be a factor leading to the development of emphysema-tous changes. Venous obstruction results in dilatation and rupture of venules, chronic low-grade hemorrhage, and, ultimately, hemosiderosis. Both estrogen and progesterone cell-surface receptors have been demonstrated in the lung.

Pulmonary manifestations are the most common presenting symptoms in patients with LAM. Of the 230 patients enrolled in the NHLBI Lymphangioleiomyomatosis Registry, spontaneous pneumothorax was the event that led to the diagnosis of LAM in approximately one-third of the patients. The average age at onset of symptoms was 39 years (range 18–76 years) and 41 years for the average age at diagnosis. TSC was present in approximately 15%. Progressive dyspnea and recurrent pneumothorax are the most common presentations. Other symptoms include wheezing, cough, and chylous pleural effusion.

Pneumothorax presents in approximately 70% of patients. Of these, more than 70% recur with an average of 4.4. Pleurodesis is recommended after the first pneumothorax in a patient known to have LAM due to the high recurrence rate. With conservative therapy (chest tube drainage or aspiration), the recurrence rate is approximately 66%; with surgical or chemical pleurodesis, the recurrence rate decreases to 32% and 27%, respectively.

Chylous pleural effusions occur bilaterally or unilaterally in about 33% of patients. Other clinical manifestations include hemoptysis (30%), ascites (11%), pericardial effusion (6%), chyloptysis (7%), and chyluria (3%). With abdominal lymphatic obstruction, chylous ascites can develop. Occasionally, communication between dilated retroperitoneal lymphatics and a kidney or ureter result in chyluria. Patients presenting with angiomyolipoma and pulmonary symptoms should be evaluated for LAM by chest CT scan, because the two are associated. Some patients may be asymptomatic at diagnosis.

The physical examination frequently is not revealing until late in the clinical course, when end-inspiratory rales, diminished lower-lobe breath sounds, scattered rhonchi, hyperinflation, signs of pleural effusion and/or ascites, and intra-abdominal or lymphatic masses are present. Abrupt exacerbation of dyspnea may signal the development of pneumothorax. Clubbing is rare.

LAM can be discovered by abnormal HRCT scan evidence of thin-walled cystic changes. Less commonly, it may be discovered on biopsy of an abdominal or retroperitoneal mass thought to be lymphoma or ovarian cancer. The chest roentgenogram initially may be normal or demonstrate reticulonodular interstitial opacities or severe emphysematous changes with hyperinflation in advanced disease. Occasionally, small cysts coalesce to form large blebs. This occurs predominantly at the lung bases. HRCT scan is more useful than the chest radiograph in assessing the presence and extent of cysts. HRCT typically demonstrates numerous small (2–20 mm) thin-walled cysts throughout both lungs. Greater morphologic and physiologic correlation is seen with the HRCT scan than with the chest radiograph.

Laboratory findings of complete blood count, serum chemistry, and liver enzyme levels are nonspecific except for chyluria. Pulmonary function tests (PFTs) most commonly reveal mild to severe airflow obstruction, followed by reduced diffusion capacity. Bronchodilator response is present in 17% of patients reported in the NHLBI Lymphangioleiomyomatosis Registry. PFTs were normal in approximately 34% of Registry patients. Hypoxemia (worsened by exertion), reduced flows and D_{LCO}, and progressive increase in plethysmographic lung volume also are characteristic. Significant functional impairment usually precedes any radiographic abnormality (other than pneumothorax). Diminished exercise capacity is seen, most likely caused by ventilatory limitation. Serial exercise testing has been suggested as a means to monitor disease progression and screen for exertional hypoxemia.

The diagnosis of LAM is likely in a young female presenting with dyspnea, emphysematous changes on the chest radiograph, recurrent pneumothorax, and/or chylous pleural effusion associated with renal tumors; PFTs may be normal or abnormal. The radiographic distribution and nature of the lesions are highly characteristic. Biopsy is generally necessary to confirm the diagnosis. Of 75 lung specimens obtained by transbronchial and open-lung biopsy, only LAM showed HMB45-positive cells. It has been suggested that if only a transbronchial biopsy is available, this marker can assist in confirming the diagnosis. A study assessing the diagnostic usefulness of the serologic test for vascular endothelial growth factor-D (VEGF-D) demonstrated its potential as a biomarker. This may eventually eliminate the need for biopsy. VEGF-D is a lymphangiogenic growth factor, and serum VEGF-D levels are higher in women with S-LAM than in women with other cystic lung diseases. Serum VEGF-D levels are significantly higher in women with TSC-LAM compared to women with TSC alone. Serum VEGF-D levels greater than 600 pg/mL were highly associated with the diagnosis of LAM; values greater than 800 pg/mL were diagnostically specific in a study of 48 women presenting with cystic lung disease.

The differential diagnosis includes pulmonary Langerhans cell histiocytosis (PLCH), emphysema, Sjögren syndrome, follicular bronchiolitis, lymphocytic interstitial pneumonitis, hypersensitivity pneumonitis, amyloidosis, bronchopulmonary dysplasia, metastatic endometrial stromal cell sarcoma, leiomyosarcomas, and Birt–Hogg–Dubé (BHD) syndrome. Low-grade sarcomas metastatic to the lung have rarely been misdiagnosed as LAM.

Mediastinal and pulmonary lymphangiomyomas are resistant to radiation therapy. Surgical or chemical obliteration (pleurodesis) of the pleural space should be performed with the first pneumothorax in known LAM due to recurrent effusion or pneumothorax. Symptomatic therapy for bronchospasm or cor pulmonale may be required. Corticosteroids and cytotoxic agents appear to offer no benefit. Hormonal manipulation can affect muscle proliferation in this disease. Pregnancy and estrogen therapy can worsen the disease, and remission of the disease can occur after menopause. Oophorectomy or tamoxifen with progesterone therapy (or both) has been successful in some cases.

Pregnancy for patients with LAM is associated with an increased risk of pneumothorax and chylothorax. There may be increased risk of bleeding from angiomyolipoma during pregnancy. While it is the patient's decision to become pregnant, patients with LAM are at increased risk of disease deterioration. Educating the patient prior to pregnancy and close monitoring through pregnancy are recommended. It may be appropriate to discourage pregnancy for patients with severe lung involvement.

Because of reports of pneumothorax associated with air travel, patients with LAM have been cautioned not to travel by air. However, for patients with minimal symptoms and mild disease, discouraging air travel is not recommended. If new respiratory symptoms develop, it is best not to travel by air until the situation has been evaluated. Patients with advanced disease should be evaluated for the need of supplemental oxygen during flight. Patients with a history of pneumothorax who have not received pleurodesis also should be cautioned about the risk of air travel.

Treatment with progesterone and antiestrogen agents has produced improvement or stabilization in a subset of patients. One study of 36 patients receiving hormonal manipulation therapy reported a survival rate of 90% at 10 years compared to 20% for historical controls. Some patients do not respond to hormonal manipulation. It may be that the presence of advanced disease limits response at the time therapy is instituted. Other investigators found that treatment with hormonal therapy was associated with an increased risk of death/transplant (hazard ratio 2.93), particularly with progesterone therapy (hazard ratio 2.17). There have been no controlled trials of progesterone in LAM. Because of the increased risk associated with the use of progesterone, its routine use is not recommended.

Mortality from LAM is approximately 10% to 20% at 10 years from the onset of symptoms and 30% at 10 years from the time of lung biopsy. However, this varies widely in individual patients. The LAM Foundation has estimated 10-year survival transplant-free of 86%. Estimated median transplant-free survival time for USA LAM patients is 29 years from onset of symptoms and 23 years from the time of diagnosis.

A clinical trial with sirolimus in the largest number of LAM patients to date has shown promise. In a 1-year-long prospective randomized study, sirolimus stabilized lung function, reduced serum VEGF-D levels, reduced symptoms, and improved quality of life. Sirolimus inhibits rapamycin (mTOR) signaling, which regulates cellular growth and lymphangiogenesis. Given the significant side effects of sirolimus, its use in LAM patients should only be considered in consultation with physicians familiar with the drug. At this time, there are no long-term data on outcome in these patients, and its use should generally be limited to those who show progressive decline in lung function.

Lung transplantation is a viable alternative for patients with end-stage disease. Criteria for transplantation include (1) progression despite medical therapy; (2) severe functional defects (e.g., forced expiratory volume in 1 second/forced vital capacity [FEV_1/FVC] <50%, total lung capacity >130% predicted, FEV_1 <30% predicted); and (3) severe cystic disease on HRCT scans. Both single and bilateral lung transplants have been performed in patients with LAM. However, given the relatively young age and risk of pneumothorax in the native lung, bilateral transplant is generally preferred. Patients with LAM/TSC may have more comorbidities than S-LAM. This should not preclude these patients from transplant, but it will need to be evaluated during the assessment for candidacy. Two-year survival is similar to outcomes observed following transplantation for other lung diseases. Recurrence of LAM in the transplanted lung has been reported, but in most cases this is not functionally important. History of pleurodesis may not be an absolute contraindication to transplantation, although there may be an increase in surgical difficulties and postoperative complications.

Patients with extensive cystic changes and hyperinflation usually survive only 3 to 10 years following the onset of symptoms. A few with primarily mediastinal LAM with minimal parenchymal involvement survive longer.

TUBEROUS SCLEROSIS

Tuberous sclerosis (Bourneville disease) is an autosomal dominant, hereditary, neurocutaneous disease. There are angiomyolipomas or tubers in the skin (adenoma sebaceum), brain, retina, kidneys, heart, and lungs. It has a broader systemic constellation of complications than LAM, but the pulmonary component of this disease appears identical to that in LAM. Approximately 30% of patients with TSC have LAM (TSC-LAM).

Seizures, intellectual disability, and skin lesions occur commonly in early childhood. Renal angiomyolipomas and lung involvement (pulmonary lymphangioleiomyomatosis, LAM) in tuberous sclerosis generally develop later. Lung involvement occurs principally in women in the fourth decade of life, rarely occurring before age 20. Dyspnea worsens rapidly, and cor pulmonale develops within years of its onset. This differs from classic tuberous sclerosis, in which no gender predilection is seen. Pregnancy exacerbates both diseases. Both disorders also are associated with renal angiofibrolipomatous tumors.

Tuberous sclerosis is a rare disease, occurring in 1 in 100,000 to 170,000 people in the general population. Two genes responsible for tuberous sclerosis (*TSC1, TSC2*) have been identified on chromosomes 9 and 16. Mutations in TSC1 or TSC2 are characterized by activation of mTOR signaling and TSC tumors. The classic triad in this disease includes intellectual disability, seizures, and dermal angiofibroma (adenoma sebaceum). Clinical features, however, can vary. When pulmonary disease accompanies TSC, the classic clinical triad is uncommon, that is, intellectual ability may be normal.

The primary features of TSC have been described to include central nervous system (CNS) lesions of cortical and subependymal tubers, ungual fibromas, and facial angiofibromas (sebaceous adenomas). Secondary lesions include shagreen patches, cerebral tubers, retinal hamartomas, multiple renal tumors, sclerotic bone lesions, and cardiac rhabdomyomas.

In a National Institutes of Health (NIH) observational cohort study of 79 adult women with TSC, 45 females were diagnosed with TSC in adulthood. Of these, 21 presented with LAM, 19 with renal angiomyolipomas, and 10 with seizures. Thirty of the 45 women with TSC met clinical criteria for this diagnosis in childhood, but remained undiagnosed for a median of 21.5 years. Fifteen women were greater than 18 years of age before meeting the clinical criteria for TSC. Whether the patient with TSC was diagnosed in childhood or adulthood, the occurrence of pneumothorax, shortness of breath, hemoptysis, nephrectomy and death were similar for both groups.

Pulmonary involvement in tuberous sclerosis is rare, with estimates varying widely from 1% to 50% of patients. HRCT scans of asymptomatic females with TSC revealed that 52% had abnormal findings. Abnormalities include interstitial opacities, honeycomb changes, and hyperinflation. HRCT scans also reveal diffuse, homogeneous, small thin-walled cysts. Pulmonary manifestations appear later than cutaneous and neurologic ones. Pulmonary disease develops most often in women of childbearing age without any CNS disease. When pulmonary disease is present, it usually dominates the clinical picture and can be the cause of death from either cor pulmonale or pneumothorax. However, the most common causes of death are renal disease and brain tumors. Lymph-node involvement and chylous effusions have been reported rarely. Pneumothorax and pulmonary insufficiency are common. Exertional dyspnea is the major symptom. Chronic cough and hemoptysis occur frequently. Lung histology, chest radiograph and CT scan findings, pulmonary presentation, and clinical course are similar to LAM.

In suspected cases, thorough cutaneous and ophthalmologic examinations should be performed. The diagnostic workup should include cranial CT scan, renal ultrasound, and skeletal radiographs, in addition to chest radiograph, chest HRCT scan, and pulmonary physiology studies. A rare but early indicator of tuberous sclerosis is an unusual, but characteristically expanded, dense rib deformity. These bony lesions can be mistaken for fibrous dysplasia or Paget disease.

Genetic counseling is important in the management of patients with this disease. Estrogen receptors have been demonstrated in the lungs of patients with TSC. Tamoxifen and progesterone therapy have slowed the pulmonary disease in some cases of tuberous sclerosis, similar to descriptions for LAM. However, hormonal therapy has not been shown to be of proven benefit.

In a phase 2, multicenter trial of 36 patients with TSC or TSC/LAM, sirolimus (an mTOR inhibitor) diminished the size of angiomyolipomas in 44% of patients (16/36 partial response), with 47% (17/36) maintaining stable disease and 8% (3/36) not evaluable. There was a 30% mean regression in kidney tumor size, 26% regression in mean diameter brain tumor size (7/11 patients), 32% mean decrease in longest diameter liver angiomyolipomas (4/5 patients), and 57% subjective improvement in facial angiofibromas. Lung function remained stable in women with TSC/LAM (15 patients). Serum VEGF-D levels decreased from elevated baseline values. The serum VEGF-D level correlated with the kidney angiomyolipoma size. Once therapy was stopped, kidney angiomyolipomas increased in size. The regression response appeared to persist in those patients with continued therapy for more than 52 weeks. Serum VEGF-D levels may be a useful biomarker for monitoring kidney angiomyolipoma size.

Both grade 1 to 2 (>20% frequency) and grade 3 drug toxicities ($n = 3$) were reported with sirolimus. For the former, this included stomatitis, joint pain, hypertriglyceridemia, hypercholesterolemia, bone marrow suppression with anemia, mild neutropenia, leukopenia, and proteinuria. For the latter, this included lymphopenia, headache, and weight gain.

Lung transplantation is a consideration in eligible patients. Other organ involvement with tuberous lesions will need to be assessed during the evaluation for candidacy.

FURTHER READING

1. Zamora AC, Collard HR, Wolters PJ, et al. Neurofibromatosis-associated lung disease: a case series and literature review. *Eur Respir J.* 2007;29:210–214.

   A retrospective review of 55 patients with NF1 at one medical center and a review of the literature to define DLD in this patient population. Medical records, radiographs, and HRCT scan were reviewed. Three patients among the 55 patients had NF-DLD. The literature review identified 61 additional cases. The authors conclude DLD is a definable clinical entity. Upper-lobe cystic and bullous disease with lower-lobe fibrosis is the characteristic finding. The association with smoking remains unclear.

2. Ryu JH, Parambil JG, McGrann PS, et al. Lack of evidence for an association between neurofibromatosis and pulmonary fibrosis. *Chest.* 2005;128:2381–2386.

   Findings of a single-center, retrospective analysis of 70 patients with NF1 by review of chest radiographs, CT scans, and medical records. A description of the findings is reported. Only three patients were found to have interstitial infiltrates. All three had a history of other potential causes for the development of these findings. Thus, leading the authors to conclude there is no association of the development of interstitial infiltrates in NF1 patients. These investigators question if previous reports of such an association represented other etiologies, including smoking-induced changes.

3. Montani D, Coulet F, Girerd B, et al. Pulmonary hypertension in patients with neurofibromatosis Type 1. *Medicine*. 2011;90:201–211.

   The association of PH with NF1 is discussed. Eight patients with known NF1 were evaluated and found to have PH. Clinical, functional, radiologic, and hemodynamic characteristics are described. No other risk factors for pulmonary hypertension were identified. Treatments prescribed and outcomes are reviewed.

4. Stewart DR, Cogan JD, Kramer MR, et al. Is pulmonary arterial hypertension in neurofibromatosis type 1 secondary to a plexogenic arteriopathy? *Chest*. 2007;132:798–808.

   Four patients with NF1-PAH were studied with radiographic findings of mosaic pattern of lung attenuation consistent with underlying vasculopathy. One autopsy findings are described. The pulmonary vasculature findings were similar to other severe types of PAH. The plexiform lesions were not plexiform neurofibromas, tumors distinctive in NF1.

5. Oikonomou A, Vadikolias K, Birbilis T, et al. HRCT findings in the lungs of non-smokers with neurofibromatosis. *Eur J Radiol*. 2011;80:e520–e523.

   Because of the question of smoking contributing to interstitial disease in neurofibromatosis, six never-smokers were evaluated by HRCT scan. The findings of two radiologists' interpretations are reported.

6. Johnson SR, Cordier JF, Cottin V, et al. European respiratory society guidelines for the diagnosis and management of lymphangioleiomyomatosis. *Eur Respir J*. 2010;35:14–26.

   The LAM Task Force produced an evidence-based, consensus guideline for the diagnosis, assessment, and treatment of patients with LAM. Recommendations are provided. A very good reference article to understand the current management of LAM.

7. McCormack FX. Lymphangioleiomyomatosis: a clinical update. *Chest*. 2008;133:507–516.

   A review article updated with additional investigative findings contributing to an understanding of LAM. The natural history of LAM, diagnostic findings, air travel, pregnancy, treatment, and clinical trials are reviewed.

8. Ryu JH, Moss J, Beck GJ, et al. The NHLBI Lymphangioleiomyomatosis Registry: characteristics of 230 patients at enrollment. *Am J Respir Crit Care Med*. 2006;173:105–111.

   An informative report of 230 women enrolled in the NHLBI Lymphangioleiomyomatosis Registry over a 3-year period. This analysis reports on patient demographics, lung function, quality of life, and pulmonary manifestations.

9. Moss J, DeCastro R, Patronas NJ, et al. Meningiomas in lymphangioleiomyomatosis. *JAMA*. 2001;286:1879–1881.

   A screening study which demonstrated that women with LAM have a high prevalence of meningiomas. Because meningiomas have a reported mitogenic response to progesterone, the authors recommend that LAM patients be screened with CNS MRI prior to the initiation of therapy with progesterone.

10. Ryu JH, Doerr CH, Fisher SD, et al. Chylothorax in lymphangioleiomyomatosis. *Chest*. 2003;123:623–667.

    A retrospective review of 79 LAM patients, 8 of whom developed chylothorax. LAM patients with chylothorax had a variable clinical course. Management options for these patients with chylothorax are discussed.

11. Abbott GF, Rosado-de-Christenson ML, Frazier AA, et al. From the archives of the AFIP: lymphangioleiomyomatosis: radiologic-pathologic correlation. *Radiographics*. 2005;25:803–828.

    Thirty-three patients with LAM were retrospectively reviewed, three of which have TSC-LAM. Clinical, plain radiograph, CT results and histopathology findings are described in detail. A good overall review.

12. Schiavina M, Contini P, Fabiani A, et al. Efficacy of hormonal manipulation in lymphangioleiomyomatosis: a 20-year-experience in 36 patients. *Sarcoidosis Vasc Diffuse Lung Dis*. 2007;24:39–50.

    A review of 36 women with LAM evaluated over a 10-year period, were treated with hormonal therapy. Lung function, radiographic studies, and survival were assessed. A marked improvement in survival is demonstrated with the use of hormonal therapy at 10 years compared to the historical survival for LAM prior to the initiation of hormonal therapy. The authors attribute the hormonal therapy as a mainstay of treatment for LAM.

13. Taveira-DaSilva AM, Stylianou MP, Hedin CJ, et al. Decline in lung function in patients with lymphangioleiomyomatosis treated with or without progesterone. *Chest*. 2004;126:1867–1874.

A retrospective review of 275 patients with LAM followed longitudinally at the NIH. Lung function was compared between groups receiving oral progesterone, IM progesterone, or no progesterone. The findings suggest that progesterone does not slow the decline in lung function in LAM.

14. Taveira-DaSilva AM, Stylianou MP, Hedin CJ, et al. Maximal oxygen uptake and severity of disease in lymphangioleiomyomatosis. *Am J Respir Crit Care Med.* 2003;168:1427–1431.

    Cardiopulmonary exercise testing (CPET) was performed in 217 LAM patients and exercise data was correlated with clinical markers of severity, CT scans, PFTs, and histology. In this study, CPET documented the presence of exercise-induced hypoxemia and assisted in the grading of disease severity and determination of supplemental oxygen requirements in LAM patients.

15. Hancock E, Osborne J. Lymphangioleiomyomatosis: a review of the literature. *Respir Med.* 2002;96:1–6.

    A comprehensive review of LAM looking at clinical features and treatment of the disease.

16. Johnson SR, Tattersfield AE. Clinical experience of lymphangioleiomyomatosis in the UK. *Thorax.* 2000;55:1052–1057.

    A report on the experience of a large cohort of patients (50) in the United Kingdom that includes a discussion of the management of pneumothorax and LAM in pregnancy.

17. Johnson SR, Whale CI, Hubbard RB, et al. Survival and disease progression in UK patients with lymphangioleiomyomatosis. *Thorax.* 2004;59:800–803.

    A survival and disease-progression study of individuals with LAM enrolled in the United Kingdom LAM Registry. Improved survival is reported with contributing factors discussed, including the findings of hormonal therapy. This objective report's findings add to controversy of the role of hormonal therapy.

18. Yu J, Parkhitko A, Henske EP. Mammalian target of rapamycin signaling and autophagy. *Proc Am Thorac Soc.* 2010;7:48–53.

    A good review of the basic science associated with LAM and TSC on a genetic level, activated pathways' effects on clinical manifestations seen in LAM and TSC, and an understanding of the significance of the biomarker, serum VEGF-D level, and therapy investigations in progress.

19. Young LR, VanDyke R, Gulleman PM, et al. Serum vascular endothelial growth factor-D prospectively distinguishes lymphangioleiomyomatosis from other diseases. *Chest.* 2010;138:674–681.

    A report by the investigators' assessment of the role of serum VEGF-D levels. This prospective study assessed the diagnostic usefulness of serum VEGF-D levels in S-LAM, TSC-LAM, TSC alone, and other causes of cystic lung disease. Elevated levels greater than 800 pg/mL associated with typical cystic lung changes by HRCT scan was diagnostic for S-LAM and identified women with TSC in this study. A negative level, however, did not exclude the diagnosis of LAM.

20. McCormack FX, Inoue Y, Moss J, et al. Efficacy and safety of sirolimus in lymphangioleiomyomatosis. *N Engl J Med.* 2011;364:1595–1606.

    A randomized, double-blind, prospective trial of sirolimus with placebo for a 12-month period, followed by a 12-month observational period involving 89 patients with LAM. The primary end point of the study was to assess the difference between the placebo and treatment arms in the rate of change in the FEV_1. The study results show promise for this medication while treatment was ongoing.

21. Bissler JJ, McCormack FX, Young LR, et al. Sirolimus for angiomyolipoma in tuberous sclerosis complex or lymphangioleiomyomatosis. *N Engl J Med.* 2008;358:140–151.

    The authors conducted a 24-month, nonramdomized, open-label trial to assess the role of sirolimus therapy in reducing angiomyolipoma size. The drug was administered only for the first 12 months. Serial MRI and CT scan studies and lung function were performed throughout the 24-month period. The effect of the drug use for adverse reactions and objective study results are reported.

22. Pechet TT, Meyers BF, Guthrie TJ, et al. Lung transplantation for lymphangioleiomyomatosis. *J Heart Lung Transplant.* 2004;23:301–308.

    A retrospective review of 14 patients with LAM during and after single or bilateral lung transplant. The diagnosis of LAM did not preclude transplant, though postoperative complications unique to LAM occurred.

23. Kpodonu J, Massad MG, Chaer RA, et al. The US experience with lung transplantation for pulmonary lymphangioleiomyomatosis. *J Heart Lung Transplant.* 2005;24:1247–1253.

    A retrospective analysis of 79 patients with LAM who underwent lung transplantation. Patient demographics and outcomes posttransplant are discussed.

24. Crino PB, Nathanson KL, Henske EP. The tuberous sclerosis complex. *N Engl J Med.* 2006;355:1345–1356.

 A concise review article of the clinical presentation for TSC by organ and diagnostic study findings. The genetic and molecular factors leading to the clinical manifestations are explained. Management and therapeutic developments are provided.

25. Moss J. Prevalence and clinical characteristics of lymphangioleiomyomatosis (LAM) in patients with tuberous sclerosis complex. *Am J Respir Crit Care Med.* 2001;164:669–671.

 The true prevalence of LAM associated with TSC is unknown. The investigators assessed 48 patients with TSC and no prior history of known LAM. Thirty-eight of the 48 patients were found to have LAM, all females. No males with TSC were found to have LAM. The prevalence of LAM in women with TSC was found to be 34%.

26. Curatolo P, Bombardieri R, Jozwiak S. Tuberous sclerosis. *Lancet.* 2008;372:657–668.

 A valuable review article describing the genetic multisystem disorder, its characteristics, genetic factors, affected molecular pathways leading to clinical manifestations, the developing therapies, and management.

27. Dabora SL, Franz DN, Ashwal S, et al. Multicenter phase 2 trial of sirolimus for tuberous sclerosis: kidney angiomyolipomas and other tumors regress and VEGF-D levels decrease. *PLoS One.* 2011;6(9):e23379. doi:10.1371/journal.pone.0023379.

 Thirty-six patients with TSC or TSC/LAM were treated with daily sirolimus in a phase 2 multicenter trial to evaluate the efficacy and adverse events of this mTOR inhibitor on the treatment of kidney angiomyolipomas. Treatment for 52 weeks demonstrated a partial regression or stable disease with treatment. The serologic biomarker, serum VEGF-D level, decreased with treatment.

28. Seibert D, Hong CH, Takeuchi F, et al. Recognition of tuberous sclerosis in adult women: delayed presentation with life-threatening consequences. *Ann Intern Med.* 2011;154(12):806–813.

 An interesting study of 45 women diagnosed with TSC in adulthood with a review of their medical history to assess for the presence of clinical criteria of disease presence in childhood. Thirty of the 45 women met clinical criteria for TSC in childhood that was undiagnosed for a median of 21.5 years. Fifteen women were greater than 18 years of age before meeting the clinical criteria to establish the diagnosis of TSC. Whether diagnosis occurred in childhood or adulthood, the occurrences of clinical manifestations of the disease were similar.

29. Davies DM, deVries PJ, Johnson SR, et al. Sirolimus therapy for angiomyolipoma in tuberous sclerosis and sporadic lymphangioleiomyomatosis: a phase 2 trial. *Clin Cancer Res.* 2011;17:4071–4081.

 A report of a prospective phase 2, multicenter, open-label drug trial with sirolimus therapy for up to 2 years in 16 patients with TSC or S-LAM with renal angiomyolipomas. The primary outcome was to assess a change in size of the renal angiomyolipomas; secondary outcomes were drug safety, neurocognitive function, and pulmonary function. Forty-one of 48 angiomyolipomas were smaller at the last measurement when compared to baseline size. Pulmonary function changed little; recall memory improved in seven of eight TSC patients. Ongoing investigation of sirolimus is needed for understanding of the findings.

30. Ryu JH, Sykes AM, Lee AS, et al. Cystic lung disease is not uncommon in men with tuberous sclerosis complex. *Respir Med.* 2012;106:1586–1590.

 This retrospective study assessed 29 men with known TSC to learn the frequency of pulmonary involvement over a 13-year period. Other characteristics are described. The investigators conclude that LAM/ TSC in males may not be as rare as first thought but is milder in severity.

31. Collins J. CT signs and patterns of lung disease. *Radiol Clin North Am.* 2001;39:1115–1135.

 A good review of CT appearance in LAM, TS, and other ILD.

32. Costello LC, Hartman TE, Tyu JH. High frequency of pulmonary lymphangioleiomyomatosis in women with tuberous sclerosis complex. *Mayo Clin Proc.* 2000;75:591–594.

 A retrospective cohort study demonstrating that the frequency of lung involvement (26%) in 78 women with TSC is substantially higher than previously suspected. This study supports routine screening chest CT scans in women with TSC.

99 Pulmonary Alveolar Proteinosis

Angela C. Wang

Pulmonary alveolar proteinosis (PAP) is a heterogeneous group of rare diseases characterized by the accumulation of eosinophilic, periodic acid-Schiff (PAS)-positive material within alveoli, and distal airways resulting in restrictive pulmonary function that can progress to respiratory failure and death. Two general categories of PAP exist: autoimmune and non-autoimmune. The latter can be further classified into hereditary and secondary.

PATHOPHYSIOLOGY

More than 90% of PAP cases are caused by defective granulocyte macrophage colony-stimulating factor (GM-CSF) signaling due to high levels of circulating autoantibodies that prevent GM-CSF binding to its receptor (autoimmune PAP). GM-CSF is a hematopoietic cytokine that regulates the clearance of surfactant lipids and proteins by alveolar macrophages. Impaired host defense results from decreased surfactant catabolism and impaired microbicidal activity by neutrophils. In congenital cases, inherited GM-CSF receptor mutations prevent GM-CSF signaling. All forms result in decreased surfactant catabolism and the accumulation of large, foamy, surfactant-filled macrophages within alveoli. Because GM-CSF also regulates multiple neutrophil functions, PAP also is associated with defective alveolar macrophage- and neutrophil-mediated host defense. Thus, patients are prone to pulmonary and systemic infections.

Three main etiologies of secondary PAP have been identified: (1) lung infections, including *Pneumocystis carinii* pneumonia in patients with and without AIDS; (2) hematologic malignancies and other immune-altering conditions; and (3) exposure to inhaled chemicals and minerals. Several toxic insults to the lung (e.g., silica, NO_2, ozone, and ONOO-) can result in alveolar proteinosis. PAP has also been produced in laboratory animals by inhalation of inert dusts of extremely fine particulate matter. Presumably, these exposures result in impaired macrophage function.

DIAGNOSIS

PAP occurs in all ethnic groups. The peak age of onset of autoimmune PAP is between 30 and 50 years; however, the disease has been described in all ages. In adults, the male to female ratio is approximately 4:1 and is associated with past or current history of smoking. Although some patients are asymptomatic at the time of diagnosis, PAP most commonly presents insidiously with increasing dyspnea and cough. However, abrupt onset also can occur, usually in the setting of a concomitant respiratory infection. Often, patients present with bilateral, community-acquired pneumonia that fails to clear with antibiotics.

Sputum production is usually scant but on occasion has been described as containing small chunks of material. Other much less-common symptoms include weight loss, weakness, chest pain, and hemoptysis. Physical findings, if present, are nonspecific. Fever usually implies superinfection, although a low-grade fever is present occasionally. Inspiratory crackles occur in up to 50% of patients; in severe cases, cyanosis and clubbing are observed.

The most common laboratory finding is a mildly elevated serum lactate dehydrogenase (LDH). Although nonspecific, LDH may be used to follow disease activity and severity. Patients with severe disease may have secondary polycythemia. The leukocyte count is normal or slightly increased. Serum protein electrophoresis may reveal increased globulins. Pulmonary function tests may be normal but usually reveal a restrictive pattern with decreased static lung compliance and decreased carbon monoxide diffusing capacity (DLCO). Arterial blood gases demonstrate hypoxemia and a widened alveolar–arterial oxygen gradient.

Chest radiographs typically show diffuse, finely nodular, soft infiltrates in a perihilar butterfly pattern, similar in appearance to pulmonary edema; however, other signs of left ventricular failure (cardiomegaly, Kerley B lines) are absent. A miliary, interstitial, or multinodular pattern and lobar consolidation also can be seen. Hilar adenopathy, pleural effusions, and cavitation are rare and suggest superimposed infection. The presence of patchy ground-glass opacities with lobular septal thickening ("crazy paving") on high-resolution chest CT is highly characteristic of PAP, but may be absent, particularly in patients with secondary PAP. Furthermore, "crazy paving" is not pathognomonic for PAP and can also be seen in alveolar sarcoidosis, lipoid pneumonia, and mucinous bronchoalveolar carcinoma.

The differential diagnosis includes any disease that can produce a diffuse acinar-filling pattern on chest roentgenogram, including cardiogenic and noncardiogenic pulmonary edema, toxic inhalations, pulmonary hemorrhage, viral pneumonia, and *P. carinii* infection. One of the clues to the diagnosis of PAP is the disparity between extensive radiographic abnormalities and minimal clinical symptomatology. When chest roentgenograms reveal a predominant interstitial pattern, the diagnosis becomes more difficult.

Although open-lung biopsy was previously used as the gold standard for diagnosing PAP, the diagnosis can now be established via bronchoscopy with bronchoalveolar lavage (BAL), combined with appropriate clinical and radiographic findings and the presence of autoantibodies against GM-CSF in BAL fluid/serum. Serum concentration of less than 10 μg/mL has been reported to have good negative predictive value. Typically, the BAL fluid in PAP appears opaque and milky and is PAS-positive. Microscopically, few alveolar macrophages are seen and these cells appear large and foamy. Increased lymphocytes may be seen. Large eosinophilic bodies appear amidst a background of PAS-positive granular debris. The presence of the phospholipid or proteinaceous material within alveoli correlates with a ground-glass appearance.

TREATMENT

Whole-lung lavage (WLL) remains the treatment of choice for all three forms of PAP, despite the lack of consensus on its performance or randomized controlled trials to determine optimal strategy. Large-volume WLL usually requires the use of a double-lumen endotracheal tube for selective lavage of each lung. The procedure can take up to 3 hours and use 15 to 20 L of saline for a single lung. Contraindications include uncorrectable hypoxemia, convulsions, and fever which may indicate the presence of infection. Fiberoptic bronchoscopy has also been used to lavage multiple segments or lobes and has the advantage of requiring local anesthesia. Multiple sessions can be carried out over 2 to 3 days. Treatment options for autoimmune PAP also include subcutaneous or aerosolized GM-CSF. Plasmapheresis also has been reported to result in transient improvement, presumably by decreasing levels of systemic snit-GM-CSF antibodies. In some cases, immunosuppression using rituximab to deplete B cells has resulted in improved oxygenation, total lung capacity, and HRCT scan findings. Although corticosteroids may be helpful in the treatment of autoimmune PAP, they are relatively contraindicated because of the high incidence of associated infection. Treatment of secondary PAP focuses on the underlying condition (e.g., the inciting hematologic malignancy).

The possibility of spontaneous resolution of PAP has made clinical decision-making regarding the need for and frequency of WLL less clear. In one series from the Cleveland Clinic, 46% of patients followed over a prolonged period never required WLL. Another 29% required repeated WLL for recurring signs and symptoms of PAP. However, lavage may improve survival overall: in one group of 146 patients, mean survival (±SD) at 5 years was 94 ± 2% with lavage versus 85 ± 5% without lavage. Radiographic evidence alone is probably not sufficient to warrant the procedure. Patients who require repeated alveolar lavages have a poorer prognosis and greater rate of progression to fibrosis.

Lung transplantation has been considered an option for some patients, but its role in acquired PAP needs careful evaluation because the disease can recur. Bone marrow transplantation also can be considered in patients with hereditary PAP if a suitable donor can be found.

COMPLICATIONS

The major complication in PAP is infection, both pulmonary and systemic. Bacterial, mycobacterial, and fungal infections have been reported frequently. Disease exacerbations often respond to antibiotics without a definite bacteriologic diagnosis. *Nocardia asteroides* and *Mycobacterium tuberculosis* have appeared most often in case reports. In one large series, *M. avium–intracellulare* was isolated from lavage fluid in 42% of cases. Other complications include pulmonary fibrosis, cor pulmonale, and spontaneous pneumothorax.

PROGNOSIS

The course of PAP is variable. Three categories of disease prognosis have been described: spontaneous improvement, stable but with persistent symptoms, and progressive deterioration. A recent review found that approximately 8% fell into the first category. Another study demonstrated a 5-year survival of approximately 75%. The majority of deaths in the latter study were from respiratory failure from PAP, with about 20% from infection. Although the prognosis in infants remains grave, with most deaths occurring between 3 and 6 months of age, long-term survival following WLL has been reported.

FURTHER READING

1. Abraham J, McEuen D. Inorganic particulates associated with pulmonary alveolar proteinosis: SEM and X-ray microanalysis results. *Appl Pathol*. 1986;4:138.

   The lungs of 24 patients with PAP were studied with light microscopy, scanning electron microscopy, and radiographic analysis and found to have increased amounts of small inorganic particulate matter.

2. Altose M, Hicks R, Edwards M. Extracorporeal membrane oxygenation during bronchopulmonary lavage. *Arch Surg*. 1976;111:1148.

   Describes the technical aspects of membrane oxygenation with pulmonary lavage.

3. Campo I, Kadija Z, Mariani F, et al. Pulmonary alveolar proteinosis: diagnostic and therapeutic challenges. *Multidiscip Respir Med*. 2012;7:4.

   An excellent overview of disease and method of WLL.

4. Carrey B, Trapnell BC. The molecular basis of pulmonary alveolar proteinosis. *Clin Immunol*. 2010;135:223–235.

   A comprehensive review of the molecular pathogenesis of PAP and the role of GM-CSF in regulating myeloid cell immune function.

5. Corrin B, King E. Pathogenesis of experimental pulmonary alveolar proteinosis. *Thorax*. 1970;25:230.

   Rats exposed to aluminum powder or pure fine quartz developed pathologic changes identical to those of PAP.

6. Dranoff G, Crawford AD, Sadelain M, et al. Involvement of granulocyte-macrophage colony-stimulating factor in pulmonary homeostasis. *Science*. 1994;264:713.

   One of two original articles describing the development of PAP in GM-CSF–deficient mice.

7. Frazier AA, Franks TJ, Cooke EO, et al. From the archives of the AFIB: pulmonary alveolar proteinosis. *Radiographics*. 2008;28:883–899.

   A review of the radiographic patterns of PAP.

8. Hammon W, McCaffree R, Cucchiara A. A comparison of manual to mechanical chest percussion for clearance of alveolar material in patients with pulmonary alveolar proteinosis (phospholipidosis). *Chest*. 1993;103:1409.

   Manual chest percussion is superior to mechanical chest percussion or no percussion in clearance of alveolar material.

9. Kariman K, Kylstra J, Spock A. Pulmonary alveolar proteinosis: prospective clinical experience in 23 patients for 15 years. *Lung*. 1984;162:223.

   Of patients, 24% had spontaneous remission, 48% improved after lung lavage, and 13% did not improve after lung lavage.

10. Kavuru MS, Bonfield TL, Thomassen MJ. Plasmapheresis, GM-CSF, and alveolar proteinosis. *Am J Respir Crit Care Med.* 2003;167:1036.

    A case report of a patient with PAP successfully treated with plasmapheresis.

11. Leth S, Bendstrup E, Vestergaard H, et al. Autoimmune pulmonary alveolar proteinosis: treatment options in the year 2013. *Respirology.* 2013;18(1):82–91.

    An excellent summary of current treatment options, including staging and treatment algorithm.

12. Nhieu J, Vojtek AM, Bernaudin JF, et al. Pulmonary alveolar proteinosis associated with *Pneumocystis carinii. Chest.* 1990;98:801.

    An analysis of BAL fluid from 26 patients with P. carinii *pneumonia showed surfactant-like material consistent with PAP.*

13. Parker LA, Novotny DB. Recurrent alveolar proteinosis following double lung transplantation. *Chest.* 1997;111:1457.

    A case report describing disease recurrence in a patient who underwent double lung transplantation for PAP.

14. Presneill JJ, Nakata K, Inoue Y, et al. Pulmonary alveolar proteinosis. *Clin Chest Med.* 2003;25: 593–613, viii.

    An excellent review.

15. Riker J, Wolinsky H. Trypsin aerosol treatment of pulmonary alveolar proteinosis. *Am Rev Respir Dis.* 1973;108:108.

    A report of a patient who appeared to respond to aerosolized trypsin on three occasions.

16. Rosen S, Castleman B, Liebow A. Pulmonary alveolar proteinosis. *N Engl J Med.* 1958;258:1123.

    The classic article that first described this disease.

17. Sakagami T, Uchida K, Carey BC, et al. Human GM-CSF autoantibodies and the reproduction of pulmonary alveolar proteinosis. *N Engl J Med.* 2009;351:2679–2681.

    Administration of highly purified GM-CSF autoantibodies derived from a patient with idiopathic PAP results in PAP in healthy nonhuman primates.

18. Selecky P, Wasserman K, Benfield JR, et al. The clinical and physiological effect of whole lung lavage in pulmonary alveolar proteinosis: a ten-year experience. *Ann Thorac Surg.* 1977; 24:451.

    Describes the technique of massive pulmonary lavage and reviews the response of 18 patients; found that heparin or acetylcysteine is not needed in the lavage fluid.

19. Seymour JF, Presneill JJ. Pulmonary alveolar proteinosis: progress in the first 44 years. *Am J Respir Crit Care Med.* 2002;166:215–235.

    An analysis detailing the clinical presentation, demographics, and clinical course of 410 patients with PAP.

20. Singh G, Katyal SL, Bedrossian CW, et al. Pulmonary alveolar proteinosis: staining for surfactant apoprotein in alveolar proteinosis and in conditions simulating it. *Chest.* 1983;83:82.

    Intra-alveolar material in patients with primary PAP stained uniformly for surfactant-specific apoprotein, whereas the staining was focal in patients with secondary PAP.

21. Spock A. Long-term survival of paediatric patients with pulmonary alveolar proteinosis treated with lung lavage. *Eur Respir J.* 2005;25:1127.

    Describes the use of lung lavage in pediatric PAP.

22. Stanley E, Lieschke GJ, Grail D, et al. Granulocyte/macrophage colony-stimulating factor–deficient mice show no major perturbation of hematopoiesis but develop a characteristic pulmonary pathology. *Proc Natl Acad Sci U S A.* 1994;91:5592.

    Original article describing the unexpected development of a PAP-like disease in mice in which the GM-CSF gene was knocked out.

23. Suzuki T, Sakagami T, Young LR, et al. Hereditary pulmonary alveolar proteinosis: pathogenesis, presentation, diagnosis, and therapy. *Am J Respir Crit Care Med.* 2010;182:1292–1304.

    Describes the presentation, diagnosis, and treatment of eight patients with various CSF2RA mutations causing PAP.

24. Uchida K, Nakata K, Trapnell BC, et al. High-affinity autoantibodies specifically eliminate granulocyte-macrophage colony-stimulating factor activity in the lungs of patients with idiopathic pulmonary alveolar proteinosis. *Blood.* 2004;103:1089.

A study demonstrating that anti-GM-CSF antibodies present in the lungs of patients with acquired PAP abrogate GM-CSF bioactivity.

25. Venkateshiah SB, Yan TD, Bonfield TL, et al. An open-label trial of granulocyte-macrophage colony stimulating factor therapy for moderate symptomatic pulmonary alveolar proteinosis. *Chest.* 2006;130:227–237.

Administration of GM-CSF improved oxygenation and other clinical and quality of life parameters in 12 of 25 patients (48%) with moderate symptomatic disease. The serum anti-GM-CSF antibody titer correlated with disease activity and was a predictor for responsiveness to therapy.

26. Witty L, Tapson V, Piantadosi A. Isolation of mycobacteria in patients with pulmonary alveolar proteinosis. *Medicine (Baltimore).* 1994;73:103.

M. avium–intracellulare *was isolated from the lavage fluid in 8 of 19 consecutive patients with PAP.*

27. Xipell J, Ham KN, Price CG, et al. Acute silicolipoproteinosis. *Thorax.* 1977;32:104.

Presents a case of acute silicosis in which the lung showed areas of fibrotic nodules, interstitial fibrosis, and alveolar filling of a PAS-positive material similar to that in PAP.

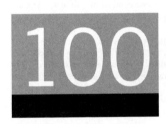

100 Bronchial Carcinoids and Benign Neoplasms of the Lung

David H. Kupferberg

Bronchial carcinoids and benign neoplasms of the lung account for less than 10% of all primary pulmonary neoplasms. Many are discovered incidentally due to the increasing use and availability of computed tomography (CT) scanning. The symptoms and diagnosis of these lesions depend very much on their location; most are asymptomatic. When centrally located, they may not be visible on chest radiographs and slowly cause progressive airway obstruction, resulting in focal wheezing, postobstructive pneumonia, or hemoptysis, and even may be confused with chronic airways disease. When peripheral, these tumors are usually clinically silent but still pose the diagnostic challenge typical of any solitary pulmonary nodule. Ultimately, the diagnosis of many of these lesions is obtained at the time of surgery performed to definitively exclude malignancy. Work-up and evaluation relies on clinical suspicion of malignancy, imaging modalities, including positron emission tomography (PET) scanning, and patient's risk and preference for surgical intervention.

Carcinoid tumors are classified as malignant tumors due their potential for metastases, although "typical" carcinoids have a growth pattern and behavior similar to benign tumors of the lung. Hamartomas are the most common benign pulmonary neoplasms. Leiomyomas, true bronchial adenomas, lipomas, chondromas, inflammatory myofibroblastic tumors, endometriosis, and even teratomas also occur.

BRONCHIAL CARCINOIDS

Bronchial carcinoids comprise the second largest group of lung tumors behind bronchogenic carcinomas and are responsible for approximately 0.5% to 2% of all bronchial tumors.

They occur with a small increased frequency in women and at an earlier average age of onset (40–60 years old) compared with noncarcinoid bronchogenic malignancies. Some studies suggest a greater incidence in Caucasians than in African Americans. The link between smoking and the development of carcinoid tumors is unclear and has not been firmly established. While more than 90% of cases are sporadic, there is an association with multiple endocrine neoplasia (MEN type 1) as well as a reported familial non-MEN1 incidence.

Bronchopulmonary carcinoid tumors account for 25% of all carcinoid tumors, which occur primarily in the gastrointestinal tract. The bronchial type tends to develop centrally, in the large airways and can be visualized easily with bronchoscopy. Macroscopically, they can grow primarily either as a polypoid lesion or as a predominantly infiltrative process, with only minimal protrusion into the bronchial lumen (known as *iceberg tumor*). Growth is largely submucosal, and the surface epithelium is usually intact, although frequently metaplastic. Carcinoids have a wide histologic spectrum; most commonly appearing as clumps of small, uniformly staining cells with a rich vascular stroma. Some form acini and produce mucin; others appear highly malignant and may bear a striking resemblance to small-cell carcinoma. They can be classified along a spectrum as follows: (1) typical carcinoid with the best prognosis and bland-appearing histology; (2) atypical carcinoid with 2 to 10 mitoses per high-power field and necrosis; (3) large-cell neuroendocrine carcinoma with a higher mitotic rate, greater atypia, and necrosis; and (4) small-cell carcinoma, the most aggressive. Immunohistochemistry-identifying synaptophysin, neuron-specific enolase, and chromogranin are often used to support the neuroendocrine origin of cells. The tumor is capable of elaborating a wide spectrum of neuroendocrine products. Atypical carcinoid may be misclassified with bronchoscopic biopsies because of difficulty with mitotic counts on limited sampling.

The clinical manifestations of bronchial carcinoid tumors depend on the site of the tumor. Approximately 80% are central and can produce symptoms and signs of bronchial obstruction, including cough, fever, chest pain, and often a localized wheeze. Hemoptysis is present in approximately 50%, reflecting both their central origin and hypervascularity. Peripheral carcinoids most often are asymptomatic and usually detected fortuitously by radiographic imaging. Regional lymph node metastasis is present in approximately 10% of typical carcinoids at presentation, compared with 30% to 50% of atypical carcinoids.

Rarely, there are associated paraneoplastic findings. The most common is Cushing syndrome, which can even predate visualization of a lung nodule. Acromegaly has also been reported with significantly elevated levels of growth hormone even without overt acromegalic features. The carcinoid syndrome occurs infrequently with an incidence as low as 0% to 3%. Production of high levels of 5-hydroxytryptamine and other substances (e.g., bradykinin, prostaglandins) can enter the systemic circulation causing flushing, wheezing, anxiety, vomiting, and hypotension. In addition, cardiac valvular damage can develop in the left heart in bronchial carcinoid syndrome, as opposed to the right heart with the abdominal variety. This syndrome always reflects metastasis of the carcinoid tumor, usually to the liver. Other neuroendocrine manifestations include the Zollinger–Ellison syndrome, hyperinsulinemia, and an association with MEN type I.

Radiographic findings depend on the site of the tumor. Central tumors may cause bronchial obstruction and result in pneumonitis, atelectasis, bronchiectasis, and collapse. Nonobstructive central and peripheral tumors may appear as a solitary pulmonary nodule, usually 4 cm or less in diameter, and are often slightly lobulated. Atypical carcinoids tend to be larger. Calcification may be present. CT scanning is helpful in identifying endobronchial lesions as well as lymph node enlargement. Because carcinoid tumors tend to be highly vascular, there is marked enhancement with intravenous contrast. Newer localization modalities include radiolabeled somatostatin analog scintigraphy, which has been reported to find up to 85% of all primary and metastatic carcinoid lesions. PET scanning may yield false-negative results because of hypometabolic activity.

Pulmonary function testing is usually normal unless central obstruction occurs, in which case flow obstruction may be demonstrated. Serum or urine hormone levels can be elevated in association with the aforementioned neuroendocrine syndromes.

Differential diagnosis includes all causes of solitary pulmonary nodules and obstructing airway lesions. The diagnosis of central tumors is usually made at bronchoscopy; the diagnosis of peripheral tumors often requires other methods (CT-guided biopsy, video-assisted thoracoscopic surgery [VATS] or thoracotomy). Treatment for bronchial carcinoids is surgical. Lung-sparing procedures, which have been shown to yield similar survival results for typical carcinoids, should be attempted when possible. Lymph node dissection should be performed with atypical carcinoids or when higher grade lesions are suspected. Surgical treatment in those cases should be similar to resection of non–small-cell lung cancer with at least lobectomy. Lobectomy is often necessitated by bronchiectasis and parenchymal necrosis distal to an obstructing tumor. In such cases, the prognosis is excellent. There may be a role for Nd:YAG laser resection in typical carcinoid, particularly when patients are not good surgical candidates, though local recurrence rates are slightly higher. Survival in cases of nonmetastatic typical carcinoid is approximately 90%. Atypical carcinoid has a 5- and 10-year survival of 60% and 40%, respectively. Positive lymph nodes, age greater than 60 years, and larger tumor size correlate with poorer overall prognosis. Chemotherapy and radiation have limited benefit for metastatic disease although platinum-etoposide regimens can be offered. Metastatic liver lesions have been treated successfully with hepatic artery embolization and local direct chemotherapeutic instillation. Interferon and octreotide have been reported to temporarily stabilize tumor growth, yet rarely produce any decrease in tumor size. Cushing syndrome can be well controlled with octreotide with significant improvement in symptoms. Targeted therapies (i.e., involving mammalian target of rapamycin pathway) are currently being investigated.

PULMONARY HAMARTOMAS

Pulmonary hamartomas, the largest group of benign pulmonary neoplasms, occur more frequently in men than in women (3:1), with a peak incidence in the sixth to seventh decade. They are uncommon before age 30. Pathologically, they contain a mixture of tissues normally present in lung (i.e., smooth muscle, collagen, and, rarely, cartilage); however, these components are totally disorganized. Ultrastructural studies indicate that pulmonary hamartomas represent a histologic spectrum of mesenchymal neoplasms derived from peribronchial connective tissue. Although pulmonary hamartomas can become extremely large, they remain benign.

Hamartomas are clinically silent because of their peripheral location. Hemoptysis is rare. Radiographically, they appear as well-circumscribed, solitary pulmonary nodules, usually less than 4 cm in diameter; occasionally, they can be large, nearly filling the hemithorax. Calcification, resembling a kernel of popped popcorn, occurs in 5% to 15% of cases. CT scan of the lung may suggest the diagnosis. Multiple tumors rarely occur. Unless the imaging and clinical course are classic, the diagnosis is usually made at the time of surgical excision because other methods fail to exclude carcinoma.

OTHER BENIGN NEOPLASMS

Infrequently, primary lung involvement may occur in other benign neoplasms. Signs and symptoms depend on the location, ranging from no clinical findings with peripheral lesions to cough, hemoptysis, or recurrent pneumonia from bronchial involvement. Radiographically, findings may be consistent with bronchial obstruction or only solitary or multiple nodules. True bronchial adenomas are benign tumors that arise from bronchial mucous glands and are quite rare. They can cause symptoms by obstructing airways. Leiomyomas arise from smooth muscle in the lung and are usually endobronchial. Most cases are asymptomatic. Women are affected slightly more often than men, and the average age at presentation is 37 years. There appears to be a distinct entity in which multiple pulmonary fibroleiomyomas occur in women who have had uterine fibroids. Although such tumors are histologically and clinically benign, controversy exists regarding their in situ or metastatic origin. Lipomas are usually endobronchial (80%) and can occur on either side of the bronchial cartilage. They can change shape roentgenographically, as the individual assumes different positions. Chondromas are extremely rare. Unlike hamartomas, they derive exclusively from formed bronchial cartilage. Teratoma is a relatively common tumor of the mediastinum, but is rarely found in lung tissue. Pulmonary teratomas may contain tissue from any germ layer. On imaging, they may contain calcifications or even well-formed teeth. Expectoration of hair (trichoptysis) has been reported. Endometriosis can occur in the lung as a solitary nodule. The origin of this lung tumor is unclear; some consider it of metastatic origin, whereas others feel it arises from pluripotential pulmonary tissue. Recurrent pneumothorax, particularly on the right side, or hemoptysis associated with menstruation should suggest the diagnosis.

FURTHER READING

1. Myers JL, Giordano TJ. Benign lung tumors. In: Mason RJ, Broaddus VC, Martin T, et al, eds. *Murray and Nadel's Textbook of Respiratory Medicine.* 5th ed. Philadelphia, PA: WB Saunders; 2010:1171–1185.

   A thorough chapter review with workup algorithm and pathology.

2. Bertino EM, Confer PD, Colonna JE, et al. Pulmonary neuroendocrine/carcinoid tumors. *Cancer.* 2009;115:4434–4441.

   A concise review of carcinoid histology types and chemotherapeutic options.

3. Cao C, Yan TD, Kennedy C, et al. Bronchopulmonary carcinoid tumors: long-term outcomes after resection. *Ann Thorac Surg.* 2011;91:339–343.

   The findings in a 25-year database and literature comparison identifying age greater than 60 and atypical carcinoid as predictors of poorer survival.

4. Naaslund A. Carcinoid tumors–incidence, treatment and outcomes: a population based study. *Eur J Cardiothorac Surg.* 2011;39:565–569.

   Twelve-year review of Norway's lung cancer registry. One percent were carcinoid tumors. They found 92% typical carcinoid and 66% atypical carcinoid 5-year survival. Recurrence rates and metastases at time of diagnosis three times more likely for atypical carcinoid.

5. Fraser RS, Muller NL, Colman NC, et al, eds. *Fraser and Paré's Diagnosis of Diseases of the Chest.* 4th ed. Philadelphia, PA: WB Saunders; 1999.

   A thorough, in-depth chapter with particular focus on pathology and histology.

6. Detterbeck FC. Management of carcinoid tumors. *Ann Thorac Surg.* 2010;89:998–1005.

   A review that also highlights the importance of mediastinoscopy for lymph node sampling in upstaging the diagnosis to atypical carcinoid.

7. Erasmus JJ, Macapinlac HA. Low-sensitivity FDG-PET studies: less common lung neoplasms. *Semin Nucl Med.* 2012;42:255–260.

   Highlights limitation of FDG-PET scanning in carcinosis and atypical lung lesions. Novel tracers, such as somatostatin for neuroendocrine tumors discussed.

8. Gridelli C, Rossi A, Airoma G, et al. Treatment of pulmonary neuroendocrine tumours: state of the art and future developments. *Cancer Treat Rev.* 2013;39(5):466–472. http://dx.doi.org/10.1016/j.ctrv.2012.06.012.

   A deeper review of chemotherapeutic avenues being explored in neuroendocrine tumors.

9. Guo W, Zhao YP, Jiang YG, et al. Surgical treatment and outcome of pulmonary hamartoma: a retrospective study of 20-year experience. *J Exp Clin Cancer Res.* 2008;27:8.

   Surgery often needed to make the diagnosis of hamartoma.

10. Huang Y, Xu Dm, Jirapatnakul A, et al. CT and computer-based features of small hamartomas. *Clin Imaging.* 2011;35(2):116–122.

   Newer CT modalities may help define and diagnose hamartomas reliably.

11. Bhatia K, Ellis S. Unusual lung tumours: an illustrated review of CT features suggestive of this diagnosis. *Cancer Imaging.* 2006;6:72–82.

   Looks at CT approach and features of many less-common pulmonary lesions.

12. Smith MA, Battafarano RJ, Meyers BF, et al. Prevalence of benign disease in patients undergoing resection for suspected lung cancer. *Ann Thorac Surg.* 2006;81:1824–1829.

   Confirms that using the modern modalities available pre-op (CT, PET, needle biopsy) the incidence of benign lesions is about 10%.

13. Li X, Zhang W, Wu X, et al. Mucoepidermoid carcinoma of the lung: common findings and unusual appearances on CT. *Clin Imaging.* 2012;36:8–13.

   A radiologic review of the CT and pathologic findings of this endobronchial tumor.

14. Rao N, Colby TV, Falconieri G, et al. Intrapulmonary solitary fibrous tumors, clinicopathologic and immunohistochemical study of 24 cases. *Am J Surg Pathol.* 2012;37:155–166.

   While typically these tumors arise from the pleura, a case series of intrapulmonary lesions is described.

15. Hammas N, Chbani L, Rami M, et al. A rare tumor of the lung: inflammatory myofibroblastic tumor. *Diagn Pathol.* 2012;7:83–86.

    Known by many names (inflammatory pseudotumor, plasma-cell granuloma, histiocytoma or fibroxanthoma), the pathology, radiologic findings, and clinical presentations are discussed.

16. Carney JA, Aidan MD. Gastric stromal sarcoma, pulmonary chondroma, and extra-adrenal paraganglioma (Carney triad): natural history, adrenocortical component and possible familial occurrence. *Mayo Clin Proc.* 1999;74:543.

    Reviews 79 patients with Carney triad, which includes pulmonary chondromas. Tumors can be separated by years (mean 8.4, longest 26).

17. Ishida T, Oka T, Nishino M, et al. Inflammatory pseudotumor of the lung in adults: radiographic and clinicopathological analysis. *Ann Thorac Surg.* 1989;48:90–95.

    Discusses patients with such tumors. Intraoperative gross appearance can resemble lung cancer, but this is a benign lesion.

18. Esteban JM, Allen WM, Schaerf RH. Benign metastasizing leiomyoma of the uterus: histologic and immunohistochemical characterization of primary and metastatic lesions. *Arch Pathol Lab Med.* 1999;123:960–962.

    Describes the pathologic connection and association between uterine leiomyoma proven to be benign and similar lung findings.

19. Turna A, Ozqul A, Kahraman S, et al. Primary pulmonary teratoma: report of a case and the proposition of "bronchotrichosis" as a new term. *Ann Thorac Cardiovasc Surg.* 2009;15:247–249.

    Coughing up hair as a sign of a primary pulmonary teratoma.

20. Erkilic S, Kocer NE, Tuncozgur B. Peripheral intrapulmonary lipoma: a case report. *Acta Chir Belg.* 2007;107:700–702.

    While most lipomas are endobronchial, a few case reports of peripheral have been described.

21. Kuo E, Bharat A, Bontumasi N, et al. Impact of video-assisted thoracoscopic surgery on benign resections of solitary pulmonary nodules. *Ann Thorac Surg.* 2012;93:266–272.

    A nice study looking at the increased use of VATS over a 15-year period and its new role in the resection of benign tumors.

22. Gjevre JA, Myers JL, Prakash UB. Pulmonary hamartomas. *Mayo Clin Proc.* 1996;71:14–20.

    A 17-year review of 215 patients, 98% asymptomatic.

23. Nistal M, Hardisson D, Riestra ML. Multiple pulmonary leiomyomatous hamartomas associated with a bronchogenic cyst in a man. *Arch Pathol Lab Med.* 2003;127:e194–e196.

    Describes a case of occurring in a man.

24. Cassina PC, Hauser M, Kacl G, et al. Catamenial hemoptysis: diagnosis with MRI. *Chest.* 1997;111:1447–1450.

    A diagnosis of pulmonary endometriosis by magnetic resonance imaging in a 24-year-old woman.

25. Lin YS, Tu CY. Thoracic endometriosis. *CMAJ.* 2011;183:E758.

    A classic case report and image.

26. Cavaliere S, Foccoli P, Farina P. Nd: YAG laser bronchoscopy. *Chest.* 1988;94:15–21.

    A 5-year experience with 1,396 applications in 1,000 patients. This treatment was curative in almost all cases of benign tumor and in many carcinoid tumors as well. This should be considered in the approach to endobronchial benign tumors of the lung.

27. Erasmus JJ, Connolly JE, McAdams HP, et al. Solitary pulmonary nodules, part I: morphologic evaluation for differentiation of benign and malignant lesions. *Radiographics.* 2000;20:43–58.

    Part I of 2-part series describing CT findings to help differentiate benign and malignant lesions, although indeterminate findings are often the case.

28. Gimenez A, Franquet T, Prats R, et al. Unusual primary lung tumors: a radiologic-pathologic overview. *Radiographics.* 2002;22:601–619.

    A very nice CT and pathologic correlation for rare benign and malignant tumors.

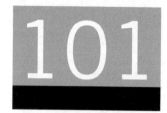

101

Lung Cancer: Diagnosis, Staging, and Prognosis

Samir S. Makani and Mark M. Fuster

CLINICAL PRESENTATION

Patients with lung cancer most often present with signs and symptoms heralding local or metastatic disease. Less commonly, an incidental radiographic finding in an asymptomatic patient triggers workup and diagnosis. This may change with more widespread use of low-dose CT-based imaging strategies. Rarely, patients may present with a paraneoplastic syndrome. How an individual presents is more often a function of (1) the site of origin (central versus peripheral airways), (2) the inherent biologic activity of the neoplasm, and (3) the presence of comorbid conditions. Even with early stage disease, signs and symptoms of local tumor growth, including cough, dyspnea, wheezing, or hemoptysis, frequently are encountered. Additionally, patients may present with purulent sputum, fever, and chills from a postobstructive pneumonia. More ominous signs and symptoms of local tumor growth include superior vena cava syndrome, Horner syndrome, dysphagia, odynophagia, hoarseness (recurrent laryngeal nerve involvement), elevated hemidiaphragm (phrenic nerve impingement), dyspnea and chest pain (pleural effusion), and dyspnea and hemodynamic compromise (pericardial involvement).

Metastatic disease usually is accompanied by malaise and anorexia; weight loss also may be present. Other symptoms reflect the site(s) of metastases: supraclavicular and cervical lymph nodes, brain, bone, liver, and adrenal glands are the most common. The presence of a paraneoplastic syndrome does not necessarily imply metastatic disease. The most common systems involved are endocrine-metabolic, neuromuscular, hematologic-vascular, dermatologic, and skeletal/connective tissue.

DIAGNOSIS

A tissue diagnosis is essential to distinguish non–small-cell lung carcinoma (NSCLC) from small-cell lung carcinoma (SCLC), and ideally is carried out with the least invasive means to accurately establish the diagnosis and extent of disease. For solitary pulmonary nodules (defined as lesions <3 cm in diameter), the initial challenge is to distinguish a benign from a malignant lesion. In some cases, the lesion is sufficiently proximal or localized to the central airways and bronchoscopic diagnosis resolves the diagnosis via direct visualization with bronchoscopic biopsy or fluoroscopically guided transbronchial biopsy. The examination of bronchoscopic brushings and washings increases the diagnostic yield. The diagnostic capability of bronchoscopy is well defined: the yield is over 90% for airway-visualized lesions, over 80% for non-visualized lesions greater than 4 cm in size, and greater than 60% for non-visualized lesions 2 to 4 cm in size. Peripheral lung lesions generally require a CT-guided transthoracic needle aspiration for the highest diagnostic yield. Regardless of the modality, a "negative" biopsy should be regarded as non-diagnostic, especially when the pretest probability of malignancy is moderate to high, and cannot be used to exclude the possibility of cancer. Unless a specific diagnosis is obtained, thoracotomy may be indicated for excisional biopsy and definitive anatomic resection in the same operative setting. In exceptional cases, patients who are high-risk for surgery (e.g., due to severe emphysema) may require empiric radiotherapy to treat a lesion that is highly suspicious but otherwise not safely accessible by biopsy.

While techniques such as conventional diagnostic bronchoscopy and transthoracic needle aspiration may often yield the tissue diagnosis, they are generally limited in the accurate evaluation of suspicious mediastinal lymphadenopathy. The latter may first appear on CT scans, though CT scans are limited in sensitivity and specificity in this setting for mediastinal lymphadenopathy greater than 1 cm in size in short axis (approximately 60% and 80%, respectively). In addition to a careful clinical survey for possible distant sites of metastases, two additional modalities have now become valuable additions to our diagnostic capability: these include positron emission tomography (PET) scanning, which relies on the specific uptake of radiolabeled glucose, and endobronchial ultrasound (EBUS), which has become especially useful in the tissue diagnosis of mediastinal lymphadenopathy. While PET scanning and EBUS now serve very important roles in staging of the mediastinum, one may often obtain the first tissue diagnosis of lung cancer through EBUS–fine-needle aspiration (FNA; i.e., positive lymph node[s], primary lesion, or both). For solitary pulmonary nodules, PET achieves approximately 94% sensitivity and 83% specificity, provided nodule size is 8 mm or greater, while for mediastinal lymphadenopathy the values are in the 85% to 90% range. For diagnosing carcinoma involvement of mediastinal lymph nodes, several analyses now combine the use of PET/CT and EBUS, increasing sensitivity to approximately 92%, while specificity approaches 100%.

The use of PET increasingly is combined in one procedure with CT, as a "PET/CT," and is integrated into the staging algorithm for any primary lesion that is either suspicious or even proven to be lung cancer, as it both strongly modifies the pretest probability of cancer and aids in assessing stage. There are, however, some important diagnostic caveats for PET/CT. First, its sensitivity falls off markedly for lesions less than 0.8 cm in mean diameter; thus, for subcentimeter lesions one cannot rely on modifying the probability of cancer with PET, and other algorithms for radiographic tracking and biopsy decisions such as the Fleischner Radiological Society guidelines, 2005 must be applied for any lesion likely to be lung cancer. Second, one must consider the fact that a highly suspicious primary lesion on chest X-ray or CT imaging that is greater than 0.8 cm may represent a slow-growing carcinoma even in the face of a negative or "cold" PET scan. This may occur, for example, with low-mitotic activity lung adenocarcinomas, including adenocarcinoma in situ (formerly known as "bronchoalveolar carcinoma") or with carcinoid tumors. Thus, one must be careful not to ignore supracentimeter PET-negative lesions that are otherwise suspicious for carcinoma by CT and (or) have other concerning clinical characteristics.

STAGING

For non–small-cell lung cancer, the international lung cancer staging system is used (see Table 101-1). This relies on TNM definitions that are carefully outlined. Several classification changes have been made since the last revision, including (1) multiple nodules or "satellite" lesions in the same lobe as the primary tumor are defined as T3 (and thus potentially resectable); (2) size matters in terms of prognosis, so T1 and T2 subdivisions (a and b) exist and a lesion greater than 7 cm is considered T3; (3) T4 tumors include satellite lesions found in more than one lobe but confined to one/ipsilateral lung; (4) satellite nodules in both lungs represent M1 disease; (5) malignant pleural effusion is considered M1 disease; and (6) T4N0M0 or T4N1M0 lesions are now classified as stage IIIA. Nodal stage definitions remain unchanged.

To define the T (tumor) characteristics of a lesion, chest radiograph, CT scanning, PET, magnetic resonance imaging (MRI), and bronchoscopy may all be helpful. MRI may be particularly useful in assessing patients with possible T3 or T4 lesions and for specific assessment of brachial plexus involvement (i.e., superior sulcus tumors) and/or chest wall invasion. In some cases, video-assisted thoracoscopic (VATS) techniques may be needed to assess or better define T4 disease.

To accurately define the N (nodal) status of a lesion, combining PET/CT with EBUS now allows for improved identification as well as access to multiple lymph node stations, beyond (and including) those that have traditionally been accessed via mediastinoscopy. Regardless of the approach, transbronchial needle aspiration (TBNA) of any lymph node should be assessed for lymphocyte yield (i.e., negative without lymphocytes has a higher false-negative likelihood); when positive, there is a risk of contamination by nearby extranodal tumor during sampling. Other approaches that may be required for nodal staging include ultrasound-guided transesophageal needle biopsy, mediastinotomy (e.g., to diagnose aortopulmonary or anterior mediastinal adenopathy), thoracoscopy, or thoracotomy (i.e., with node sampling/definition at resection). In general, nodes that are enlarged on CT and positive on PET require tissue confirmation, except when gross mediastinal invasion by tumor (T4) is obvious. In either case, tissue diagnosis will be required for appropriate treatment. Finally, a patient should not be denied potentially curative

TABLE 101-1	Staging of Non–Small-Cell Lung Cancer—TNM Definitions According to the IASLC 7th Edition

Primary tumor (T)

TX	Occult carcinoma (status not able to be assessed)
T0	No evidence of primary tumor
Tis	Carcinoma in situ
T1	Tumor ≤3 cm in greatest dimension, surrounded by lung or visceral pleura, and without bronchoscopic evidence of invasion proximal to a lobar bronchus. T1a versus T1b discriminates lesions lesser or greater than 2 cm.
T2	A tumor >3 cm in greatest dimension but ≤7 cm, or a tumor of any size that either invades the visceral pleura or has associated atelectasis or obstructive pneumonitis that extends to the hilar region; at bronchoscopy, proximal extent of demonstrable tumor must be at least 2 cm distal to the main carina; any associated atelectasis or obstructive pneumonitis must involve less than an entire lung. T2a versus T2b discriminate lesions lesser or greater than 5 cm.
T3	Tumor >7 cm; or tumor of any size with direct extension into the chest wall (including superior sulcus tumors), diaphragm, phrenic nerve, mediastinal pleura, or parietal pericardium without involving the heart, great vessels, trachea, esophagus, or vertebral bodies; or a tumor in the main bronchus within 2 cm of main carina without involving it; or atelectasis/obstructive pneumonitis of the entire lung; or separate tumor nodules in the same lobe.
T4	A tumor of any size with invasion of the mediastinum or involving the heart, great vessels, trachea, esophagus, recurrent laryngeal nerve, vertebral bodies, or main carina; or separate tumor nodules in a different ipsilateral lobe

Nodal involvement (N)

NX	Occult carcinoma
N0	No regional lymph node metastasis
N1	Metastasis of lymph nodes in the ipsilateral peribronchial and/or perihilar regions, and intrapulmonary nodes, including involvement by direct extension
N2	Metastatic involvement of ipsilateral mediastinal lymph nodes and/or subcarinal lymph nodes
N3	Metastatic involvement of contralateral mediastinal lymph nodes, contralateral hilar nodes; or the involvement of any scalene or supraclavicular nodes

Distant metastatic involvement (M)

M0	No (known) distant metastatic involvement
M1a	Separate tumor nodules in a contralateral lobe; or malignant pleural involvement; or pleural tumor nodules
M1b	Distant metastasis

Modified from Detterbeck FC, Boffa DJ, Tanoue LT. The new lung cancer staging system. *Chest.* 2009;136:260–271.

surgery based solely on radiographic criteria. In this regard, PET/CT may assist in identifying patients with enlarged lymph nodes on CT but PET-negative in the mediastinum: Such patients, with a high probability of false-positive nodes on CT, should be considered for EBUS–TBNA for staging the mediastinum or definitive resection with nodal sampling at the time of surgery.

TABLE 101-2	New International Revised Stage Grouping
Stage	**TNM Subset**
0	Carcinoma in situ
IA	T1a, bN0M0
IB	T2aN0M0
IIA	T1a, bN1M0
	T2aN1M0
	T2bN0M0
IIB	T2bN1M0
	T3N0M0
IIIA	T1–3N1M0
	T3N1M0
	T4N0,1M0
IIIB	T4N2M0
	T1–4N3M0
IV	T *any* N *any* M1a,b

Modified from Detterbeck FC, Boffa DJ, Tanoue LT. The new lung cancer staging system. *Chest.* 2009;136:260–271.

The M (metastasis) characteristics of a lesion may be defined through history and physical examination, chemistry panel, liver function tests, and imaging studies, including assessment of liver and adrenal glands on CT and whole-body PET to guide further sampling. Questions and examination focused on neurologic signs/symptoms and/or bony pain may guide brain (CT or MRI) or bone scanning. Guidelines by the National Comprehensive Cancer Network (NCCN) now recommend an MRI brain scan for any stage II or higher NSCLC patient, as the risk of occult brain metastasis becomes significant (up to 10% for adenocarcinoma), and may thus markedly influence the treatment plan. Finally, whole-body PET studies indicate that unsuspected metastatic disease may often be found (11%–29% of patients in one series). More investigation is needed to determine the role of alternative radiolabeled uptake analogs as well as single-photon emission CT (SPECT) imaging in evaluating local/regional and distant disease in lung cancer.

Stages of lung cancer are defined by combining the TNM components (see Table 101-2). Stage I includes those patients with no lymph node involvement (N0) and no invasion of structures (T1,2). Stage II includes patients with either no invasion (T1,2) and hilar (N1) lymph node metastases or patients with chest wall invasion or even satellite lesions in one lobe, but no lymph node involvement (T3N0; stage IIB). Stage III is divided into those with potentially resectable disease (IIIA) and those with unresectable disease (IIIB). With the possibility of multiple advanced T and N combinations, stage III (and even IIIA) remains particularly heterogeneous. Stage IV disease is confined to those patients with metastasis to distant sites.

While the staging system continues to be refined by advances in detection technology, biological understanding, and therapy, it remains critical to make a strong effort to accurately stage patients using the current system. Determination of the N (nodal) status remains one of the most challenging aspects of thoracic TNM staging for NSCLC. Use of the American Joint Committee on Cancer (AJCC) regional lymph node map allows for uniform reporting of patient data. This is also important for the design and implementation of new clinical trials.

For SCLC, once a tissue diagnosis is made, the disease is staged as limited versus extensive stage. Limited-stage SCLC is limited to one hemithorax (i.e., disease that can be contained in a "tolerable" radiation field or port). Extensive-stage SCLC involves metastasis beyond the hemithorax.

PROGNOSIS

The stage of NSCLC at presentation correlates strongly with lung cancer survival. With surgery, the 5-year survival for clinical TNM stages IA, IB, and IIA/IIB disease is approximately 50%, 43%, and 36%/25%, respectively. For pathologic stages IA, IB, and IIA/IIB, 5-year survivals are 73%, 56%, and 46%/36%, respectively. Stage III patients are highly heterogeneous with 5-year survival ranging from less than 25% in the majority up to 30% to 40% in some select patients, depending on the particular TNM status and treatment modalities employed (see Chapter 104). Patients with clinical stage IV disease have a 1-year survival of 20% to 30% and 5-year survival of less than 5%. Occasionally, patients with stage IV disease who respond well to chemotherapy may survive 2 to 3 years or longer.

The patient's performance status at diagnosis, according to the Eastern Cooperative Oncology Group (ECOG) scale, also carries significant prognostic weight and influences treatment decisions (see Chapter 103). Finally, while a number of histologic and biologic molecular markers are not formally integrated into the anatomic-based TNM scale, several of these markers are now being employed in the selection of molecular-targeted therapies, and appear to have significant prognostic significance. Further work may integrate some of these into future prognostic algorithms.

Survival is limited to weeks to months in untreated SCLC. Current treatment of limited-stage SCLC is associated with median survival of 18 to 24 months and 5-year survival of 20% to 25%. For extensive-stage disease, median survival of 8 to 10 months is typically observed. Survival analyses of SCLC patients using the IASLC database show that TNM staging for SCLC also has prognostic significance, and should be incorporated in clinical trials of early stage disease. For now, it is sensible to provide TNM data on SCLC to the tumor registry while clinically staging and treating patients according to the limited versus extensive-stage definition.

FURTHER READING

1. Detterbeck FC, Boffa DJ, Tanoue LT. The new lung cancer staging system. *Chest.* 2009;136:260–271.

   A publication outlining the current 7th edition IASLC lung cancer staging system with detailed descriptors for T, N, and M; and prognoses for descriptors as well as clinical- and pathologic stages.

2. Lababede O, Meziane J, Rice T. Seventh edition of the cancer staging manual and stage grouping of lung cancer: quick reference chart and diagrams. *Chest.* 2011;139:183–189.

   Helpful diagrams and descriptions of 7th edition IASLC staging system that may be used as a reference that accompanies the paper summarizing current staging system (Detterbeck et al., 2009).

3. Maeda R, Yoshida J, Ishii G, et al. Prognostic impact of histology on early-stage non-small cell lung cancer. *Chest.* 2011;37:2798–2800.

   This publication provides compelling data highlighting the importance of how microanatomic predictors (such as histologic differentiation, vessel invasion, and visceral pleural invasion) might be used alone or as a group to refine prediction/prognosis for any given stage. It focuses on early stage NSCLC, and emphasizes the utility (and possible future incorporation) of measures beyond our macroscopic T and N descriptors as an additional prognostic guide.

4. MacMahon H, Austin JH, Gamsu G, et al. Guidelines for management of small pulmonary nodules detected on CT scans: a statement from the Fleischner Society. *Radiology.* 2005;237:395–400.

   Fleischner society statement/guidelines on management of subcentimeter nodules on CT imaging. Used as a common guide for decisions on the frequency of imaging follow-up as modified by the state of cancer risk factors.

5. Sher T, Dy GK, Adjei AA. Small cell lung cancer. *Mayo Clin Proc.* 2008;83:355–367.

   A comprehensive review that includes overview of the practical treatment-oriented staging approach as well as prognoses for limited and extensive small-cell lung cancer.

6. Chandra S, Nehra M, Agarwal D, et al. Diagnostic accuracy of endobronchial ultrasound-guided transbronchial needle biopsy in mediastinal lymphadenopathy: a systematic review and meta-analysis. *Respir Care.* 2012;57:304–391.

   A comprehensive review and meta-analysis of 14 recent studies utilizing EBUS-TBNA.

102 Lung Cancer: Classification, Epidemiology, and Screening

Philippe R. Montgrain

CLASSIFICATION

The term *lung cancer* comprises a number of specific malignancies (Table 102-1). The four major histologic types of lung cancer are squamous cell carcinoma, adenocarcinoma, large-cell carcinoma, and small-cell carcinoma. Historically, clinicians have been concerned primarily with the division of lung cancer into small-cell lung carcinoma (SCLC) and non–small-cell lung carcinoma (NSCLC). These two major groups have very different clinical presentations, metastatic potential, and responses to therapy. However, in the past decade, there has been increased emphasis on the precise classification of NSCLC since molecular testing and potential therapies now depend on histology. For example, adenocarcinomas are more likely to harbor epidermal growth factor receptor (EGFR) mutations that respond to specific targeted inhibitors. As a result of this need for more precision, the classification of lung adenocarcinoma was further refined in 2011, as shown in Table 102-1. One major change is that the term bronchioloalveolar carcinoma (BAC) is no longer used. The four major histologic types of lung cancer are discussed below.

Squamous cell carcinoma accounts for about 20% to 25% of all lung cancers in the United States. It used to be the most common type of lung cancer, but for unclear reasons its incidence has dropped, and it is now surpassed by adenocarcinoma. Historically, the majority of squamous cell carcinomas presented as central tumors. However, more recent data suggest an increasing percentage of peripheral tumors. Cavitation is not uncommon. Morphological features include intercellular bridging, squamous pearl formation, and keratinization. Squamous cell carcinoma typically arises from altered bronchial epithelium and is preceded by years of progressive mucosal changes that include squamous metaplasia, dysplasia, and carcinoma in situ. In its early stages of growth, the tumor may appear as a small, red, granular plaque or as a focus of leukoplakia. Later, it may appear as a large exophytic endobronchial mass.

Adenocarcinoma is the most common histologic type, representing 40% to 50% of all lung cancers in the United States. Adenocarcinomas are classically peripheral tumors arising from the peripheral airways and alveoli, but they may also arise proximally from the epithelium or submucosal glands. Cavitation is rare. Morphologically, they appear as cuboidal or columnar cells forming gland-like structures that may or may not produce mucin. Some adenocarcinomas display a lepidic growth pattern, meaning growth restricted to neoplastic cells along preexisting alveolar structures without invasion. These preinvasive or minimally invasive lesions carry a better prognosis. The new 2011 classification of adenocarcinoma introduced many changes, some of which are worth highlighting. First, the term bronchioloalveolar carcinoma was discontinued and further divided into new terms (Table 102-1). Second, new concepts of adenocarcinoma in situ and minimally invasive adenocarcinoma were introduced. Third, micropapillary adenocarcinoma was added as a new subtype with poor prognosis. Finally, new terminology and diagnostic criteria for small biopsies and cytology specimens were proposed. These changes will assist in determining patient therapy and predicting outcome.

SCLC comprises about 15% of all lung cancers. It has a distinct clinical presentation, with a very aggressive course and frequent metastases at presentation. Paraneoplastic syndromes are common. Though chemoresponsive, SCLC has a very poor prognosis. About two-thirds

TABLE 102-1	Histologic Classification of Lung Cancer

Squamous cell carcinoma

Variants: papillary, clear cell, small cell, basaloid

Small-cell carcinoma

Variant: combined small-cell carcinoma

Adenocarcinoma

Adenocarcinoma in situ (formerly BAC)

Minimally invasive adenocarcinoma (≤3 cm lepidic predominant tumor with ≤5 mm invasion)

Invasive adenocarcinoma
• Lepidic predominant (formerly nonmucinous BAC pattern, with >5 mm invasion)
• Acinar predominant
• Papillary predominant
• Micropapillary predominant
• Solid predominant with mucin production

Variants of invasive adenocarcinoma
• Invasive mucinous adenocarcinoma (formerly mucinous BAC)
• Colloid
• Fetal (low and high grade)
• Enteric

Large-cell carcinoma

Variants: large-cell neuroendocrine carcinoma, basaloid carcinoma, lymphoepithelioma-like carcinoma, clear-cell carcinoma, large-cell carcinoma with rhabdoid phenotype

Sarcomatoid carcinoma

Variants: pleomorphic carcinoma, spindle cell carcinoma, giant cell carcinoma, carcinosarcoma, pulmonary blastoma, other

Carcinoid tumor

Variants: typical carcinoid, atypical carcinoid

Carcinomas of salivary gland type

Variants: mucoepidermoid carcinoma, adenoid cystic carcinoma, epimyoepithelial carcinoma

Adenosquamous carcinoma

of SCLC present as a perihilar mass, though it can present as a solitary pulmonary nodule in up to 5% of cases. Extensive lymph node metastases are common, and the tumor often causes bronchial obstruction by extrinsic compression. Tumor cells are small, with a round to fusiform shape, scant cytoplasm, and absent or faint nucleoli. Nuclear molding and smearing of nuclear chromatin as a result of crush artifact can be seen. Extensive necrosis is common. Staining for neuroendocrine markers, such as CD56, chromogranin, and synaptophysin, can aid in diagnosis.

Large-cell carcinoma represents about 3% to 9% of all lung cancers. The majority are peripheral tumors, often quite large and necrotic. Histologically, they often consist of sheets and nests of large polygonal cells with vesicular nuclei and prominent nucleoli. The presence of squamous or glandular differentiation must be excluded to make the diagnosis. Thus, large-cell carcinoma cannot be diagnosed in small biopsies and cytology specimens. A resection specimen is required. Large-cell carcinomas are a heterogeneous group of poorly differentiated tumors.

Several variants exist, some of which are associated with a worse prognosis, such as large-cell neuroendocrine carcinoma.

EPIDEMIOLOGY

Lung cancer is the leading cause of cancer mortality worldwide. The disease became an epidemic in the last century, as incidence and mortality rose dramatically. More than 1.5 million new cases are diagnosed annually throughout the world. Incidence in the United States alone is estimated to be 226,160 cases in 2012. Though historically a disease of men, lung cancer now affects the sexes equally, with 116,470 new cases in men and 109,690 new cases in women expected in 2012. Mortality remains very elevated for lung cancer. 2012 US estimated deaths are 87,750 in men and 72,590 in women. This represents 29% and 26% of all cancer deaths in men and women, respectively. Lung cancer kills more people than breast, prostate, and colon cancers combined. Age, racial, and socioeconomic disparities also exist. Lung cancer is a disease of the aging, with 60% of cases diagnosed in persons over the age of 65. Incidence and mortality are higher in Caucasians and African Americans than in other ethnic groups in the United States, and socioeconomic status correlates inversely with lung cancer mortality.

Risk factors for lung cancer can be divided into genetic factors, behavioral factors, and environmental factors. By far the most important risk (and causal) factor is behavioral: tobacco smoking. Smoking causes about 85% of lung cancer cases in the United States. Smokers have about a 20-fold increase in lung cancer risk compared to never-smokers. There is a direct dose–response relationship between cigarettes smoked and lung cancer risk. Tobacco smoke contains about 4,000 chemicals, of which at least 60 are known carcinogens. These carcinogens and their metabolites lead to the formation of DNA adducts. Along with free-radical damage, these adducts can lead to carcinogenesis. Carcinogenic risk in former smokers declines progressively following smoking cessation. Lung cancer risk falls by greater than 70% after 15 years of smoking cessation. The risk will eventually approach that of a never-smoker, though some residual risk remains and that risk depends upon the intensity of the precessation smoking history (e.g., pack-years, inhalation, and age at initiation).

Secondhand smoke exposure is now recognized as a cause of lung cancer among nonsmokers. A dose–response relationship has been confirmed; there is no safe level of secondhand smoke exposure. Nonsmokers who live with a smoker have a 20% to 30% increased risk of lung cancer. Secondhand, or passive, smoking is estimated to cause 3,000 lung cancer deaths per year in the United States alone.

Other environmental risk factors for lung cancer include radon, indoor and outdoor air pollution, and certain occupational exposures. Radon is the second leading cause of lung cancer, responsible for 10% of lung cancer deaths. The amount of radon found in homes varies, and radon testing kits are easily available. Homes with radon levels of 4 pCi/L or higher should undergo interventions to reduce levels. Occupational exposures known to cause lung cancer include ionizing radiation, arsenic, chromium, nickel, asbestos, tar, and soot. Many of these exposures are additive or synergistic with cigarette smoke in the induction of pulmonary malignancies.

There may be significant individual susceptibility to lung cancer. Having a positive family history of lung cancer is associated with a 1.7-fold increased risk of the disease. Even in nonsmokers, the risk is elevated at 1.4-fold. A positive family history in two or more relatives is associated with a 3.6-fold increased risk. Variant alleles of several genes are associated with increased susceptibility to lung cancer. Some of these genes are involved in the metabolism of tobacco carcinogens; others are involved in DNA repair. Genome-wide association studies have also identified polymorphisms that predispose to lung cancer. These host factors are areas of active research.

Preexisting lung disease has also been implicated to increase the risk of lung cancer. Chronic obstructive pulmonary disease, pulmonary fibrosis, tuberculosis, pneumoconioses, and systemic sclerosis have all been associated with an increased risk. Other host factors like HIV infection may also be important. Finally, there is consistent evidence that dietary intake of fruits and vegetables lowers the risk of lung cancer. High consumption of β-carotene has been associated with a 50% reduction in the risk of lung cancer in comparison to low consumption. However, three prospective, randomized, controlled intervention trials found no benefit or *increased* lung cancer mortality in those patients given β-carotene as a dietary supplement.

SCREENING

The basic principles of any good screening program are (1) diagnose disease early in asymptomatic patients; (2) detect diseases that respond better to early versus late treatment; and (3) ensure that the benefits of treating the few patients who will be diagnosed with the disease outweigh the harms associated with screening the large number without the disease. Lung cancer, the leading cause of cancer mortality worldwide, would certainly be a good candidate for screening. Currently, only about 30% of lung cancer is diagnosed at an early, potentially curable stage. This could improve with screening. Multiple studies in the 1970s and 1980s evaluated lung cancer screening with chest radiography (CXR) and sputum cytology. These studies showed that one could diagnose more lung cancers with CXR screening, but lung cancer mortality was not affected. In 2011 the Prostate, Lung, Colon and Ovary (PLCO) screening trial, the largest US screening trial ever done, published the results of its lung cancer screening arm. Over 150,000 subjects were randomized to usual care or annual CXR. After 13 years of follow-up, there was no difference in lung cancer deaths, stage, or histology between the two groups. It is now clear that CXR should not be used for lung cancer screening.

Radiographic chest imaging has advanced substantially since the 1970s. Current computed tomography (CT) scanners can detect lesions in the 2-mm range. Several large observational studies demonstrated that annual CT screening of high-risk populations yields a substantial number of asymptomatic lung cancers, most at an early stage. These advances rekindled enthusiasm for lung cancer screening. The National Lung Screening Trial (NLST), supported by the National Cancer Institute, randomized over 50,000 high-risk subjects to annual low-dose CT versus annual CXR (note that CXR was used in the control group because the PLCO trial results were not yet known). Subjects were aged 55 to 74 years and current or former smokers with at least 30 pack-years; if former smokers, they must have quit within 15 years. After 6 years of follow-up, the low-dose CT screening group had a 20% reduction in lung cancer mortality. The number needed to screen was 320 to prevent one lung cancer death. This compares very favorably with other established screening programs. Following NLST, multiple medical societies and the US Preventive Services Task Force now recommend lung cancer screening with annual low-dose CT in high-risk patients. Screening patients outside of the inclusion criteria for NLST (age 55–74, smoked ≥30 pack-years) is controversial and not recommended by many societies.

Many questions and uncertainties remain about low-dose CT screening for lung cancer. Will screening be cost-effective? Some studies suggest it will be, but data on cost-effectiveness from NLST are still pending. How long or until what age should patients be screened? What is the risk of overdiagnosis (diagnosing a low-grade cancer that would not have killed the patient)? What are the long-term radiation risks? The average radiation dose of low-dose CT is 1.5 millisieverts (mSv). To put that in context, a standard diagnostic CT is about 8 mSv, and background radiation exposure after a year living on earth is about 3 mSv. So the radiation dose is clearly low, but the cumulative exposure of repeated screens may not be negligible. Another question is whether the elevated false-positive rate (about 94% of positive screens) can be lowered, perhaps by using biomarkers to select patients at even higher risk of lung cancer. Also, in what setting should screening be performed, and what infrastructure will be required? Ideally, screening will be carried out in settings with multidisciplinary, specialized care with close surveillance and follow-up. However, real-world implementation may not always be so ideal. These questions, and others, will need to be addressed over the coming years.

In summary, we can now reduce lung cancer mortality by 20% with low-dose CT screening. This benefit is limited to a specific, high-risk population (age 55–74 years and 30 or more pack-years of smoking). Data cannot and should not be extrapolated to other "risky" populations at this time. Ideally, screening should be a multidisciplinary effort that includes smoking cessation, and implemented carefully and with appropriate resources.

FURTHER READING

1. The Alpha–Tocopherol, Beta-Carotene Cancer Prevention Study Group. The effect of vitamin E and β-carotene on the incidence of lung cancer and other cancers in male smokers. *N Engl J Med.* 1994;330:1029–1035.

   In a randomized, double-blind, placebo-controlled trial, the β-carotene arm had an 18% increased incidence of lung cancer.

2. Auerbach O, Stout AP, Hammond EC, et al. Changes in bronchial epithelium in relation to lung cancer. *N Engl J Med.* 1961;265:253–267.

   One of the major pathologic studies supporting epidemiologic data linking cigarette smoking and the development of lung cancer.

3. Bach PB, Mirkin JN, Oliver TK, et al. Benefits and harms of CT screening for lung cancer: a systematic review. *JAMA.* 2012;307:2418–2429.

   An excellent review that discusses the benefits of low-dose CT screening, but also the uncertainty about potential harms and generalizability.

4. Cohen MH. Natural history of lung cancer. *Clin Chest Med.* 1982;3:229–241.

   A comprehensive, well-referenced review of the natural history of lung cancer.

5. Cone JE. Occupational lung cancer. *Occup Med.* 1987;2:273–295.

   A comprehensive review of the subject.

6. de Groot P, Munden RF. Lung cancer epidemiology, risk factors, and prevention. *Radiol Clin North Am.* 2012;50:863–876.

   A comprehensive review of lung cancer epidemiology.

7. Hammond EC, Horn D. Smoking and death rates: report on 44 months follow-up of 187,783 men. *JAMA.* 1958;166:1294–1308.

   A classic early epidemiologic paper linking cigarette smoking to an increased risk of death from lung and other cancers and from cardiovascular disease.

8. Hennekens CH, Buring JE, Manson JE, et al. Lack of effect of long-term supplementation with beta carotene on the incidence of malignant neoplasms and cardiovascular disease. *N Engl J Med.* 1996;334:1145–1149.

   A randomized, double-blind, placebo-controlled trial found no difference in incidence or death rates from lung cancer with β-carotene supplementation.

9. Knekt P, Jarvinen R, Seppanen R, et al. Dietary antioxidants and the risk of lung cancer. *Am J Epidemiol.* 1991;134:471–479.

   The relationship between the intake of retinoids, carotenoids, vitamins E and C, and selenium and the subsequent risk of lung cancer was investigated in a large series of men followed up for 20 years.

10. Midthun DE. Screening for lung cancer. *Clin Chest Med.* 2011;32:659–668.

    A comprehensive review of lung cancer screening.

11. National Lung Screening Trial Research Team. Reduced lung-cancer mortality with low-dose computed tomographic screening. *N Engl J Med.* 2011;365:395–409.

    A pivotal trial showing a 20% reduction in lung cancer mortality with annual low-dose CT screening in a high-risk population.

12. Omenn GS, Goodman GE, Thornquist MD, et al. Effects of a combination of beta carotene and vitamin A on lung cancer and cardiovascular disease. *N Engl J Med.* 1996;334:1150–1155.

    This randomized, double-blind, placebo-controlled trial showed a 28% increased incidence of lung cancer in β-carotene arm and study was stopped 21 months earlier than planned.

13. *Smoking and Health: A Report of the Surgeon General.* Washington, DC: US Department of Health, Education, and Welfare; 1979. Publication no [PHS] 79-50066.

    A reiteration of the 1964 report linking cigarette smoking to the development of lung cancer.

14. *The Health Consequences of Smoking: Cancer. A Report of the Surgeon General.* Rockville, MD: US Department of Health and Human Services; 1982. Publication no DHHS [PHS] 82-50179.

    The most comprehensive review of the subject by the federal government's watchdog agency.

15. Siegel R, Naishadham D, Jemal A. Cancer statistics, 2012. *CA Cancer J Clin.* 2012;62:10–29.
    Updated cancer statistics, including incidence and mortality.
16. Travis WD. Pathology of lung cancer. *Clin Chest Med.* 2011;32:669–692.
    An excellent review of the histologic classification of lung cancer. Includes the updated classification of adenocarcinomas.
17. Travis WD, Brambilla E, Noguchi M, et al. International Association for the Study of Lung Cancer/American Thoracic Society/European Respiratory Society international multidisciplinary classification of lung adenocarcinoma. *J Thorac Oncol.* 2011;6:244–285.
    Presents the new classification of lung adenocarcinoma. Also proposes classification system for small biopsies and cytology specimens.

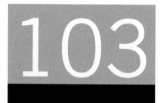

103 Lung Cancer: Treatment

Mark M. Fuster

While overall survival for patients diagnosed with lung cancer remains poor (16%–18% 5-year survival), clinical and basic research over the last 10 to 15 years has led to the incorporation of adjuvant therapies as well as targeted therapies that may significantly improve outcomes in select groups of patients. The approach to treatment is now guided by a combination of histology (small-cell versus non–small cell) and stage of disease as well as the presence of molecular signatures that permit individualized therapy. The treatment approach also must take into consideration a patient's general performance status and pulmonary function. The involvement of a multidisciplinary team (pulmonary, medical and radiation oncology, thoracic surgery, radiology, pathology, palliative care, and nursing specialists) in making integrated treatment decisions helps to provide state-of-the-art care. For non–small-cell lung cancer (NSCLC), the most basic decision at the time of diagnosis is whether the patient has *early stage* and potentially resectable disease (if the patient is deemed operable) or *advanced-stage* disease. For small-cell lung cancer (SCLC), the treatment approach depends on whether disease is *limited* versus *extensive* in anatomic extent, features that determine whether and how radiation is paired with chemotherapy as a basic form of treatment. Most of the chapter, and the following sections, will focus on NSCLC.

OPERABILITY, RESECTABILITY, AND ADJUVANT THERAPY FOR STAGE I AND STAGE II NSCLC

Surgical resection should be the first consideration for possible cure of stage I or stage II NSCLC. A patient must be operable to undergo resection. This assessment requires routine cardiovascular evaluation as well as pulmonary function and arterial blood gas testing. In general, a predicted postoperative forced expiratory volume in 1 second (FEV_1) or diffusing capacity of the lung for carbon monoxide (D_{LCO}) of less than 40% indicates significant risk of perioperative complications or death following anatomic/lobar resections. D_{LCO} is particularly important when imaging reveals diffuse parenchymal lung disease or in the setting of dyspnea on exertion. When pulmonary function results are marginal, cardiopulmonary exercise testing (with Vo_2 max < 15 mL/kg/min indicating increased perioperative risk) and/or quantitative ventilation–perfusion lung scanning may greatly assist in decision-making regarding operability. The lung scan occasionally may weight a decision toward surgery in a patient with marginal FEV_1 if a tumor-affected lobe contributes minimally to ventilation (or perfusion). In general, decisions must be individualized and often rely on integrating physiologic testing data.

Once a patient is deemed operable, the assessment of resectability depends upon stage. Stages I and II patients are candidates for resection. Following a lobar resection, adjuvant chemotherapy has been found to improve outcomes in patients with pathological stage II disease, although there is still no role for adjuvant therapy following resection of a lesion that is pathological stage IA. Finally, when compromised lung function precludes anatomic resection, a curative attempt with radiotherapy is generally employed, with sublobar resection (for stage IA) a less frequent approach. Radiotherapy for stage IA lesions has evolved to incorporate the use of higher-dose, hypofractionated programs (i.e., stereotactic body radiotherapy [SBRT]) that have markedly improved local control rates and curability. Studies on outcomes using SBRT for early stage disease are ongoing; however, more conventional radiation therapy for early stage lesions still produce significantly lower cure rates than that achieved by anatomic surgical resection. Following definitive therapy, surveillance imaging (i.e., CT thorax) is typically carried out twice yearly for 2 years, and yearly thereafter.

ADVANCED-STAGE NSCLC: CHEMOTHERAPY, RADIOTHERAPY, AND COMBINED-THERAPY APPROACHES

Stage IIIA disease is very heterogeneous. Most patients (e.g., with bulky N2/mediastinal adenopathy) are not resection candidates, and benefit most from a combination of chemotherapy and radiation. Standard chemotherapy is platinum-based and involves the use of two agents. Some stage IIIA patients (e.g., T3N1 superior sulcus tumor) may benefit from a "neoadjuvant" approach, wherein surgery following a good response to induction chemotherapy/radiation offers 5-year survival rates that exceed 30%. Neoadjuvant therapy, however, remains an area of investigation; for some patients, toxicity of this approach may be significant, and its use should generally remain within the context of a protocol. Occasionally, patients are found to have pathologic stage IIIA disease upon postoperative pathological review following lobar resection of what appeared to be clinical stage I or II; adjuvant chemotherapy has improved outcomes for such patients. Adjuvant radiotherapy may also be employed in patients found to have advanced-stage (III) disease at time of resection (or when resection results in positive surgical margins for any stage), with its major benefit a reduction in local–regional recurrence. For stage IIIB or stage IV disease, chemotherapy is the main form of therapy for patients with good-performance status. Concurrent delivery of chemotherapy and radiotherapy may be employed in the aggressive treatment of stage III patients, although toxicity may limit this approach. Sequential use of these modalities is a frequently used alternative. For stage IV NSCLC disease in patients with good-performance status, unless radiation is necessary for palliation, treatment is limited to chemotherapy. Stage IV disease is mostly noncurable with overall 5-year survival in the range of 10% to 15% for pathologic stage IV; however, patients with good-performance status may have 2-year survival rates of 30% to 40%. Survival in such patients may be further modified in responders to novel targeted therapies. Limited performance should be recognized, however, with appropriate and early institution of palliative measures to improve quality of life.

TARGETED TREATMENT FOR NSCLC: TAILORING THERAPY TO TARGETS AND THE INDIVIDUAL

In the last decade, a number of growth receptors have been identified as important contributors to tumor growth and spread. Some of these have surfaced curiously in unique demographic groups with distinct histology. To date, the best such characterized target is the epidermal growth factor receptor (EGFR), which has been found to have a kinase-domain mutation in lung adenocarcinomas predominating in nonsmoking females (including higher probability among individuals of Asian descent). Tumors bearing a specific group of EGFR mutations (e.g., δ-LRE, L858R, G719X) respond well to small-molecule tyrosine kinase inhibitors, such as erlotinib, which may be used as a main form of (targeted) drug therapy for appropriate patients. It is reasonable to suspect such mutations in any non- or remote former smoker with lung adenocarcinoma, and needle-biopsy or histology specimens should be submitted for pathologic testing in such individuals. Treatment with erlotinib may also benefit advanced-stage patients who have not responded to first- or second-line chemotherapy. Nevertheless, primary as well as acquired resistance mutations have also been described, and may limit length of therapy. Another recently discovered target involves a gene fusion (EML4-ALK) that activates anaplastic lymphoma kinase (ALK), which is highly oncogenic and present in approximately 3% to 6% of NSCLC. It also appears with highest frequency in younger never-smokers with adenocarcinoma. Responses to targeted ALK inhibitors in this group appear promising. It should be noted that expression of KRAS mutations predicts lack of response to EGFR or ALK inhibitors, and may identify patients who are unlikely to benefit from EGFR (and possibly ALK) kinase inhibitors.

SMALL-CELL LUNG CARCINOMA

This lung cancer is aggressive, highly metastatic, and very rapidly fatal without treatment. In terms of therapy, limited-stage disease (LD-SCLC), limited to the hemithorax, or "contained" within a port of radiation, has median survival of approximately 18 to 24 months, and should be distinguished from extensive, or metastatic, disease (ED-SCLC). Patients with LD-SCLC can be treated with combined chemotherapy and radiation with curative intent, achieving 5-year survivals of up to 20% to 25%. However, patients with ED-SCLC typically have a median survival of only 8 to 10 months with therapy. They should generally be offered chemotherapy, with the use of palliative radiotherapy targeted to symptomatic sites, as needed. Surgery does not play a primary role in the treatment of SCLC; however, rarely an early stage lesion may be resected during thoracotomy for a solitary pulmonary nodule. In that setting, adjuvant chemotherapy is generally recommended. Prophylactic cranial irradiation (PCI) should also be offered to patients with disease remission, since this significantly lowers the development of central nervous system (CNS) metastases and has also been shown to improve survival, even in ED-SCLC patients responsive to chemotherapy. The risk of late CNS toxicity from PCI is associated with radiation fractions of 2.5 Gy (or total radiation doses of >30 Gy).

PALLIATIVE TREATMENT

There are multiple modalities for palliation of symptoms that may be applied to advanced-stage disease, recurrent disease, or disease that is unresectable or inoperable. Radiation may be used to palliate airway compression, cough, obstructive pneumonia/atelectasis, hemoptysis, pain (e.g., bony metastases), brain metastases, or superior vena cava obstruction, among other localized tumor-mediated problems. Endobronchial stenting may be used for central airway obstruction (e.g., extrinsic main-stem bronchus compression); other modalities may be used to alleviate endobronchial disease, such as laser therapy via the rigid bronchoscope (e.g., exophytic growth into the airway, hemoptysis) or endobronchial radiation (brachytherapy). Other treatment modalities that may be used for palliating central airway disease include electrocautery, balloon dilatation, cryotherapy, and photodynamic therapy. The goal of such palliative approaches is to alleviate symptoms and improve patient's quality of life. In patients with metastatic NSCLC, integrating early palliative care with standard oncologic care may improve both quality of life and mood as well as extend survival.

FURTHER READING

1. Alberts WM. Follow up and surveillance of the patient with lung cancer: what do you do after surgery? *Respirology*. 2007;12:16–21.

   Considerations on optimum surveillance imaging following definitive treatment for lung cancer. The use of CT scanning for 2 years at 6-monthly intervals is considered, followed by yearly imaging.

2. Arriagada R, Bergman B, Dunant A, et al. Cisplatin-based adjuvant chemotherapy in patients with completely resected non–small-cell lung cancer. *N Engl J Med*. 2004;350:351–360.

   One of the major trials that helped establish the importance of adjuvant chemotherapy for a group of predominantly stage II and III postresection NSCLC patients.

3. Belderbos J, Sonke JJ. State-of-the-art lung cancer radiation therapy. *Expert Rev Anticancer Ther*. 2009;9:1353–1363.

   A review of important basic radiotherapy delivery principles for lung cancer patients, and discussion of efficacy.

4. Cheng H, Xu X, Costa DB, et al. Molecular testing in lung cancer: the time is now. *Curr Oncol Rep*. 2010;12:335–348.

A comprehensive review of new molecular markers that are being used to individualize therapy for lung cancer, including EGFR and EML4-ALK mutations and small-molecule inhibitors as tailored therapy.

5. Colice GL, Shafazand S, Griffin JP, et al. Physiologic evaluation of the patient with lung cancer being considered for resectional surgery: ACCP evidenced-based clinical practice guidelines (2nd edition). *Chest*. 2007;132:161S–177S.

An essential review of pulmonary function testing, lung perfusion testing, and exercise considerations during the preoperative evaluation for lung cancer resection.

6. Detterbeck FC, Boffa DJ, Tanoue LT. The new lung cancer staging system. *Chest*. 2009;136:260–271.

A highly important summary of the latest (IASLC 7th edition) staging system for lung cancer. This summarizes current staging definitions, including T, N, M, and their integration into current stages as well as prognosis with tables and helpful diagrams. The data is the essential basis for making treatment decisions at this time.

7. Herbst RS, Heymach JV, Lippman SM. Lung cancer. *N Engl J Med*. 2008;359:1367–1380.

An excellent review of the molecular origins of lung cancer and the basis for now considering the importance of histology in the basic treatment of NSCLC.

8. Jemal A, Siegel R, Xu J, et al. Cancer statistics, 2010. *CA Cancer J Clin*. 2010;60:277–300.

Highlights current outcomes for lung cancer among other carcinomas, tabulated by demographic groups and overall statistics.

9. Kvale PA, Selecky PA, Prakash UB. Palliative care in lung cancer: ACCP evidence-based clinical practice guidelines (2nd edition). *Chest*. 2007;132:368S–403S.

An important discussion of multiple palliative modalities for advanced lung cancer patients, including specifics on pain control, palliating airway involvement, and multiple other palliative care issues.

10. Nath SK, Sandhu AP, Kim D, et al. Locoregional and distant failure following image-guided stereotactic body radiation for early-stage primary lung cancer. *Radiother Oncol*. 2011;99:12–17.

Demonstration of institutional experience and promising local control rates using SBRT approach for irradiation of early stage lung cancers in nonsurgical patients.

11. Onishi H, Araki T, Shirato H, et al. Stereotactic hypofractionated high-dose irradiation for stage I non–small-cell lung carcinoma: clinical outcomes in 245 subjects in a Japanese multi-institutional study. *Cancer*. 2004;101:1623–1631.

One of the earlier studies employing SBRT as a new hypofractionated radiotherapy modality in Japan.

12. Reungwetwattana T, Eadens MJ, Molina JR. Chemotherapy for non–small-cell lung carcinoma: from a blanket approach to individual therapy. *Semin Respir Crit Care Med*. 2011;32:78–93.

A comprehensive review of chemotherapy programs and targeted therapy as they are applied to patients in the adjuvant postoperative setting and in the setting of advanced unresectable lung cancer.

13. Rusch VW, Giroux DJ, Kraut MJ, et al. Induction chemoradiation and surgical resection for superior sulcus non–small-cell lung carcinomas: long-term results of Southwest Oncology Group Trial 9416 (Intergroup Trial 0160). *J Clin Oncol*. 2007;25:313–318.

An experience showing success of neoadjuvant approach to the treatment of superior sulcus tumors in advanced-stage NSCLC patients.

14. Scagliotti GV, Parikh P, von Pawel J, et al. Phase III study comparing cisplatin plus gemcitabine with cisplatin plus pemetrexed in chemotherapy-naive patients with advanced-stage non–small-cell lung cancer. *J Clin Oncol*. 2008;26:3543–3551.

A trial showing unique responsiveness of adenocarcinoma to pemetrexed-based platinum treatment, and distinguishing this from distinct histology (i.e., squamous cell carcinoma) that may respond better to other therapeutic combinations with platinum. Histology now matters for multiple reasons.

15. Scott WJ, Howington J, Feigenberg S, et al. Treatment of non-small cell lung cancer stage I and stage II: ACCP evidence-based clinical practice guidelines (2nd edition). *Chest*. 2007;132: 234S–242S.

The basic ACCP guidelines for the management of early stage lung carcinoma.

16. Sher T, Dy GK, Adjei AA. Small-cell lung cancer. *Mayo Clin Proc.* 2008;83:355–367.

    An excellent review of all aspects of small-cell lung cancer, from limited versus extensive staging outcomes, treatment, and prophylactic cranial irradiation.

17. Simon GR, Turrisi A. Management of small-cell lung cancer: ACCP evidence-based clinical practice guidelines (2nd edition). *Chest.* 2007;132:324S–339S.

    The ACCP guidelines for management of small-cell lung cancer—with comprehensive recommendations and grades of evidence.

18. Socinski MA, Crowell R, Hensing TE, et al. Treatment of non–small cell lung cancer, stage IV: ACCP evidence-based clinical practice guidelines (2nd edition). *Chest.* 2007;132:277S–289S.

    A review of treatment options for advanced-stage lung cancer.

19. Vergnon JM, Huber RM, Moghissi K. Place of cryotherapy, brachytherapy and photodynamic therapy in therapeutic bronchoscopy of lung cancers. *Eur Respir J.* 2006;28:200–218.

    An overview of some of the multiple modalities used to treat airway involvement in lung cancer, along with associated technical challenges and complications.

20. Winton T, Livingston R, Johnson D, et al. Vinorelbine plus cisplatin vs. observation in resected non–small-cell lung cancer. *N Engl J Med.* 2005;352:2589–2597.

    A classic article showing marked (up to 15%) improvement in 5-year survival for postresection stage II lung cancer patients who received adjuvant chemotherapy. This contributed to the literature supporting adjuvant therapy for stage II and III lung carcinoma patients postresection.

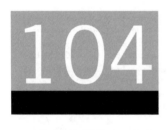

104 Extrathoracic and Endocrine Manifestations of Lung Cancer

Shari A. Brazinsky

The extrathoracic manifestations of bronchogenic carcinoma can be categorized into those related to local spread, those related to metastases, and those that are independent of cancer spread, namely, the paraneoplastic syndromes.

MANIFESTATIONS OF LOCAL SPREAD

Local spread, which causes extrathoracic manifestations, is most often caused by superior sulcus tumors involving the eighth cervical and first thoracic nerves. Patients complain of pain in the shoulder and along the ulnar distribution of the arm. Paravertebral involvement of the sympathetic chain can cause a Horner syndrome. Tumor also can involve the recurrent laryngeal nerve and produce hoarseness. Superior vena cava syndrome is caused by tumor compression anywhere along the course of this vessel. Other extrathoracic symptoms may result from spread into the mediastinum, with involvement of the heart and esophagus.

METASTATIC DISEASE

Although metastatic disease is common in patients dying of lung cancer (96%), symptomatic disease is less frequent. Metastases are most common in lymph nodes (70%), liver (49%), brain (30%), adrenals (25%), bone (30%), and kidneys (18%), although they can involve any organ or tissue. Lymph node, adrenal, and renal metastases are rarely symptomatic. Bony metastases can produce local pain and even spinal cord compression if the vertebral bodies are involved. The diagnosis and treatment of spinal cord compression is a medical emergency and should always be considered in this setting, particularly if neurologic symptoms are present. Liver involvement is generally asymptomatic but can cause abdominal discomfort. Brain metastases can mimic cerebrovascular disease or primary intracranial neoplasm.

PARANEOPLASTIC SYNDROMES

The paraneoplastic syndromes can be characterized as (1) constitutional, (2) hematologic, (3) skeletal, (4) neuromuscular, (5) cutaneous, (6) vasculitic, and (7) endocrine. The most common constitutional syndromes are weight loss, anorexia, and fatigue. Tumor size alone does not explain the presence or magnitude of symptoms, and their cause(s) is unknown. Cachexia is a significant prognostic factor in the course of lung cancer. Recent studies suggest that cytokines such as tumor necrosis factor-α, interleukin (IL)-6 and IL-1β influence cachexia, as well as loss of muscle mass and adipose tissue. Megestrol acetate, a synthetic progestin, has been found to improve well-being, as well as allow weight gain, in many types of lung cancer.

Normochromic, normocytic anemia occurs in less than 10% of patients with bronchogenic carcinoma and is unrelated to marrow infiltration or therapy. A number of coagulopathies are associated with lung cancer. They include migratory thrombophlebitis (Trousseau syndrome), disseminated intravascular coagulation, chronic hemorrhagic diathesis, nonbacterial thrombotic endocarditis, and arterial embolization. Trousseau syndrome often involves unusual sites such as the upper extremities or the vena cava and is frequently unresponsive to anticoagulant therapy. Non–small-cell carcinomas have also been associated with tumor-related leukocytosis, which is cytokine mediated and carries an ominous prognosis.

Hypertrophic pulmonary osteoarthropathy occurs in 4% to 12% of patients with lung cancer, most commonly with epidermoid carcinoma and only rarely with small-cell carcinoma (5%). It consists of periosteal new bone formation in the long bones, with digital clubbing and symmetric arthritis. Vasomotor instability is often present with episodic blanching, swelling, and diaphoresis of the hands and feet. The ankles, wrists, and long bones can be very painful and tender. Although new bone growth is present, the syndrome does not seem to be caused by ectopic human growth hormone production, but it may be mediated by autonomic reflexes. It usually regresses after tumor removal, vagotomy, or thoracotomy without tumor resection. Prognosis does not appear to be altered if this syndrome is present, and tumor recurrence is frequently accompanied by recurrent osteopulmonary arthropathy. Unilateral facial pain and cluster headaches can be referred pain, or caused by hypertrophic osteopathy or paraneoplastic circulating humoral factors. Pain can be relieved by radiotherapy, tumor resection with vagotomy or medical treatment with nonsteroidal anti-inflammatory agents or a bisphosphonate.

An increasing number of neuromuscular syndromes have been associated with bronchogenic carcinoma, most commonly small-cell carcinoma. These syndromes may precede the clinical appearance of the tumor by months to years. The most potentially devastating are cerebral encephalopathy and cortical cerebellar degeneration, both of which can occur precipitously. Peripheral neuropathies, usually sensorimotor and often presenting as pain and paraesthesias of the lower extremities, occur in up to 15% of patients with lung cancer. This can be followed by the gradual onset of a neuropathic arthropathy. Lambert–Eaton myasthenic syndrome (LEMS) occurs in 6% of patients with small-cell carcinoma and differs from myasthenia gravis primarily by an increase in the muscle action potential on repetitive stimulation and the lack of improvement in muscle strength with anticholinesterases. Studies suggest the antibodies associated with LEMS may confer a survival advantage, as the median survival with small-cell lung carcinoma was prolonged by more than 10 months in patients who tested positive for it. SOX1 antibodies presence in LEMS predicts the presence of small-cell carcinoma of the lung. Symmetric proximal muscle neuromyopathy associated with muscle wasting is also common. Non–small-cell tumors have been reported with a paraneoplastic necrotizing myopathy. Paraneoplastic encephalomyelitis, frequently associated with small-cell carcinoma, is characterized by inflammatory infiltrates and neuronal loss. A rapidly progressive binocular vision loss, termed *cancer-associated retinopathy,* has been described in patients with small-cell carcinoma. Also associated with small-cell carcinoma is an adult-onset opsoclonus–myoclonus syndrome. There is no specific immunoreactivity, and the paraneoplastic variety has a worse prognosis than if idiopathic. If the tumor is treated effectively, significant neurologic recovery is noted.

The cause of these neuromuscular paraneoplastic syndromes is generally not known. Evidence has been found, however, for an autoimmune basis for several of these syndromes. In these cases, antibodies have been found that cross-react with tumor and normal tissue antigens. In LEMS, the antibodies cross-react with presynaptic voltage-gated calcium channels at the neuromuscular junction. In cancer-associated retinopathy, antibodies to a tumor antigen cross-react with a subset of retinal ganglion cells (to the photoreceptor protein recoverin). Prednisone therapy has been reported to reduce antibody titers and stabilize visual fields. A heterogeneous group of cases including of paraneoplastic encephalomyelitis, cerebellar degeneration, LEMS, and sensory neuronopathy with small-cell carcinoma associated with a specific antibody in the serum or cerebral spinal fluid is considered part of the anti-Hu syndrome (bearing the name of the first patient in whom the antibody was discovered). These include the presence of high titers of Hu antibody associated with more severe cerebellar degeneration than in the subset without the antibody. An anti-Purkinje cell antibody has also been found in some patients with paraneoplastic cerebellar degeneration. In patients with lung cancer, however, the antibody is rarely found, and the clinical picture is less severe and slower to develop than when the syndrome is associated with other types of cancer. Lower motor neuron disease as a paraneoplastic syndrome has also been seen with anti-Hu antibody. In terms of early diagnosis of malignancy, presence of paraneoplastic neuronal autoantibodies is associated with successful positron emission tomography (PET)–CT directed cancer search in 18% of patients.

Some studies have found more than one antibody present in patients with paraneoplastic syndrome, raising the possibility of multimodal autoantibody production. Such autoantibodies are found to be associated with other paraneoplastic syndromes. Gastrointestinal motor dysfunction is known to be associated with small-cell carcinoma (with multiple paraneoplastic autoantibodies) and can precede the recognition of tumor by months to years. Dysfunction includes delayed gastric emptying, esophageal dysmotility, and abnormal autonomic reflexes.

Cutaneous manifestations include features of dermatomyositis, hyperpigmentation caused by ectopic production of melanocyte-stimulating hormone, and acanthosis nigricans. The last is a hyperkeratotic, hyperpigmented dermatosis with small papillomatous lesions giving the skin a velvety texture. It is symmetric and prominent in skin folds. When it occurs after age 40, it is almost always associated with cancer (90% intra-abdominal, 5% lung). Dermatomyositis has been associated with an autoantibody to a nuclear complex of unknown function. Other rare manifestations include erythema gyratum (thickened, bandlike urticarial plaques imparting a "knotty pine" appearance) with small-cell carcinoma, universal hypertrichosis lanuginosa with epidermoid carcinoma, and rapidly progressive digital necrosis with small-cell carcinoma. Recently, benign dermatosis granuloma annulare, interstitial granulomatous dermatitis, tripe palms, and subacute cutaneous lupus erythematosus were reported as being temporally associated with carcinoma of the lung, and regressed with successful treatment of the malignancy.

Non–small-cell carcinomas have been associated with cutaneous vasculitis and purpura rheumatica. Disseminated vasculitis has now been reported with small-cell carcinoma of the lung. A nonsystemic subacute vasculitic neuropathy called *paraneoplastic vasculitic neuropathy* has been described with small-cell carcinoma of the lung. The neuropathy, which varies from a mononeuropathy multiplex to a symmetric polyneuropathy, is associated with an elevated erythrocyte sedimentation rate and high cerebrospinal fluid protein count. Both chemotherapy and immunotherapy for vasculitis are effective in this disorder.

Many endocrine and metabolic syndromes are associated with bronchogenic carcinoma; they are primarily, but not exclusively, associated with small-cell carcinoma. It is theorized that lung cells embryologically derived from neural crest cells with the ability for amine precursor uptake and decarboxylation undergo malignant derepression and secrete one or more peptide hormones. Overt clinical syndromes appear in approximately 10% of patients with lung cancer, although subclinical hormone production is more common. The hormones produced are peptides and include adrenocorticotropic hormone (ACTH), melanocyte-stimulating hormone, parathyroid hormone, antidiuretic hormone (ADH), human chorionic gonadotropin, prolactin, serotonin, insulin, glucagon, corticotropin-releasing factor, and calcitonin. Most is known about ectopic ACTH, parathyroid hormone, and ADH.

Probably the most commonly produced ectopic hormone is ACTH (50% of patients with small-cell carcinoma), although Cushing syndrome is seen rarely with bronchogenic carcinoma. Tumors appear to elaborate both active ACTH in small amounts and an immunoreactive, but biologically weak "big ACTH," which can be a precursor molecule. Big ACTH was evaluated as a marker for lung cancer, because it is present in more than 80% of all patients who have lung cancer. It is not, however, specific, because it also occurs in a significant number of patients with chronic obstructive pulmonary disease. When Cushing syndrome does occur in association with tumor ACTH secretion, it is a virulent disease with poor prognosis. Ketoconazole, an inhibitor of adrenal steroid synthesis secondary to its inhibitory effects on the cytochrome P-450 enzyme system, has been reported to significantly suppress serum cortisol levels in a patient with Cushing syndrome caused by small-cell carcinoma.

Hypercalcemia occurs in at least 12% of patients with lung cancer, mainly with epidermoid carcinomas. Although small-cell carcinoma frequently metastasizes to bone, it rarely causes hypercalcemia. Ectopic parathyroid hormone production is one cause of hypercalcemia that usually responds to therapy. Some cases may be caused by tumor-secreted prostaglandin E. The hypercalcemia in these patients can be suppressed by aspirin or indomethacin. Other cases may be caused by tumor production of a peptide with significant structural homology to parathyroid hormone, but without immunologic cross-reactivity.

The syndrome of inappropriate ADH (SIADH) results from ectopic ADH secretion. It occurs in 11% of patients with small-cell carcinoma and, although hyponatremia can be severe, symptoms occur in only about 25% of patients with tumor-induced SIADH. It usually resolves within 3 weeks of the initiation of chemotherapy. Retrospective studies reveal hyponatremia is associated with a poorer prognosis in small-cell cancer of the lung, as is failure to normalize serum sodium after two chemotherapy cycles. Occasionally, severe SIADH can occur in the first 5 days following the start of chemotherapy; thus, patients should be monitored carefully during this time. Preliminary studies have used ^{131}I-labeled antibodies against vasopressin-associated neurophysin to localize tumors using radio imaging.

Other causes of hyponatremia associated with lung cancer are much less common. Renal tubular dysfunction in association with glycosuria and aminoaciduria has been reported, as has sodium loss associated with massive bronchorrhea in bronchoalveolar cell carcinoma. In addition, some hyponatremic patients with lung cancer who have normal levels of ADH have been found to have increased messenger RNA levels for atrial natriuretic factor as a possible mechanism for their deranged sodium homeostasis.

Gonadotropin production occurs predominantly with large-cell carcinoma and can cause gynecomastia, which can be unilateral. Gynecomastia in a man should be evaluated with hCG testing. Prolactin production by anaplastic tumors can cause lactation in women. Rarely, epidermoid carcinomas have been associated with the production of vasoactive intestinal peptides, resulting in a syndrome of watery diarrhea, hypokalemia, and achlorhydria. In addition, bronchogenic carcinomas have been found to produce small, biologically active amines or peptides, including serotonin, histamine, and a substance resembling eosinophilic chemotactic factor of anaphylaxis.

Currently, most of these hormones represent curiosities. In the future, some may become useful markers of disease or response to therapy, and the mechanisms of their production may provide insights into the behavior of carcinoma.

A retrospective study of 40 years of reports in the literature found that 13% of patients with resectable non–small-cell lung cancer had a paraneoplastic syndrome. The authors suggested that recent onset arthritis and arthralgias, without other explanations, should be considered as early clues to possible lung cancer. PET appears to be useful in localizing (particularly small-cell) carcinoma in patients presenting with paraneoplastic syndromes. Increasing recognition of new paraneoplastic syndromes, many of which are felt to be immunologically mediated, has been accompanied by frequently disappointing trials of therapy with steroids, immunoglobulins, and plasmapheresis. Ongoing study of immunoadsorption with protein A for paraneoplastic neurologic syndromes has shown some initial success and merits further trials.

FURTHER READING

1. Amital H, Applbaum YH, Vasiliev L, et al. Hypertrophic pulmonary osteoarthropathy: control of pain and symptoms with pamidronate. *Clin Rheumatol.* 2004;23(4):330–332.

   A case report of complete pain resolution with a single dose of pamidronate.

2. Antoine JC, Absi L, Honnorat J, et al. Antiamphiphysin antibodies are associated with various paraneoplastic neurological syndromes and tumors. *Arch Neurol.* 1999;56:172.

   These antibodies, which are not specific for one tumor type or one neurologic syndrome, can be part of a multimodal autoantibody production.

3. Bataller L, Graus F, Sarz A, et al. Clinical outcome in adult onset idiopathic or paraneoplastic opsoclonus-myoclonus. *Brain.* 2001;124(pt 2):437.

   A comparison of patients with idiopathic and paraneoplastic presentations of this rare syndrome with very different outcomes.

4. Batchelor TT, Platten M, Hochberg FH. Immunoadsorption therapy for paraneoplastic syndromes. *J Neurooncol.* 1998;40:131.

   A report of 13 patients treated with protein A immunoadsorption with promising results (75% with complete or partial response).

5. Beck C, Burger HG. Evidence for the presence of immunoreactive growth hormone in cancers of the lung and stomach. *Cancer.* 1972;30:75.

   Growth hormone was found in 7 of 18 lung tumors. The patients were not symptomatic.

6. Campanella N, Moraca A, Pergolini M, et al. Paraneoplastic syndromes in 68 cases of resectable non-small cell carcinoma: can they help in early detection? *Med Oncol.* 1999;16:129.

   A compilation of prior publications suggesting that recent onset of unexplained arthralgias and arthritis could be early clues of lung cancer.

7. Chester KA, Lang B, Gill J, et al. Lambert–Eaton syndrome antibodies: reaction with membranes from a small cell lung cancer xenograft. *J Neuroimmunol.* 1988;18:97.

   Reviews evidence for an IgG-mediated reduction in the number of presynaptic voltage-gated calcium channels at neuromuscular junctions in LEMS.

8. Crotty E, Patz EF Jr. FDG-PET imaging in patients with paraneoplastic syndromes and suspected small cell lung cancer. *J Thorac Imaging.* 2001;16:89–93.

   New imaging techniques help to locate tumors in suspected paraneoplastic syndromes.

9. Dimopoulos MA, Fernandez JF, Samaan NA, et al. Paraneoplastic Cushing's syndrome as an adverse prognostic factor in patients who die early with small cell lung cancer. *Cancer.* 1992;69:66.

   Of patients with Cushing syndrome, 82% died within 14 days of initiation of chemotherapy compared with 25% of the control patients. Median survival was halved, and 45% of the deaths were caused by opportunistic infection in the patients with Cushing syndrome. Biochemical control of Cushing syndrome before initiation of chemotherapy may ameliorate the poor prognosis.

10. Gewirtz G, Yalow RS. Ectopic ACTH production in carcinoma of the lung. *J Clin Invest.* 1974;53:1022.

    "Big" ACTH was found in primary tumor and metastases in all types of lung cancer examined.

11. Grunwald GB, Kornguth SE, Towfighi J, et al. Autoimmune basis for visual paraneoplastic syndrome in patients with small cell lung carcinoma. *Cancer.* 1987;60:780.

    Describes the visual paraneoplastic syndrome and the antibodies to tumor antigens that cross-react with the subset of retinal ganglions involved in the syndrome.

12. Hansen O, Sorensen P, Hansen KH. The occurrence of hyponatremia in SCLC and the influence on prognosis: a retrospective study of 453 patients treated in a single institution in a 10-year period. *Lung Cancer.* 2010;68(1):111–114.

    Hyponatremia was shown to be a poor prognostic indicator in SCLC, as was the failure to correct hyponatremia after two cycles of chemotherapy.

13. Heckmayr M, Gatzemeier U. Treatment of cancer weight loss in patients with advanced lung cancer. *Oncology.* 1992;49(suppl 2):32.

    Megestrol acetate is an effective therapy for weight gain and well-being of patients with lung cancer cachexia.

14. Hoffman DM, Brigham B. The use of ketoconazole in ectopic adrenocorticotropic hormone syndrome. *Cancer.* 1991;67:1447.

    Ketoconazole therapy resulted in significant suppression of serum cortisol levels.

15. Holling H, Brody R, Boland H. Pulmonary hypertrophic osteoarthropathy. *Lancet.* 1961;2:1269.

    An old, but excellent, review of the clinical features of this paraneoplastic syndrome.

16. Kasuga I, Makino S, Kiyokawa H, et al. Tumor-related leukocytosis is linked with poor prognosis in patients with lung carcinoma. *Cancer.* 2001;92:2399.

    Reports of a paraneoplastic syndrome associated with large-cell carcinomas and mediated by hematopoietic cytokines.

17. Keltner JL, Thirkill CE, Tyler CE, et al. Management and monitoring of cancer-associated retinopathy. *Arch Ophthalmol.* 1992;110:48.

    Discusses the efficacy of prednisone to stabilize visual fields in cancer-associated retinopathy. Includes a case report where antibody titers were followed to make clinical decisions regarding institution of steroid therapy.

18. Lee HR, Lennon VA, Camilleri M, et al. Paraneoplastic gastrointestinal motor dysfunction: clinical and laboratory characteristics. *Am J Gastroenterol.* 2001;96:373–379.

    Gastrointestinal symptoms preceded the diagnosis of small-cell carcinoma, and was associated with anti-Hu and other paraneoplastic autoantibodies.

19. Levin KH. Paraneoplastic neuromuscular syndromes. *Neurol Clin.* 1997;15:597.

    A good review of neuromuscular paraneoplastic syndromes.

20. Levin MI, Mozaffar T, Al-Lozi MT, et al. Paraneoplastic necrotizing myopathy: clinical and pathological features. *Neurology.* 1998;50:764.

    Describes a rapidly progressive, symmetric, proximal muscle weakness associated with non–small-cell carcinoma.

21. List AF, Hainsworth JD, Davis BW, et al. The syndrome of inappropriate secretion of antidiuretic hormone (SIADH) in small cell lung cancer. *J Clin Oncol.* 1986;4:1191.

    A comprehensive review of the clinical aspects of this syndrome in lung cancer.

22. Maddion P, Lang B. Paraneoplastic neurological autoimmunity and survival in small-cell lung cancer. *J Neuroimmunol.* 2008;201:159–162.

    Median survival improved from 8.9 to 19.6 months for patients who tested positive for anti-LEMS antibodies.

23. Marchioli CC, Graziano SL. Paraneoplastic syndromes associated with small cell lung cancer. *Chest Surg Clin N Am.* 1997;7:65.

    An excellent general review of the topic.

24. Mason WP, Graus F, Lang B, et al. Small-cell lung cancer, paraneoplastic cerebellar degeneration and the Eaton–Lambert myasthenic syndrome. *Brain.* 1997;120:1279.

    A more detailed discussion of the anti-Hu syndrome and neuromuscular paraneoplastic syndromes.

25. Matsubara S, Yamaji Y, Fujita T, et al. Cancer-associated retinopathy syndrome: a case of small cell lung cancer expressing recoverin immunoreactivity. *Lung Cancer.* 1996;14:265.

    The presence of recoverin immunoreactivity supports that cancer-retina immunologic cross-reaction leads to visual loss.

26. McKeon A, Apiwattanakul M, Lachance DH, et al. Positron emission tomography-computed tomography in paraneoplastic neurologic disorders: systematic analysis and review. *Arch Neurol.* 2010;67(3):322–329.

    A validation of the use of newer forms of technology for earlier diagnosis in elusive paraneoplastic syndromes which predate diagnosis of the malignancy.

27. Merrill WW, Bondy PK. Production of biochemical marker substances by bronchogenic carcinomas. *Clin Chest Med.* 1982;3:307.

    A good review with extensive references.

28. Miller FW. Myositis-specific autoantibodies. *JAMA.* 1993;270:1846.

    Divides myositis into groups based on autoantibodies that have clinical and prognostic significance.

29. Mortin D, Itabashi H, Grimes D. Nonmetastatic neurologic complications of bronchogenic carcinoma: the carcinomatous myopathies. *J Thorac Cardiovasc Surg.* 1966;51:14.

    Chest radiographs were normal in one-third of the patients presenting with this syndrome. It was more common in small-cell carcinoma (2.5:1).

30. Moses AM, Scheinman SJ. Ectopic secretion of neurohypophyseal peptides in patients with malignancy. *Endocrinol Metab Clin North Am.* 1991;20:489.

    A good review of SIADH, including pathogenesis and therapy.

31. Oh SJ. Paraneoplastic vasculitis of the peripheral nervous system. *Neurol Clin.* 1997;15:849.

    Discusses potentially treatable neuropathy associated with small-cell cancer of the lung.

32. Patel AM, Davila DG, Peters SG. Paraneoplastic syndromes associated with lung cancer. *Mayo Clin Proc.* 1993;68:278.

    An excellent general review including mechanisms, diagnosis, and treatment.

33. Richardson GE, Johnson BE. Paraneoplastic syndromes in lung cancer. *Curr Opin Oncol.* 1992;4:323.

    Reviews recent literature on humoral hypercalcemia, autoimmune paraneoplastic syndromes, and cancer cachexia.

34. Rosen SW, Becker CE, Schlaff S, et al. Ectopic gonadotropin production before clinical recognition of bronchogenic carcinoma. *N Engl J Med.* 1968;279:640.

    Gynecomastia appeared 1 year before the discovery of the carcinoma.

35. Sack G, Levin J, Bell W. Trousseau's syndrome and other manifestations of chronic disseminated coagulopathy in patients with neoplasm. *Medicine* (Baltimore). 1977;56:1.

    In this review of 182 cases, 20% were associated with lung cancer, second only to pancreatic carcinoma (24%).

36. Sarlani E, Schwartz AH, Greenspan JD, et al. Facial pain as first manifestation of lung cancer: a case of lung cancer-related cluster headache and a review of the literature. *J Orofac Pain.* 2003;17:262–267.

    A summary of 32 cases of facial pain suggesting that with atypical or refractory facial pain should include lung cancer in the possible etiologies.

37. Schiller JH, Jones JC. Paraneoplastic syndromes associated with lung cancer. *Curr Opin Oncol.* 1993;5:335.

    Reviews recent advances in the diagnosis and treatment of endocrinologic and neurologic manifestations of lung cancer syndromes.

38. Seyberth HW, Segre GV, Morgan JL, et al. Prostaglandins as mediators of hypercalcemia associated with certain types of cancer. *N Engl J Med.* 1975;293:1278.

    An increased urinary level of a prostaglandin metabolite was associated with hypercalcemia that was reversed by prostaglandin inhibitors.

39. Silva OL, Becker KL, Primack A, et al. Ectopic secretion of calcitonin by oat-cell carcinoma. *N Engl J Med.* 1974;290:1122.

    The patients were not symptomatic, and their calcium levels were normal.

40. Yatura S, Harrara E, Nopajaroonsri C, et al. Gynecomastia attributable to human chorionic gonadotropin-secreting giant cell carcinoma of lung. *Endocr Pract.* 2003;9:233–235.

    hCG-secreting carcinoma can present as painful gynecomastia, which responds to treatment of the tumor.

105 Neoplastic Disease of the Pleura

Henri G. Colt

ETIOLOGY AND PATHOPHYSIOLOGY

Neoplastic disease of the pleura can be primary, arising from the cellular elements of the pleural surface (e.g., mesothelial tissue), or metastatic, arising from either thoracic or extrathoracic sites. Metastatic pleural tumors comprise most pleural neoplasms. These resemble the primary tumor histologically and are usually associated with roentgenographically apparent pleural effusion or thickening.

Primary tumors of the pleura are rare. They are classified as benign mesotheliomas (i.e., solitary or localized fibrous) or diffuse malignant mesotheliomas. Solitary fibrous tumors of the pleura occur equally in men and women with a peak incidence in the fourth to sixth decades. Tobacco smoking and exposure to asbestos do not appear to increase the risk for these benign tumors, which are usually grossly well encapsulated and histologically composed of fibrous elements. Similar lesions have been reported as postinflammatory tumors of the pleura, leading to speculation that they are part of a spectrum of mesothelial cell response to a variety of stimuli. Immunohistochemical, ultrastructural, and tissue culture studies were previously felt to support a mesenchymal origin, but most agree now that these tumors derived from fibroblasts have the potential for multidirectional differentiation.

Malignant pleural mesothelioma (MPM), on the other hand, while also rare, has a well-described relationship with occupational exposures, noted in about 80% of patients with MPM, most of whom report exposure to asbestos. The pathogenesis of other metastatic malignant pleural disease, also referred to as pleural carcinomatosis or secondary pleural metastasis, is less clear. Most frequently caused by lung, breast, and gastrointestinal adenocarcinomas, the prognosis for these tumors is poor, with median survivals of only about 9 months. Other less-common primary tumors are those of the ovary, pancreas, liver, kidney, uterus, adrenal glands, testis, larynx, and thyroid. In addition, benign pelvic tumors can be associated with pleural effusion and ascites (Meigs–Salmon syndrome) that subside following tumor resection. The prognosis for patients with malignant pleural disease from non–small-cell lung cancer is even worse, prompting a recent change in TNM staging from T4 to M1.

CLINICAL PRESENTATION AND DIAGNOSIS

Clinically, 30% to 40% of patients with pleural tumors are asymptomatic at the time of diagnosis; others complain of chest pain, cough, dyspnea, and weight loss in decreasing frequency. Tumors can reach enormous size. They can be attached to the pleura by a pedicle and lead to a sensation of something moving about in the chest after a positional change. Other times they may affect diaphragmatic surfaces. Rarely, they cause lobar collapse or superior vena caval obstruction. They may present as wide-based parietal pleural abnormalities, as well as pleural thickening noted on chest radiographs or computed tomography (CT) scans. Infrequently, tumors involve the visceral pleural surface, presenting radiographically as solitary pulmonary nodules. Secondary pleural metastases are frequently noted at post mortem examinations in patients from cancer but without pleural effusions. These deposits probably result from hematogenous spread, although some investigators emphasize a role for lymphatic obstruction in view of frequently noted swollen lymphatics along the posterior and inferior costal parietal pleura during thoracoscopic inspection.

In patients with benign disease, physical examination is usually unrewarding but may show evidence of clubbing (<20%), or osteoarthropathy or arthropathy (<15%) simulating rheumatoid arthritis. The chest roentgenogram usually reveals a localized mass; pleural effusion occurs in fewer than 15% of cases. In some patients with large tumors, hypoglycemia has been reported. Needle biopsy, pleural fluid cytology, or pleural biopsy may suggest the diagnosis, but definitive diagnosis of solitary fibrous tumors of the pleura usually requires thoracoscopy, CT-guided cutting needle biopsy, or thoracotomy. Preoperative differential diagnoses include malignant mesothelioma, metastatic carcinoma, sarcomas, and bizarre pseudotumors related to the organization of a pleural exudate. Surgical resection is usually curative but can be difficult in cases of gross invasion of contiguous vascular, neural, or mediastinal structures. Recurrences may not appear for years following initial resection. Often, the arthropathy disappears with tumor resection but can recur with regrowth. It can then be relieved by further resection.

In patients with suspected malignant mesothelioma, tissue diagnosis is required after obtaining a good occupational history. Pleural fluid cytology results are often equivocal. Recent studies suggest a role for serum mesothelin-related proteins and osteopontin, but these may only support a presumptive diagnosis. Mesothelioma is rare, accounting for less than 1% of all cancer deaths in the general population; however, its incidence is rising because of (1) the delayed effects of an increase in the occupational exposure to asbestos; (2) increased awareness by pathologists of this disease; and (3) more accurate diagnostic methods, such as electron microscopy and immunohistochemistry. Today, it is felt that approximately 2,000 cases are diagnosed yearly in the United States. Tumors must be distinguished from other neoplasms such as soft-tissue sarcoma and leukemia or lymphoma involving the pleura.

Malignant mesotheliomas also occur as primary tumors of the peritoneum and tunica vaginalis of the testes; simultaneous occurrence of pleural mesothelioma with mesothelioma at these other sites has not been described, although patients may have both pleural and peritoneal involvement during the course of their illness. Pathologically, MPM tumor appears early as single or multiple, small, white or gray lesions; later it may produce a thick, gelatinous, gray–pink sheath enveloping the affected lung. It is noteworthy that thoracoscopic appearance can be misleading. Parietal pleura can appear normal, as is often the case in stage 1A malignant mesothelioma, or appear as a conglomeration of small or large nodules involving parietal, visceral, or both pleural surfaces.

Histologically, tumors are composed of epithelial and mesenchymal (fibrosarcomatous) elements and are classified as epithelial (54%), fibrosarcomatous (21%), or mixed (25%). Epithelial mesotheliomas are the most frequently diagnosed histologic type. Seven types of epithelial mesotheliomas are seen, the most common of which is tubulopapillary. Sarcomatoid mesotheliomas account for approximately 20% of mesotheliomas, and are usually positive on keratin staining. This is unlike most sarcomas. Twenty percent of epithelial mesotheliomas produce hyaluronic acid, which can be identified by specific stains. The presence of hyaluronic acid contributes to the increased viscosity often noted in pleural fluid from patients with mesothelioma. Carcinoembryonic antigen (CEA) has been reported as negative in 88% of mesotheliomas. This immunostaining procedure can be helpful in excluding mesothelioma from the diagnosis. Immunohistochemical and ultrastructural analysis of pleural neoplasms can lead to an accurate diagnosis of mesothelioma in most cases, although a careful review of an entire battery of tests often including CEA, *Leu*-M1, and mucicarmine staining is necessary. Electron microscopy is also helpful when abnormalities such as long, slender microvilli are noted. Increasingly, biologic markers of pleural malignancy are being studied, and differential gene expression between MPM, adenocarcinoma, and normal or benign mesothelium are being assessed.

In some patients, diagnosis can only be made retrospectively after careful review of the exposure history, clinical history, immunohistochemical stains and ultrastructural analyses, clinical and radiographic progressions of disease (usually one of gradual entrapment of the lung with associated pleural thickening, and dyspnea), and autopsy findings. Although the pathogenesis of malignant mesothelioma is unclear, asbestos is the single most important causative agent. This conclusion is based on (1) retrospective studies showing a strikingly higher incidence (300×) of malignant mesothelioma among asbestos workers; (2) studies showing a significantly higher incidence of asbestos exposure among new mesothelioma cases versus controls; and (3) direct measurements of significantly increased asbestos fiber content of the lungs of patients with mesothelioma (95%) with respect to controls. A shift has occurred in exposure history from primary users to end-users of asbestos (handlers of asbestos products, such as workers in the construction industry). A threshold amount of asbestos exposure necessary to induce mesothelioma is unknown but presumed. Cigarette smoking is not a risk factor for malignant mesothelioma, but the addition of smoking to asbestos exposure significantly increases risk for lung cancer. Histologic, biologic, and cellular prognostic factors such as microvessel density of tumor specimens, overexpression of COX-2, levels of MIB-1, and role for Simian SV40 virus (a DNA virus shown to induce mesothelioma in up 100% of hamsters after intrapleural injection) remain controversial.

Asbestos exposure can occur occupationally, as in textile, shipyard, mining, insulation, and construction industries, or it can occur environmentally, as with persons living near asbestos mines and mills. Significant exposure can also occur when family members of asbestos workers handle the workers' clothing (paraoccupational). Thus, the level of exposure may seem inconsequential and the fiber burden may be less than expected to cause asbestosis. Fiber size can be important in that fibers that are long and thin have been found to be more tumorigenic than shorter, thicker fibers, although all types of asbestos can induce mesotheliomas. The various types of asbestos vary in tumorigenicity. Fibers with the longest length:diameter ratio are the most carcinogenic, but the carcinogenic potential of short fibers cannot be ruled out. It appears that amphiboles, particularly crocidolite (but also amosite, anthophyllite, tremolite, and actinolite), are more frequently associated with malignancy than serpentine fibers such as chrysotile asbestos.

A direct relationship exists between intensity and duration of exposure with tumor incidence. Intensity of exposure is related inversely to time of presentation. The mean time between exposure and presentation (latency period) is approximately 29 years for factory workers and 48 years for those exposed environmentally. Asbestos fibers are inhaled and deposited at the level of smaller bronchioles and alveoli, where they are ingested by pulmonary alveolar macrophages and coated with a ferrous proteinaceous material. Asbestos fibers are believed to be both promoters and initiators of malignant transformation. Once inhaled, asbestos fibers cannot be destroyed or removed; thus, the lifetime risk for mesothelioma increases over time.

Other nonasbestos causes of mesothelioma are also seen, including naturally occurring fibrous silicate minerals called *erionite,* a fibrous zeolite. Individuals living in small villages in central Turkey where this mineral was used in building materials have had the highest incidence of mesothelioma in the world. Most artificial fibers (e.g., ceramic fibers, glass wool, and rock wool) have not been clearly shown to cause mesothelioma, although results from at least one study suggest that genetic predisposition influences man-made mineral fiber (erionite) carcinogenesis.

While CT scans and a conventional TNM staging system are commonly used at diagnosis, the staging system of the International Mesothelioma Interest Group is commonly used subsequently to identify extent of disease after treatment and determine prognosis. Increasingly, magnetic resonance imaging and CT scans are used to help accurately stage patients, and results from recent studies suggest the benefit from ^{18}F-fluorodeoxyglucose positron emission tomography (FDG-PET) for differentiating MPM from benign disease, staging, and detecting recurrence. According to a recent ERS–ESTS guideline, an international panel of experts could not agree on a common classification system (at least five different ones exist and are being used). Regardless, authors of these guidelines note that performance status and histopathological subtype are the only clinical factors of importance in terms of disease management.

In contrast to patients with solitary fibrous tumors of the pleura, almost all patients with malignant mesothelioma are symptomatic at the time of diagnosis, although presentation as an incidental radiographic finding of pleural effusion is increasingly common. Chest pain (43%) of a constant gnawing character is a frequent complaint. Occasionally positional, it is rarely pleuritic in nature. Dyspnea is another frequent symptom (27%), with or without chest pain at presentation. Cough (19%), weight loss (13%), and fever (7%) also occur. Weight loss is a poor prognostic sign.

The physical examination frequently reveals evidence of pleural effusion. Clubbing is infrequent (<5%). Auscultation of the chest may reveal decreased breath sounds unilaterally, coarse crackles, squeaks, or pleuropericardial rubs. Horner syndrome, hoarseness, or tumor extending through the chest wall in the tract of a previous needle tract or incision site are infrequently noted today. The chest roentgenogram typically reveals a unilateral pleural effusion, pleural nodularity or thickening, or a localized mass lesion. A massive effusion without mediastinal shift away from the side of the fluid collection should raise suspicions for mesothelioma, especially with a history of asbestos exposure. Rib destruction may be present adjacent to the pleural lesion. Interstitial fibrotic changes or diaphragmatic pleural calcifications suggest prior asbestos exposure and are not indicative of MPM. CT scan may demonstrate pleural calcifications, a distinct pleural mass, invasion of contiguous structures, or abdominal extension not otherwise apparent radiographically.

The tissue diagnosis of malignant mesothelioma can be difficult. Sputum cytology is negative, and bronchoscopy usually reveals no endobronchial lesions, although extrinsic bronchial compression caused by mediastinal pleural thickening, a large pleural effusion, or entrapped lung with volume loss is observed occasionally. The pleural fluid from a thoracentesis is usually straw colored but can be serosanguinous or bloody in 30% to 50% of cases. Typically, the protein level is elevated, ranging from 3.5 to 5.5 g/dL and lactic acid dehydrogenase is high. Cytology is of limited value because benign and malignant mesothelial cells closely resemble each other.

Abrams or Cope needle pleural biopsy may confirm the diagnosis, but usually provides insufficient tissue. CT-guided pleural biopsy provides greater diagnostic yield. Thoracoscopy provides tissue and allows complete evacuation of pleural effusion, a thorough examination of parietal and visceral pleural surfaces, assessment of lung expandability, and visually guided biopsy of both normal and abnormal appearing areas of the costal and diaphragmatic parietal pleura. Procedures are almost always diagnostic, although false negatives may occur. If intrapleural chemotherapy is not planned, patients can undergo thoracoscopic talc pleurodesis, which is successful in preventing fluid reaccumulation in more than 80% of instances. Rarely, open thoracotomy is necessary for definitive diagnosis, but should probably not be performed unless an open parietal pleural biopsy has been unsuccessful. An independent panel of pathologist should be convened to review tissues in case of doubt and in patients enlisted for clinical trials.

Malignant mesothelioma is an unrelenting, progressively fatal disease. As disease progresses, patients may present with obstruction of the superior or inferior vena cava (or both) or pericardial involvement. Involvement of the soft tissues of the chest cage, ipsilateral lung, contralateral pleura, supraclavicular nodes, and peritoneal cavity is also seen. Distant metastases to bone, liver, or brain rarely occur. There is limited evidence supporting debulking surgery. Aggressive surgical resection, radiation therapy, and chemotherapy have all yielded poor results. Newer regimens using combined treatment modalities are under evaluation but have yet to significantly alter prognosis (median survival 20–24 months). Radical surgery (extrapleural pneumonectomy) in the setting of a multimodality therapy protocol has reached reasonably low mortality (5%) in experienced centers, but morbidity remains high. Combination chemotherapy can be administered at diagnosis, but at least one British Thoracic Society study has reported no survival benefit over best supportive care. Novel gene therapy protocols are still in the experimental stage and have not been shown to alter outcome significantly. Palliative radiation therapy may be beneficial for pain control, but radiation dose must be carefully controlled. The value of prophylactic radiation to prevent thoracoscopy, thoracotomy, or chest tube tract tumor seeding is unclear.

Secondary metastatic pleural involvement is the most common form of neoplastic pleural disease. It usually presents as a pleural effusion that can be pathogenically related to visceral or parietal pleural implants, peripheral or mediastinal lymphatic and venous obstruction, thoracic duct obstruction, or a combination of these mechanisms. Tumor lymphatic obstruction, thoracic duct invasion, or both can also result in chylothorax.

The clinical manifestations of metastatic pleural tumors relate to the primary neoplastic process and the size of the effusion. Dyspnea can be severe if a large amount of fluid accumulates. Roentgenographically, the findings of mediastinal shift toward the side of the pleural effusion (implying atelectasis), an underlying parenchymal or mediastinal mass, or rib erosions suggest a malignant cause. In many of these cases, flexible bronchoscopy is warranted to exclude bronchial obstruction before performing thoracoscopy or chest tube insertion. The diagnosis of pleural carcinomatosis is based on evaluation of the pleural fluid, pathologic evaluation of biopsied specimens, or both. Characteristically, the fluid is an exudate and is often blood tinged. In longstanding effusions, the glucose can be low and the pH less than 7.35. The white cell count is typically low and predominantly lymphocytic. Cytologic examination can identify the primary site in up to 70% of cases. Not surprisingly, repeated thoracenteses increase the yield, as the pleural fluid malignant cell burden can increase over time, and as the malignant disease itself progresses.

Closed-needle pleural biopsy yields a diagnosis in up to 50% of cases and, when combined with cytology, in close to 90%. Thoracoscopy almost always makes the diagnosis (the only false-negative findings being in patients with early malignant mesothelioma), and provides an opportunity for pleurodesis or insertion of an indwelling pleural catheter. Treatment of recurrent effusions has included intrapleural instillation of sclerosing agents, such as quinacrine, *Corynebacterium parvum*, nitrogen mustard, mitoxantrone, doxycycline, minocycline, tetracycline (no longer commercially available), iodine, bleomycin, and pleural abrasion or pleurectomy. Small bore chest tube insertion followed by pleurodesis in preferred over repeated aspiration except in patients with survival measured in weeks. Asbestos-free, sterile talc powder is the most effective and least expensive pleurodesis agent available, and appears to be equally effective whether administered as a slurry or by insufflations. Pleuritic chest pain and fever are its most frequent adverse effects. Patient rotation is not necessary after chest tube instillation of slurry. In case of trapped lung, intrapleural indwelling chest tube insertion may be warranted. This technique also results in a substantial number of favorable results for patients with recurrent symptomatic malignant effusions who are not candidates for pleurodesis or who wish to avoid hospitalization.

FURTHER READING

1. Baas P. Predictive and prognostic factors in malignant pleural mesothelioma. *Curr Opin Oncol.* 2003;15:127–130.

    A recent review of established prognostic factors as well as a summary of recent developments in molecular biology and potential place for SV40.

2. Berghmans T, Paesmans M, Lalami Y, et al. Activity of chemotherapy and immunotherapy on malignant mesothelioma: a systematic review of the literature with meta-analysis. *Lung Cancer.* 2002;38:111–121.

    Concluding that the most effective single agent for chemotherapeutic treatment of malignant mesothelioma remains cisplatin, and proposing that the combination cisplatin and doxorubicin be used as control arm of future randomized clinical trials.

3. Britton M. The epidemiology of mesothelioma. *Semin Oncol.* 2002;29:18–25.

    A nice review of the fiber controversy surrounding mesothelioma.

4. Bourdes V, Boffetta P, Pisani P. Environmental exposure to asbestos and risk of pleural mesothelioma: review and meta-analysis. *Eur J Epidemiol.* 2000;16:411–417.

    An excellent and timely review.

5. Colt HG. Thoracoscopic management of malignant pleural effusions. *Clin Chest Med.* 1995;16:505.

    A detailed review of diagnostic and treatment roles as well as techniques of this minimally invasive procedure that is increasingly used in patients with pleural disease.

6. Dogan AU, Baris YI, Dogan M, et al. Genetic predisposition of fiber carcinogenesis causes a mesothelioma epidemic in Turkey. *Cancer Res.* 2006;66:5063–5068.

    Raises the question of genetics in at-risk populations.

7. Eibel R, Tuengerthal S, Schoenberg SO. The role of new imaging techniques in diagnosis and staging of malignant pleural mesothelioma. *Curr Opin Oncol.* 2003;15:131–138.

    A description of the most recently developed staging system from the International Mesothelioma Interest Group in addition to a careful description of the utility of contrast-enhanced magnetic resonance imaging as well as advantages and disadvantages of positive emission tomography in this patient population.

8. England DM, Hochholzer L, McCarthy MJ. Localized benign and malignant fibrous tumors of the pleura: a clinicopathologic review of 223 cases. *Am J Surg Pathol.* 1993;17:876.

    In this study, 223 tumors of the pleura were reviewed: 141 benign and 82 malignant. The presenting symptoms were chest pain, dyspnea, and cough. One-fourth of the patients had hypoglycemia, clubbing, or a pleural effusion. Two-thirds of tumors involved the visceral pleura. Neoplasms were seen in atypical sites, such as fissure and inverted into the peripheral lung. Of the malignant tumors, 45% were cured by surgical excision. These lesions primarily were pedunculated or well circumscribed. Resectability, therefore, is the single most important indicator of clinical outcome.

9. Francis RJ, Byrne MJ, van der Schaaf AA, et al. Early prediction of response to chemotherapy and survival in malignant mesothelioma using a novel semiautomated 3-dimensional volume based analysis of serial ^{18}F-FDG PET scans. *J Nucl Med.* 2007;48:1449–1458.

   A promising future for FDG-PET, but future studies are needed, especially to see whether this technique can be used for both diagnosis and measuring disease progression or recurrence.

10. International Mesothelioma Interest Group. A proposed new international TNM staging system for malignant mesothelioma. *Chest.* 1995;108:1122.

    Reviews and describes previously used staging systems and proposes a new classification system that might provide a framework for analyzing results of prospective clinical trials.

11. Janssen JP, Collier G, Astoul P. Safety of pleurodesis with talc poudrage in malignant pleural effusion: a prospective cohort study. *Lancet.* 2007;369:153–159.

    A landmark study demonstrating the success and safety of talc poudrage.

12. Marchevsky AM, Wick MR. Current controversies regarding the role of asbestos exposure in the causation of malignant mesothelioma: the need for an evidence-based approach to develop medicolegal guidelines. *Ann Diagn Pathol.* 2003;7:321–332.

    A well-written review of the asbestos controversy as causation of mesothelioma.

13. Mitchell JD. Solitary fibrous tumor of the pleura. *Semin Thorac Cardiovasc Surg.* 2003;15:305–309.

    A review of the clinical presentation, imaging aspects, and surgical treatment of these benign tumors derived from mesenchymal cells.

14. Mohanty SK, Dey P. Serous effusions: diagnosis of malignancy beyond cytomorphology: an analytic review. *Postgrad Med J.* 2003;79:569–582.

    An interesting overview of newer cytopathology techniques for differential diagnosis of pleural carcinomatosis, including flow cytometry, immunofluorescence, telomerase activity, polymerase chain reaction, and oncogene products.

15. Powers A, Carbone M. The role of environmental carcinogens, viruses, and genetic predisposition in the pathogenesis of mesothelioma. *Cancer Biol Ther.* 2002;1:348–353.

    Focuses on potential new research fronts including simian virus 40 and other genetic factors.

16. Rahman NM, Ali NJ, Brown G, et al. Local anaesthetic thoracoscopy: British Thoracic Society pleural disease guideline 2010. *Thorax.* 2010;65:ii54–ii65.

    An excellent review, but introducing a new terminology (local anesthetic thoracoscopy).

17. Roberts ME, Neville E, Berrisford RG. Management of a malignant pleural effusion: British Thoracic Society pleural disease guideline 2010. *Thorax.* 2010;65(suppl 2):ii32–ii40.

    Another excellent review with lots of references.

18. Scherpereel A, Astoul P, Baas P, et al. Guidelines of the European Respiratory Society and the European Society of Thoracic Surgeons for the management of malignant pleural mesothelioma. *Eur Respir J.* 2010;35:479–495.

    A must-read with many references.

19. Stahel RA, Weder W, Felip E. Malignant pleural mesothelioma: ESMO clinical recommendations for diagnosis and follow-up. *Ann Oncol.* 2008;19:ii43–ii44.

    Another set of "guidelines."

20. Stathopoulos GT. Translational advances in pleural malignancies. *Respirology.* 2011;16:53–63.

    An excellent and understandable review of advances in translational research.

21. Tomek S, Emri S, Krejcy K, et al. Chemotherapy for malignant pleural mesothelioma: past results and recent developments. *Br J Cancer.* 2003;88:167–174.

    A nice summary of previously conducted clinical trials and results suggesting favorable effects of antimetabolites such as pemetrexed in combination with platinum compounds.

22. Van Ruth S, Bass P, Zoetmulder FA. Surgical treatment of malignant pleural mesothelioma. *Chest.* 2003;123:551–561.

    A concise review of the questionable survival benefits for patients undergoing surgical resection, including a discussion of intracavitary therapies.

Index

Pages followed by *f* indicate figures; pages followed by *t* indicate tables.

A

Absolute hypoventilation, 191
"Absolute" lung volumes, 15
Acanthosis nigricans, with lung cancer, 596
Acapella™, 68
Acceleration, 107
Acetazolamide, 115, 469
Acetylcysteine, nebulized, for COPD, 374
Acid–base homeostasis, 25–31
  acidoses and alkalosis, approaches to, 27–31
  anion gap, 26–27
  disturbances, causes for, 29–30, 30*t*
  Hendersen–Hasselbalch equation in, 26, 26*f*, 28
  interpretation approaches for, 30–31, 31*t*
  respiratory derangements of, 28–29, 29*t*
Acidosis
  approaches to, 27–32
  common causes of, 29–30, 30*t*
  as consequence of hypercapnia, 192–193
  in hypercapnic respiratory failure, 192–193
Acinetobacter pneumonia, 253–259. *See also* Pneumonia, gram-negative bacilli
Acquired immune deficiency syndrome (AIDS). *See also* Human immunodeficiency virus (HIV) infection
  cryptococcosis with, 326
  disseminated *M. avium* complex infection and, 293
  histoplasmosis with, 304–305
  infection in, 167, 168–169
Acromegaly, 576
Actinomyces hypersensitivity pneumonitis, 213*t*
Actinomycetales, 320–323
Actinomycosis, 322–323
  pulmonary, 322
  thoracic, 322
Activated factor X, 399
Active disease, 494
Activin-like kinase 1 (ALK1), 421
Acute chest syndrome (ACS), 439–440
  causes of, 440
  characteristics of, 439
  treatment for, 440
Acute interstitial pneumonia, 533–534
Acute mountain sickness, 113, 114–115
Acute radiation syndrome (ARS), 76–77
Acute rejection, after lung transplantation, 436

Acute respiratory distress syndrome (ARDS), 174–175, 378–383
  definition and epidemiology of, 378
  etiology of, 378–379, 378*t*
  management of, 381–383
  pathophysiology of, 379–381, 380*t*
  prognosis in, 383
Acute respiratory failure, 190
Acyclovir, for varicella-zoster virus, 275
Adaptive servo-ventilation therapy, in central sleep apnea, 469
Addison disease, 282
Adenocarcinoma, of lung, 585, 586*t*. *See also* Lung cancer
Adenoma, bronchial, 577
Adenosine, 126, 426
Adenosquamous carcinoma, 586*t*
Adenovirus pneumonia, 275
Adrenocorticotropic hormone ectopic production, in lung cancer, 596–597
Adriamycin, 505
Aerobic metabolism, 20
Aerosolized nebulizer therapy, for burn injury patients, 490–491
Aerosolized radiolabeled particles, 5
Aerospace Medical Association, 111
African Americans
  pulmonary testing for, 10
  sarcoidosis among, 512
Aggravation, 107
Aggressive pulmonary physiotherapy, for intubated burn patient, 490
Aging lung, 367
Air embolism, venous, 414–415
Air-entrainment masks, 66
Air leaks, after pulmonary resection, 144–145
Air travel, 110–113
Airway
  clearance, in neuromuscular disorders, 460–461
  diseases
    pharmacotherapy of, 50–52
    in rheumatoid arthritis, 543
  obstruction, 25, 185–189
    cause of, 186
    evaluation of, 186–187
    fixed obstruction, 187
    flow-volume loop, 187–189
    location and types of, 186*t*

Airway (*continued*)
  variable extrathoracic obstruction,
    187–188
  variable intrathoracic obstruction,
    188–189
  oscillation devices, 68
  patency, 490–491
  preoperative physical examination,
    components of, 208*t*
  resistance, 185
  secretions, in neuromuscular
    disorders, 460–461
  smooth muscle, 62
  stents, 436
  vesicants (mustards), disaster management
    of, 78
Airway-pressure release ventilation
  (APRV), 87
Albendazole
  for echinococcosis, 337, 338
  for nematode infection, 331, 333
Albuterol, for asthma, 50
Alemtuzumab, for lung
  transplantation, 437
Alkalosis
  approaches to, 27–32
  causes of, 29–30, 30*t*
Allergic bronchoconstriction, 485
Allergic bronchopulmonary aspergillosis
  (ABPA), 198–199, 200, 229
  clinical stages in, 314–315
  in cystic fibrosis, 448
  diagnosis of, 314
  pathogenesis of, 314
  treatment of, 315
Alopecia, 300
α-hemolysin, 241
α_1-antiprotease deficiency, emphysema
  from, 366
α_1 antitrypsin deficiency, 432
α_1-proteinase inhibitor, 478
Alveolar echinococcosis, 338
Alveolar gas equation, 64
Alveolar hemorrhage diffuse, in rheumatoid
  arthritis, 543
Alveolar hypoventilation, 190
  clinical manifestations of, 469
  definition of, 469
  syndrome of primary, 469
Alveolar ventilation, 191
Alveolar–arterial gradient, in
  hypoxemia, 191–192
Alveolitis, extrinsic allergic, 493–496.
  See also Hypersensitivity pneumonitis
Alveolo-interstitial edema, 36

Alzheimer's disease, aspiration pneumonia
  in, 157
Amantadine, for viral pneumonia, 275
Ambrisentan
  for asthma, 53
  for pulmonary hypertension, 427
Amebiasis, 335–336
Amebic pleuropulmonary disease, 336
American College of Chest Physicians
  (ACCP), 97, 111–112
  Antithrombotic and Thrombolytic
    Therapy, 463
  guidelines, for antithrombotic treatment of
    VTEs, 399–400
American Medical Association (AMA)
  *Guides to the Evaluation of Permanent
    Impairment*, 108
American Society of Anesthesiologists (ASA)
  Difficult Airway Algorithm, 206,
    207*f*, 208
American Thoracic Society (ATS), 481
Amifostine, 507
Amikacin
  for gram-negative bacilli pneumonias, 256
  for nocardiosis, 321
  for nontuberculous mycobacterial
    infections, 292, 293, 294
  for tuberculosis, 278, 287
Aminoglycoside
  for cystic fibrosis, 446
  for gram-negative bacilli pneumonias, 256
  for KPC-producing strains, 251
Amniotic fluid embolism (syndrome), 163,
  415–416
Amosite, 481
Amoxicillin-clavulanate
  for anaerobic pneumonia, 264
  for chronic obstructive pulmonary
    disease, 374
  for gram-negative bacilli pneumonias, 257
  for *Haemophilus influenzae*
    infection, 247
  for nocardiosis, 321
  for tuberculosis, 287
Amphetamines, on lungs, 175. *See also* Drug
  abuse
Amphibole asbestos, 480
Amphotericin B
  for aspergilloma, 315
  for blastomycosis, 310
  for coccidioidomycosis treatment,
    299–300
  for cryptococcosis, 327, 328
  for histoplasmosis, 305
  for immunocompromised host, 167

Ampicillin
  for anaerobic pneumonia, 264
  for chronic obstructive pulmonary
    disease, 374
  for *Haemophilus influenzae* infection, 247
  for hypercapnic respiratory failure, 195
Amyl nitrate, for cyanide poisoning, 489
Amyotrophic lateral sclerosis (ALS), 462
Anaerobic lung infections, 263–265
  antibiotic treatment for, 264
  diagnosis of, 264
Anaerobic metabolism, 20
Anaerobic threshold, 20
Anaplastic lymphoma kinase (ALK)
  inhibitors, 592
Anastomotic dehiscence, after lung
  transplantation, 436
Anastomotic stenosis, after lung
  transplantation, 436–437
Ancylostoma duodenale, 331
Anechoic image, 33
Anemia, normochromic, normocytic,
  in lung cancer, 595
Anesthesia, as postoperative risk factor, 45
Angiography
  for chronic thromboembolic pulmonary
    hypertension, 408
  for pulmonary embolism, 389
Angioscopy, pulmonary, for chronic
  thromboembolic pulmonary
  hypertension, 409
Angiotensin-converting enzyme (ACE)
  inhibitor therapy, 128–129
Angiotensin II converting enzyme inhibitors
  (ACE-I), 507
Angiotensin receptor blockers (ARB), 507
Ankylosing spondylitis (AS), 450–451
Anthracofibrosis, 477
Anthracosilicosis, 477
Anthracosis, 477
Anthrax, disaster management of, 79–80
Anti-CD 52 antibodies, for lung
  transplantation, 437
Anti-Hu syndrome, 596
Anti-inflammatory therapy, in cystic
  fibrosis, 446
Anticholinergic agents. *See also specific agents*
  for asthma, 51, 357
  for chronic obstructive pulmonary
    disease, 373
Anticoagulation
  in acute treatment of VTE, 399, 400
  with air travel, 112
  complication of, 401
  goal of, 399

Antigenic drift, 274
Antigenic shift, 274
Antiglomerular basement membrane
  antibody (AGBMA) disease, 521–523
Antihistamines. *See also specific agents*
  aspiration pneumonia and, 156
  pulmonary embolism from abuse of, 417
Antimicrobial treatment, of pneumonia, 183
Antineutrophil cytoplasmic
  antibodies (ANCA), in Wegener's
  granulomatosis, 516
Antinuclear antibodies, 478
Antisynthetase syndrome, 552
Antithrombin, 399
Apical fibrobullous disease, 451
Apical fibrocavitary disease, 292
  in rheumatoid arthritis, 544
Apical lordotic views, 2
Apixaban, for thromboembolic disease
  prophylaxis, 395
Apnea
  central sleep, 467
  mixed sleep, 467
  obstructive sleep, 466–469
    as postoperative risk factor, 46
  types of, 467
Apnea/Hypopnea Index (AHI), 467
Apportionment, basis for, 109
Areflexia, 461
Arformoterol, for asthma, 50
Argon plasma coagulation, 62
Arterial blood gas (ABG) evaluation, 23–31
  acid–base homeostasis in (*See* Acid–base
    homeostasis)
  carbon dioxide in, 25
  oxygen in, 24–25
  pH in, 26, 27t
  preoperative, 46
  for pulmonary hypertension, 426
  sample collection in, 23
Arterial hypoxemia, 191–192
Arterial pH, 25
"Artificial nose," 67
Asbestos, 480, 481
  mesothelioma from, 481, 602–603
  related disease, 480–482, 602–603
Ascaris lumbricoides, 228, 331
Aspergilloma, 312–313
Aspergillosis (*Aspergillus* lung disease),
  311–317
  allergic bronchopulmonary, 314–315
  aspergilloma in, 312–313
  chronic invasive (semi-invasive)
    pulmonary, 312–313
  chronic necrotizing, 312–313

Aspergillosis (*Aspergillus* lung disease)
(*continued*)
in HIV-infected, 343
hypersensitivity pneumonitis in, 313
IgE-mediated asthma in, 313
in immunocompromised, 167
invasive pulmonary, acute, 315–317
species of, 312
tracheobronchial, 317
Aspergillus galactomannin, 170
Aspergillus infection, after lung
transplantation, 437
Aspiration
definition of, 155
from drug abuse, 174
risk factors for, 155
upper respiratory tract, drug abuse in, 174
Aspiration pneumonia, 155–158
clinical features of, 157
definition of, 156
oral and dental hygiene in, 156–157
treatment, 157–158
Aspiration pneumonitis
definition of, 156
management of, 156
with scleroderma, 551
Aspirin, 41
Asthma, 11, 90, 128, 129, 186, 188,
353–361, 441
air travel with, 111
aspirin-sensitive, 360
clinical presentation of, 355–356
definition of, 353
diagnosis of, 356, 485–486
epidemiology of, 353
etiology, 353–354, 484
exercise-induced, 360
IgE-mediated, from *Aspergillus*, 313
intrinsic, 353
laryngeal (vocal-cord) dysfunction *vs.*, 356
management of, 356–357
allergens and irritants in, 357
hospital, 357
patient education in, 357
in status asthmaticus, 359
vaccination in, 357
medications for, 357
occupational, 212, 213*t*, 484
pathogenesis, 485
pathophysiology of, 353–354
persistent nocturnal, 360
pharmacotherapy for, 50–53, 357–358
airway diseases, 50–52
anticholinergic, 51, 357
beta-2 agonists, 50–51, 358–360

calcium channel blockers, 52
corticosteroids, 50–52, 357–359
cromolyn sodium, 51
cromolyn sodium and nedocromil, 358
endothelin-receptor antagonists, 53
inhalational, 50
leukotriene modifiers, 51, 360
macrolide antibiotics, 52
mast cell stabilizers, 51
methylxanthines, 51
omalizumab, 52, 358
phosphodiesterase-5 inhibitors, 53
pulmonary vascular diseases, 52–53
theophylline, 51, 358, 359, 360
in postoperative pulmonary
complications, 46
in pregnancy, 160, 161*t*, 360
respiratory complications during and after
surgery, 360–361
surgery in, 360
symptoms of, 354–355
treatment, 486
triad, 354
work-related, 484–486
Asthmatic bronchitis, 356, 365
Atelectasis
pleural effusion from, 132
after pulmonary resection, 143
rounded, 482
Atmospheric pressure (P_{baro}), 110, 111*t*
Atovaquone, 340*t*, 341*t*
Atropine sulfate, 79
AVA-Biothrax vaccine, 80
Avian flu (H5N1), 273
Azathioprine
for idiopathic interstitial pneumonias, 537
for idiopathic pulmonary
hemosiderosis, 528
for interstitial pneumonitis, with
rheumatoid arthritis, 541
for sarcoidosis, 514
for systemic lupus erythematosus, 549
for Wegener's granulomatosis, 518
Azithromycin, 201, 446
for atypical pneumonia, 28
for cystic fibrosis, 446
for *Haemophilus influenzae* infection, 247
for lung transplantation, 437
for nontuberculous mycobacterial
infections, 292, 293
Aztreonam
for gram-negative bacilli pneumonias, 256
for *Haemophilus influenzae*
infection, 247
Aztreonam lysate, for cystic fibrosis, 446

B

B-readers, 3
Bacillus anthracis, 79, 80
Bacillus Calmette-Guérin (BCG)
    vaccination, for TB prevention, 279
Bacterial infections, after lung
    transplantation, 437. *See also
    specific infections*
Bacterial pneumonia, 167, 170, 182
    in HIV-infected, 342
    in pregnancy, 160
Bacteroides melaninogenicus, 263
Balloon dilation, 436
Barcode sign, in ultrasound, 36
Barotrauma, from mechanical
    ventilation, 90–91
"Batwing" sign, in thoracic ultrasound, 33
Beclomethasone
    for asthma, 50, 358, 360
    in pregnancy, 360
Benfluorex, pulmonary hypertension, 422
Benzimidazole, for echinococcosis, 337
Benzonatate, 130
β_2-agonists, 490–491. *See also specific agents*
    for asthma, 50–51, 354, 357–358,
        358–360
    for chronic obstructive pulmonary
        disease, 373
β-hemolytic streptococci, classification
    of, 242
β-lactam/β-lactamase inhibitor, for anaerobic
    lung infections, 264
Bicarbonate, 25
    transport, in cystic fibrosis, 445
Bilateral (sequential) lung transplant
    (BLT), 435
Bilateral pneumothorax, 151
Bilevel positive airway pressure (BiPAP), 209
Bilevel ventilation, 87
Biologic agents, disaster management of
    anthrax, 79–80
    plague, 80
    ricin, 81
    smallpox, 80
Biopsies. *See also specific disorders*
    closed pleural, 35
    kidney, 522
    open lung, 182
    for pleural effusion, 134
    surgical lung, 536–537
    thoracic ultrasound in, 34–35
    transbronchial, 536
    transthoracic, of lung lesions, 36–37
Bioterrorism, 137, 138
Bisphosphonate, 595

Black Lung Benefits Program, 478
Blastomyces dermatitidis infection,
    308–310, 343
Blastomycosis, 308–310
    diagnosis of, 310
    disseminated, 309
    in HIV-infected, 343
    in pregnancy, 310
    transmission of, 309
Bleb, in pneumothorax, 149
Bleomycin, 505
    for malignant pleural disease, 605
Blood gas evaluation, arterial, 23–31. *See
    also* Arterial blood gas (ABG) evaluation
Blue bloater, 370
BMPR2 gene mutations, in pulmonary
    hypertension, 421
Bone scans, for coccidioidomycosis, 298
Bone tuberculosis, 284
Borg Dyspnea Index, 122
Bosentan (Tracleer®)
    for asthma, 53
    for pulmonary hypertension, 427
Botulinum, 79
Bourneville disease. *See* Tuberous sclerosis
Brachytherapy, for malignant airway
    lesions, 62
Brain natriuretic peptide (BNP), 121
Brain tissue embolism, pulmonary, 417
Breath sequence, in mandatory
    ventilation, 85–86
Breathing
    normal tidal, 460
    reducing work of, 86 (*See also* Ventilation,
        mechanical)
    retraining techniques for, in
        COPD, 375
British Thoracic Society (BTS)
    guidelines, 182, 183
Bronchial alveolar lavage, for pneumonia
    diagnosis, 182
Bronchial artery embolization (BAE), 139
    for chronic invasive pulmonary
        aspergillosis, 313
    for hemoptysis, 139
Bronchial carcinoids, 575–577
Bronchial challenge testing, 355–356
Bronchial hygiene therapy, 293
    in pulmonary therapeutics, 67–68
Bronchial obstruction, 195–196
    pneumothorax from, 149
Bronchial stenosis, in radiation-induced lung
    injury, 506
Bronchial stump integrity, after pulmonary
    resection, 145, 146

Bronchial thermoplasty
for asthma, 62–63
in interventional pulmonology, 62–63
Bronchiectasis, 68, 197–202
cause of, 199
complication of, 199
cylindrical, 198
in cystic fibrosis, 445
definition of, 197
diagnostic testing, 200–201
diffuse, 199
drug abuse in, 177
focal, 199
medical management, 201
microbes cultured from, 198
pathogenesis of, 199–200
presentation of, 198–199
in rheumatoid arthritis, 543
saccular, 198
surgical management, 201–202
traction, 198
treatment for, 201–202
varicose, 198
Bronchiolar obstruction, in
lymphangioleiomyomatosis, 564
Bronchiolitis, 189
Bronchiolitis obliterans syndrome
(BOS), 168, 436, 437
Bronchiolitis obliterans with organizing
pneumonia (BOOP), 494, 506
drug abuse in, 176
in rheumatoid arthritis, 543
in systemic lupus erythematosus, 547
Bronchitis, 485
acute, 174, 356
asthmatic, 356
chronic, 11 (*See also* Chronic obstructive
pulmonary disease (COPD))
definition and clinical description
of, 363
drug abuse in, 176
hemoptysis from, 138
eosinophilic, 129
industrial, 213*t*, 478
Bronchoalveolar carcinoma, 581
Bronchoalveolar lavage fluid (BALF), 494
Bronchoconstriction, allergic, 485
Bronchodilators. *See also specific agents*
for aspiration pneumonia, 156, 157
for chronic obstructive pulmonary
disease, 373
for cystic fibrosis, 447
Bronchogenic carcinoma,
in HIV-infected, 344
Broncholithiasis, from histoplasmosis, 304

Bronchopleural fistula, after pulmonary
resection, 145–146
Bronchopulmonary carcinoid tumors, 576
Bronchoscopic confirmation, of airway
injury, 488
Bronchoscopic pulmonary toilet, 490
Bronchoscopy, 182
endobronchial ultrasound, 41–42
flexible
fiberoptic, 40–41
for hemoptysis, 139
for pneumonia diagnosis, 182
for hemoptysis, 139
navigational, 42–43
rigid, with advanced therapeutic
techniques, 61–62
Bronchospasm, 355, 360
drug-induced, 176
exercise-induced, 19
treatment of, 195
Bronchus-associated lymphoid tissue, 495
"Bronchus sign" in navigational
bronchoscopy, 43
Bubbler device, 67
Budesonide, for asthma, 50
Bullous lung disease, drug abuse in, 176
Bupropion, 70
Burkholderia cepacia type III, 431
Burning injury, patients with
chronic obstructive pulmonary disease and
facial burns, 489
in intubation, 489–490
pneumonia in, 491
pulmonary injury in, 488–491
pulmonary toilet and airway
patency, 490–491
smoke inhalation injury, 488–489
"BURP" maneuver, 210
Busulfan, 505
Butyrophilin-like 2 (BTNL2), 512

C

C-reactive protein (CRP), 181, 183, 258
Calcium channel blockers, for asthma, 52
Cancer-associated retinopathy, with lung
cancer, 595–596
Candida albicans, 167
Canine blastomycosis, 309
Caplan syndrome, 478, 542
Capreomycin, for tuberculosis, 278, 287
Carbapenem, 250. *See also specific agents*
for anaerobic lung infections, 264
for gram-negative bacilli pneumonias, 256
Carbon dioxide, arterial measurement of, 25

Carbon monoxide, 77
Carcinoembryonic antigen (CEA), 602
Carcinoid tumor, 586t
Carcinoids, bronchial, 575–577
Carcinoma, bronchogenic, in
   HIV-infected, 344
Cardiac arrhythmias, 195
Cardiac herniation, after pulmonary
   resection, 146
Cardiopulmonary exercise testing, 122
Cardiovascular conditions, contraindications
   for commercial flights, 112–113
Caspofungin, for acute invasive pulmonary
   aspergillosis, 317
Catheterization, right-heart, 421, 426
   for chronic thromboembolic pulmonary
      hypertension, 408
   in evaluation of pulmonary vascular
      disease, 126–127
   for pulmonary arterial hypertension, 440
Causation, 107
Cefepime, for gram-negative bacilli
   pneumonias, 256
Cefotaxime
   for *Haemophilus influenzae* infection, 247
   for nocardiosis, 321
   for pneumococcal pneumonia, 235
Cefoxitin, for nontuberculous mycobacterial
   infections, 294
Ceftaroline, for streptococcal
   pneumonia, 241, 242
Ceftazidime, for gram-negative bacilli
   pneumonias, 256
Ceftobiprole, for streptococcal
   pneumonia, 241
Ceftriaxone
   for nocardiosis, 321
   for pneumococcal pneumonia, 235
   for streptococcal pneumonia, 242
Cefuroxime axetil, for *Haemophilus
   influenzae* infection, 247
Cell-mediated immunity, 304
Cellulose, pulmonary embolism from, 417
Central airway obstruction, 187
Central alveolar hypoventilation, 469
   pulmonary hypertension in, 423
Central sleep apnea, 467
Central venous catheter (CVC)
   access, using ultrasound, 37
   intervention to eliminate, 101–102,
      103, 104
Cephalosporin, 440
   for streptococcal pneumonia, 241, 242
Cerebellar cortical degeneration, with lung
   cancer, 595

Cerebral edema, high-altitude, 113, 114
Cerebral encephalopathy, with lung
   cancer, 595
Cerebrospinal fluid (CSF), 284
Cestode infections, 331
Check valve, in pneumothorax, 149
Chemical exposure, disaster management of
   biologic agents
      anthrax, 79–80
      plague, 80
      ricin, 81
      smallpox, 80
   inhalational toxins
      airway vesicants (mustards), 78
      direct respiratory irritants (chlorine,
         phosgene), 77–78
   neurotoxic agents, 79
Chemiluminescent DNA probes, 292
Chest drain insertion, thoracic
   ultrasound in, 35
Chest drainage catheters, thoracic
   ultrasound, 34–35
Chest films, 1. *See also* Radiography
Chest physiotherapy, 57, 446, 447, 450
Chest radiography
   for asthma, 486
   computer-aided diagnosis in, 3
   for diaphragm disorders, 454
   for fat embolism, 415
   for hypersensitivity pneumonitis, 494
   for pulmonary hypertension, 425, 426
   for submersion-induced pulmonary
      edema, 501
Cheyne–Stokes ventilation, 469
Chickenpox, 80
Chlamydia trachomatis, 268
Chlamydophila pneumoniae, 267–271
Chlamydophila psittaci pneumonia, 267–271
Chloramphenicol, 80, 235, 322
Chlorine, disaster management of, 77
Chloroquine, 336, 514, 528
Chondromas, 577
Chronic allograft rejection, after lung
   transplantation, 437
Chronic interstitial pneumonitis, in systemic
   lupus erythematosus, 547
Chronic invasive pulmonary
   aspergillosis, 312–313
Chronic obstructive pulmonary disease
   (COPD), 77, 90, 434, 489, 126,
   186, 188. *See also* Bronchitis, chronic;
   Emphysema
   air travel with, 111
   clinical and laboratory manifestations
      of, 369

Chronic obstructive pulmonary disease
(COPD) (*continued*)
consequences of, 191
definition and clinical description
of, 363–365
diaphragmatic disorders in, 456
epidemiology of, 365
hypercapnic respiratory failure in, 191 (*See
also* Hypercapnic respiratory failure)
management of, 372–375
antibiotics in, 374
anticholinergics in, 373
breathing retraining techniques in, 375
bronchodilators in, 373
corticosteroids in, 374
goals of, 372
hydration and mucolytic agents in, 374
influenza and pneumococcal vaccination
in, 373
occupational-environmental pollutant
reduction in, 373
oxygen therapy in, 375
patient education in, 373
pulmonary rehabilitation in, 57–58, 375
smoking cessation in, 372
steroids in, inhaled, 374
surgery in, 375
theophylline in, 373
pathophysiology of, 370
pharmacotherapy of asthma and, 50
on postoperative pulmonary
complications, 46
prognosis in, 370
pulmonary hypertension from, 423
from smoking, 366
theophylline for, 51
types of, 370
Chronic thromboembolic pulmonary
hypertension (CTEPH), 6–7, 126–127,
406–411, 422t, 423, 425. *See also*
Pulmonary hypertension, chronic
thromboembolic
Chrysotile, 480
Churg–Strauss syndrome, 51, 231, 232
Chylothorax, 144, 563
Chylous pleural effusions, 564
Cigarette smoking. *See* Smoking
Cimetidine, 373
Ciprofloxacin, 80, 373
for gram-negative bacilli pneumonias,
256, 257
for hypercapnic respiratory failure, 195
for nontuberculous mycobacterial
infections, 294
for pneumonic plague, 138

Cisplatin, 505
Cisternal injections, for
coccidioidomycosis, 300
Clarithromycin, 448
for community-acquired pneumonia, 183
for cystic fibrosis, 446
for nocardiosis, 321
for nontuberculous mycobacterial
infections, 292, 293
Clindamycin, 80
for actinomycosis, 322
for anaerobic pneumonia, 264
for pneumonia
aspiration, 157
streptococcal, 242
Clinical quality improvement, techniques
for, 100–105
background, 100–101
examples for system improvement,
101–103
key concepts for successful, 103–104, 103t
Clofazimine, for tuberculosis, 287
Clonidine, 70
Closed pleural biopsy, thoracic ultrasound
in, 35
CO poisoning, 488
treatment for, 489
Coagulopathies, in lung cancer, 595
Coal Act. *See* Federal Coal Mine Health and
Safety Act
Coal macule, 477
Coal workers' pneumoconiosis (CSP). *See*
Pneumoconiosis
Cobb angle, 449
Cocaine, on lungs, 173. *See also* Drug abuse
Coccidioides immitis infection, 297–300,
343. *See also* Coccidioidomycosis
Coccidioides posadii infection, 297–300.
See also Coccidioidomycosis
Coccidioidomycosis, 297–300
clinical presentation, 297–298
control and prevention of, 300
diagnosis of, 299
epidemiology, 297
etiology and pathogenesis of, 297
in HIV-infected, 343
microbiology of, 297
prognosis in, 298
serological tests in, 299
treatment of, 299–300
Cold agglutinin-induced hemolysis,
267–268
Colistin
for gram-negative bacilli pneumonias, 257
for KPC-producing strains, 251

Combivent RESPIMAT®, 50
Comfortflow™, 66
Community-acquired pneumonia (CAP), 180
  biomarkers for management of, 183
  incidence of, 180
Compression ultrasonography, for deep venous thrombosis, 387
Compressive devices, intermittent pneumatic, for venous thromboembolism prophylaxis, 395–396
Computed radiography (CR), digital, 2–3
Computed tomography (CT), 507–508. *See also specific disorders*
  for allergic bronchopulmonary aspergillosis, 314
  for chronic thromboembolic pulmonary hypertension, 408
  for cryptogenic organizing pneumonia, 534
  for idiopathic pulmonary hemosiderosis, 528
  for immunocompromised host, 171
  for invasive pulmonary aspergillosis, 316
  for lung cancer, 580–581, 588
  for mediastinal masses, 223–224
  for pneumothorax, 149, 150–151
  for pulmonary embolism, 5, 389
  for solitary pulmonary nodule, 217
  for thoracic spine disorders, 450
  for Wegener's granulomatosis, 517
Computer-aided diagnosis (CAD), in chest radiography, 3
Congenital heart disease, pulmonary hypertension in, 421
Congestive heart failure, pleural effusion from, 131–132
Continuation-phase therapy, for drug-susceptible tuberculosis, 287
Continuous intravenous prostenoid therapy, 427
Continuous positive airway pressure (CPAP), 209
  for sleep apnea, 468
Contraceptives, oral, smoking and, 69
Contrast venography, for deep venous thrombosis, 387–388
Coronary angiography, for chronic thromboembolic pulmonary hypertension, 408–409
Cortical cerebellar degeneration, with lung cancer, 595
Corticosteroids, 544. *See also specific agents*
  for AGBMA disease (Goodpasture's), 523
  for airways disease, in rheumatoid arthritis, 543
  for asthma, 50–52, 357–359, 357–358
  for chronic obstructive pulmonary disease, 374
  for cryptogenic organizing pneumonia, 534
  for cystic fibrosis, 446
  for hypercapnic respiratory failure, 195
  for hypersensitivity pneumonitis, 495
  for idiopathic pulmonary hemosiderosis, 528
  for interstitial pneumonitis, in rheumatoid arthritis, 541
  for *Pneumocystis carinii* pneumonia with HIV infection, 341, 343
  for polymyositis, 552
  pulse IV, for lung transplantation, 436
  for radiation pneumonitis, 507
  systemic, agents for asthma, 51
  for systemic lupus erythematosus, 549
  for tuberculosis, 288
Corynebacterium parvum, for malignant pleural disease, 605
Cotrimoxazole
  for Q fever pneumonia, 269
  for Wegener's granulomatosis, 518
Cough
  chronic, 128–130
    cigarette smokers and, 128
    idiopathic, 129
    immunosuppressed patients and, 128
  hypersensitivity syndrome, 129
  postinfectious, 128
  psychogenic, 129
  reflex, with cervical spinal cord injury, 463
  subacute, 128
  variant asthma, 129
CoughAssist Mechanical Insufflation/Exsufflation™, 67–68
Coxiella burnetii pneumonia, 267–271
Crack cocaine, on lung, 174–175. *See also* Drug abuse
Crack lung, 175
CREST syndrome, 549
Cricothyroidotomy, 211
Cristobalite, 474
Critical care patients, aspiration pneumonia in, 157
Cromolyn sodium, for asthma, 51, 357
Cryotherapy, for management of central airway obstruction, 62

Cryptococcal polysaccharide antigen (CRAG) testing for cryptococcosis, 327
Cryptococcosis (*Cryptococcus neoformans* infection), 309, 325–328
  diagnosis of, 326–327
  management of, 327–328
  microbiology and epidemiology of, 325–326
  pathogenesis and clinical manifestations of, 326
  treatment of, 327–328
Cryptococcus gattii infection, 325, 328
Cryptogenic organizing pneumonia (COP), 343, 534, 548
CURB-65, 182
"Curtain sign", in thoracic ultrasound, 33
Cushing syndrome, 597
Cutaneous vasculitis, with lung cancer, 596
Cyanide poisoning, 488–489
Cyclophosphamide, 505
  for AGBMA disease (Goodpasture's), 523
  for interstitial pneumonitis, with rheumatoid arthritis, 541
  for progressive systemic sclerosis, 552
  for systemic lupus erythematosus, 549
  for Wegener's granulomatosis, 518
Cycloserine, for tuberculosis, 287
Cyclosporine, for asthma, 53
Cylindrical bronchiectasis, 198
Cystic dilatation, diffuse, 563
Cystic fibrosis (CF), 68, 200, 444–448
  clinical presentation, 445
  complications of, 447–448
  diagnosis of, 445
  etiology and pathophysiology of, 444–445
  management of, 446–447
  ongoing research, 448
  in pregnancy, 162
Cystic fibrosis transmembrane conductance regulator (CFTR), 444
Cystic fibrosis–related diabetes (CFRD), 448
Cytomegalovirus (CMV), 168, 169, 276, 436

D

D-penicillamine, in rheumatoid arthritis, 544
Dabigatran, 395, 400–401
Dactinomycin, 505
Dalteparin, 394, 400
Dapsone, 340*t*
Deep venous thrombosis (DVT). *See also* Pulmonary embolism (PE)
  from air travel, 111
  diagnosis of, 388
  epidemiology of, 385–386
  natural history of, 386
  in pregnancy, 162
  prophylaxis against, 393–396
    drugs in, 394
    intermittent pneumatic compressive devices in, 395–396
    options and strategies in, 393–394
  risk factors for, 386
  signs and symptoms of, 387
  treatment of, 399–402
Deoxyribonuclease (DNase)
  for chronic obstructive pulmonary disease, 374
  for cystic fibrosis, 446
Dermatomyositis, 552
  with lung cancer, 596
Desquamative interstitial pneumonia (DIP), 534–535
Dexamethasone, 114
Dextromethorphan (DM), 130
Diabetes, with cystic fibrosis, 448
Diameter-defined Strahler model, 420
Diaphragm
  eventration of, 455
  fatigue of, 456
    in systemic lupus erythematosus, 547
  functional disorders of, 456
  herniation of, 455
  paralysis of, 454–455
  pleural effusion and contour of, 132
  tears and rupture of, 456
Diaphragmatic flutter, 456
Diazepam, 79
Difficult airway, 206–211
  algorithm, 207*f*
  etiology of, 209
  mask ventilation, optimal positioning for, 209
  preparation and environment, 206–208
  recognition and intervention in, 208
  secure airway, obtaining, 209–210
Diffuse alveolar hemorrhage (DAH). *See* Goodpasture's syndrome
Diffuse bronchiectasis, 199
Diffuse cutaneous systemic sclerosis (dcSSc), 549
Diffuse cystic dilatation, 563
Diffuse panbronchiolitis, 189
Digital chest radiography, 2–3
Dilatational therapy, for benign airway stenosis, 62
Diloxanide furoate, for amebiasis, 336

Diphenylhydantoin, for diaphragmatic flutter, 456
Diphosgene, 78
Direct arterial gas embolism, 414
Direct laryngoscopy, 188, 210
Direct respiratory irritants (chlorine, phosgene), disaster management of, 77–78
Direct thermal injury, of smoke inhalation, 489
Directly observed therapy (DOT), for tuberculosis, 288
Dirofilaria immitis, 332
Dirty bomb. *See* Radiation dispersal device (RDD)
Disability, 106–109
  basis for apportionment in, 109
  definition of, 106
  diagnosis in, 107–108
  evaluation reports for, 107, 107*t*
  evidence and severity of impairment in, 108
  need for further treatment in, 109
  presence of, 108
  vocational retraining in, 109
  work-relatedness in, 107–108
Disaster management, by pulmonologist, 74–81
  acute radiation syndrome, 76–77
  airway vesicants (mustards), 78
  anthrax, 79–80
  biologic agents, 79–81
  chemical exposure, 77–81
  direct respiratory irritants (chlorine, phosgene), 77–78
  earthquakes, 75
  inhalational toxins, 77–79
  ionizing radiation exposure, 76–77
  neurotoxic agents, 79
  plague, 80
  planning for, 74
  ricin, 81
  smallpox, 80
  surge capacity and, 74–75
Disease-modifying therapy, for idiopathic pulmonary arterial hypertension (IPAH), 411
Distal airways disease, in rheumatoid arthritis, 543
Diuretics, 191, 209, 427. *See also specific agents*
Diving accidents, 498–501
Diving, scuba, 500–501
Dog heartworm, 332
Donor selection, for lung transplantation, 434–435

Dopamine, for cryptococcosis, 326
Doppler effect, in sound waves, 33
Doripenem, 526
Dornase alpha, 491
Dorsalis pedis artery, 23
Doxycycline, 80
  for atypical pneumonia, 269, 270
  for *Haemophilus influenzae* infection, 247
  for *Legionella* pneumonia, 270
  for malignant pleural disease, 605
  for nontuberculous mycobacterial infections, 294
  for pneumonic plague, 138
  for Q fever pneumonia, 269
Drowning, 498–501
  clinical manifestations of, 498–499
  complications in, 499
  dry, 498
  management of, 499
  near-, 498–501
  pathophysiology of, 498
  prognosis, 499–500
Drug abuse, 173–177. *See also specific drugs*
  aspiration in, 174
  bronchiectasis with, 177
  bronchiolitis obliterans with organizing pneumonia with, 176
  bronchitis with
    acute, 174
    chronic, 176
  bronchospasm with, 176
  bullous lung disease with, 176
  crack lung with, 175
  fungal pulmonary infections with, 174
  interstitial lung disease with, 176
  lung cancer with, 177
  pneumonia with
    community-acquired, 174
    with heroin overdose, 174
  pneumothorax or pneumomediastinum with, 177
  pulmonary complications and, 173*t*
  pulmonary edema with, noncardiogenic, 175
  pulmonary embolism with
    noninfectious, 417–418
    septic, 174, 416
  pulmonary hemorrhage with, 175
  pulmonary hypertension with, 175
  pulmonary tuberculosis with, 174
  respiratory failure with, 177
  talcosis with, 176
  thermal epiglottitis with, 176
  thermal injury with, 176
  tracheal stenosis with, 176

Drug-induced pulmonary disease,
in rheumatoid arthritis, 541–542
Dry drowning, 498
DuoNeb®, 50
Dyspnea, 120–122
clinical presentation, 120–121
definition of, 120
differential diagnoses, 121–122, 121t
etiology of, 121
on exertion, 19
in neurofibromatosis type 1, 562–563
in pregnancy, 160
quantification of, 122

E

Earthquakes, disaster management, 75
Eastern Cooperative Oncology Group
(ECOG) scale, 584
Echinocandins, for acute invasive pulmonary
aspergillosis, 315, 317
Echinococcosis, 336–338
Echinococcus granulosus infection, 336–338
Echinococcus multilocularis infection,
336–338
Echocardiography, for pulmonary
hypertension, 426
Efavirenz-based antiretroviral therapy, 289
Effusion
complicated parapneumonic, 134
parapneumonic, 134 (*See also* Empyema)
pleural (*See* Pleural effusion)
Embolectomy, acute pulmonary, 402
Embolism
amniotic fluid, 163, 415–416
from brain tissue, 417
direct arterial gas, 414
fat, 415
pulmonary (*See* Pulmonary embolism)
septic, 416
from tumor, 416–417
venous air, 414–415
Emphysema, 11. *See also* Chronic
obstructive pulmonary disease (COPD)
compensatory, 367
congenital lobar, 366–367
definition and clinical description of, 364
diaphragmatic disorders in, 456
epidemiology of, 366
pathophysiology of, 370
senile, 367
Empiric therapy, 181
Empyema, 133, 236, 241, 264–265
in rheumatoid arthritis, 541
thoracic ultrasound in, 35

Encephalomyelitis, paraneoplastic, with lung
cancer, 595
Encephalopathy, cerebral, with lung
cancer, 595
Endobronchial ablative therapy, 61–62
Endobronchial stents, in airway patency, 62
Endobronchial ultrasound (EBUS), 37
benefits of, 42
bronchoscopy, in interventional
pulmonology, 41–42
Endobronchial ultrasound with guided
transbronchial needle aspiration
(EBUS-TBNA), 42, 224
Endoglin (ENG), 421
Endoluminal radiotherapy, for malignant
airway lesions, 62
Endometriosis, 577
Endoscopic ultrasound with fine needle
aspiration (EUS-FNA), 224
Endotracheal intubation, 206, 210, 211
Endotracheal tubes, aspiration pneumonia
from, 157
Engraftment syndrome, 169
Enoxaparin, 394, 400
Entamoeba histolytica infection, 335–336
Enterobacter pneumonia, 253–259. *See also*
Pneumonia, gram-negative bacilli
Environmental lung disease,
occupational, 212–214, 213t. *See also*
Asthma; *specific diseases*
Enzyme-linked immunosorbent assay
(ELISA) test, 299
Eosinophilia, tropical pulmonary, 332
Eosinophilic lung disease, 228–232. *See also*
Eosinophilic pneumonias
drug-and-toxin-induced, 229–230
helminthic and fungal
infection-associated, 228–229
Eosinophilic pneumonias, 228
approach to diagnosis, 232
of known etiology, 228–229
of unknown etiology, 230
acute eosinophilic pneumonia,
176, 230, 232
chronic eosinophilic pneumonia,
231, 232
Churg–Strauss syndrome, 231
idiopathic hypereosinophilic
syndrome, 231
Eosinophilic vasculitis, 356
Epidermal growth factor receptor
(EGFR), 591
Epiglottitis, thermal, drug abuse in, 176
Epithelial anion transport, modulators
of, 448

Epoprostenol, 52, 126, 426, 427
Epstein–Barr virus, 169
Erionite, 603
Erlotinib, 591–592
Error reduction techniques, 100–105
Ertapenem, for gram-negative bacilli
  pneumonias, 256
Erythromycin, 373, 442
  for actinomycosis, 322
  for chronic obstructive pulmonary
    disease, 373
Escherichia coli pneumonia, 253–259.
  See also Pneumonia, gram-negative bacilli
Etanercept, 304, 514, 518, 542
Ethambutol, 448
  for cystic fibrosis, 446
  for nontuberculous mycobacterial
    infections, 292, 293, 294
  in pregnancy, 289
  for tuberculosis, 280, 287–289
Ethionamide, 287
Eventration, of diaphragm, 455
Exercise
  capacity, in postoperative pulmonary
    complications, 47
  higher level, 20
  -induced asthma, 360
  low-level, 20
  in patients with lung diseases, 20
  testing, 16, 19–21, 122
  training, for COPD, 57–58
Expert Panel Report III, 354
Expiratory central airway collapse, 188
Expiratory positive airway pressure (EPAP),
  for OHS, 471
Extended-spectrum azole antifungals, for
  coccidioidomycosis, 299
Extensively drug-resistant (XDR)
  tuberculosis, 288
Extrapulmonary dissemination, 298
Extrinsic allergic alveolitis, 493–496. *See also*
  Hypersensitivity pneumonitis
Exudative phase, 380
EZ Pap™, 68

F

Facial burns, 489
Facial edema, during resuscitation phase of
  burn injury, 490
Fat embolism, 415, 440
Federal Coal Mine Health and Safety
  Act, 478
Federal Mine Safety and Health Act of
  1977, 478

Fenfluramine, for pulmonary
  hypertension, 422
Fiberoptic bronchoscopy
  flexible, 40–41
  for solitary pulmonary nodule,
    218–219
  standard, 218
Fibrinolysis, 386
Fibroleiomyomas, 577
Fibrosing mediastinitis, from
  histoplasmosis, 304
Fibrosis
  from histoplasmosis, 305
  idiopathic pulmonary, 531–532
  interstitial
    with scleroderma, 549–550
    in systemic lupus erythematosus, 547
  pleural, 482
  progressive massive, 477
Filariasis, 332
Filters, inferior vena caval, 402, 408
Flatworm infections, 333
Flesh-eating bacteria, 242
Flow–volume loop, 14–15, 15*f*
Fluconazole
  for coccidioidomycosis, 300
  for cryptococcosis, 327
  for histoplasmosis, 305
Flucytosine, 327, 328
Fludeoxyglucose positron emission
  tomography (FDG-PET), 506
Fluke infections, 333
Flunisolide, for asthma, 50
Fluoroquinolone-clindamycin, for anaerobic
  lung infections, 264
Fluoroquinolones
  for atypical pneumonia, 269
  for cystic fibrosis, 446
  for *Haemophilus influenzae* infection, 247
  for *Legionella* pneumonia, 270
  for nocardiosis, 321
  for pneumococcal pneumonia, 235
  for streptococcal pneumonia, 241
  for tuberculosis, 278, 287
Fluoroscopy, 2
Fluticasone, for asthma, 50
Flutter Valve™, 68
Focal bronchiectasis, 199
Follicular bronchiolitis, in rheumatoid
  arthritis, 543
Fondaparinux
  prophylaxis against, 394
  for thromboembolic disease, 399–400
Food and Drug Administration (FDA),
  70, 237, 316, 437

Foramen of Morgagni, herniation through the, 455
Forced expiratory volume (FEV), 450
Forced vital capacity (FVC), 450
Formoterol, for asthma, 50
Fraction of inspired oxygen, 110
Francisella tularensis, 138
Frequencer™, 68
Friedlander's pneumonia, 250–251
Fulminant psittacosis, 268
Function testing. *See* Pulmonary function tests
Functional imaging, of lung injury, 506
Functional residual capacity (FRC), 450, 460
Fungal infections. *See also specific infections*
   drug abuse in, 174
   in HIV-infected, 343
   in immunocompromised host, 167–168
   after lung transplantation, 437
Fungus ball, 312–313
Fusobacterium nucleatum, 263

G

G5 Percussor™, 67
Gabapentin, 130
Galactomannan, 316
Gallium-67 (^{67}Ga) lung scanning, 7
Ganciclovir, for cytomegalovirus pneumonia, 276
Gastric colonization, in hospital-acquired pneumonia, 348
Gastroesophageal reflux disease (GERD), 128, 129, 432
Gastrointestinal hemorrhage, 195
Gatifloxacin, for *Haemophilus influenzae* infection, 247
Gefitinib, 507
Gemcitabine, 505
Genetic counseling, for tuberous sclerosis, 567
Genistein, 507
Genitourinary tuberculosis, 284
Genome-wide scans, 512, 587
Gentamycin
   for gram-negative bacilli pneumonias, 256
   for tularemia, 138
Germ cell tumors (GCT), 224, 225–226
Global Initiative for Asthma (GINA) 2010, 354
Global Initiative for Chronic Obstructive Lung Disease (GOLD), 372
Glomerulonephritis. *See* Goodpasture's syndrome
Glottic and subglottic extra/intra thoracic obstruction, 186*t*
Glycerol, iodinated, for COPD, 374

Gold, interstitial pneumonitis from, 543
Goodpasture's syndrome, 15, 521–523
   clinical manifestations of, 521–522
   diagnosis of, 522
   etiology of, 521
   histopathological examination of, 522
   pathogenicity of, 522
   prognosis of, 523
   in rheumatoid arthritis, 543
   treatment of, 523
Gram-negative bacilli pneumonia, 253–259.
   See also Pneumonia, gram-negative bacilli; *specific organisms*
   background and etiology of, 253–254
   clinical presentations of, 254–255
   diagnosis of, 255–256
   prevention of, 258–259
   prognosis with, 258
   treatment of, 256–258
Granulocyte macrophage colony-stimulating factor (GM-CSF), 571
Granulomatosis with polyangiitis (GPA), 516–518
   diagnosis of, 517
   prognosis of, 518
   radiographic findings, 517
   treatment for, 518
Ground glass opacities (GGOs), 217–218
Guanylate cyclase (BAY 41-2272), 423
Guillain–Barré syndrome (GBS), 461–462
Gynecomastia, with lung cancer, 597

H

Haemophilus influenzae type B vaccines, 247
Haemophilus influenzae infection, 245–247, 274, 373
   etiology and epidemiology of, 245
   in HIV-infected, 342
   natural history and transmission of, 246
   pathogenesis and clinical manifestations of, 246
   risk factors for, 245–246
   in sickle cell disease, 442
   treatment of, 247
Halo sign, 316
Haloperidol, aspiration pneumonia and, 156
Hamartomas, pulmonary, 577
Hamman–Rich syndrome. *See* Acute interstitial pneumonia
Hantavirus pulmonary syndrome (HPS), 276
Health-care-associated pneumonia (HCAP), 180, 183
Healthy worker effect, 479, 484
Heart disease, congenital, pulmonary hypertension in, 421

Heart failure, congestive, pleural effusion from, 131–132
Heart–lung transplantation, 427, 435
Heat moisture exchanger (HME), 67
Heerfordt syndrome, 513
Heimlich maneuver, 158
Helminthic infections, 331–334
  nematode, 331–334
  trematode, 333
Hemagglutinin (H) glycoproteins, influenza A virus and, 274
Hematopoietic stem cell transplants, acute invasive pulmonary aspergillosis in, 315–316
Hematopoietic syndrome, 76–77
Hemithorax, 583
Hemodynamic compromise, from mechanical ventilation, 90–91
Hemoptysis, 137–141, 199, 202, 388
  in ankylosing spondylitis, 450
  causes of, 137
  chest radiograph, 138
  in cystic fibrosis, 447
  diagnostic approaches, 138–139
  evaluation of, 138–139
  therapy for, 140–141
Hemorrhage, pulmonary
  alveolar
    in rheumatoid arthritis, 543
    in systemic lupus erythematosus, 548
  drug abuse in, 175
  resection, 143–144
Hemosiderosis, idiopathic pulmonary, 527–528
Hemothorax, 151–152
Hendersen–Hasselbalch equation, 26, 26f, 28
Heparin
  for pulmonary embolism, 401
  for thromboembolic disease, 399–401
    prophylaxis against, 394
"Hepatization sign" in ultrasound, 35
Herd immunity, 247
Hernia, hiatal, 455
Herniation
  cardiac, 146
  diaphragm, 455
  through the foramen of Morgagni, 455
Heroin, on lungs, 174, 175, 176. *See also* Drug abuse
Herpes simplex virus (HSV), 276
Hiatal hernia, 455
Hiccup, 456
High-altitude cerebral edema (HACE), 113, 114
High-altitude illness, 113–116
High-altitude pulmonary edema (HAPE), 113, 114–115

High-frequency oscillating ventilation (HFOV), 87
High-performance liquid chromatography (HPLC), 292
High-resolution computed tomography (HRCT), 426, 517
Highly active antiretroviral therapy (HAART), 326, 339, 342–344
Hilar lymph node, endobronchial ultrasound bronchoscopy for, 42
Histoplasma capsulatum infection, 303–306, 343. *See also* Histoplasmosis
Histoplasmosis, 303–306, 309
  clinical presentation of, 303
  diagnosis of, 305
  etiology and epidemiology of, 303
  with HIV/AIDS, 304–305, 343
  immunocompromised patients with, 304–305
  inflammatory reaction to, 303
  natural history and pathophysiology of, 303–304
  other manifestations, 304
  progressive disseminated, 303–304
  pulmonary, 303
    acute, 303
    chronic, 303
  treatment of, 305–306
HMB45 antibody, 564
Hodgkin disease, mediastinal masses and, 226
Hookworm, 331
Horner syndrome, 223
Hospital-acquired pneumonia (HAP), 180, 253, 347–350
Human immunodeficiency virus (HIV) infection. *See also* Acquired immune deficiency syndrome (AIDS)
  aspergillosis, 343
  bronchogenic carcinoma, 344
  Haemophilus influenzae, 342
  Kaposi's sarcoma, 343, 344
  Mycobacterium avium complex, 343
  Mycobacterium kansasii, *M. xenopi*, *M. gordonae*, 343
  pneumonia
    bacterial, 342
    fungal, 343
    Pneumocystis carinii, 340–342, 340t, 341t
    Streptococcus pneumoniae, 342
  pulmonary hypertension, 344
  pulmonary infections and complications in, 339–344
  tuberculosis, 284, 342–343
    prophylaxis against, 280
    treatment of, 287

Human neutrophil elastase, 366
Humidification, 67
Hydatid disease, 336–338
Hydration. *See also specific disorders*
  for chronic obstructive pulmonary
    disease, 374
  for hypercapnic respiratory failure, 195
  hypothesis, 445
Hydropneumothorax, 151, 152
Hydroxychloroquine, in rheumatoid
  arthritis, 544
Hydroxycobalamin (CYANOKIT), for
  cyanide poisoning, 489
Hygiene hypothesis, 353
HYPER therapy, for drowning, 500
Hyperbaric oxygen therapy, for CO
  poisoning, 489
Hypercalcemia, with lung cancer, 597
Hypercapnia, 25, 190
  acidosis from, 192
  chronic, 369
Hypercapnic respiratory failure, acute,
  190–196
  acidosis in, 192–193
  complications of, 195–196
  definition of, 190
  diagnosis of, 191–192
  management of, 193–195
    mechanical ventilation in, 193–194
    oxygen supplementation in, 193
    symptomatic treatment in, 195
    underlying cause in, 194
Hypercarbia, preoperative evaluation
  and, 46
Hyperechoic image, 33
Hyperpigmentation, with lung
  cancer, 596
Hypersensitivity pneumonitis (HP), 213*t*,
  493–496
  from *Aspergillus*, 313
  diagnosis of, 494–495
  etiology of, 493
  pathophysiology of, 495
  prognosis with, 496
  treatment of, 495
Hypertension, pulmonary. *See* Pulmonary
  hypertension
Hypertrophic pulmonary osteoarthropathy,
  in lung cancer, 595
Hypocapnia, 25
Hypoechoic image, 33
Hyponatremia, 282
  with lung cancer, 597
Hypoventilation. *See also specific disorders*
  absolute and relative, 191

alveolar, 190 (*See also* Hypercapnic
    respiratory failure)
  central, 469
    pulmonary hypertension in, 423
  primary, 469
  in neuromuscular disorders, 460
  obesity in, 469–471
    pulmonary hypertension in, 423
Hypoxemia, 190, 369, 41. *See also specific
  disorders*
  acute reversible, in systemic lupus
    erythematosus, 549
  in aspiration pneumonia, 157
  assessment guidelines for, 24*t*
  cause of PH in COPD, 423
  classification of, 24
  in drowning, 498
  exercise-induced, with chronic obstruction
    pulmonary disease, 58
  in neurofibromatosis type 1, 563
  in rheumatoid arthritis, 549
Hypoxia-altitude simulation test
  (HAST), 112–113

I

Iatrogenic pneumothorax, 148, 150
Ibuprofen
  for cystic fibrosis, 446
  interstitial pneumonitis from, 542
Iceberg tumor, 576
Idiopathic hypereosinophilic syndrome, 231
Idiopathic interstitial pneumonias
  (IIP), 530–538. *See also* Pneumonia,
  idiopathic interstitial
  classification, 530–531
  clinical, radiographic, and histologic
    features, 531–536
    acute interstitial pneumonia, 533–534
    cryptogenic organizing pneumonia, 534
    desquamative interstitial
      pneumonia, 534–535
    idiopathic pulmonary fibrosis, 531–532
    lymphoid interstitial pneumonia, 535–536
    nonspecific interstitial pneumonia,
      532–533
    respiratory bronchiolitis interstitial lung
      disease, 535
  diagnosis of, 536–537
    flexible bronchoscopy, bal, and
      transbronchial biopsy, 536
    imaging studies, 536
    serologic testing, 536
    surgical lung biopsy, 536–537
  treatment, 537–538

Idiopathic kyphoscoliosis, 450
Idiopathic pulmonary arterial hypertension
  (IPAH), 6–7, 411, 421
Idiopathic pulmonary fibrosis (IPF), 434,
  531–532
Idiopathic pulmonary hemosiderosis
  (IPH), 527–528
  clinical findings, 528
  diagnosis, 528
  etiology, 527
  presentation, 527
  treatment and prognosis, 528
IgE-mediated asthma, in aspergillosis, 313
Iloprost
  for asthma, 52
  for pulmonary hypertension, 427
Imipenem
  for nocardiosis, 321
  for nontuberculous mycobacterial
    infections, 294
  for pneumonia
    gram-negative bacilli, 256
    pneumococcal, 235
  for tuberculosis, 287
Imipenem-cilastatin
  for actinomycosis, 322
  for *Haemophilus influenzae* infection, 247
Immune Reconstitution Inflammatory
  Syndrome (IRIS), 342
Immunocompromised host, 167–171. *See
  also specific disorders*
  bacterial infection in, 167
  diagnosis in, 169–171
  fungal infection in, 167–168
  non-infectious etiologies in, 169–170
  viral infection in, 168
Immunoglobulins, for asthma, 355. *See also
  specific immunoglobulins*
Immunotherapy, passive, for gram-negative
  bacilli pneumonias, 258
Impedance plethysmography (IPG), for deep
  venous thrombosis, 387, 399
Indacaterol, for asthma, 50
Industrial bronchitis, 213*t*, 478
Infection. *See also specific disorders and
  organisms*
  anaerobic lung, 263–265
    antibiotic treatment for, 264
    diagnosis of, 264
  in aspiration pneumonia, 156–157
  cestode, 331
  fungal (*See* Fungal infections)
  in immunocompromised host, 167–170
    (*See also* Immunocompromised host)
  after lung transplantation, 437

from mechanical ventilation, 91
  hospital-acquired pneumonia in, 348
  nematode, 331–334
  after pulmonary resection, 145, 146
  respiratory, neuromuscular disorders,
    460–461
  of respiratory tract in pregnancy, 160
  in sickle cell disease, 442
  tapeworm, 331
  trematode, 333
  viral (*See specific infections*)
Infectious Diseases Society of America/
  American Thoracic Society (IDSA/
  ATS), 181, 182, 183
Inferior vena cava filters, 396,
  402, 408
Inflammatory bronchoconstriction, 485
Infliximab
  for interstitial pneumonitis, in rheumatoid
    arthritis, 542
  for sarcoidosis, 514
Influenza. *See also Haemophilus influenzae*
  infection
  pneumonia from, 274–275 (*See also*
    Pneumonia, viral)
  vaccine against, 274–275
    for chronic obstructive pulmonary
      disease prophylaxis, 373
    in pregnancy, 160
  viruses, 274
Inhalation injury, smoke. *See* Smoke
  inhalation injury
Inhalational toxins, 77–78. *See also specific
  toxins*
Inhaled corticosteroids agents, for
  asthma, 50–51
Inspiratory positive airway pressure
  (IPAP), 471
Institute for Healthcare Improvement
  (IHI), 349
Institute of Medicine (IOM)
  To Err Is Human, 100–101
Intensity modulated radiation therapy
  (IMRT), in lung cancer treatment, 507
Interferon-gamma release assays
  (IGRAs), 282–283
  for tuberculosis, 279
Intermittent pneumatic compressive
  devices, for venous thromboembolism
  prophylaxis, 395–396
Intermittent Positive Pressure Breathing
  (IPPB), 68
Interstitial fibrosis
  in scleroderma, 549–550
  in systemic lupus erythematosus, 547

Interstitial lung disease (ILD), 442
  drugs in, 176
  pulmonary hypertension from, 423
  respiratory bronchiolitis in, 535
Interstitial pneumonia
  acute, 533–534
  chronic, 547
  desquamative, 534–535
  idiopathic, 530–538 (*See also* Idiopathic
    interstitial pneumonias)
  lymphoid, 535–536
  nonspecific, 532–533
Interstitial pneumonitis
  in neurofibromatosis type 1, 562–563
  in rheumatoid arthritis, 541
    drug-related, 541–542
  in systemic lupus erythematosus,
    547–549
Interventional pulmonology, 61–63
  advanced diagnostic procedures
    endobronchial ultrasound
      bronchoscopy, 41–42
    flexible fiberoptic bronchoscopy, 40–41
    navigational bronchoscopy, 42–43
  therapeutic procedures
    bronchial thermoplasty, 62–63
    rigid bronchoscopy with advanced
      therapeutic techniques, 61–62
Intraconazole, 305
Intravenous immunoglobulin, for Guillain–
  Barré syndrome, 462
Intrinsic asthma, 353
Intubation, burning injury patients in,
  489–490
Invasive pulmonary aspergillosis (IPA),
  311–312
  acute, 315–317
  clinical presentation of, 316
  epidemiology of, 316
Inverse ratio ventilation (IRV), 86
Iodinated glycerol, for chronic obstructive
  pulmonary disease, 374
Iodine, for malignant pleural disease, 605
Iodoquinol, for amebiasis, 336
Ionizing radiation exposure, disaster
  management, 76
  acute radiation syndrome, 76–77
Ipratropium, 50
Ipratropium bromide, 358, 360
Isoechoic image, 33
Isoniazid
  for tuberculosis, 286–289
  in pregnancy, 289
  prevention of, 279–280
Isoproterenol, for asthma, 50

Itraconazole
  for allergic bronchopulmonary
    aspergillosis, 315
  for aspergillosis
    allergic bronchopulmonary, 313
    chronic invasive pulmonary, 313
    chronic necrotizing aspergillosis, 313
  for blastomycosis, 310
  for coccidioidomycosis, 300
  for cryptococcosis, 327
Ivermectin, for nematode infection, 332

J

Joint tuberculosis, 284

K

Kalydeco™, 448
Kanamycin, for tuberculosis, 278, 287
Kaposi's sarcoma, in HIV-infected, 343, 344
Kartagener syndrome, 200
Katayama fever, 414. *See also* Schistosomiasis
Ketoconazole
  for coccidioidomycosis, 300
  on cortisol levels, 597
Keystone Project, 101–102, 103, 104
Kidney biopsy, for AGBMA disease, 522
Klebsiella pneumonia, 250–251
  etiology of, 250
  pathophysiology of, 251
Klebsiella pneumoniae carbapenemase
  (KPC), 250–251
Kyphoscoliosis, 449–450
Kyphosis, 449–450

L

Lady Windermere syndrome, 200, 292
Lambert–Eaton myasthenic syndrome
  (LEMS), 595
Langerhans' cell, 559
Langerhans cell histiocytosis,
  pulmonary, 558–560
Laparoscopy *vs.* open techniques, as
  postoperative risk factor, 45
Large-cell carcinoma, of lung, 586, 586t.
  See also Lung cancer
Large volume entrainment nebulizer, 66
Laryngeal (vocal-cord) dysfunction, 356
Laryngeal mask airway (LMA), 210–211, 490
Leeuwenhoek disease, 456
Leflunomide
  interstitial pneumonitis from, 543
  for Wegener's granulomatosis, 518

Legionella pneumonia, 267–271
Legionnaires' disease, 267–271
Leiomyomas, 577
Lemierre syndrome, 416
Leukotriene modifiers. *See also specific agents*
  for asthma, 51, 357, 360
Levalbuterol, for asthma, 50
Levofloxacin, 80
  for gram-negative bacilli pneumonias, 256
  for *Haemophilus influenzae* infection, 247
  for pneumonia
    atypical, 268, 269
    gram-negative bacilli, 256, 257
  for tuberculosis, 287
Liberation, from mechanical ventilation,
  89, 91–92
Lidocaine, for cough suppression, 130
Light's criteria, in pleural effusion, 133
Limited cutaneous systemic sclerosis
  (lcSSc), 549
Linezolid
  for nocardiosis, 321
  for streptococcal pneumonia, 241
  for tuberculosis, 287
Lipomas, 577
Liposomal formulations, 300
Liquid-based culture media, use of, 291–292
Liquid mustard, 78
Liver cells, pulmonary embolism from, after
  abdominal trauma, 417
Living donor transplantation, 435
Lobar torsion, after pulmonary
  resection, 146
Lobectomy, for bronchial carcinoids, 577
Löffler's syndrome, 228, 331
Löfgren syndrome, 513
Logistic regression model, for
  hypersensitivity pneumonitis, 494
Long-acting beta-2 agonists (LABAs), for
  asthma, 50
Lorazepam, 79
Low-flow oxygen systems, 64–66
Low-molecular-weight heparin (LMWH),
  for thromboembolic disease, 399–401
  prophylaxis against, 394
Lung
  aging, 367
  in drug abuse, 173–177
  lesions, transthoracic biopsies of, 36–37
  microbial agents in, 181
  nodules, guidelines for follow-up, 218*t*
Lung allocation score (LAS), 434
Lung cancer, 213*t*, 585–588
  from asbestos, 481, 602–603
  classification of, 585–587, 586*t*

clinical presentation of, 580
diagnosis and staging of, 580–583, 582*t*, 583*t*
drug abuse in, 177
epidemiology of, 587–588
local spread of, 594
metastatic, 594–595
paraneoplastic syndromes from, 595–597
prognosis in, 584, 590
risk factors for, 587
screening for, 588
  on mortality rates, 588
  radiographic, 3–4
  small lesions on outcome in, 588
  on smoking cessation, 588
  usefulness of, 588
treatment of, 590–592
  chemotherapy and radiotherapy in, 591
  operability, resectability, and adjuvant
    therapy for stage I and stage II
    NSCLC, 590–591
  palliative, 592
  for small-cell lung carcinoma, 592
  tailoring therapy, 591–592
Lung disease, radiation-induced, 504–508
  clinical presentation, 505–507
    acute radiation pneumonitis, 506
    chronic radiation fibrosis, 506
    radiographic changes, 506–507
  complications, 507
  conformal techniques in
    radiotherapy, 507–508
  future directions of, 508
  pathophysiology, 505
  prevention and treatment, 507
Lung expansion therapy, in pulmonary
  therapeutics, 68
Lung resection. *See also specific disorders*
  for hemoptysis, 139, 140–141
  preoperative evaluation in, 47
Lung transplantation, 411, 430–437
  for cystic fibrosis, 446
  donor selection in, 434–435
  guidelines for selected diseases, 432–433*t*
  indications for, 430
  lung allocation score, 434
  for lymphangioleiomyomatosis, 566
  patient selection, 430–434
    exclusion criteria, 431–432
    inclusion criteria, 432–434
  posttransplant complications, 436–437
    acute rejection, 436
    anastomotic complications, 436–437
    chronic rejection, 437
    infection, 437
    primary graft dysfunction, 436

Lung transplantation (*continued*)
  pregnancy following, 162
  for pulmonary alveolar proteinosis, 572
  for pulmonary hypertension, 427
  tracheobronchial aspergillosis after, 317
  types of, 435
Lung ventilation and perfusion (V/Q)
  scanning, 5
Lymphangiography, 144
Lymphangioleiomyomatosis (LAM),
  563–566
  in pregnancy, 161–162
Lymphangiomatosis, 563–566
Lymphoid interstitial pneumonia
  (LIP), 535–536
Lymphomas, mediastinal masses and,
  223, 226

M

Macrolide antibiotics, 243, 270. *See also
  specific agents*
  for asthma, 52
  for cystic fibrosis, 292, 446
  for tuberculosis, 287
Macrophage inflammatory protein, 553
Magnesium sulfate, for status
  asthmaticus, 359
Magnetic phrenic nerve stimulators, for
  diaphragm paralysis, 455
Magnetic resonance imaging (MRI). *See also
  specific disorders*
  for chronic thromboembolic pulmonary
    hypertension, 408
  for deep venous thrombosis, 387
  for pulmonary embolism, 389
Mahler Dyspnea Score, 122
Malignant airway obstruction, 61
Malignant mesothelioma
  from asbestos, 602–603
  pleural, 601–605 (*See also* Mesothelioma,
    pleural)
Malignant pleural mesothelioma
  (MPM), 601
Mandatory ventilation, 84–86
Marijuana, on lungs, 173–177. *See also*
  Drug abuse
Mask ventilation, 209
Mast cell stabilizers (cromolyn), for
  asthma, 51
Maximum expiratory pressure (MEP),
  16, 460
Maximum inspiratory pressure (MIP),
  16, 460
Maximum mid-expiratory flow rate, 14

Measles (rubeola), pneumonia from, 276
Mebendazole
  for echinococcosis, 337, 338
  for nematode infection, 331
Mechanical insufflation and exsufflation
  devices, 67–68
Mechanical ventilation. *See* Ventilation,
  mechanical
Mediastinal crunch, in pneumothorax, 150
Mediastinal developmental cysts, 226
Mediastinal granuloma, 303
Mediastinal masses, 222–226
  clinical presentation of, 223
  diagnosis of, 223–224
  etiology of, 224–226
  infections, 226
  location of, 222–223
Mediastinal ultrasound, 37
Mediastinoscopy, 41–42
Mediastinum
  endobronchial ultrasound bronchoscopy
    for, 42
  location of, 222–223
  lymphomas in, 223
  thymomas, 223
Medicolegal evaluation, 106–109
  basis for apportionment in, 109
  diagnosis in, 107–108
  evidence and severity of impairment in, 108
  need for further treatment in, 109
  presence of disability in, 108
  reports in, 106–107, 107*t*
  vocational retraining in, 109
  work-relatedness in, 107–108
Meig syndrome, 132
Meigs–Salmon syndrome, 601
Mendelson syndrome, 155, 156
Meningitis
  coccidioidal, 298, 300
  tuberculous, 284
Meningoencephalitis, 325
Meperidine abuse, pulmonary embolism
  from, 417
Meropenem
  for nocardiosis, 321
  for pneumonia gram-negative bacilli, 256
Mesothelioma, pleural, 601–605
  from asbestos, 602–603
  clinical presentation of, 601
  diagnosis of, 602–603
  etiology and pathophysiology of, 601
  treatment and prognosis of, 605
Metaproterenol, for asthma, 50
Metered-dose inhalers (MDIs), for
  asthma, 50, 357, 359, 360, 373

Methacholine, for asthma, 486
Methadone, on lungs, 175. *See also* Drug abuse
Methamphetamine, 175
Methicillin-resistant *Staphylococcus aureus* (MRSA), 241
Methotrexate
  for interstitial pneumonitis, in rheumatoid arthritis, 541–542
  pulmonary toxicity of, 542
  for Wegener's granulomatosis, 518
Methylphenidate (hydrochloride)
  on lungs, 175, 176 (*See also* Drug abuse)
  pulmonary embolism from, 417
Methylprednisolone
  for asthma, 51, 359
  for histoplasmosis, 305
  for hypercapnic respiratory failure, 195
Methylxanthines, for asthma, 51
Metronidazole
  for amebiasis, 336
  for aspiration pneumonia, 157
Microbial agents, in lungs, 181
Microbiology, 291–292
Microimmunofluorescence (MIF) assay, 269
Microvascular tumor embolism, 416–417
Miliary tuberculosis, 284
Mine Act. *See* Federal Mine Safety and Health Act of 1977
Minocycline
  for malignant pleural disease, 605
  for nocardiosis, 321
Minute ventilation, 20, 191
Mitomycin, 505
Mitoxantrone, for malignant pleural disease, 605
Mixed connective tissue disease (MCTD), 553–554
Monoclonal antibodies, 77
Montelukast, for asthma, 51
Moraxella catarrhalis, 373
Mounier-Kuhn syndrome, 200
Moxifloxacin
  for anaerobic pneumonia, 264
  for *Haemophilus influenzae* infection, 247
  for atypical pneumonia, 268
  for tuberculosis, 287
Mucolytic agents, 491. *See also specific agents*
  for chronic obstructive pulmonary disease, 374
  for hypercapnic respiratory failure, 195
Mustard gas, 78
Mycetoma, 312–313
Mycobacterial infection, non-TB, with silicosis, 477

Mycobacterium abscessus, 293–294
Mycobacterium avium, 291, 292
  complex, 292
    treatment, 292–293
  infection and AIDS, disseminated, 293
Mycobacterium avium-intracellulare complex (MAC), 169. *See also* Mycobacterial infection, non-TB, with silicosis
  in HIV-infected, 343
Mycobacterium gordonae, in HIV-infected, 343
Mycobacterium intracellulare, 292
Mycobacterium kansasii, 169, 291, 294
  in HIV-infected, 343
Mycobacterium massiliense, 294
Mycobacterium tuberculosis (MTB), 168–169, 278, 282–284, 512, 573
Mycobacterium xenopi, in HIV-infected, 343
Mycophenolate, for idiopathic interstitial pneumonias, 537
Mycophenolate mofetil
  for progressive systemic sclerosis, 552
  for Wegener's granulomatosis, 518
Mycoplasma pneumoniae pneumonia, 267–271
Myeloperoxidase (MPO), 517

N

N-acetylcysteine, 78, 491
N-terminal pro-brain natriuretic peptide (NT-pro-BNP), 121
Naloxone, 175
Narcotics, illicit. *See also* Drug abuse; *specific drugs*
  on lungs, 175, 177
Nasal cannulas device, 65
Nasogastric feeding tubes (NGT), hospital-acquired pneumonia from, 348
Nasogastric tubes, aspiration pneumonia from, 157
National Asthma Education and Prevention Program (NAEPP) 2007, 354
National Institutes of Health (NIH) observational cohort study, 566
National Lung Cancer Screening Trial (NLST), 3–4, 216
Navigational bronchoscopy, 219
  interventional pulmonology, 42–43
  for solitary pulmonary nodule, 219
Near-drowning, 498–501
Nebulizers
  for asthma, 50
  heparin, 491
  sodium carbonate, 77

Necator americanus, 331
Nematode infections, 331–334
Neoplastic disease, of pleura, 601–605. *See also*
Pleura, neoplastic disease of; *specific cancers*
Nerve agents, 79
Neurofibromatosis type 1 (NF1), 562–563
Neurogenic tumors, mediastinal masses
and, 225
Neuromuscular disorders, 459–462. *See also*
specific disorders
amyotrophic lateral sclerosis, 462
Guillain–Barré syndrome, 461–462
hypoventilation in, 460
respiratory infections in, 460–461
sleep-related breathing problems in, 461
Neuropathic arthropathy, with lung
cancer, 595
Neurotoxic agents, 79
Neutrophilic alveolitis, in hypersensitivity
pneumonitis, 494
NF1 gene, 562
Nicotine, 70, 79
Nitrogen mustard, for pleural disease,
malignant, 605
Nocardiosis (Nocardia infection), 320–322
acute, 321
chronic, 321
clinical manifestations of, 321
diagnosis of, 321
microbiology and epidemiology, 320–321
treatment of, 321–322
Nocturnal hypoventilation, in neuromuscular
diseases, 461
Nocturnal nasal oxygen therapy, for
obstructive sleep apnea, 468
Nodule, solitary pulmonary, 215–220.
See also Solitary pulmonary nodule
Non-Hodgkin lymphoma, mediastinal
masses and, 226
Noninvasive ventilation, hospital-acquired
pneumonia in, 348
Nonpulmonary disease, caused by NTM
species, 294–295
Non–small-cell lung carcinoma (NSCLC)
advanced-stage, 591
operability, resectability, and adjuvant
therapy for stage I and stage II, 590–591
stereotactic body radiation therapy
for, 508
targeted treatment for, 591–592
Nonspecific interstitial pneumonia
(NSIP), 532–533
Nonsteroidal antiinflammatory drugs
(NSAIDs), 229
for cystic fibrosis, 446

Nontuberculous mycobacterial (NTM)
infections, 291–295. *See also*
Mycobacterial infection, non-TB, with
silicosis
diagnosis of, 291
microbiology, 291–292
Mycobacterium abscessus, 293–294
Mycobacterium avium complex, 292
infection and AIDS, disseminated, 293
treatment, 292–293
Mycobacterium kansasii, 294
nonpulmonary disease caused by, 294–295
North American blastomycosis. *See*
Blastomycosis
Nosocomial pneumonia, 180
Novel coronavirus pneumonia, 275
Nucleic acid amplification (NAA) test, for
tuberculosis, 283

O

Obesity-hypoventilation syndrome
(OHS), 469–471
pulmonary hypertension in, 423
Obliterative bronchiolitis, 188–189
with organization pneumonia. *See*
Bronchiolitis obliterans with organizing
pneumonia (BOOP)
in rheumatoid arthritis, 543
Obstructive sleep apnea (OSA), 461,
466–469
characteristics of, 466
diagnosis of, 467
as postoperative risk factor, 46
treatment of, 468–469
Occupational asthma, 212, 213*t*, 484
Occupational-environmental lung disease
(OELD), 212–214, 213*t*
examples of, 213*t*
general approach to patient of, 213*t*
historical features of, 213, 214*t*
radiographic screening for, 3
Ochroconis gallopavum, 167, 168
Omalizumab, for asthma, 52, 358
Ondine curse, 469
Open lung biopsy, 182
Opiates, pulmonary embolism from abuse
of, 417. *See also specific opiates*
Optiflow™, 66
Oral contraceptives, smoking and, 69
Oral hygiene, in aspiration
pneumonia, 156–157
Organizing pneumonia. *See* Bronchiolitis
obliterans with organizing pneumonia
(BOOP)

Oseltamivir, 275
Osteoarthropathy, hypertrophic pulmonary, in lung cancer, 595
Osteomyelitis, in sickle cell disease, 442
Oxygen
  arterial measurement of, 24
  for burning injury patients, 491
  delivery, 64–66, 65t
Oxygen therapy
  for acute respiratory distress syndrome, 381
  for chronic obstructive pulmonary disease, 375
  for hypercapnic respiratory failure, 193
Oxymizer, 65

P

2-PAM (Protopam chloride), 79
p-Aminosalicylic acid (PAS), for tuberculosis, 287
Paclitaxel, 505
Panbronchiolitis, diffuse, 189
Pancreatic malabsorption, in cystic fibrosis, 446
Panton–Valentine leukocidin (PVL), 241
Papanicolaou, for blastomycosis, 310
Paradoxical reaction, 289
Paragonimus westermani, 333–334
Parainfluenza virus, 275
Paraneoplastic encephalomyelitis, with lung cancer, 595
Paraneoplastic syndromes, 595–597
Paraneoplastic vasculitic neuropathy, with lung cancer, 596
Parapneumonic effusion, complicated, 134
Parenchyma, pulmonary hypertension in diseases of, 423
Parenteral prostanoids, for asthma, 52
Paromomycin, for amebiasis, 336
Partial pressure of inspired oxygen, 110, 111t
Particulate matter, smoke inhalation injury and, 488
Patent airway, verification of, 211
Patient-driven protocols, 96
Penicillin, 442
  for actinomycosis, 322
  for streptococcal pneumonia, 241, 242
Penicillin G, for pneumococcal pneumonia, 235
Pentamidine, for P. carinii pneumonia with HIV, 340t, 341t
  prophylaxis against, 340t
Pentazocine abuse, pulmonary embolism from, 417

Pentoxifylline, 77, 507
Percutaneous transthoracic lung aspiration, for pneumonia diagnosis, 182
Perfusion scans, 5–7
  application of, 6
  for pulmonary embolism, 389
  for thromboembolic pulmonary hypertension, 408
Pericardial tuberculosis, 284
Peripheral neuropathy, in lung cancer, 595
Peromyscus maniculatus, 276
Persistent pulmonary hypertension of the newborn (PPHN), 423
pH, 26, 27t
Pharmacologic bronchoconstriction, 485
Phenothiazines. See also specific agents
  aspiration pneumonia and, 156
Phenylephrine, 402
Phosgene, 78
Phosphodiesterase-5, 423
  for asthma, 53
  for pulmonary hypertension, 427
Pickwickian syndrome, 469
Picture archiving and communication system (PACS), 3
Pilocarpine iontophoresis, in cystic fibrosis, 445
Pink puffer, 370
Piperacillin
  for gram-negative bacilli pneumonias, 256
  for Haemophilus influenzae infection, 247
Piperacillin-tazobactam (pip/tazo), for gram-negative bacilli pneumonias, 256
Pirbuterol, for asthma, 50
Plague, disaster management of, 79, 80
"Plankton sign", in thoracic ultrasound, 34
Plasmapheresis
  for AGBMA disease (Goodpasture's), 523
  for Guillain–Barré syndrome, 462
Plethysmography, 15
Pleura, neoplastic disease of, 601–605
  clinical presentation of, 601
  diagnosis of, 601–605
  etiology and pathophysiology of, 601
  metastatic, 604
  treatment and prognosis of, 605
Pleural carcinomatosis, 601, 604
Pleural effusion, 131–134
  causes of, 131–132
  chest roentgenogram for, 132
  definition of, 131
  differential diagnosis of, 133
  fluid analysis in, 133–134
  open biopsy for, 134
  parenchymal abnormalities with, 132–133

Pleural effusion (*continued*)
physical examination findings in, 132–133
pleural ultrasonography for, 132
after pulmonary resection, 144
in radiation-induced lung injury, 506
in rheumatoid arthritis, 541
thoracoscopy for, 134
treatment of, 134
ultrasound in, 34
Pleural fibrosis, 482
Pleural fluid, analysis of, 131, 133–134
Pleural tear, pneumothorax from, 149
Pleural ultrasonography, for pleural effusion, 132
Pleuritic chest pain, 388
Pleuritis
in scleroderma, 551
in systemic lupus erythematosus, 547
Pleurodesis, 134, 152
for lymphangioleiomyomatosis, 564
talc, 605
"Pneumobelt", 461
Pneumococcal pneumonia. *See* Pneumonia, pneumococcal
Pneumococcal vaccine, for COPD prophylaxis, 373
Pneumococcus, 167. *See also Streptococcus pneumoniae*
Pneumoconiosis, 213*t*
coal workers', 477–479
impairment and disability, 478–479
pathogenesis of, 477–478
pathophysiology of, 477
regulations and risk of, 478
Pneumocystis carinii, 168, 381
Pneumocystis carinii pneumonia (PCP)
with HIV, 339–344, 340*t*, 341*t*
with pulmonary alveolar proteinosis, 571
Pneumocystis jiroveci, 168
Pneumomediastinum, 149
drug-induced, 177
spontaneous, 552–553
Pneumonia, 180–184
Acinetobacter, 253–259 (*See also* Pneumonia, gram-negative bacilli)
antimicrobial treatment of, 183
aspiration, 155–158
atypical, 267–271
bacterial, in HIV-infected, 342
in burn patients, 491
Chlamydophila (*Chlamydia*), 267–271
clinical presentation of, 180
colonization pattern in, 180, 181
community-acquired
drug abuse in, 174
gram-negative, 253

cryptogenic organizing, 534
diagnosis of, 181–182
Enterobacter, 253–259 (*See also* Pneumonia, gram-negative bacilli)
Escherichia coli, 253–259 (*See also* Pneumonia, gram-negative bacilli)
etiology of, 180, 181
fungal, in HIV-infected, 343
general considerations in, 180–184
gram-negative bacilli, 253–259
background and etiology of, 253–254
clinical presentations of, 254–255
diagnosis of, 255–256
prevention of, 258–259
prognosis with, 258
treatment of, 256–258
hematogenous or embolic causes of, 181
heroin use in, 174
hospital-acquired (nosocomial), 347–350
choice of antibiotic regimens for, 350
definition and epidemiology of, 347
diagnosis of, 349–350
gram-negative, 253–259 (*See also* Pneumonia, gram-negative bacilli)
in immunocompetent host, 347
pathogenesis of, 347–348
prevention of, 348–349
treatment of, 350
idiopathic interstitial, 530–538
acute interstitial, 534–535
cryptogenic organizing, 534
desquamative interstitial, 534–535
idiopathic pulmonary fibrosis, 531–532
lymphoid interstitial, 535–536
nonspecific interstitial, 532–533
respiratory bronchiolitis interstitial lung disease, 535
incidence of, 180
interstitial (*See* Interstitial lung disease; Interstitial pneumonia)
Klebsiella, 250–251 (*See also Klebsiella pneumonia*)
Legionella, 267–271
management of, initial antibiotics in, 181–182
Mycoplasma pneumoniae, 267–271
nomenclature, 180
nonspecific interstitial, 532–533
pathogenesis of, 181
pneumococcal, 233–237, 242
clinical manifestations of, 234
complications of, 236
diagnosis of, 234–235
etiology and pathogenesis of, 234
natural history of, 235

treatment of, 236
vaccines against, 236–237, 243
prevention of, 184
Proteus, 253–259 (*See also* Pneumonia, gram-negative bacilli)
Pseudomonas aeruginosa, 253–259 (*See also* Pneumonia, gram-negative bacilli)
Q fever, 267–271
Serratia, 253–259 (*See also* Pneumonia, gram-negative bacilli)
staphylococcal, 240–243
streptococcal, 240–243
ventilator-associated, 347–350
gram-negative, 253–259 (*See also* Pneumonia, gram-negative bacilli)
viral, 273–276
adenovirus, 275
bacterial coinfection with, 274
cytomegalovirus, 276
diagnosis of, 274
factors of, 273
hantavirus pulmonary syndrome, 276
herpes simplex virus, 276
influenza, 274–275
measles (rubeola), 276
neurological sequelae of, 274
novel coronavirus, 275
parainfluenza, 275
respiratory syncytial virus (RSV), 275
rhinovirus, 275
severe acute respiratory syndrome, 273, 275
varicella-zoster virus (VZV), 275–276
Pneumonia Patient Outcomes Research Team (PORT), 182
Pneumonia Severity Index (PSI), 103, 182
Pneumonic plague, 80, 138
Pneumonitis, 180. *See also* Pneumonia
aspiration, with scleroderma, 551
chronic interstitial, in systemic lupus erythematosus, 547–548
hypersensitivity, 213*t*, 493–496 (*See also* Hypersensitivity pneumonitis)
interstitial
in neurofibromatosis type 1, 562–563
in rheumatoid arthritis, 541
drug-related, 541–542
in systemic lupus erythematosus, 547
presentation of, 493–494
Pneumothorax, 90, 148–153, 195
air travel and, 111
categories of, 148–150
iatrogenic, 148, 150
primary spontaneous, 149
secondary spontaneous, 149

spontaneous (idiopathic), 148, 149–150
traumatic, 148, 150
clinical manifestations/physical findings in, 150
complications of, 151–152
bilateral, 151
hemothorax, 151–152
pyothorax, 152
tension, 151
in cystic fibrosis, 447
diagnosis of, 150–151
drug-induced, 177
hydropneumothorax with, 151, 152
management of, 152–153
radiography for, 2
risk factors for, 149
thoracic ultrasound using, 36
thoracotomy for, 153
Polymerase chain reaction (PCR), 267, 273, 283
Polymyositis, 552–553
Polymyxin B, for gram-negative bacilli pneumonias, 257
Polymyxin E, for gram-negative bacilli pneumonias, 257
Polysaccharide vaccine, in pneumococcal pneumonia, 236
Polysomnography
for chronic lung disease in sickle cell disease, 442
for pulmonary hypertension, 426
Portopulmonary hypertension (PoPH), 421
Posaconazole
for coccidioidomycosis, 299
for cryptococcosis, 328
Positive end-expiratory pressure (PEEP), 86
for acute respiratory distress syndrome, 381–382
use of, 86
Positron emission tomography (PET)
for lung cancer, 581
solitary pulmonary nodule, 217
Postinfectious cough, 128
Postoperative pulmonary complications, 45–47. *See also specific disorders*
impact of increasing age on, 45
risk factor for, 45
Postpneumonectomy syndrome, 146–147
Posttransplant lymphoproliferative disease, 169
Potassium hydroxide (KOH), for blastomycosis, 310
Pott's disease, 284, 289. *See also* Tuberculosis (TB)

Pralidoxime chloride (2-PAM or Protopam chloride), 79
Praziquantel
  for paragonimiasis, 334
  for schistosomiasis, 334
Precipitation, 107
Prednisone
  for allergic bronchopulmonary aspergillosis, 315
  for asthma, 51, 359
  for chronic obstructive pulmonary disease, 374
  for histoplasmosis, 305
  for progressive systemic sclerosis, 553
  taper, for lung transplantation, 436
  for Wegener's granulomatosis, 518
Pregnancy, 159–164
  asthma in, 160–161, 360
  bacterial pneumonia in, 160
  blastomycosis in, 310
  cystic fibrosis in, 162
  deep venous thrombosis in, 162
  drugs in, 161, 289
  dyspnea in, 160
  influenza vaccination, 160
  following lung transplantation, 162
  lymphangioleiomyomatosis, 161–162
  medications, pulmonary, 163–164t
  pulmonary edema in, 163
  pulmonary embolism in, 162
  pulmonary function tests in, 160
  pulmonary hypertension in, 162–163
  radiography in, 160
  respiratory tract infection in, 160
  sarcoidosis in, 162
  sleep disordered breathing in, 162
  tidal volume in, 160
  tuberculosis in, 160, 289
  varicella pneumonia in, 160
  venous thromboembolism in, 162
  viral pneumonia in, 160
  vital capacity in, 160
"Pregnancy category X," 53
Preoperative pulmonary evaluation, 45–47
Primaquine-clindamycin, for *P. carinii* pneumonia with HIV, 341t
Primary alveolar hypoventilation, 469
Primary graft dysfunction (PGD), 436
Primary or metastatic pleural tumors, 34
Primary pulmonary hypertension. *See* Idiopathic pulmonary arterial hypertension (IPAH)
Procalcitonin, 181, 182, 183, 258
Prodromal symptoms, 76
Progesterone

for lymphangioleiomyomatosis, 565
for tuberous sclerosis, 567
Progressive disseminated histoplasmosis, 303–304
Progressive massive fibrosis, 477
Progressive systemic sclerosis, 549–552
Prominent hilar adenopathy, 282
Prophylaxis, 501
  mechanical, 395–396
  pharmacologic, 394–395
  risk assessment, 393
Propionibacterium acnes, 512
Proportional assist ventilation, 87
Propoxyphene, on lungs, 175. *See also* Drug abuse
Prostacyclin receptor agonists therapy, for pulmonary hypertension, 427
Prostanoids, for asthma, 52
Protected brush specimen (PBS), 182
Protein-conjugate vaccines, 243
Proteinase 3 (PR3), 517
Protein–calorie malnutrition, in cystic fibrosis, 446
Proteus pneumonia, 253–259. *See also* Pneumonia, gram-negative bacilli
Protocol-driven care, in respiratory therapy, 96–98
  advantages of, 97–98
  considerations, 98
  development of, 97
  success of, 96
Protopam chloride (2-PAM), 79
Proximal muscle neuromyopathy, symmetric, with lung cancer, 595
Pseudomonas aeruginosa, 180, 431
Pseudomonas aeruginosa pneumonia, 253–259. *See also* Pneumonia, gram-negative bacilli
Pseudotumor, pleural effusion and, 132
Psittacosis, 268
Psychogenic cough, 129
Puffing, 370
Pulmonary actinomycosis, 322
Pulmonary alveolar hemorrhage, in systemic lupus erythematosus, 548
Pulmonary alveolar proteinosis (PAP), 571–573
  complications of, 573
  diagnosis of, 571–572
  pathophysiology of, 571
  prognosis in, 573
  treatment of, 572
Pulmonary arterial hypertension (PAH), 124, 421, 422t, 440–441. *See also* Pulmonary hypertension
  diagnosis of, 421–422

etiology of, 440–441
obstructive sleep apnea and, 467
oral arginine supplementation effects, in SCD patients with, 441
with scleroderma, 550
treatment of, 126–127, 423
WHO classification of, 125*t*
Pulmonary arterial obstruction, 6
Pulmonary artery pressure (PAP), 124, 421
Pulmonary barotrauma, with cerebral air embolism, 500
Pulmonary capillaritis, in rheumatoid arthritis, 543
Pulmonary capillary hemangiomatosis (PCH), 423
Pulmonary disease, 291
  caused by NTM
    diagnosis of, 291
    microbiologic criteria, 291
  and cryptococcosis, 325
  HIV-negative patients with, 292
Pulmonary edema, 188
  drug-induced, 175
  high-altitude, 113, 114–115
  in pregnancy, 163
  reperfusion, 410
Pulmonary embolism (PE), 385–402
  from air travel, 111
  amniotic fluid, 415–416
  brain tissue, after head trauma, 417
  diagnosis of, 389
    perfusion scans in, 5, 6, 389
    radioisotopic techniques for, 5
  from drug abuse, noninfectious, 417–418
  epidemiology of, 385
  fat, 415
  liver cell, after abdominal trauma, 417
  lower extremity deep veins in, 386
  natural history of, 386
  pathophysiology of, 386
  in pregnancy, 162
  prophylaxis against, 393–396
    drugs in, 394
    intermittent pneumatic compressive devices in, 395–396
    options and strategies in, 393–394
  from pulmonary embolism, 413–414
  septic, 416
    drug-induced, 174, 416
  submersion-induced, 501
  from thromboembolic disease, 385–390
    (*See also* Venous thromboembolism (VTE))
  treatment of, 401–402
  trophoblastic tissue, 417
    from tumor, 416–417
      microvascular, 416–417
    venous air, 414–415
      direct arterial gas, 414
Pulmonary evaluation, preoperative, 45–47
Pulmonary fibrosis, 77
  idiopathic, 531–532
Pulmonary function tests (PFTs), 9–17, 57, 460, 513
  in asthma, 486
  in diaphragmatic paralysis, 454
  exercise testing in, 16
  flow-volume loop in, 14–15, 15*f*
  gas dilution techniques in, 15
  for hypersensitivity pneumonitis, 494
  normal values for, 10–11, 10*t*
  in pregnancy, 160
  preoperative, 46–47
  for pulmonary hypertension, 426
  for radiation pneumonitis, 505
  sleep studies in, 17
  spirometry in, 12–15*f*, 14
Pulmonary hamartomas, 577
Pulmonary hemosiderosis, idiopathic, 527–528
Pulmonary histoplasmosis, 303–304
Pulmonary hydatid cyst, 336, 337
Pulmonary hypertension (PH), 46, 124, 420–423
  air travel with, 111
  classes of, 422*t*
  with cor pulmonale, in rheumatoid arthritis, 548
  detection of, 124–125
  diagnosis and treatment of, 420–421, 425–427
  Doppler echocardiography for, 426
  drug-induced, 175
  endothelin antagonists for, 427
  in HIV-infected, 344
  hypoventilation syndromes in, 423
  owing to left heart disease, 422, 422*t*
  owing to lung diseases and/or hypoxia, 422*t*
  pathogenesis and etiology of, 420–423
  in pregnancy, 162–163
  pulmonary arterial hypertension, 421, 422*t*
  in pulmonary Langerhans cell histiocytosis, 560
  in rheumatoid arthritis, 543
  from schistosomiasis, 414
  with unclear multifactorial mechanisms, 422*t*
  WHO classification of, 125*t*

Pulmonary hypertension, chronic
  thromboembolic, 406–411, 422*t*, 423
  diagnosis of, 406–408
  epidemiology of, 406
  imaging of, 408
  pathophysiology and predisposing factors
    in, 406
  treatment of, 409–411
    postoperative management in, 409–410
    pulmonary thromboendarterectomy
      in, 409–411
    reperfusion pulmonary edema in, 410
Pulmonary impairment, 478–479
Pulmonary infarction, from embolism, 386
Pulmonary injury, in burn patients,
  488–491
Pulmonary Langerhans cell histiocytosis
  (PLCH), 558–560
  clinical presentation, 558
  diagnosis of, 558–559
  treatment, 559–560
Pulmonary macrophage, in
  pneumoconiosis, 477–478
Pulmonary nodules
  in rheumatoid arthritis, 542–543
  solitary (*See* Solitary pulmonary nodule)
Pulmonary rehabilitation (PR), 57–58
  for chronic obstructive pulmonary
    disease, 375
  goal of, 57
Pulmonary resection, complications
  of, 143–147
  air leaks, 144–145
  atelectasis, 143
  bronchial stump integrity, 145, 146
  bronchopleural fistula, 145–146
  cardiac herniation, 146
  hemorrhage, 143–144
  infection, 145, 146
  lobar torsion, 146
  pleural effusion, 144
  postpneumonectomy syndrome, 146–147
  postresectional space, 145
  preoperative preparation in, 143
Pulmonary therapeutics, 64–68
  bronchial hygiene, 67–68
  humidification, 67
  lung expansion, 68
  oxygen delivery, 64–66, 65*t*
Pulmonary thromboendarterectomy,
  409–411
  postoperative management in, 409–410
    intensive care, 410
  reperfusion pulmonary edema in, 410
Pulmonary toilet, 489, 490–491

Pulmonary tuberculosis, drug abuse in, 174
Pulmonary vascular disease, 124–127
  asthma, 52–53
  epidemiology of, 125–126
  pharmacologic treatment of, 52–53
  pulmonary hypertension, detection
    of, 124–125
  in rheumatoid arthritis, 543
  right heart catheterization in evaluation
    of, 126–127
Pulmonary vascular resistance (PVR), 421
Pulmonary vasodilator therapy, 124, 126
Pulmonary veno-occlusive disease
  (PVOD), 423
Pulmonary venous pressure, pleural effusion
  from, 131–132
Pulse oximeter, 24
Pulsus paradoxus, 355
Purpura rheumatica, with lung cancer, 596
Pyothorax, 152
Pyrazinamide, for tuberculosis, 286–289
  in HIV-infected, 280
  in pregnancy, 289

Q

Q fever pneumonia, 267–271
  diagnosis of, 269
  treatment of, 269
QuantiFeron-TB test (QFT), 279
Quantitative scans, for lung, 6
Quartz, 474
Quick-relief asthma medications, 357
Quinacrine, for malignant pleural
  disease, 605

R

Radial artery, 23
Radial endobronchial ultrasound (EBUS)
  bronchoscopy, 218, 219
Radial probe endobronchial ultrasound
  (RP-EBUS), with navigational
  bronchoscopy, 43
Radiation dispersal device (RDD), 76
Radiation fibrosis, chronic, 506
Radiation Injury Treatment Network
  (RITN), 77
Radiation pneumonitis
  acute, 505, 506
  chronic, 506
Radiography, 1–4. *See also specific disorders*
  chest
    digital, 2–3
    for lung cancer, 588

error in, 4
for pleural effusions, 133
in pregnancy, 160
for screening, 3–4
studies in, supplemental, 2
technique for, 1–2
Radioisotopic techniques, 5–7
pulmonary embolism
diagnosis of, 5
Radiology. *See* Radiography
Rapid eye movement (REM), 461
Rapid sequence intubation (RSI), 210
Rasmussen aneurysm, 282
Raynaud phenomenon, in rheumatoid
arthritis, 548
Reactive airways dysfunction syndrome
(RADS), 485
Reasonable medical probability, 107
Recombinant human vascular endothelial
growth factor (rhVEGF), 423
Reflex bronchoconstriction, 485
Rehabilitation, pulmonary, 57–58
for chronic obstructive pulmonary
disease, 57–58, 375
goal of, 57
Rejection, after lung transplantation
acute, 436
chronic, 437
Relative hypoventilation, 191
Renal tubular dysfunction, with lung cancer, 597
Reperfusion pulmonary edema, 410
Residual disease, 494
Respiratory bronchiolitis interstitial lung
disease (RB-ILD), 535
Respiratory care protocol, 96–98
Respiratory distress. *See* Acute respiratory
distress syndrome (ARDS); *specific disorders*
Respiratory effort related arousals (RERAs), 467
Respiratory failure
acute, 190
drug abuse in, 177
Respiratory infections, in neuromuscular
disorders, 460–461
Respiratory muscle weakness, in systemic
lupus erythematosus, 548
Respiratory myoclonus, 456
Respiratory syncytial virus (RSV)
pneumonia, 168, 275
Respiratory tract infection. *See also specific
infections*
in pregnancy, 160
Respiratory viral infections, 168
Retinopathy, cancer-associated, with lung
cancer, 595–596
Reverberation artifacts, 33–34

Reversible hypoxemia, acute, in systemic
lupus erythematosus, 549
Rheumatoid arthritis, 540–544
airways disease in, 543
apical fibrocavitary disease in, 544
drug-related pulmonary disease in, 541–542
interstitial pneumonitis in, 541
pleural disease in, 540–541
pulmonary nodules in, 542–543
pulmonary vascular disease in, 543
Rhinovirus pneumonia, 275
Rhodococcus equi, 167
Ribavirin, for respiratory syncytial virus, 275
Ricin, disaster management of, 79, 81
Rifabutin, for tuberculosis with HIV, 280, 289
Rifampin, 80, 278, 448
for asthma, 53
for cystic fibrosis, 446
for nontuberculous mycobacterial
infections, 292, 293, 294
in pregnancy, 289
for tuberculosis, 283, 286–289
in HIV-infected, 280, 287
prevention of, 280
Right heart catheterization
in evaluation of pulmonary vascular
disease, 126–127
for pulmonary hypertension, 440–441
Rigid bronchoscopy, with advanced
therapeutic techniques, 61–62
Riluzole, 462
Rimantadine, 53, 275
Ritonavir, for asthma, 53
Rituximab, for polymyositis, 553
Rivaroxaban, 395, 400–401
Roentgen, Wilhelm, 1
Roflumilast (Daliresp®), for asthma, 51
Rounded atelectasis, 482
Rubeola pneumonia, 276

S

Saccular bronchiectasis, 198
Salivary gland type, carcinomas of, 586*t*
Salmeterol, for asthma, 50
Sampling techniques, in flexible fiberoptic
bronchoscopy, 41
Samter syndrome. *See* Triad asthma
San Joaquin Valley Fever, 298
Sarcoidosis, 512–514
clinical presentation of, 513
diagnosis of, 513
pathophysiology of, 512–513
prognosis of, 514
treatment of, 513–514

Sarcomatoid carcinoma, 586*t*
Scar, venous, 386
Schistosomiasis, 333
  cardiopulmonary, 414
  pulmonary embolism from, 413–414
Scoliosis, 449–450
  infantile, 450
  juvenile, 450
Screening
  for lung cancer, 3, 588 (*See also* Lung
    cancer, screening for)
  for occupational-environmental lung
    disease, 3
  radiography in, 3–4
  for tuberculosis, 3
Scuba diving, 500–501
"Seashore sign", in thoracic
  ultrasound, 33
Second-hand smoke, 366
Secondary pleural metastasis, 601
Secretion clearance. *See* Bronchial hygiene
  therapy, in pulmonary therapeutics
Secure airway
  advantage of, 209–210
  alternative modes of, 210–211
  definition of, 209
Selective decontamination of the digestive
  tract (SDD), for ventilator-associated
  pneumonia prevention, 349
Septic pulmonary embolism, 174, 416
  drug-induced, 174, 416
Serratia pneumonia, 253–259. *See also*
  Pneumonia, gram-negative bacilli
Severe acute respiratory syndrome
  (SARS), 168, 273, 275
Short-acting beta-2 agonists (SABAs), for
  asthma, 50
Shrinking lung syndrome, 548
Shuttle walk test (SWT), 21
  endurance, 21
  incremental, 21
Sickle cell disease (SCD), pulmonary
  manifestations of, 439–442
  acute chest syndrome in, 439–440
    causes of, 440
    characteristics of, 439
    treatment for, 440
  asthma in, 441
  chronic lung disease in, 441–442
  infection in, 442
  pulmonary arterial hypertension in,
    440–441
    etiology of, 440–441
    oral arginine supplementation effects
     with, 441

Sildenafil, 423
  for asthma, 53
  for pulmonary hypertension, 427
Silica, 477
  free, 474
Silicoproteinosis, 475
Silicosis, 474–476
  clinical presentations of, 475
  diagnosis of, 576
  management, 576
Simian SV40 virus, 603
Simple masks, 65
Sin Nombre virus (SNV), 276
Single lung transplant (SLT), 435
Single photon emission computed
  tomography (SPECT), 7, 506
Sirolimus, for lung transplantation,
  436, 437
Skin testing, 299
Sleep apnea
  central, 467
  mixed, 467
  obstructive, 466–469
    as postoperative risk factor, 46
Sleep disordered breathing, 466–469
  in neuromuscular disorders, 461
  in pregnancy, 162
  with sickle cell disease, 442
Sleep studies, 17
"Sliding sign", in thoracic ultrasound, 33
Small airways disease, 186*t*
  in rheumatoid arthritis, 543
Small-cell carcinoma of lung, 583, 585–586,
  586*t*, 592, 595. *See also* Lung cancer
Smallpox, disaster management of, 79, 80
Smoke inhalation injury, 488–489
  clinical signs and symptoms of, 488
  due to particulate matter, 488
  due to toxic byproducts of
    combustion, 488–489
Smoking
  in asthma, 485
  chronic obstructive pulmonary disease
    from, 366
  control of, 69–72
    for chronic obstructive pulmonary
     disease, 372
    lung cancer screening on, 588
    for pulmonary Langerhans cell
     histiocytosis, 559
  lung cancer from, 587
  on postoperative pulmonary
    complications, 46
  for pulmonary impairment, 478
  spontaneous pneumothorax from, 149

Solitary fibroma, of pleura, 601–605
Solitary pulmonary nodule (SPN),
    215–220, 580
  clinical and radiographic evaluation
    of, 216–217
  diagnosis of, 215
  etiologies of, 216
  guidelines for follow-up lung
    nodules, 218*t*
  intervention, 218–219
  management of, 217
  surveillance imaging of, 217–218
SOX1 antibodies, with lung cancer, 595
Spinal cord injury, 462–463
Spirometry, 12–15*f*, 14, 186–187, 357, 369
Spleen, 442
Spontaneous (idiopathic)
    pneumothorax, 148, 149–150
Spontaneous or aerosol-induced sputum
    sampling, 283
Squamous cell carcinoma of lung, 585,
    586*t*. *See also* Lung cancer
Standard electrocautery, 62
Standard fiberoptic bronchoscopy, for
    solitary pulmonary nodule, 218
Staphylococcal pneumonia, 240–243
Staphylococci, 240
Staphylococcus aureus infections, 180,
    241–242, 274
  in cystic fibrosis, 446, 447
  after lung transplantation, 437
Staphylococcus aureus pneumonia, 240–242
Staphylococcus epidermidis, 240
Staphylococcus saprophyticus, 240
Status asthmaticus, 359
STEER protocol, 92–93
Stents, 436–437
  migration, 62
Stereotactic body radiation therapy
    (SBRT), 219
  in lung cancer treatment, 507–508
Steroids. *See* Corticosteroids; *specific agents*
  in cystic fibrosis, 446
  for mixed connective tissue disease, 553
  for radiation pneumonitis, 507
  for Wegener's granulomatosis, 518
Storage phosphor plates, 2–3
Strahler model, 420
Stratosphere sign, in ultrasound, 36
Streptococcal pneumonia, 240–243
Streptococcus agalactiae pneumonia, 241, 242
Streptococcus pneumoniae, 240–243, 250,
    274, 373
  in HIV-infected, 342
  in sickle cell disease, 442

Streptococcus pyogenes pneumonia, 241, 242
Streptomycin
  for nontuberculous mycobacterial
    infections, 292
  in pregnancy, 289
  for tuberculosis, 287, 289
Stroke, aspiration pneumonia in, 156
Strongyloides stercoralis, 332
Subacute cough, 128
Subacute pulmonary histoplasmosis, 303
Subglottic suctioning, for aspiration
    pneumonia, 157
Submersion-induced pulmonary embolism
    (SIPE), 501
Substance abuse. *See* Drug abuse; *specific
    drugs*
Sucralfate, 348–349
Sulfur mustard, 78
Supplemental oxygen, 112
Supraglottic upper airway obstruction, 186*t*
Surge capacity
  definition of, 74
  and management in disaster
    planning, 74–75
Swallowing provocation test, 157–158
Swine flu (H1N1), 273, 274
Symmetric proximal muscle neuromyopathy,
    with lung cancer, 595
Syndrome of inappropriate ADH (SIADH),
    with lung cancer, 597
Systemic corticosteroids agents, for
    asthma, 51
Systemic lupus erythematosus (SLE),
    547–549
Systemic scleroderma, 549–552
Systolic pressure, pulmonary arterial, 426

T

T-lymphocytes, 436
Tadalafil (Adcirca®)
  for asthma, 53
  for pulmonary hypertension, 427
Talc
  for malignant pleural disease, 605
  pulmonary embolism from, 417
Talc pleurodesis, 605
Talcosis, drug abuse in, 176
Tamoxifen, for tuberous sclerosis, 567
Tapeworm infections, 331
Taurine, 507
Technetium-99m (^{99m}Tc), 5
Telephone counseling services, 70, 71
Tension pneumothorax, 151
Teratoma, 577

Terbutaline, for asthma, 50
Tetracycline
  for actinomycosis, 322
  for chronic obstructive pulmonary
    disease, 374
  for hypercapnic respiratory failure, 195
  for KPC-producing strains, 251
  for malignant pleural disease, 605
  for pneumonia, atypical, 271
ThairapyVest™, 68
Theophylline
  for asthma, 51, 357, 358, 359, 360
  for chronic obstructive pulmonary
    disease, 373
Therapeutic procedures, interventional
  pulmonology
  bronchial thermoplasty, 62–63
  rigid bronchoscopy with advanced
    therapeutic techniques, 61–62
Thermal epiglottitis, drug abuse in, 176
Thermal injury
  direct, of smoke inhalation, 489
  drug abuse in, 176
Thermoplasty, bronchial
  for asthma, 62–63
  in interventional pulmonology, 62–63
Thin film transistor (TFT), light-sensitive, 3
Thoracentesis
  for pleural effusion, 133, 134
  pneumothorax from, 151–152
  thoracic ultrasound in, 34–35
Thoracic actinomycosis, 322
Thoracic spine disorders, 449–451
  ankylosing spondylitis, 450–451
    treatment of, 451
  kyphoscoliosis, 449–450
    idiopathic, 450
  kyphosis, 449–450
  scoliosis, 449–450
    infantile, 450
    juvenile, 450
Thoracic ultrasound, 32–37
  biopsies, 34–35
  central venous catheter access, 37
  chest drain insertion, 35
  chest drainage catheters, 34–35
  closed pleural biopsy, 35
  mediastinal ultrasound, 7
  normal findings, 33–34
  preparing for examination, 33
  in specific lung diseases, 35–36
    alveolo-interstitial edema, 36
    consolidation, 35–36
    pneumothorax, 36
  technical aspects and physics of, 33

thoracentesis, 34–35
  transthoracic biopsies, of lung
    lesions, 36–37
Thoracoscopy, for pleural effusion, 134
Thoracotomy, for pneumothorax, 153
Thromboembolic disease, 385–402. *See
  also* Deep venous thrombosis (DVT);
  Pulmonary embolism (PE); Pulmonary
  hypertension, chronic thromboembolic
  chronic pulmonary, 6
  diagnosis of, 388
  epidemiology of, 385–386
  natural history of, 386
  prophylaxis against, 393–396
    drugs in, 394
    intermittent pneumatic compressive
      devices in, 395–396
    options and strategies in, 393–394
  signs and symptoms of, 387
  therapy for, 399–402
    duration and follow-up of, 402
    fondaparinux in, 399–400
    goals of, 399
    heparin in, 399–401
Thromboendarterectomy, pulmonary,
  409–411
  postoperative management in, 409–410
    intensive care, 410
  reperfusion pulmonary edema in, 410
Thrombolytic agents. *See also specific agents*
  for pulmonary embolism, 402
Thymomas, mediastinal masses and,
  223, 225
Tidal volume, in pregnancy, 160
Tigecycline, 252, 269, 270
Tinzaparin, 400
Tiotropium, for asthma, 50
TNF-α antagonists, in histoplasmosis, 304
Tobacco. *See* Smoking
Tobramycin
  for bronchiectasis in cystic fibrosis, 446
  for gram-negative bacilli pneumonias, 256
"Tongue" sign, in thoracic ultrasound, 34
Total body surface area (TBSA), 491
Total lung capacity (TLC), 450
Toxocara canis, 332
Toxocara cutis, 332
Toxocariasis, 332–333
Tracheal stenosis, drug abuse in, 176
Tracheobronchial aspergillosis, 317
Tracheobronchomalacia, 62, 188
Tracheostomy, in amyotrophic lateral
  sclerosis, 462
Traction bronchiectasis, 198
Traditional asthma, 129

Transcription-mediated amplification, for tuberculosis, 283
Transforming growth factor-β (TGF-β), 505
Transthoracic biopsies, of lung lesions, thoracic ultrasound in, 36–37
Transthoracic needle aspiration (TTNA), for solitary pulmonary nodule, 219
Trauma
  pneumothorax from, 150
  pulmonary embolism from, 417
Traumatic pneumothorax, 148, 150
Travel, air, 110–113
Trematode infections, 333
Treprostinil (Remodulin®)
  for asthma, 52
  for pulmonary hypertension, 427
Triad asthma, 354
Triamcinolone, for asthma, 50, 51
Triazoles, 300
Trichoptilosis, 577
Tricothecene mycotoxin, 138
Tridymite, 474
Trimethoprim-sulfamethoxazole (TMP-SMX)
  for chronic obstructive pulmonary disease, 374
  for *Haemophilus influenzae* infection, 247
  for hypercapnic respiratory failure, 195
  for nocardiosis, 321
  for pneumonia
    P. carinii prophylaxis, 340*t*
    P. carinii with HIV, 340*t*, 341*t*
Trophoblastic tissue embolism, pulmonary, 417
Tropical pulmonary eosinophilia (TPE), 229, 332
Trousseau syndrome, in lung cancer, 595
Tuberculin skin test (TST), 278–279, 282–283
Tuberculosis (TB), 278–280
  bone and joint, 284
  clinical manifestations of, 282–284
  diagnosis of, 278–280, 282–284
  epidemiology of, 278
  extrapulmonary, 283
    treatment of, 288
  genitourinary, 284
  in HIV-infected, 284, 342–343
    prophylaxis against, 280
    treatment of, 288–289
  in immunocompromised host, 169
  large airway (endobronchial), 283–284
  laryngeal, 283–284
  meningeal, 284
  miliary, 284

  pathophysiology of, 282
  pericardial, 284
  pleural, 284
  in pregnancy, 160
  prevention of, 279–280
  primary, 182
  radiographic screening for, 3
  reactivation of, 282
  with silicosis, 475
  treatment of, 286–289
    adverse reactions from, 289
    in children, 287, 289
    directly observed therapy in, 288
    first-line agents in, 286–287
    with HIV, 287, 288–289
    latent infection in, 279–280
    monitoring response to, 288
    phases of, 287
    in pregnancy, 289
    second-line agents in, 287
    third-line drugs in, 287
    using drugs, 286–287
Tuberculous meningitis, 284
Tuberous sclerosis, 566–567
Tularemia, 79, 138
Tumor. *See specific tumors*
Tumor embolism, 416–417
Tumor necrosis factor (TNF), importance of, 512
Tumor necrosis factor-α (TNF-α), 495, 505
Tyrosine kinase inhibitors, for pulmonary hypertension, 427

U

Ultrasonography, 2. *See also specific disorders*
Ultrasound (US), thoracic, 32–37
  biopsies, 34–35
  central venous catheter access, 37
  chest drain insertion, 35
  chest drainage catheters, 34–35
  closed pleural biopsy, 35
  mediastinal, 7
  normal findings, 33–34
  preparing for examination, 33
  in specific lung diseases, 35–36
    alveolo-interstitial edema, 36
    consolidation, 35–36
    pneumothorax, 36
  technical aspects and physics of, 33
  thoracentesis, 34–35
  transthoracic biopsies, of lung lesions, 36–37
Ultrasound transducer, for diaphragm paralysis, 455

Unfractionated heparin (UFH), for thromboembolic disease, 399
Upper airway cough syndrome (UACS), 128, 129, 461
Upper airway resistance syndrome, 467
Upper airways involvement, in rheumatoid arthritis, 543
USA300 strain, 241

V

Vaccines
for *Haemophilus influenzae*, 246–247
against infections, 442
influenza, 246–247, 274–275
for COPD prophylaxis, 373
pneumococcal pneumonia, 236–237
for COPD prophylaxis, 373
13-valent pneumococcal conjugate vaccine, 237
Valganciclovir, 437
for cytomegalovirus pneumonia, 276
Vancomycin, for pneumonia
pneumococcal, 235
staphylococcus, 241
streptococcal, 241
Varenicline, 70
Variable extrathoracic obstruction, 187–188
Variable intrathoracic obstruction, 188–189
Varicella pneumonia, in pregnancy, 160
Varicella-zoster virus (VZV) pneumonia, 275–276
Varicose bronchiectasis, 198
Variola virus, 80
Vascular endothelial growth factor-D (VEGF-D), 565
Vasculitis
cutaneous, with lung cancer, 596
disseminated, with lung cancer, 596
in rheumatoid arthritis, 548
Venography, contrast, for deep venous thrombosis, 387–388
Venous air embolism, 414–415
Venous scar, 386
Venous thromboembolism (VTE), 102–103, 104, 385–402. *See also* Pulmonary embolism (PE)
diagnosis of, 388
radioisotopic techniques for, 5
epidemiology of, 385–386
inferior vena caval filter for, 396
natural history of, 387, 393–394
in pregnancy, 162

prophylaxis against, 393–396
drugs in, 394
intermittent pneumatic compressive devices in, 395–396
options and strategies in, 393–394
risk factors for, 386
signs and symptoms of, 387
therapy for
duration and follow-up of, 402
fondaparinux in, 399–400
goals of, 399
heparin in, 399–401
treatment of, 399–402
Ventilation
alveolar, 190
for burning injury patients, 491
minute, 191
for pulmonary embolism, 389
scans, 5–7
Ventilation, mechanical, 84–87, 89–93, 184
for acute respiratory distress syndrome, 381
airway–pressure release, 87
barotrauma from, 90–91
bilevel, 87
breath sequence, 85–86
complications of, 90–91
discontinuation of, 91–93
hemodynamic compromise, 90–91
high-frequency oscillating, 87
for hypercapnic respiratory failure, 193–194
indications, 92
infection from, 91
hospital-acquired pneumonia in, 348
inhalation and exhalation, duration of, 86
inverse ratio ventilation in, 86
models of, 84–85
positive end-expiratory pressure in, 86
procedure, 92
proportional assist ventilation in, 87
reducing workload in, 86
triggering inhalation, 86
volume *vs.* pressure, control, 84–85
Ventilation–perfusion lung scanning. *See also* Perfusion scans
for chronic thromboembolic pulmonary hypertension, 408
for pulmonary hypertension, 426
Ventilator-associated pneumonia (VAP), 180, 347–350. *See also* Pneumonia, hospital-acquired (nosocomial); Pneumonia, ventilator-associated
gram-negative, 253–259 (*See also* Pneumonia, gram-negative bacilli)

VentiMask, 66
Venturi effect, 66
Video-assisted thoracoscopic surgery
(VATS), 219, 536, 559
Vincristine, 505
Viral encephalitides, 79
Viral infections. *See also specific infections*
in immunocompromised host, 168–169
after lung transplantation, 437
Viral pneumonia, 273–276
bacterial coinfection with, 274
cytomegalovirus, 276
diagnosis of, 274
factors of, 273
hantavirus pulmonary syndrome, 276
herpes simplex virus, 276
neurological sequelae of, 274
novel coronavirus, 275
parainfluenza, 275
in pregnancy, 160
rhinovirus, 275
Virtual map, drawback of, 44
Visceral larvae migrans, 332–333
Visual Analogue Scale, 122
Vital capacity (VC), 450, 460, 461
in pregnancy, 160
Vitamin C, for mustard gas, 77
Vitamin K antagonists, 394, 400
Vocal cord dysfunction, 187–188, 485
Vocational retraining, 109
Volume *vs.* pressure, control, in mechanical
ventilation, 84–85
Volutrauma, 90–91
von Recklinghausen disease. *See*
Neurofibromatosis type 1 (NF1)
Voriconazole
for aspergillosis
acute invasive pulmonary, 315, 317
chronic invasive pulmonary, 313
chronic necrotizing aspergillosis, 313
for blastomycosis, 310
for coccidioidomycosis, 299
for cryptococcosis, 328

W

Walk-Pulmonary Hypertension and Sickle
Cell Disease with Sildenafil Therapy
(Walk-PHaSST) study, 441
"Walking pneumonia," 267
Warfarin, 41, 400
for asthma, 51, 53
for pulmonary hypertension, 427
for thromboembolic disease
prophylaxis, 394–395
Weaning, from mechanical ventilation, 89, 91–92
Wegener's granulomatosis. *See*
Granulomatosis with polyangiitis (GPA)
Weibel model, 420
Williams-Campbell syndrome, 200
Woolsorter disease, 79

X

Xa factor, 399
Xenon-133 (^{133}Xe) gas, 5–6

Y

Yellow Nail Syndrome, 200
Yellow rain. *See* Tricothecene mycotoxin
Yersinia pestis, 80, 138
Young syndrome, 200

Z

Zafirlukast, 51
Zanamivir, 275
Zileuton, 51
Zinc, 253